BASIC SCIENCES

DENTOGIST
MCQs in Dentistry

WITH EXPLANATORY ANSWERS

BASIC SCIENCES

DENTOGIST
MCQs in Dentistry

WITH EXPLANATORY ANSWERS

Seventh Edition

Revised by
Anand Mohatta BDS MDS
Academics Incharge, Target Educare Pvt Ltd.
Mumbai, Maharashtra, India

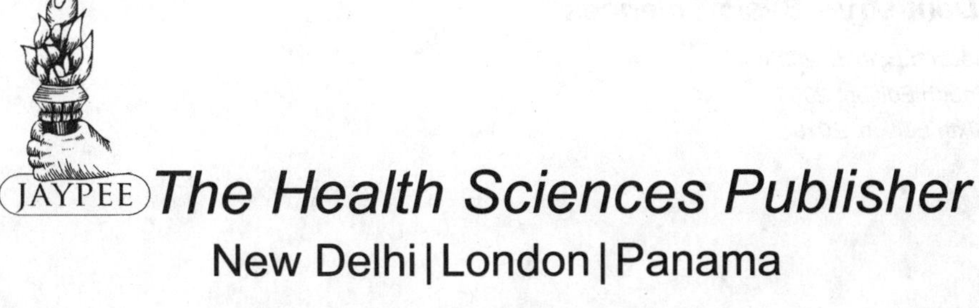

New Delhi | London | Panama

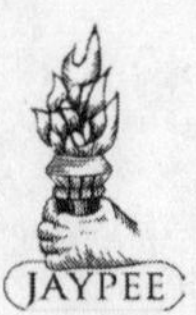

Jaypee Brothers Medical Publishers (P) Ltd

Headquarters
Jaypee Brothers Medical Publishers (P) Ltd.
4838/24, Ansari Road, Daryaganj
New Delhi 110 002, India
Phone: +91-11-43574357
Fax: +91-11-43574314
E-mail: jaypee@jaypeebrothers.com

Overseas Offices
JP Medical Ltd.
83, Victoria Street, London
SW1H 0HW (UK)
Phone: +44-20 3170 8910
Fax: +44(0)20 3008 6180
E-mail: info@jpmedpub.com

Jaypee-Highlights Medical Publishers Inc.
City of Knowledge, Bld. 235, 2nd Floor, Clayton
Panama City, Panama
Phone: +1 507-301-0496
Fax: +1 507-301-0499
E-mail: cservice@jphmedical.com

Jaypee Brothers Medical Publishers (P) Ltd.
17/1-B, Babar Road, Block-B, Shyamoli
Mohammadpur, Dhaka-1207
Bangladesh
Mobile: +08801912003485
E-mail: jaypeedhaka@gmail.com

Jaypee Brothers Medical Publishers (P) Ltd.
Bhotahity, Kathmandu, Nepal
Phone: +977-9741283608
E-mail: kathmandu@jaypeebrothers.com

Website: www.jaypeebrothers.com
Website: www.jaypeedigital.com

Dentogist: MCQs in Dentistry—Basic Sciences

First Edition: 1996 *Second Edition: 2000*
Third Edition: 2003 *Fourth Edition: 2005*
Fifth Edition: 2008 *Sixth Edition: 2010*
Seventh Edition: **2017**

ISBN: 978-93-86150-42-4

Printed at Sanat Printers

Dedicated to

My mother, Smt. Asha Mohatta
My sister, Dr Archana Mohatta Borase
and the Students…

Preface

Success is an art which not only requires a lot of grey matter but also needs an intense will to succeed, lot of devotion, a positive attitude, and above all, a firm determined constant effort in the right direction with proper strategy.

We feel elated in bringing out the latest edition of "Dentogist: MCQs in Dentistry" (7th edition). It has been in the market for more than two decades now. It is time-tested and has been a hallmark for Dental PG entrance preparation. It contains all the basic and clinical subjects to help all the aspirants to study in a systematic way.

"Change is the rule of life" for everything and everybody, and with this edition, the book undergoes a well-deserved rejuvenation in every sense. The book has been modified significantly with the incorporation of a concept of "comprehensive learning". It is not the lack of literature but its availability in an overwhelming abundance that makes the search for a precise explanation a tedious job. The inherent form of the book has been maintained and the questions are arranged in a logical and sequential manner, so as to minimize the burden of reading unwanted things for entrance preparation. The questions covers all the important topics of a subject. The explanations are given in a simple and lucid language. Students can analyze the topics of weakness and revert to reading textbook where needed.

It has been stressed time and again that the topics from previous papers are always repeated. The questions are usually based on a specific set of often-repeated topics. It is noteworthy that NBE takes immense pleasure in introducing subtle changes in the questions which leads to drastic changes in the answer. This is their endeavor to discourage mugging up of answers. Instead they try to inculcate an analytical and clinical approach in combating the challenges, integral in the field of medical and dental science. This book will surely help you tackle such subtle changes in question substance by providing concepts and clues, which will prove to be the key in solving difficult questions.

I believe that this edition is the most comprehensive text of its kind. Previous issues have stood the test of time and I am sure this trend will continue. This book would be useful for not just students but also for the practicing dentists.

Remember it is not just the last-minute preparation that counts but the knowledge of your complete graduation time.

I recommend you to read this book thoroughly twice or thrice, highlighting the important points and facts while reading, and then restrict your reading to only these highlighted portions in future revisions, so as to save your precious time at the end. Always read the relevant textbooks at the time of solving MCQs.

Friends, remember that even the brightest of bright students are jumpy and unsure of their preparation as, being sufficient, we could never find anyone who could say with conviction that he was well-prepared for the exams. Only the one who holds his/her nerves in the last few days and more, so in the final 3 hours is sure to come out triumphant.

Finally, remember problem-solving is an art. You may not have read a topic and still you may be able to solve questions on it keeping your cool and scrutinizing the options well enough. Remember that the answer is in front of you, you just have to have a discerning eye to get hold of it.

At the end I would like to say:

"There is no substitute to make your career bright. Even a small negligence can descent your merit. Hence, you must make proper use of your time."

Inspite of all our efforts, some imperfections and errors are bound to remain. Your invaluable suggestions to further improve this book are always welcome.

Please communicate with me for any enquiry regarding entrance exams and problems in study.

Best of luck for your exams and your bright future.

Anand Mohatta BDS MDS
E-mail: anand.mohatta@gmail.com

Acknowledgments

At the very outset, I fail to find adequate words with limited vocabulary at my command to express my emotions to my mother, Smt. Asha Mohatta and my sister, Dr Archana Mohatta Borase for their constant undemanding love, dedication, inspiring guidance, affection, encouragement and never-ending enthusiasm, without which this book would not have seen the light of the day.

An ostentatious use of words will not be sufficient to express my heartiest thanks to my uncles, Shri Pannalalji Mohatta and Shri Kishorji Mohatta, who have supported me in thick and thin and have stood by me as a pillar of strength, shielding and taking care of all my weaknesses. This book bears an indelible imprint of them on my life. Words are not enough when it comes to say thanks to people who are important to you. My special thanks to my brother-in-law, Dr Shri Pradeep Borase; elder brother, Shri Pankaj Mohatta; sister, Neha Somani Garg; brother-in-law, Shri Abhayji Garg; my aunt, Smt. Shailjaji Somani; my uncles, Shri Ravibhai Kothari, Shri Rajeshji Kothari and Shri Sanjayji Kothari; my younger brother, Shrikant Kothari and all the members of Mohatta and Kothari families, without whose support this marathon task was impossible. A very special thanks to Shri Shirishji Upadhyay for his unwavering support and guidance.

I was indeed lucky to have Dr Mansing Pawar Sir, Dean, Government Dental College and Hospital, Mumbai, Maharashtra; President, Maharashtra State Dental Council; Member, Dental Council of India; Ex-Joint Director, Directorate Medical Education and Research; Ex-Dean, Dental Faculty, MUHS, Nashik, Maharashtra, India who was not only my guide but was also a pillar during my ups and downs. His constant support and motivation kept me on track during my postgraduate and professional life. It is a great honor and pleasure to be his student.

A very special thanks to Dr Neha Jain, without whose hard work and meticulous proofreading, this book would have never been possible.

This book is possible due to the efforts of Target Educare team and its Chief, Dr Praveen Bansal, whose constant support, guidance and enthusiasm as always pushed me to go beyond my limits.

A very special thanks to Dr Rajeev Chitguppi, Academic Director, Target Educare, who has been an icon to the PG aspirants and a positive force for me to excel.

I am highly obliged to Shri Jitendar P Vij (Group Chairman), Mr Ankit Vij (Group President), Ms Chetna Malhotra Vohra (Associate Director—Content Strategy) and the team at Jaypee Brothers Medical Publishers (P) Ltd, New Delhi, who took keen interest in this project and due to their untiring efforts, this book has seen the light of the day.

Last but not least, a very special thanks to all the students who push me to work beyond my limits.

Contents

1 General Anatomy

OSTEOLOGY OF HEAD AND NECK

1. **All of the following characteristics differentiate a typical cervical vertebra from a thoracic vertebra *except* that:** *(AIIMS May 2009)*
   a. It has a triangular vertebral canal
   b. It has a foramen transversarium
   c. Superior articular facet is directed backwards and upwards
   d. It has a large vertebral body

2. **Infraorbital nerve exits through the:** *(AIIMS May 2009)*
   a. Foramen ovale
   b. Foramen spinosum
   c. Foramen magnum
   d. Inferior orbital fissure

3. **Early fusion of the coronal suture results in:** *(AIIMS May 2008, AIPG 2007)*
   a. Oxycephaly   b. Scaphocephaly
   c. Brachycephaly   d. Trigonocephaly

4. **Middle constrictor is attached to the:** *(AIIMS May 2007, AIPG 2007, 2010)*
   a. Hyoid bone
   b. Pterygomandibular raphe
   c. Ramus of the mandible
   d. Maxillary tuberosity

5. **The infrahyoid muscles are supplied by:** *(AIIMS Nov 2006)*
   a. The vagus nerve
   b. The cervical plexus
   c. The brachial plexus
   d. The supraclavicular nerve

6. **The number of fontanelle present at birth is:** *(AIPG 2007)*
   a. 4   b. 6
   c. 8   d. 10

7. **Palatine aponeurosis is:** *(AIPG 2005)*
   a. Tendon of levator veli palatine muscle
   b. Tendon of tensor veli palatine muscle
   c. A part of muscle uvulae
   d. A modification of palatal periosteum

8. **Arterial supply to floor of the mouth and suprahyoid muscle:** *(AIPG 2012)*
   a. Lingual artery
   b. Maxillary artery
   c. Inferior alveolar artery
   d. Facial artery

9. **Facial vein communicates with cavernous sinus through:** *(COMED 2012)*
   a. Posterior facial vein
   b. Common facial vein
   c. Deep facial vein
   d. Posterior auricular vein

10. **Mandibular fossa is a part of:** *(COMED 2012)*
    a. Mandible bone   b. Maxilla bone
    c. Sphenoid bone   d. Temporal bone

11. **Infection from the dangerous area of the face spread through one of the following veins?** *(COMED 2011)*
    a. Maxillary
    b. Retromandibular vein
    c. Superficial temporal vein
    d. Ophthalmic vein

12. **One of the following nerves is the motor nerve for occipital belly of occipitofrontalis?** *(COMED 2011)*
    a. Greater auricular   b. Lesser occipital
    c. Third occipital   d. Posterior auricular

13. **The type of suture represented by sagittal suture of the cranial vault is:** *(COMED 2010)*
    a. Serrate   b. Denticulate
    c. Squamous   d. Plane

14. Blood supply of coronoid process of mandible is primarily from: *(COMED 2006)*
a. Inferior alveolar artery
b. Deep temporal artery
c. Facial artery
d. Middle meningeal artery

15. Skull at birth has: *(COMED 2006)*
a. 22 bones b. 34 bones
c. 45 bones d. 54 bones

16. The medial surface of the neck of the mandible is related to the: *(KCET 2006)*
a. Inferior alveolar nerve
b. Lingual nerve
c. Auriculotemporal nerve
d. Chorda tympani nerve

17. Median cleft of the upper lip occurs as results of defective formation of the: *(KCET 2009)*
a. Frontonasal prominence
b. Lateral nasal prominence
c. Lens placode
d. Mandibular prominence

18. The joint between the atlas and axis is: *(KCET 2010)*
a. Synovial
b. Closely related to the first cervical nerves
c. Allow rotation of the head
d. Supported by the alar ligaments

19. Which part of body is underdeveloped at birth? *(KCET 2010)*
a. Eyes b. Ears
c. Face d. Brain

20. Located medical to the third molar at the junction of the maxilla and the horizontal plate of the palatine bone: *(KCET 2012)*
a. Posterior nasal spine
b. Mylohyoid line
c. Pterygoid hamulus
d. Grater palatine foramen

21. What is the number of bones a neonate has in the skeleton? *(KCET 2013)*
a. 270
b. 250
c. 230
d. 206

22. Through which foramen middle meningeal artery passes? *(MH 2012)*
a. Foramen rotundum
b. Foramen ovale
c. Foramen spinosum
d. Supra orbital foramen

23. All is/are false about vertebral artery *except*? *(MH 2011)*
a. It is a branch of the first part of subclavian artery
b. It lies in suboccipital region
c. It enters vertebral column through C7 vertebra
d. It is divided into 4 parts

24. Which of the following is present in the posterior cranial fossa in a five year old child? *(PGI 2011)*
a. Foramen rotundum
b. Foramen lacerum
c. Jugular foramen
d. Foramen spinosum

25. Which out of the following bone ossify first? *(PGI 2008)*
a. Mandible b. Nasal bone
c. Vomer d. Occipital

26. The hyoid bone lies in the midline at the front of the neck at the level of the: *(BHU 2012)*
a. Third cervical vertebra
b. Fourth cervical vertebra
c. Fifth cervical vertebra
d. Seventh cervical vertebra

27. The orbital opening is somewhat: *(BHU 2012)*
a. Quadrangular
b. Oval
c. Oblong
d. Circular

SCALP TEMPLE AND FACE

28. Danger layer of scalp is: *(AIIMS May 2013)*
a. Perostium b. Connective tissue
c. Loose areolar tissue d. Aponeurosis

29. Right anterior quadrant of the scalp is supplied by the following arteries *except*: *(COMED 2012)*
a. Right supraorbital artery
b. Right supratrochlear artery
c. Right superficial temporal artery
d. Right maxillary artery

SIDE OF NECK

30. The deepest layer of cervical fascia is: *(AIPG 2010)*

a. Vertebral
b. Carotid sheath
c. Deep fascia
d. Prevertebral fascia

31. Gonial angle at birth is: *(AIPG 2007)*

a. 110°
b. 140°
c. 175°
d. 200°

32. The anterior triangle occupies the side of the neck in front of sternomastoid muscle. Each triangle presents boundary in front: *(COMED 2005)*

a. Anterior median line of the neck extending from symphysis menti to suprasternal notch
b. The midline of the neck
c. Midline of the neck upto the sternoclavicular joint
d. Posterior border of thyroid gland

33. Suprasternal space does not contain which of the following structures? *(COMED 2006)*

a. Jugular arch
b. Anterior jugular vein
c. Sternal head of sternocleidomastoid
d. External jugular vein

34. 'Wry neck' deformity is due to the damage of: *(KCET 2007)*

a. Platysma
b. Sternohyoid
c. Sternocleidomastoid
d. Omohyoid

CRANIAL CAVITY

35. Which is not a branch of the cavernous part of the internal carotid artery? *(AIPG 2009)*

a. Cavernous branch
b. Inferior hypophyseal
c. Meningeal artery
d. Ophthalmic artery

36. Infection from dangerous area of face goes to cavernous sinus through: *(AIIMS May 2013, Nov 2011, 2013,)*

a. Pterygoid plexus
b. Ethmoid
c. Maxillary sinus
d. Submental lymph nodes

37. Cavernous sinus thrombosis from face occurs due to: *(AIPG/NEET 2013)*

a. Veins have valves to allow back flow
b. Facial vein communicate with superior ophthalmic vein
c. Injury to the facial tissues
d. Lymphatic drainage

38. Nerve of the pterygoid canal is formed by the union of: *(COMED 2006)*

a. Deep petrosal nerve with greater petrosal nerve
b. Deep petrosal nerve with lesser petrosal nerve
c. Greater petrosal and lesser petrosal nerves
d. Greater petrosal and external petrosal nerves

39. The artery that passes forwards through cavernous sinus is: *(KCET 2006)*

a. Supratrochler
b. Supraorbital artery
c. Internal carotid artery
d. Anterior ethmoidal artery

40. Accessory meningeal artery enters cranial cavity through: *(KCET 2006)*

a. Foramen lacerum
b. Foramen rotundum
c. Foramen spinosum
d. Foramen ovale

41. Nerve passing through the center of cavernous sinus is: *(KCET 2005)*

a. Occulomotor nerve
b. Trochler nerve
c. Abducent nerve
d. Maxillary nerve

42. Facial vein communicates with the cavernous sinus through: *(KCET 2007)*

a. Retromolar vein and internal jugular vein
b. External jugular vein and internal jugular vein
c. Internal jugular vein and retomandibular vein
d. Superior ophthalmic vein and pterygoid venous plexus

43. Rathke's pouch gives origin to all *except*? *(MH 2011)*

a. Pars tuberalis
b. Pars intermedia
c. Pars posterior
d. Pars distalis

44. The transverse venous sinus continuous as: *(IGNOU 2010)*

a. Straight sinus
b. Cavernous sinus
c. Sigmoid sinus
d. Ethmoidal sinus

CONTENTS OF ORBIT

45. Anterior ethmoidal nerve supplies all *except*: *(AIPG 2011)*
a. Maxillary sinus
b. Interior of nasal cavity
c. Dural sheath of anterior cranial fossa
d. Ethmoidal air cells

46. Lacrimal gland secretion is affected by injury of: *(AIPG 2010)*
a. Greater petrosal b. Nasociliary
c. Nasopalatine d. Infraorbital

47. Pain sensation from ethmoid sinus is transmitted by: *(AIPG/NEET 2013)*
a. Nasociliary nerve b. Supratrochlear nerve
c. Lacrimal nerve d. Frontal nerve

48. Intrinsic muscle of eyeball are all, *except*: *(AIPG/NEET 2013)*
a. Levator palpebrae b. Ciliary
c. Sphincter pupillae d. Dilator papillae

49. Which of these is not a part of ethmoid bone (which of the following does not contribute to ethmoid bone)? *(AIIMS Nov 2013)*
a. Agger nasi
b. Inferior turbinate
c. Uncinate process
d. Cribriform plate (crista galli)

50. Loss of lacrimation due to injury to which nerve? *(AIPG 2012)*
a. Greater petrosal nerve
b. Lesser petrosal nerve
c. Sphenopalatine nerve
d. Nasociliary nerve

51. Pain in ethmoid sinusitis is carried by: *(AIPG 2012)*
a. Nasociliary
b. Infratrochlear
c. Lacrimal
d. Middle meningeal nerve

52. Dacryocystitis is interruption in the drainage of: *(COMED 2007)*
a. Submandibular gland
b. Parotid gland
c. Lacrimal gland
d. Sublingual gland

53. Injury to one of the following arteries results in extradural hematoma: *(KCET 2009)*
a. Middle meningeal artery
b. Facial artery
c. Temporal artery
d. Anterior cerebral artery

54. Which of the following is the weakest part of the orbit? *(KCET 2009)*
a. Medial wall
b. Lateral wall
c. Floor of the orbit
d. Roof of the orbit

ANTERIOR TRIANGLE OF NECK

55. Common carotid artery bifurcates: *(AIPG 2010, AIPG 2007)*
a. At the upper border of thyroid cartilage
b. At the lower border of thyroid cartilage
c. Below cricoid cartilage
d. At the level of C6 vertebra

56. Following are the branches of external carotid artery *except*: *(COMED 2013)*
a. Facial artery
b. Lingual artery
c. Occipital artery
d. Middle meningeal artery

57. All the following structures are contents of the carotid sheath *except*: *(KCET 2008)*
a. Vagus nerve
b. Internal jugular vein
c. Common carotid artery
d. Sympathetic trunk

58. The following arteries provide a rich blood supply to the face, *except* the: *(KCET 2009)*
a. Buccal artery
b. Mental artery
c. Posterior auricular artery
d. Infraorbital artery

59. A muscle with dual nerve supply is? *(MH 2011)*
a. Masseter
b. Medial pterygoid
c. Digastricus
d. Buccinator

PAROTID REGION

60. All the following are true regarding duct of parotid *except*: *(AIPG 2007)*
a. That it pierces masseter
b. That it pierces the buccinator
c. That it opens in buccal vestibule opposite lower second molar
d. That it can be palpated externally

61. Muscle responsible for lateral movement of mandible: *(AIIMS Nov 2013)*
a. Medial and lateral pterygoid
b. Masseter and lateral pterygoid
c. Masseter and medial pterygoid
d. Masseter

62. Parotid duct traverse: *(COMED 2006)*
a. Masseter
b. Buccinator
c. Medial pterygoid
d. Lateral pterygoid

63. The structures that does not traverse parotid gland is: *(COMED 2006)*
a. Superficial temporal artery
b. Posterior auricular artery
c. External carotid artery
d. Internal carotid artery

64. Orifice of the parotid duct opens opposite to: *(KCET 2010)*
a. Upper third molar
b. Upper second molar
c. Lower 2nd molar
d. Lower incisor

65. Inferior salivary nucleus supplies: *(KCET 2005)*
a. Lacrimal gland
b. Parotid gland
c. Submandibular salivary gland
d. Sublingual salivary gland

66. During inferior alveolar nerve block the needle of LA syringe is penetrated into parotid gland which of the following structure is most likely to be penetrated? *(PGI 2006)*
a. Lingual nerve
b. Lingual artery
c. Internal carotid artery
d. External carotid artery

TEMPORAL OR INFRATEMPORAL REGION

67. Sensory nerve supply of capsule of temporomandibular joint (TMJ) is: *(AIIMS Nov 2010, May 2012)*
a. Auriculotemporal nerve
b. Facial nerve
c. Masseteric nerve
d. Auricular nerve

68. Which of the following muscles causes the forward movement of the condyle in the glenoid fossa? *(AIIMS May 2008)*
a. Masseter b. Temporalis
c. Medial pterygoid d. Lateral pterygoid

69. Mylohyoid nerve, the nerve which supplies the anterior belly of digastric, is a branch of? *(AIIMS May 2008, AIPG 2007)*
a. Anterior trunk of mandibular nerve
b. Inferior alveolar nerve
c. Auriculotemporal nerve
d. Facial nerve

70. The muscle that is attached to the disc of TMJ and that brings about its forward movement is: *(AIIMS May 2007, AIPG 2007)*
a. Medial pterygoid b. Lateral pterygoid
c. Masseter d. Temporalis

71. Lateral movement of condyle takes place by: *(AIIMS Nov 2006)*
a. Contralateral lateral pterygoid
b. Ipsilateral lateral pterygoid
c. Same side medial pterygoid
d. Both medial and lateral pterygoid

72. All the following muscles are grouped together as muscle of mastication *except*: *(AIIMS May 2006)*
a. Buccinator
b. Masseter
c. Temporalis
d. Pterygoids

73. The floor of mouth and suprahyoid muscles are supplied by: *(AIIMS Nov 2005)*
a. Lingual nerve
b. Inferior alveolar nerve
c. Maxillary nerve
d. Facial nerve

74. The only sensory branch of anterior division of mandibular nerve is: *(AIPG 2011)*

a. Auriculotemporal nerve
b. Lingual nerve
c. Long buccal nerve
d. Buccal nerve

75. Sensory branch of mandibular nerve are all, *except*: *(AIPG 2009)*

a. Mylohyoid b. Lingual
c. Temporal d. Buccal nerve

76. The middle meningeal artery is a branch of: *(AIPG 2006)*

a. External carotid artery
b. Internal maxillary artery
c. Superficial temporal artery
d. Middle cerebral artery

77. Temporomandibular joint develops at: *(AIIMS May 2013)*

a. 10 weeks b. 2 weeks
c. 20 weeks d. 22 weeks

78. Muscle of mastication derives from: *(AIPG/NEET 2013)*

a. First arch b. Second
c. Third d. Sixth

79. Muscle responsible for lateral movement of mandible: *(AIIMS Nov 2013)*

a. Medial and lateral pterygoid
b. Masseter and lateral pterygoid
c. Masseter and medial pterygoid
d. Masseter

80. Opening of mouth is directed by: *(AIIMS Nov 2013, AIPG 2012, COMED 2007)*

a. Lateral pterygoid
b. Medial pterygoid
c. Temporalis
d. Masseter

81. Nerve supply of buccinators muscle: *(AIIMS May 2012)*

a. V b. VII
c. IX d. XII

82. All are supplied by anterior division of the mandibular nerve *except*: *(AIPG 2012)*

a. Medial pterygoid b. Lateral pterygoid
c. Masseter d. Temporalis

83. Inferior alveolar nerve and vessels course along: *(COMED 2012)*

a. Mandibular canal b. Mylohyoid groove
c. Sublingual fossa d. Submandibular fossa

84. All of the following canals open on the posterior wall of the pterygopalatine fossa *except*: *(COMED 2012, 2011)*

a. Greater palatine canal
b. Foramen rotundum
c. Pterygoid canal
d. Palatovaginal canal

85. Masseter muscle is a powerful muscle because of: *(COMED 2005)*

a. Bipennate arrangement of fibers
b. Multipennate arrangements of fibers
c. It has multiple tendinous septa
d. Its attachment to bone is unique

86. Among the muscle of TMJ , the following muscle opposes, stabilizes and antagonizes muscle forces as far as the disc is concerned: *(COMED 2006)*

a. Medial pterygoid
b. Temporalis
c. Lateral pterygoid
d. Masseter

87. Protraction of the mandible is brought about by: *(COMED 2007)*

a. Lateral pterygoid b. Medial pterygoid
c. Temporalis d. Masseter

88. Accessory meningeal artery enters cranial cavity through: *(KCET 2006)*

a. Foramen lacerum b. Foramen rotundum
c. Foramen spinosum d. Foramen ovale

89. The following muscles are supplied by mandibular nerve *except*: *(KCET 2006)*

a. Tensor tympani
b. Tensor veli palatini
c. Levator veli palatini
d. Mylohyoid

90. Depression of the mandible during the opening of the mouth is caused by: *(KCET 2008)*

a. Medial pterygoid
b. Lateral pterygoid
c. Temporalis
d. Masseter

91. Which of the following muscle is attached to posterior part of pterygomandibular raphes? *(KCET 2011, 2012)*

a. Lateral pterygoid
b. Buccinator
c. Superior constrictor
d. Medial pterygoid

92. Which of the following accessory ligaments of the TMJ is likely to have significance upon mandibular movements? *(KCET 2013)*

a. Sphenomandibular
b. Stylomandibular
c. Pterygomandibular
d. All of the above

93. Which of the following arteries is not a branch of the first part of the internal maxillary artery? *(KCET 2013)*

a. Anterior tympanic
b. Middle meningeal
c. Deep auricular
d. Infraorbital

94. Medial pterygoid muscle is supplied by: *(KCET 2007)*

a. Branch from trunk of mandibular nerve
b. Branch from anterior division of mandibular nerve
c. Branch from posterior division of mandibular nerve
d. Branch from maxillary nerve

95. Protrusion of the jaws is brought about by? *(MH 2011, MH 2010)*

a. Buccinator
b. Mylohyoid
c. Temporalis
d. Lateral pterygoid

96. The disk of TMJ in the center: *(MH 2010)*

a. Has maximum blood supply and nerve supply
b. Has no blood supply and nerve supply
c. Has nerve supply but no blood supply
d. Has minimum blood supply and nerve supply

97. All of the following supply TMJ *except*: *(AP 2011)*

a. External carotid artery
b. Internal maxillary artery
c. Transverse facial artery
d. Branches supplying lateral pterygoid

SUBMANDIBULAR REGION

98. Sublingual salivary gland lies: *(AIIMS May 2007, AIPG 2007)*

a. Superior to mylohyoid
b. Inferior to mylohyoid
c. Deep to geniohyoid
d. In the vestibule

99. The muscle that is supplied by the facial and mandibular nerves is: *(AIIMS May 2005)*

a. Masseter
b. Digastric muscle
c. Medial pterygoid
d. Buccinators

100. The branch of the facial nerve that passes through the submandibular salivary gland, divides it into two parts, travels along the lower border of the mandible is: *(AIPG 2008)*

a. Angular
b. Submental
c. Inferior labial
d. Marginal mandibular

101. Sublingual gland is separated from submandibular gland by: *(AIIMS Nov 2012)*

a. Genioglossus and geniohyoid
b. Fibers of mylohyoid
c. Submandibular space
d. Body of mandible

102. During surgery on the submandibular gland: *(COMED 2010)*

a. Damage to the lingual nerve will cause loss of sensation to the posterior third of the tongue
b. The submandibular gland is seen to wrap around the posterior border of mylohyoid
c. The facial artery and vein are usually divided as they course through the deep part of the gland
d. The hypoglossal nerve is seen to loop under the submandibular duct

103. Deep surface hyoglossus is related to: *(COMED 2006)*

a. Lingual nerve
b. Hypoglossal nerve
c. Submandibular ganglion
d. Glossopharyngeal nerve

104. Deep part of submandibular salivary gland is in relation to: *(COMED 2006)*

a. Facial nerve
b. Lingual nerve
c. Accessory nerve
d. Mandibular nerve

105. Structures related to the medial surface of the hyoglossus muscle include the following *except*: *(COMED 2008)*
a. Glossopharyngeal nerve
b. Stylohyoid ligament
c. Lingual artery
d. Hypoglossal nerve

106. Which one of the following nerves is not encountered during submandibular gland resection? *(COMED 2008)*
a. Lingual nerve b. Hypoglossal nerve
c. Accessory nerve d. Facial nerve

107. The nerve which lies in associations to Wharton duct is: *(KCET 2006)*
a. Facial b. Spinal accessory
c. Hypoglossal d. Lingual

108. Submandibular gland is related medially to the following structure: *(MH 2012)*
a. Digastric and medial pterygoid muscle
b. Hyoglossus, mylohyoid, and digastric muscle
c. Hyoglossus, mylohyoid muscle
d. Hyoglossus, digastric muscle

109. Submandibular spaces are considered to be anterior extension of which space? *(MH 2012)*
a. Parapharyngeal space
b. Infratemporal space
c. Buccal space
d. Pterygomandibular space

110. Which of the following is not present on the medial surface of a submandibular gland? *(PGI 2011)*
a. Styloglossus b. Mylohyoid
c. Facial thyroid d. Hypoglossus

DEEP STRUCTURE OF NECK

111. Which of the following is not attached laterally to thyroid cartilage, or all the following muscles are attached to the oblique line of thyroid cartilage *except*: *(AIIMS Nov 2008)*
a. Sternothyroid b. Thyrohyoid
c. Superior constrictor d. Inferior constrictor

112. All muscles attach to oblique line of thyroid cartilage *except*: *(AIIMS Nov 2011)*
a. Thyrohyoid
b. Middle constrictor
c. Superior constrictor
d. Sternohyoid

113. Carotid artery can be plated at: *(AIPG 2012)*
a. Upper border of thyroid cartilage
b. Lower border of thyroid
c. Cricoid cartilage
d. Hyoid bone

114. Inferior thyroid artery is a branch of: *(COMED 2006)*
a. External carotid artery
b. Internal carotid artery
c. Common carotid artery
d. Subclavian artery

115. Facial sheath for thyroid gland is provided by: *(KCET 2008)*
a. Investing layer of deep cervical fascia
b. Prevertebral fascia
c. Pretracheal fascia
d. Carotid sheath

116. Recurrent laryngeal nerve close relation to: *(KCET 2012)*
a. Superior thyroid artery
b. Middle thyroid vein
c. Inferior thyroid artery
d. Inferior parathyroid

117. Hassall's corpuscles are seen in: *(KCET 2005)*
a. Prostate
b. Spleen
c. Thymus
d. Liver

118. All the following are tributaries of internal jugular vein (IJV) *except*:
a. Inferior petrosal sinus
b. Pharyngeal vein
c. Lingual vein
d. Inferior cerebral vein

MOUTH AND PHARYNX

119. Sensory fibers from the taste buds in the hard and soft palate travel along: *(AIIMS May 2005)*
a. The trigeminal nerve
b. The facial nerve
c. The glossopharyngeal nerve
d. The vagus nerve

120. The palatine tonsil receives its arterial supply from all of the following, *except*: *(AIIMS May 2005)*
a. Facial
b. Ascending palatine
c. Sphenopalatine
d. Dorsal lingual

121. The sensory supply of the palate is through all of the following, *except*: *(AIPG 2011)*
a. The facial nerve
b. The vagus nerve (hypoglossal according to some students)
c. The glossopharyngeal nerve
d. The trigeminal nerve

122. Tensor palati is supplied by: *(AIIMS Nov 2012)*
a. Facial nerve b. Trigeminal
c. Vagus d. Hypoglossal

123. All the following muscles are supplied by cranial accessory except (muscles spared, if spinal accessory nerve is damaged): *(AIIMS Nov 2012,AIPG 2012)*
a. Stylopharyngeus
b. Salpingopharyngeus
c. Palatopharyngeus
d. Cricopharyngeus

124. Hypoglossal nerve supplies all of these muscles *except*? *(COMED 2011)*
a. Styloglossus b. Genioglossus
c. Palatoglossus d. Hyoglossus

125. Lymphatics of upper gums drain into: *(COMED 2006)*
a. Lingual nodes
b. Retropharyngeal nodes
c. Submandibular nodes
d. Submental nodes

126. Palatine tonsil develops from: *(KCET 2008)*
a. Dorsal part of II pharyngeal pouch
b. Ventral part of II pharyngeal pouch
c. Dorsal part of III pharyngeal pouch
d. Ventral part of I pharyngeal pouch

127. Structure passing through superior constrictor muscle and base of skull are: *(KCET 2005)*
a. Stylopharyngeus and glossopharyngeal nerve
b. Auditory tube and levator palati muscle
c. Internal laryngeal nerve and superior laryngeal vessels
d. Recurrent laryngeal nerve and inferior laryngeal vessels

128. Lymphatic drainage of tonsils taken into which lymph node? *(MH 2012)*
a. Jugulodigastric lymph nodes
b. Submandibular lymph node
c. Omohyoid lymph node
d. Jugulo-omohyoid lymph node

129. Location of palatine tonsils is in? *(MH 2011)*
a. Oropharynx b. Nasopharynx
c. Laryngopharynx d. Fossa of Rosenmuller

130. Mandibular gingival drains into lymph nodes: *(MH 2011)*
a. Submental b. Submandibular
c. Sublingual d. Jugulo-omohyoid

131. Quinsy is caused due to suppuration of: *(MH 2010)*
a. Pericoronal abscess
b. Pharyngeal abscess
c. Peritonsillar abscess
d. Retropharyngeal abscess

NOSE AND PARANASAL SINUSES

132. Supply to nasal cavity is by: *(AIPG/NEET 2013)*
a. Trigeminal b. Facial
c. Glossopharyngeal d. Facial

133. Inferior meatus of nasal cavity contain the opening of: *(KCET 2006)*
a. Maxillary sinus b. Middle ethmoidal sinus
c. Nasolacrimal duct d. Frontal sinus

134. The epithelial lining of the maxillary air sinus is: *(KCET 2006)*
a. Simple squamous
b. Simple cuboidal
c. Ciliated columnar
d. Stratified squamous non keratinized

135. Which of the following paranasal sinuses is formed before birth ? *(KCET 2005)*
a. Maxillary sinus b. Frontal sinus
c. Ethmoid sinus d. Mastoid air sinus

136. The maxillary air sinus opens into middle meatus at: *(KCET 2007)*
a. Infundibulum b. Summit of infundibulum
c. Bulla ethmoidalis d. Hiatus semilunaris

137. Maxillary sinus extends in body: *(MH 2010)*
a. Fundus b. Isthmus
c. Recess d. Cleft

138. All of the following open in Hiatus semilunaris *except*: *(MH 2009)*
a. Ant. ethmoidal sinus b. Post ethmoidal sinus
c. Maxillary sinus d. Frontal sinus

139. Middle conchae of nose are a part of: *(PGI 2008)*
a. Nasal bone b. Ethmoid
c. Vomer d. Maxilla

LARYNX

140. All are extrinsic ligament of larynx, *except*: *(AIPG/NEET 2013)*
a. Cricothyroid b. Stylohyoid
c. Hyoepiglottic d. Thyrohyoid muscles

141. Nerve supply to the vocal cords is by: *(COMED 2010)*
a. Internal laryngeal nerve
b. Recurrent laryngeal nerve
c. Superior laryngeal nerve
d. Internal and recurrent laryngeal nerve

142. The abductors of the vocal cords are: *(COMED 2009)*
a. Transverse arytenoid
b. Oblique arytenoid
c. Lateral thyroarytenoid
d. Posterior cricoarytenoid

143. Sensory innervation of larynx as far as the vocal folds is by: *(COMED 2006)*
a. External laryngeal nerve
b. Recurrent laryngeal nerve
c. Internal laryngeal nerve
d. Glossopharyngeal nerve

TONGUE

144. Tongue movement has its effect primarily on: *(AIIMS May 2010, 2008, AIPG 2007)*
a. Lip b. Cheek
c. Palatoglossal arch d. Facial musculature

145. Insertion of hyoglossus is at: *(AIPG 2010)*
a. Side of tongue b. Tip of tongue
c. Base of tongue d. Dorsum of tongue

146. Action of styloglossus muscle: *(AIPG 2010)*
a. Protrusion
b. Sidewise
c. Upwards and backwards pull of tongue
d. Retraction and depression tongue

147. Motor supply of tongue is by: *(AIPG 2009)*
a. Hypoglossal b. Glossopharyngeal
c. Vagus d. Facial

148. Posterior one-third of the tongue is innervated by: *(AIPG 2007)*
a. The vagus nerve
b. The glossopharyngeal nerve
c. The hypoglossal nerve
d. The lingual nerve

149. Which of the following is the normal arrangement of lingual nerve and vessels in the tongue from medial to lateral? *(AIPG 2005)*
a. Nerve, artery and vein
b. Artery, nerve and vein
c. Vein, artery and nerve
d. Nerve, artery. and vein

150. All the following cranial nerves transmit taste sensation to the brain *except*? *(AIIMS May 2013, AIPG 2012)*
a. 9 b. 10
c. 5 d. 7

151. Which of the following nerve carries taste sensation from circumvallate papillae? *(AIIMS May 2013, COMED 2005)*
a. Lingual nerve
b. Glossopharyngeal nerve
c. Chorda tympani nerve
d. Hypoglossal nerve

152. Which of the following lymphatics does not drain the tongue: *(AIIMS Nov 2013)*
a. Posterior vessels b. Central vessels
c. Marginal vessels d. Ventral vessels

153. Unilateral paralysis of hypoglossal nerve leads to: *(COMED 2009)*
a. Deviation of tongue to normal side
b. Deviation of tongue to paralysed side
c. No change in position of tongue
d. Retraction of tongue

154. Genioglossus muscle is attached in the posterior surface of symphysis menti in the: *(COMED 2005)*
a. Mental spines
b. Superior genial tubercle
c. The inferior genial tubercle
d. Just above the lower border of mandible

155. Mental spines provide attachment to: *(COMED 2007)*

a. Genioglossus and geniohyoid
b. Anterior and posterior bellies of digastric
c. Mylohyoid
d. Superior constrictor of pharynx

156. Lingual nerve, supplying tongue, is a branch of: *(COMED 2007)*

a. Facial nerve b. Hypoglossal nerve
c. Mandibular nerve d. Maxillary nerve

157. The mucosa of the posterior one-third of the tongue is supplied by: *(KCET 2009)*

a. Facial nerve b. Trigeminal nerve
c. Mandibular nerve d. Glossopharyngeal nerve

158. Taste functions are primarily mediated by: *(KCET 2009)*

a. Lingual nerve b. Chorda tympani
c. Hypoglossal nerve d. Glossopharyngeal nerve

159. Which of the following is called as the safety muscle of the tongue? *(KCET 2013)*

a. Styloglossus b. Stylopharyngeus
c. Genioglossus d. Hypoglossus

160. Hypoglossal nerve supplies all, *except*: *(MH 2010, AP 2006)*

a. Palatoglossus b. Genioglossus
c. Hyoglossus d. Styloglossus

161. The tongue: *(PGI 2006)*

a. Separated from the epiglottis by glossoepiglottic folds
b. Contains foramen caecum which is present on the dorsum of frenulum
c. Contains 6 to 10 circumvallate papilla located posterior to sulcus terminals
d. Embryologically derives from 1st branchial arch only

162. Base of the tongue is attached to the: *(PGI 2006)*

a. Hyoid bone
b. Mandible
c. Hyoid bone and mandible

EAR AND VESTIBULAR NERVE

163. Ceruminous glands present in the ear are: *(AIIMS May 2005)*

a. Modified eccrine glands
b. Modified apocrine glands
c. Mucous gland
d. Modified holocrine glands

164. What is the type of joint between the ossicles of ear? *(AIPG 2009)*

a. Fibrous joint
b. Primary cartilaginous
c. Secondary cartilaginous
d. Synovial joint

165. The following statements concerning chorda tympani nerve are true, *except*: *(AIPG 2005)*

a. That it carries secretomotor fibers to the submandibular gland
b. That it joins lingual nerve infratemporal fossa
c. That it is a branch of the facial nerve
d. That it contains postganglionic parasympathetic fibers

166. Which blood vessel does not supply pharyngotympanic tube? *(AIIMS May 2012, AIPG 2012)*

a. Ascending pharyngeal
b. Ascending palatine
c. Middle meningeal
d. Artery of pterygoid canal

167. One of the bones named below reaches its adult size of birth? *(AIPG 2012)*

a. Ear ossicles
b. Parietal bone
c. Mastoid process
d. Maxilla

168. Posterior ethmoidal air sinus opens into: *(COMED 2012)*

a. Superior meatus
b. Middle meatus
c. Inferior meatus
d. Sphenoethmoidal recess

169. Which of the following venous sinuses is more likely to be affected with thrombosis in chronic otitis media and mastoiditis? *(COMED 2010)*

a. Cavernous b. Inter-cavernous
c. Sigmoid d. Superior petrosal

EYEBALL

170. Horner's syndrome include all *except*: *(COMED 2009)*

a. Enophthalmos b. Miosis
c. Exophthalmos d. Ptosis

EMBRYOLOGY

171. Which of the following is not a neuroectodermal derivative? *(AIPG 2010)*
a. Paneth cells b. Neurons
c. Schwann cells d. Odontoblasts

172. Which of the following bone is not derived from viscerocranium? *(AIPG 2010)*
a. Sphenoid b. Lacrimal
c. Vomer d. Zygomatic

173. Primitive streak is maintained by: *(AIPG 2008)*
a. Brachyury gene b. Nodal gene
c. BMPR IV d. Fibroblast growth factor VIII

174. Intrinsic muscles of the tongue are derived from: *(AIPG 2008, COMED 2006)*
a. Cervical somites
b. Occipital somites
c. Pharyngeal arch mesoderm
d. Second branchial cleft

175. Component from 2nd branchial arch is: *(AIIMS May 2012)*
a. Mandible
b. Muscle of mastication
c. Muscle of facial expression
d. TMJ

176. During which time of intrauterine life Neural tube formation occurs? *(MH 2012, COMED 2013)*
a. 18-23 days b. 17th day
c. 90-30 days d. 10-15 days

177. Which of the following muscle is not a derivative of second pharyngeal arch? *(COMED 2013)*
a. Buccinator muscle b. Stapedius
c. Platysma d. Anterior belly of digastric

178. Failure of descent of thyroid anlage can be seen in the tongue: *(COMED 2012, 2008)*
a. In anterior 2/3 of dorsal aspect
b. In posterior 1/3 of dorsal aspect
c. Near the base of tongue close to foramen caecum
d. In anterior 2/3 of inferior surface

179. Meiotic division of male germ cells commences: *(COMED 2010)*
a. During intrauterine life
b. Just before birth
c. By around 6 years after birth
d. By around 16 years

180. The first evidence of cartilage getting converted to bone in craniofacial skeleton occurs during: *(COMED 2010)*
a. 4th postnatal week b. 8th prenatal week
c. 4th prenatal week d. 8th postnatal week

181. Umbilical cord contains: *(COMED 2009)*
a. Three arteries and one vein
b. One artery and three veins
c. One artery and one vein
d. Two arteries and one vein

182. Muscles of face are derived from the mesoderm of: *(COMED 2005)*
a. 1st branchial arch
b. 2nd branchial arch
c. 3rd branchial arch
d. 2nd and 3rd branchial arch

183. Derivative of 2nd pharyngeal arch is: *(COMED 2006)*
a. Sphenomandibular ligament
b. Stylomandibular ligament
c. Anterior ligament of malleus
d. Stylohyoid ligament

184. Development of mandible is by: *(COMED 2008)*
a. I branchial arch b. II branchial arch
c. IV branchial arch d. III branchial arch

185. Hyoid bone is a derivative of: *(COMED 2007)*
a. 1st pharyngeal arch
b. 1st and 2nd pharyngeal arches
c. 2nd and 3rd pharyngeal arches
d. 4th pharyngeal arch

186. Which of the following is a derivative of the second branchial pouch: *(KCET 2009)*
a. Tympanic cavity b. Meckel's cartilage
c. Palatine tonsil d. Tongue base

187. At which stage congenital defects are more pronounced, especially when certain teratogenic agents interfere during the development of embryo? *(KCET 2010)*
a. 4th to 8th week
b. Initiation stage before 4th week
c. 5th to 6th month of intrauterine life
d. All of the above

188. The Meckel's cartilage is derived from the: *(KCET 2010)*

a. 1st branchial arch b. 2nd branchial arch
c. 3rd branchial arch d. 4th branchial arch

189. Philtrum of upper lip develops from: *(KCET 2011, 2012)*

a. Mandibular process
b. Maxillary process
c. Frontonasal process
d. Palatal process

190. Which of the following is not a derivative of Meckel's cartilage? *(KCET 2013)*

a. Incus
b. Malleus
c. Stapes
d. Sphenomandibular ligament

191. Schwan cells are delivered from: *(KCET 2007)*

a. Neural crest cells b. Mesoderm
c. Endoderm d. Ectoderm

HISTOLOGY

192. All of the following cells are of connective tissue origin *except*: *(AIIMS May 2008, AIPG 2010)*

a. Macrophages b. Fibroblasts
c. Clara cells d. Melanocytes

193. The cells belonging to which of the following types of epithelium are provided with extra reserve of cell membrane? *(AIIMS May 2006)*

a. Transitional b. Stratified squamous
c. Stratified cuboidal d. Stratified columnar

194. Which of the following is not present in the basal lamina? *(AIPG 2008)*

a. Rhodopsin b. Entactin
c. Laminin d. Nidogen

195. All of the following are true about pericytes *except*: *(AIPG 2008)*

a. That they are undifferentiated mesenchymal cells
b. That they are present outside the endothelium of capillaries
c. That they differentiate into fibroblasts in response to injury
d. None of the above

196. Hard tissues are developed from: *(AIPG 2008)*

a. The endoderm
b. The endoderm and ectoderm
c. The mesoderm
d. The ectoderm and mesoderm

197. Urothelium lines all of the following *except*: *(AIPG 2008)*

a. The collecting duct
b. The minor calyx
c. The urinary bladder
d. The ureter

198. Barr body is found in which of the following phase of the cell cycle? *(AIPG 2005)*

a. Interphase b. Metaphase
c. GI phase d. Telophase

199. Most of the structure of oral cavity is derived from: *(AIPG/NEET 2013)*

a. Ectodermal b. Endodermal
c. Mesoderm d. None of the above

200. The lingual surface of epiglottis is lined by: *(COMED 2010)*

a. Stratified squamous epithelium
b. Simple squamous epithelium
c. Stratified columnar epithelium
d. Pseudostratified epithelium

201. The cortex of lymph node contains: *(KCET 2012)*

a. Cords of billroth
b. Hassall's corpuscles
c. Lymphatic nodules
d. White pulp

BRAIN

202. The area that lies immediately lateral to the anterior perforating substance is: *(AIIMS May 2011)*

a. The orbital gyrus
b. The uncus
c. The optic chiasma
d. The limen insulae

203. Geniculate neuralgia is associated with which cranial nerve? *(AIIMS Nov 2010)*

a. Facial
b. Glossopharyngeal
c. Trigeminal
d. Hypoglossal

204. Broca's area is concerned with: *(AIIMS May 2009)*
a. Word formation b. Comprehension
c. Repetition d. Reading

205. Proprioception is carried from head and neck by all, *except*: *(AIIMS May 2009)*
a. Trigeminal
b. Facial
c. Glossopharyngeal
d. Spinal accessory

206. Which of the following cells are not present in the cortex? *(AIIMS May 2008, AIPG 2010)*
a. Purkinje b. Cajal
c. Stellate d. Pyramidal

207. Which of the following is true about chorda tympani? *(AIIMS May 2008)*
a. It enters the pterygoid canal
b. It carries preganglionic secretomotor fibers to the submandibular gland
c. It is the nerve of the tympanic membrane
d. It contains postganglionic parasympathetic fibers

208. The tingling sensation felt in the nose just before sneezing is carried by: *(AIIMS May 2008)*
a. Glossopharyngeal nerve
b. Facial nerve
c. Nasopalatine nerve
d. Nasociliary nerve

209. The cortical nuclei are connected to the subcortical nuclei through fibers: *(AIIMS May 2008)*
a. Collateral b. Commissural
c. Projection d. Association

210. Which one of the following is a junction of frontal, parietal, temporal and greater wing of sphenoid bone? *(AIIMS Nov 2007, AIPG 2006)*
a. Pterion b. Lambda
c. Vertex d. Inion

211. All of the following are supplied by pharyngeal plexus of nerve *except*: *(AIIMS Nov 2006)*
a. Musculus uvulae
b. Palatoglossus
c. Palatopharyngeus
d. Tensor veli palate

212. All of the following statements about the vagus nerve are true *except*: *(AIIMS Nov 2005)*
a. That it supplies heart and lung
b. That it carries postganglionic parasympathetic fibers
c. That it innervates right two-third of transverse colon
d. That it stimulates peristalsis and relaxes sphincters

213. Lining of the blood vessels in blood brain barrier is formed of: *(AIPG 2010)*
a. Astrocytes b. Endothelial cells
c. Oligodendrocytes d. Microglial cells

214. Which nerve originates from the dorsal surface of brain? *(AIPG 2010)*
a. Trochlear b. Glossopharyngeal
c. Oculomotor d. Abducens

215. About blood brain barrier all are true, *except*: *(AIPG 2010)*
a. Solutes can be dissolved and move outside through membrane
b. There is high junction between astrocyte and endothelial cells so that no solute can pass through it
c. Less transcytotic activity exists for the most lipid-soluble substances
d. It is almost totally impermeable to plasma protein

216. Which of the following nerves is not efferent? *(AIPG 2008)*
a. Trochlear b. Facial
c. Abducens d. Oculomotor

217. Posterior cerebral artery is a branch of: *(AIPG 2007)*
a. Internal carotid b. External carotid
c. Subclavian d. Basilar artery

218. Which of the following is not a branch of trigeminal nerve? *(AIPG 2007)*
a. Maxillary b. Mandibular
c. Ophthalmic d. Carotid

219. In adults, the spinal cord normally ends at: *(AIPG 2006)*
a. The lower border of L1
b. The lower border of L3
c. The lower border of S1
d. The lower border of L5

220. Afferent component of corneal reflex is mediated by: *(AIPG 2006)*
a. The vagus nerve
b. The facial nerve
c. The trigeminal nerve
d. The glossopharyngeal nerve

221. All carry proprioceptive impulse, *except*: *(AIPG 2006)*

a. Glossopharyngeal b. Facial
c. Trigeminal d. Abducens

222. Facial nerve is located: *(AIIMS Nov 2012)*

a. Superficial to SMAS and superficial to parotidomasseteric fascia
b. Superficial to SMAS and deep to parotidomasseteric fascia
c. Deep to SMAS and superficial to parotido-masseteric
d. Deep to SMAS superficial to buccal pad of fat

223. Damage to ambiguus nucleus effects all *except*: *(AIIMS Nov 2012)*

a. Muscles of pharynx
b. Muscles of larynx
c. Parotid gland
d. Cardiac nucleus (ganglia)

224. All the following are true about facial nerve, *except*? *(AIIMS May 2013)*

a. It is secretomotor to the submandibular gland
b. It supplies anterior belly of digastric
c. It has a large motor and small sensory root
d. Parasympathetic innervations to palatal and nasal gland

225. Damage to facial nerve just above branching of chorda tympani causes all, *except*? *(AIIMS May 2013, AIPG 2012)*

a. Hyperacusis
b. Decrease salivation
c. Loss of taste from tongue
d. Paralysis of muscles of facial expression

226. Motor nerve likely to be damaged when excessive pressure at angle of mandible during establishment of patent airway damages: *(AIIMS Nov 2012, AIPG/NEET 2013)*

a. Trigeminal
b. Facial
c. Occulomotor
d. Glossopharyngeal

227. Occulomotor nerve palsy causes all, *except*: *(AIPG/NEET 2013)*

a. Miosis
b. Ptosis
c. Outward eye deviation
d. Diplopia

228. Premaxillary part supplied by: *(AIIMS Nov 2013)*

a. Nasopalatine b. Glossopharyngeal
c. Greater palatine d. Anterior pharyngeal

229. Nervus intermedius does not carry? *(AIIMS May 2012)*

a. Special visceral efferent
b. Special visceral afferent
c. General somatic afferent
d. General visceral efferent

230. Which of the following is not a branch of the occulomotor nerve? *(AIPG 2012)*

a. Nerve to superior rectus
b. Nerve to medial rectus
c. Twigs to ciliary ganglion
d. Lacrimal nerve

231. Glossopharyngeal nerve passes through: *(COMED 2013)*

a. Foramen ovale b. Jugular foramen
c. Foramen rotundum d. Foramen spinosum

232. Epicritic perception of pain occurs at the level of: *(COMED 2010)*

a. Thalamus b. Area 3, 1, 2
c. Area 5, 7 d. Pulvinar

233. CSF is directly returned to venous system by: *(COMED 2009)*

a. Choroid plexus b. Cerebral veins
c. Arachnoid villi d. Emissary veins

234. Cricothyroid muscle is supplied by: *(COMED 2005)*

a. External laryngeal nerve
b. Internal laryngeal nerve
c. Recurrent laryngeal nerve
d. A direct branch from vagus nerve

235. Pterygopalatine ganglion is functionally related to: *(COMED 2006)*

a. Facial nerve
b. Mandibular nerve
c. Glossopharyngeal nerve
d. Maxillary nerve

236. Which of the following lobes of cerebrum is related to the inferior horn of the lateral ventricle: *(COMED 2008)*

a. Frontal b. Parietal
c. Temporal d. Occipital

237. The branch of facial nerve that conveys the secretomotor impulse involved in lacrimation is: *(COMED 2008)*
a. Chorda tympani nerve
b. Deep petrosal nerve
c. Greater petrosal nerve
d. Lesser petrosal nerve

238. Mastoid air sinus is posteriorly related to: *(KCET 2006)*
a. Cavernous sinus b. Sigmoid sinus
c. Straight sinus d. Sphenoparietal sinus

239. Posterior belly of digastric muscle is supplied by: *(KCET 2008)*
a. Mandibular nerve b. Maxillary nerve
c. Ansa cervicalis d. Facial nerve

240. During surgery of submandibular gland following cranial nerve may get injured: *(KCET 2008)*
a. Glossopharyngeal nerve
b. Accessory nerve
c. Hypoglossal nerve
d. Trigeminal nerve

241. Bell's palsy results in the inflammation of one of the following nerves: *(KCET 2009)*
a. Hypoglossal nerve b. Accessory nerve
c. Facial nerve d. Glossopharyngeal nerve

242. Secretomotor fibers for the parotid gland are relayed in one of the following ganglia: *(KCET 2009)*
a. Otic ganglion b. Submandibular ganglion
c. Ciliary ganglion d. Pterygopalatine ganglion

243. All the cranial nerves provide innervations for the structures in the head and neck *except* one that additionally supplies the thorax and abdomen: *(KCET 2010)*
a. Glossopharyngeal b. Spinal accessory
c. Vagus d. Hypoglossal

244. Hypoglossal nerve is: *(KCET 2010)*
a. Purely sensory b. Purely motor
c. Mixed d. Spinal nerve

245. Cardiac pain may be transmitted to the jaw due to the overlapping of: *(KCET 2012)*
a. 5th cranial nerve, third cervical nerve and first thoracic nerve
b. 7th cranial nerve, third cervical nerve and first thoracic nerve
c. 5th cranial nerve, second cervical nerve and first thoracic nerve
d. 7th cranial nerve, second cervical nerve and first thoracic nerve

246. Which of the following is not a part of the greater wing of the sphenoid bone? *(KCET 2013)*
a. Foramen rotundum
b. Foramen spinosum
c. Optic canal
d. Canaliculus innominatus

247. Which of the following is false about otic parasympathetic ganglion? *(KCET 2013)*
a. Secretomotor supply for parotid gland
b. Situated at the floor of the infratemporal fossa
c. Has parasympathetic, sympathetic and sensory fibers
d. All of the above

248. The preganglionic parasympathetic fibers for otic ganglion commence at: *(KCET 2007)*
a. Superior salivatory nucleus
b. Inferior salivatory nucleus
c. Nucleus of tractus solitarius
d. Lacrimatory nucleus

249. After leaving posterior cranial fossa facial nerve enters into: *(MH 2012)*
a. Internal acoustic meatus
b. Stylomastoid foramen
c. Foramen ovale
d. Foramen lacerum

250. Broca's area is present in: *(MH 2009)*
a. Inferior frontal gyrus
b. Pre-central gyrus
c. Post-central gyrus
d. Superior temporal gyrus

251. Ptosis may occur due to damage to: *(MCET 2007)*
a. Trochlear nerve
b. Occulomotor
c. Trigeminal nerve
d. Superior oblique muscle

252. All cranial nerves are confined to the head and neck with exception of: *(BHU 2012)*
a. One
b. Two
c. More than two
d. None of the above

MISCELLANEOUS

253. The largest organ of the body is: *(AIIMS Nov 2010)*
a. Liver b. Lung
c. Kidney d. Heart

254. Which of the following is categorized in the list of obligate carriers having disease with recessive trait? *(AIIMS Nov 2010)*
a. Phenotypically normal woman with affected brother and son but normal daughter
b. Phenotypically diseased woman with affected husband and daughter but normal son
c. Phenotypically normal woman with diseased husband and son but normal daughter
d. Phenotypically diseased woman with diseased husband and affected son and daughter

255. Which of the following oropharyngeal function is not involuntary? *(AIIMS May 2010)*
a. Tongue position b. Gagging
c. Respiration d. Speech

256. All of the following are true regarding heart muscle, *except*: *(AIIMS May 2009)*
a. That it acts as syncytium
b. That it has multiple nuclei
c. That it has gap junctions
d. That it has branching

257. Which of the following is known as musician's nerve? *(AIIMS May 2008)*
a. Ulnar b. Median
c. Radial d. Mucocutaneous

258. The right heart border in a 10-year-old is formed by all *except*: *(AIIMS May 2008)*
a. VC b. SVC
c. RA d. Ascending aorta

259. A nonsynovial joint with dense connective tissue between two bony surfaces is termed as: *(AIIMS Nov 2007, May 2006)*
a. Synchondrosis b. Syndesmosis
c. Symphysis d. Suture

260. The lymphatics from the lower lip first enter the blood stream through: *(AIIMS May 2007, AIPG 2007, 2010, Nov 2011)*
a. Inferior labial artery
b. Inferior labial vein
c. Brachiocephalic vein
d. Pterygoid plexus of veins

261. The cell junctions allowing the exchange of cytoplasmic molecules between two cells are called: *(AIIMS May 2006)*
a. Gap junctions
b. Tight junctions
c. Anchoring junctions
d. Focal junctions

262. The ducts of all the following glands consist of stratified cuboidal epithelium, *except*: *(AIIMS May 2005)*
a. Sweat glands b. Sebaceous glands
c. Salivary glands d. Pancreas

263. Neuroepithelial type of sensory receptors is present in which of the following system? *(AIIMS May 2005)*
a. Visual b. Auditory
c. Gustatory d. Olfactory

264. Following statements are true regarding the SA node, *except*: *(AIIMS May 2005)*
a. That it is located at the right border of the ascending aorta
b. That it contains specialized nodal cardiac muscle
c. That it is supplied by the atrial branches of the right coronary artery
d. That it initiates cardiac conduction

265. Slightly movable articulations in which the contiguous bony surfaces are either connected by broad, flattened disk of fibrocartilage or united by interosseous ligaments are known as: *(AIPG 2010)*
a. Gomphosis b. Enarthrosis
c. Diarthrosis d. Amphiarthrosis

266. Routine technique for karyotyping using light microscopy is: *(AIPG 2010)*
a. C-banding
b. G-banding
c. Q-banding
d. B-V-skinning

267. A person showing two cell lines derived from a single zygote is called as: *(AIPG 2010)*
a. Chimerism b. Mosaicism
c. Segregation d. Pseudodominance

268. Which are composite muscles? *(AIPG 2009)*
a. Pectineus b. Biceps femoris
c. Adductor magnus d. All of the above

269. In skin, which of the following is true? *(AIPG 2008)*
a. Keratoepithelial cells/keratosomes account for 50% of all the epithelial cells
b. Keratoepithelial cells/keratosomes provide protection against UV rays
c. Epidermis provides support for cutaneous vessels
d. Keratoepithelial cells reduce moisture loss

270. Slight movable joint which is joined by fibers is: *(AIPG 2007)*
a. Amphiarthrosis b. Gomphosis
c. Synostosis d. Synchondrosis

271. All of the following physiological processes occur during the growth at the epiphyseal plate, *except*: *(AIPG 2005)*
a. Proliferation and hypertrophy
b. Calcification and ossification
c. Vasculogenesis and erosion
d. Replacement of red bone marrow with yellow marrow

272. Which of the following is a pneumatic bone is: *(PGI June 2013, AIPG 2012)*
a. Maxilla b. Mandible
c. Nasal d. Occipital

273. All muscles retract scapulae, *except*: *(AIPG/NEET2013)*
a. Trapezius b. Rhomboid major
c. Rhomboid minor d. Levator scapulae

274. Which of the following is dangerous area for oromaxillofacial infections? *(AIIMS Nov 2011)*
a. Carotid sheath
b. Space post to carotid sheath in the post triangle
c. Posterior to prevertebral area
d. Between the alar plate and prevertebral fascia

275. Area of skin supplied by single nerve: *(AIPG 2012)*
a. Dermatome b. Dermoid
c. Pedicle d. Graft

276. Following factor delay the wound healing *except*: *(COMED 2013)*
a. Vitamin C deficiency
b. Infection
c. Anemia
d. Immobilization

277. Liver is devided into: *(COMED 2005)*
a. Couinaud segments
b. Couinaud segments
c. Couinaud segments
d. Couinaud segments

278. Basic metabolic unit of bone is: *(KCET 2006)*
a. Osteon b. Osteoblast
c. Osteocyte d. Osteoclast

279. What is the type of joint formed between the tooth and the alveolar socket? *(KCET 2011, 2012)*
a. Gomphosis b. Syndesmosis
c. Suture d. Synovial

280. The classic karyotype of klinefelter syndrome is: *(KCET 2011)*
a. 45, XO b. 47, XXY
c. Trisomy 18 d. Trisomy 21

281. Multipennate order is not seen in which of the following muscle: *(PGI June 2013)*
a. Masseter b. Deltoid
c. Medial pterygoid d. Temporalis

282. Primary teeth having prominent transverse ridge joining mesiobuccal mesiolingual cusp is: *(PGI June 2013)*
a. Maxilla 1st molar b. Maxilla 2st molar
c. Mandible 1st molar d. Mandible 2st molar

283. Most common missing permanent teeth: *(PGI June 2013)*
a. Mandibular second premolar
b. Mandibular 1st molar
c. Maxillary 1st molar
d. Mandibular central incisors

284. Dental lamina arise from which part of gum pad: *(PGI JUNE 2013)*
a. Transverse groove b. Dental groove
c. Labial groove d. Lingual groove

285. The nerve supply of deltoid muscle is by? *(MH 2011)*
a. Radial b. Axillary
c. Median d. Subscapular

286. Anteriorly, which organ is related to the right kidney? *(MH 2011)*
a. Jejunum b. Spleen
c. Liver d. Ureter

287. Parotid duct opening is seen opposite: *(MH 2010)*
a. Near maxillary 2nd molar
b. Near mandibular 2nd molar
c. Near maxillary 1st molar
d. Near mandibular 1st molar

288. A nodule is seen in: *(MH 2010)*
a. Epithelium
b. Basal layer
c. Deep in dermis
d. Superficial dermis

289. Number of muscle in human body to propel the skeleton are: *(MH 2009)*
a. 439
b. 639
c. 739
d. 839

290. Nerve injured due to carrying heavy loads on shoulder is: *(MH 2009)*
a. Suprascapular nerve
b. Nerve to serratus anterior
c. Lateral pectoral nerve
d. Thoracodorsal nerve

Answers with Explanations

OSTEOLOGY OF HEAD AND NECK

1. Ans. (d) It has a large vertebral body *Ref: BDC 5th ed. p 40*

Characteristics of typical cervical vertebrae:

- Transverse process is dorsomedial to the foramen transversarium.
- Vertebral foramen is larger than the body.
- The body of cervical vertebrae is small and broader from side to side.

Size of vertebral body:

Cervical (Broad from side to side) < Thoracic (Heart shape) < Lumbar (Kidney shape).

2. Ans. (d) Inferior orbital fissure *Ref: BDC 5th ed. p 28*

- Inferior orbital fissure transmits the following nerve:
  - Zygomatic nerve
  - Orbital branch of pterygopalatine ganglion
  - Infraorbital nerve and vessels.
- Infraorbital nerve exits through the inferior orbital fissure and enters into the orbit.
- Infraorbital nerve supply to the skin and subcutaneous tissue of the face below and nasal to the orbit.

3. Ans. (c) Brachycephaly *Ref: Freyschmidt's "Koehler/Zimmer's Borderland of Normal and Early Pathological Finding in Skeletal Radiography 5th ed. p 392*

Fusion of different suture leads to different patterns of growth of the skull.

Example:

Trigonocephaly - Fusion of metopic suture.

Brachycephaly - Fusion of coronal suture.

Dolichocephaly - Fusion of sagittal suture.

Plagiocephaly - Unilateral premature closure of lambdoid and coronal suture.

Oxycephaly - Fusion of coronal and lambdoidal suture.

Acrocephaly - Multiple suture closure.

4. Ans. (a) Hyoid bone *Ref: Gray's Anatomy 2nd ed. p 988,989*

- The middle pharyngeal constrictor is a fan shaped muscle located in the neck.
- It is innervated by the branch of vagus nerve through the pharyngeal plexus.
- The middle pharyngeal constrictor muscle attaches anteriorly to the hyoid bone and the stylohyoid ligament.
- It inserts posteriorly into the medial pharyngeal raphe.

5. Ans. (b) The cervical plexus *Ref: Anatomy for Dental Students by Martin Atkinson 4th ed. p 226*

- The infrahyoid muscle (strap muscle) are a group of four pairs of muscles in the anterior part of the neck.
- The four infrahyoid muscle are- the sternohyoid, sternothyroid, thyrohyoid, and omohyoid muscle.
- The infrahyoid muscles either originates from or insert on to the hyoid bone.

- The infrahyoid muscles are innervated by the ansa cervicalis from the cervical plexus (C1-C3) except the thyrohyoid muscle which is innervated by fiber only from the first cervical spinal nerve travelling with the hypoglossal nerve.
- Its function is to depress the hyoid bone and larynx during swallowing and speech.

6. Ans. (b) 6 *Ref: BDC 5th ed. p 30*

- A fontanelle (or fontanel) (colloquially, soft spot) is an anatomical feature on an infant's skull comprising any of the soft membranous gaps between the incompletely formed cranial bones of a fetus or an infant.
- Fontanelles allow for rapid stretching and deformation of the cranium as the brain expands faster than the surrounding bone can grow.
- Fontanelles are soft spots on a baby's head which, during birth, enable the bony plates of the skull to flex, allowing the child's head to pass through the birth canal. The ossification of the bones of the skull causes the anterior fontanelle to close over by 9 to 18 months. The sphenoidal and posterior fontanelles close during the first few months of life. The closures eventually form the sutures of the neurocranium. Other than the anterior and posterior fontanelles, the mastoid fontanelle and the sphenoidal fontanelle are also significant.
- At birth, the skull features a small posterior fontanelle, an open area covered by a tough membrane, where the two parietal bones adjoin the occipital bone (at the lambda). This fontanelle usually closes during the first two to three months of an infant's life. This is called intramembranous ossification. The mesenchymal connective tissue turns into bone tissue.
- The much larger, diamond-shaped anterior fontanelle where the two frontal and two parietal bones join generally remains open until the child is about two years of age, however, in cleidocranial dysostosis it is often late in closing or may never close. Examination of an infant includes palpating the anterior fontanelle.
- Two smaller fontanelles are located on each side of the head, more anteriorly the sphenoidal or anterolateral fontanelle (between the sphenoid, parietal, temporal, and frontal bones) and more posteriorly the mastoid or posterolateral fontanelle (between the temporal, occipital, and parietal bones).

7. Ans. (b) Tendon of tensor veli palatine muscle *Ref: Gray's Anatomy for Student 2nd ed. p 1048*

- Palatine aponeurosis is the expanded interlacing tendons of the tensor veli palatini muscles in the anterior two thirds of the soft palate to which the other palatine muscles attach.
- The tensor veli palatini is innervated by the medial pterygoid nerve, a branch of mandibular nerve, the third branch of the trigeminal nerve (CN V) - the only muscle of the palate not innervated by the vagus nerve.

8. Ans. (a) Lingual artery *Ref: Gray's Anatomy for Student 2nd ed. p 1041*

- The lingual artery arises from the external carotid artery between the superior thyroid artery and facial artery. It can be located easily in tongue
- Branch of lingual artery:
  - Suprahyoid branch
  - Dorsal lingual branch
  - Deep lingual branch
  - Sublingual branch.
- Lingual artery supply the entire tongue, floor of the mouth, lingual gingiva, a portion of soft palate, tonsil and the supra hyoid muscle.

9. Ans. (c) Deep facial vein *Ref: BDC 5th ed. p 62 and Gray's Anatomy 2nd ed. p 871*

- Facial veins communicates with veins passing into deeps region of the face, i.e. The deep facial vein connecting with the pterygoid plexus of veins.

- Hence deep facial veins connected with the intracranial cavernous sinus through emissary veins that connect intracranial and extracranial veins.
- There is no value in the facial vein or any other venous channel in the head so the injection of the face should be handled with great care.

10. Ans. (d) Temporal bone *Ref: Gray's anatomy 2nd ed. p 821*

- Mandibular fossa is a part of temporal bone
- A concavity in the temporal bone where the head of the mandible articulates with the base of the skull
- The prominent articular tubercle is an important feature of this articulation it is the downward projection of the anterior border of the mandibular fossa.

11. Ans. (d) Ophthalmic vein *Ref: B.D. Chaurasia's 5th ed. p 46*

Dangerous area of face—

Facial vein communicates with the cavernous sinus through:

- Communication between the supraorbital vein and superior ophthalmic vein.
- Through pterygoid plexus of vein via deep facial vein.
- Infection involves cavernous sinus by spreading through this path which is most likely to occur when the lower part of nose and upper lips is the source of infection.
- The danger triangle of the face consists of the area from the corners of the mouth to the bridge of the nose, including the nose and maxilla. Due to the special nature of the blood supply to the human nose and surrounding area, it is possible (although very rare) for retrograde infections from the nasal area to spread to the brain.
- This is possible because of venous communication (via the ophthalmic veins) between the facial vein and the cavernous sinus. The cavernous sinus lies within the cranial cavity, between layers of the meninges and is a major conduit of venous drainage from the brain.

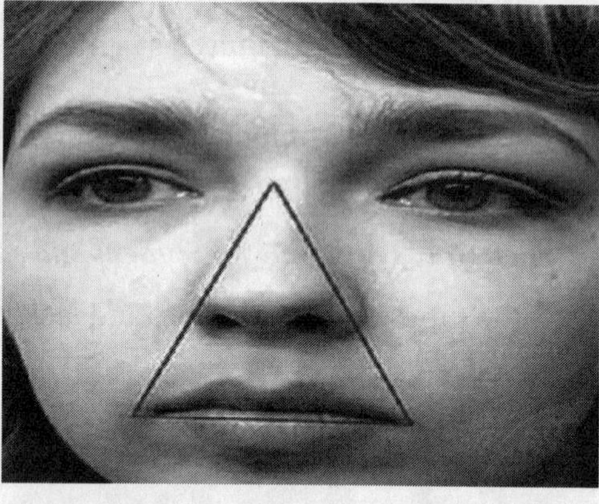

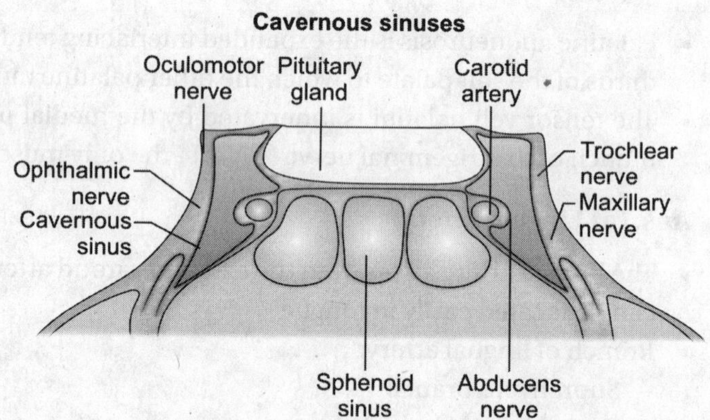

12. Ans. (d) Posterior auricular *Ref: B.D. Chaurasia's 5th ed. p 39*

Occipitofrontalis:

- Has two bellies frontal and occipital.
- Now as we all know that all the facial muscles are developed from 2nd branchial arch hence supplied by the nerve of same arch which is the facial nerve.
- Fontal belly is partially joined in midline and supplied by temporal branch of facial nerve.
- Occipital bellies are separate and are supplied by posterior auricular branch of facial nerve.

13. Ans. (a) Serrate *Ref:B.D. Chaurasia's 5th ed. p 127*

Sutures:

- *Coronal suture*: This is placed between the frontal bone and the two parietal bones. The suture crosses the cranial vault from side to side and runs downwards and forwards.
- *Sagittal suture*: It is placed in the median plane between the two parietal bones. It is an example of serrate suture.
- *Lambdoid suture*: It lies posteriorly between the occipital and the two parietal bones, and it runs downwards and forwards across the cranial vault.
- *Metopic suture*: This is occasionally present in about 3 to 8% individuals. It lies in the median plane and separates the two halves of the frontal bone.

Sutures are unique to the skull and are classified as fibrous joints. There are several types of sutures:

- **Serrate sutures** are characterized by edges that interdigitate in a serrated fashion, with the teeth of the interdigitations tapering slightly e.g. sagittal suture.
  - It is also known as dentate suture, this configuration allows gapping of the joint.
- **Denticulate sutures** are similar to serrate suture but exhibit a "dovetail" effect, with the teeth widening toward the ends, which more effectively lock the suture, e.g. lamboid suture.
- Squamous suture are characterized by overlapping bones such as the temporal and parietal, which are reciprocally beveled.
  - Mainly of two types:
    - Limbous sutures have mutual ridges or sensation
    - Plane suture which exhibit less structured surfaces which are mutually roughened. For example:
      Termporoparietal suture
      Suture between two maxillae
      Meeting of zygomatic and palatine bone.

14. Ans. (b) Deep temporal artery *Ref: Plastic Surgery 3rd ed. p 107*

- The deep temporal artery is a branch of internal maxillary artery.
- The deep temporal artery provides the primary blood supply for the temporalis muscle. The temporalis muscle have its insertion site on the coronoid process of the mandible. In this way the deep temporal artery primarily supply to the coronoid process of mandible.

15. Ans. (c) 45 bones *Ref: Oxford Handbook of Dental Nursing p 40*

- The skull can be separated into 4 areas: the mandible, the maxilla, the cranial bone and the facial bones.
- The primary function of skull is to protect the brain.
- At birth, the skull has 45 bones.

16. Ans. (c) Auriculotemporal nerve *Ref: Grays Anatomy for Students p 933*

The auriculotemporal nerve is a branch of the mandibular nerve that runs with the superficial temporal artery and vein, and provides sensory innervation to various regions on the side of the head.

Origin:

The auriculotemporal nerve arises as two roots from the posterior division of the mandibular nerve. The mandibular nerve is a branch of the trigeminal nerve, and the mandibular nerve exits the skull through the foramen ovale.

Course:

The auriculotemporal nerve passes between the neck of the mandible and the sphenomandibular ligament, gives off parotid branches and then turns superiorly, posterior to its head and moving anteriorly, gives off anterior branches to the auricle. It then crosses over the root of the zygomatic process of the temporal bone, deep to the superficial temporal artery.

17. Ans. (a) Frontonasal prominence *Ref: Orban's, 12th ed p 9, 10; B.D. Chaurasia's for Dental Students, p 322*

- Failure of local fusion of one maxillary process with the corresponding premaxillary region, leading to a persistent.
- Fissure between the philtrum and lateral part of the upper lip on that side, is called a cleft lip.
- If the palatal shelves fail to fuse across the midline and with the nasal septum a cleft palate is produced.

18. (a, c, d) Synovial, Allow rotation of the head, Supported by the alar ligaments *Ref: Gray's Anatomy p 31-33*

Atlas and axis - vertebra CI (the atlas) articulates with the head. Its major distinguishing feature is that it lacks a vertebral body. When viewed from above the atlas is ring-shaped and composed of two lateral masses interconnected by an anterior arch and a posterior arch.

- Each lateral mass articulates above with an occipital condyle of the skull and below with the superior articular process of vertebra CII (the axis). The superior articular surfaces are bean shaped and concave, whereas the inferior articular surfaces are almost circular and flat.
- The atlantooccipital joint allows the head to nod up and down on the vertebral column.
- The posterior surface of the anterior arch has an articular facet for the dens, which projects superiorly from the vertebral body of the axis. The dens is held in position by a strong transverse ligament of atlas posterior to it and spanning the distance between the oval attachment facets on the medial surfaces of the lateral masses of the atlas.
- The transverse process of the atlas are large and protrude further laterally than those of the other cervical vertebrae and act as levers for muscle action, particularly for muscles that move the head at the atlantoaxial joints.
- The axis is characterized by the large tooth-like dens, which extends superiorly from the vertebral body. The anterior surface of the dens has an oval facet for articulation with the anterior arch of the atlas.
- The two superolateral surfaces of the dens possess circular impressions that serve as attachment sites for strong alar ligaments, one on each side, which connect the dens to the medial surfaces of the occipital condyles. These alar ligaments check excessive rotation of the head and atlas relative to the axis.

19. Ans. (c) Face *Ref: William R. Proffit, 4th ed p 76-78*

- Face is underdeveloped at birth.

20. Ans. (d) Grater palatine foramen *Ref: B.D. Chaurasia 3rd, p 9*

- Greater palatine foramen located medial to the third molar at the junction of the maxilla and the horizontal palate of the palatine bone.
- Greater palatine foramen transmits descending palatine vessels and palatine nerve.

21. Ans. (a) 270 *Refer: Shobha Tandon 2nd, p 51*

- The neonate has 270 bones as compared to an adult which has 206 bones. Similarly skull bones in neonate are 45 and in the adult 22.

22. Ans. (c) Foramen spinosum *Ref: B.D. Chaurasia's 5th ed. p 45*

(a) **Foramen ovale (O):**	Mandibular nerve (CN V3), Accessory meningeal artery, Lesser petrosal nerve.
(b) **Foramen rotundum:**	Maxillary nerve (CN V2)
(c) **Foramen spinosum (s):**	Middle meningeal artery and vein meningeal branch of mandibular nerve (CN V3)
(d) **Superior orbital fissure**	**Lateral part, middle part, medial part**
• Lateral part	Lacrimal and frontal nerves, branch of ophthalmic nerve, trochlear nerve, superior ophthalmic vein, meningeal branch of lacrimal artery; anastomotic branch of middle meningeal artery, which anastomoses with recurrent branch of lacrimal artery.
• Middle part	Upper and lower divisions of oculomotor nerve (CN III), nasociliary nerve, abducent nerve (CN VI).
• Medial part	Inferior ophthalmic vein; sympathetic nerve from plexus around internal carotid artery.

23. Ans. (c) It enters the vertebral column through C7 vertebrae *Ref: B. D. Chaurasia's 3rd ed. p 168*

- The vertebral arteries are major arteries of the neck. They branch from the subclavian arteries and merge to form the single midline basilar artery in a complex called the vertebrobasilar system, which supplies blood to the posterior part of the circle of Willis and thus significant portions of the brain.
- The vertebral arteries arise from the subclavian arteries, one on each side of the body, then enter deep to the transverse process of the level of the 6th cervical vertebrae (C6), or occasionally (in 7.5% of cases) at the level of C7. They then proceed superiorly, in the transverse foramen (foramen transversarium) of each cervical vertebra. Once they have passed through the transverse foramen of C1 (also known as the atlas), the vertebral arteries travel across the posterior arch of C1 and through the suboccipital triangle before entering the foramen magnum.
- It is divided into 4 parts:
  - The 1st, part extends from the origin to the transverse process of the 6th cervical vertebra.
  - It runs through the foramina of the upper6 cervical vertebrae.
  - 3rd part of the artery lies in the occipital triangle.

24. Ans. (c) Jugular foramen *Ref: BDC 5th ed p 45*

- **The posterior cranial fossa is part of the intracranial cavity, located between the foramen magnum and tentorium cerebelli. It contains the brainstem and cerebellum.**
- **This is the most inferior of the fossae. It houses the cerebellum, medulla and pons. Anteriorly it extends to the apex of the petrous temporal. Posteriorly it is enclosed by the occipital bone. Laterally portions of the squamous temporal and mastoid part of the temporal bone form its walls.**
- **It consists of:**
  - **Foramen magnum**
  - **Jugular foramen**
  - **Anterior condylar canal**
  - **Internal acoustic meatus**
  - **External opening of vestibular aqueduct**
  - **Posterior condylar canal**
  - **Mastoid foramen.**

Jugular foramen

Lies between the inferior edge of the petrous temporal bone and the adjacent occipital bone and transmits the internal jugular vein (actually begins here), the glossopharyngeal (IX), the vagus (X) and the accessory (XI) nerves.

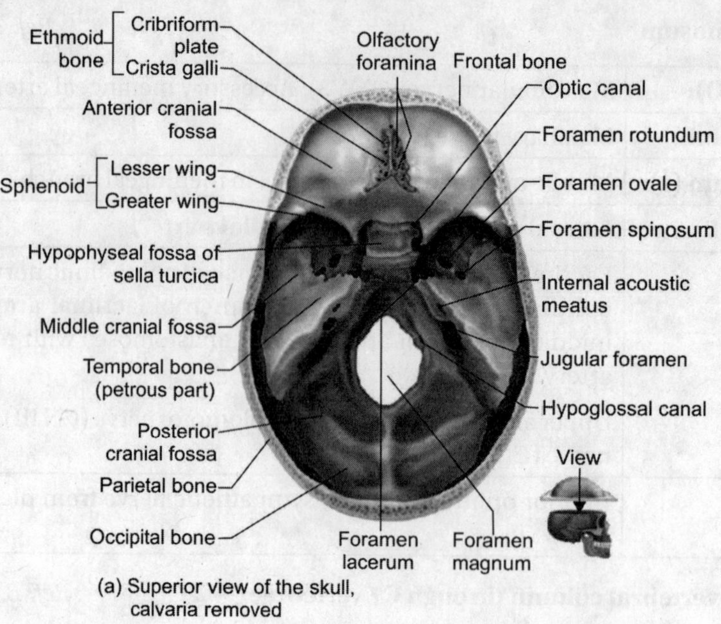

(a) Superior view of the skull, calvaria removed

25. Ans. (a) Mandible *Ref: BDC 5th ed. p 34*

The very first bone in human body which is ossified is clavicle and the mandible is the second bone which is ossify.

26. Ans. (a) Third cervical vertebra *Ref: BDC 5th ed. p 39*

- The hyoid bone (lingual bone) is a horseshoe-shaped bone situated in the anterior midline of the neck between the chin and the thyroid cartilage.
- At rest, it lies at the level of the base of the mandible in the front and the third cervical vertebra (C3) behind.
- Unlike other bones, the hyoid is only distantly articulated to other bones by muscles or ligaments.
- The hyoid is anchored by muscles from the anterior, posterior and inferior directions, and aids in tongue movement and swallowing.
- The hyoid bone provides attachment to the muscles of the floor of the mouth and the tongue above, the larynx below, and the epiglottis and pharynx behind.

Muscle attachments

The following muscles are attached to the hyoid:

Superior
- Middle pharyngeal constrictor muscle
- Hyoglossus muscle
- Digastric muscle
- Stylohyoid muscle
- Geniohyoid muscle
- Mylohyoid muscle

Inferior
- Thyrohyoid muscle
- Omohyoid muscle
- Sternohyoid muscle

27. Ans. (a) Quadrangular *Ref: BDC 5th ed p 7*

- The orbits are conical or four-sided pyramidal cavities, which open into the midline of the face and point back into the head. Each consists of a base, an apex and four walls. They protect the eye from mechanical injury.
- Orbital opening is somewhat quadrangular anterior entrance to the orbit that forms the base of the pyramidal orbital cavity. It is bounded by the sharp supraorbital, infraorbital, and lateral orbital margins and a less obvious medial margin on each side of the upper nose.

- It is bounded by the following four margin:
  - Superior margin: frontal bone
  - Inferior margin: maxilla, palatine and zygomatic
  - Medial margin: frontal, lacrimal and ethmoid
  - Lateral margin: zygomatic and sphenoid.

SCALP TEMPLE AND FACE

28. Ans. (D) Aponeurosis *Ref: Textbook of Forensic Medicine and Toxicology 4th ed. p 352*

Areolar tissue loosely connects the epicranial aponeurosis to the pericranium and allows the superficial 3 layers of the scalp to move over the pericranium. Scalp flaps are elevated along a relatively avascular plane in craniofacial and neurosurgical procedures. However, certain emissary veins traverse this layer, which connects the scalp veins to the diploic veins and intracranial venous sinuses.

The clinically important layer is the aponeurosis. Scalp lacerations through this layer mean that the "anchoring" of the superficial layers is lost and gaping of the wound occurs; this requires suturing. This can be achieved with simple or vertical mattress sutures using a nonabsorbable material, which are subsequently removed at around days 7-10. So it is a dangerous layer of scalp.

29. Ans. (d) Right maxillary artery *Ref: Gray's Anatomy 2nd ed. p 876*

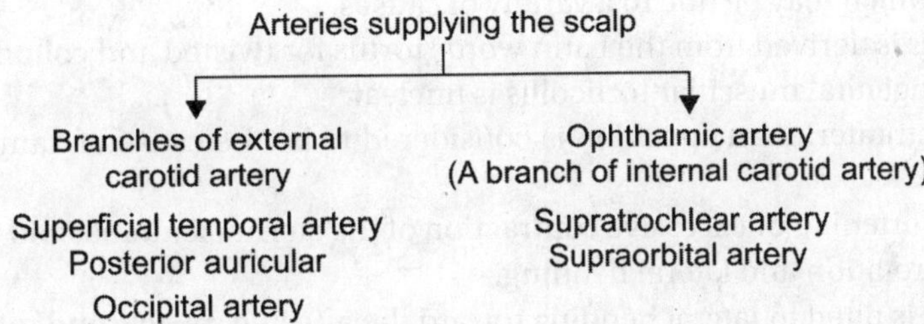

SIDE OF NECK

30. Ans. (d) Prevertebral fascia *Ref: BDS 5th ed. p 70*

The arrangement of layers from outside to inside is:

a. Pretracheal fascia b. Investing fascia c. Prevertebral fascia

- The prevertebral fascia extends medially behind the carotid vessels, where it assists in forming there sheath and passes in front of prevertebral muscles.

31. Ans. (b) 140° *Ref: BDC 5th ed. p 34*

The angle of the mandible (gonial angle) is located at the posterior border at the junction of the lower border of the ramus of the mandible.

Izard G in 1927 cited the following averages of the variability in the gonial angle:

- 135 to 150 degrees at birth
- 135 to 140 degrees when the first dentition is finished
- 120 to 130 degrees up to the time of eruption of the second molars
- and 120 to 150 degrees in old age.

32. Ans. (a) Anterior median line of the neck extending from symphysis menti to suprasternal notch *Ref: Gray's Anatomy 2nd ed. p 954*

- Anterior triangle of the neck bounded by:
  - Medially: Anterior median line of the neck
  - Laterally: Anterior margin of sternocleidomastoid
  - Superiorly: Inferior border of the mandible
  - Apex: at the manubrium sterni.
- The anterior triangle is subdivided into:
  - Submental triangle
  - Submandibular triangle
  - Carotid triangle
  - Muscular triangles.

33. Ans. (d) External jugular vein *Ref: Textbook of Anatomy with Color Atlas by Inderbir Singh p 800*

- Suprasternal space contains the sterna head of the right and left sternocleidomastoid muscle, the interclavicular ligament the jugular arch joining the right and left anterior jugular veins and a lymph node.
- Suprasternal space is a narrow interval between the deep and superficial layers of the cervical fascia above the manubrium of the sternum through which pass the anterior jugular veins.

34. Ans. (c) Sternocleidomastoid *Ref: BDC 5th ed. p 79*

- Torticollis, also known as wry neck or loxia, is a dystonic condition defined by an abnormal, asymmetrical head or neck position, which may be due to a variety of causes.
- The term torticollis is derived from the Latin words tortus for twisted and collum for neck.
- The etiology of congenital muscular torticollis is unclear.
- Birth trauma or intrauterine malposition is considered to be the cause of damage to the sternocleidomastoid muscle in the neck.
- This results in a shortening or excessive contraction of the sternocleidomastoid muscle, which curtails its range of motion in both rotation and lateral bending.
- The head typically is tilted in lateral bending toward the affected muscle and rotated toward the opposite side.

CRANIAL CAVITY

35. Ans. (d) Ophthalmic artery *Ref: BDC 5th ed. p 109*

The internal carotid artery can be divided into four portion based on its course:

- Cervical part:
  - No branches.
- Petrous part:
  - Caroticotympanic arteries.
- Cavernous part:
  - Cavernous branch
  - Hypophyseal branch
  - Meningeal branch.
- Cerebral part:
  - Anterial choroidal
  - Posterior communicating
  - Middle cerebral
  - Ophthalmic artery
  - Anterior cerebral.

Contd...

Bone	*Cranial fossa*	*Foramina*	*Vessels*	*Nerves*
Maxilla	—	**Incisive foramen/ incisive canal**	Sphenopalatine artery	Nasopalatine nerve (V2)
Palatine	—	Greater palatine foramen	Greater palatine artery, greater palatine vein	Greater palatine nerve
Palatine and maxilla	—	Lesser palatine foramina	Lesser palatine artery lesser palatine vein	Lesser palatine nerve
Sphenoid and maxilla	—	Inferior orbital fissure	Inferior ophthalmic veins infraorbital artery Infraorbital vein	Zygomatic nerve and infraorbital nerve of maxillary nerve (V2) orbital branches of pterygopalatine ganglion
Maxilla	—	Infraorbital foramen	Infraorbital artery Infraorbital vein	Infraorbital nerve
Sphenoid	Middle cranial fossa	Foramen ovale	Accessory meningeal artery	Mandibular nerve (V3) lesser petrosal nerve (occasionally)
Sphenoid	Middle cranial fossa	Foramen spinosum	Middle meningeal artery	Meningeal branch of the mandibular nerve (V3)
Sphenoid	Middle cranial fossa	Foramen lacerum	Internal carotid artery, artery of pterygoid canal	Nerve of pterygoid canal
Temporal	Posterior cranial fossa	Internal acoustic meatus	Labyrinthine artery	Facial nerve (VII), vestibulo cochlear nerve(VIII)

41. Ans. (c) Abducent nerve *Ref: BDC 5th ed. p 102*

The cavernous sinus (or lateral sellar compartment), is a large collection of thin- walled veins creating a cavity bordered by the temporal bone of the skull and the sphenoid bone, lateral to the sella turcica.

Each cavernous sinus (one for each hemisphere of the brain) contains the following: vertically, from superior to inferior (within the lateral wall of the sinus).

- Oculomotor nerve (CN III)
- Trochlear nerve (CN IV)
- Ophthalmic nerve, the V1 branch of the trigeminal nerve (CN V)
- Maxillary nerve, the V2 branch of CN V.

Unlike the nerves listed above, the abducens nerve (CN VI) does not run within the lateral wall of the cavernous sinus; rather, it runs through the middle of the sinus alongside the internal carotid artery.

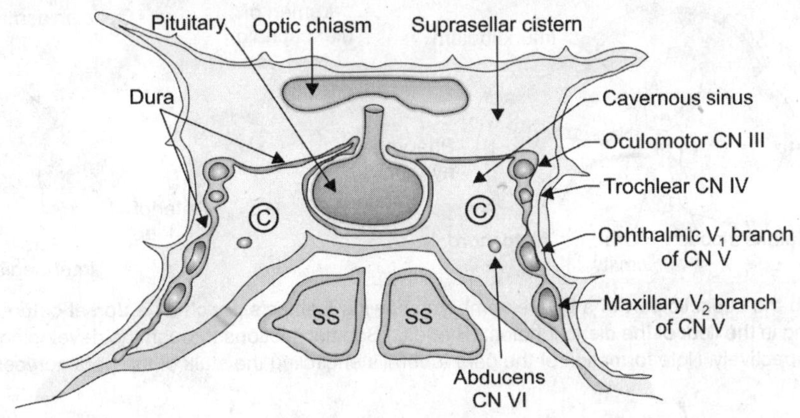

These nerves, with the exception of CN V2, pass through the cavernous sinus to enter the orbital apex through the superior orbital fissure. The maxillary nerve, division V2 of the trigeminal nerve travels through the lower portion of the sinus and exits via the foramen rotundum.

42. Ans. (d) Superior ophthalmic vein and pterygoid venous plexus *Ref: BDC 5th ed. p 102*

- The pterygoid plexus is a venous plexus of considerable size, and is situated between the temporalis muscle and lateral pterygoid muscle, and partly between the two pterygoid muscles.
- This plexus communicates freely with the anterior facial vein; it also communicates with the cavernous sinus, by branches through the foramen Vesalii, foramen ovale, and foramen lacerum. Due to its communication with the cavernous sinus, infection of the superficial face may spread to the cavernous sinus, causing cavernous sinus thrombosis.
- Facial vein communicates with the cavernous sinus also through Superior ophthalmic vein and pterygoid venous plexus, emissary vein.

43. Ans. (c) Pars posterior *Ref: B.D. Chaurasia's 3rd, p 77*

- In embryogenesis, Rathke's pouch is a depression in the roof of the developing mouth in front of the bucco-pharyngeal membrane. It gives rise to the anterior pituitary (adenohypophysis), a part of the endocrine system.
- Appears in 3rd week of intrauterine life.
- The pouch eventually loses its connection with the pharynx giving rise to the anterior pituitary. The anterior wall of Rathke's pouch proliferates; filling most of the pouch to form pars distalis and pars tuberalis. The posterior wall forms pars intermedia.
- In some organisms, the proliferating anterior wall does not fully occupy Rathke's pouch, leaving a remnant (Rathke's cleft) between the pars distalis and pars intermedia.
- Rathke's pouch may develop benign cysts. Craniopharyngioma is a neoplasm which can arise from the epithelium within the cleft.

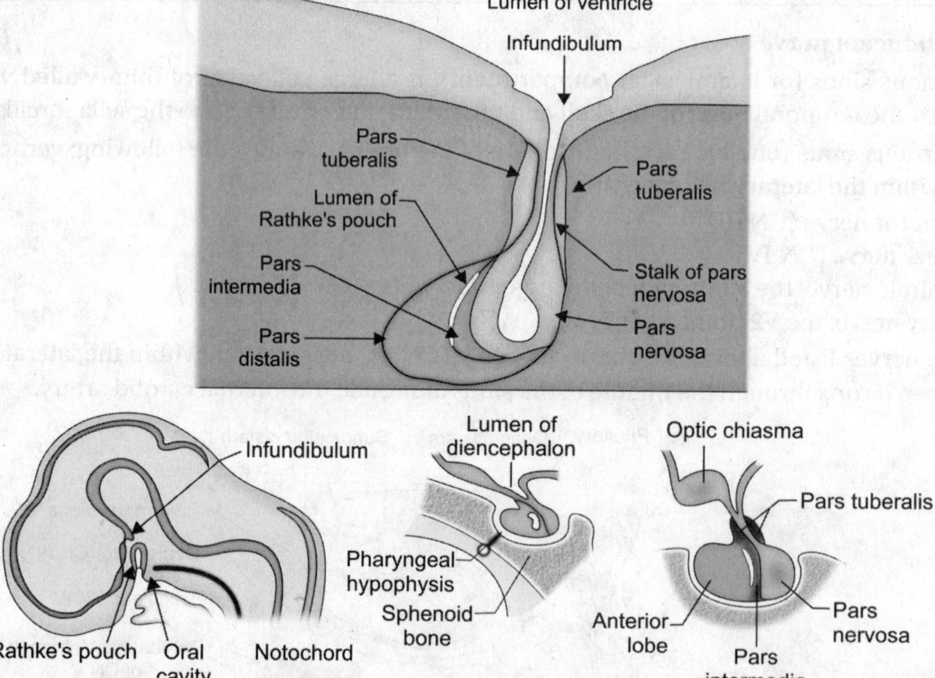

(A) Sagittal section through the cephalic part of a 6-week embryo showing Rathke's pouch as a dorsal outpocketing of the oral cavity and the infundibulum as a thickening in the floor of the diencephalon. (B and C) Sagittal sections through the developing hypophysis in the 11th and 16th weeks of development, respectively. Note formation of the pars tuberalis encircling the stalk of the pars nervosa.

44. Ans. (c) Sigmoid sinus *Ref: BDC 5th ed. p 104*

- The right and left transverse sinus is a continuation of the superior sagittal sinus and straight sinus respectively.
- Each right and left sigmoid sinus is the direct continuation of the transverse sinus.

CONTENTS OF ORBIT

45. Ans. (a) Maxillary sinus *Ref: Oxford-Textbook of Anaesthesia for Oral and Maxillofacial Surgery Lan Shaw p 75*

- Anterior ethmoidal nerve exits through the anterior ethmoid foramen.
- It supplies:
  - The anterior and middle ethmoidal air cells
  - Some of the mucosa covering nasal septum
  - Lateral wall of the nose
  - Dura of the anterior cranial fossa.
- Nerve supply for maxillary sinus is from the infraorbital and superior alveolar branches of the maxillary nerve.

46. Ans. (a) Greater petrosal *Ref: Walsh and Hoyt's Clinical Neuro-Ophthalmology 6th ed. p 701*

- Parasympathetic innervations of the lacrimal gland occurs via the greater superficial petrosal nerve.
- Greater petrosal nerve transverse via petrous portion of temporal bone, middle cranial fossa, pterygoid canal and pterygopalatine fossa in order to supply the lacrimal gland.
- Defect of greater petrosal nerve may be tested with Schirmer's test for secretory function of the lacrimal gland.

47. Ans. (a) Nasociliary nerve *Ref: BDC 5th ed. p 353*

Trigeminal nerve have 3 branches as:

- Ophthalmic
- Maxillary
- Mandibular.

Ophthalmic nerve is sensory. Its branches are:

- Frontal
- Nasociliary
- Lacrimal.

Nasociliary branches of ophthalmic nerve gives following branches.

- Posterior ethmoidal from ethmoid sinus
- Long ciliary
- Nerve to ciliary ganglion
- Infratrochlear
- Anterior ethmoidal.

Nasociliary nerve carry pain sensation from ethmoid sinus through posterior ethmoidal nerve.

48. Ans. (a) Levator palpebrae *Ref: Gray's Anatomy for Student 2nd ed. p 887*

Extrinsic muscle of eyeball

- Superior rectus
- Inferior rectus
- Medial rectus
- Lateral rectus
- Superior oblique
- Inferior oblique.

Muscle of eye lids:

- Levator palpebrae superioris
- Orbicularis oculi

Intrinsic muscle of eye:

- Sphincter papillae
- Dilator papillae
- Ciliary.

49. Ans. (b) Inferior turbinate *Ref: Grays Anatomy for Students 2nd ed. p 1016*

- The ethmoid bulla is a protrusion under the middle nasal concha. It has the opening of the middle ethmoidal air cells in it. The agger nasi is a landmark used to mark the location of the anterior ethmoid air cells.
- The olfactory sulcus of the cerebrum should be located just above the agger nasi.
- The uncinate process is a projection of the ethmoid bone below the middle nasal concha. It is located anterior to the ethmoid bulla and the semilunar hiatus.
- The ethmoid bone forms a large portion of the lateral wall of the nasal cavity including the middle and superior concha, the uncinate process, the ethmoid bulla and the cribiform plate superiorly.

50. Ans. (a) Greater petrosal nerve *Ref: Neurosurgical Emergencies by Christopher 2nd ed. p 143, 144*

- **The greater (superficial) petrosal nerve is a nerve** in the skull that branches from the facial nerve; it forms part of a chain of nerves that innervate the lacrimal gland. The fibers have synapses in the pterygopalatine ganglion.
- The greater (superficial) petrosal nerve carries gustatory (taste) and parasympathetic fibers. Postganglionic parasympathetic fibers from pterygopalatine ganglion supply lacrimal gland and the mucosal glands of the nose, palate, and pharynx.
- The gustatory fibers do not relay in the ganglion and are distributed to the palate.

51. Ans. (a) Nasociliary *Ref: Atlas of Head and Neck Pathology Bruce M. Wenig p 5*

Somatic nerve supply:

- **Sphenoid and ethmoid** sinuses are both innervated by posterior ethmoidal branch of nasociliary nerve (which come off ophthalmic division of trigeminal nerve). So the transmission of pain in ethmoidal sinusitis is through nasociliary nerve.
- **Maxillary sinus** is innervated maxillary division of trigeminal nerve. More specifically, maxillary is innervated by superior alveolar and infraorbital branches of maxillary division of trigeminal nerve.
- **Frontal sinus** is innervated by supraorbital branch of ophthalmic division of trigeminal nerve.

52. Ans. (c) Lacrimal gland *Ref: BDC 5th ed p 65*

- The functional purpose of the lacrimal excretory system is to drain tears from the eye into the nasal cavity. Stagnation of tears in a pathologically closed lacrimal drainage system can result in dacryocystitis.
- Dacryocystitis can be acute or chronic. Acute dacryocystitis is heralded by the sudden onset of pain and redness in the medial canthal region.
- An insidious onset of epiphora is characteristic of chronic inflammation or infection of the lacrimal sac.
- Dacryocystitis has long been noted to occur more frequently on the left side than on the right side. In many instances, the nasolacrimal duct and lacrimal fossa formed a greater angle on the right side than on the left side.

53. Ans. (a) Middle meningeal artery *Ref: B.D. Chaurasia's for Dental Students 1st ed p 133. 212*

- Epidural or extradural hematoma (haematoma) is type of traumatic brain injury in which a buildup of blood occurs between the duramater (the tough outer membrane of the central nervous system) and the skull. The duramater also covers the spine, so epidural bleeds may also occur in the spinal column. Often due to trauma, the condition is potentially dead, because the buildup of blood may increase pressure in the intracranial space and compress delicate brain tissue. The condition is present in one to three percent of head injuries.

- Epidural hematoma commonly results from a blow to the side of the head. **The pterion region which overlies the middle meningeal artery is relatively weak and prone to injury.** This, only 20 to 30% of epidural hematomas occur outside the region of the temporal bone.
- Epidural hematoma is usually found on the same side of the brain that was impacted by the blow, but on very rare occasions, it can be due to a contrecoup injury.

54. Ans. (a) Medial wall *Ref: B.D. Chaurasia's for Dental Students p 148*

Medial wall

It is very thin. From before backwards it is formed by:

- The frontal process of the maxilla.
- The lacrimal bone.
- The orbital plate of the ethmoid.
- The body of the sphenoid bone.

ANTERIOR TRIANGLE OF NECK

55. Ans. (a) At the upper border of thyroid cartilage *Ref: BDC 5th ed. p 134*

- The common carotid artery is a paired structure, meaning that there are two in the body, one for each half.
- The left and right common carotid arteries follow the same course with the exception of their origin. The right common carotid originates in the neck from the brachiocephalic trunk. The left arises from the aortic arch in the thoracic region.
- The bifurcation into the external and internal carotid arteries occurs at the upper border of the thyroid cartilage, at around the level of the fourth cervical vertebra (C4).
- The left and right common carotid arteries are arteries that supply the head and neck with oxygenated blood.

56. Ans. (d) Middle meningeal artery *Ref: B. D. Chaurasia 5th ed. p 134, 135*

External carotid artery:

- External carotid artery is one of the terminal branches of the common carotid artery. In general, it lies anterior to the internal carotid artery it supply to structures in the front of the neck and face.

Branches

The external carotid artery gives off eight branches which may be grouped as follows:

Anterior

- Superior thyroid
- Lingual
- Facial.

Posterior

- Occipital
- Posterior auricular.

Medial

- Ascending pharyngeal.

Terminal

- Maxillary
- Superficial temporal.

57. Ans. (d) Sympathetic trunk *Ref: Gray's Anatomy, p 901*

- Each **Carotid sheath** is a column of fascia that surrounds the common carotid artery, the internal carotid artery, the internal jugular vein, and the vagus nerve as these structures pass through the neck.
- It receives contributions from the investing, prevertebral, and pretracheal layers, though the extent of each component's contribution varies.

58. Ans. (c) Posterior auricular artery *Ref: B.D. Chaurasia's for Dental Students, p 174-176*

- **Arteries of the face:** The face is richly vascular. It is supplied by: (1) The facial artery, (2) the transverse facial artery, and (3) arteries that accompany the cutaneous nerves.
- **Arteries accompanying cutaneous nerves:** These arteries are infraorbital, mantel, buccal, supraorbital, and supratrochlear. These also supply the muscles.
- The back of the scalp is supplied by the posterior auricular and occipital arteries.

59. Ans. (c) Digastric *Ref: B.D. Chaurasia's 3rd ed. p 128*

- The digastric muscle (also digastricus) (named digastric as it has two bellies) is a small muscle located under the jaw. The term "digastric muscle" refers to this specific muscle. However, other muscles that have two separate muscle bellies include the ligament of treitz, omohyoid,occipitofrontalis.
- It lies below the body of the mandible, and extends, in a curved form, from the mastoid process to the symphysis menti. It belongs to thesuprahyoid muscles group.
- A broad aponeurotic layer is given off from the tendon of the digastricus on either side, to be attached to the body and greater cornu of the hyoid bone; this is termed the suprahyoid aponeurosis.
- The anterior belly arises from a depression on the inner side of the lower border of the mandible called the Digastric Fossa, close to the symphysis, and passes downward and backward.
- The anterior body is supplied by the trigeminal via the mylohyoid nerve, a branch of the inferior alveolar nerve, itself a branch of the mandibular division of the trigeminal nerve. It originates from the first pharyngeal arch.
- The posterior belly, longer than the anterior belly, arises from the mastoid notch which is on the inferior surface of the skull, medial to the mastoid process of the temporal bone. The mastoid notch is a deep groove between the mastoid process and the styloid process. The mastoid notch is also referred to as the digastric groove or the digastric notch.
- The posterior belly is supplied by the digastric branch of facial nerve.

PAROTID REGION

60. Ans. (c) That it opens in buccal vestibule opposite lower second molar *Ref: Gray's Anatomy for Student 2nd ed. p 863*

The **ducts of the salivary** glands allow the passage of salivary juice from the glands to the oral cavity:

- Parotid duct (Stensen's duct): Connects the parotid gland to the buccal mucosa, adjacent to maxillary second molar.
- Submandibular duct (Wharton's duct): Connects the submandibular gland to the floor of the mouth.
- Duct of Rivinus: The sublingual gland drains through numerous small ducts all of which open into the floor of the mouth and are collectively termed the duct of Rivinus; the largest is the major duct of the sublingual salivary gland called Bartholin's duct.

Parotid duct:

- The parotid duct or Stensen duct is a duct and the route that saliva takes from the major salivary gland, the parotid gland into the mouth.
- It passes through the buccal fat, buccopharyngeal fascia, and buccinator muscle then opens into the vestibule of the mouth across from the maxillary second molar tooth on the inner surface of the buccal mucosa at the parotid papilla.
- Running along with the duct superiorly is the transverse facial artery and upper buccal nerve; running along with the duct inferiorly is the lower buccal nerve.

61. Ans. (a) Medial and lateral pterygoid *Ref: Gray's Anatomy for Students 2nd ed. p 925*

There are four muscle of mastification:

- Masster- Elevation of mandible
- Temporalis- Elevation and retraction of mandible

- Medial pterygoid- Elevation of mandible side to side movement of mandible
- Lateral pterygoid- Protrusion of mandible side to side movement of mandible.

62. Ans. (b) Buccinator *Ref: BDC 5th ed. p 144*

- The parotid duct or Stensen duct is a duct and the route that saliva takes from the major salivary gland, the parotid gland into the mouth.
- It passes through the buccal fat, buccopharyngeal fascia, and buccinator muscle then opens into the vestibule of the mouth across from the maxillary second molar tooth on the inner surface of the buccal mucosa at the parotid papilla.
- The buccinator acts as a valve that prevents inflation of the duct during blowing. Running along with the duct superiorly is the transverse facial artery and upper buccal nerve; running along with the duct inferiorly is the lower buccal nerve.

63. Ans. (d) Internal carotid artery *Ref: Gray's Anatomy 2nd ed. p 864*

The parotid gland is a major salivary gland in humans. It is a bilateral structure, and the largest of the salivary glands. It is wrapped around the mandibular ramus, and secretes saliva through Stensen duct (or parotid duct) into the oral cavity, to facilitate mastication and swallowing and to begin the digestion of starches. The word 'parotid' (para-aortic) literally means around the ear.

Structures that pass through the gland:

(1) Facial nerve
(2) Retromandibular vein
(3) External carotid artery
(4) Superficial temporal artery
(5) branches of the great auricular nerve
(6) Posterior auricular artery

64. Ans. (b) Upper second molar *Ref: B.D. Chaurasia's for Dental Students, p 245*

- **Parotid Duct:** It is thick walled and is about 5 cm long. It emerges for the middle of the anterior border of the gland.
- It runs forwards and slightly downwards on the masseter. Here it's relations are:
  - Superiorily:
    - Accessory parotid gland,
    - Upper buccal branch of the facial nerve,
  - The transverse facial vessels.
  - Inferiorly: The lower buccal branch of the facial nerve.
- At the anterior border of the masseter, it turns medially and pierces:
  - The buccal pad of fat.
  - The buccopharyngeal fascia, and
  - The buccinators (obliquely). Because of the oblique course of the duct through the buccinators inflation of the duct is prevented during blowing.
- The duct runs forwards for a short distance between the buccinators and the oral mucosa. Finally, the duct turns medially and opens into the vestibule of the mouth (gingivobuccal vestibule) opposite the crown of the upper second molar tooth.

65. Ans. (b) Parotid gland *Ref: BDC 5th ed. p 339*

- The **inferior salivatory nucleus** is a cluster of neurons controlling the parasympathetic input to the parotid gland.
- It is a type of general visceral efferent nuclei situated at the lower part of pons below the superior nucleus.
- Glossopharyngeal nerve send the fiber of inferior salivary nucleus to the otic ganglion in order to supply the parotid gland.
- While the superior salivatory nucleus send its fiber through facial nerve and chorda tympani in order to supply the submandibular and sublingual nerve.

66. Ans. (d) External carotid artery *Ref: BDC 5th ed. p 143*

Structures that pass through the gland

These are from lateral to medial:

- Facial nerve
- Retromandibular vein
- External carotid artery
- Superficial temporal artery
- Branches of the great auricular nerve.

TEMPORAL OR INFRATEMPORAL REGION

67. Ans. (a) Auriculotemporal nerve *Ref: Burkitt's Oral Medicine 11th ed. p 228*

- The temporal mandibular joint is the joint of the jaw and is frequently referred to as TMJ.
- The capsule is a dense fibrous membrane that surrounds the joint and incorporates the eminence. It attaches to the articular eminence, the articular disc and the neck of the mandibular condyle.
- The only sensory innervations of the TMJ is derived from the auriculotemporal and masseteric branches of V3 or mandibular branch of trigeminal nerve.
- The auriculotemporal nerve provides most of the innervations to the joint capsule.
- The sympathetic innervations of TMJ is from superior cervical ganglion.
- The ratio of sensory nerve to sympathetic is approximately 1:3 in the TMJ.
- Blood supply of TMJ- superficial temporal maxillary artery.

68. Ans. (d) Lateral pterygoid *Ref: BDC 5th ed. p 149*

- The lateral pterygoid muscle has two heads, one arising from the outer part of the lateral pterygoid plate and other from the base of sphenoid bone. The two heads come together and are inserted into the neck of the condyle.
- The main function of this muscle is to draw both the head of the condyle and the disc forward during opening movement.
- Lateral pterygoid muscles cause the forward movement of the condyle into the glenoid fossa.

69. Ans. (d) Facial nerve *Ref: BDC 5th ed. p 159*

- The mylohyoid nerve is a nerve that innervates the mylohyoid muscle and the anterior belly of the digastrics muscle.
- The mylohyoid nerve branches from the inferior alveolar nerve (a branch of mandibular nerve, the 3rd part of trigeminal nerve) just before it enters the mandibular foramen.
- The mylohyoid nerve have all the motor fibers of the posterior division of the inferior alveolar nerve.

70. Ans. (b) Lateral pterygoid *Ref: BDC 5th ed. p 149*

- Lateral pterygoid is the muscle of mastication having 2 part- upper head and lower head.
- Upper head is inserted into pterygoid fovea on the anterior surface of neck of mandible.
- Lower head is inserted into anterior margin of articular disc of TMJ.

71. Ans. (a) Contralateral lateral pterygoid *Ref: Human Evolutionary Anatomy, Leslie Aiello 1st ed. p 95*

- Lateral movement of condyle is due to the contraction of contralateral lateral pterygoid:
  - Contraction of right lateral pterygoid- Left lateral working movement.
  - Contraction of the right lateral pterygoid- Right lateral working movement.

72. Ans. (a) Buccinator *Ref: BDC 5th ed. p 148, 149*

- Buccinator muscle helps to keep the food in the correct position during mastication and in this way it assists the muscle of mastication and termed as accessory muscle of mastication.
- It aids whistling and smiling and in neonates it is used to suckle.
- It is important not to classify it as a proper muscle of mastication(like masseter, temporalis, medial pterygoid and lateral pterygoid) because it is not supplied by the mandibular nerve.

73. Ans. (b) Lingual nerve *Ref: Gray's Anatomy 2nd ed. p 955*

- The suprahyoid muscles are those which connects the hyoid bone to the skull.
- It includes digastrics, Stylohyoid, Mylohyoid and geniohyoid.
- All suprahyoid muscle contribute to the floor of the mouth but the actual muscle plate which bridges between the two rami of mandible is formed by the mylohyoid muscle and it is supplied by the inferior alveolar nerve.

74. Ans. (c) Long buccal nerve *Ref: BDC 5th ed. p 157, 354*

The mandibular nerve gives off the following branches:

- **From the main trunk of the nerve (before the division):**
  - muscular branches, which are efferent nerves for the medial pterygoid, tensor tympani, and tensor veli palatini muscles (motor)
  - meningeal branch (a sensory nerve).
- **From the anterior division:**
  - masseteric nerve (motor)
  - deep temporal nerves, anterior and posterior (motor)
  - buccal nerve (a sensory nerve)
  - lateral pterygoid nerve (motor).

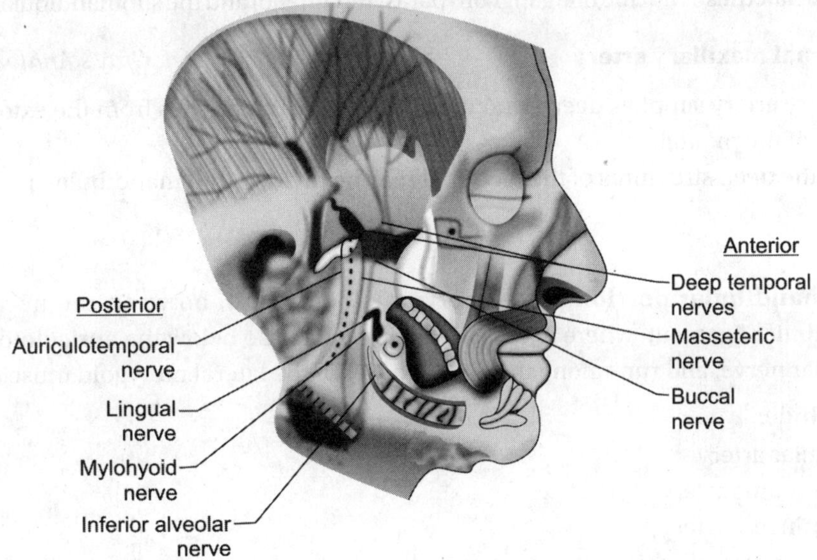

Branches from the posterior and anterior divisions (except lateral pterygoid nerve)

- **From the posterior division:**
  - auriculotemporal nerve (a sensory nerve)
  - lingual nerve (a sensory nerve)
  - inferior alveolar nerve (a sensory nerve)
  - motor branch to mylohyoid and anterior belly of digastric muscles (mylohyoid nerve).

To remember the sensory branches of V3:

- **B** - Buccal nerve (should be long buccal nerve because buccal nerve is the motor branch off of CN VII)
- **A** - Auriculotemporal nerve
- **I** - Inferior Alveolar nerve
- **L** - Lingual nerve

75. Ans. (a) Mylohyoid *Ref BDC 5th ed.*

Mandibular Nerve (V3) - This nerve exits the cranial cavity via foramen ovale carrying both motor and sensory fibers. It is composed of anterior and posterior divisions:

- **Anterior Division** - a motor root with one sensory nerve:
  - Anterior/Posterior deep temporal branches - motor to temporalis muscle
  - Masseteric nerve - motor to masseter
  - Lateral/Medial pterygoid nerves - motor to medial/lateral pterygoid muscles
  - Nerve of tensor veli palatini - motor nerve
  - Nerve to tensor tympani - motor nerve to inner ear muscle (Long)
  - Buccal nerve - sensory to buccal mucosa on inner cheek.
- **Posterior Division** - a sensory root with one motor nerve:
  - Meningeal branch - to cranial cavity
  - Auriculotemporal nerve - cutaneous sensory to the lateral side of the head (identifiable as the nerve which loops around the middle meningeal artery. Also carries parasympathetic information to the parotid gland.
  - Lingual nerve associated with chorda tympani and general sensory from the anterior two thirds of the tongue.
  - Inferior alveolar nerve - enters mandibular foramen and is sensory to the mandibular teeth (terminal branch is the mental nerve serving as sensory to the lower third of the face)
  - Mylohyoid nerve - branch off the inferior alveolar nerve, motor to mylohyoid muscle.
  - V3 is associated also with the otic ganglion (parasympathetic) and the submandibular ganglion (parasympathetic).

76. Ans. (b) Internal maxillary artery *Ref: Gray's Anatomy for Student 2nd ed. p 936*

- The maxillary artery supplies deep structures of the face. It branches from the external carotid artery just deep to the neck of the mandible.
- It supplies the deep structures of the face, and may be divided into mandibular, pterygoid, and pterygopalatine portions.

First portion:

The first or **mandibular portion** passes horizontally forward, between the neck of the mandible and the sphenomandibular ligament, where it lies parallel to and a little below the auriculotemporal nerve; it crosses the inferior alveolar nerve, and runs along the lower border of the lateral pterygoid muscle.

Branches include:

- Deep auricular artery
- Anterior tympanic artery
- Middle meningeal artery
- Inferior alveolar artery which gives off its mylohyoid branch just prior to entering the mandibular foramen
- Accessory meningeal artery.

Second portion:

The second or **pterygoid portion** runs obliquely forward and upward under cover of the ramus of the mandible and insertion of the temporalis, on the superficial (very frequently on the deep) surface of the lateral pterygoid muscle; it then passes between the two heads of origin of this muscle and enters the fossa.

Branches include:

- Masseteric artery
- Pterygoid branches
- Deep temporal arteries (anterior and posterior)
- Buccal artery.

Third portion:

The third or **pterygopalatine portion** lies in the pterygopalatine fossa in relation with the pterygopalatine ganglion. This is considered the terminal branch of the maxillary artery.

Branches include:

- Sphenopalatine artery (nasopalatine artery is the terminal branch of the maxillary artery)
- Descending palatine artery
- Infraorbital artery
- Posterior superior alveolar artery
- Artery of pterygoid canal
- Pharyngeal artery
- Middle superior alveolar (a branch of the infraorbital artery)
- Anterior superior alveolar arteries (a branch of the infraorbital artery).

77. Ans. (a) 10 weeks *Ref: Craniofacial Embryogenesis and Development 2nd ed. p 161*

- Formation of the TMJ occurs at around 12 weeks in utero when the joint spaces and the articular disc develop.
- At approximately 10 weeks the component of the fetus future joint becomes evident in the mesenchyme between condylar cartilage of the mandible and the developing temporal bone.
- Two slits like joint cavities and intervening disk make their appearance in this region by 12 weeks. The mesenchyme around the joint begins to form the fibrous joint capsule.
- The developing superior head of the lateral pterygoid muscle attaches to the anterior portion of the fetal disk. The disk also continues posterior through the petrotympanic fissure and attaches to the malleus of middle ear.

A growth center is located in the head of each mandibular condyle before an individual reaches maturity. This growth center consists of hyaline cartilage underneath the periosteum on the articulating surface of the condyle. This is the last growth center of bone in the body and is multidirectional in its growth capacity, unlike a typical long bone. This area of cartilage within the bone grows in length by appositional growth as the individual grows to maturity.

78. Ans. (a) First arch *Ref: BDC 5th ed. p 148*

- There are four classical muscles of mastication
- The masseter
- The temporalis (the sphenomandibularis is considered a part of the temporalis by some sources, and a distinct muscle by others)
- The medial pterygoid
- The lateral pterygoid.

Each of these primary muscles of mastication is paired, with each side of the mandible possessing one of the four:

- The muscles of mastication are all innervated by the trigeminal nerve (or CN V). More specifically, they are innervated by the mandibular branch, or V3.

Muscle of mastication origin from the first branchial arch.

79. Ans. (a) Medial and lateral pterygoid *Ref: Gray's Anatomy for Students 2nd ed. p 925*

There are four muscle of mastication:

- Masster- Elevation of mandible
- Temporalis- Elevation and retraction of mandible

- Medial pterygoid- Elevation of mandible side to side movement of mandible
- Lateral pterygoid- Protrusion of mandible side to side movement of mandible.

80. Ans. (a) Lateral pterygoid *Ref: Thieme, Atlas of Anatomy (Head and Neuroanatomy) p 48*

Lateral Pterygoid

Origin:

- Superior head from inferior surface of greater wing of sphenoid
- Inferior head from lateral surface of lateral pterygoid plate.

Insertion:

- Superior head-articular disc of TMJ
- Inferior head-pterygoid fovea on neck of mandibular condyle.

Action:

- Protrude mandible
- Opening of mouth
- Moving the articular disc forward.

Innervation:

Lateral pterygoid nerve, a branch of the mandibular division of CN V3.

81. Ans. (b) VII *Ref: Gray's Anatomy for Student 2nd ed. p 1035*

- The **buccinators** is a thin quadrilateral muscle, occupying the interval between the maxilla and the mandible at the side of the face.
- It forms the anterior part of the cheek or the lateral wall of the oral cavity.
- Its purpose is to pull back the angle of the mouth and to flatten the cheek area, which aids in holding the cheek to the teeth during chewing.
- Motor innervation is from the buccal branch of the facial nerve (cranial nerve VII).
- Sensory innervation is supplied by the buccal branch (one of the muscular branches) of mandibular nerve (cranial nerve V3).

82. Ans. (a) Medial pterygoid *Ref: Gray's Anatomy for Student 2nd ed. p 931, 932*

Mandibular nerve:

- It is the largest branch of trigeminal nerve
- It is motor as well as sensory in nature
- It's motor branch is originated in the infratemporal fossa. While sensory parts originates from the trigeminal ganglion in the middle cranial fossa.
- **Branches from the anterior trunk are:**
  - Buccal
  - Masseteric
  - Deep temporal.
- **Branches from posterior trunk are:**
  - Auriculotemporal
  - Lingual
  - Inferior alveolar.
- **Buccal nerve:**
  - Carry motor innervations to lateral pterygoid and temporalis.
- **Masseteric nerve:**
  - Supply masseter muscle.

- **Deep temporal nerve:**
  - Supply temporalis muscle.

83. Ans. (b) Mylohyoid groove *Ref: Gray's Anatomy 2nd ed. p 1059*

- The inferior alveolar nerve along its accompanying vessels enter the mandibular foramen. Just before entering the mandibular foramen it gives origin to the nerve to mylohyoid, which lies in the mylohyoid groove inferior to the foramen.
- The lower teeth are all innervated by branches from the inferior alveolar nerve which originates in the infratemporal fossa from the mandibular nerve.

84. Ans. (a) Greater palatine canal *Ref: Gray's Anatomy 2nd ed. p 941*

Structures open onto the pterygopalatine fossa:

- The foramen rotundum and pterygoid canal communicate with the middle cranial fossa and open onto the posterior wall
- A small palatovaginal canal opens onto the posterior wall and leads to the nasopharynx
- The pterygoid canal is a bony canal opening onto the posterior surface of the pterygoid process.

Apart from it:

- Palatine canal opens inferiorly
- Sphenopalatine foramen opens in the medial wall
- Inferior orbital fissure from floor of orbit opens in anterior wall.

85. Ans. (b) Multipennate arrangements of fibers *Ref: BDC 5th ed. p 149*

- Masseter muscle is a powerful muscle of mastication because of its multipennate arrangement of fibers.
- The masseter muscle extends from the zygomatic arch to the ramus and body of mandible. The fibers of this muscle is broad extending from the region of 2nd molar on the surface of the mandible to the surface of the ramus.
- The muscle is divided into 2 parts- Superficial and deep.

Origin:

- Superficial- anterior 2/3 of lower border of zygomatic arch and zygomatic process of maxilla.
- Middle- anterior 2/3 of deep surface and posterior 1/3 of lower border of zygomatic arch.
- Deep layer- deep surface of zygomatic arch.

86. Ans. (c) Lateral pterygoid *Ref: BDC 5th ed. p 149*

When left and right lateral pterygoid muscle contract together, the condyle is pulled forward and slightly downward. The upper head is used to pull the articular disc forward when the jaw is opened.

87. Ans. (a) Lateral pterygoid

Refer Ans. 80

88. Ans. (d) Foramen ovale *Ref: BDC 5th ed. p 153*

Accessory meningeal artery: Foramen ovale
Middle meningeal artery: Foramen spinosum
Inferior alveolar artery: Mandibular Foramen.

89. Ans. (c) Levator veli palatini *Ref: Gray's Anatomy For Students 2nd ed. p 852*

Mandibular Nerve:

The motor fiber innervative:

- Muscle of mastication is masseter, buccinators, lateral and medical pterygoid.
- Tensor tympani

- The tensor veli palatine
- Anterior belly of digastric
- Mylohyoid muscles.

It receive sensory branches from the skin of the lower face cheek, lower lip, anterior part of external ear, part of external acoustic meatus and temporal region.

90. Ans. (b) Lateral pterygoid *Ref B. D. Chaurasia for Dental Students, p 154*

- The lateral pterygoid muscle is inserted into the pterygoid fovea on the anterior aspect of the neck. The muscle is related to the medial surface of the ramus, above the mandibular foramen.
- Depression of mandible is caused by following muscles:
  - Lateral pterygoid-main muscle
  - Suprahyoid
  - Infrahyoid.

91. Ans. (c) Superior constrictor *Ref: Gray's 39th, p 629*

Superior constrictor:

Pterygomandibular raphe gives attachment posteriorly to the superior constrictor of the pharynx, and anteriorly the central part of buccinators.

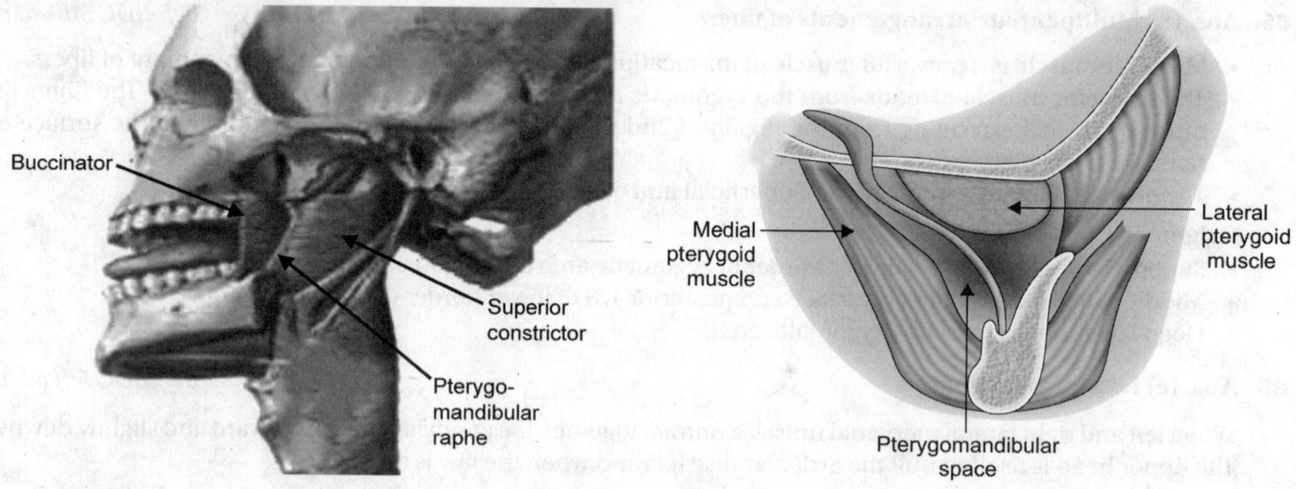

92. Ans. (a) Sphenomandibular *Ref Scott-Brown's Otorhinolaryngology: Head and Neck Surgery 7 ed. Vol 3, p 1810*

- Like the accessory ligaments around all joints, those around the TMJ help to stabilize it by keeping the joint surface in optimal anatomic contact.
- The sphenomandibular, stylomandibular, and pterygomandibular ligaments, considered accessory ligaments, support and protect the joint during wide excursion.
- Stretching of these ligaments is associated with disunity of the articular disk and the condyle, hypermobility,and temporomandibular dislocation.
- However, only the sphenomandibular ligament is likely to have any significant influence upon mandibular movement.

93. Ans. (d) Infraorbital *Ref: BDC 5th ed. p 153*

- The maxillary artery supplies deep structures of the face. It branches from the external carotid artery just deep to the neck of the mandible.

First portion

The **first or mandibular portion** passes horizontally forward, between the neck of the mandible and the sphenomandibular ligament, where it lies parallel to and a little below the auriculotemporal nerve; it crosses the inferior alveolar nerve, and runs along the lower border of the lateral pterygoid muscle.

Branches include:

- Deep auricular artery
- Anterior tympanic artery
- Middle meningeal artery
- Inferior alveolar artery which gives off its mylohyoid branch just prior to entering the mandibular foramen
- Accessory meningeal artery.

Second portion

The second or pterygoid portion runs obliquely forward and upward under cover of the ramus of the mandible and insertion of the temporalis, on the superficial (very frequently on the deep) surface of the lateral pterygoid muscle; it then passes between the two heads of origin of this muscle and enters the fossa.

Branches include:

- Masseteric artery
- Pterygoid branches
- Deep temporal arteries (anterior and posterior)
- Buccal artery.

Third portion

The third or pterygopalatine portion lies in the pterygopalatine fossa in relation with the pterygopalatine ganglion. This is considered the terminal branch of the maxillary artery.

Branches include:

- Sphenopalatine artery (nasopalatine artery is the terminal branch of the maxillary artery)
- Descending palatine artery
- Infraorbital artery
- Posterior superior alveolar artery
- Artery of pterygoid canal
- Pharyngeal artery
- Middle superior alveolar (a branch of the infraorbital artery)
- Anterior superior alveolar arteries (a branch of the infraorbital artery).

94. Ans. (a) Branch from trunk of mandibular nerve *Ref: BDC 5th ed p 149*

- The medial pterygoid (or internal pterygoid muscle), is a thick, quadrilateral muscle of mastication.
- The mandibular branch of the fifth cranial nerve, the trigeminal nerve, innervates the medial pterygoid muscle.
- Unlike the lateral pterygoid and all other muscles of mastication which are innervated by the anterior division of the mandibular branch of the trigeminal nerve, the medial pterygoid is innervated by the main trunk of the mandibular branch of the trigeminal nerve (V), before the division.

Its functions include:

- Elevation of the mandible (closes the jaw)
- Minor contribution to protrusion of the mandible
- Assistance in mastication
- Excursion of the mandible; contralateral excursion occurs with unilateral contraction.

95. Ans. (d) Lateral pterygoid *Ref: B.D. Chaurasia's 3rd ed. p 124*

- **Protrusion:**
  - By lateral and medial pterygoids of both side.

- **Elevation:**
  - By masseter, the temporalis, the medial pterygoids of both sides.
- **Retraction:**
  - By posterior fibers of the temporalis.
- **Depression:**
  - Primary muscle-lateral pterygoid mainly
  - Secondary muscle-digastrics, geniohyoid and mylohyoid helps when the mouth is opened wide.
- **Side to side movement:**
  - Medial and lateral pterygoids of each side acting alternatively.

96. Ans. (b) Has no blood supply and nerve supply *Ref: http://emedicine.mesp ace.com/article/385129-overview*

- The nerve fibers primarily follow the vascular supply and terminate as free nerve endings
- Thus, the capsule, subsynovial tissue and periphery of the disk are innervated
- The articular cartilage and the central part of the disk contain no nerves
- Myelinated and nonmyelinated nerves are seen in TMJ
- The retrodiscal bilaminar zone has a rich neurovascular supply and is the source of proprioception.

97. Ans. (c) Transverse facial artery *Ref: BDC 5th ed. p 156*

- Its arterial blood supply is provided by branches of the external carotid artery, predominately the superficial temporal branch.
- Other branches of the external carotid artery namely: the deep auricular artery, anterior tympanic artery, ascending pharyngeal artery, and maxillary artery- may also contribute to the arterial blood supply of the joint.

SUBMANDIBULAR REGION

98. Ans. (a) Superior to mylohyoid *Ref: Salivary Gland Disease, Robert L.Witt p 14*

Sublingual salivary gland:

- It is the smallest among all major salivary glands.
- It is the almond shape gland that lies in between the mylohyoid and the side of the tongue.

Relation:

- Superiorly, the sublingual gland is related to the mucosa of floor of the mouth.
- Inferiorly, it is related to the mylohyoid muscle.
- Posteriorly, it is related to the deep part of submandibular gland.
- Laterally, it is related to the sublingual fossa of mandible.
- Medially, the submandibular duct and lingual nerve are related.

99. Ans. (b) Digastric muscle *Ref: BDC 5th ed. p 164*

- The digastrics muscle is the small muscle located under the jaw.
- The two bellies of the digastrics muscle have different embryological origin and are supplied by different cranial nerves.
- The posterior belly is supplied by the digastrics branch of facial nerve while anterior belly is supplied by trigeminal via the mylohyoid nerve, a branch of the inferior alveolar nerve.
- Anterior belly originates from the first pharyngeal arch where as posterior belly originates from the second pharyngeal arch.
- Digastric muscle contracts, to elevate the hyoid bone.

100. Ans. (d) Marginal mandibular *Ref: Burkitt Essential Surgery, p 690/ BDC 5th ed. p 358*

- There are five branches of facial nerve named a temporal (or frontal), zygomatic, buccal, marginal mandibular and cervical.
- Frontal and marginal mandibular are at higher risk during the surgery.
- The fascia of submandibular is clinically relevant because the marginal mandibular branch of the facial nerve.
- The marginal mandibular branch of the facial nerve passes forward beneath the platysma and depressor anguli oris, supplying the muscles of the lower lip and chin and communicating with the mental branches of the inferior alveolar nerve.

101. Ans. (b) Fibers of mylohyoid *Ref: BDC 5th ed. p 166*

- Sublingual gland is separated from submandibular gland by Fibers of mylohyoid.

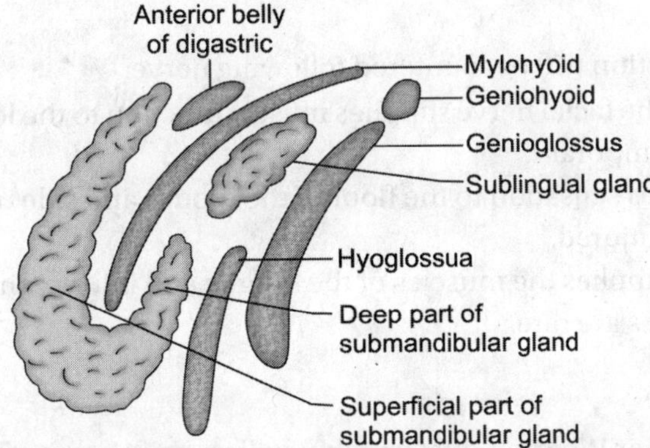

102. Ans. (b) The submandibular gland is seen to wrap around the posterior border of mylohyoid
Ref: B. D. Chaurasia's 5th ed. p 266

- The mylohyoid muscle is a paired muscle running from the mandible to the hyoid bone, forming the floor of the oral cavity. It is named after its two attachments near the molar teeth ("mylo" comes from the Greek word for "molar").These muscles are mesodermal in embryologic origin. The mylohyoid muscle is derived from the first pharyngeal arch.
- The mylohyoid muscle separates the sublingual space from the submandibular space, which communicate in a lateral gap between the mylohyoid and geniohyoid muscles.
- The submandibular gland wraps around the edges of the mylohyoid, and is divided into superficial and deep lobes above and below the muscle.

103. Ans. (d) Glossopharyngeal nerve *Ref: BDC 5th ed. p 165*

Relation of hyoglossus:

Superficial	*Deep*
Lingual nerve	Inferior longitudinal muscle of tongue
Styloglossus	Genioglossus
Submandibular ganglion	Middle constrictor of the pharynx
Deep part of submandibular gland	Glossopharyngeal
Submandibular duct	Stylohyoid ligament
Hypoglossal nerve	Lingual artery

104. Ans. (b) Lingual nerve *Ref: BDC 5th ed. p 166*

- The submandibular gland is usually just palpable. It has a larger superficial part (body) and a smaller deep process.
- It has three surfaces: inferior (covered by skin and platysma), lateral (related to the medial surface of the mandible), and medial (related to the mylohyoid, hyoglossus, and digastric muscles).
- The deep process lies between the mylohyoid and hyoglossus muscles the submandibular duct, which is crossed by the lingual nerve, runs anterior from this process.

105. Ans. (d) Hypoglossal nerve *Ref: BDC 5th ed. 165*

Hyoglossus muscle—it is the key muscle of the submandibular region. It is a quadrate muscle having superficial (lateral surface) and deep (medial surface) posterior margin and anterior margin.

106. Ans. (c) Accessory nerve *Ref: BDC 5th ed. 166,169*

Submandibular gland resection will encountered following nerve:

- The marginal branch of the facial nerve supplies muscle function to the lower lip is the nerve most at risk. Injury to this nerve is usually temporary.
- The lingual nerve supplies sensation to the floor of the mouth and side of the tongue. Numbness of these areas will occur if the nerve is injured.
- The hypoglossal nerve supplies the muscles of the tongue and injury can involve deviation of the tongue to one side. Both of these injuries are rare.

107. Ans. (d) Lingual *Ref: BDC 5th ed p 167*

- The submandibular duct or Wharton duct or submaxillary duct is one of the salivary excretory ducts.
- It is about 5 cm long, and its wall is much thinner than that of the parotid duct.
- At the anterior border of hyoglossus, the submandibular duct is crossed by lingual nerve.
- It is supplied by following nerve from the submandibular ganglion:
  - Secretomotor fibers
  - Lingual nerve
  - Vasomotor sympathetic fibers from plexus on the facial artery.

108. Ans. (b) Hyoglossus, mylohyoid, and digastric muscle *Ref: B.D. Chaurasia 5th ed. p 166*

Relations of Submandibular gland

The inferior surface is covered by:

- Skin
- Platysma
- Cervical branch of the facial nerve
- Deep fascia
- Facial vein
- Submandibular lymph nodes.

The lateral surface is related to:

- The submandibular fossa on the mandible
- Insertion of the medial pterygoid
- The facial artery.

The medial surface is related to:

- Mylohoid, hyoglossus and styloglossus muscles from before backwards
- Inferiorly, it overlaps stylohoid and the posterior belly of the digastrics.

109. Ans. (a) Parapharyngeal space *Ref: Oral and Maxillofacial Infection by Top Azian 4th ed. p 82*

Submandibular space:

- The submandibular space is a fascial space of the head and neck (sometimes also termed fascial spaces or tissue spaces). It is a potential space, and is paired on either side, located on the superficial surface of the mylohyoid muscle between the anterior and posterior bellies of the digastric muscle.
- The submandibular spaces are considered to be the anterior extension of parapharyngeal space.

Communications

The communications of the submandibular space are:

- Medially and anteriorly to the submental space (located medial to the paired submandibular spaces, separated from them by the anterior bellies of the digastric muscles).
- Posteriorly and superiorly to the sublingual space (located above the mylohyoid muscle).
- Inferiorly to the lateral pharyngeal space.

110. Ans. (c) Facial thyroid *Ref: BDC 5th ed. p 166*

- Medial surface of submandibular gland is related to:
  - Styloglossus (option A)
  - Mylohyoid (option B)
  - Hyoglossus (option D)

  } from before backward

It overlaps posterior belly of digastrics and stylohyoid inferiorly.

- Inferior surface is covered by:
  - Submandibular lymph node
  - Facial vein
  - Skin
  - Platysma
  - Deep fascia
  - Cervical branch of facial nerve.
- Lateral surface of submandibular gland is related to:
  - Facial artery
  - Insertion of medial pterygoid
  - Submandibular fossa of mandible.

DEEP STRUCTURE OF NECK

111. Ans. (c) Superior constrictor *Ref: Gray's Anatomy 2nd ed. p 999*

- Larynx is composed of nine cartilage out of which 3 are paired and 3 unpaired.
- Paired—Arytenoids, corniculates and cuneiforms. Unpaired—Thyroid, cricoids, epiglottis.
- Thyroid cartilage is the largest cartilage of larynx.
- On the lateral surface of thyroid cartilage three extrinsic laryngeal muscle are connects to it as:
  - Sternohyoid
  - Thyrohyoid
  - Inferior pharyngeal constrictor.

112. Ans. (c) Superior constrictor *Ref: Gray's Anatomy for Student 2nd ed. p 999*

- Muscle attached to the oblique line of the thyroid cartilage:
  - Thyrohyoid
  - Inferior constrictor of pharynx
  - Sternothyroid.

- Muscle attached to the posterior border of the lamina of the thyroid cartilage:
  - Salpingopharyngeus
  - Palatopharyngeus
  - Stylopharyngeus

113. Ans. (a) Upper border of thyroid cartilage *Ref: Gray's Anatomy for Student 2nd ed. p 806*

- In human anatomy, the left and right common carotid arteries are arteries that supply the head and neck with oxygenated blood; they divide in the neck to form the external and internal carotid arteries.
- The common carotid artery is a paired structure, meaning that there are two in the body, one for each half. The left and right common carotid arteries follow the same course with the exception of their origin. The right common carotid originates in the neck from the brachiocephalic trunk. The left arises from the aortic arch in the thoracic region. The bifurcation into the external and internal carotid arteries occurs at the upper border of the thyroid cartilage, at around the level of the fourth cervical vertebra (C4).
- The common carotid artery is often used in measuring the pulse, especially in patients who are in shock and who lack a detectable pulse in the more peripheral arteries of the body.
- The pulse is taken by palpating the artery just deep to the anterior border of the sternocleidomastoid muscle at the level of the superior border of the thyroid cartilage.
- Presence of a carotid pulse has been estimated to indicate a systolic blood pressure of more than 40 mm Hg, as given by the 50% percentile.

114. Ans. (d) Subclavian artery *Ref: General Anatomy and Musculoskeletal System p 333*

Branches of subclavian artery:

- Thyrocervical trunk with the inferior thyroid artery, suprascapular artery, and transverse cervical artery.
- Vertebral artery.
- Internal thoracic artery.
- Costocervical trunk.

115. Ans. (c) Pretracheal fascia *Ref: BD Chaurasia for Dental Students p 276*

Capsules of thyroid:

- The true capsule is the peripheral condensation of the connective tissue of the gland. The false capsule is derived from the pretracheal layer of the deep cervical fascia. It is thin along the posterior border of the lobes, but thick on the inner surface of the gland where it forms a suspensory ligament (of Berry), which connects the lobe to the cricoid cartilage.

116. Ans. (c) Inferior thyroid artery *Ref: BD Chaurasia 5th ed. p 174*

Inferior thyroid artery:

- The terminal part of inferior thyroid artery is related to the recurrent laryngeal nerve, while its proximal part is away from the nerve.
- It is a branch of thyrocervical trunk.

117. Ans. (c) Thymus *Ref: BDC 5th ed. p 177*

- **Arthur Hill Hassall** discovered thymic corpuscles in 1849 and named as Hassall's corpuscles.
- It is seen in the medulla of human thymus.
- It is formed from eosinophilic type IV epithelial reticular cells arranged concentrically.
- It is known that, Hassall's corpuscles are a potent source of the cytokine TSLP. In vitro TSLP directs the maturation of dendritic cells.
- Hassall's corpuscles are vary in size with diameter from 20 - >100 micro meters and tend to grow larger with age.

118. Ans. (d) Inferior cerebral vein *Ref: BDC 4th ed. Vol. III p 180*

Tributaries of IJV are:
- Inferior petrosal sinus
- Common facial vein
- Lingual vein
- Pharyngeal vein
- Superior thyroid vein
- Middle thyroid vein
- Occipital vein (sometimes).

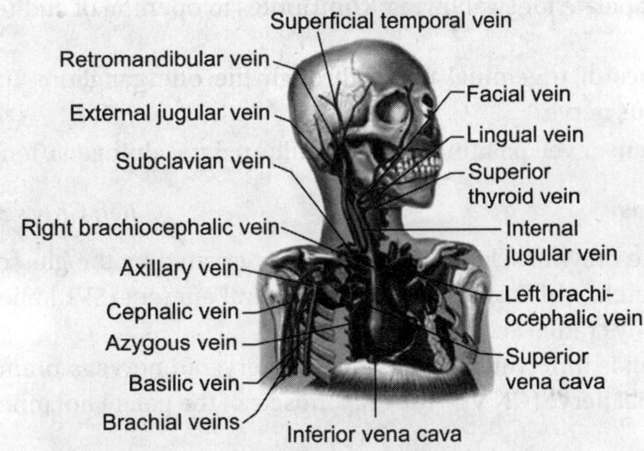

MOUTH AND PHARYNX

119. Ans. (b) The facial nerve *Ref: BDC 5th ed. p 212*

- At the border of the soft and hard palate, taste buds are present. Taste sensation is passed through lesser palatine nerves to sphenopalatine ganglion.
- The further course of the taste sensation is via the greater petrosal nerve, facial nerve, geniculate ganglion and nerves intermedius and terminates at the nucleus of the tractus solitarius.

120. Ans. (c) Sphenopalatine *Ref: BDC 5th ed. p 216*

- Palatine tonsils, occasionally called the faucial tonsils.
- These are seen on the left and right side at the back of the throat.
- The palatine tonsil are located inside the oropharynx between two mucosa covered pillars on the lateral side of the cavity, the anterior being the palatoglossal arch and the posterior being the palate pharyngeal arch.
- Blood supply is provided by tonsillar branch of 5 arteries:
  - Dorsal lingual artery (of the lingual artery)
  - Ascending palatine artery (of the facial artery)
  - Tonsillar branch (of the facial artery)
  - Ascending pharyngeal artery (of external carotid artery)
  - Lesser palatine artery (of the descending palatine artery).

121. Ans. (b) The vagus nerve (hypoglossal according to some students) *Ref: Gray's Anatomy for Student 2nd ed. p 1054*

Palate is supplied by general as well as special sensory nerve:
- Special sensory nerve:
  - Facial nerve

- General sensory nerve:
  - Glossopharyngeal nerve
  - Middle and posterior (lesser) palatine nerve. (A branch of maxillary nerve)

122. Ans. (b) Trigeminal *Ref: BDC 5th ed. p 210-212*

Tensor palati muscle that tenses the soft palate, so that the tongue may compress the food bolus against it during swallowing, forcing the mass into the oropharynx;

- *Origin*, scaphoid fossa of sphenoid, cartilaginous and membranous part of pharyngotympanic (auditory) tube and spine of sphenoid;
- *Insertion*, posterior border of hard palate and aponeurosis of soft palate;
- *Action*, tenses the soft palate for swallowing; contributes to opening of auditory tube to enable equilibration of pressure;
- *Nerve supply*, branches of trigeminal nerve through the otic ganglion. The only muscle of the palate not innervated by the vagus nerve.

Synonym(s): musculus tensor veli palatini [TA], musculus palatosalpingeus, tensor (muscle) of soft palate

123. Ans. (a) Stylopharyngeus *Ref: Gray's Anatomy for Student 2nd ed. p 990*

- Stylopharyngeus is the only muscle in the pharynx innervated by the glossopharyngeal nerve (CN IX) and is done by its motor branch, which supplies special visceral efferent (SVE) fibers to it, while all other muscles of pharynx are supplied by cranial accessory nerve.
- The tensor veli palatini is innervated by the medial pterygoid nerve, a branch of mandibular nerve, the third branch of the trigeminal nerve (CN V)—the only muscle of the palate not innervated by the vagus nerve (cranial accessory nerve).

124. Ans. (c) Palatoglossus *Ref: B.D. Chaurasia's p 213-214*

- All muscles of the tongue, both extrinsic and intrinsic are supplied by hypoglossal nerve except palatoglossus.
- Palatoglossus is being supplied by the cranial part of accessory nerve via pharyngeal plexus.

All muscles of	*Supplied by*	*Except*	*Which is supplied by*
Pharynx	Pharyngeal plexus (IX, X and sympathetic)	Stylopharyngeus	Glossopharyngeal (IX)
Palate	Pharyngeal plexus (IX, X and sympathetic)	Tensor veli palatini	Nerve to medial pterygoid (VC)
Tongue	Hypoglossal (XII)	Palates/occur	Pharyngeal plexus (IX, X and sympathetic)
Facial expression and buccinator	Facial (VII)	Levator palpebrae superioris	Oculomotor (III)
Mastication	Mandibular division of trigeminal (Vc)	Buccinator	Facial (VII)
Larynx	Recurrent laryngeal	Cricothyroid	External branch of superior laryngeal nerve (X)

125. Ans. (c) Submandibular nodes *Ref: BDC 5th ed. p 206*

- The gingiva cover the alveolar process and roots of the teeth.
- Externally, the gingiva are related to the lips and cheeks, separated by the oral vestibule.

Arterial Supply

- The buccal gingivae of both the maxilla and mandible are supplied by branches of the buccal artery (a branch of the 2nd part of the maxillary artery), as well as branches of the posterior superior alveolar artery.
- The palatine gingivae are supplied by branches of the greater palatine artery.
- The mandibular labial gingivae receive blood from the incisive artery and mental artery (terminal branches of the inferior alveolar artery).
- The maxillary labial gingivae are supplied by branches of the anterior superior alveolar artery and the labial branches of the infraorbital nerve. Finally, the lingual gingivae are supplied by the lingual artery and the lingual branch of the inferior alveolar artery.

Lymphatic Drainage

- Lymph drainage from the gingivae depends on the site. With the exception of the labial gingivae of the mandible, the labial, buccal and palatine gingivae drain to submandibular lymph nodes. The labial gingivae of the mandible drains to the submental nodes. The lingual gingivae drains directly to superior deep cervical nodes.

Innervation

- The mandibular gingivae are innervated by various branches of the mandibular division of the trigeminal nerve (lingual nerve, buccal nerve, inferior alveolar nerve and its two terminal branches).
- The maxillary gingivae are wholly innervated by branches of the maxillary nerve, including the nasopalatine, greater palatine, anterior/middle/posterior superior alveolar and infraorbital nerves.

126. Ans. (b) Ventral part of II pharyngeal pouch *Ref: B.D Chaurasia for Dental Students, p 326*

- Development of palatine tonsil.
- The epithelium over the tonsil develops from ventral part of second pharyngeal pouch. The lymphocytes are mesodermal in origin.
- The second pharyngeal pouch is largely obliterated as the palatine tonsil develops. A part of this pouch remains as the tonsillar sinus (fossa).

127. Ans. (b) Auditory tube and levator palati muscle *Ref: BDC 5th ed. p 219*

- The superior pharyngeal constrictor muscle is a muscle of pharynx.
- The muscle is divided into 4 parts i.e. Pterygopharyngeal
  - Mylopharyngeal
  - Buccopharyngeal
  - Glossopharyngeal.
- The interval between the upper border of the muscle and the base of the skull is closed by the pharyngeal aponeurosis and is known as the Sinus of Morgagni. Structure passing through this interval are:
  - Auditory tube
  - Levator veli palate muscle
  - Ascending palatine artery.
- Structure passing through gap between the superior and middle constrictor:
  - Stylopharyngeus
  - Glossopharyngeal nerve.
- Structure passing through gap between the middle and inferior constrictor:
  - Internal laryngeal nerve
  - Superior laryngeal nerve.
- Structure passing through gap between the lower border of inferior constrictor and esophagus:
  - Recurrent laryngeal nerve
  - Internal laryngeal nerve.

128. Ans. (a) Jugulodigastric lymph nodes *Ref: BD Chaurasia's 5th ed. p 216*

Arterial Supply of Tonsil

- Main source: Tonsillar branch of facial artery.
- Additional sources:
  - Ascending palatine branch of facial artery
  - Dorsal lingual branches of the lingual artery
  - Ascending pharyngeal branch of the external carotid artery
  - The greater palatine branch of the maxillary artery.

Venous Drainage

One or more veins leave the lower part of deep surface of the tonsil, pierce the superior constrictor, and join the palatine, pharyngeal, or facial veins.

Lymphatic Drainage

Lymphatics pass to jugulodigastric node.

Nerve Supply

Glossopharyngeal and lesser palatine nerves.

129. Ans. (a) Oropharynx *Ref: BD Chaurasia 3rd ed. p 184*

- Palatine tonsils, occasionally called the faucial tonsils, are the tonsils that can be seen on the left and right sides at the back of the throat.
- The palatine tonsil is one of the mucosa-associated lymphoid tissues (MALT), located at the entrance to the upper respiratory and gastrointestinal tracts to protect the body from the entry of exogenous material through mucosal sites. In consequence it is a site of, and potential focus for, infections, and is one of the chief immunocompetent tissues in the oropharynx. It forms part of the Waldeyer's ring, which comprises the nasopharyngeal tonsil or adenoid (NT), the paired tubal tonsils (TT), the paired palatine tonsils (PT) and the lingual tonsil (LT). From the pharyngeal side, they are covered with a stratified squamous epithelium, whereas a fibrous capsule links them to the wall of the pharynx. Through the capsule pass trabeculae that contain small blood vessels, nerves and lymphatic vessels. These trabeculae divide the tonsil into lobules.
- The palatine tonsils are located inside the oropharynx between two mucosa-covered pillars on the lateral sides of the cavity, the anterior being the palatoglossal arch, and the posterior being thepalatopharyngeal arch. Collectively they are referred to as the fauces. Between these arches is the tonsillar bed, within which lie the palatine tonsils and the nervous and arterial structures that supply them.

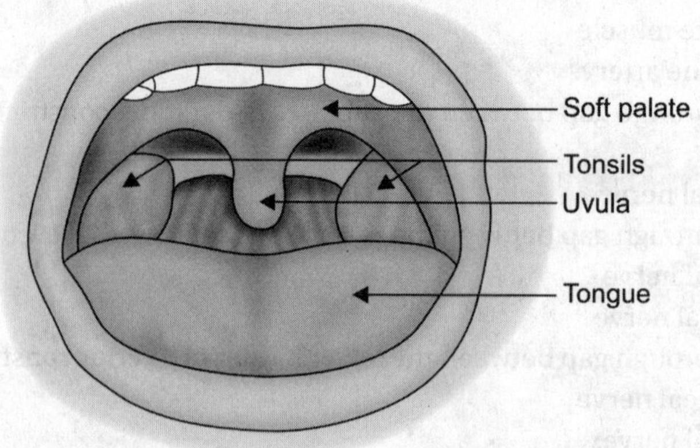

130. Ans. (b) Submandibular *Ref: BD Chaurasia's 3rd ed. p 175-177*

Lymphatic drainage of lip

- Central part by submental lymph node
- Rest part lower and upper lip by submandibular lymph node

Lymphatic drainage of cheek

- Mainly by submandibular and preauricular nodes
- By buccal and mandibular node partially

Lymphatic drainage from oral cavity proper

- Anterior part submandibular
- Hard palate and soft palate by retropharyngeal and upper deep cervical

Lymphatic drainage of gums

- Anterior part of lower gum submental
- Posterior part of lower and complete upper gum in submandibular.

131. Ans. (b) Peritonsillar abscess *Ref: BDC, 4th ed. Vol. III, p 145*

- The tonsils are frequently sites of infection, especially in children
- Infection may spread to surrounding tissue forming a peritonsillar abscess
- Suppuration of peritonsillar area is called as quinsy

NOSE AND PARANASAL SINUSES

132. Ans. (a) Trigeminal *Ref: Grays Anatomy for Student 2nd ed. p 852*

- The ophthalmic nerve (V1) is one of the three branches of the trigeminal nerve, the fifth cranial nerve. The ophthalmic nerve carries only sensory fibers
- The ophthalmic nerve supplies branches to the cornea, ciliary body, and iris; to the lacrimal gland and conjunctiva; to the part of the mucous membrane of the nasal cavity; and to the skin of the eyelids, eyebrow, forehead and nose.
- It is the smallest of the three divisions of the trigeminal, and arises from the upper part of the trigeminal ganglion as a short, flattened band, about 2.5 cm. long, which passes forward along the lateral wall of the cavernous sinus, below the oculomotor and trochlear nerves; just before entering the orbit, through the superior orbital fissure, it divides into three branches, lacrimal, frontal, and nasociliary.

133. Ans. (c) Nasolacrimal duct *Ref: BDC 5th ed. p 228*

- The nasolacrimal duct (sometimes called the tear duct) carries tears from the lacrimal sac into the nasal cavity.
- The opening of the nasolacrimal duct into the inferior nasal meatus is partially covered by a mucosal fold. Excess tears flow through nasolacrimal duct which drains into the inferior nasal meatus.
- This is the reason the nose starts to run when a person is crying or has watery eyes from an allergy, and why one can sometimes taste eye drops.
- Like the lacrimal sac, the duct is lined by stratified columnar epithelium containing mucus-secreting goblet cells, and is surrounded by connective tissue.

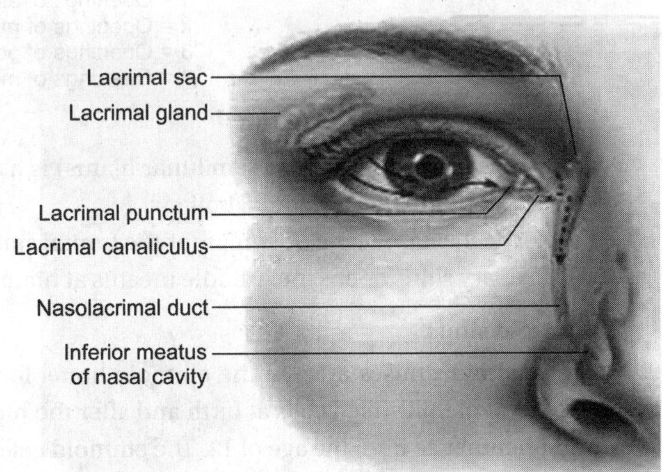

134. Ans. (c) Ciliated columnar *Ref: Oral and Maxillofacial Surgery by Laskin, Vol: 1, 1st ed. p 20, 21*

- The pyramid-shaped maxillary sinus (or antrum of highmore) is the largest of the paranasal sinuses, and drains into the middle meatus of the nose
- Found in the body of the maxilla, this sinus has three recesses: an alveolar recess pointed inferiorly, bounded by the alveolar process of the maxilla; a zygomatic process pointed laterally, bounded by the zygomatic bone; and an infraorbital recess pointed superiorly, bounded by the inferior orbital surface of the maxilla. The medial wall is composed primarily of cartilage
- The sinus is lined with mucoperiosteum, with cilia that beat toward the ostia. This membrane is also referred to as the "Schneiderian membrane", which is histologically a bilaminar membrane with ciliated columnar epithelial cells on the internal (or cavernous) side and periosteum on the osseous side.

135. Ans. (c) Ethmoid sinus *Ref: Clinical Anatomy for Students by Neeta V Kulkarni 1st ed. p 502*

The paranasal sinuses are air-filled spaces located within the bones of the skull and face. They are centered on the nasal cavity and have various functions, including lightening the weight of the head, humidifying and heating inhaled air, increasing the resonance of speech, and serving as a crumple zone to protect vital structures in the event of facial trauma.

Four sets of paired sinuses exist: maxillary, frontal, sphenoid, and ethmoid.

136. Ans. (d) Hiatus semilunaris *Ref: BDC 5th ed. p 231*

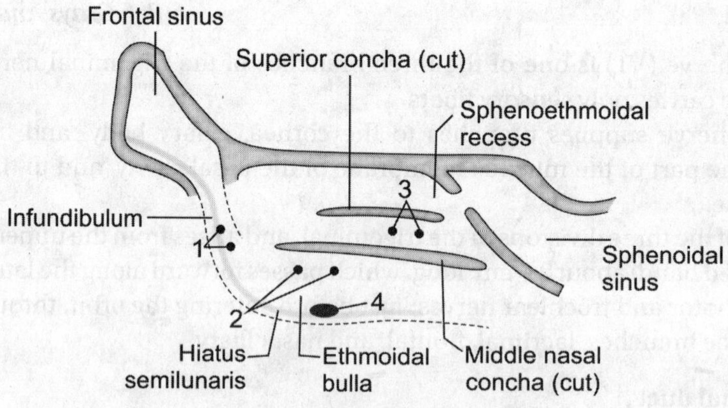

1 = Openings of anterior ethmoidal sinuses
2 = Openings of middle ethmoidal sinuses
3 = Openings of posterior ethmoidal sinuses
4 = Openings of maxillary sinus

- The hiatus semilunaris (or semilunar hiatus) is a crescent-shaped groove in the lateral wall of the nasal cavity just inferior to the ethmoidal bulla.
- It is the location of the openings for the frontal sinus, maxillary sinus, and anterior ethmoidal sinus.
- Maxillary sinus opens into middle meatus at hiatus semilunaris.

Ethmoid sinus

The ethmoid sinuses arise in the ethmoid bone, forming several distinct air cells between the eyes. They are a collection of fluid-filled cells at birth and after the birth ethmoidal air cells are converted into bony cavity. It grow and pneumatize until the age of 12. The ethmoid cells are shaped like pyramids and are divided by thin septa.

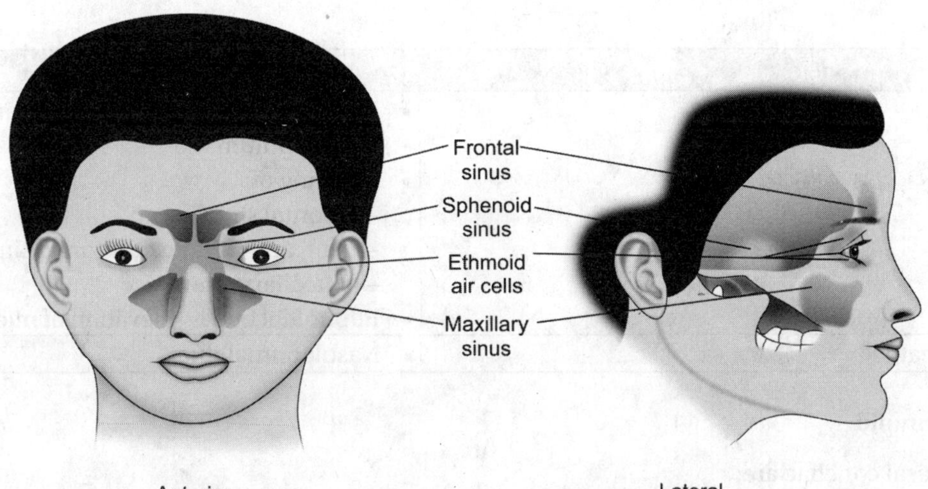

137. Ans. (c) Recess *Ref http://en.wikip edia.org/wiki/maxillary-sinus*

- Found in the body of the maxilla, the sinus has 3 recess:
  - An alveolar recess pointed inferiorly bounded by the alveolar process of the maxilla
  - A zygomatic recess pointed laterally, bounded by the zygomatic bone and
  - An infraorbital recess pointed superiorly. Bounded by the inferior orbital surface of the maxilla
- The medial wall is composed primarily of cartilage
- The size of sinuses varies in different skulls, and even on 2 sides of the same skull

138. Ans. (b) Post ethmoidal sinus *Ref: BDC 4th ed. Vol. III, p 231 and Dhingra, 3rd ed. p 16*

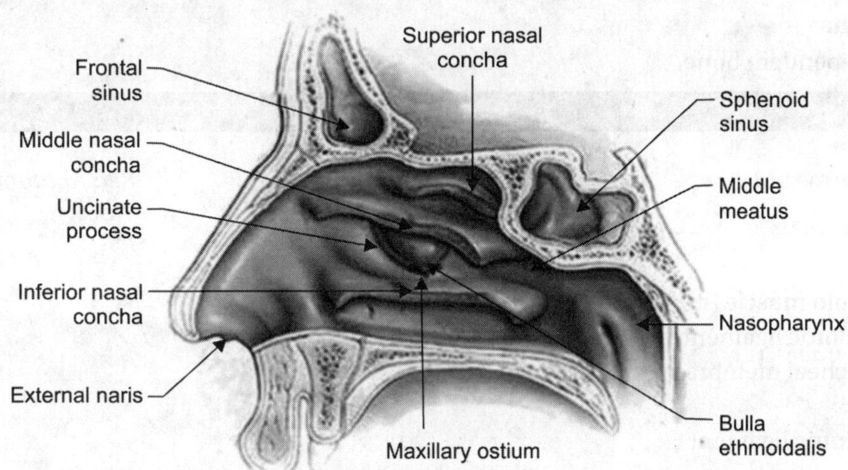

Meatus	*Opening*
Sphenoethmoidal Recess (Above sup. Conchae)	Sphenoid sinus
Superior meatus Below sup. conchae; shortest and shallowest Middle meatus (Below middle conchae) (Mnemonic – Hi-flame)	Postethmoidal sinus

Contd...

Contd...

Meatus	*Opening*
	• Hiatus semilunaris – semicircular sulcus below bulla • Infundibulum • Opening of: – Frontal sinus – Ant. and middle ethmoidal sinus – Maxillary sinus • Ethmoidal bulla—elevation of middle ethmoidal cells
Inferior meatus	• Nasolacrimal duct

139. Ans. (b) Ethmoid *Ref: BDC 5th ed. p 228*

The three nasal conchae are:

Superior concha:

- The back part of the medial surface of the labyrinth of ethmoid is subdivided by a narrow oblique fissure, the superior meatus of the nose, bounded above by a thin, curved plate, the superior nasal concha.
- The bone found in superior nasal concha is part of the ethmoid bone.

Middle concha:

- The medial surface of the labyrinth of ethmoid consists of a thin lamella, which descends from the under surface of the cribriform plate, and ends below in a free, convoluted margin, the middle nasal concha
- It is rough, and marked above by numerous grooves, directed nearly vertically downward from the cribriform plate; they lodge branches of the olfactory nerves, which are distributed to the mucous membrane covering the superior nasal concha.

Inferior concha:

- It is an independent bone.

LARYNX

140. Ans. (a) Cricothyroid *Ref: Anatomy by S Mitra Vol. 2, p 121*

Ligaments of Larynx

- Extrinsic:
  - Thyrohyoid muscle (membrane)
  - Hyoepiglottic ligament
  - Cricotracheal membrane.
- Intrinsic:
  - Aryepiglottic ligament
  - Vestibular ligament
  - Vocal ligament
  - Cricothyroid ligament
  - Thyroepiglottic ligament.

While stylohyoid is an extrinsic muscle of larynx and cricothyroid is the intrinsic.

141. Ans. (d) Internal and recurrent laryngeal nerve *Ref: BD Chaurasia's 5th ed. p 347*

- Recurrent laryngeal nerve (RLN) is a branch of the vagus nerve (cranial nerve X) that supplies all the intrinsic muscles of the larynx, with the exception of the cricothyroid muscles. The recurrent laryngeal nerves supply sensation to the larynx below the vocal cords. The recurrent laryngeal nerves are the nerves of the sixth pharyngeal arch.

- The internal laryngeal nerve is the internal branch (ramus internus) of the superior laryngeal nerve. Above the vocal folds the sensory innervation of the larynx is via the internal laryngeal nerve.
- Hence, the vocal fold itself receives dual innervation from both nerves.

142. Ans. (d) Posterior cricoarytenoid *Ref: BD Chaurasia's 5th ed. p 346*

Muscles acting on the larynx

Movement	*Muscles*
1. Elevation of larynx	Thyrohyoid, mylohyoid
2. Depression of larynx	Sternothyroid, sternohyoid
3. Opening inlet of larynx	Thyroepiglottic
4. Closing inlet of larynx	Aryepiglotticus
5. Abductor of vocal cords	Posterior cricoarytenoid only
6. Adductor of vocal cords	Lateral cricoarytenoid transverse, oblique arytenoids
7. Tensor of vocal cords	Cricothyroid
8. Relaxor of vocal cords	Thyroarytenoid

143. Ans. (c) Internal laryngeal nerve *Ref: BD Chaurasia's 5th ed. p 347*

Refer Ans 141

TONGUE

144. Ans. (c) Facial musculature *Ref: BDC 5th ed. p 252*

Palatoglossus:

- Palatoglossus is an extrinsic muscle of tongue, it originates from the oral surface of palatine aponeurosis.
- Palatoglossus connects the tongue to the palate.
- It descends in the palatoglossal arch, to the side of the tongue, at the junction of oral and pharyngeal part.
- Palatoglossus pulls up the root of tongue, approximates the palatoglossal arches and thus closes the oropharyngeal isthmus.

145. Ans. (a) Side of tongue *Ref: BDC 5th ed. p 252*

Hyoglossus muscle: it is a thin, quadrilateral muscle:

- Origin: body and greater cornu of hyoid bone.
- Insertion: side of tongue.
- Innervation: hypoglossal nerve.
- Action: depress and retracts tongue.

146. Ans. (c) Upwards and backwards pull of tongue *Ref: BDC 5th ed. p 252*

The four major extrinsic muscles of the tongue are:

- The mylohyoid muscle, which is responsible for raising the body of the tongue in high vowels and velar consonants.
- The hyoglossus, which pulls it downwards (and slightly backwards).
- The styloglossus, which pulls the tongue upwards and backwards.
- The genioglossus, which forms the bulk of the inferior part of the tongue and pulls the body of the tongue forwards.

147. Ans. (a) Hypoglossal *Ref: BDC 5th ed. p 252*

Nerve Supply of Tongue

The tongue is divided into the anterior two thirds and a posterior third when discussing its innervation. It is supplied via sensory and motor pathways to both sections.

The Anterior two-thirds are innervated by:

- Sensory branches of the lingual nerve (CN V/III - trigeminal nerve, mandibular branch) and the chorda tympani branch of CN VII - facial nerve for taste.
- Motori branches of the hypoglossal nerve (CN XII).

The Posterior third is innervated by:

- Sensory branches of the glossopharyngeal nerve (CN IX), for sensation and taste.
- Motori branches of the hypoglossal nerve (CN XII).

The hypoglossal nerve (CN XII) provides motor innervation to all the extrinsic and intrinsic muscles of the tongue except the palatoglossus muscle which is innervated by the vagus nerve (CN X).

148. Ans. (b) The glossopharyngeal nerve *Ref: BDC 5th ed. p 252*

Innervation of tongue:

Nerves which supply the sensation and taste of the tongue differ between the anterior and posterior parts:

- Anteriorly, the sensation of taste is passed along the chorda tympani, a branch of the facial nerve. Sensation is passed along the lingual nerve, a branch of the trigeminal nerve.
- Posteriorly, both taste and sensation are passed along the glossopharyngeal nerve. All intrinsic and extrinsic muscles of the tongue are supplied by the hypoglossal nerve, with the exception of the palatoglossus. The palatoglossus is innervated by the vagus nerve.
- The average length of the human tongue from the oropharynx to the tip is 10 cm (4 in).

149. Ans. (b) Artery, nerve and vein *Ref: Gavilan Functional and Selective Neck Dissection p 47*

The normal arrangement of lingual nerve and vessels in the tongue from medial to lateral is:

Deep lingutal artery → Lingual nerve → Deep lingual vein

150. Ans. (b) 10 *Ref: BDC 5th ed. p 252, 253*

Nerves which supply the sensation and taste of the tongue differ between the anterior and posterior parts:

- Anteriorly, the sensation of taste is passed along the chorda tympani, a branch of the facial nerve. Sensation is passed along the lingual nerve, a branch of the trigeminal nerve.
- Posteriorly, both taste and sensation are passed along the glossopharyngeal nerve.

All intrinsic and extrinsic muscles of the tongue are supplied by the hypoglossal nerve, with the exception of the palatoglossus. The palatoglossus is innervated by the vagus nerve.

151. Ans. (b) 10 *Ref: BDC 5th ed. p 253*

- Circumvallate papillae are sunken papillae, with a trough separating them from surrounding wall.
- The taste buds are in tiers within the trough of the papillae. They are situated on the circumvallate line and confer a sour/bitter sensitivity to the posterior 2/3 of the tongue.
- Innervated by the glossopharyngeal (IX cranial) nerve.
- 3-13 circumvallate papillae per tongue with 252 taste buds per papillae, total = 2200 circumvallate taste buds per tongue.

152. Ans. (a) Posterior vessels *Ref: Anatomy for Dental Students p 264*

Four lymph vessel drain from the tongue

Apical vessels	Drain from the tip of the tongue It pierces the mylohyoid muscle and goes into submental nodes
Marginal vessel	Drain the margins of the anterior 2/3 of the tongue It is done unilaterally through mylohyoid muscle and some goes into submandibular nodes and finally to the jugulo-omohyoid node
Central vessel	Drain the central portion of the anterior 2/3 of the tongue on either side of median raphe It drain to the submental and jugulo-omohyoid nodes, which drain into the deep cervical nodes
Basal vessels	Drain the posterior 1/3 of the tongue Then it goes to the jugulo-digastric nodes

153. Ans. (b) Deviation of tongue to paralysed side *Ref: BD Chaurasia's 5th ed. p 296, 297*

- The hypoglossal nerve is the twelfth cranial nerve (XII), leading to muscles of the tongue. It is called hypoglossal nerve because it is below the tongue. It controls tongue movements of speech, food manipulation, and swallowing.

Testing of hypoglossal nerve

To test the function of the nerve, a patient is asked to stick their tongue straight out. If there is a loss of innervation to one side, the tongue will curve toward the affected side, due to unopposed action of the opposite genioglossus muscle. If this is the result of a lower motor neuron lesion, the tongue will be curved toward the damaged side, combined with the presence of fasciculations or atrophy. However, if the deficit is caused by an upper motor neuron lesion, the tongue will be curved away from the side of the cortical damage, without the presence of fasciculations or atrophy.

154. Ans. (b) Superior genial tubercle *Ref: Gray's Anatomy 2nd ed. p 1039*

- A mental spine is a small projection of bone on the posterior aspect of the mandible (jaw bone) in the midline. There are usually four mental spines: two superior and two inferior. Collectively they are also known as the genial tubercle.
- The inferior mental spines are the points of origin of the geniohyoid muscle, one of the suprahyoid muscles.
- The superior mental spines are the origin of the genioglossus muscle, one of the muscles of the tongue.
- In this way, genioglossus muscle is attached in the posterior surface of symphysis menti in the superior genial tubercle.

155. Ans. (a) Genioglossus and geniohyoid

Same as above

156. Ans. (c) Mandibular nerve *Ref: BDC 5th ed. p 154*

- The lingual nerve is a branch of the mandibular division of the trigeminal nerve (CN V3), which supplies sensory innervation to the tongue. It also carries fibers from the facial nerve, which return taste information from the anterior two thirds of the tongue.
- The lingual nerve supplies general somatic afferent innervation from the mucous membrane of the anterior two-thirds of the tongue.
- It also carries nerve fibers that are not part of the trigeminal nerve, including the chorda tympani nerve of the facial nerve, which provides special sensation (taste) to the anterior 2/3 part of the tongue as well as parasympathetic and sympathetic fibers.
- The submandibular ganglion is suspended by two nerve filaments from the lingual nerve.

157. Ans. (d) Glossopharyngeal nerve *Ref: BD Chaurasia's for Dental Students, p 274*

Parts of the tongue

Nerve supply	*Anterior two-thirds*	*Posterior one-third*	*Posterior most part or vallecula*
Sensory	Lingual	Glossopharyngeal	Internal laryngeal branch of vagus
Taste	Chorda tympani except vallate papillae	Glossopharyngeal including the vallate papillae	Internal laryngeal branch of vagus
Development of epithelium from endoderm	Lingual swellings of 1 arch tuberculum impart which soon disappears	Third arch which forms large ventral part of hypobranchial eminence	Fourth arch which forms small dorsal part of hypobranchial eminence

158. Ans. (b) Chorda tympani and (d) Glossopharyngeal nerve *Ref: BD Chaurasia's for Dental Students, p 274*

Same as above.

159. Ans. (a) Styloglossus *Ref: BDC 5th ed. p 252*

Genioglossus:

- Fan shaped muscle, which form the main bulk of tongue.
- Upper fibers retract the lip, middle fibers depress the tongue and lower fibers protrude the tongue.
- Also known as safety muscle of tongue because it prevent the tongue from falling backward and blocking (chocking) the airway.

160. Ans. (d) Styloglossus *Ref: BDC, 4th ed. Vol. III, p 252*

- All the intrinsic (superior and inferior longitudinal, transverse, vertical) and extrinsic (genioglossus, hyoglossus and styloglossus) muscles except palatoglossus are supplied by hypoglossal nerve.
- The palatoglossus is supplied by the cranial root of the accessory nerve through the pharyngeal plexus.

161. Ans. (a) Separated from the epiglottis by glossoepiglottic folds *Ref: BDC 5th ed. p 250*

- The anterior or lingual surface of the epiglottis is curved forward, and covered on its upper, free part by mucous membrane which is reflected on to the sides and root of the tongue, forming a median and two lateral glossoepiglottic folds; the lateral folds are partly attached to the wall of the pharynx.
- The median glossoepiglottic fold connects the base of the tongue to the lingual surface of the epiglottis.

162. Ans. (c) Hyoid bone and mandible *Ref: BDC 5th ed. p 250*

- The root of the tongue rests on the floor of the mouth and is attached to the mandible and soft palate above and hyoid bone below.

EAR AND VESTIBULAR NERVE

163. Ans. (b) Modified apocrine glands *Ref: BDC 5th ed. p 258*

- Ceruminous gland are located in the external auditory canal of human ear.
- It is modified apocrine gland or modified sweat gland.
- It is simple, coiled tubular glands made up of an inner secretary layer of cells and an outer myoepithelial layer of cells.

- It produce cerumen or earwax, by mixing their secretion with sebum and dead epidermal cells.
- Cerumen keep the eardrum pliable, lubricates and clean the external auditory canal, waterproof the canal, kills bacteria and serves as a barrier to trap foreign particles (dust, fungal spores, etc) by coating the guard cells of the ear and making them sticky.

164. Ans. (d) Synovial joint *Ref: BDC 5th ed. p 264*

The auditory ossicles consist of three small bones found within a space (the tympanic cavity) in the temporal bone of the skull. The bones (which are named for their shape) are connected by synovial joints. Resting against the oval window of inner ear is the stapes (stirrup), which articulates with the middle ossicle called the incus (anvil). The incus articulates with the malleus (hammer), whose "handle" is attached to the internal surface of the tympanic membrane (eardrum).

165. Ans. (d) That it contains postganglionic parasympathetic fibers *Ref: Gray's Anatomy for Student 2nd ed. p 935*

- The chorda tympani is a nerve that originates from the taste buds in the front of the tongue, runs through the middle ear, and carries taste messages to the brain. It joins the facial nerve (cranial nerve VII) inside the facial canal, at the level where the facial nerve exits the skull via the stylomastoid foramen.
- The chorda tympani carries two types of nerve fibers from their origin with the facial nerve to the lingual nerve that carries them to their destinations:
  - **Special sensory fibers** providing taste sensation from the anterior two-thirds of the tongue.
  - **Presynaptic parasympathetic fibers** to the submandibular ganglion, providing secretomotor innervation to two salivary glands: the submandibular gland and sublingual gland and to the vessels of the tongue, which when stimulated, cause a dilation of blood vessels of the tongue.

166. Ans. (b) Ascending palatine *Ref: Gray's Anatomy for Student 2nd ed. p 909*

Middle ear and nasopharynx are connected by the pharyngotympanic tube

It equalizes the pressure on both side of tympanic membrane

It receive its arterial supply from several sources as:

- Ascending pharyngeal artery
- Middle meningeal artery artery of the pterygoid plexus
- Venous drainage is through pterygoid plexus of vein.

It is innervated by tympanic nerve, a branch of the glossopharyngeal nerve (IX)

167. Ans. (a) Ear ossicles *Ref: Clinical Neuroembryology by Hans and Martin p 287*

- The ears are composed of external, middle, and internal anatomical parts. The external and middle parts of the ears regulate the transference of sound waves from the exterior to the internal ears; this process converts the sound waves into nerve impulses. The internal ears are concerned with both hearing and balance.
- The middle ear is formed by tympanic cavity and ear ossicles, i.e. malleus, incus, and stapes.
- The malleus and the incus develop from the cartilage of the first pharyngeal arch, whereas the stapes develops from the cartilage of the second arch.
- Before birth the middle ear reaches its adult size as the ossification of the entire chain is started by the 16th week of gestation.

168. Ans. (a) Superior meatus *Ref: BDC 5th ed. p 231*

Ethmoidal sinuses are numerous small intercommunication spaces which lie within the labyrinth of the ethmoid bone.

Ethmoidal sinus divided into:

	Made up of	*Opens into*	*Supplied by*	*Lymphatics drain*
Anterior	1–11 air cells	Anterior part of hiatus semilunaris of nose	Anterior ethmoid nerve and vessels	Submandibular nodes
Middle	1–7 air cells	Middle meatus of nose	Posterior ethmoid nerve and vessels and orbital branch of pterygopalatine ganglion	Submandibular nodes
Posterior	1–7 air cells	Superior metaus of nose	Posterior ethmoid nerve and vessels and orbital branch of pterygopalatine ganglion	Posterior ethmoid nerve and vessels and orbital branch of pterygopalatine ganglion

169. Ans. (c) Sigmoid *Ref: BD Chaurasia's 5th ed. p 208*

Sigmoid sinus thrombosis can due to the infection such as acute otitis media, acute mastoiditis or apical petrositis. The sigmoid sinus is separated from the middle ear through a thin plate of bone. In chronic inflammation, the erosion of this thin plate will occur and it leads to sigmoid sinus thrombosis

EYEBALL

170. Ans. (c) Exophthalmos *Ref: BD Chaurasia's 5th ed. p 299*

- Horner's syndrome (also Horner syndrome, Bernard-Horner syndrome, Claude Bernard-Horner syndrome or as oculosympathetic palsy) is the combination of drooping of the eyelid (ptosis) and constriction of the pupil (miosis), sometimes accompanied by decreased sweating (anhidrosis) of the face on the same side; redness of the conjunctiva of the eye is often also present.
- Apparent enophthalmos is also a frequent symptom.
- It indicates a problem with the sympathetic nervous system, a part of the autonomic nervous system.
- Medical imaging and response to particular eye drops may be required to identify the location of the problem and the underlying cause

EMBRYOLOGY

171. Ans. (a) Paneth cells *Ref: Inderbir Singh 8th ed. p 320*

Structure derived from neural crest:

- Neuron
- Odontoblast
- Schwann cell
- Glial cells
- Melanocytes
- Arachnoid and piamater
- Adrenal medulla
- C-cells of thyroid
- Muscle connective tissue of face and neck
- Facial cartilage
- Ciliary body of eye
- Ganglia of ANS

Structure derived from neural tube:

- Spinal cord and motor neurons
- Retina
- Posterior pituitary
- Brain (Rhombencephalon, mesencephalon, and prosencephalon).

172. Ans. (a) Sphenoid *Ref: Human Embryology and Development Biology by Bruce M Carlson 5th ed. p 177 by Bruce M Carlson*

- The part of the skull formed by viscerocranium that makes the face.
- The viscerocranium consist of two division is:
  - Cartilaginous viscerocranium
  - Membranous viscerocranium.
- The viscerocranium is made by 14 bones out of which 6 are paired and 2 are unpaired. They are named as:
  - Maxillae
  - Zygomatic bones
  - Nasal bones
  - Lacrimal bones
  - Palatine bones
  - Mandible
  - Vomer
  - Squamous part of temporal.

173. Ans. (b) Nodal gene *Ref: Human Embryology by Inderbir Singh 8th ed. p 42*

- The primitive streak is a structure that forms in the blastula during the early stages of avian, reptilian and mammalian embryonic development
- The formation of the primitive streak in the blastocyst involves the coordinated movement and rearrangement of cells in the epiblast. Even before the streak is visible, epiblast cells have started to move
- The formation of the primitive streak relies on a complex network of signaling pathways that work together to ensure that this process is highly-regulated. Activation of various secreted factors (Vg1, Nodal, Wnt8C, FGF8 and Chordin) and transcription factors (Brachyury and Goosecoid) adjacent to the site of streak formation is required for this process
- Nodal a known mesodermal inducer of the TGFB superfamily, has been implicated in streak formation.

174. Ans. (b) Occipital somites *Ref: Human Embryology by Inderbir Singh 8th ed.*

Development of the Tongue from Pharyngeal Arches 1 through 4 and the Occipital Somites as:

Embryonic precursor	*Intermediate structure*	*Adult structure*	*Innervation*
Pharyngeal arch 1	Median tongue bud	Overgrown by lateral lingual swellings	Lingual branch (sensory) of mandibular division of trigeminal nerve (V)
	Lateral lingual swellings	Mucosa of anterior two-thirds of tongue	Chorda tympani from facial nerve (VII; innervating arch 2) (innervates all taste buds except vallate papillae)
Pharyngeal arch 2	Copula	Overgrown by other structures	
Pharyngeal arch 3	Large, ventral part of hypopharyngeal eminence	Mucosa of most of posterior one-third of tongue	Sensory branch of glossopharyngeal nerve (IX) (also supplies vallate papillae)

Contd...

Contd...

Embryonic precursor	*Intermediate structure*	*Adult structure*	*Innervation*
Pharyngeal arch 4	Small, dorsal part of hypopharyngeal eminence	Mucosa of small region on dorsal side of posterior one-third of tongue	Sensory fibers of superior laryngeal branch of vagus nerve (X)
Occipital somites	Myoblasts	Intrinsic muscles of tongue	Hypoglossal nerve (XII)
Head mesoderm	Myoblasts	Palatoglossus muscle	Pharyngeal plexus of vagus nerve (X)

175. Ans. (c) Muscle of facial expression *Ref: Head and Neck Anatomy by Eric Baker for Dental Medicine p 61*

Refer Ans. 177

176. Ans. (a) 18-23 days *Ref: Shobha Tandon 2nd ed. p 48*

During the 4th week of intrauterine life following structures are formed:

- Neural tube is formed
- Embryonic disc assumes a C-shape as the head, tail and lateral folds form
- All major organs and systems of the body start developing from the 3 germ layers
- Formation of the foregut, midgut and hindgut takes place
- By the 24th day, 3 pairs of branchial arches are present
- Dental lamina too formed

177. Ans. (d) Anterior belly of digastric *Ref: BD Chaurasia, 5th ed. p 150*

Pharyngeal arch	*Muscular contributions*	*Skeletal contributions*	*Nerve*	*Artery*
1st (also called mandibular arch)	Muscles of mastication, anterior belly of the digastric, mylohyoid, tensor tympani, tensor veli palatini	Maxilla, mandible (only as a model for mandible not actual formation of mandible), the incus and malleus of the middle ear, also Mecker's cartilage	Trigeminal nerve (V2 and V3)	Maxillary artery, external carotid artery
2nd (also called the hyoid arch)	Muscles of facial expression, buccinator, platysma, stapedius, stylohyoid, posterior belly of the digastric	Stapes, temporal styloid process, hyoid (lesser horn and upper part of body), Reichert's cartilage	Facial nerve (VII)	Stapedial artery, hyoid artery
3rd	Stylopharyngeus	Hyoid (greater horn and lower part of body), thymus, inferior parathyroids	Glossopharyngeal nerve (IX)	Common carotid, internal carotid

Contd...

Contd...

Pharyngeal arch	*Muscular contributions*	*Skeletal contributions*	*Nerve*	*Artery*
4th	Cricothyroid muscle, all intrinsic muscles of soft palate including levator veli palatini	Thyroid cartilage, superior parathyroids, epiglottic cartilage	Vagus nerve (X), superior laryngeal nerve	Right 4th aortic arch: subclavian artery Left 4th aortic arch: aortic arch
6th	All intrinsic muscles of larynx except the cricothyroid muscle	Cricoid cartilage, arytenoid cartilages, corniculate cartilage	Vagus nerve (X), recurrent laryngeal nerve	Right 6th aortic arch: pulmonary artery Left 6th aortic arch: pulmonary artery and ductus arteriosus

178. Ans. (c) Near the base of tongue close to foramen caecum *Ref: Shafer's 6th ed. p 32*

Lingual thyroid nodule:

- From the ventral floor of the pharynx, thyroid gland is developed during embryo
- Tongue is formed at same time and closely linked with thyroid anatomically. Foramen caecum is the lingual remnant of it
- Failure of the primitive thyroid anlage to descend are the cause of lingual thyroid nodule
- It is manifested near the base of the tongue in general vicinity of the foramen caecum

179. Ans. (d) By around 16 years *Ref: IB Singh Embryology 7th ed p 23*

Meiosis in the male does not begin until after puberty.

Meiotic division of male germ cells commences during the puberty ie, 13-16 years of age.

Biologic characteristics of normal human spermatozoa:

- Length: 65 mm
- Number: 100 million per ml of semen
- Motile at emission: more than 80%
- Rate of movement in the genital tract: 5 mm per minute
- Survival in the genital tract: 3 to 4 days.

180. Ans. (b) 8th prenatal week *Ref: William R Proffit's, 4th ed p 40*

Bone formation begins about the 8th week of gestation and involves the delivery of bones cell precursors to the site of bone formation:

- During early fetal life, the fetal skeleton is mainly of hyaline cartilage that eventually undergoes ossification and bone formation
- The formation of bones from cartilage continues until to thin strips remain at the end of the bones (epiphyseal palate)

181. Ans. (d) Two arteries and one vein *Ref: Inderbir Singh 7th ed. p 250*

- In placental mammals, the umbilical cord (also called the navel string, birth cord or funiculus umbilicalis) is a conduit between the developing embryo or fetus and the placenta.
- During prenatal development, the umbilical cord is physiologically and genetically part of the fetus and (in humans) normally contains two arteries (the umbilical arteries) and one vein (the umbilical vein), buried within Wharton's jelly.

- The umbilical vein supplies the fetus with oxygenated, nutrient-rich blood from the placenta. Conversely, the fetal heart pumps deoxygenated, nutrient-depleted blood through the umbilical arteries back to the placenta.
- The blood flow through the umbilical cord is approximately 35 ml/min at 20 weeks, and 240 ml/min at 40 weeks of gestation.

182. Ans. (b) 2nd branchial arch *Ref: BDC 5th ed. p 55*

The facial muscles are a group of striated skeletal muscles innervated by the facial nerve (cranial nerve VII) that, among other things, control facial expression. These muscles are also called mimetic muscles.

Innervation

- The facial muscles are innervated by facial nerve (cranial nerve VII), with each nerve serving one side of the face. In contrast, the nearbymasticatory muscles are innervated by the mandibular nerve, a branch of the trigeminal nerve (V) cranial nerve.

Development

- The facial muscles are derived from the second branchial/pharyngeal arch.

List of muscles

The facial muscles include:

- Occipitofrontalis muscle
- Temporoparietalis muscle
- Procerus muscle
- Nasalis muscle
- Depressor septi nasi muscle
- Orbicularis oculi muscle
- Corrugator supercilii muscle
- Depressor supercilii muscle
- Auricular muscles (anterior, superior and posterior)
- Orbicularis oris muscle
- Depressor anguli oris muscle
- Risorius
- Zygomaticus major muscle
- Zygomaticus minor muscle
- Levator labii superioris
- Levator labii superioris alaeque nasi muscle
- Depressor labii inferioris muscle
- Levator anguli oris
- Buccinator muscle
- Mentalism.

183. Ans. (d) Stylohyoid ligament *Ref: Human Embryology by Indervir Singh 8th ed. p 108*

The second pharyngeal arch or hyoid arch (or second branchial arch) assists in forming the side and front of the neck.

Derivative

Skeletal elements

From the cartilage of the second arch arises:

- Stapes,
- Temporal styloid process,
- Stylohyoid ligament, and
- Lesser cornu of the hyoid bone.

Muscles

- Muscles of face
- Occipitofrontalis muscle
- Platysma
- Stylohyoid muscle
- Posterior belly of digastric
- Stapedius muscle
- Auricular muscles.

Nerve supply

- Facial nerve.

184. Ans. (a) I branchial arch *Ref: BDC 5th ed. p 32*

The first branchial arch, also called the first pharyngeal arch and mandibular arch, is the first of six pharyngeal arches that develops in fetal life during the fourth week of development. It is located between the stomodeum and the first pharyngeal groove. The skeletal elements and muscles are derived from mesoderm of the pharyngeal arches.

Derivatives of the first arch:

Skeletal elements

- Malleus and incus of the middle ear
- Maxilla and mandible
- Spine of sphenoid bone
- Sphenomandibular ligament
- Palatine bone
- Squamous part of temporal bone
- Anterior ligament of malleus.

Muscles

- Muscles of mastication (chewing)
- Masseter
- Medial and lateral pterygoid muscles
- Temporalis muscles
- Mylohyoid muscle
- Digastric muscle, anterior belly
- Tensor palati muscle
- Tensor tympani muscle.

Other derivatives

Mucous membrane and glands of the anterior two thirds of the tongue are derived from ectoderm and endoderm of the arch.

185. Ans. (c) 2nd and 3rd pharyngeal arches *Ref: BDC 5th ed. p 39*

Refer Ans 177

186. Ans. (c) Palatine tonsil *Ref: BD Chaurasia's for Dental Students, p 150*

Derivatives of endodermal pouches

Pharyngeal pouch	*Derivatives*
Dorsal ends of I and II pouches form tubotympanic recess	Proximal part of tubotympanic recess gives rise to auditory tube. Distal part gives rise to tympanic cavity and mastoid antrum. Mastoid cells develop at about two years of age.

Contd...

Contd...

Pharyngeal pouch	*Derivatives*
Ventral part of II pharyngeal pouch	Epithelium covering the **palatine tonsil** and tonsillar crypts, lymphoid tissue is mesodermal in origin.
III pharyngeal pouch	Thymus and interior parathyroid gland or parathyroid III. Thymic epithelial reticular cells and Hassall's corpuscles are endodermal Lymphocytes are derived from hemopoietic stem cells during 12th week
IV pharyngeal pouch	Superior parathyroid or parathyroid IV
V pharyngeal pouch (ultimobranchial body)	Parafollicular or 'C' cells of the thyroid gland

187. Ans. (a) 4th to 8th week *Ref: KD Tripathi (Essentials of Pharmacology for Dentistry), p 61*

Drugs can affect the fetus at three stages:

- Fertilization and implantation-conception to 17 days-failure of pregnancy which often goes unnoticed.
- Organogenesis—18 to 55 days of gestation-most vulnerable period, deformities is produced.
- Growth and development-56 days onwards-developmental and functional abnormalities can occur, e.g. ACE inhibitors can cause hypoplasia of organs, especially lungs and kidneys; NSAIDs may induce premature closure of ductus arteriosus.

188. Ans. (a) 1st branchial arch *Ref: BD Chaurasia for Dental Students, p 150*

Refer Ans 177.

189. Ans. (c) Frontonasal process *Ref: Inderbir Singh 7th ed. p 139*

- The lips and palate originate from three areas of the baby's developing face.
- Central or frontal nasal prominence: normally grows to become the forehead, nose, middle portion of the upper lip (philtrum or Cupid's bow) and the primary palate (part of the upper jaw that holds the middle four teeth)
- Left and right maxillary prominences: grow and become the lower face, lower lip and jaw, all but the middle portion of upper lip and jaw, and the secondary palate (behind the four upper middle teeth to back of mouth.

These three prominences on the child's developing face grow towards the center of the face and fuse together during the 6th to 13th weeks of pregnancy. When this happens correctly, the child's lips, mouth, and palate develop normally. But sometimes this growth process is disturbed in some way and the prominences do not meet. When this happens, the lips and mouth do not form properly, leaving a cleft or split in the lip.

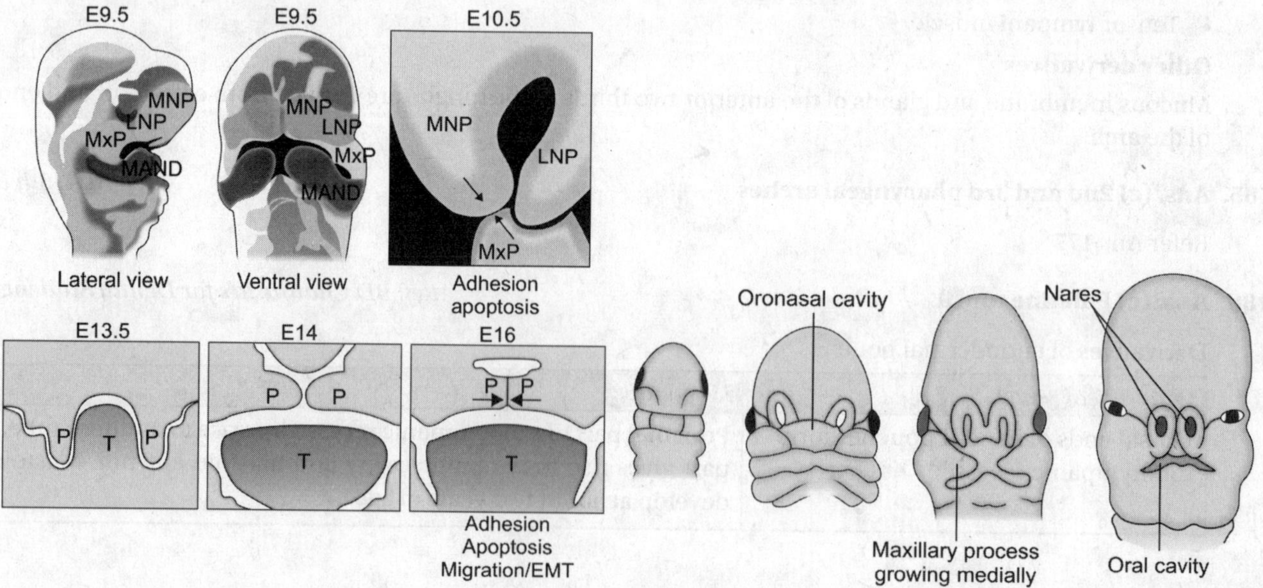

190. Ans. (c) Stapes *Ref: Human Embryology by Inderbir Singh 8th ed. p 1o7*

- A major portion of the Meckel's cartilage disappears during growth and the remaining part develops into the following structures:
  - The mental ossicles
  - Incus and malleus
  - Spine of sphenoid bone
  - Anterior ligament of malleus
  - Sphenomandibular ligament.
- The dorsal end of each cartilage is connected with the ear-capsule and is ossified to form the malleus and incus.
- The intervening part of the cartilage disappears; the portion immediately adjacent to the malleus is replaced by fibrous membrane, which constitutes the sphenomandibular ligament.

191. Ans. (a) Neural crest cells *Ref: Human Embryology, Inderbir Singh 8th ed. p 272*

Neural crest derivative:

- **Mesoectoderm**: Odontoblasts, dental papillae, the chondrocranium (nasal capsule, Meckel's cartilage, scleral ossicles, quadrate, articular, hyoid and columella), tracheal and laryngeal cartilage, lower vertebrates, pericytes and smooth muscle of branchial arteries and veins, tendons of ocular and masticatory muscles, connective tissue of head and neck glands (pituitary, salivary, lachrymal, thymus, thyroid) dermis and adipose tissue of calvaria, ventral neck and face.
- **Endocrine Cells**: Chromaffin cells of the adrenal medulla, parafollicular cells of the thyroid, glomus cells type I/II.
- **Peripheral nervous system**: Sensory neurons and glia of the dorsal root ganglia, cephalic ganglia (VII and in part, V, IX, and X), Rohon-Beard cells, some Merkel cells in the whisker, Satellite glial cells of all autonomic and sensory ganglia, Schwann cells of all peripheral nerves.
- **Melanocytes and iris pigment** cells.

HISTOLOGY

192. Ans. (c) Clara cells *Ref: Textbook of Human Histology by Inderbir Singh 5th ed. p 65-69*

- From all the three layer, i.e. endoderm, mesoderm and ectoderm. Mesoderm is responsible for the formation of connective tissues.
- Cells of connective tissue are fibroblast, undifferentiated mesenchymal cell, pigment cell, macrophages, mast cells, etc.
- Cells of respiratory system derived from:
  - Ectoderm- Neural components (ANS).
  - Mesoderm- Fibroblast, vascular endothelium, smooth muscle cells.
  - Endoderm- Kulchitsky cells, Clara cells. Goblet and serous cells, ciliated cells, alveolocytes.

Clara cells

- It is dome shaped cell with short microvilli found in the small airways (bronchioles) of the lungs.
- These cells secrete glycosaminoglycans to protect the bronchiole lining.
- They are also known as 'Club cells' and 'bronchiolar exocrine cells'.

193. Ans. (a) Transitional *Ref: Textbook of Human Histology by Inderjit Singh 5th ed. p 50,51*

Transitional epithelium:

- It has several layers of cells of varying shape in the absence of stretching and tension.

- As tension increases, the epithelium sheet is extended and the number of observable cell layer will decrease and cell shape will change.
- The ability to transitional epithelium to stretch protects the distensible structures that it lines from tearing when stretched with great force.

194. Ans. (a) Rhodopsin *Ref: Histology by Michael H Rose p 126*

The basal lamina (lamina - layers), also known as the basement membrane, is a specialized form of extracellular matrix. The basal lamina can be organized in three ways:

- It can surround cells (for example muscle fibers have a layer of basal lamina around them);
- It lies underneath sheets of epithelial cells
- It separates two sheets of cells, such as the endothelial cells of blood vessels and epithelial cells of another tissue. This type of arrangement is found in the kidney glomerulus, where the basal lamina acts as a permeability barrier or sieve.

The basal lamina consists of a mixture of collagens, laminin (glycoprotein), perlecan (heparan sulphate glycoprotein), entactin (glycoprotein). These proteins can bind to each other to make a highly crosslinked extracellular matrix.

- Laminins are major proteins in the basal lamina. The laminins are an important and biologically active part of the basal lamina, influencing cell differentiation, migration, and adhesion, as well as phenotype and survival.
- Entactin is a member of the nidogen family of basement membrane glycoproteins. The protein interacts with several other components of basement membranes. Structurally it (along with perlecan) connects the networks formed by collagens and laminins to each other, It may also play a role in cell interactions with the extracellular matrix

195. Ans. (d) None of the above *Ref: Histology a Text and Atlas Corelated Cell Biology by Michael Ross p 172, 173*

Pericytes: Pericytes are imp ortant cellular constituents of the Cap Illaries and Post Cap Illary Venules and are located Albuminal to the endothelial cells and luminal to parenchymal astrocytes.

- A broad flat cell with slender projections, have a prominent round muscles.
- A pericyte is a mesenchymal like cell, associated with the walls of small blood
- vessels. As a relatively undifferentiated cell it serves to support these vessels.
- It can be differentiated into a fibroblast, smooth muscle cell or macrophage as well, if required.
- Also known as Roughet cell or mural cells.

196. Ans. (c) The mesoderm *Ref: Human Embroyology by Inderbir Singh 8th ed. p 320*

Derivatives of mesoderm:

Hard tissues are developed from

- Adipose tissue, reticular tissue, cartilage and bone.
- Ligaments, tendons, aponeurosis, and dermis of skin.
- Dentine of tissue.
- Heart, all blood cells, vessels and lymphatics.
- Urinary system including kidney.
- Reproductive system.
- Mesothelium.
- Substance of cornea, sclera, choroid, ciliary body and iris.
- Duramater, microglia.

197. Ans. (a) The collecting duct *Ref: Histology by Micheal H Ross p 100-101*

- On leaving the collecting ducts at the area cribrosa, the urine enters a series of structures that do not modify it but are specialized to store and pass the urine to the exterior of the body. The urine flows sequentially to a minor calyx, a major calyx, and the renal pelvis, and leaves each kidney through the ureter to the urinary bladder, where it is stored. The urine is finally voided through the urethra.

- Transitional epithelium (urothelium) lines the excretory passages leading from the kidney. This stratified epithelium is essentially impermeable to salts and water. The epithelium begins in the minor calyces as two cell layers and increases to an apparent four to five layers in the ureter and as many as six or more layers in the empty bladder. However, when the bladder is distended, as few as three layers are seen.

198. Ans. (a) Interphase *Ref: Histology by Micheal H Ross p 74*

- A Barr body (named after discoverer Murray Barr) is the inactive X chromosome in a female somatic cell or the inactive Z in a male rendered inactive in a process called lyonization, in those species (including humans) in which sex is determined by the presence of the Y or W chromosome rather than the diploidy of the X or Z.
- The Lyon hypothesis states that in cells with multiple X chromosomes, all but one are inactivated during mammalian embryogenesis. This happens early in embryonic development at random in mammals, except in marsupials and in some extra-embryonic tissues of some placental mammals, in which the father's X chromosome is always deactivated.
- In men and women with more than one X chromosome, the number of Barr bodies visible at interphase is always one less than the total number of X chromosomes. For example, men with a 47,XXY karyotype have a single Barr body, whereas women with a 47,XXX karyotype have two Barr bodies. Barr bodies can be seen on the nucleus of neutrophils

199. Ans. (a) Ectodermal *Ref: Oral Development and Histology 3rd ed. p 244*

The surface ectoderm (or external ectoderm) forms the following structures:

- Skin (only epidermis; dermis is derived from mesoderm) (along with glands, hair, and nails)
- **Epithelium of the mouth** and nasal cavity salivary glands, and glands of mouth and nasal cavity
- **Tooth enamel** (as a side note, dentin and dental pulp are formed from ectomesenchyme which is derived from ectoderm (specifically neural crest cells and travels with mesenchymal cells)
- Epithelium of anterior pituitary
- Lens, cornea, lacrimal gland, tarsal glands and the conjunctiva of the eye
- Apical ectodermal ridge inducing development of the limb buds of the embryo
- Sensory receptors in epidermis.

200. Ans. (a) Stratified squamous epithelium *Ref: BD Chaurasia's 5th ed. p 345*

- The epiglottis is a flap that is made of elastic cartilage tissue covered with a mucous membrane, attached to the entrance of the larynx.
- It projects obliquely upwards behind the tongue and the hyoid bone, pointing dorsally.
- There are taste buds on the epiglottis.
- The epiglottis has two surfaces, a lingual and a laryngeal surface, related to the oral cavity and the larynx respectively.
- The entire lingual surface and the apical portion of the laryngeal surface (since it is vulnerable to abrasion due to its relation to the digestive tract) are covered by stratified squamous non-keratinized epithelium. The rest of the laryngeal surface on the other hand, which is in relation to the respiratory system, has respiratory epithelium: pseudostratified, ciliated columnar cells and mucus secreting Goblet cells.

201. Ans. (c) Lymphatic nodules *Ref: Histology by Indervir Singh 5th ed. p 187*

- The cortex of lymph mode contains lymphatic nodules
- Lymph node is consist of 3 parts, i.e.:
  - Capsule
  - Cortex
  - Medulla

BRAIN

202. Ans. (d) The limen insulae *Ref: Practical Neuroangiography 2nd ed. p 218*

- The limen insulae forms the junction point between anterior posterior stem of the sylvian fissure.
- It is the lateral most limit of the anterior perforated substance and the starting point of the insular cortex.
- It is the tongue shaped area of cortex that lies at the apex of insula.
- Anterior perforated substance is an irregularly quadrilateral area in front of the optic tract and behind the olfactory tract.

203. Ans. (a) Facial *Ref: Gray's Anatomy 2nd ed. p 852*

- Geniculate ganglionitis or geniculate neuralgion (GN) also called nervus intermedius neuralgia, is a rare disorder that involves severe pain deep in the ear, mastoid or eye region.
- The pain of GN is sharp, shooting, burning and can last for hours.
- GN may caused by compression of somatic sensory branch of cranial nerve VII i.e. facial nerve which goes through nervus intermedius.
- GN may also develop following herpes zoster oticus (Ramsay Hunt Syndrome), where cold sores occur on the ear drum.
- Ganglia associated with cranial nerves are:
  - Facial nerve geniculate ganglion.
  - Trigeminal nerve trigeminal ganglion
  - Occulomotor nerve- ciliary ganglion.
  - Glossopharyngeal nerve superior ganglion, inferior ganglion, otic ganglion.
  - Vestibulocochlear nerve- Spiral ganglion, vestibular ganglion.

204. Ans. (a) Word formation *Ref: Guyton and Hall 11th ed. p 687*

- Broca's area constitute the motor speech area no. 44,45
- Wernicke's area is responsible for the generation of words situated at area no. 22 and these words are transmitted to Broca's area via arcuate fasciculus.
- The motor plans for the formation of words is in Broca's area.
- Broca's area is a region in the frontal lobe of the hemisphere of the hominid brain with function linked to speech production.

Broca's Asphasia:

- Damage to Broca's area.
- In this condition, words are not coming out properly formed, slowed or slurred speech, prevention of producing words and possibility of not being able to comprehend language.

Wernicke's Asphasia:

- Damage to Wernicke's area.
- It result in people suffering from the loss of ability to comprehend language and also the ability to speak word clearly but the inability to properly put them together.

205. Ans. (d) Spinal accessory *Ref: Lippincott's Neuroscience 1st ed. p 175*

- Proprioception from muscle of mastication—trigeminal nerve.
- Proprioception from muscle of facial expression—facial nerve.
- Proprioception from muscle of pharynx—glossopharyngeal nerve
- Proprioception from muscle that move the head, neck and shoulders cranial accessory

Spinal accessory nerve is purely motor in nature it supplies motor fibers to the sternocleidomastoid and trapezius muscle.

206. Ans. (a) Purkinje *Ref: BDC 5th ed. p 392*

Purkinje cell:

- It is the characteristic cell of cerebellum.
- It is a large neuron with many branching extension.
- Most of it secrete a neurotransmitter GABA which exerts inhibitory action on certain neuron and there by reduces the transmission of nerve impulse.
- The loss of or damage to purkinje cells can give rise to certain neurological disease. During embryonic growth purkinje cells can be permanently destroyed by exposure to alcohol, there be contributing to the development of fetal alcohol syndrome.
- The loss of purkinje cells has been observed in children with autism and in individual with Neimann-Pick disease.

207. Ans. (b) It carries preganglionic secretomotor fibers to the submandibular gland *Ref: Gray's Anatomy 2nd ed.p 935*

- The chorda tympani is a nerve that originates from the taste buds in the front part of the tongue, runs through the middle ear, and carries taste message to the brain.
- The chorda tympani carries two types of nerve fibers from their origin with the facial nerve to the lingual nerve that carries them to their destination:
  - Special sensory fibers providing taste sensation from the anterior two third of the tongue.
  - Presynaptic parasympathetic fibers to the submandibular ganglion, providing secretomotor innervations to 2 salivary glands, i.e. submandibular gland and sublingual gland.

208. Ans. (c) Nasopalatine nerve *Ref: Gray's Anatomy 2nd ed. p 1029*

- The nasopalatine nerve is one of the largest nasal nerve from the 7 nasal nerves, passes through medial wall of nasal cavity.
- It passes anteriorly down to supplies the bulk of nasal septum.
- It gives out nasal branches, which supply the nasal mucosa.
- Hence, it is the nerve, which gives tingling sensation in the nose just before sneezing.

209. Ans. (c) Projection *Ref: Clinical Neuroscience 2nd ed. p 206*

The great bulk of the cerebral hemisphere is formed by white matter. It consist of nerve fibers interconnecting different parts of the brain.

There are three types of nerve fibers:

- Projection fibers—It connects the cerebral cortex to the lower level of nervous system.
- Association fibers—These fibers connects the area of the same hemisphere.
- Commisural fibers—These cross the median plane in order to connect the similar structure and function of two hemisphere.

210. Ans. (a) Pterion *Ref: Gray's Anatomy 2nd ed. p 814*

- The pterion is the area, where four bones, i.e. the parietal, the frontal, the greater wing of the sphenoid bone and the squamous part of the temporal bone are approach each other.
- The pterior is the weakest part of the skull.
- The lambda is the meeting point of sagittal and lambdoid suture.
- The vertex is the meeting point of four bone, i.e. the frontal, the two parietal and the occipital bone. It is the highest point of skull.
- Inion is the external occipital protuberance.

211. Ans. (d) Tensor veli palate *Ref: BDC 5th ed. p 365*

- The pharyngeal plexus is a network of nerve fibers innervating most of the palate, larynx and pharynx.
- It is located on the surface of the middle pharyngeal constrictor muscle.
- This include the following muscle—palatopharyngeus, palatoglossus, musculus uvulae. The pharyngeal constrictors, salpingopharyngeus.

212. Ans. (b) That it carries postganglionic parasympathetic fibers *Ref: BDC 5th ed. p 363-367*

Branches of vagus nerve

- Auricular nerve
- Pharyngeal nerve
- Superior laryngeal nerve
- Superior cervical cardiac branches of vagus nerve
- Inferior cervical cardiac branch
- Recurrent laryngeal nerve
- Thoracic cardiac branches
- Branches to the pulmonary plexus
- Branches to the esophageal plexus
- Anterior vagal trunk
- Posterior vagal trunk
- Hering-Breuer reflex in alveoli

The vagus runs posterior to the common carotid artery and internal jugular vein inside the carotid sheath.

Functional component of vagus nerve

- The vagus nerve carries axons of type GVE, general visceral efferent, which provides parasympathetic innervation to glands of mucous membranes of the pharynx, larynx, organs in the neck, thorax, and abdomen.
- The vagus nerve also carries axons of type GVA, general visceral afferent, which carries information from the thoracic and abdominal viscera; aortic body and arch.
- The vagus nerve also carries axons of type SVA, special visceral afferent, which carry taste of the epiglottis region of the tongue.
- The vagus nerve also carries axons of type GSA, general somatic afferent, which carry sensation from the external auditory meatus and tympanic membrane.
- The vagus nerve also carries axons of type SVE, special visceral efferent, which innervate skeletal muscle of the pharynx and larynx.

Parasympathetic innervation of the heart is controlled by the vagus nerve.

213. Ans. (b) Endothelial cells *Ref: BDC 5th ed. p 445*

- The blood brain barrier (BBB) between the intracerebral blood vessels and the brain parenchyma formed by tight junction between the endothelial cells of the blood vessels and the surrounding astroglial endfeet.
- The barrier between the blood and brain was discovered by Paul Ehrlich.
- The endothelial cells that line CNS blood vessels differ from those outside the nervous system and help to differentiate the brain and non-brain capillaries.

214. Ans. (a) Trochlear *Ref: Gray's Anatomy for Students 2nd ed. p 894*

- The trochlear nerve (the fourth cranial nerve) is a motor nerve (a "somatic efferent" nerve) that innervates a single muscle: the superior oblique muscle of the eye.
- The trochlear nerve emerges from the dorsal aspect of the brainstem at the level of the caudal mesencephalon

- The trochlear nerve carries axons of type GSE, general somatic efferent, which innervate skeletal muscle of the superior oblique muscle.
- It is the smallest nerve in terms of the number of axons it contains. It has the greatest intracranial length.

215. Ans. (c) Less transcytotic activity exists for the most lipid-soluble substances *Ref: Ganongs 23rd ed. p 572-574*

- The blood brain barrier (BBB) is a dynamic interface that separates the brain from the circulatory system and protects the central nervous system (CNS) from potentially harmful chemicals while regulating transport of essential molecules and maintaining a stable environment.
- The endothelial cells forming the blood-brain barrier are highly specialized to allow precise control over the substances that enter or leave the brain.
- The bloodbrain barrier is composed of high-density cells restricting passage of substances from the bloodstream much more than endothelial cells in capillaries elsewhere in the body Astrocyte cell projections called astrocytic feet (also known as "glia limitans") surround the endothelial cells of the BBB, providing biochemical support to those cells.
- The bloodbrain barrier acts very effectively
- It is almost totally impermeable to plasma protein to protect the brain from many common bacterial infections. Thus, infections of the brain are very rare.

216. Ans. (b) Facial *Ref: BDC 5th ed. p 354*

Trochlear nerve (IV)

The trochlear nerve is part of the cranial nerve group responsible for innervation of the muscles of the head. The trochlear nerve originates from the dorsal mid-brain and is a motor nerve. It is composed of general somatic efferent fibers and is the smallest of the cranial nerves. The nerve is specifically responsible for the 'dorsal oblique muscle' muscle of the eye and also passes through the orbital fissure.

Abducent nerve (VI)

The abducent nerve is part of the cranial nerve group responsible for innervation of the muscles of the head. The abducent nerve originates from the medulla oblongata and is a motor nerve. It is composed of general somatic efferent fibers which are responsible for controlling the 'lateral rectus' muscle and the 'retractor bulbi' muscle of the eye. The nerve passes through the orbital fissureand can be found within the same layer of the meninges as the opthalmic branch (V1) of the trigeminal nerve (V).

Oculomotor nerve (III)

The oculomotor nerve is part of the group of cranial nerves responsible for innervating the muscles of the head. The nerves originate from the ventral midbrain and is a motor nerve. It is composed ofgeneral somatic efferent fibers and general visceral efferent fibers. The general somatic efferent fibers of the oculomotor nerve are responsible for the motor function of four of the six external muscles of the eyeball; the 'dorsal rectus', 'medial rectus', 'ventral rectus', 'ventral oblique' and 'levator of the upper eyelid'. The general visceral efferent fibers of the oculomotor nerve are responsible for the control of pupil diameter and therefore control the 'spincter pupillae' muscle and the 'ciliaris' muscle.

Facial nerve (VII)

The facial nerve is part of the cranial nerve group responsible for the innervation of structures originating from the branchial arches. It originates from the medulla oblongata and from the second branchial arch. It has a common dura sheet with the opthalmic (V1) branch of the trigeminal nerve. The facial nerve is of a mixed composite and is made up of a number of different fibre types. It has a general somatic efferent fibre within the ear canal, a general visceral efferent fiber acting under parasympathetic control to some salivary glands, lacrimal glands, nasal cavity and palate, a special visceral afferent fiber providing taste to the anterior 2/3 of the tongue and finally it has a general somatic efferent fibre supplying motor function to the muscles of facial expression.

217. Ans. (d) Basilar artery *Ref: Gray's Anatomy for Student 2nd ed. p 837*

At the level of the midbrain the basilar artery bifurcates to form the two posterior cerebral arteries (PCA). The posterior cerebral artery (PCA) is one of a pair of blood vessels that supply oxygenated blood to the posterior aspect of the brain (occipital lobe) in human anatomy.

- The branches of the posterior cerebral artery are divided into two sets, ganglionic and cortical.
- The PCA is divided into four segments named P1 to P4:
  - P1—from it origin at the termination of the basilar artery to posterior communicating artery (PCOM), within interpeduncular cistern.
  - P2—from the PCOM around the mid-brain, divided into P2A (anterior) and P2P (posterior) subsegments. P2A is within crural cistern which then bridges to the P2P segement in ambient cistern (thus ambient segment)
  - P3—quadrigeminal segment (segment with the quadrigeminal cistern)
  - P4—cortical segment (e.g., calcarine artery, within the calcarine fissure).

218. Ans. (d) Carotid *Ref: BDC 5th ed. p 351*

- The trigeminal nerve is a nerve responsible for sensation in the face and certain motor functions such as biting and chewing.
- It is the largest of the cranial nerves.
- Its name ("trigeminal" = tri- or three, and -geminus or twin, or thrice twinned) derives from the fact that each trigeminal nerve, one on each side of the pons, has three major branches: the ophthalmic nerve (V1), the maxillary nerve (V2), and the mandibular nerve (V3).
- The ophthalmic and maxillary nerves are purely sensory. The mandibular nerve has both cutaneous and motor functions.
- The sensory function of the trigeminal nerve is to provide the tactile, proprioceptive, and nociceptive afference of the face and mouth. The motor function activates the muscles of mastication, the tensor tympani, tensor veli palatini, mylohyoid, and anterior belly of the digastric.

219. Ans. (a) The lower border of L1 *Ref: Gray's Anatomy for Student 2nd ed. p 101*

- The spinal cord is a long, thin, tubular bundle of nervous tissue and support cells that extends from the brain (the medulla oblongata specifically). The brain and spinal cord together make up the central nervous system (CNS).
- At birth, the spinal cord terminates at the lower border of the third lumbar vertebra.
- In adults, the spinal cord is between 42 and 45 cm in length, weighs about 35 gm, and usually terminates at the level of the intervertebral disk between L1 and L2.
- The spinal cord is the main pathway for information connecting the brain and peripheral nervous system
- The spinal cord is supplied with blood by three arteries that run along its length starting in the brain, and many arteries that approach it through the sides of the spinal column. The three longitudinal arteries are called the anterior spinal artery, and the right and left posterior spinal arteries.

220. Ans. (c) The trigeminal nerve *Ref: Neurology in Clinical Practice by Walter G Bradley p 514*

The corneal reflex, also known as the blink reflex, is an involuntary blinking of the eyelids elicited by stimulation of the cornea (such as by touching or by a foreign body), or bright light, though could result from any peripheral stimulus.

The reflex is mediated by:

- The nasociliary branch of the ophthalmic branch (V1) of the 5th cranial nerve (trigeminal nerve) sensing the stimulus on the cornea, lid, or conjunctiva (i.e. it is the afferent).
- The temporal and zygomatic branches of the 7th cranial nerve (facial nerve) initiating the motor response (i.e. it is the efferent).
- Possibly mediated by a medullary center (citation needed).

221. Ans. (d) Abducens *Ref: Gray's Anatomy for Student 2nd ed. p 852,895*

- Proprioceptive impulse is carried from the muscle of mastication facial muscle and extra ocular muscle through trigeminal nerve.
- Abducent nerve does not have any proprioceptive impulse.

222. Ans. (d) Deep to SMAS superficial to buccal pad of fat *Ref: Aesthetic Plastic Surgery 2009 p 88*

- The structural planes of the face include skin; subcutaneous tissue; the superficial musculoaponeurotic system (SMAS) and mimetic muscles; the deep facial fascia; and the plane containing the facial nerve, parotid duct, and buccal fat pad.
- These muscle actions are transmitted to the skin by ligamentous attachments located between the SMAS and the dermis. The SMAS is also connected to the underlying bone by a network of fibrous septa and ligaments. Thus, facial support is transmitted from the deep fixed structures of the face to the overlying dermis.
- Two major components of this system are the osteocutaneous ligaments (orbitomalar, zygomatic, and mandibular) and the ligaments formed by a condensation of superficial and deep facial fasciae (parotidocutaneous and masseteric).

223. Ans. (c) Parotid gland *Ref: Anatomy for Dental Students by Martin Atkinson 4th ed. p 178, 179*

- The nucleus ambiguus is a region of histologically disparate cells located just dorsal (posterior) to the inferior olivary nucleus in the lateral portion of the upper (rostral) medulla. It receives upper motor neuron innervation directly via the corticobulbar tract.
- The nucleus ambiguus is a motor nucleus.
- Cells in the nucleus ambiguus are very difficult to see (hence the name), and innervate striated muscle throughout the neck and thorax.
- This includes some muscles of the palate and pharynx, muscles of the larynx, and the parasympathetic innervation of the heart.
- So, damage to ambiguus nucleus effects all its normal function.

224. Ans. (b) It supplies anterior belly of digastric *Ref: BDC 5th ed. p 354-356*

The two bellies of the digastric muscle have different embryological origins, and are supplied by different cranial nerves.

Posterior belly

- The posterior belly, longer than the anterior belly, arises from the mastoid notch which is on the inferior surface of the skull, medial to the mastoid process of the temporal bone.
- The posterior belly is supplied by the digastric branch of facial nerve.

Anterior belly

- The anterior belly arises from a depression on the inner side of the lower border.
- of the mandible called the Digastric Fossa, close to the symphysis, and passes downward and backward.
- The anterior body is supplied by the trigeminal via the mylohyoid nerve, a branch of the inferior alveolar nerve, itself a branch of the mandibular division of the trigeminal nerve.
- It originates from the first pharyngeal arch.

225. Ans. (a) Hyperacusis *Ref: BDC 5th ed. p 356*

- Hyperacusis: It is a health condition characterized by an over sensitivity to certain frequency and volume ranges of sound.
- A lesion higher to the origin to stapedius nerve can cause hyperacusis.
- It is the lesion of lower motor neuron.
- Hence, it is not occurs when the damage of facial nerve just above the branching of chorda tympani.

226. Ans. (b) Facial

Ref: BDC 5th ed. p 358

- The facial nerve is the seventh cranial nerve emerges from the brainstem between the pons and medulla
- It also supplies preganglionic parasympathetic fibers to several head and neck ganglia
- Five major extracranial branches of the facial nerve (in parotid gland)-from top to bottom is—
  - Temporal
  - Zygomatic
  - Buccal
  - Marginal mandibular
  - Cervical
- When excessive or prolonged pressure is applied at angle of mandible during establishment of patent airway may damages facial nerve (marginal mandibular branch). As it run below angle of mandible deep to the platysma
- Muscles of lower lip and chin are supplied by it.

227. Ans. (a) Miosis

Ref: Thieme, Atlas of Anatomy (Head and Neuroanatomy) p 72

- Oculomotor nerve palsy is an eye condition resulting from damage to the third cranial nerve or a branch thereof. As the name suggests, the oculomotor nerve supplies the majority of the muscles controlling eye movements.
- Thus, damage to this nerve will result in the affected individual being unable to move his or her eye normally. In addition, the nerve also supplies the upper eyelid muscle (Levator palpebrae superioris) and the muscles responsible for pupil constriction (sphincter pupillae).
- The eye will be displaced outward and displaced downward; outward because the lateral rectus (innervated by the sixth cranial nerve) maintains muscle tone in comparison to the paralyzed medial rectus. The eye will be displaced downward, because the superior oblique(innervated by the fourth cranial or trochlear nerve), is unantagonized by the paralyzed superior rectus, inferior rectus and inferior oblique.
- The affected individual will also have a ptosis, or drooping of the eyelid, and mydriasis (pupil dilation).

228. Ans. (a) Nasopalatine

Ref: Grays Anatomy for Students 2nd ed. p 943

Premaxilla:

- It is an anterior hard palate
- It is comprised of the anterior nasal spine and alveolar segment in the maxilla, which fold and support anterior four teeth
- Formed by the palatine process of the maxilla
- Blood supply of premaxilla is nasopalatine branch of the Sphenopalatine artery via incisive foramen and it is innervated by the nasopalatine nerve.

229. Ans. (a) Special visceral efferent

Ref: De Jong's The Neurological Examination p 250

The Nervus Intermedius:

The sensory and autonomic component of facial nerve is the nerve intermedius It contains the two sensory and one parasympathetic fiber of the facial nerve special sensory fiber carry taste from the anterior 2/3 of the tongue. The two sensory cells located in the geniculate ganglion are:

- General somatic afferent
- Special visceral afferent.

The parasympathetic fiber have general visceral afferent. They are secretomotor to the lacrimal sublingual and submandibular glands as well as to the paranasal sinus mucosa of nose and the hard and soft palate.

230. Ans. (d) Lacrimal nerve

Ref: Gray's Anatomy for Student 2nd ed. p 850

- The oculomotor nerve is the third cranial nerve.
- It enters the orbit via the superior orbital fissure and controls most of the eye's movements, including constriction of the pupil and maintaining an open eyelid by innervating the levator palpebrae superioris muscle.

- The oculomotor nerve include axons of type GSE, general somatic efferent, which innervate skeletal muscle of the levator palpebrae superioris, superior rectus, medial rectus, inferior rectus, and inferior oblique muscles.
- The nerve also includes axons of type GVE, general visceral efferent, which provide preganglionic parasympathetics which synapse (twigs) to the ciliary ganglion.

231. Ans. (b) Jugular foramen *Ref: Gray's 2nd ed. p 812*

Glossopharyngeal nerve

- The glossopharyngeal nerve, known as the ninth cranial nerve, is a mixed nerve that carries afferent sensory and efferent motor information.
- From the medulla oblongata, the glossopharyngeal nerve passes laterally across the flocculus, and leaves the skull through the central part of the jugular foramen,in a separate sheath of the dura mater, lateral to and in front of the vagus and accessory nerves.

Functions

There are a number of functions of the glossopharyngeal nerve:

- Receives general sensory fibers from the tonsils, the pharynx, the middle ear and the posterior 1/3 of the tongue
- Receives special sensory fibers (taste) from the posterior one-third of the tongue
- Receives visceral sensory fibers from the carotid bodies
- Supplies parasympathetic fibers to the parotid gland via the otic ganglion
- Supplies motor fibers to stylopharyngeus muscle, the only motor component of this cranial nerve
- Contributes to the pharyngeal plexus.

232. Ans. (b) Area 3, 1, 2 *Ref: BD Chaurasia's 5th ed. p 352*

There are two sensory stimuli in the sensory system they are epicritic and protopathic:

- Epicritic carry proprioceptive vibratory and fine touch sensation. It occurs at the level of area 3,2,1.
- Protopathic carry diffuse touch and temperature sensation. It occurs at the level of thalamus.

233. Ans. (c) Arachnoid villi *Ref: BD Chaurasia's 5th ed. p 399*

- CSF is produced partly by an active secretory process and partly by passive diffusion.
- It is a colorless fluid containing little protein and few cells.
- The volume of CSF in the combined ventricular and subarachnoid spaces is approximately 150 mL. CSF is produced continuously, at a rate sufficient to fill these spaces several times each day.
- This means that an efficient mechanism is required for the circulation of CSF and its reabsorption.
- Arachnoid granulations (or arachnoid villi) are small protrusions of the arachnoid (the thin second layer covering the brain) through the dura mater (the thick outer layer).
- They protrude into the venous sinuses of the brain, and allow cerebrospinal fluid (CSF) to exit the subarachnoid space and enter the blood stream.

234. Ans. (a) External laryngeal nerve *Ref: Gray's Anatomy 2nd ed. p 1006 Table 8.19*

- The cricothyroid muscle is the only tensor muscle of the larynx, aiding with phonation.
- It attaches to the anterolateral aspect of the cricoid and the inferior cornu and lower lamina of the thyroid cartilage, and its action tilts the thyroid forward to help tense the vocal cords.
- Not to be confused with the posterior cricoarytenoid muscles, which are the only muscles directly responsible for opening (abducting) the space between the vocal cords to allow for sound production.
- This muscle is the only laryngeal muscle supplied by the branch of the vagus nerve known as the external branch of the superior laryngeal nerve(rather than the recurrent laryngeal nerve.

235. Ans. (a) Facial nerve *Ref: BDC 5th ed. p 294*

- The pterygopalatine ganglion (Meckel's ganglion, nasal ganglion or sphenopalatine ganglion) is a parasympathetic ganglion found in the pterygopalatine fossa.
- It is largely innervated by the greater petrosal nerve (a branch of the facial nerve); and its axons project to the lacrimal glands and nasal mucosa.
- Functionally it is related to the facial nerve while topographically it is related to maxillary nerve.
- In the pterygopalatine ganglion, the preganglionic parasympathetic fibers from the greater petrosal branch of the facial nerve synapse with neurons whose postganglionic axons, vasodilator, and secretory fibers are distributed with the deep branches of the trigeminal nerve to the mucous membrane of the nose, soft palate, tonsils, uvula, roof of the mouth, upper lip and gums, and upper part of the pharynx. It also sends postganglionic parasympathetic fibers to the lacrimal nerve (a branch of the Ophthalmic nerve, also part of the trigeminal nerve) via the zygomatic nerve, a branch of the maxillary nerve (from the trigeminal nerve), which then arrives at the lacrimal gland.

236. Ans. (c) Temporal *Ref: BDC 5th ed. p 430*

- The lateral ventricles are part of the ventricular system of the brain. Classified as part of the telencephalon, they are the largest of the ventricles.
- The lateral ventricles connect to the central third ventricle through the interventricular foramen of Monro

Each lateral ventricle has three horns:

- The anterior or frontal horn extends into the frontal lobe
- The posterior or occipital horn into the occipital lobe
- The inferior or temporal horn into the temporal lobe.

237. Ans. (c) Greater petrosal nerve *Ref: BDC 5th ed. p 356,65*

- The lacrimal glands are paired almond-shaped glands, one for each eye, that secrete the aqueous layer of the tear film.
- They are situated in the upper, outer portion of each orbit, in the lacrimal fossa of the orbit formed by the frontal bone.
- Inflammation of the lacrimal glands is called dacryoadenitis.
- The lacrimal gland produces tears which then flow into canals that lead to the lacrimal sac. From this sac, the tears drain through the lacrimal duct into the nose.
- The lacrimal nerve, derived from the ophthalmic nerve, supplies the sensory component of the lacrimal gland.
- The greater petrosal nerve, derived from the facial nerve, supplies the parasympathetic autonomic component of the lacrimal gland. The greater petrosal nerve travels alongside branches of the V1 and V2 divisions of the trigeminal nerve.

238. Ans. (b) Sigmoid sinus *Ref: Manual of Middle Ear Surgery Vol. 2 Mikro p 55*

Mastoid air sinus is bounded by:

- Anteriorly- epitympanic recess through auditory meatus
- Posteriorly-sigmoid sinus
- Laterally- squamous part of temporal bone
- Medially petrous temporal bone
- Superiorly-temporal lobe of cerebrum and tegmen tympani
- Inferiorly- mastoid process containing mastoid air cell.

239. Ans. (d) Facial nerve *Ref: BD Chaurasia for Dental Students p 267*

Suprahyoid Muscles

Muscle	*Proximal attachment*	*Fibers*	*Distal attachment*	*Nerve supply*	*Actions*
Digastric (DG) has two bellies united by an intermediate tendon	• Anterior belly (DGA): from digastric fossa of mandible • Posterior belly (DGP): from mastoid notch of temporal bone	• Anterior belly runs downwards and backwards • Posterior belly runs downwards and forwards	Both bellies meet at the intermediate tendon which perforates SH and is held by a fibrous pulley to the hyoid bone	• Anterior belly by nerve to mylohyoid • Facial nerve	• Depresses mandible when mouth is opened widely or against resistance; it is secondary to lateral pterygoid • Elevates hyoid bone

240. Ans. (c) Hypoglossal nerve *Ref: BD Chaurasia for Dental Students p 266-269*

The contents of submandibular triangle are:

- Mylohyoid muscle;
- Submandibular gland;
- Lymph nodes;
- Wharton's duct;
- Sublingual gland;
- Submandibular ganglion;
- Lingual nerve;
- Nerve to mylohyoid;
- Hypoglossal nerve;
- Facial artery and vein;
- Submental arteries and nerve and facial nerve

Hypoglossal nerve may get injured during surgery of submandibular gland, as it is present in the close vicinity of submandibular salivary gland.

241. Ans. (c) Facial nerve *Ref: BD Chaurasia's for Dental Students p 382*

Clinical Anatomy:

- Bell's palsy: Sudden paralysis of facial nerve at the stylomastoid foramen. Result is symmetry of corner of mouth. Inability to close the eye, disappearance of nasolabial fold and loss of wrinkling of skin of forehead on the same side.
- Lesion above the origin of chorda tympani nerve will show symptoms of Bell's palsy plus loss of taste from anterior two-thirds of tongue except vallate papillae.
- Lesion above the origin of nerve to stapedius will cause symptoms 1 and 2 and further causes hyperacusis.

Lesions 1, 2 and 3 are lower motor neuron type. Upper motor neuron paralysis will not affect the upper part of face, i. e. orbicularis oculi, only lower half of opposite side of face is affected. The upper half of face has bilateral representation. Whereas lower half has only ipsilateral representation.

242. Ans. (a) Otic ganglion *Ref: B.D. Chaurasia's for Dental Students, p 245-247*

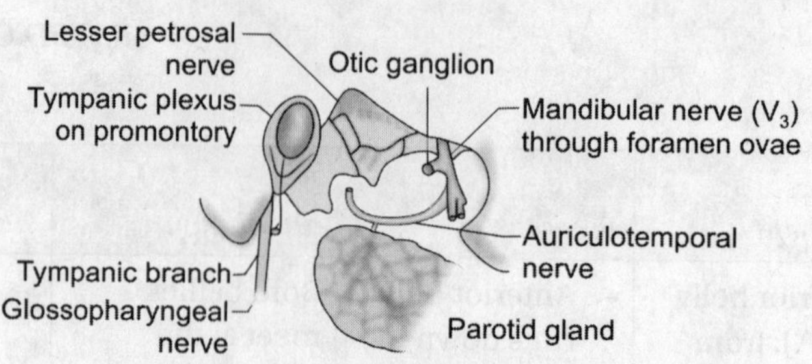

Parasympathetic nerve supply to the parotid gland.

- Parasympathetic nerves are secretomotor. They reach the gland through the auriculotemporal nerve. The preganglionic fibers being in the inferior salivatory nucleus; pass through the glossopharyngeal nerve, its tympanic branch, the tympanic plexus and the lesser petrosal nerve and relay in the otic ganglion. The postganglionic fibers pass through the auriculotemporal nerve and reach the gland.
- Sympathetic nerves are vasomotor, and are derived from the plexus around the external carotid artery.
- Sensory nerves to the gland come from the auriculotemporal nerve, but the parotid fascia is innervated by the sensory fibers of the great auricular nerve.

243. Ans. (c) Vagus *Ref: BD Chaurasia for Dental Students p 292*

Vagus nerve is the tenth cranial nerve. It is so called because of its extensive (vague) course, through the head, the neck, the thorax and the abdomen. The fibers of the cranial root of the accessory nerve are also distributed through it.

244. Ans. (b) Purely motor *Ref: BD Chaurasia's for Dental Students p 296*

- Hypoglossal is the twelfth cranial nerve. It supplies the muscles of the tongue.
- **Functional Components**/Nuclear columns:
  - General somatic efferent column. The fibers arise from the hypoglossal nucleus which lies in the medulla. In the floor of the fourth ventricle deep to the hypoglossal triangle.
  - General somatic afferent column. The nucleus is mesencephalic nucleus of cranial nerve V where proprioceptive fibers from tongue end.
- **Nucleus** - The hypoglossal nucleus, 2 cm long, lies in the floor of fourth ventricle beneath the hypoglossal triangle. It is divided into parts for individual muscles innervated:
  - Connection of the nucleus with opposite pyramidal tract forms supranuclear pathway of the nerve. It is also connected to cerebellum, reticular formation of medulla, sensory nuclei of 5th nerve, and the nucleus of tractus solitarius.

245. Ans. (a) 5th cranial nerve, third cervical nerve and first thoracic nerve *Ref: Ingle's 5th ed. p 316*

Cardiac pain may be transmitted to the joint due to the overlapping of 5th cranial nerve, third cervical nerve, and first thoracic nerve.

246. Ans. (c) Optic canal *Ref: Gray's Anatomy for Student's 2nd ed. p 825*

The greater wing of the sphenoid bone, or alisphenoid, is a bony process of the sphenoid bone; there is one on each side, extending from the side of the body of the sphenoid and curving upward, laterally, and backwards:

- The foramen rotundum is a circular aperture at its anterior and medial part; it transmits the maxillary nerve.
- The foramen ovale is behind and lateral to this; it transmits the mandibular nerve, the accessory meningeal artery, and sometimes the lesser petrosal nerve.

- The sphenoidal emissary foramen is occasionally present; it is a small aperture medial to the foramen ovale, opposite the root of the pterygoid process; it opens below near the scaphoid fossa, and transmits a small vein from the cavernous sinus.
- The foramen spinosum, in the posterior angle near to and in front of the spine; it is a short canal which transmits the middle meningeal vessels and a recurrent branch from the mandibular nerve.
- The foramen petrosum, (Canaliculus innominatus) a small occasional opening, between the foramen spinosum and foramen ovale, for transmission of the lesser petrosal nerve.

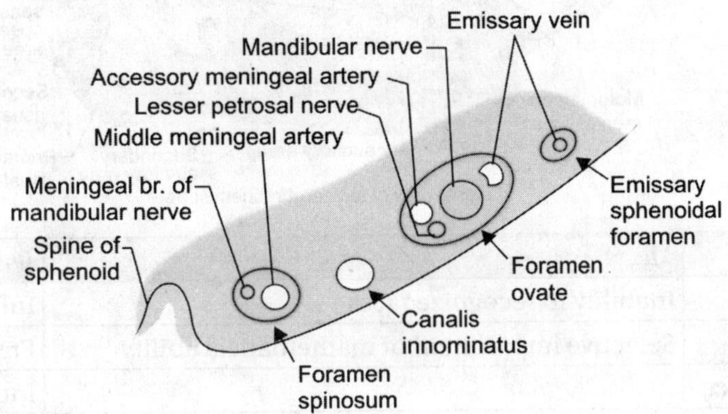

247. Ans. (b) Situated at the floor of the infratemporal fossa *Ref: BDC 5th ed. p 294*

- The otic ganglion is a small, oval shaped, flattened parasympathetic ganglion of a reddish-gray color, located immediately below the foramen ovale in the infratemporal fossa. It gives innervation to the parotid gland for salivation.
- It has sensory, sympathetic, secretomotor, and motor roots.
- Its Secretomotor fiber supply for parotid gland

248. Ans. (b) Inferior salivatory nucleus *Ref: BDC 5th ed.p 339*

- The Preganglionic parasympathetic fibers for otic ganglion commence at Inferior Salivatory nucleus.
- The otic ganglion is a small, oval shaped, flattened parasympathetic ganglion of a reddish-gray color, located immediately below the foramen ovale in the infratemporal fossa.
- It gives innervation to the parotid gland for salivation.
- It is one of four parasympathetic ganglia of the head and neck (the others are the submandibular ganglion, pterygopalatine ganglion, and ciliary ganglion).

249. Ans. (a) Internal acoustic meatus *Ref: Head and Neck Trauma by Arne Ernst p 86*

Facial nerve:

- It is the 7th cranial nerve.
- It emerges from the brainstem between the pons and the medulla, and controls the muscles of facial expression, and functions in the conveyance of taste sensations from the anterior two-thirds of the tongue and oral cavity.
- It also supplies preganglionic parasympathetic fibers to several head and neck ganglia.
- The motor root medial to sensory root.
- The sensory attached midway between the motor root (medially) and the vestibulocochlear nerve (laterally). It is therefore called the nervus intermedius.
- From this attachment the motor and sensory roots pass forward laterally and leave the posterior cranial fossa by entering the internal acoustic meatus (on the posterior aspect of petrous temporal bone).

250. Ans. (a) Inferior frontal gyrus *Ref: Ganong, 21st ed. p 273-280 and Guyton, 10th ed. p 686*

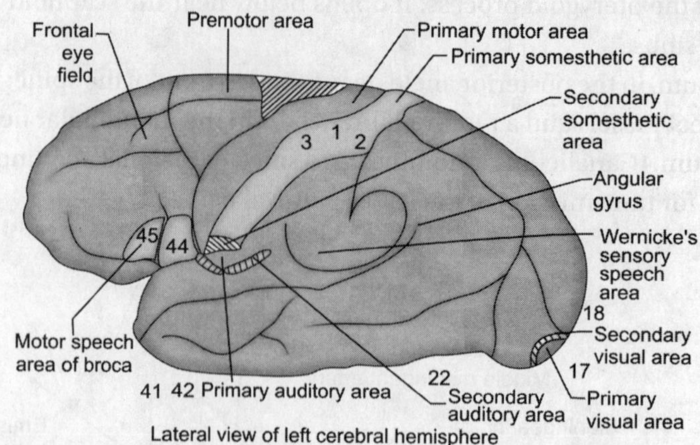

Lateral view of left cerebral hemisphere

Functional disability	*Meaning*	*Found in lesions of*
Prosopagnosia	Inability to recognize faces	Inferior temporal lobes (rt.>lt.)
Acalculia	Selective impairment of mathematical ability	Frontal lobe
Finger counting defect		Intra-parietal sulci of parietal lobe
Navigation defect	• Right hippocampus is concerned with learning where places are located • Right caudate nucleus facilitate movements to the places	Hippocampus, caudate nucleus (right)
Agnosia	Inability to recognize objects by a particular sensory modality even though the sensory modality itself is intact.	Parietal lobe
Unilateral inattention and neglect	Patient ignore stimuli from Contralateral half of body, e.g. Shaving half face, dressing half body, reading half of each page • Treatment is wearing glasses that contain prisms.	Inferior parietal lobule (post part of parietal lobe that is close to occipital lobe)
Non fluent Aphasia **Fluent aphasia**	Interpretation is normal but expression in words is poor. Fails to comprehend the meaning of spoken or written words. Speech itself is normal. However what they say is full of jargon and neologism.	**Broca's area** **Wernicke's area**
Conduction aphasia	Patient speak relatively well and have good auditory comprehension but can't put parts of words together	• Arcuate fasciculus • Lesion in and around auditory cortex (area 40, 41, 42)
Anomic aphasia	• No difficulty in speech and understanding auditory information but there is trouble in understanding written language or pictures, because visual information is not processed	Angular gyrus
Dyslexia	Impaired ability to read	Angular gyrus
Deja-vu-phenomenon	An in appropriate feeling of familiarity with new events or in new surroundings	• Temporal lobe epilepsy • From time to time in normal
Confabulation	Describe events that have never occurred, i.e. "honest lying"	Ventromedial frontal lobe

- Amygdala is concerned with encoding emotions related to memories. Lesions make animals less fearful. Hippocampus is most medial portion of temporal lobe. Lesion in it is associated with antegrade amnesia both for verbal and symbolic type.
- Superior temporal gyrus (Brodmann's area 41) is auditory cortex.
- Wernicke's area (post end of superior temporal gyrus = area 22) is concerned with comprehension of auditory and visual information.
- Broca's area (in frontal lobe just in front of inferior end of motor cortex, area 44) processes the information received from Wernicke's area into a detailed and coordinated pattern for vocalization.
- Angular gyrus behind Wernicke's area processes information obtained from reading in such a way that it is converted into auditory form of words in Wernicke's area.
- Arcuate fasciculus projects information from Wernicke's area to Broca's area.
- In 96% of right handed persons left hemisphere is dominant of categorical hemisphere. In 70% of left handed persons left hemisphere is dominant hemisphere.

251. Ans. (b) Occulomotor *Ref: BDC 5th ed. p 370*

- Ptosis is a drooping or falling of the upper or lower eyelid. The drooping may be worse after being awake longer, when the individual's muscles are tired. This condition is sometimes called "lazy eye".
- Ptosis may be caused by damage/trauma to the muscle which raises the eyelid, damage to the superior cervical sympathetic ganglion or damage to the nerve [3rd cranial nerve (oculomotor nerve)] which controls this muscle.

252. Ans. (a) One *Ref: BDC 5th ed. p 363*

- The vagus nerve is one of 12 cranial nerves.
- It extends from the brain stem to the abdomen, via various organs including the heart, esophagus and lungs.
- Also known as cranial nerve X, the vagus forms part of the involuntary nervous system and commands unconscious body procedures, such as keeping the heart rate constant and controlling food digestion.
- It is so called due to its vague course.

MISCELLANEOUS

253. Ans. (a) Liver *Ref: Gray's Anatomy 2nd ed. p 316*

- Liver is the largest and heaviest of all organs of the body.
- The body of the liver is reddish brown with four lobes of unequal size and shape.
- The human liver weighs about 1.44-1.66 kg (3.2 to 3.7 lb).
- It is both the largest internal organ (the skin being the largest organ overall) and the largest gland in the human body.

Things to remember

- Arterial supply - hepatic artery.
- Venous supply - hepatic vein and hepatic portal vein.
- Nerve supply - celiac ganglion and vagus nerve.
- Precursor - foregut.

254. Ans. (a) Phenotypically normal woman with affected brother and son but normal daughter *Ref: Internet*

- Option A-X linked recessive trait.
- Option B-X linked dominant trait.
- Option C-Y linked or holandric trait.
- Option D-Autosomal dominant trait.

255. Ans. (d) Speech *Ref: Plastic Surgery: Craniofacial, Head and Neck 3rd ed. 3 Vol*

- Tongue position, gagging and respiration are the involuntary oropharyngeal function.
- Speech is the only voluntary function from the given option, sometime speech is also involuntary action but only during pathological condition.
- Apraxia of speech: It is a condition where speech becomes involuntary in nature, it is an acquired oral motor speech disorder affecting an individual ability to translate conscious speech plans into motor plans.
- Apraxia of speech only affects volitional (willful or purposeful) movements pattern.

256. Ans. (b) That it has multiple nuclei *Ref: Guyton and Hall 11th ed. p 103,104*

- Cardiac muscle cells are known as cardiomyocytes or myocardiocytes contains only one unique nucleus.
- Cardiac muscle exhibits cross striations formed by alternating segments of thick and thin protein filaments.
- In cardiac muscle, T tubules are larger and broader and run along the Z-discs, but fewer in number in comparison to skeletal muscle.
- Cardiac muscle fibers branch and anastomose to form a network.
- Intercalated discs, if cardiac muscle consist of 3 different type of cell to cell junction, i.e. adherence junctions, desmosomes and gap junctions.
- Intercalated disc are complex adhering structures that connects single cardiac myocytes to an electrochemical syncytium and are responsible for force transmission during muscle contraction.

257. Ans. (a) Ulnar *Ref: Ashalata- Textbook of Anatomy and Physiology p 96-97*

Ulnar Nerve:

- The ulnar nerve is a nerve which runs near the ulna bone. It is the largest unprotected nerve in the human body (not protected by muscle or bone). So injury is common.
- The ulnar nerve controls the hand intrinsic movements and thus controls all the fine movements of the hand.
- Ulnar nerve is termed as Musician's nerve because it supplies the muscles that are responsible for the finger movements in the persons who play guitar, sitar or piano.
- It is most common in the Guitar player.

258. Ans. (d) Ascending aorta *Ref: Gray's Anatomy 2nd ed. p 181*

Here,
IVC - Inferior vena cava}
SVC - Superior vena cava
RA - Right atrium

} All are the structure present in right heart border.

259. Ans. (d) Suture *Ref: Coloring Guide to Human Anatomy 3rd ed. p 37*

Synchondrosis:

- Cartilagenous joint (structural)
- Permits no movement.

Syndesmosis:

- Fibrous joint (structural)
- Permits a little movement.

Symphysis:

- Cartilagenous joint (structural)
- Permits a little movement.

Suture:

- Fibrous joint

- Permits no movement
  - Suture occurs only in the skull, where adjacent bones are attached by a layer of dense connective tissue.

260. Ans. (c) Brachiocephalic vein *Ref: BDC 5th ed. p 63, Woelfel's Dental Anatomy 7th ed. p 69*

Lymphatic nodes are categorized into several groups:

- Parotid lymph nodes- from the side of face and scalp.
- Submandibular lymph node from upper lip and part of lower lip and most of oral cavity.
- Submental lymph node from the chin and center of lower lip.
- Lymph from these lymph nodes eventually drains into the deep cervical lymph nodes and then into the jugular lymphatic trunk, which joins the internal jugular vein and brachiocephalic vein on the right side and thoracic duct on the left side.

261. Ans. (a) Gap junctions *Ref: Guyton and Hall 11th ed. p 559,771 Gap Junction*

- A gap junction or nexus is a specialized intercellular connection between a multitude of human cell.
- It directly connects the cytoplasm of two cells, through which ions and molecules can pass freely between cells.
- Gap junctions are analogous to the plasmodesmata that join plant cells.

Anchoring junction

- It holds neighboring cells in a tissue together.

Focal junctions

- It contacts the cell to extracellular matrix.

Tight junctions

- It prevents materials diffusing in the intercellular space between two cells.

262. Ans. (b) Sebaceous glands *Ref: Dermato pathology By Klaus J Busam p 5*

- Sweat glands are lined by stratified cuboidal epithelium.
- Sebaceous glands are lined by stratified squamous epithelium.

263. Ans. (d) Olfactory *Ref: Regeneration of Vertebrate Sensory Receptor Cells p 6*

Receptors are classified as epithelial, neuronal, and neuroepithelial.

Neuroepithelial receptors:

- It is a neuron with a soma.
- It is situated near the sensory surface and an axons that carries the sensory signals via synapsing on a second order neuron into the CNS.
- Example of this is the only olfactory epithelium sensory neuron in man.
- This system is evolutionary primitive.
- Example of neuronal receptor is all cutaneous sensors (except merkel cells) and proprioceptors.
- Epidermal Merkel cells, auditory receptor and taste buds are the example of epithelial receptor system.

264. Ans. (a) That it is located at the right border of the ascending aorta *Ref: Guyton and Hall 11th ed. p 116*

- SA node is situated on the wall of the right atrium, near to the entrance of superior vena cava.
- It is the generator of normal sinus rhythm.
- It receives blood supply from SA node artery
- Occlusion of the arterial blood supply to SA node can cause ischemia and cell death and results MI.
- SAN has the highest rate of autorhythmicity (pacemaker of heart), 70 to 80/min.

265. Ans. (d) Amphiarthrosis *Ref: Anatomy and Physiology by Martini 2007, p 190*

- **Structural classification of joints**
  - Fibrous joint

- Cartilaginous joint
- Synovial joint.

- **Functional classification**
  - Synarthrosis (immovable)
  - Amphiarthrosis (slightly movable)
  - Diarthrosis (synovial Joint).

Amphiarthrosis

- Slight movement is possible
- Pad of cartilage lies between the bone surface
- Fibrous capsule hold the bone and cartilage
- Cartilage act as shock absorber, e.g. intervertebral disc between vertebrae.

266. Ans. (b) Genomics proteomics the nervous system *Ref: James D Clelland/p 179*

- A karyotype is the number and appearance of chromosome in the nucleus of a eukaryotic cell.
- The term is also used for the complete set of chromosome in a species, or an individual organisms.
- G-banding is the technique used to produce an individual's karyotype from GHR, for chromosome analysis.
- Giemsa-stain is used to produce a series of dark and light band, with each chromosome displaying a unique banding pattern under light microscope.
- This technique is relatively inexpensive and is a good first line test for individuals with dysmorphic features, growth patterns, learning disability or multiple congenital anomalies.
- One of the major limitations of this technique is the ability to detect small deletions or rearrangements.

267. Ans. (b) Mosaicism *Ref: Essence of Pediatrics by MR Khan 4th ed. p 424*

Mosaic:

- An individual who has two or more genetically different cells lines derived from a single zygote (because of fresh mutation or chromosomal mishap).
- It is generally seen in Down's syndrome and turners syndrome.
- Also termed as chromosomal mosaicism.

Chimerism:

- It is a condition where two different cell population arise from two different zygote. The organisms are composed of two genetically distinct tissue (such as partly male and partly female).

268. Ans. (d) All of the above *Ref: Gray's Anatomy 38th ed. p 873-875*

Composite muscle - A muscle is called as a composite muscle when it is innervated by two nerves or when it is derived from two embryological environment, for example:

- Adductor magnus
- Biceps femoris
- Pectineus
- **Adductor magnus** - Innervated by obturator nerve and the tibial division of sciatic nerve (L2,3,4)
- **Biceps femoris** - Innervated by sciatic nerve (L5,S1 and 2) long head through the tibial division of and short head through the common peroneal division reflecting the composite derivation from flexor and extensor muscle
- **Pectineus** - Innervated by the femoral nerve, L2 and 3 and accessory obturator L3 when present.

269. Ans. (d) Keratoepithelial cells reduce moisture loss *Ref: Textbook of Human Histology with Color Atlas 5th ed. p 199-201, 204*

- Skin is the soft outer covering of vertebrates.

- The epidermis is composed of the outermost layers of the skin. It forms a protective barrier over the body's surface, responsible for keeping water in the body and preventing pathogens from entering, and is a stratified squamous epithelium, composed of proliferating basal and differentiated suprabasal keratinocytes. The epidermis also helps the skin regulate body temperature.
- Keratinocyte are the major cells, constituting 95% of the epidermis while Merkel cells, melanocytes and Langerhans cells are also present. The epidermis can be further subdivided into the following strata or layers (beginning with the outermost layer).
- Stratum corneum.
- Stratum lucidum (only in palms and soles).
- Stratum granulosum.
- Stratum spinosum.
- Stratum germinativum (also called the stratum basale).
- During that process keratinocytes will become highly organized, forming cellular junctions (desmosomes) between each other and secreting keratin proteins and lipids which contribute to the formation of an extracellular matrix and provide mechanical strength to the skin, hence it reduces the moisture loss. Keratinocytes from the stratum corneum are eventually shed from the surface.

270. Ans. (b) Gomphosis *Ref: Gray's Anatomy for Student 2nd ed. p 22*

- Gomphosis is a joint that binds the teeth to bony sockets (dental alveoli) in the maxillary bone and mandible. The fibrous connection between a tooth and its socket is a periodontal ligament. Specifically, the connection is made between the maxilla or mandible to the cementum of the tooth.
- The motion of a gomphosis is minimal, though considerable movement can be achieved over time the basis of using braces to realign teeth. The joint can be considered a synarthrosis.
- The gomphosis is the only joint-type in which a bone does not join another bone, as teeth are not technically bone. In modern, more anatomical, joint classification, the gomphosis is simply considered a fibrous joint because the tissue linking the structures is ligamentous.
- A gomphosis is a specialized fibrous joint in which a conical process or peg of one bone fits into a hole or socket in another bone (gomphos is a Greek word meaning bolt). Small quantity of fibrous tissue holds the bones together.

271. Ans. (d) Replacement of red bone marrow with yellow marrow *Ref: Epiphyseal Growth Plate Fracture by Hamlet A Peterson p 12-16*

- Skeletal growth at the epiphyseal plate is an active and dynamic process. The epiphyseal growth plate, being a highly specialized layer of cartilage where chondrocytes proliferate and differentiate, brings forth longitudinal bone growth. The epiphyseal growth plate can be divided into three main chondrocyte subpopulations: the resting, proliferating and hypertrophic chondrocytes.
- Longitudinal bone growth occurs in the epiphyseal growth plate through a process called endochondral bone formation and ossification.
- Endochondral bone formation is a process where resting zone chondrocytes are recruited to start active proliferation and then undergo differentiation, followed by mineralization.
- Endochondral bone development leading at the epiphyseal growth plate contributes to longitudinal bone growth through a process through which undifferentiated mesenchymal cells differentiate into chondrocytes, which then undergo well-ordered and controlled phases of proliferation, hypertrophic differentiation, death, blood vessel invasion, and finally replacement of cartilage with bone.
- The newly formed cartilage is invaded by blood vessels and bone cells that remodel the newly formed cartilage into bone tissue.

272. Ans. (a) Maxilla *Ref: Dental Anatomy and Tooth Morphology 1st ed. p 50*

Pneumatic Bone

- Pneumatic bone are those bone which have an air filled cavity within them, e.g. maxilla, frontal, sphenoid and ethmoid.

Maxillary sinus the antrum of highmore is present in the maxilla in this way it will have the cavity and hence, it is characterized as a pneumatic bone.

273. Ans. (d) Levator scapulae *Ref: Gray's Anatomy for Student 2nd ed. p 678*

Muscle which produce scapular adduction (retraction):

- Rhomboid major
- Rhomboid minor
- Trapezius
- Latissimus dorsi.

274. Ans. (d) Between the alar plate and prevertebral fascia *Ref: Oral and Maxillofacial Infection 4th ed. p 207*

- The danger space is a region of the neck.
- It is bounded superiorly by the skull base, anteriorly by the alar fascia and posteriorly by the prevertebral fascia.
- It comes to an end at the level of the diaphragm.
- It gets its common name from the risk that an infection in this space can spread directly to the thorax, it is sometimes also referred to as the Alar space. It is a median space without a midline raphe and hence infection can spread easily to either side.
- It extents superiorly from the base of the skull to the diaphragm inferiorly.

275. Ans. (a) Dermatome *Ref: Gray's Anatomy for Student 2nd ed. p 38*

- A dermatome is the skin are that is mainly supplied by a single spinal nerve.
- Each and every spinal nerve carry sensory information on the surface of the body from a specific area of skin.
- Pain dermatomes are narrower and overlap with each other less than touch dermatome. So the level of a spinal cord lesion cause sensory impairment is easier to determine by pinprick testing than by light touch (the opposite is true for peripheral nerve lesion).

276. Ans. (d) Immobilization *Ref: Love and Bailey 25th ed. p 267,1216*

Wound healing is delayed in following:

- In malnourished
- Vitamin C deficiency or vitamin A deficiency
- Deficiency of copper and other trace elements administered these deficient agents, to aid healing.
- Steroids also inhibit the adequate healing of wounds
- Wound infection is the most common postoperative complication occurring in 5-10% of all patients.

Treatment is by wound drainage and antibiotics when required. The organisms responsible are usually a mixture of Gram negative bacilli and anaerobic bacteria, predominantly bacteroides species and anaerobic streptococci.

277. Ans. (a) Couinaud segments *Ref:Malignant Liver Tumor by Pierre Alain 3rd ed.*

- Claude Couinaud was a French surgeon and anatomist who made significant contributions in the field of hepatobiliary surgery. He is best known for his detailed anatomic studies of the liver and was the first to describe its segmental anatomy.
- The Couinaud classification of liver anatomy divides the liver into eight functionally independent segments.

Each segment has its own vascular inflow, outflow and biliary drainage.

In the center of each segment there is a branch of the portal vein, hepatic artery and bile duct.

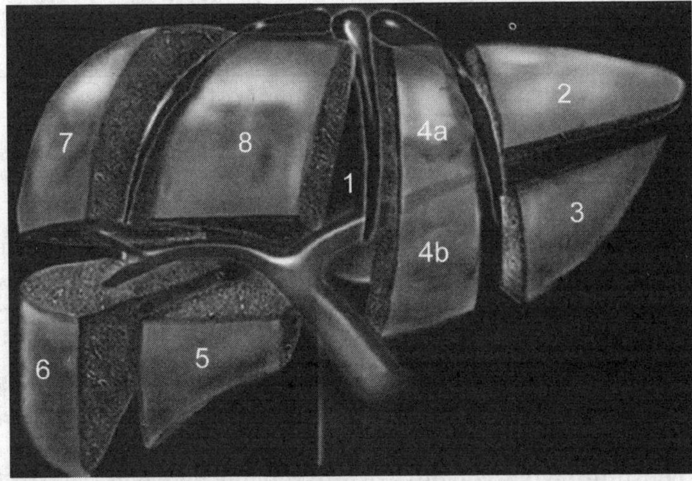

In the periphery of each segment there is vascular outflow through the hepatic veins.

- **Right hepatic vein** divides the right lobe into anterior and posterior segments.
- **Middle hepatic vein** divides the liver into right and left lobes (or right and left hemiliver). This plane runs from the inferior vena cava to the gallbladder fossa.
- **Left hepatic vein** divides the left lobe into a medial and lateral part.
- **Portal vein** divides the liver into upper and lower segments.

The left and right portal veins branch superiorly and inferiorly to project into the center of each segment.

278. Ans. (a) Osteon *Ref: Orban's Oral Histology and Embryology 13th ed. p 209*

- The osteon or haversian system is the fundamental functional unit of bone.
- Osteons are roughly cylindrical structures that are typically several millimeters long and around 0.2 mm in diameter. They are present in many bones of most mammals and some bird, reptile, and amphibian species.
- Each osteon consists of concentric layers, or lamellae, of compact bone tissue that surround a central canal, the haversian canal. The haversian canal contains the bone's nerve and blood supplies. The boundary of an osteon is the cement line.
- Osteons are connected to each other and the periosteum by oblique channels called Volkmann's canals or perforating canals.

279. Ans. (a) Gomphosis *Ref: BD Chaurasia's 3rd ed. p 50*

- Gomphosis is a joint that binds the teeth to bony sockets (dental alveoli) in the maxillary bone and mandible. The fibrous connection between a tooth and its socket is a periodontal ligament. Specifically, the connection is made between the maxilla or mandible to the cementum of the tooth.
- The motion of a gomphosis is minimal, though considerable movement can be achieved over time the basis of using braces to realign teeth. The joint can be considered a synarthrosis.
- The gomphosis is the only joint-type in which a bone does not join another bone, as teeth are not technically bone. In modern, more anatomical, joint classification, the gomphosis is simply considered a fibrous joint because the tissue linking the structures is ligamentous.
- A gomphosis is a specialized fibrous joint in which a conical process or peg of one bone fits into a hole or socket in another bone (gomphos is a Greek word meaning bolt). Small quantity of fibrous tissue holds the bones together. No movement is possible at such peg-and-socket joints.

Structural classification of joints:

Fibrous joints	*Cartilaginous joints*	*Synovial joints*
Sutures,	Primary (synchondrosis)	
Syndesmosis and	Secondary (symphysis)	
Gomphosis (e.g. tooth in its socket)		

280. Ans. (b) 47, XXY *Ref: Inderbir Singh 7th ed. p 24*

- Klinefelter syndrome or Klinefelter's syndrome is the set of symptoms resulting from additional X genetic material in males. Also known as 47, XXY or XXY, is a genetic disorder in which there is at least one extra X chromosome to a standard human male karyotype, for a total of 47chromosomes rather than the 46 found in genetically normal humans.
- While females have an XX chromosomal makeup, and males an XY, individuals with Klinefelter syndrome have at least two X chromosomes and at least one Y chromosome. Because of the extra chromosome, individuals with the condition are usually referred to as "XXY males", or "47,XXY males".
- This chromosome constitution (karyotype) exists in roughly between 1:500 to 1:1000 live male births but many of these people may not show symptoms. If the physical traits associated with the syndrome become apparent, they normally appear after the onset of puberty.
- In humans, 47,XXY is the most common sex chromosome aneuploidy in males and the second most common condition caused by the presence of extra chromosomes. Other mammals also have the XXY syndrome, including mice.
- Principal effects include hypogonadism and sterility. A variety of other physical and behavioral differences and problems are common, though severity varies and many XXY boys have few detectable symptoms.

281. Ans. (d) Temporalis *Ref: Human Evolutionary Anatomy by Christopher Dean p 23*

- A pennate or pinnate muscle (also called a penniform muscle) is a muscle with fascicles that attach obliquely (in a slanting position) to its tendon. These types of muscles generally allow higher force production but smaller range of motion. When a muscle contracts and shortens, the pennation angle increases.
- If all the fascicles are on the same side of the tendon, the pennate muscle is called unipennate. Examples of this include certain muscles in the hand.
- If there are fascicles on both sides of the central tendon, the pennate muscle is called bipennate. The rectus femoris, a large muscle in the quadriceps, is example.
- If the central tendon branches within a pennate muscle, the muscle is called multipennate as seen in the masseter, medial pterygoid, and deltoid muscle in the shoulder.

282. Ans. (c) Mandible 1st molar *Ref: Dental Anatomy by Woelfel 8th ed. p 185*

Mandibular first deciduous molar:

- This tooth dose not resemble any other tooth. It is unique into itself
- There are two roots
- There is a strong bulbous enamel bulge buccally at the mesial
- The mesiolingual cusp on this tooth is the highest and largest of the cusps
- It has a prominent transverse ridge joining mesiobuccal and mesiolingual cusp in its occlusal table
- It also has a prominent cervical ridge.

283. Ans. (a) Mandibular second premolar *Ref: Pediatric Dentistry by Richard Welbury p 254*

- Anodontia, the complete failure of teeth to develop, is extremely rare. Hypodontia (partial anodontia) is more common.
- The most frequently absent teeth in children are mandibular second premolars, maxillary lateral incisors and maxillary second premolars.

- The congenitally missing teeth may be bilateral or unilateral.
- If a primary tooth is missing the permanent tooth will usually be missing. However, even if a primary tooth is present a permanent tooth can be missing.
- Prevalence of congenitally missing teeth was totally 45.7% and 34.8% for third molars. The most frequent congenitally missing teeth was mandibular second premolars (23.34%) followed by maxillary second premolars (22.02%).
- Upper jaw showed significantly higher number of congenitally missing teeth.

284. Ans. (b) Dental groove *Ref: Essentials of Pedodontics by TN Tilakraj 1st ed. p 36*

- In the development of dentition dental lamina plays very important role. It originates all the teeth in oral cavity by:
  - Direct proliferation give rise primary teeth
  - Distal proliferaction develops to permanent molars
  - Lingual extension develops those permanent teeth that replace the primary ones.
- At the time of birth, the alveolar process is termed as gum pads.
- The gum pads have labial buccal and lingual portion which is separated from each other by a dental groove which is the site of origin of dental lamina.

285. Ans. (b) Axillary *Ref: BD Chaurasia's 3rd ed. p 70*

- In human anatomy, the deltoid muscle is the muscle forming the rounded contour of the shoulder. Anatomically, it appears to be made up of three distinct sets of fibers though electromyography suggests that it consists of at least seven groups that can be independently coordinated by the central nervous system.
- **The deltoid is innervated by the axillary nerve.** The axillary nerve originates from the ventral rami of the C5 and C6 cervical nerves, via the superior trunk, posterior division of the superior trunk, and the posterior cord of the brachial plexus.
- The axillary nerve is sometimes damaged during operations on the axilla, such as for breast cancer. It may also be injured by anterior dislocation of the head of the humerus.
- The deltoid is supplied by the posterior **circumflex humeral artery.**

286. Ans. (c) Liver *Ref: BD Chaurasia's 3rd ed. p 124*

- The superior border of the right kidney is adjacent to the liver; and the spleen, for the left kidney. Therefore, both move down on inhalation.
- Anteriorly the right kidney is related to the Liver, duodenum and hepatic flexure of ascending colon.
- Anteriorly the left kidney is related to stomach, jejunum, pancreas, spleen and descending colon.
- Adrenal gland is superior and anterior to the kidneys.
- The kidney is surrounded by a distinct layer of fascia (perirenal fascia) that separates the fat surrounding the kidney into the perinephric and paranephric fat. Kidneys lie in a fatty cushion of perinephric fat.
- Right kidney is related to the 12th rib posteriorly resting on diaphragm.
- The left kidney rises to as high as the 11th thoracic rib posteriorly, extending from T11-L3, resting on diaphragm.

287. Ans. (a) Near maxillary 2nd molar *Ref: BDC 4th ed. Vol. III p 137*

- **At the anterior border of the masseter, it turns medially and pierces**
  - Buccal pad of fat
  - The buccopharyngeal fascia
  - The buccinators (obliquely).
- Because of the oblique course of the duct through the buccinators inflation of the duct is prevented during blowing.
- The duct runs forwards for a short distance between the buccinators and the oral mucosa.
- Finally, the duct turns medially and opens into the vestibule of the mouth (gingivobuccal vestibule) opposite the crown of upper 2nd molar tooth.

288. Ans. (c) Deep in dermis *Ref: http://www.histop athology_india.net/Gran.htm*

- Nodule is located deep in dermis, subcutis and rarely deep soft tissue.
- Area of necrobiosis is larger than the superficial type.
- Granulation tissue and lymphoid aggregates may be present near palisaded granuloma.
- Eosinophils are more common in this variant.

289. Ans. (b) 639 *Ref: Principles of General Anatomy, AK Dutta, 1st ed. p 82-84*

- There are approximately 639 skeletal muscles in human body.
- Out of this 639, 30 are facial muscle.

290. Ans. (b) Nerve to serratus anterior *Ref: Principles of General Anatomy, AK Dutta, 1st ed. p 82-84*

- According to the text "Principles of Anatomy and Physiology" by Tortora and Grabowski, 7th ed there are nearly 639-640 skeletal muscles in the human body.
- "There are around 640 named muscles in human body" (www.ivy-rose.co.uk).
- There are more than 639 skeletal muscles in the human body. Some sources will say 640. On average, 40% of body weight is muscles. Out of 639/640 muscles, 30 of them are facial muscles" (www.drstandley.com).
- **Voluntary Muscle:** Form about 42% of the total body weight. They act on joints producing movements. Only 20% of the energy set free during movements is expressed as work, and the remainder is utilized to produce heat.
- Part of voluntary muscle It presents two parts. Fleshy and fibrous:
  - The fleshy part of the muscle is contractile, highly vascular with higher metabolic rate, and cannot withstand pressure of friction.
  - The fibrous part may be tendinous or aponeurotic. The tendons are non-elastic, less vascular and resistant to friction. When a muscle presses on unyielding structure, the fleshy part is replaced by tendon. If a tendon is subjected to friction a bursa or synovial sheath is interposed.

Classification of voluntary muscles:

According to the color - The muscles are of two types red and white. The color depends on capillary density and on the amount of myohemoglobin in the sarcoplasm of the muscle cells. In red muscle, the myohemoglobin is more abundant.

Red and while muscles present the following differences:

Red muscles	*White muscles*
• It is more primitive, presents less cross-striation and more sarcoplasm. • Contraction is slow, but more sustained. • Red muscles contain high concentrations of mitochondria and enzymes associated with oxidative metabolism. A dense capillary network surrounds each muscle fibre. • The red fibers are normally utilized for dexterous movements requiring large numbers of small motor units and for postural stance requiring sustained contractions. • The red fibers are found in deep muscles and deeper aspects of superficial, muscles. • The antigravity muscles of the trunk and the one-joint brachialis and soleus muscles are examples of red muscles.	• It is more recent, presents more cross-striation and less sarcoplasm. • Contraction is rapid, but less sustained. Fatigue develops early. • White muscles possess abundant sarcoplasmic reticulum and T-system of tubules, high levels of glycogen and glycolytic enzymes, and few mitochondria. A poor capillary network surrounds each fiber. Their rapid fatigability is associated with their anaerobic metabolism. Therefore, red fibers are called the 'oxidative' fibers and white fibers the 'glycolytic' fibers. • The white fibers contract in response to sudden and transient demands requiring extra activity. • The white fibers are found in superficial muscles. • The phasic two-joint biceps brachii, hamstring and gastrocnemius muscles are examples of white muscles.

2 General Physiology

CELLULAR AND MOLECULAR BASIS FOR MEDICAL PHYSIOLOGY

1. **All of the following use only CAMP as a second messenger, *except*:** *(AIIMS Nov 2010)*
   a. Corticotrophin b. Dopamine
   c. Glucagon d. Vasopressin

2. **Components of innate immunity that are active against viral cells include:** *(AIIMS May 2008)*
   a. Natural killer (NK) cells
   b. Cytotoxic T cells
   c. Suppressor T cells
   d. B cells

3. **All of the following about nitric oxide is true, *except*:** *(AIIMS Nov 2007)*
   a. That it causes penile erection
   b. That it acts via cAMP
   c. That it decreases the vasomotor tone
   d. That it is present in cigarette smoke

4. **Fluoride is transported in blood through:** *(AIIMS Nov 2006)*
   a. Plasma b. RBCs
   c. RBCs and plasma d. WBCs

5. **Which of the following acts as a cytoplasmic inclusion?** *(AIIMS Nov 2006)*
   a. Endoplasmic reticulum
   b. Golgi bodies
   c. Ribosomes
   d. Glycogen

6. **The buffering capacity of a buffer is maximum at pH equal to:** *(AIIMS May 2006)*
   a. 0.5 pKa
   b. pKa
   c. pKa + 1
   d. 2 pKa

7. **Transformation of cell from one type to another is called:** *(AIIMS Nov 2005)*
   a. Dysplasia b. Anaplasia
   c. Metaplasia d. Hyperplasia

8. **The most potent stimulator of naive T cells is:** *(AIIMS Nov 2005)*
   a. B cell b. Mature dendritic cells
   c. Epithelial cells d. Macrophages

9. **Why do fetal cells continue to divide but terminally differentiated adult cells do not divide?** *(AIPGEE 2009)*
   a. There are many cyclin inhibitors that prevent cells to enter into S phase in adult
   b. Phosphatase is absent in fetal cells
   c. Proteinase is absent in fetus
   d. CD kinase is absent

10. **The normal range of serum osmolality is (in mOsm/L):** *(AIPGEE 2006)*
    a. 270285 b. 300320
    c. 350375 d. 200250

11. **Golgi bodies are responsible for** *(AIPGEE 2005)*
    a. The synthesis of polypeptides
    b. The formation of glycoproteins only
    c. The modification and sorting of glycoproteins
    d. Lipid and steroid synthesis

12. **The blood cells responsible for humoral immunity are:** *(AIPGEE 2005)*
    a. T cells
    b. B cells
    c. No cells only antibodies
    d. Mostly B cells and sometimes T cells

13. **Which of the following minerals is found in the highest amount in human body?** *(AIPGEE 2005)*
    a. Sodium b. Calcium
    c. Phosphorus d. Iron

14. Cellular and flagellar movement is carried out by all of the following *except*: *(AIPGEE 2005)*
a. Intermediate filaments
b. Actin
c. Tubulin
d. Myosin

15. The membrane protein clathrin is involved in: *(AIPGEE 2005)*
a. Cell motility
b. Receptor-mediated endocytosis
c. Exocytosis
d. Cell shape

16. The Chief cation in extracellular fluid: *(KCET 2006)*
a. Sodium b. Potassium
c. Calcium d. Magnesium

17. The total number of ATP molecules that are generated per molecule of glucose under aerobic conditions is: *(KCET 2010)*
a. 38 b. 2
c. 36 d. 40

18. The fluid mosaic model of membrane structure was proposed by: *(KCET 2010)*
a. Watson and Crick b. Edward Angle
c. G.V. Black d. Singer and Nicolson

19. All cells do not divide at the same rate. Events in which phase of the cell cycle determine when a cell is going to replicate: *(COMEDK 2005)*
a. M phase b. G1 phase
c. S phase d. G2 phase

20. In the physiologic system, Nitric oxide is known to act through: *(COMEDK 2009)*
a. Cyclic AMP b. Calcium ions
c. Cyclic GMP d. Prostacyclins

21. Ubiquitin involved in? *(COMEDK 2011)*
a. Intracellular proteolysis
b. Electron transport chain
c. Transport of ATP
d. Protein folding

PHYSIOLOGY OF NERVE AND MUSCLE CELLS

22. The main cause of increased blood flow to exercising muscles is: *(AIIMS May 2011)*
a. Raised blood pressure
b. Vasodilation due to local metabolites
c. increased sympathetic discharge to peripheral vessels
d. Increased heart rate

23. Muscle spindle detects: *(AIIMS May 2011)*
a. Tension b. Length
c. Proprioception d. Stretch

24. Glucose transporter in myocyte stimulated by insulin is: *(AIIMS Nov 2010)*
a. GLUT-1 b. GLUT-2
c. GLUT-3 d. GLUT-4

25. Which nerve fiber has the largest diameter and fastest conduction velocity? *(AIIMS Nov 2010)*
a. A-α b. A-β
c. A-γ d. A-δ

26. The order of sensitivity of nerve fibers to LA in decreasing order is:
a. Pain (C&Aδ), preganglionic sympathetic (B), motor
b. Preganglionic sympathetic (B), pain (C&Aδ), motor
c. Pain (C&Aδ) sensory, motor, preganglionic sympathetic (B)
d. Preganglionic sympathetic (B), sensory, motor, (pain C&Aδ)

27. The most outer covering of the nerve fibers is called: *(AIIMS Nov 2006)*
a. Neurilemma
b. Perineurium
c. Axolemma
d. Myelin sheath

28. Synaptic potentials can be recorded by: *(AIIMS May 2005)*
a. Patch clamp technique
b. Voltage clamp technique
c. Microelectrode
d. EEG

29. Which of the following is true of substance P? *(AIPGEE 2011)*
a. It mainly mediates pain sensation at primary neurons
b. It has inhibitory effect in the descending pathways that modulate pain
c. Substance P is a neurotransmitter that acts as a regulator of pain in brain
d. All of the above

30. Synaptic stripping: *(AIPGEE 2010)*
a. Does not cause hyperexcitability of neurons
b. Is that postinflammation microglia remove the branches from nerve near the damaged tissue
c. Causes leakage of neurotransmitter to the surrounding neuron at neuromuscular junction
d. Occurs in the peripheral nerve

31. Excitation contraction coupling is cardiac muscle:
a. ↑ Na^+ in ECF b. ↑ K^+ in ECF
c. ↑ Ca^{+2} in ECF d. ↑ Sarcoplasmic Ca^{+2}

32. Increase in the threshold level on applying subthreshold, slowly rising stimulus is known as: *(AIPGEE 2009)*
a. Adaptation b. Accommodation
c. Refractoriness d. Electrotonus

33. The axon, after axonotmesis, following an injury does not regenerate due to: *(AIPGEE 2008)*
a. Inhibitory stimulus by glial cells
b. Schwann cells stop growing
c. Damage to basal lamina
d. Sprouting after injury is minimal in adult axon

34. For first axonal transport, all of the following are involved *except*: *(AIPGEE 2008)*
a. Kinesin b. Microfilaments
c. Dynein d. Neurofilaments

35. All of the following are sarcolemmal proteins *except*: *(AIPGEE 2007)*
a. Dystrophin b. Dystroglycan
c. Sarcoglycan d. Dysmorphin

36. Which cells form the myelin sheath in the CNS? *(KCET 2008) (KCET 2010)*
a. Astrocytes
b. Oligodendrocytes
c. Microglia
d. Schwann cells

37. The contribution of operation of sodium potassium electrogenic pump for the development of net-90 millivolt of resting membrane potential is: *(KCET 2010)*
a. Minus 4 millivolt
b. Minus 80 millivolt
c. Minus 70 millivolt
d. Plus 4 millivolt

38. ________ is an example for rapidly acting neurotransmitter: *(KCET 2010)*
a. Stomatostatin b. Calcitonin
c. Substance P d. Glycine

39. The number of muscle fibers in a motor unit is least in: *(COMEDK 2005)*
a. Laryngeal muscles
b. Pharyngeal muscles
c. Muscles of middle ear
d. Extraocular muscles

40. Which one of the following is a regulatory protein of the muscle? *(COMEDK 2008)*
a. Troponin b. Myosin
c. Actin d. Protein-C

41. The absolute refractory period of an action potential is due to: *(COMEDK 2009)*
a. Insufficient neurotransmitter
b. Depletion of intracellular Na^+
c. Inactivation Na^+-K^+ ATPase
d. Voltage inactivation of the Na^+ channel

42. Axon hillock is a part of the soma of neuron which: *(COMEDK 2009)*
a. Has dense Nissl granules
b. Has no Nissl granules
c. Is at commencement of dendrites
d. Is round in shape

43. Contraction in smooth muscles is initiated when calcium binds to? *(COMEDK 2011)*
a. Calbindin b. Calmodulin
c. Troponin d. Tropomyosin

44. In a nerve, the magnitude of the action potential overshoot is normally a function of the? *(COMEDK 2011)*
a. Magnitude of the stimulus
b. Intracellular potassium concentration
c. Extracellular sodium concentration
d. Resting membrane potential

45. Small packets of acetylcholine released randomly from the nerve cell membrane at rest produces: *(COMEDK 2013)*
a. End plate potential
b. Miniature end plate potential
c. Action potential
d. Inhibitory postsynaptic potential

CENTRAL AND PERIPHERAL NEUROPHYSIOLOGY

46. Which of the following is true for electric transduction of visual cycle? *(AIIMS May 2011)*
a. Repolarization
b. Depolarization
c. Hyperpolarization
d. None of the above

47. Lesions of the lateral cerebellum cause all of the following, *except*: *(AIIMS Nov 2010) (COMEDK 2009) (KCET 2009)*
a. Incoordination b. Intention tremor
c. Resting tremor d. Ataxia

48. The nucleus involved in Papez circuit is: *(AIIMS May 2010)*
a. Pulvinar
b. Intralaminar
c. VPL nucleus
d. Anterior nucleus of thalamus

49. Delta waves are seen in: *(AIIMS May 2010)*
a. Deep sleep b. REM sleep
c. Awake state d. Stage I NREM sleep

50. Broca's area: *(AIIMS May 2010), (AIIMS May 2009) (AIIMS May 2008)*
a. Is concerned with word formation
b. Comprehends language not speaking
c. Is present in the posterior part of the temporal lobe
d. Is the confluence of somatic, auditory and visceral area

51. The conversion of short-term memory into long-term memory is done in: *(AIIMS May 2010)(AIPGEE 2010)*
a. Prefrontal cortex
b. Hippocampus
c. Neocortex
d. Amygdale

52. The mechanism of hearing and memory includes all *except*: *(AIIMS May 2010)*
a. Changes in level of neurotransmitter at synapse
b. Increasing protein synthesis
c. Recruitment by multiplication of neurons
d. Spatial reorganization of synapse

53. The most commonly used objective method to assess pain in patients is: *(AIIMS Nov 2008)*
a. Facial pain scale
b. Knee jerk
c. H jerk
d. R jerk

54. When a person is exposed to extremely hot environment, cutaneous vasodilatation occurs by all *except*: *(AIIMS May 2008)*
a. Direct effect of temperature
b. Noradrenaline mediated
c. Reduced parasympathetic supply to skin
d. No role of sympathetic system

55. Which one of the following is true after exercise? *(AIIMS Nov 2007) (AIPGEE 2008)*
a. Cerebral blood flow increases if there is an increase in systolic blood pressure
b. Blood flow to muscle increases in 30 seconds
c. Body temperature increases
d. Lymphatic flow to the muscle decreases

56. Which one of the following statements is true when a normal person lies down? *(AIIMS Nov 2007) (AIPGEE 2008)*
a. The heart rate settles above that of normal
b. There is an immediate increase in the venous return
c. Cerebral blood flow increases
d. Blood flow to apex of the lung decreases

57. Merkel cells act as *(AIIMS Nov 2006)*
a. Tactile receptors
b. Inflammatory receptors
c. Visceroreceptors
d. Osmoreceptors

58. The pathway of pain and temperature is carried by: *(AIIMS Nov 2006) (AIPGEE 2009)*
a. Corticospinal tract
b. Corticocerebral tract
c. Lateral spinothalamic tract
d. Ventral spinothalamic tract

59. Group A nerve fibers are most susceptible to: *(AIIMS May 2005)*
a. Pressure
b. Hypoxia
c. Local anesthetics
d. Temperature

60. Phantom limb sensations are best described by: *(AIIMS May 2005)*
a. Weber-Fechner law
b. Power law
c. Bell-Magendie law
d. Law of projection

61. Which of the following is true regarding the Golgi tendon organ? *(AIPGEE 2009)*
a. It senses the dynamic length of muscle
b. It is involved in reciprocal innervations
c. It sends signals through alpha motor neuron on stimulation
d. It senses muscle tension

62. Pain and temperature sensations are carried by: *(AIPGEE 2008) (AIIMS Nov 2006)*
a. Corticospinal tract
b. Lateral spinothalamic tract
c. Ventral spinothalamic tract
d. Corticocerebral tract

63. Which of the following is not interpreted in the posterior column? *(AIPGEE 2008)*
a. Pressure b. Temperature
c. Vibration d. Motion

64. Which of the following hormones has decreased secretions at night? *(AIPGEE 2008)*
a. GH b. ACTH
c. Melatonin d. Insulin

65. Pain perception is decreased with repetitive painful stimulus because: *(AIPGEE 2008)*
a. Pain threshold decreases
b. Receptive area decreases
c. Reflex action is faster
d. Of stimulation of large diameter fibers

66. Which of the following is an inhibitory neurotransmitter? *(AIPGEE 2007)*
a. Aspartate b. GABA
c. Acetylcholine d. Glutamate

67. During moderate level exercise, blood flow to brain: *(AIPGEE 2007)*
a. Remains constant b. Increases
c. Decreases d. No relation

68. The lining of blood vessels in brain is by: *(AIPGEE 2007)*
a. Oligodendrocytes b. Astrocytes
c. Ependymal cells d. None

69. Afferent component of corneal reflex is mediated by: *(AIPGEE 2006)*
a. The vagus nerve
b. The facial nerve
c. The trigeminal nerve
d. The glossopharyngeal nerve

70. The first physiological response to high environmental temperature is: *(AIPGEE 2005)*
a. Sweating
b. Vasodilatation
c. Decrease in heat production
d. Nonshivering thermogenesis

71. The feature of slow pain is: *(KCET 2006)*
a. No projection to reticular nucleus
b. Carried by A(alpha) fibers
c. Poor localization
d. Glutamate is the neurotransmitter

72. Delta waves of electroencephalogram have frequency of: *(KCET 2007)*
a. More than 14 cycles per second
b. Between 8 and 13 cycles per second
c. Less than 3.5 cycles per second
d. Between 4 and 7 cycles per second

73. All the following features are seen in cerebellar dysfunction *except*: *(KCET 2009) (COMEDK 2009)*
a. Static tremor
b. Dysmetria
c. Scanning speech
d. Rebound phenomenon

74. The condition, in which the person can see near objects but not the far object, is? *(KCET 2011)*
a. Hypermetropia b. Myopia
c. Presbyopia d. Astigmatism

75. Sensory receptors for pain are: *(COMEDK 2005)*
a. Pacinian corpuscles
b. End organs of raffini
c. End bulbs of Krause
d. Free nerve endings

76. The receptor cells of the olfactory epithelium are: *(COMEDK 2008)*
a. Bipolar neurons
b. Unipolar neurons
c. Multipolar neurons
d. Stellate cells

77. Which of the following fibers are responsible for conduction of pain impulse? *(COMEDK 2009)*

a. A alfa
b. A beta
c. A delta
d. A gamma

78. Which of the following events DO NOT occur in rods in response to light? *(COMEDK 2009)*

a. Structural changes in rhodopsin
b. Activation of transducin
c. Decreased intracellular cGMP
d. Opening of Na^+ channels

79. All of the following are signs of cerebellar disease *except*: *(COMEDK 2009) (KCET 2009) except (AIIMS Nov 2010)*

a. Resting tremors
b. Past pointing
c. Nystagmus
d. Ataxic gait

80. Which of the following is used to measure pain intensity? *(COMEDK 2009)*

a. Visual analogue scale
b. Visual anesthesia score
c. Verifiable assessment of soreness
d. Visual assessment of soreness

81. Sudden loud sound is more likely to damage the cochlea than a prolonged sounds because: *(COMEDK 2010)*

a. Basilar fibers are sensitive to sudden sounds but adapt to prolonged sounds
b. A sudden sound carries more energy
c. Tympanic membrane becomes flaccid during prolonged loud sounds
d. There is a latent period before the attenuation reflex occurs

82. Following are the change during accommodation *except*: *(COMEDK 2013)*

a. Constriction of pupil
b. Dilatation of pupil
c. Convergence of eye ball
d. Increase in the anterior curvature of lens

83. The feature of lower motor neuron lesion is: *(COMEDK 2013)*

a. Hypertonia
b. Hyperactive stretch reflex
c. Muscular atrophy
d. Abnormal plantar extensor reflex (Babinski's sign)

84. All the following cranial nerves transmit taste sensation to the brain *except*: *(COMEDK 2013)*

a. Facial nerve
b. Glossopharyngeal nerve
c. Vagus nerve
d. Hypoglossal nerve

ENDOCRINE AND REPRODUCTIVE PHYSIOLOGY

85. Which one of the following is not secreted by the neuroendocrine cells? *(AIIMS May 2011) (AIIMS May 2008) (AIPGEE 2010)*

a. Intrinsic factor
b. Motilin
c. Secretin
d. Gastric peptide

86. Noradrenaline increases blood pressure by: *(AIIMS May 2008)*

a. Vasoconstriction
b. Increasing HR
c. Increasing preload
d. Increasing myocardial contractility

87. Which of the following hypothalamic nucleus is mainly involved in the secretion of antidiuretic hormone (ADH)? *(AIPGEE 2011)*

a. Preoptic
b. Supraoptic
c. Paraventricular
d. Suprachiasmatic

88. Somatomedin mediates: *(AIPGEE 2011)*

a. The deposition of chondroitin sulfate
b. Lipolysis
c. Gluconeogenesis
d. Decreased rate of glucose uptake by cells

89. Which of the following does not have a corresponding releasing hormone from hypothalamus? *(AIPGEE 2011)*

a. FSH
b. TSH
c. ACTH
d. Prolactin

90. Genes for sex determination is: *(AIPGEE 2010)*

a. SHH
b. SRY
c. AZF
d. HOX

91. Inhibin B is secreted by: *(AIPGEE 2010)*

a. Increase in sperm number
b. FSH
c. Sertoli cell activity
d. Cells of Leydig

92. FSH, LH and TSH acts through which mechanism? *(AIPGEE 2010)*

a. Cyclic AMP　b. cGMP
c. NO　d. Cytoplasmic receptor

93. All of the following are cause of adrenal deficiency *except*: *(AIPGEE 2010)*

a. Hypoglycemia
b. Hypocalcemia
c. Hypotension
d. Hyponatremia

94. Which is seen in acromegaly? *(AIPGEE 2009)*

a. Large tongue
b. Hypoglycemia
c. Crowding of tooth
d. All of the above

95. Which of the following does not have a releasing hormone from the hypothalamus? *(AIPGEE 2008)*

a. FSH　b. TSH
c. ACTH　d. Prolactin

96. Calcitonin is secreted by:

a. Thyroid gland
b. Parathyroid gland
c. Adrenal gland
d. Ovaries

97. All of the following hormones have cell-surface receptors *except*: *(AIPGEE 2005)*

a. Adrenalin　b. Growth hormones
c. Insulin　d. Thyroxine

98. Osteoclasts are inhibited by: *(AIPGEE 2005)*

a. Parathyroid hormone
b. Calcitonin
c. 1,25-dihydroxycholecalciferol
d. Tumor necrosis factor

99. Secretions of the parafollicular cells of the thyroid gland are stimulated by: *(KCET 2006)*

a. Increase in serum calcium
b. Increase in serum thyroxin
c. Decrease in serum calcium
d. Decrease in serum thyroxin

100. Parathyroid hormone increases the blood level of: *(KCET 2007)*

a. Copper　b. Calcium
c. Iron　d. Sodium

101. Glycosylated hemoglobin assay is helpful in the monitoring of patients with: *(KCET 2007)*

a. Addison's disease
b. Diabetes mellitus
c. Cushing's disease
d. Graves' disease

102. Insulin increases the following pathways in the liver *except*: *(KCET 2009)*

a. Fatty acid synthesis
b. Glycogen synthesis
c. Protein synthesis
d. Glucose synthesis

103. Gestation period consists of the following *except*: *(KCET 2010)*

a. Germinal period　b. Embryonic period
c. Fertilization period　d. Fetal period

104. Parathyroid hormone: *(KCET 2011)*

a. Decreases the intestinal calcium absorption
b. Stimulates bone resorption
c. Stimulates osteoblasts
d. Increases renal excretion of calcium

105. The acrosome reaction occurs when the sperm: *(KCET 2011)*

a. Enters the uterine cavity
b. Comes in contact with zona pellucida
c. Penetrates corona radiata
d. Penetrates cell membrane of oocyte

106. The male sex hormone testosterone is produced by: *(KCET 2011)*

a. Sertoli cells
b. Epithelial cells
c. Interstitial cells of leydig
d. Primitive germ cells

107. Which of the following hormones modify and regulate the activity of osteoclasts? *(KCET 2011)*

a. Calcitonin
b. Thyroid
c. Insulin
d. Pituitary

108. Parathormone in normal parathyroid gland is secreted by: *(COMEDK 2010)*

a. Fat cells
b. Glandular cells
c. Chief cells
d. Water clear cells

109. A positive Chvostek's sign is suggestive of: *(COMEDK 2010) (COMEDK 2011)*
a. Hypercalcemia
b. Hypocalcemia
c. Hyperkalemia
d. Acidosis

110. Ultimobronchial body forms? *(COMEDK 2011)*
a. 'C' cells of thyroid gland
b. Principal cells of parathyroid gland
c. Acidophils of pituitary gland
d. Pituicytes of pituitary gland

111. All the following hormones bind to cell surface receptors of the target tissue *except*? *(COMEDK 2011)*
a. TSH b. Glucagon
c. Estrogen d. Epinephrine

112. Removal of parathyroid gland produces the following changes *except*: *(COMEDK 2013)*
a. Decline plasma calcium level
b. Decrease in plasma phosphate level
c. Neuromuscular hyperexcitability
d. Hypocalcemic tetany

113. Sjogren's syndrome affected: *(COMEDK 2013)*
a. Exocrine glands
b. Paracrine glands
c. Endocrine glands
d. Autocrine glands

114. Beginning of adolescent growth in boys is with: *(COMEDK 2013)*
a. Pubic hair growth
b. Feminine fat distribution
c. Facial hair on chin and lip
d. Facial hair on upper lip only

115. Growth hormone function is carried/mediated by: *(MHCET 2012)*
a. Somatomedin C
b. Stomatostatin C
c. Somatomedin and Stomatostatin C
d. None of the above

GASTROINTESTINAL PHYSIOLOGY

116. Intrinsic factor of castle is secreted by which of the following cells in gastric glands? *(AIIMS May 2011)*
a. Chief cells
b. Parietal cells
c. Enterochromaffin cells
d. B cells

117. Average number of bacteria present in saliva is: *(AIIMS Nov 2010)*
a. 500 million/mL b. 750 million/mL
c. 850 million/mL d. 900 million/mL

118. Chief cells are seen at: *(AIIMS Nov 2009), (AIIMS May 2009)*
a. Fundus b. Pylorus
c. Cardiac d. Body

119. Which of the following is stable at acidic pH? *(AIIMS May 2009)*
a. Pepsin b. Trypsin
c. Chymotrypsin d. Carboxypeptidase

120. If bile acid pool is small, recycling is: *(AIPGEE 2011)*
a. Fast b. Slow
c. Normal d. There will be no recycling

121. Decreased BMR is seen in: *(AIPGEE 2011)*
a. Obesity b. Hyperthyroidism
c. Feeding d. Exercise

122. In an obese person, body mass index (BMI) is: *(AIPGEE 2009)*
a. >10 b. >20
c. >30 d. >40

123. Which of the following papilla does not contain taste buds? *(AIPGEE 2008)*
a. Foliate b. Fungiform
c. Filiform d. Circumvallate

124. Which of the following is the correct pair? *(AIPGEE 2008)*
a. A: Insulin b. D: Glucagon
c. B: Somatostatin d. G: Gastrin

125. All of the following are true about intestinal motility *except*: *(AIPGEE 2008)*
a. It does not depend upon gastric motility
b. It increases by distention of the small intestine
c. It increases by acetylcholine
d. It increases by cholecystokinin

126. Buffering capacity of saliva is against: *(AIPGEE 2008)*
a. Acidogenic bacteria
b. Intracellular bacteria

c. Polymorphic bacteria
d. Anaerobic bacteria

127. Which of the following vitamins requires an intrinsic factor for absorption? *(AIPGEE 2008)*
a. Vitamin B1 b. Vitamin B12
c. Vitamin B2 d. Vitamin B3

128. The geniculate ganglion is associated with: *(AIPGEE 2008)*
a. Acoustic sensation
b. Taste sensation
c. Olfactory function
d. Vision pathways

129. Which of the following organs is not involved in calcium homeostasis? *(AIPGEE 2006)*
a. Kidneys
b. Skin
c. Intestines
d. Lungs

130. Which of the following secretions has a very high pH? *(AIPGEE 2006)*
a. Gastric juice
b. Pancreatic juice
c. Bile in the gall bladder
d. Saliva

131. Calcium absorption is increased by: *(KCET 2005)*
a. Increased Na^+ absorption
b. Hypercalcemia
c. Iron over load
d. 1,25- dihydroxycholecalciferol

132. In infants, defecation often follows a meal. The cause of colonic contraction in this situation is: *(KCET 2005)*
a. The gastroileal reflex
b. The enterogastric reflex
c. Gastrocolic reflex
d. Increased circulatory levels of C.C.K

133. Principle cation (+) require for absorption of D-glucose is: *(KCET 2005)*
a. K^+ b. Na^+
c. Ca^{++} d. Mg^{++}

134. Cephalic phase on gastric secretion can be demonstrated by the following experiment: *(KCET 2007)*
a. Heidenhain's pouch
b. Condition reflex
c. Pavlov's pouch
d. None of the above

135. Trypsin is an activator of all the following enzymes *except*: *(KCET 2007)*
a. Chymotrypsinogen
b. Pepsinogen
c. Proelastase
d. Procolipase

136. Which of the following is a gastrointestinal hormone? *(KCET 2008)*
a. Pepsin b. Ptyalin
c. Cholecystokinin d. Trypsin

137. All the following cause the secretion of gastric juice during cephalic phase *except*: *(KCET 2009)*
a. Food in the mouth
b. Sight of food
c. Food in the stomach
d. Thought of food

138. The PH of gastric juice is about: *(KCET 2011)*
a. 1 b. 6
c. 9 d. 7

139. Ceruloplasmin is a protein containing? *(KCET 2011)*
a. Iron b. Copper
c. Manganese d. Magnesium

140. After secretion of trypsinogen into the duodenum, the enzyme is converted into its active form trypsin by: *(COMEDK 2005)*
a. Enteropeptidase
b. Procarboxypeptidase
c. Pancreatic lipase
d. Previously secreted trypsin

141. Function of hepatic Kupffer cells is: *(COMEDK 2005)*
a. Formation of sinusoids
b. Vitamin A storage
c. Increases blood perfusion
d. Phagocytosis

142. The normal brown red color of feces results from the presence of: *(COMEDK 2005)*
a. Heme b. Stercobilin
c. Biliverdin d. Bilirubin diglucuronide

143. Supporting cells of taste buds are: *(COMEDK 2005)*
a. Sustentacular cells b. Taste cells
c. Von ebner cells d. Acini

144. Glucose tolerance test is usually done to access: *(COMEDK 2005)*

a. Acute pancreatitis
b. Carcinoma of head and pancreas
c. Acinar function of the pancreas
d. Endocrine dysfunction of the pancreas

145. Glycemic control over the previous 6–8 weeks in patients with diabetes mellitus is best assessed by the estimation of: *(COMEDK 2008)*

a. Fasting blood glucose
b. Glycated hemoglobin
c. Fasting C peptide
d. Fasting plasma insulin

146. Intrinsic factor in the stomach is secreted by: *(COMEDK 2008)*

a. Oxyntic cells b. Chief cells
c. Mast-like cells d. D-cells of antrum

147. Vitamin B12 is absorbed in: *(COMEDK 2009)*

a. Stomach b. Duodenum
c. Jejunum d. Ileum

148. Type I diabetes mellitus is associated with: *(COMEDK 2010)*

a. Insulin resistance
b. Defect in mitochondrial DNA
c. Islet cell autoantibodies
d. Beta cell dysfunction

149. The most important action of secretion is to: *(COMEDK 2010)*

a. Neutralize the acid from the stomach
b. Increase secretion of bicarbonate by pancreas
c. Decrease gastric secretion
d. Cause contraction of pyloric sphincter

150. Daily loss of iron in a healthy adult per day is? *(COMEDK 2011)*

a. 0.06 mg
b. 0.6 mg
c. 60 mg
d. 600 mg

151. Parietal cells secrete_____in the body of stomach: *(MHCET 2012)*

a. HCI
b. Intrinsic factor
c. HCI and intrinsic factor
d. None of the above

152. Gag reflex is stimulated by which of the following nerve? *(MHCET 2012)*

a. Accessory nerve
b. Hypoglossal nerve
c. Facial nerve
d. Gloss pharyngeal nerve

CARDIOVASCULAR PHYSIOLOGY

153. The site of RBC formation in a 20-year-old healthy male is: *(AIIMS May 2010)* *(AIIMS May 2008) (AIPGEE 2010)*

a. Flat bones b. Long bones
c. Liver d. Yolk sac

154. Prothrombin time (PT) is increased in: *(AIIMS Nov 2008)*

a. von Willebrand's (vW's) disease
b. Hemophilia
c. Warfarin therapy
d. Liver disease

155. All of the following statements are true regarding cardiac muscle, *except*: *(AIIMS Nov 2008)*

a. Functional syncytium
b. Multiple nuclei
c. Gap junctions
d. Shows branching

156. Lysis of fibrin is brought about by: *(AIIMS Nov 2007)*

a. Plasmin b. Hyaluronidase
c. Collagenase d. Coagulase

157. Normal hemoglobin in adults is designated as: *(AIIMS May 2008)*

a. HbH b. HbS
c. HbA d. HbF

158. A complex factor mucopolysaccharide present in the lung and liver that also prevents coagulation of blood is: *(AIIMS Nov 2007)*

a. Heparin b. Plasmin
c. Acetylsalicylic acid d. Histamine

159. Vitamin K-dependent clotting factors are: *(AIIMS May 2007) (AIPGEE 2010) (AIPGEE 2007)*

a. 2, 7, 9, 10
b. 3, 7, 9, 10
c. 7, 9, 10, 12
d. 3, 6, 8, 10

160. Which of the following does not participate in the coagulation process? *(AIIMS Nov 2006)*
a. Thrombin b. Vitamin K
c. Plasmin d. Fibrin

161. The velocity of blood is maximum in: *(AIIMS May 2005)*
a. Large veins b. Small veins
c. Venules d. Capillaries

162. Differential leukocyte count is used for the diagnosis of: *(AIPGEE 2011)*
a. Anemia b. Leukocytosis
c. Leukopenia d. Eosinophilia

163. Christmas disease occurs due to the deficiency of: *(AIPGEE 2011)*
a. Factor IX b. Factor X
c. Factor XI d. Factor VII

164. All of the following have defects in clotting mechanism *except*? *(AIPGEE 2011)*
a. Christmas disease
b. Von Willebrand disease
c. Patients on brufen
d. Thalassemia

165. Hematopoietic stem cells differ from committed progenitor cells by: *(AIPGEE 2011)*
a. Long-term reconstitution of bone marrow
b. High differentiating capacity than progenitor cell
c. Self-renewal
d. All of the above

166. For the second heart sound, true is: *(AIPGEE 2010)*
a. Longer duration than first
b. End of diastole
c. It is split sound
d. Louder than the first heart sound

167. Fibrin degradation products are utilized in: *(AIPGEE 2010)*
a. Disseminated intravascular coagulation (DIC)
b. von Willebrand's disease
c. Hemophilia
d. Platelet dysfunction disorder

168. Primary hemostasis is due to:
a. Platelet destruction
b. Aggregation of platelets at damaged blood vessels
c. Deposition of fibrosis mesh
d. Activation of coagulation system

169. Pernicious anemia is due to the deficiency of: *(AIPGEE 2010)*
a. Folic acid b. Cyanocobalamin
c. Riboflavin d. Pyridoxine

170. Which of the following increases turbulence in blood flow?
a. Reynolds number less than 2000
b. When velocity is decreased
c. When density of blood decreases
d. When diameter of blood vessels increases

171. Pulmonary circulation differs from systemic circulation in: *(AIPGEE 2009)*
a. Pulmonary vasodilation in hypoxia
b. Pulmonary vasoconstriction in hypoxia
c. Decreased blood volume during systole
d. Increased basal vasoconstrictor tone

172. Which of the following is also known as hemophilia B, is inherited and has clinical findings identical to hemophilia A? *(AIPGEE 2008)*
a. Thrombocytopenia
b. vW disease
c. Christmas disease
d. Rendu Osler Weber disease

173. Erythropoiesis in adults takes place in: *(AIPGEE 2008)*
a. Long bones b. Liver
c. Flat bones d. spleen

174. Iron is transported in: *(AIPGEE 2008)*
a. Free form b. Ferritin form
c. Ferrous form d. Ion form

175. Which of the following is required for the conversion of prothrombin to thrombin? *(AIPGEE 2007)*
a. Stable factor
b. Labile factor
c. Fibrinogen
d. Factor VIII

176. The most abundant plasma protein is: *(AIPGEE 2007)*
a. Fibrinogen b. Albumin
c. Erealinine d. Globulin

177. Heme is converted to bilirubin mainly in: *(AIPGEE 2005)*
a. Kidney b. Liver
c. Spleen d. Bone marrow

178. Both vitamins K and C are involved in: *(AIPGEE 2005)*
a. The synthesis of clotting factors
b. Posttranslation modifications
c. Antioxidant mechanisms
d. The microsomal hydroxylation

179. Sinoatrial node acts as a pacemaker of the heart because of the fact that it: *(AIPGEE 2005)*
a. Is capable of generating impulses spontaneously
b. Has rich sympathetic innervations
c. Has poor cholinergic innervations
d. Generates impulses at the highest rate

180. Distribution of blood flow is mainly regulated by the: *(AIPGEE 2005)*
a. Arteries b. Arterioles
c. Capillaries d. Venules

181. When the radius of the resistance vessels is increased, which of the following is increased? *(KCET 2005)*
a. Capillary blood flow
b. Systolic blood pressure
c. Diastolic blood pressure
d. Hematocrit

182. Which of the following has the greatest effect on the ability of blood to transport oxygen? *(KCET 2005)*
a. CO_2 content of red blood cells
b. PH of plasma
c. Amount of hemoglobin in the blood
d. Capacity of the blood to dissolve oxygen

183. Cyanosis is bluish discoloration of skin due to more than ... gm/100 ml blood of deoxygenated hemoglobin: *(KCET 2006)*
a. 2 b. 5
c. 8 d. 10

184. Normal blood flow pattern is: *(KCET 2006)*
a. Predominantly streamline
b. Predominantly turbulent
c. Streamline and turbulent in equal ratio
d. None of above

185. Coronary blood flow to the left ventricle is predominantly from: *(KCET 2006)*
a. Right coronary artery and during diastole
b. Right coronary artery and during systole
c. Left coronary artery and during systole
d. Left coronary artery and during diastole

186. Platelets adhere to the subendothelial collagen through one of the following: *(KCET 2006)*
a. Platelet factor 4
b. Fibronectin
c. Von wille brands factor
d. None of above

187. The tissue macrophages are derived from the: *(KCET 2007)*
a. Neutrophil b. Eosinophil
c. Monocyte d. All of the above

188. Bilirubin is formed from: *(KCET 2009)*
a. Cholic acid b. Cholesterol
c. Heme d. Purines

189. Test of primary hemostasis is: *(KCET 2009)*
a. Coagulation time
b. Bleeding time
c. Prothrombin time
d. Platelet count

190. In an emergency which of the following blood groups can be transfused without cross matching? *(KCET 2009)*
a. B positive b. AB positive
c. O positive d. O negative

191. The vitamin K-dependent proteins C and S are characterized by their ability to inactivate factor: *(KCET 2010)*
a. VIII a and V a b. VIII a
c. V a d. None of the above

192. The first heart sound is due to: *(KCET 2011)*
a. Sudden closure of mitral and tricuspid valve
b. Sudden closure of semilunar valves
c. Ventricular systole
d. Atrial systole

193. Which one of the following is a vasodilator? *(KCET 2011)*
a. Bradykinin b. Nor-epinephrine
c. Epinephrine d. Angiotensin II

194. Citrate is a useful anticoagulant because of its ability to: *(COMEDK 2005)*
a. Buffer basic groups of coagulation factors
b. Bind factor XII

c. Bind vitamin K
d. Chelate calcium

195. Ventricular muscle receives impulses directly from the: *(COMEDK 2005)*
a. Purkinje system
b. Bundle of his
c. Right and left bundle branches
d. AV node

196. The hemoglobin oxygen saturation of blood entering the right ventricle is approximately: *(COMEDK 2005)*
a. 97% b. 85%
c. 75% d. 53%

197. The normal pH of human blood is: *(COMEDK 2005)*
a. 7.0 b. 7.2
c. 7.35 to 7.40 d. 7.6

198. The following factors increase the cardiac output *except*: *(COMEDK 2005)*
a. Preload
b. Afterload
c. Heart rate
d. Myocardial contractility

199. Normal myeloid—erythroid ratio is: *(COMEDK 2005)*
a. 3:1 b. 1:3
c. 4:1 d. 6:1

200. Isovolumetric relaxation ends immediately after: *(COMEDK 2008)*
a. AV valve closes
b. Ventricular pressure falls below aortic pressure
c. Ventricular pressure falls below atrial pressure
d. None of the above

201. The most common coagulation disorders Hemophilia A and Von Willebrand's disease are due to: *(COMEDK 2009)*
a. Factor IX deficiency
b. Vitamin K deficiency
c. Factor X deficiency
d. Factor VIII deficiency

202. Increased levels of hemoglobin A2 is characteristic of HbA2: *(COMEDK 2009)*
a. Sickle cell trait
b. Beta-thalassemia trait
c. Glucose-6-phosphate dehydrogenase deficiency
d. Alpha-thalassemia

203. The prothrombin time is high in a patient with liver disease. However, the prothrombin time is normalized after the injection of vitamin K. This is a feature in: *(COMEDK 2009)*
a. Severe hepatocellular disease
b. Chronic alcoholic liver disease
c. Deficiency of hepatic g-carboxylase
d. Cholestatic liver disease

204. Thrombocytosis is seen in: *(COMEDK 2009)*
a. Osteopetrosis
b. Disseminated intravascular coagulation
c. Hemolytic anemia
d. Thiazide therapy

205. Starling's law of the heart: *(COMEDK 2009)*
a. Does not operate in the failing heart
b. Does not operate during exercise
c. Explains the increase in cardiac output that occurs when venous return is increased
d. Explains the increase in the cardiac output when the sympathetic nerves supplying the heart are stimulated

206. Primary cause of bleeding disorder in liver damage is due to: *(COMEDK 2010)*
a. Decreased level of prothrombin
b. Lack of vitamin K
c. Platelet deficiency
d. Lack of vitamin B

207. Administration of folic acid in pernicious anemia will largely: *(COMEDK 2010)*
a. Correct the anemia but not the neurological symptoms
b. Correct the anemia and the neurological symptoms
c. Correct the neurological symptoms but not the anemia
d. Correct neither neurological symptoms nor anemia

208. The velocity of conduction in purkinje fibers of the heart: *(COMEDK 2010)*
a. 1–4 m/sec
b. 5 to 8 m/sec
c. 9–12 m/sec
d. More than 12 m/sec

209. The second heart sound is produced due to: *(COMEDK 2013)*

a. Closure of semilunar valves
b. Closure of atrioventricular valves
c. Ventricular filling
d. Opening of semilunar valves

210. Activation of which one of the following coagulation factor is not essential for hemostasis: *(COMEDK 2013)*

a. XII b. XI
c. IX d. X

211. Plasma oncotic pressure is mainly due to: *(MHCET 2010)*

a. Albumin b. Globulin
c. Ceruloplasmin d. Hemoglobin

RESPIRATORY PHYSIOLOGY

212. A patient presents the following parameters: pH = 7.5, PCO_2 = 30 mm Hg, PO_2 = 102 mm Hg and HCO_2 = 16 meq/L. Which of the following correctly describes the compensatory mechanism? *(AIIMS Nov 2010)*

a. Respiratory alkalosis
b. Metabolic alkalosis
c. Respiratory acidosis
d. Metabolic acidosis

213. Stability of alveoli is maintained by: *(AIIMS Nov 2010)*

a. Compliance of the lungs
b. Residual air in alveoli
c. Negative intrapleural pressure
d. Reduced surface tension by surfactant

214. Transection at mid-pons level results in: *(AIIMS Nov 2010)*

a. Apneusis
b. Asphyxia
c. Hyperventilation
d. Rapid and shallow breathing

215. Carbon monoxide has limited diffusion because: *(AIIMS Nov 2010)*

a. It has high affinity for hemoglobin
b. Alveolar membrane is impermeable to CO
c. Diffusion is dependent on the blood flow
d. All of the above

216. Which of the following adaptations will be apt to increase the work capacity at high altitude? *(AIIMS May 2009) (AIPGEE 2010)*

a. Increasing workload, decreasing duration of exercise
b. Increasing workload, increasing duration of exercise
c. Decreasing workload, increasing duration of exercise
d. Decreasing workload, decreasing duration of exercise

217. What is the most acute effect of smoking cessation? *(AIIMS May 2005)*

a. Shift of oxyhemoglobin curve to the right
b. Increased ciliary function
c. Decreased mucus production
d. Decreased incidence of postoperative pneumonia

218. Hypercapnia results due to: *(AIPGEE 2011) (AIPGEE 2010)*

a. Low blood pH
b. Low H^+ ion concentration
c. Decrease in CO_2 tension
d. Hyperventilation

219. Bronchial circulation is associated with: *(AIPGEE 2011) (AIPGEE 2010)*

a. Air conditioning
b. Drug absorption
c. Gaseous exchange
d. Reserve volume

220. Pulmonary endothelium is not concerned with which of the following? *(AIPGEE 2011)*

a. Lipoprotein lipase
b. Plasminogen activator
c. Thrombin
d. Factor X

221. CO poisoning causes: *(AIPGEE 2011) (AIPGEE 2010)*

a. Hypoxic hypoxia
b. Shift of oxygen dissociation curve to left
c. Cyanosis
d. Reduction in the diffusion capacity of lungs

222. An important nonrespiratory function of lung is: *(AIPGEE 2011)*

a. Anion balance b. Sodium balance
c. Potassium balance d. Calcium balance

223. In bronchial circulation, there is: *(AIPGEE 2010)* *(AIPGEE 2011)*

a. Gaseous exchange
b. Pulmonary reserve
c. Absorption of drug from lungs
d. Used for blood gas analysis

224. In hypercapnia, there is: *(AIPGEE 2010)* *(AIPGEE 2011)*

a. ↑ pH of blood
b. ↓ pH of blood
c. ↑ O_2 concentration in blood
d. ↓ O_2 concentration of blood

225. Cells that are not found in the lungs are: *(AIPGEE 2009)*

a. Brush
b. Clara
c. Kulchitsky
d. Langerhans

226. The most common cause of pulmonary embolism is: *(AIPGEE 2009)*

a. Lymphangitis
b. Endarteritis
c. Thrombosis
d. Buerger's disease

227. All of the following cells are of connective tissue origin *except*: *(AIPGEE 2007)*

a. Macrophages
b. Fibroblast
c. Melanocytes
d. Clara cells

228. CO_2 is primarily transported in the arterial blood as: *(AIPGEE 2005)*

a. Dissolved CO_2
b. Carbonic acid
c. Carbaminohemoglobin
d. Bicarbonate

229. In which of the following does a reduction in arterial oxygen tension occur? *(AIPGEE 2005)*

a. Anemia
b. CO poisoning
c. Moderate exercise
d. Hypoventilation

230. Shifting of the oxygen dissociation curve to the right is caused by the following factors *except*: *(KCET 2008)*

a. Increased 2,3-biphosphoglycerate
b. Increased temperature
c. Increased concentration of carbon dioxide
d. Increased concentration of oxygen

231. Energy expenditure during normal breathing is: *(KCET 2008)*

a. 25–50 percent of the total energy spent
b. 50–75 percent of the total energy spent
c. 15–20 percent of the total energy spent
d. 2–3 percent of the total energy spent

232. Which of the following acts as lung surfactant? *(KCET 2008)*

a. Lysolecithin
b. Cephalin
c. Dipalmitoyl lecithin
d. None of the above

233. A pulmonary disorder causes the alveoli to break-down and coalesce into large air spaces. The lungs also lose elasticity and compliance is increased. A person who suffers from this disease will have: *(KCET 2009)*

a. Increased dead air space
b. Increased vital capacity
c. Decreased PCO_2
d. Decreased anteroposterior diameter

234. The normal value of intrapleural pressure at the base of the lungs at the start of inspiration is: *(COMEDK 2009)*

a. Minus 6 mm Hg
b. Minus 2.5 mm Hg
c. Plus 2.5 mm Hg
d. Plus 6 mm Hg

235. The work of breathing is: *(COMEDK 2010)*

a. Inversely related to lung compliance
b. Remains constant during exercise
c. Not affected by respiratory rate
d. Decrease in lying posture

236. At rest the normal intrapleural pressure is: *(MHCET 2010)*

a. 14 mm
b. 4 mm
c. +4 mm
d. +14 mm

237. Tachypnea is defined as: *(MHCET 2012)*

a. Increase in respiratory rate
b. Increase in pulse rate
c. Increase in heart rate
d. Decrease in respiratory rate

RENAL PHYSIOLOGY

238. The tubuloglomerular feedback is mediated by: *(AIPGEE 2010)*
a. Sensing of Na^+ concentration in the macula densa
b. Sensing of Cl concentration in macula densa
c. Sensing NaCl concentration in the macula densa
d. Opening up of voltage-gated Na^+ channels in the afferent arteriole

239. Test for elimination of urea and creatinine is for determining which of the following? *(AIPGEE 2008)*
a. Renal failure detection
b. Tubular excretion
c. Glomerular filtration rate (GFR)
d. None of the above

240. Renin is secreted by: *(KCET 2005)*
a. Cells in proximal tubules
b. Cells in distal tubules
c. Macula densa
d. Juxtaglomerular cells

241. Normal glomerular filtration rate is: *(KCET 2008)*
a. 125 L/day
b. 650 mL/minute
c. 180 mL/minute
d. 125 mL/minute

242. Renin release is inhibited by: *(COMEDK 2005)*
a. PGI2
b. Atrial natriuretic peptide
c. Epinephrine
d. Decreased glomerular filtration

243. In clinical practice, GFR is estimated using the plasma clearance value of: *(COMEDK 2005)*
a. Inulin b. PAH
c. Glucose d. Creatinine

244. Which of the following is called countercurrent exchanger? *(COMEDK 2008)*
a. Loop of Henle
b. Vasa recta
c. Collecting duct
d. Proximal convoluted tubule

245. Tubular maximum for glucose is: *(COMEDK 2010)*
a. 180 mg/dl b. 325 mg/min
c. 375 mg/min d. 375 mg/dl

246. The normal GFR is: *(MHCET 2009)*
a. 125 ml/min b. 250 ml/min
c. 600 ml/min d. 900 ml/min

247. Calcium binding protein that can bind four calcium atoms at times is: *(MHCET 2009)*
a. Calmodulin b. Calcitonin
c. Calcitriol d. Calnexin

Answers with Explanations

CELLULAR AND MOLECULAR BASIS FOR MEDICAL PHYSIOLOGY

1. Ans. (d) Vasopressin *Ref: Introduction to Endocrinology By Negi (Table 2.5) http://books.google.co.in/books?id=olMiuZwj63cC&pg=PA31&dq=cAMP+as+a+second+messenger+Cor ticotropin,+dopamine+and+glucagon+ vasopressin&hl=en&sa=X&ei=n9L1UpWhJ4a3iQeWgIE4&ved= 0CCoQ6AEwAA#v=onep&q=cAMP% 20as%20a%20second%20messenger%20Corticotropin%2C%2 0dopamine%20and%20glucagon%20vasopressin&f=false*

Some signals that use cAMP as second messenger	
Corticotropin (ACTH)	Melanocyte-stimulating hormone (MSH)
Corticotropin-releasing hormone (CRH)	Odorants (Many)
Dopamine (D-1, D-2)*	Parathyroid hormone (PTH)
Epinephrine (β-adrenergic)	Prostaglandins E_1, E_2
Follicle-stimulating hormone (FSH)	(PGE_1, PGE_2)
Glucagon	Serotonin (5-HT-1a. 5-HT-2b)*
Histamine (H-2)*	Somatostatin
Luteinizing hormone (LH)	Tastants (sweet, bitter)
	Thyroid-stimulating hormone (TSH)

2. Ans. (a) Natural killer (NK) cells *Ref: Anantnarayan*

3. Ans. (b) That it acts via cAMP *Ref: Ganong, 23rd ed., p 563564*

Nitric oxide acts via cGMP to relax smooth muscles of the vessels and not through camp. All other statements are true.

4. Ans. (c) RBCs and plasma *Ref: http://imsear.hellis.org/bitstream/123456789/145019/1/ijeb2010v48n7p666.pdf. Indian Journal of Experimental Biology, Vol. 48, July 2010, p. 671. Arsenic and Fluoride: Two Major Ground Water Pollutants*

Fluoride is converted to HF in stomach and when absorbed is unevenly distributed to plasma and RBCs. More concentration of fluoride is in plasma than RBCs.

5. Ans. (d) Glycogen *Ref: Ham's histology book http://en.wikipedia.org/wiki/cytoplasmic_inclusion*

Glycogen is the most common cytoplasmic inclusion mostly found in muscle and liver cells. When required this glycogen is converted into glucose to gain energy. All other options are cell organelles and not inclusions.

6. Ans. (b) pKa *Ref: Ganong Review of Medical Physiology, 23rd ed. p 4*

pH is negative logarithm of H_+. According to Henderson Hasselbach equation------. For acid HApH = pKa + log [A-]/[HA] where Ka is a constant [Ka =(H+)(A-)/(HA)]. From the above equation, we can conclude that the buffering capacity of the weak acid (HA) will be best when pKa of that acid is equal to pH of that acid. As [A-] = [HA], Then pH= pKa

7. Ans. (c) Metaplasia *Ref:Robbins Basic Pathology, 8th ed. p 5*

- Metaplasia meta-transform into, plasia-growth: One adult cell (epithelial or mesenchymal) changes to other adult cell.

- Dysplasia: Dys-abnormal, plasia-growth—Abnormal uncoordinated growth
- Anaplasia-Ana-Up or backward, plasia-growth (literally means to form backward). Lack of differentiation, cell does not show features of normal completely formed cell
- Hyperplasia-Hyper-increase in, plasia-growth—Increase in number of cells.

8. Ans. (b) Mature dendritic cells *Ref: http://mcb.berkeley.edu/courses/mcb150/Lecture15/Lecture15%286%29.pdf*

- Dendritic cell express both MHC I and MHC II
- They start in right place (tissues) and end up in the right place (lymph nodes)
- Immature dendritic cells are most effective at taking antigen
- When matured these cells present antigen to naïve T cells.

9. Ans. (a) There are many cyclin inhibitors that prevent cells to enter into S phase in adult *Ref: Robbins Basic Pathology, 8th ed. p 28,190.*

There are many proposed reasons for this as mentioned below:

- Cell division is mainly assisted by cyclin dependent kinases (CDKs). While cyclins arouse CDKs, their inhibitors (CDKIs), of which there are many, silence the CDKs and exert negative control over the cell cycle, e.g. p27, p57 etc.
- As cells grow old, there is constant DNA damage. Most of it is repaired but not all of it is repaired.
- Telomere and Telomerase length: As cells divide, they lose some part of the telomere each time. This part is repaired by telomerase. With age telomerase loses its function and hence loses the ability to divide.

10. Ans. (a) 270285 *Ref: Harper's Biochemistry, 28th ed., p 647. http://www.webmd.com/a-to-z-guides/serum- osmolality? p=2 http://www.webmd.com/a-to-z-guides/serum-osmolality*

Serum osmolality is measured to:

- Check the balance between the water and the chemicals dissolved in blood.
- Find out if severe dehydration or overhydration is present.
- Check to see if the hypothalamus is producing enough antidiuretic hormone (ADH).

Normal:	275:295 milliosmoles per kilogram (mOSm/kg) of water (278–300 mmol/kg of water)

11. Ans. (c) The modification and sorting of glycoproteins *Ref: Textbook of Human Histology by Inderbir Singh, 5th ed. Ganong Review of Medical Physiology, 23rd ed. p 40*

The Golgi complex is an organelle found in most eukaryotic cells. Golgi is composed of stacks of membrane-bound structures known as cisternae. Protein material formed in roughendoplasmic reticulum is then transferred to Golgi complex where it is modified, sorted out and packed properly to either send out of the cell as a secretion or might be used in the cell for its own benefit.

12. Ans. (b) B cells *Ref:Ganong Review of Medical Physiology, 23rd ed. p 70*

Human immunity system can be divided into innate immunity and acquired immunity. Innate immunity provides first line of defense. Acquired immunity is the second line of defense and it can be divided into 1. Humoral immunity and 2. Cellular immunity humoral immunity mainly involves immunoglobulin antibodies secreted by modified B lymphocyte cells called as plasma cells while cellular immunity is mediated by T lymphocyte. This cellular immunity is mainly involved in delayed allergic reactions and rejection of transplants of foreign tissues.

13. Ans. (b) Calcium *Ref: Satyanarayana Biochemistry, 3rd ed. p 404*

Calcium is the most abundant among the minerals in the body. Total content in adult male is 1-1.5 kg 99% of it is present in bones and teeth. A small fraction found outside the skeletal tissues performs numerous functions. Recommended dietary allowance—0.8-1 g/d.

14. Ans. (a) Intermediate filaments *Ref: Ganong Review of Medical Physiology, 23rd ed. p 35-37*

All cells have cytoskeleton not only to maintain their structure but also to change their shape and for movement of the cell itself or the movement of the molecules inside the cell. This cytoskeleton is made up primarily by:

- Microfilaments—7 nm wide—e.g. actin
- Intermediate filament—10 nm wide, e.g. keratin
- Microtubule—25 nm wide, e.g. tubulin out of these 3 actin along with myosin (which is a motor unit present in the cell to cause movement of the molecule) work for cellular and flagellar movement. Tubulin is a type of microtubule which is responsible for movement of chromosomes during mitosis. Intermediate filament is mainly responsible for maintaining the structure of the cell hence doesn't take part in movement of the cell.

15. Ans. (b) Receptor-mediated endocytosis *Ref: Ganong Review of Medical Physiology, 23rd ed. p 43. http://en.wikipedia.org/wiki/clathrin*

Clathrin is a protein that plays a major role in the formation of coated vesicles.

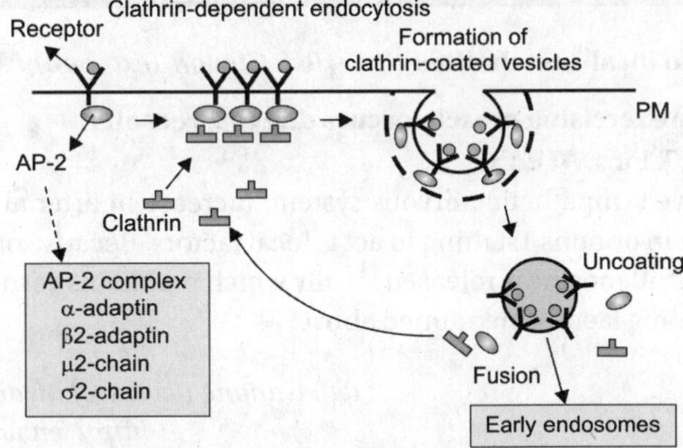

16. Ans. (a) Sodium *Ref: Ganong Review of Medical Physiology, 23rd ed. p 2, 3*

Extracellular fluid

Main cations:

- Sodium (Na^+ = 136145 mEq/L), potassium (K^+ = 3.55.5 mEq/L), Calcium (Ca^{2+} = 2.22.6 mEq/L)

Main anions:

- Chloride (Cl^- = 99109 mEq/L), hydrogen carbonate (HCO_3^- 2226 mM). It is poorer in proteins, as compared to intracellular fluid.
- Ionic composition Na^+ 150 (mM), K^{+5} (mM), Cl^- 110 (mM)

17. Ans. (a) 38 *Ref: Satyanarayana Biochemistry, 3rd ed. p 249*

In aerobic respiration, one molecule of glucose yields 38 ATP molecules, eight produced during glycolysis, six from the link reaction and 24 from the Krebs cycle. The net gain is 36 ATP, as two of the ATP molecules produced from glycolysis are used up in the re-oxidation of the hydrogen carrier molecule NAD.

18. Ans. (d) Singer and Nicolson *Ref: http://en.wikipedia.org/wiki/cell_membrane#fluid_mosaic_model*

According to the fluid mosaic model of SJ Singer and GL Nicolson (1972), which replaced the earlier model of Davson and Danielli, biological membranes can be considered as a two-dimensional liquid in which lipid and protein molecules diffuse more or l00000000.ess easily.

19. Ans. (b) G1 phase *Ref: Morgan, David. The Cell Cycle: Principals of Control. London: New Science Press LTD, 2007. http://en.wikipedia.org/wiki/G1_phase*

G1 phase is particularly important in the cell cycle because it determines whether a cell commits to division or to leaving the cell cycle. If a cell is signaled to remain undivided, instead of moving onto the S phase, it will leave the G1 phase and move into a state of dormancy called the G0 phase.

20. Ans. (c) Cyclic GMP *Ref: Ganong Review of Medical Physiology, 23rd ed. p 563-564*

NO acts through the stimulation of the soluble guanylate cyclase, which is a heterodimeric enzyme with subsequent formation of cyclic-GMP. Cyclic-GMP activates protein kinase G, which causes reuptake of Ca^{2+} and the opening of calcium-activated potassium channels. The fall in concentration of Ca^{2+} ensures that the myosin light-chain kinase (MLCK) can no longer phosphorylate the myosin molecule, thereby stopping the cross bridge cycle and leading to relaxation of the smooth muscle cell.

21. Ans. (a) Intracellular proteolysis *Ref: Ganong Review of Medical Physiology, 23rd ed. p 18*

Ubiquitination is a post-translational modification, where ubiquitin is attached to a substrate protein. The addition of ubiquitin can affect proteins in many ways: It can signal for their degradation via the proteasome, alter their cellular location, affect their activity, and promote or prevent protein interactions.

PHYSIOLOGY OF NERVE AND MUSCLE CELLS

22. Ans. (b) Vasodilation due to local metabolites *Ref: Guyton Textbook of Medical Physiology, 11th ed. p 247*

Increased blood flow to the exercising muscle occurs due to 2 reasons

- Local factors: Adenosine, k ions, ATP, CO_2
- Nervous regulation: Active sympathetic nervous system, increase in arterial pressure and increase in cardiac output. Out of these, 2 main options 1st thing to act is local factors. Because of reduced oxygen in the exercising muscle, substance named adenosine is released locally which maintains vasodilatation of the muscle arterioles along with other vasodilating factors mentioned above.

23. Ans. (b) Length *Ref: Ganong Review of Medical Physiology, 23rd ed. p 158-160*
http://en.wikipedia.org/wiki/Muscle_spindle

Muscle spindles are sensory receptors within the belly of a muscle, which primarily detect changes in the length of this muscle. They convey length information to the central nervous system via sensory neurons. This information can be processed by the brain to determine the position of body parts.

24. Ans. (d) GLUT-4 *Ref: http://en.wikipedia.org/wiki/Glucose_transporter#Glucose_transport_in_Mammals*

Name	*Distribution*	*Notes*
GLUT1	Is widely distributed in fetal tissues. In the adult, it is expressed at highest levels in erythrocytes and also in the endothelial cells of barrier tissues, such as the blood-brain barrier. However, it is responsible for the low-level of basal glucose uptake required to sustain respiration in all cells.	Levels in cell membranes are increased by reduced glucose levels and decreased by increased glucose levels.
GLUT2	Is a bidirectional transporter, allowing glucose to flow in 2 directions. Is expressed by renal tubular cells, small intestinal epithelial cells, liver cells and pancreatic beta cells. It is also present in the basolateral membrane of the small intestine epithelium.	Is a high-capacity and low- affinity isoform. There is some evidence that GLUT 1 and 3 are actually the functional transporters in beta cells.
GLUT3	Expressed mostly in neurons (where it is believed to be the main glucose transporter isoform), and in the placenta.	Is a high-affinity isoform, allowing it to transport even in times of low glucose concentrations.
GLUT4	Found in adipose tissues and striated muscle (skeletal muscle and cardiac muscle)	Is the insulin-regulated glucose transporter. Responsible for insulin-regulated glucose storage

25. Ans. (a) A-α *Ref: Ganong Review of Medical Physiology, 23rd ed. p 89*

Fiber type	*Function*	*Fiber diameter (μm)*	*Conduction velocity (m/s)*	*Spike duration (ms)*	*Absolute refractory period (ms)*
A					
α	Proprioception: Somatic motor	12–20	70–120	0.4–0.5	0.4–1
β	Touch, pressure	5–12	30–70		
γ	Motor to muscle spindles	3–6	15–30		
d	Pain, cold, touch	2–5	12–30		
B	Preganglionic autonomic	<3	3–15	1.2	1.2
C					
Dorsal root	Pain, temperature, some mechanoreception	0.4–1.2	0.5–2	2	2
Sympathetic	Postganglionic sympathetic	0.3–1.3	0.7–2.3	2	2

26. Ans. (b) Preganglionic sympathetic (B), pain (C&Aδ), motor
Ref: Ganong Review of Medical Physiology, 23rd ed. p 89

Refer above table (Physiology of nerve and muscle cells, Section A - AIPGEE / AIIMS Q 4)

27. Ans. (b) Perineurium *Ref: Textbook of Human Histology by Inderbir Singh, 5th ed. p 152, 142*

- Nerve fiber has a central core formed by axon called as axis cylinder.
- The plasma membrane surrounding the axis cylinder is axolemma.
- It is surrounded by myelin sheath which is formed by Schwann cells. The outer layer of the cytoplasm here is called as neurilemma.
- Each nerve fiber as a whole is surrounded by endoneurium. Endoneurium holds together adjoining nerve fibers together and forms bundles or fascicule. Apart from collagen fibers, it also contains fibroblast schwann cells endothelial cells and macrophages.
- Each fasciculus is surrounded by a thicker layer of connective tissues called as perineurium. The perineurium probably controls diffusion of substances in and out of the axons.
- A very thin nerve may consist of a single fasciculus, but usually a nerve is made up of several fascicule. The fascicule are held together and surrounded by a dense layer of connective tissue called epineurium.

28. Ans. (c) Microelectrode *Ref: http://en.wikipedia.org/wiki/Synaptic_potential*

Synaptic potential refers to the difference in voltage between the inside and outside of a postsynaptic neuron. In other words, they are the 'incoming' signal of a neuron. Synaptic potential comes in two forms: excitatory and inhibitory. Excitatory postsynaptic potentials (EPSPs) depolarize the membrane and move it closer to the threshold for an action potential. Inhibitory postsynaptic potentials (IPSPs) hyperpolarize the membrane and move it farther away from the threshold. In order to depolarize a neuron enough to cause an action potential, there must be enough EPSPs to both counterbalance the IPSPs and also depolarize the membrane from its resting membrane potential to its threshold.

29. Ans. (a) It mainly mediates pain sensation at primary neurons
Ref: Ganong Review of Medical Physiology, 23rd ed. p 143

Substance P is found in high concentration in the endings of primary afferent neurons in the spinal cord, it is probably the mediator at the first synapse in the pathways for pain transmission in the dorsal horn. Also found in nigrostriatal system, where its concentration is proportional to that of dopamine, and in the hypothalamus, where it may play a role in neuroendocrine regulation.

- Substance P is an important element in pain perception. The sensory function of substance P is thought to be related to the transmission of pain information into the central nervous system. Substance P coexists with the excitatory neurotransmitter glutamate in primary afferents that respond to painful stimulation.
- Substance P has been known to stimulate cell growth in culture
- Substance P also has effects as a potent vasodilator.

30. Ans. (b) Is that postinflammation microglia remove the branches from nerve near the damaged tissue

Ref: http://en.wikipedia.org/wiki/Microglia#Synaptic_stripping

- A phenomenon first noticed in spinal lesions by Blinzinger and Kreutzberg in 1968, postinflammation microglia remove the branches from nerves near damaged tissue. This helps, promote regrowth and remapping of damaged neural circuitry.
- Post-inflammation, microglia undergo several steps to promote regrowth of neural tissue. These include synaptic stripping, secretion of anti-inflammatory cytokines, recruitment of neurons and astrocytes to the damaged area, and formation of gitter cells. Without microglial cells regrowth and remapping would be considerably slower in the resident areas of the CNS and almost impossible in many of the vascular systems surrounding the brain and eyes.

31. Ans. (d) ↑ Sarcoplasmic Ca^{+2} *Ref: Biophys J Biophysical Society, Volume 63, August 1992;497-517*

The cardiac contraction is coordinated by an electrical action potential propagated throughout the cardiac syncytium. Despite many years of research, the exact mechanism by which this electrical signal is transduced into contraction of the myofilaments is not understood. The broad outlines of the process are known: Depolarization of the sarcolemma causes influx of calcium through voltage- dependent channels; a larger amount of stored calcium is then released from the sarcoplasmic reticulum (SR). The released calcium, together with the calcium entering through the sarcolemma, binds to troponin-C and activates the myofilaments. In the past few years, calcium channels, which are believed to mediate calcium release from the SR, have been isolated from the sarcoplasmic reticulum.

32. Ans. (b) Accommodation *Ref: J Physiol (I952) I I7, 500-544, Ganong Review of Medical Physiology, 23rd ed. p 85-87 Guyton Textbook of Medical Physiology, 11th ed. p 65-70*

- Neural accommodation or neuronal accommodation occurs when a neuron or muscle cell is depolarized by slowly rising current (ramp depolarization) in vitro.
- During neuronal accommodation the slowly rişing depolarization drives the activation and inactivation, as well as the potassium gates simultaneously and never evokes action potential. Failure to evoke action potential by ramp depolarization of any strength had been a great puzzle until Hodgkin and Huxley created their physical model of action potential. Later in their life they received Noble Prize for their influential discoveries.
- Neuronal accommodation can be explained in two ways. 'First, during the passage of a constant cathodal current through the membrane, the potassium conductance and the degree of inactivation will rise, both factors raising the threshold. Secondly, the steady state ionic current at all strengths of depolarization is outward, so that an applied cathodal current which rises sufficiently slowly will never evoke a regenerative response from the membrane, and excitation will not occur.
- Electrotonus is the change in the membrane potential due to the presence of subthreshold polarizing currents known as electrotonic current. They are passive and do not generate action potential, but affect the membrane potential.
- Accommodation: Now, if a stimulus is applied slowly and the potential is allowed to rise slowly, then the recorded (final) excitatory threshold voltage will be higher than the one found with a suddenly applied stimulus. The difference shows the accommodation undergone by the nerve fibers.
- Adaptation: If a stimulus of constant strength is applied, then slowly the frequency of generation of action potential declines over a period of time. This is because the membrane gets adapted (desensitized: sensitivity reduced).
- Refractory period is the period following an action potential, when an excitable membrane does not respond to stimulus. In absolute refractory period, no stimulus (of any strength) can excite, whereas in relative refractory period stronger than normal stimuli can cause excitation.

33. Ans. (a) Inhibitory stimulus by glial cells

Ref: http://en.wikipedia.org/wiki/Neuroregeneration#Central_nervous_system_regeneration

Axonotmesis is a disruption of nerve cell axon, with Walerian degeneration occurring below and slightly proximal to the site of injury. If axons, and their myelin sheath are damaged, but schwann cells, the endoneurium, perineurium and epineurium remain intact is called axonotmesis.

- Nerve regeneration occurs rapidly in peripheral nervous system as compared to the central nervous system.
- Unlike peripheral nervous system injury, injury to the central nervous system is not followed by extensive regeneration.
- It is limited by the inhibitory influences of the glial and extracellular environment. The hostile, non-permissive growth environment is, in part, created by the migration of myelin-associated inhibitors, astrocytes, oligodendrocytes, oligodendrocyte precursors, and microglia.
- The environment within the CNS, especially following trauma, counteracts the repair of myelin and neurons. Growth factors are not expressed or re-expressed; for instance, the extracellular matrix is lacking laminins. Glial scars rapidly form, and the glia actually produce factors that inhibit remyelination and axon repair; for instance, NOGO and NI-35.

34. Ans. (d) Neurofilaments

35. Ans. (d) Dysmorphin *Ref: Ganong Review of Medical Physiology, 23rd ed. p 96*

- Dystrophin is a rod-shaped cytoplasmic protein, and a vital part of a protein complex that connects the cytoskeleton of a muscle fiber to the surrounding extracellular matrix through the cell membrane.
- In skeletal muscle, the dystroglycan complex works as a transmembrane linkage between the extracellular matrix and the cytoskeleton.
- The sarcoglycans are a family of transmembrane proteins (α, β, γ, δ or ε) involved in the protein complex responsible for connecting the muscle fiber cytoskeleton to the extracellular matrix, preventing damage to the muscle fiber sarcolemma through shearing forces.

36. Ans. (b) Oligodendrocytes *Ref: Sembulingum*

37. Ans. (a) Minus 4 millivolt *Ref: Guyton Textbook of Medical Physiology, 11th ed. p 61*

Resting membrane potentials of the large nerves when not transferring any signal is –90 mv. That means potential inside the fiber is 90 mv more negative than outside the fiber. This negativity is maintained by movement of Na^+ and K^+. This movement takes place in 3 forms. One is diffusion of K^+ (major contributor in making negative potential), diffusion of Na+ and finally active transfer by NA^+ -K+ pump. The diffusion potentials alone caused by potassium and sodium diffusion would give a membrane potential of –86 mv, almost all of it determined by potassium diffusion alone. Then additional-4 millivolts is contributed to the membrane potential by Na^+-K^+ pump.

38. Ans. (d) Glycine *Ref: Guyton Textbook of Medical Physiology, 11th ed. p 562-563*

Chemical substances which act as synaptic neurotransmitters are classified in two main groups

- Small-molecule, rapidly acting transmitters which include acetylcholines, amino acids, etc. e.g. norepinephrine, epinephrine, glycine.
- Neuropeptides of much larger molecules which act slowly comparatively, e.g. calcitonin, substance P, gastrin growth hormone and many more.

39. Ans. (d) Extraocular muscles *Ref: Ganong Review of Medical Physiology, 23rd ed. p 105*

A motor unit is made up of a motor neuron and the skeletal muscle fibers innervated by that axon. The number of muscle fibers within each unit can vary within a particular muscle and still more widely from muscle to muscle; the muscles that act on the largest body masses have motor units that contain most of the muscles fibers whereas smaller muscles consist of less muscle fibers in each unit. For instance, thigh muscles can have a thousand fibers in each unit, while extraocular muscles might have ten.

40. Ans. (a) Troponin *Ref: Guyton Textbook of Medical Physiology, 11th ed. p 76*
http://www.getbodysmart.com/ap/muscletissue/fibers/regulatoryproteins/tutorial.html

Myosin head when attached to actin (thin) filament causes contraction of the muscle fiber. But this attachment and movement is regulated by two proteins namely troponin and tropomyosin. Tropomyosin is the long thread like protein which is wound around actin/thin filament. Myosin head for movement attaches to G actin through this tropomyosin but this attachment is prevented by troponin molecule. When calcium influx happens this troponin molecule changes its conformation and allows myosin head to attach to G actin. And, this is how the muscle fiber is contracted.

41. Ans. (d) Voltage inactivation of the Na$^+$ channel *Ref: Guyton Textbook of Medical Physiology, 11th ed. p 70*

A new action potential cannot occur in the nerve fiber as long as the membrane is still depolarized from the preceding action potential. The reason for this is that shortly after action potential has been initiated the sodium channels or calcium channels or both are inactivated and no stimulus applied to these channels will now open the inactivated gates until the membrane comes back to the resting potential. Then within another small fraction of second channel gates open and new action potential can be initiated. The period when second action potential cannot be elicited is called as absolute refractory period.

42. Ans. (b) Has no Nissl granules *Ref: http://en.wikipedia.org/wiki/Nissl_body*

The axon hillock is a specialized part of the cell body (or soma) of a neuron that connects to the axon. As a result, the axon hillock is the last site in the soma where membrane potentials propagated from synaptic inputs are summated before being transmitted to the axon. A Nissl body, also known as Nissl or tigroid substance, is a large granular body found in neurons. These granules are rough endoplasmic reticulum (RER) with rosettes of free ribosomes, and are the site of protein synthesis. Nissl bodies can be demonstrated by a method of selective staining developed by Nissl (Nissl staining), using an aniline stain to label extranuclear RNA granules. This staining method is useful to localize the perikaryon, cell body, as it can be seen in the soma and dendrites of neurons, though not in the axon or axon hillock.

43. Ans. (b) Calmodulin *Ref: Ganong Review of Medical Physiology, 23rd ed. p 110*

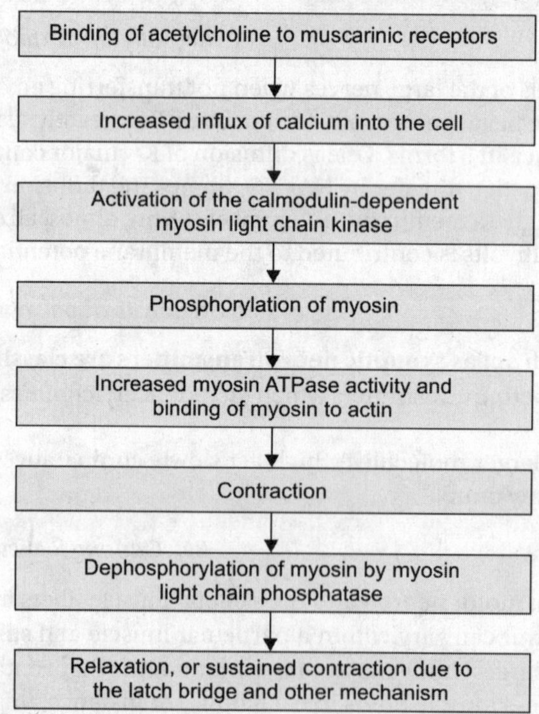

Sequence of events in contraction and relaxation of smooth muscle.

44. Ans. (c) Extracellular sodium concentration *Ref: Guyton Textbook of Medical Physiology, 11th ed. p 61-62*

Nerve signals are transmitted by actin potential, which are rapid changes in the membrane potential that spread rapidly along the nerve fiber membrane.

Action potential has following 3 stages:

- Resting stage
- Depolarization stage
- Repolarization stage: During depolarization stage, the normal polarized state of –90 mv is immediately neutralized by the inflowing positively charged sodium ions, with the potential rising rapidly in positive direction. In large nerve fibers, the great excess of sodium ions moving to the inside causes the membrane potential to actually 'overshoot' beyond the zero level and to become somewhat positive. In some smaller fibres, the potential merely approaches zero and does not overshoot to positive state. Also the necessary actor in causing both depolarization and repolarization of the nerve membrane during the action potential is the voltage gated sodium channel.

45. Ans. (b) Miniature end plate potential *Ref: Ganong Review of Medical Physiology, 23rd ed. p 124*

Small packets of acetylcholine are released randomly from the nerve cell membrane at rest termed as a miniature end plate potential, which is about 0.5 mV in amplitude. The size of the quanta of acetylcholine released varies directly with the Ca^{2+} concentration and inversely with the Mg^{2+} concentration at the end plate.

CENTRAL AND PERIPHERAL NEUROPHYSIOLOGY

46. Ans. (c) Hyperpolarization *Ref: Ganong Review of Medical Physiology, 23rd ed. p 190*

Both rods and cons contain chemical that decompose on exposure to light and in the process excite the nerve fibers leading from the eye. The light sensitive pigment in the rods is rhodopsin and, in the cones, it is cone pigments/color pigments. Composition of both is almost similar. Rods have 2 portions: One is outer segment where photoreceptor discs are located and the other is inner segment. The inner segment constantly pumps Na^+ ions from inside to outside making inside potential negative throughout the cell. In absence of light, outer segment is very leaky and allows Na^+ ions to enter inside the cell. But when exposed to light rhodopsin in this portion decomposes. This results in hindrance to enter Na^+ ions inside the cell. Hence, inside of the cell keeps on gaining negativity and hence this process is of hyperpolarization and not depolarization.

47. Ans. (c) Resting tremor *Ref: Guyton Textbook of Medical Physiology, 11th ed. p 706*

To cause serious and continuing dysfunction of the cerebellum, the cerebellar lesion usually must involve one or more of the deep cerebellar nuclei—the dentate, interposed, or fastigial nuclei.

Features of cerebellar lesions/dysfunction are as follows:

- Dysmetria
- Dysarthria
- Ataxia
- Incoordination
- Intention tremor
- Past pointing
- Hypotonia
- Cerebellar nystagmus
- Dysdiadokinesia

48. Ans. (d) Anterior nucleus of thalamus

Ref: Guyton Textbook of Medical Physiology, 11th ed. p 731. http://en.wikipedia.org/wiki/Papez_circuit

The Papez circuit is a neural pathway in the brain first described by American Neuroanatomist James Papez in 1937. Papez believed that the circuit was involved with emotions. Since the circuit's discovery, many experiments have been conducted to explore the system and how its structures work together. Recent studies show that it has a more significant role in memory functions than in emotion. The Papez circuit was later modified by American Neuroscientist and Physician Paul D. MacLean and, now, the circuit is known as the limbic system.

49. Ans. (a) Deep sleep *Ref: Ganong review of Medical Physiology, 23rd ed. p 234*

Delta waves, like other brain waves, are recorded with an electroencephalogram.

- When awake alpha rhythm (8–13 Hz) is noted on EEG.
- When attention is focused on something alpha rhythm changes to beta rhythm (13–30 Hz)
- When individual is aroused and focuses attention on something gamma oscillations (30–80 Hz) are noted.
- During sleep, there are two phases: NREM sleep and REM sleep.
- NREM sleep has 4 stages out of that in 3rd stage delta waves (0.5–4 Hz) are seen.

50. Ans. (a) Is concerned with word formation *Ref: Ganong Review of Medical Physiology, 23rd ed. p 297*
Guyton Textbook of Medical Physiology, 11th ed. p 687

Broca's area is a region in the frontal lobe of one hemisphere (usually the left) of the hominid brain with functions linked to speech production. Wernicke's area is concerned with the comprehension of auditory and visual information. Broca's area processes the information received from Wernicke's area into detailed and coordinated pattern for vocalization and then projects the pattern via speech articulation area in the insula to the motor cortex, which initiates the appropriate movements of the lips, tongue and larynx to produce. Damage to Broca's area does not prevent a person from vocalizing but makes it impossible to speak whole words.

51. Ans. (b) Hippocampus *Ref: Ganong Review of Medical Physiology, 23rd ed. p 293*

The key to memory is the alteration in the strength of selected synaptic connections. In all but the simplest of cases, the alteration involves protein synthesis and activation of genes. This occurs during the change from short-term memory to long-term memory. While the encoding process for short-term memory involves the hippocampus, long-term memories are stored in various parts of the neocortex.

52. Ans. (c) Recruitment by multiplication of neurons *Ref: Ganong Review of Medical Physiology, 23rd ed. p 293*

It is now established that, new nerve cells are not formed after birth is wrong because recently it has been found that new nerve cells are formed from stem cells and not by multiplication of existing nerve cells. This is called as neogenesis and it is formed throughout the lifetime mainly in two areas: (i) Olfactory lobe and (ii) hippocampus.

53. Ans. (a) Facial pain scale *Ref: http://en.wikipedia.org/wiki/Pain_scale*

Knee jerk: The test itself assesses the nervous tissue between and including the L2 and L4 segments. The absence or decrease of this reflex is problematic, and known as Westphal's sign. On the other hand, multiple oscillation of the leg following the tap may be a sign of a cerebellar disease. The H-reflex (or Hoffmann's reflex) is a reflectory reaction of muscles after electrical stimulation of sensory fibers (Ia afferents stemming from muscle spindles) in their innervating nerves (for example, those located behind the knee). After about 5 days in zero gravity, for instance in orbit around Earth, the h-reflex diminishes significantly. A pain scale measures a patient's pain intensity or other features. Pain scales are based on self-report, observational (behavioral), or physiological data. Self-report is considered primary and should be obtained if possible (since pain is a quale by definition, and therefore assessment based on any set scale of expected outcomes from similar cases can fail to provide useful clinical data). Pain scales are available for neonates, infants, children, adolescents, adults, seniors, and persons whose communication is impaired. Pain assessments are often regarded as 'the 5th Vital Sign.' R jerk—Not enough information available.

54. Ans. (b) Noradrenaline mediated

55. Ans. (c) Body temperature increases

Ref: Guyton Textbook of Medical Physiology, 11th ed. p 1065

Almost all the energy released by the body's metabolism of nutrients is eventually converted into body heat. And, this is also true in case of exercise, because only 20–25% of nutrient energy is used for muscle work and remaining energy is converted into heat energy. Also in that 20–25% of nutrient energy which is used for muscle work it is actually used for overcoming viscous resistance of the muscles and joints; overcoming friction of the blood flowing through the blood vessels.

56. Ans. (b) There is an immediate increase in the venous return

57. Ans. (a) Tactile receptors

Ref: Guyton Textbook of Medical Physiology, 11th ed. p 573
Ganong Review of Medical Physiology, 23rd ed. p 150

Merkel cells are expanded dendritic endings, and they respond to sustained pressure and touch.

Sensory system	*Modality*	*Stimulus energy*	*Receptor class*	*Receptor cell types*
Somatosensory	Touch	Tap, flutter 5–40 Hz	Cutaneous mechanoreceptor	Meissner corpuscles
Somatosensory	Touch	Motion	Cutaneous mechanoreceptor	Hair follicle receptors
Somatosensory	Touch	Deep pressure, vibration 60–300 Hz	Cutaneous mechanoreceptor	Pacinian corpuscles
Somatosensory	Touch	Touch, pressure	Cutaneous mechanoreceptor	Merkel cells
Somatosensory	Touch	Sustained pressure	Cutaneous mechanoreceptor	Ruffini corpuscles
Somatosensory	Proprioception	Stretch	Mechanoreceptor	Muscle spindles
Somatosensory	Proprioception	Tension	Mechanoreceptor	Golgi tendon organ
Somatosensory	Temperature	Thermal	Thermoreceptor	Cold and warm receptors
Somatosensory	Pain	Chemical, thermal, and mechanical	Chemoreceptor, thermoreceptor, and mechanoreceptor	Polymodal receptors or chemical, thermal, and mechanical nociceptors
Somatosensory	Itch	Chemical	Chemoreceptor	Chemical nociceptor
Visual	Vision	Light	Photoreceptor	Rods, cones
Auditory	Hearing	Sound	Mechanoreceptor	Hair cells (cochlea)
Vestibular	Balance	Angular acceleration	Mechanoreceptor	Hair cells (semicircular canals)
Vestibular	Balance	Linear acceleration, gravity	Mechanoreceptor	Hair cells (otolith organs)
Olfactory	Smell	Chemical	Chemoreceptor	Olfactory sensory neuron
Gustatory	Taste	Chemical	Chemoreceptor	Taste buds

58. Ans. (c) Lateral spinothalamic tract *Ref: Guyton Textbook of Medical Physiology, 11th ed. p 606*

The sensations of pain, heat, and cold sensations served by the spinothalamic pathway.

Tracts	*Characteristics*
Dorsal columns/medial lemniscus	• Convey sensations of proprioception, vibration, tactile discrimination • Fasciculus cuneatus and gracilis • Nerve fibers ascend to medulla where they cross to form medial lemniscus, ascend to thalamus, then to cortex
Spinothalamic	• Lateral conveys pain and temperature • Medical conveys crude touch • Tracts ascend one or two ipsilateral spinal cord segments, than cross to the contralateral segment of the spinal cord ascend to thalamus
Spinocerebellar	• Convey proprioception • Dorsal tracts ascend to ipsilateral cerebellum • Ventral tracts ascend to contralateral and ipsilateral cerebellum
Spinoreticular	• Convey deep and chronic pain

59. Ans. (a) Pressure *Ref: Ganong Review of Medical Physiology, 23rd ed. p 90*

Relative susceptibility of mammalian A, B, and C nerve fibers to conduction block produced by various agents.

Susceptibility to:	*Most susceptible*	*Intermediate*	*Least susceptible*
Hypoxia	B	A	C
Pressure	A	B	C
Local anesthetics	C	B	A

60. Ans. (d) Law of projection *Ref: Ganong Review of Medical Physiology, 23rd ed. p 176, 155*

In 1551, a military surgeon, Ambroise Pare, wrote, '... the patients, long after the amputation is made, say they still feel pain in the amputated part. Of this they complain strongly, a thing worthy of wonder and almost incredible to people who have not experienced this.' This is perhaps the earliest description of phantom limb pain. Between 50% and 80% of amputees experience phantom sensations, usually pain, in the region of their amputated limb. Phantom sensations may also occur after the removal of body parts other than the limbs, for example, after amputation of the breast, extraction of a tooth (phantom tooth pain), or removal of an eye (phantom eye syndrome). Numerous theories have been evoked to explain this phenomenon. No matter where a particular sensory pathway is stimulated along its course to the cortex, the conscious sensation produced is referred to the location of the receptor. This principle is called the law of projection. Cortical stimulation experiments during neurosurgical procedures on conscious patients illustrate this phenomenon. For example, when the cortical receiving area for impulses from the left hand is stimulated, the patient reports sensation in the left hand, not in the head.

61. Ans. (d) It senses muscle tension *Ref: Guyton Textbook of Medical Physiology, 11th ed. p 679*

Golgi tendon reflex: Golgi tendon organ helps control muscle tension. The Golgi tendon organ is an encapsulated sensory receptor through which muscle tendon fibers pass. About 10 to 15 muscle fibers are usually connected to each Golgi tendon organ, and the organ is stimulated when this small bundle of muscle fibers is 'tensed' by contracting or stretching the muscle. Thus, the major difference in excitation of the Golgi tendon organ versus the muscle spindle is that the spindle detects muscle length and changes in muscle length, whereas the tendon organ detects muscle tension as reflected by the tension in itself. The tendon organ, like the primary receptor of the muscle spindle, has both a dynamic response and a static response, responding intensely when the muscle tension suddenly increases (the dynamic response) but settling down within a fraction of a second to a lower level of steady-state firing that is almost directly proportional to the muscle tension (the static response). Thus, Golgi tendon organs provide the nervous system with instantaneous information on the degree of tension in each small segment of each muscle.

62. Ans. (b) Lateral spinothalamic tract *Ref: Sembulingam 4th/ed Pg 728*

63. Ans. (b) Temperature *Ref: Guyton Textbook of Medical Physiology, 11th ed. p 587*

The sensory signals are carried through one of two alternative sensory pathways:

- The dorsal (posterior) columnmedial lemniscal system or
- The anterolateral system. These two systems come back together partially at the level of the thalamus. The dorsal column medial lemniscal system is composed of large, myelinated nerve fibers that transmit signals to the brain at velocities of 30 to 110 m/sec, whereas the anterolateral system is composed of smaller myelinated fibers that transmit signals at velocities ranging from a few meters per second up to 40 m/sec.

Dorsal Column Medial Lemniscal System

- Touch sensations requiring a high degree of localization of the stimulus
- Touch sensations requiring transmission of fine gradations of intensity
- Phasic sensations, such as vibratory sensations
- Sensations that signal movement against the skin
- Position sensations from the joints
- Pressure sensations having to do with fine degrees of judgment of pressure intensity

Anterolateral System

- Pain
- Thermal sensations, including both warmth and cold sensations
- Crude touch and pressure sensations capable only of crude localizing ability on the surface of the body
- Tickle and itch sensations
- Sexual sensations

64. Ans. (d) Insulin *Ref: Guyton Textbook of Medical Physiology, 11th ed. p 909,956*
Ganong Review of Medical Physiology, 23rd ed. p 238

- Superimposed on the negative and positive feedback control of hormone secretion are periodic variations in hormone release that are influenced by seasonal changes, various stages of development and aging, the diurnal (daily) cycle, and sleep. For example, the secretion of growth hormone is markedly increased during the early period of sleep but is reduced during the later stages of sleep. In many cases, these cyclical variations in hormone secretion are due to changes in activity of neural pathways involved in controlling hormone release.
- The diurnal change in melatonin secretion may function as a timing signal to coordinate events with the light dark cycle in the environment. Melatonin synthesis and secretion are increased during the dark period of the day and maintained at a low level during daylight hours.
- The secretory rates of CRF, ACTH, and cortisol are high in the early morning but low in the late evening. The plasma cortisol level ranges between a high of about 20 mg/dl an hour before arising in the morning and a low of about 5 mg/dl around midnight. This effect results from a 24-hour cyclical alteration in the signals from the hypothalamus that cause cortisol secretion. When a person changes daily sleeping habits, the cycle changes correspondingly.

65. Ans. (d) Of stimulation of large diameter fibers

66. Ans. (b) GABA *Ref: Ganong Review of Medical Physiology, 23rd ed. p 141*

GABA is the major inhibitory mediator in the brain, including being responsible for presynaptic inhibition. GABA, which exists as β-aminobutyrate in the body fluids, is formed by decarboxylation of glutamate. GABA is the chief inhibitory neurotransmitter in the mammalian central nervous system. It plays a role in regulating neuronal excitability throughout the nervous system. In humans, GABA is also directly responsible for the regulation of muscle tone. In vertebrates, GABA acts at inhibitory synapses in the brain by binding to specific transmembrane receptors in the plasma membrane of both pre- and postsynaptic neuronal processes. This binding causes the opening of ion channels to allow the flow of either negatively charged chloride ions into the cell or positively charged potassium ions out of the cell. This action results in a negative change in the transmembrane potential, usually causing hyperpolarization.

67. Ans. (a) Remains constant *Ref: Am J Vet Res. 1983 Oct;44(10):1861-6.*

Blood flow to the brain, heart, kidneys, diaphragm, and skeletal muscles was studied at rest and during graded treadmill exercise, using radionuclide-labeled microspheres (15 microns diameter), in 11 healthy adult ponies. Hemodynamic changes brought about by exercise included marked increases in cardiac output, mean aortic pressure, left ventricular end-diastolic pressure, and right ventricular systolic and end-diastolic pressures. Blood flow to the brain stem and cerebral hemispheres was unchanged during both moderate exercise (heart rate = 154 +/- 3 beats/min) and severe exercise (heart rate = 225 +/- 7 beats/min) (Am J Vet Res. 1983 Oct; 44(10):1861-6.) The following view is more recent view but for answer of this question you write ans A refer journal address at the end of this question. Constant cerebral blood flow (CBF) is vital to human survival. Originally thought to receive steady blood flow, the brain has shown to experience increases in blood flow during exercise. Although increases have not consistently been documented, the overwhelming evidence supporting an increase may be a result of an increase in brain metabolism. Regulation of cerebral blood flow during exercise. Sports Med. 2007;37(9):765-82.

68. Ans. (b) Astrocytes *Ref: Textbook of Human Histology by Inderbir Singh 5th ed. p 172*

Astrocytes (also known collectively as astroglia, are characteristic star-shaped glial cells in the brain and spinal cord. They are the most abundant cell of the human brain. They perform many functions, including biochemical support of endothelial cells that form the blood-brain barrier, provision of nutrients to the nervous tissue, maintenance of extracellular ion balance, and a role in the repair and scarring process of the brain and spinal cord following traumatic injuries oligodendrocytes are a type of neuroglia. Their main functions are to provide support and insulation to the axons ependyma is the thin epithelium-like lining of the ventricular system of the brain and the spinal cord. Ependyma is one of the four types of neuroglia in the central nervous system (CNS). It is involved in the production of cerebrospinal fluid (CSF).

69. Ans. (c) The trigeminal nerve *Ref: en.wikipedia.org/wiki/Corneal_reflex*

The corneal reflex, also known as the blink reflex, is an involuntary blinking of the eyelids elicited by stimulation of the cornea (such as by touching or by a foreign body), or bright light, though could result from any peripheral stimulus. Stimulation should elicit both a direct and consensual response (response of the opposite eye). The reflex consumes a rapid rate of 0.1 second. The evolutionary purpose of this reflex is to protect the eyes from foreign bodies and bright lights (the latter known as the optical reflex).

The reflex is mediated by:

- The nasociliary branch of the ophthalmic branch (V1) of the 5th cranial nerve (trigeminal nerve) sensing the stimulus on the cornea, lid, or conjunctiva (i.e. it is the afferent).
- The temporal and zygomatic branches of the 7th cranial nerve (facial nerve) initiating the motor response (i.e. it is the efferent).

70. Ans. (b) Vasodilatation *Ref: Ganong Review of Medical Physiology, 23rd ed. p 563, 285*

The reflex responses activated by cold are controlled from the posterior hypothalamus. Those activated by warmth are controlled primarily from the anterior hypothalamus, although some thermoregulation against heat still occurs after decerebration at the level of the rostral midbrain. Stimulation of the anterior hypothalamus causes cutaneous vasodilation and sweating, and lesions in this region cause hyperthermia, with rectal temperatures sometimes reaching 43°C.

71. Ans. (c) Poor localization *Ref: Guyton Textbook of Medical Physiology, 11th ed. p 600, 601*

The fast sharp pain signals are elicited by either mechanical or thermal pain stimuli; they are transmitted in the peripheral nerves to the spinal cord by small type Ad fibers at velocities between 6 and 30 m/sec. Conversely, the slow-chronic type of pain is elicited mostly by chemical types of pain stimuli but sometimes by persisting mechanical or thermal stimuli. This slow-chronic pain is transmitted to the spinal cord by type C fibers at velocities between 0.5 and 2 m/sec. It is believed glutamate is the neurotransmitter most involved in transmitting fast pain into the central nervous system, and substance P is concerned with slow-chronic pain. Slow pain pathway that is paleospinothalamic pathway terminates widely in the brain stem. Only one tenth to one fourth of the fibers pass all the way to the thalamus. Instead, most terminate in one of three areas: (1) The reticular nuclei of the medulla, pons, and mesencephalon, (2) the tectal area of the mesencephalon, (3) the periaqueductal gray region surrounding the aqueduct of sylvius. Localization of pain transmitted by way of the paleospinothalamic pathway is poor. For instance, slow-chronic pain can usually be localized only to a major part of the body, such as to one arm or leg but not to a specific point on the arm or leg. This is in keeping with the multisynaptic, diffuse connectivity of this pathway. It explains why patients often have serious difficulty in localizing the source of some chronic types of pain.

72. Ans. (c) Less than 3.5 cycles per second *Ref: Ganong Review of Medical Physiology, 23rd ed. p 234*

In stage 3, a high-amplitude delta rhythm (0.54 Hz) dominates the EEG waves. Refer explanation of Chapter 3 AIPGEE Q-4

73. Ans. (a) Static tremor *Ref: Refer explanation of Chapter 3 AIPGEE Q-2*

Intention tremor. When a person who has lost the cerebellum performs a voluntary act, the movements tend to oscillate, especially when they approach the intended mark, first overshooting the mark and then vibrating back and forth several times before settling on the mark. This reaction is called an intention tremor or an action tremor, and it results from cerebellar overshooting and failure of the cerebellar system to 'damp' the motor movements.

The Holmes Rebound phenomenon is a sign of cerebellar disease. There are two ways of eliciting the sign:

- With patient having their arms outstretched, you ask the patient to keep their arms in that position as you press down on their arm. As you release your hand, their arm shoots up above the position it originally was and bounces up.
- Flex the patients elbow. Ask the patient to keep their arm in that position as you pull away, when you release the arm, the arm will hit the patient's body.

74. Ans. (b) Myopia *Ref: Guyton Textbook of Medical Physiology, 11th ed. p 619*

In myopia, or 'nearsightedness,' when the ciliary muscle is completely relaxed, the light rays coming from distant objects are focused in front of the retina. This is usually due to too long an eyeball, but it can result from too much refractive power in the lens system of the eye.

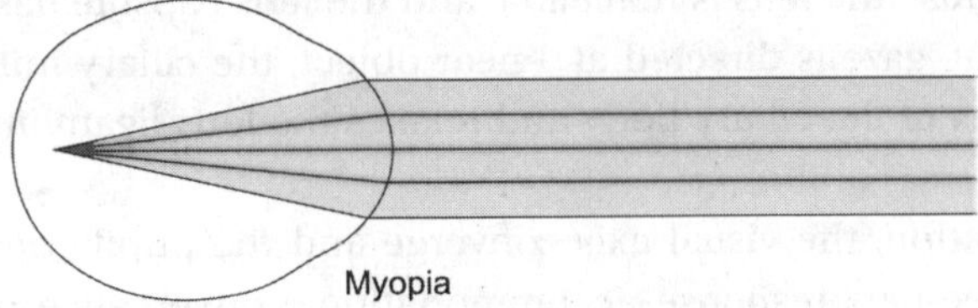

Ref: http://en.wikipedia.org/wiki/Pain_scale Visual Analog Scale and Verbal Pain Intensity Scale: From Pain Management: Theory and Practice, edited by RK Portenoy & RM Tanner, copyright 1996 by Oxford University Press, Inc. Used by permission of Oxford University Press

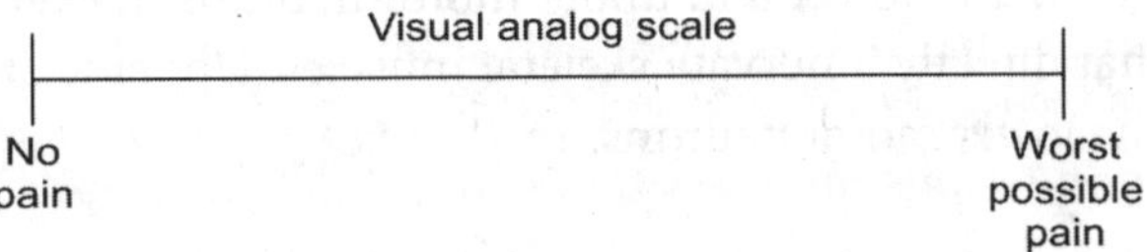

75. Ans. (d) Free nerve endings

76. Ans. (a) Bipolar neurons

77. Ans. (c) A delta

78. Ans. (d) Opening of Na^+ channels

79. Ans. (a) Resting tremors

80. Ans. (a) Visual analogue scale

81. Ans. (d) There is a latent period before the attenuation reflex occurs

Ref: Guyton Textbook of Medical Physiology, 11th ed. p 652

When loud sounds are transmitted through the ossicular system and from there into the central nervous system, a reflex occurs after a latent period of only 40 to 80 milliseconds to cause contraction of the stapedius muscle and, to a lesser extent, the tensor tympani muscle. The tensor tympani muscle pulls the handle of the malleus inward while the stapedius muscle pulls the stapes outward. These two forces oppose each other and thereby cause the entire ossicular system to develop increased rigidity, thus greatly reducing the ossicular conduction of low frequency sound, mainly frequencies below 1000 cycles per second. This attenuation reflex can reduce the intensity of lower-frequency sound transmission by 30 to 40 decibels, which is about the same difference as that between a loud voice and a whisper. The function of this mechanism is believed to be two fold:

- To protect the cochlea from damaging vibrations caused by excessively loud sound.
- To mask low-frequency sounds in loud environments. This usually removes a major share of the background noise and allows a person to concentrate on sounds above 1000 cycles per second, where most of the pertinent information in voice communication is transmitted.

82. Ans. (b) Dilatation of pupil *Ref: Ganong Review of Medical Physiology, 23rd ed. p 189*

- The process by which the curvature of the lens is increased is called accommodation. At rest, the lens is held by the lens ligaments. Because the lens is malleable and the lens capsule has elasticity, the lens is pulled into a flattened shape. When the gaze is directed at a near object, the ciliary muscle contracts. This decrease the distance between the edges of the ciliary body and relaxes the lens ligaments, so that the lens springs into a more convex shape.
- In addition to accommodation, the visual axis converge and the pupil constricts when an individual looks at a near object. This three-part response-accommodation, convergence of the visual axes, and papillary constriction, is called the near response.

83. Ans. (c) Muscular atrophy *Ref: Ganong Review of Medical Physiology, 23rd ed. p 244*

The motor system can be divided into lower and upper motor neurons. Lower motor neurons refer to the spinal and cranial motor neurons that directly innervate skeletal muscles. Upper motor neurons are those in the cortex and brainstem that activate the lower motor neurons.

Lower motor neurons

- Lower motor neurons are those whose axons terminate on skeletal muscles. Damage to these neurons is associated with flaccid paralysis, muscular atrophy, fasciculation (visible muscle twitches that appear as flickers under the skin), hypotonia (decreased muscle tone), hyporeflexia or areflexia.
- An example of a disease that leads to lower motor neuron damage is amyotrophic lateral sclerosis (ALS). This fatal disease is also known as Lou Gehrig disease because Gehrig, a famous American baseball player, died of it.

Upper motor neurons

- Upper motor neurons typically refer to corticospinal tract neurons that innervate spinal motor neurons, but they can also include brain stem neurons that control spinal motor neurons.
- Damage to these neurons initially causes muscles to become weak and flaccid but eventually leads to spasticity, hypertonia (increase resistance to passive movement), hyperactive stretch reflexes, and abnormal plantar extensor reflex (Babinski sign).

84. Ans. (d) Hypoglossal nerve *Ref: Guyton Textbook of Medical Physiology, 11th ed. p 665-666*

Taste impulses from the anterior two thirds of the tongue pass first into the lingual nerve, then through the chorda tympani into the facial nerve, and finally into the tractus solitarius in the brain stem. Taste sensations from the circumvallate papillae on the back of the tongue and from other posterior regions of the mouth and throat are transmitted through the glossopharyngeal nerve also into the tractus solitarius, but at a slightly more posterior level. Finally, a few taste signals are transmitted into the tractus solitarius from the base of the tongue and other parts of the pharyngeal region by way of the vagus nerve.

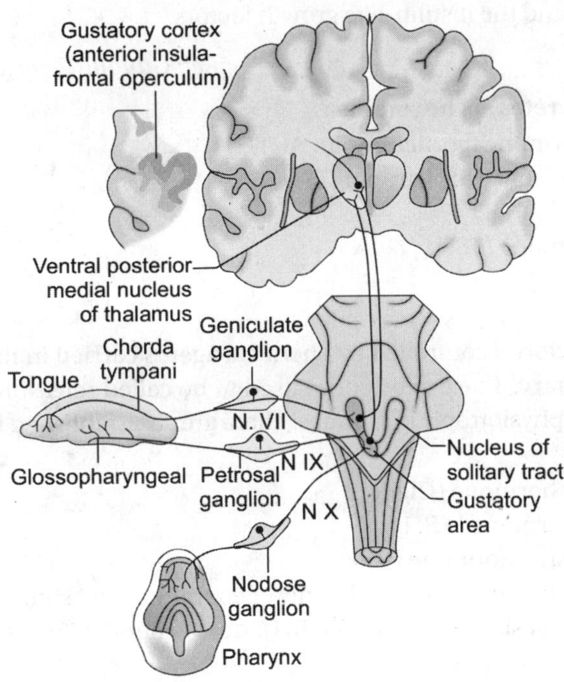

Transmission of taste signals into the central nervous system

ENDOCRINE AND REPRODUCTIVE PHYSIOLOGY

85. Ans. (a) Intrinsic factor

86. Ans. (b) Increasing HR

87. Ans. (b) Supraoptic *Ref: Guyton Textbook of Medical Physiology, 11th ed. p 928*

The posterior pituitary gland, also called the neurohypophysis, is composed mainly of glial-like cells called pituicytes. The pituicytes do not secrete hormones; they act simply as a supporting structure for large numbers of terminal nerve fibers and terminal nerve endings from nerve tracts that originate in the supraoptic and paraventricular nuclei of the hypothalamus. The nerve endings are bulbous knobs that contain many secretory granules. These endings lie on the surfaces of capillaries, where they secrete two posterior pituitary hormones: (1) antidiuretic hormone (ADH), also called vasopressin, and (2) oxytocin. ADH is formed primarily in the supraoptic nuclei, whereas oxytocin is formed primarily in the paraventricular nuclei. Each of these nuclei can synthesize about one sixth as much of the second hormone as of its primary hormone.

88. Ans. (a) The deposition of chondroitin sulfate *Ref: Ganong Review of Medical Physiology, 23rd ed. p 383*

The effects of growth hormone on growth, cartilage, and protein metabolism depend on an interaction between growth hormone and somatomedins, which are polypeptide growth factors secreted by the liver and other tissues. The first of these factors isolated was called sulfation factor because it stimulated the incorporation of sulfate into cartilage. However, it also stimulated collagen formation, and its name was changed to somatomedin. It then became clear that there are a variety of different somatomedins and that they are members of an increasingly large family of growth factors that affect many different tissues and organs. The principal (and in humans probably the only) circulating somatomedins are insulin-like growth factor I (IGF-I, somatomedin C) and insulin-like growth factor II (IGF-II).

- Comparison of insulin and the insulin-like growth factors.

89. Ans. (d) Prolactin *Ref: Ganong Review of Medical Physiology, 23rd ed. p 280*

The anterior pituitary secretes six hormones:

1. Adrenocorticotropic hormone (corticotropin, ACTH)
2. Thyroid-stimulating hormone (thyrotropin, TSH)
3. Growth hormone
4. Follicle stimulating hormone (FSH)
5. Luteinizing hormone (LH)
6. Prolactin (PRL)

Anterior pituitary secretion is controlled by chemical agents carried in the portal hypophysial vessels from the hypothalamus to the pituitary. These substances used to be called releasing and inhibiting factors, but now they are commonly called hypophysiotropic hormones. There are six established hypothalamic releasing and inhibiting hormones:

1. Corticotropin-releasing hormone (CRH)
2. Thyrotropin-releasing hormone (TRH)
3. Growth hormone-releasing hormone (GRH)
4. Growth hormone-inhibiting hormone (GIH), now generally called somatostatin
5. Luteinizing hormone-releasing hormone (LHRH), now generally known as gonadotropin-releasing hormone (GnRH)
6. Prolactin-inhibiting hormone (PIH). In addition, hypothalamic extracts contain prolactin-releasing activity, and a prolactin-releasing hormone (PRH) has been postulated to exist.

From given information, correct answer for this question can be inferred as prolactin because currently definite evidence about prolactin-releasing hormone (PRH) is not available.

90. Ans. (b) SRY *Ref: Ganong Review of Medical Physiology, 23rd ed. p 392*

Sex is determined genetically by two chromosomes, called the sex chromosomes, to distinguish them from the somatic chromosomes (autosomes). In humans and many other mammals, the sex chromosomes are called X and Y chromosomes. The Y chromosome is necessary and sufficient for the production of testes, and the testis-determining gene product is called SRY (for sex determining region of the Y chromosome). SRY is a DNA binding regulatory protein. It bends the DNA and acts as a transcription factor that initiates transcription of a cascade of genes necessary for testicular differentiation.

91. Ans. (c) Sertoli cell activity *Ref: Ganong Review of Medical Physiology, 23rd ed. p 409*

- Inhibin is a factor of testicular origin that inhibits FSH secretion.
- There are two inhibins in extracts of testes in men and in antral fluid from ovarian follicles in women.
- Both αβA (inhibin A) and αβB (inhibin B) inhibit FSH secretion by a direct action on the pituitary, though it now appears that it is inhibin B that is the FSH-regulating inhibin in adult men and women. Inhibins are produced by sertoli cells in males and granulosa cells in females.

92. Ans. (a) Cyclic AMP *Ref: Guyton Textbook of Medical Physiology, 11th ed. p 913*

Some hormones that use the adenylyl cyclase cAMP second messenger system

- Adrenocorticotropic hormone (ACTH)
- Angiotensin II (epithelial cells)
- Calcitonin
- Catecholamines (b receptors)
- Corticotropin-releasing hormone (CRH)
- Follicle-stimulating hormone (FSH)
- Glucagon
- Human chorionic gonadotropin (HCG)
- Luteinizing hormone (LH)
- Parathyroid hormone (PTH)
- Secretin
- Somatostatin
- Thyroid-stimulating hormone (TSH)
- Vasopressin (V2 receptor, epithelial cells)

93. Ans. (b) Hypocalcemia *Ref: Guyton Textbook of Medical Physiology, 11th ed. p 957*
Ganong Review of Medical Physiology, 23rd ed. p 356

Hypoadrenalism-Addison's Disease:

- Mineralocorticoid deficiency: Lack of aldosterone secretion greatly decreases renal tubular sodium reabsorption and consequently allows sodium ions, chloride ions, and water to be lost into urine in great profusion. The net result is a greatly decreased extracellular fluid volume, the plasma volume also is reduced, resulting in hypotension, circulatory insufficiency, and, eventually, fatal shock. Furthermore, hyponatremia, hyperkalemia, and mild acidosis develop because of failure of potassium and hydrogen ions to be secreted in exchange for sodium reabsorption.
- Glucocorticoid deficiency: Loss of cortisol secretion makes it impossible for a person with Addison's disease to maintain normal blood glucose concentration between meals because he or she cannot synthesize significant quantities of glucose by gluconeogenesis.
- Lack of adequate glucocorticoid secretion also makes a person with Addison's disease highly susceptible to the deteriorating effects of different types of stress, and even a mild respiratory infection can cause death.
- Melanin pigmentation: Another characteristic of most people with Addison's disease is melanin pigmentation of the mucous membranes and skin.

94. Ans. (a) Large tongue *Ref: Guyton Textbook of Medical Physiology, 11th ed. p 927*

Acromegaly is a syndrome that results when the anterior pituitary gland produces excess growth hormone (GH) after epiphyseal plate closure at puberty.

- Soft-tissue swelling visibly resulting in enlargement of the hands, feet, nose, lips and ears, and a general thickening of the skin.
- Soft-tissue swelling of internal organs, notably the heart with attendant weakening of its muscularity, and the kidneys, also the vocal cords resulting in a characteristic thick, deep voice and slowing of speech
- Generalized expansion of the skull at the fontanelle
- Pronounced brow protrusion, often with ocular distension (frontal bossing)
- Pronounced lower jaw protrusion (prognathism) with attendant macroglossia (enlargement of the tongue) and teeth gapping
- Hypertrichosis, hyperpigmentation, and hyperhidrosis may occur in these patients.
- Acrochordon (skin tags)
- Carpal tunnel syndrome

95. Ans. (d) Prolactin *Ref: Refer explanation of Chapter 4 AIPGEE Q-5*

Refer explanations of Ans 89

96. Ans. (a) Thyroid gland *Ref: Guyton Textbook of Medical Physiology, 11th ed. p 988*

- Calcitonin, a peptide hormone secreted by the thyroid gland, tends to decrease plasma calcium concentration and, in general, has effects opposite to those of PTH.
- Synthesis and secretion of calcitonin occur in the parafollicular cells, or C cells, lying in the interstitial fluid between the follicles of the thyroid gland. These cells constitute only about 0.1 per cent of the human thyroid gland and are the remnants of the ultimobranchial glands of lower animals, such as fish, amphibians, reptiles, and birds. Calcitonin is a 32-amino acid peptide with a molecular weight of about 3400.

97. Ans. (d) Thyroxine *Ref: Guyton Textbook of Medical Physiology, 11th ed. p 915*

Transcription in the cell nucleus: The thyroid hormones thyroxine and triiodothyronine cause increased transcription by specific genes in the directly with receptor proteins in the nucleus itself; these receptors are probably protein molecules located within the chromosomal complex, and they likely control the function of the genetic promoters or operators.

Two important features of thyroid hormone function in the nucleus are the following:

- They activate the genetic mechanisms for the formation of many types of intracellular proteins probably 100 or more. Many of these are enzymes that promote enhanced intracellular metabolic activity in virtually all cells of the body.
- Once bound to the intranuclear receptors, the thyroid hormones can continue to express their control functions for days or even weeks.

98. Ans. (b) Calcitonin *Ref: Guyton Textbook of Medical Physiology, 11th ed. p 988*

Calcitonin decreases blood calcium ion concentration rapidly, beginning within minutes after injection of the calcitonin, in at least two ways.

1. The immediate effect is to decrease the absorptive activities of the osteoclasts and possibly the osteolytic effect of the osteocytic membrane throughout the bone, thus shifting the balance in favor of deposition of calcium in the exchangeable bone calcium salts. This effect is especially significant in young animals because of the rapid interchange of absorbed and deposited calcium.
2. The second and more prolonged effect of calcitonin is to decrease the formation of new osteoclasts. Also, because osteoclastic resorption of bone leads secondarily to osteoblastic activity, decreased numbers of osteoclasts are followed by decreased numbers of osteoblasts. Therefore, over a long period, the net result is

reduced osteoclastic and osteoblastic activity and, consequently, very little prolonged effect on plasma calcium ion concentration. That is, the effect on plasma calcium is mainly a transient one, lasting for a few hours to a few days at most.

99. Ans. (c) Decrease in serum calcium *Ref: Guyton Textbook of Medical Physiology, 11th ed. p 988*

Synthesis and secretion of calcitonin occur in the parafollicular cells, or C cells, lying in the interstitial fluid between the follicles of the thyroid gland. Calcitonin, a peptide hormone secreted by the thyroid gland, tends to decrease plasma calcium concentration and, in general, has effects opposite to those of PTH.

100. Ans. (b) Calcium *Ref: Guyton Textbook of Medical Physiology, 11th ed. p 985*

Parathyroid hormone provides a powerful mechanism for controlling extracellular calcium and phosphate concentrations by regulating intestinal reabsorption, renal excretion, and exchange between the extracellular fluid and bone of these ions. Excess activity of the parathyroid gland causes rapid absorption of calcium salts from the bones, with resultant hypercalcemia in the extracellular fluid; conversely, hypofunction of the parathyroid glands causes hypocalcemia, often with resultant tetany.

101. Ans. (b) Diabetes mellitus *Ref: http://en.wikipedia.org/wiki/Glycated_hemoglobin*

Glycated hemoglobin (HbA1c) is a form of hemoglobin that is measured primarily to identify the average plasma glucose concentration over prolonged periods of time. It is formed in a non-enzymatic glycation pathway by hemoglobin's exposure to plasma glucose. Normal levels of glucose produce a normal amount of glycated hemoglobin. As the average amount of plasma glucose increases, the fraction of glycated hemoglobin increases in a predictable way. This serves as a marker for average blood glucose levels over the previous months prior to the measurement. In diabetes mellitus, higher amounts of glycated hemoglobin, indicating poorer control of blood glucose levels, have been associated with cardiovascular disease, nephropathy, and retinopathy. Monitoring HbA1c in type 1 diabetic patients may improve outcomes.

102. Ans. (d) Glucose synthesis *Ref: Guyton Textbook of Medical Physiology, 11th ed. p 963*

- Carbohydrates: Immediately after a high-carbohydrate meal, the glucose that is absorbed into the blood causes rapid secretion of insulin. The insulin in turn causes rapid uptake, storage, and use of glucose by almost all tissues of the body, but especially by the muscles, adipose tissue, and liver.
- One of the most important of all the effects of insulin is to cause most of the glucose absorbed after a meal to be stored almost immediately in the liver in the form of glycogen. Then, between meals, when food is not available and the blood glucose concentration begins to fall, insulin secretion decreases rapidly and the liver glycogen is split back into glucose, which is released back into the blood to keep the glucose concentration from falling too low.
- Adipose tissue: Insulin has several effects that lead to fat storage in adipose tissue. First, insulin increases the utilization of glucose by most of the body's tissues, which automatically decreases the utilization of fat, thus functioning as a fat sparer. However, insulin also promotes fatty acid synthesis. This is especially true when more carbohydrates are ingested than can be used for immediate energy, thus providing the substrate for fat synthesis. Almost all this synthesis occurs in the liver cells, and the fatty acids are then transported from the liver by way of the blood lipoproteins to the adipose cells to be stored.
- Protein: During the few hours after a meal when excess quantities of nutrients are available in the circulating blood, not only carbohydrates and fats but proteins as well are stored in the tissues; insulin is required for this to occur. The manner in which insulin causes protein storage is not as well understood.

103. Ans. (c) Fertilization period *Ref: http://en.wikipedia.org/wiki/Gestation_period http://en.wikipedia.org/wiki/Embryo http://wiki.answers.com/Q/What_happens_during_the_germinal_period_of_pregnancy?#slide=2*

The gestation period is the time in which a fetus develops, beginning with fertilization and ending at birth. In humans, it is called an embryo until about eight weeks after fertilization (i.e. ten weeks after the last menstrual period or

LMP), and from then it is instead called a fetus. The germinal period is the two week period after the sperm and the egg unite.

104. Ans. (b) Stimulates bone resorption *Ref: Guyton Textbook of Medical Physiology, 11th ed. p 986*

A much better known effect of PTH and one for which the evidence is much clearer is its activation of the osteoclasts. Activation of the osteoclastic system occurs in two stages: (1) Immediate activation of the osteoclasts that are already formed and (2) formation of new osteoclasts. Bone contains such great amounts of calcium in comparison with the total amount in all the extracellular fluids (about 1000 times as much) that even when PTH causes a great rise in calcium concentration in the fluids, it is impossible to discern any immediate effect on the bones. Prolonged administration or secretion of PTH over a period of many months or years finally results in very evident absorption in all the bones and even development of large cavities filled with large, multinucleated osteoclasts.

105. Ans. (b) Comes in contact with zona pellucida *Ref: Guyton Textbook of Medical Physiology, 11th ed. p 1000*
Ganong Review of Medical Physiology, 23rd ed. p 423

- **Sequential events in fertilization in mammals**

Sperm are attracted to the ovum, bind to the zona pellucida, release acrosomal enzymes, penetrate the zona pellucida, and fuse with the membrane of the ovum, releasing the sperm nucleus into its cytoplasm. Current evidence indicates that the side, rather than the tip, of the sperm head fuses with the egg cell membrane.

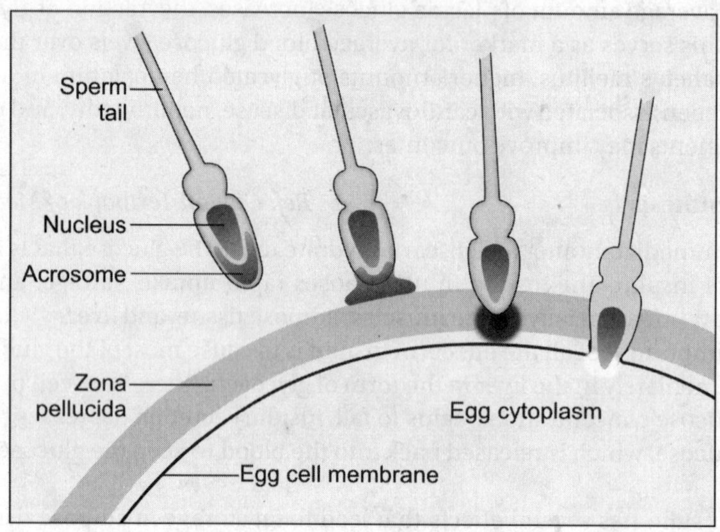

106. Ans. (c) Interstitial cells of leydig *Ref: Guyton Textbook of Medical Physiology, 11th ed. p 1003*

The testes secrete several male sex hormones, which are collectively called androgens, including testosterone, dihydrotestosterone, and androstenedione. Testosterone is so much more abundant than the others that one can consider it to be the significant testicular hormone, although as we shall see, much, if not most, of the testosterone is eventually converted into the more active hormone dihydrotestosterone in the target tissues. Testosterone is formed by the interstitial cells of Leydig, which lie in the interstices between the seminiferous tubules and constitute about 20 per cent of the mass of the adult testes.

107. Ans. (a) Calcitonin *Ref:Refer explanation of Chapter 4 AIPGEE Q-14*

Refer explanation of Answer 98

108. Ans. (c) Chief cells *Ref: Guyton Textbook of Medical Physiology, 11th ed. p 986*

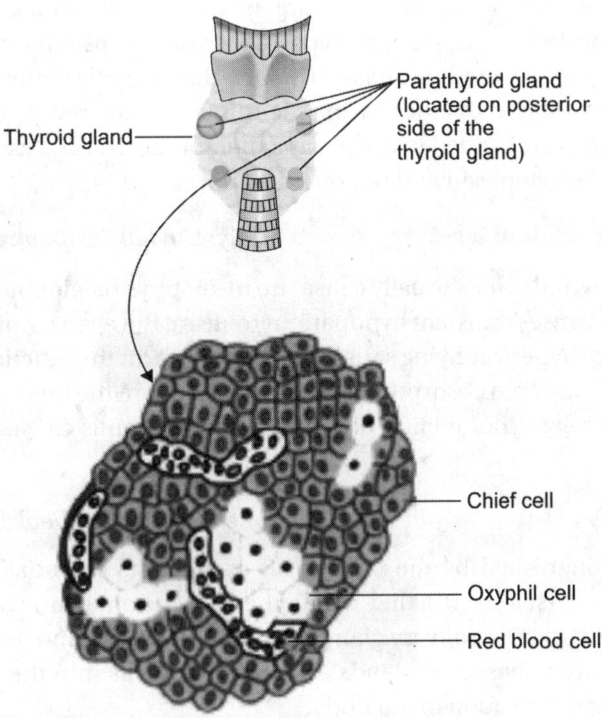

The four parathyroid glands lie immediately behind the thyroid gland. Almost all of the parathyroid hormone (PTH) is synthesized and secreted by the chief cells. The function of the oxyphil cells is uncertain, but they may be modified or depleted chief cells that no longer secrete PTH.

109. Ans. (b) Hypocalcemia *Ref: Ganong Review of Medical Physiology, 23rd ed. p 367*

It is the free, ionized calcium in the body fluids that is a vital second messenger and is necessary for blood coagulation, muscle contraction, and nerve function. A decrease in extracellular Ca^{2+} exerts a net excitatory effect on nerve and muscle cells in vivo. The result is hypocalcemic tetany, which is characterized by extensive spasms of skeletal muscle, involving especially the muscles of the extremities and the larynx. Laryngospasm can become so severe that the airway is obstructed and fatal asphyxia is produced. The signs of tetany in humans include Chvostek's sign, a quick contraction of the ipsilateral facial muscles elicited by tapping over the facial nerve at the angle of the jaw, and Trousseau's sign a spasm of the muscles of the upper extremity that causes flexion of the wrist and thumb with extension of the fingers.

110. Ans. (a) 'C' cells of thyroid gland *Ref: Guyton Textbook of Medical Physiology, 11th ed. p 988*

The ultimobranchial body is an embryological structure that gives rise to the calcitonin-producing cells also called parafollicular cells or C cells of the thyroid gland. In humans, this body is a derivative of the ventral recess of the fourth pharyngeal pouch.

111. Ans. (c) Estrogen *Ref: Guyton Textbook of Medical Physiology, 11th ed. p 910*

The locations for the different types of hormone receptors are generally the following:

- In or on the surface of the cell membrane. The membrane receptors are specific mostly for the protein, peptide, and catecholamine hormones.
- In the cell cytoplasm, the primary receptors for the different steroid hormones are found mainly in the cytoplasm.

- In the cell nucleus, the receptors for the thyroid hormones are found in the nucleus and are believed to be located in direct association with one or more of the chromosomes. The reason why steroid receptors are cytoplasmically-located is because steroids can cross the plasma membrane by themselves: they just diffuse through, because they are lipid-based (in fact, they are all synthesized from cholesterol, a membrane component). Proteins cannot cross the plasma membrane, so the receptors of proteinaceous signaling factors must be outside the cell—embedded in the plasma membrane. Natural estrogens are steroid hormones. Hence their receptors are in the cytoplasm and not on the surface.

112. Ans. (a) Decline plasma calcium level *Ref: Guyton Textbook of Medical Physiology, 11th ed. p 985*

Removal of half the parathyroid glands usually causes no major physiologic abnormalities. However, removal of three of the four normal glands causes transient hypoparathyroidism. But even a small quantity of remaining parathyroid tissue is usually capable of hypertrophying satisfactorily to perform the function of all the glands. Excess activity of the parathyroid gland causes rapid absorption of calcium salts from the bones, with resultant hypercalcemia in the extracellular fluid; conversely hypofunction of the parathyroid glands causes hypocalcemia, often with resultant tetany.

113. Ans. (a) Exocrine glands *Ref: Guyton Textbook of Medical Physiology, 11th ed. p 905*

- Exocrine gland is distinguished by the fact that it excretes its essential product by way of a duct to some environment external to itself, be it either inside the body or on a surface of the body. Examples of exocrine glands include the sweat glands, salivary glands, mammary glands, and liver.
- Endocrine hormones are released by glands or specialized cells into the circulating blood and influence the function of cells at another location in the body.
- Neuroendocrine hormones are secreted by neurons into the circulating blood and influence the function of cells at another location in the body.
- Paracrines are secreted by cells into the extracellular fluid and affect neighboring cells of a different type.
- Autocrines are secreted by cells into the extracellular fluid and affect the function of the same cells that produced them by binding to cell surface receptors.
- Cytokines are peptides secreted by cells into the extracellular fluid and can function as autocrines, paracrines, or endocrine hormones. Examples of cytokines include the interleukins and other lymphokines that are secreted by helper cells and act on other cells of the immune system.

114. Ans. (b) Feminine fat distribution *Ref: Ganong Review of Medical Physiology, 23rd ed. p 398*

There follows in all mammals a period in which the gonads of both sexes are quiescent until they are activated by gonadotropins from the pituitary to bring about the final maturation of the reproductive system. This period of final maturation is known as adolescence. It is often also called puberty, although puberty, strictly defined, is the period when the endocrine and gametogenic functions of the gonads have first developed to the point where reproduction is possible. In girls, the first event is thelarche, the development of breasts, followed by pubarche, the development of axillary and pubic hair, and then by menarche, the first menstrual period. Another event that occurs in humans at the time of puberty is an increase in the secretion of adrenal androgens. The onset of this increase is called adrenarche. It occurs at age 8 to 10 years in girls and age 10 to 12 years in boys.

115. Ans. (a) Somatomedin C *Ref: Guyton Textbook of Medical Physiology, 11th ed. p 924*

Growth hormone exerts much of its effect through intermediate substances called 'somatomedins' (also called 'insulin-like growth factors'). It has been postulated that most, if not all, of the growth effects of growth hormone result from somatomedin C and other somatomedins, rather than from direct effects of growth hormone on the bones and other peripheral tissues. It has been found that growth hormone causes the liver (and, to a much less extent, other tissues) to form several small proteins called somatomedins that have the potent effect of increasing all aspects of bone growth. Many of the somatomedin effects on growth are similar to the effects of insulin on growth. Therefore, the somatomedins are also called insulin-like growth factors (IGFs). At least four somatomedins have been isolated, but by far the most important of these is somatomedin C (also called IGF-I). The molecular weight of somatomedin C is about 7500, and its concentration in the plasma closely follows the rate of growth hormone secretion.

GASTROINTESTINAL PHYSIOLOGY

116. Ans. (b) Parietal cells *Ref: Guyton Textbook of Medical Physiology, 11th ed. p 797*

Secretion of Intrinsic Factor

The substance intrinsic factor, essential for absorption of vitamin B12 in the ileum, is secreted by the parietal cells along with the secretion of hydrochloric acid. When the acid-producing parietal cells of the stomach are destroyed, which frequently occurs in chronic gastritis, the person develops not only achlorhydria (lack of stomach acid secretion) but often also pernicious anemia because of failure of maturation of the red blood cells in the absence of vitamin B12 stimulation of the bone marrow.

117. Ans. (b) 750 million/mL

118. Ans. (a) Fundus *Ref: Ganong Review of Medical Physiology, 23rd ed. p 433*

119. Ans. (a) Pepsin *Ref: Guyton Textbook of Medical Physiology, 11th ed. p 797*

Several slightly different types of pepsinogen are secreted by the peptic and mucous cells of the gastric glands. Even so, all the pepsinogens perform the same functions. When pepsinogen is first secreted, it has no digestive activity. However, as soon as it comes in contact with hydrochloric acid, it is activated to form active pepsin. Pepsin functions as an active proteolytic enzyme in a highly acid medium (optimum pH 1.8 to 3.5), but above a pH of about 5 it has almost no proteolytic activity and becomes completely inactivated in a short time.

120. Ans. (a) Fast

121. Ans. (a) Obesity *Ref: Ganong Review of Medical Physiology, 23rd ed. p 462*

The metabolic rate determined at rest in a room at a comfortable temperature in the thermoneutral zone 12 to 14 hours after the last meal is called the basal metabolic rate (BMR). This value falls about 10% during sleep and up to 40% during prolonged starvation. The rate during normal daytime activities is, of course, higher than the BMR because of muscular activity and food intake. The maximum metabolic rate reached during exercise is often said to be 10 times the BMR, but trained athletes can increase their metabolic rate as much as 20-fold. The BMR of a man of average size is about 2000 kcal/d. Large animals have higher absolute BMRs, but the ratio of BMR to body weight in small animals is much greater.

122. Ans. (c) >30 *Ref: Guyton Textbook of Medical Physiology, 11th ed. p 872*

Obesity can be defined as an excess of body fat. A surrogate marker for body fat content is the body mass index (BMI), which is calculated as:

BMI = Weight in kg/height m^2 in clinical terms, a BMI between 25 and 29.9 kg/m^2 is called overweight, and a BMI greater than 30 kg/m^2 is called obese.

123. Ans. (c) Filiform *Ref: Guyton Textbook of Medical Physiology, 11th ed. p 665*

The taste buds are found on three types of papillae of the tongue, as follows:

- A large number of taste buds are on the walls of the troughs that surround the circumvallate papillae,which form a V line on the surface of the posterior tongue.
- Moderate numbers of taste buds are on the fungiform papillae over the flat anterior surface of the tongue.
- Moderate numbers are on the foliate papillae located in the folds along the lateral surfaces of the tongue. Additional taste buds are located on the palate, and a few are found on the tonsillar pillars, on the epiglottis, and even in the proximal esophagus. Adults have 3000 to 10,000 taste buds, and children have a few more.

124. Ans. (d) G: Gastrin *Ref: Guyton Textbook of Medical Physiology, 11th ed. p 907, 776, 961*

- Gastrin is secreted by the 'G' cells of the antrum of the stomach.
- The delta cells of the islets of langerhans secrete the hormone somatostatin.
- The beta cells, constituting about 60 percent of all the cells of the islets, lie mainly in the middle of each islet and secrete insulin and amylin, a hormone that is often secreted in parallel with insulin, although its function is unclear. The alpha cells, about 25 per cent of the total, secrete glucagon.

125. Ans. (c) It increases by acetylcholine *Ref: Guyton Textbook of Medical Physiology, 11th ed. p 785*
Ganong Review of Medical Physiology, 23rd ed. p 475.

The movements of the small intestine, like those elsewhere in the gastrointestinal tract, can be divided into mixing contractions and propulsive contractions. When a portion of the small intestine becomes distended with chyme, stretching of the intestinal wall elicits localized concentric contractions spaced at intervals along the intestine and lasting a fraction of a minute. Intestinal motility does not depend on gastric motility however gastric motility is dependent on many intestinal inhibitory factors, such as presence of chyme (acidic and fatty food or chyme) also cholecystokinin (CCK), which is released from the mucosa of the jejunum acts as an inhibitor to block increased stomach motility caused by gastrin.

126. Ans. (a) Acidogenic bacteria *Ref: Ganong Review of Medical Physiology, 23rd ed. p 431;*
Guyton Textbook of Medical Physiology 11th ed. p 794;
http://cariology.wikifoundry.com/p/Buffer+System+in+the+Saliva

The carbonic acid/bicarbonate buffer is the major buffer in stimulated saliva, with bicarbonate acting mainly to neutralize acids produced by bacteria when they digest sugars in the mouth or acids from the stomach. The concentration of the bicarbonate ion depends largely on the salivary flow rate.

127. Ans. (b) Vitamin B12 *Ref: Guyton Textbook of Medical Physiology, 11th ed. p 797*

The substance intrinsic factor, essential for absorption of vitamin B12 in the ileum, is secreted by the parietal cells along with the secretion of hydrochloric acid. When the acid-producing parietal cells of the stomach are destroyed, which frequently occurs in chronic gastritis, the person develops not only achlorhydria (lack of stomach acid secretion) but often also pernicious anemia because of failure of maturation of the red blood cells in the absence of vitamin B12 stimulation of the bone marrow.

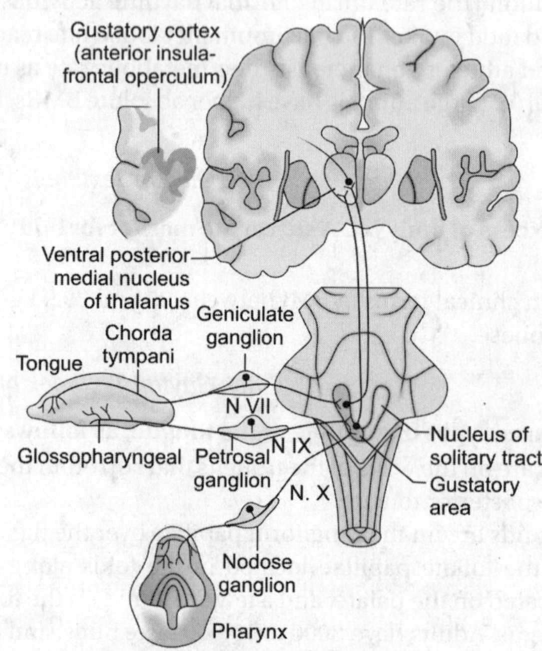

128. Ans. (b) Taste sensation *Ref: Guyton Textbook of Medical Physiology, 11th ed. p 666*

- Transmission of taste signals into the central nervous system.

129. Ans. (d) Lungs *Ref: Guyton Textbook of Medical Physiology, 11th ed. p 984*

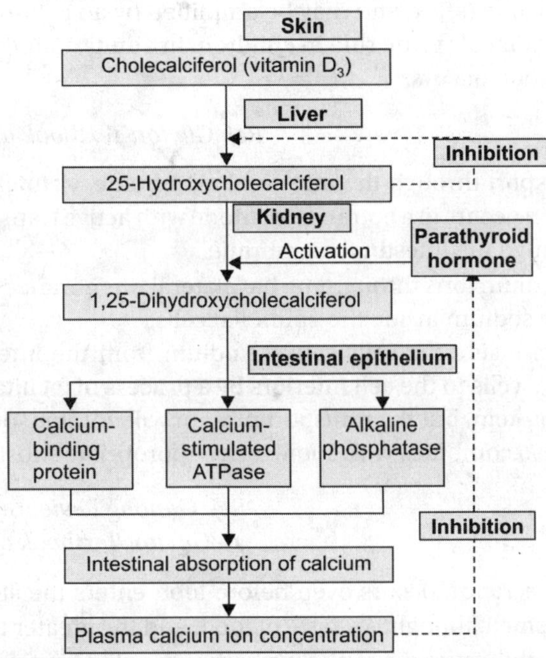

Activation of vitamin D3 to form 1,25-dihydroxycholecalciferol and the role of vitamin D in controlling the plasma calcium concentration.

130. Ans. (b) Pancreatic juice *Ref: Guyton Textbook of Medical Physiology, 11th ed. p 801*

- Gastric juice: pH of 1-2
- Bile pH 7-8
- Saliva: pH 6.2 to 7.4
- Pancreatic juice: pH about 8.8
- Bicarbonate ion secretion by the pancreas provides an appropriate pH for action of the pancreatic digestive enzymes, which function optimally in a slightly alkaline or neutral medium, at a pH of 7.0 to 8.0. Fortunately, the pH of the sodium bicarbonate secretion averages 8.0.

131. Ans. (d) 1,25- dihydroxycholecalciferol *Ref: Guyton Textbook of Medical Physiology, 11th ed. p 985*
Also refer explanation of Chapter 5 AIPGEE Q-14

1, 25-dihydroxycholecalciferol itself functions as a type of 'hormone' to promote intestinal absorption of calcium. It does this principally by increasing, over a period of about 2 days, formation of a calcium-binding protein in the intestinal epithelial cells. This protein functions in the brush border of these cells to transport calcium into the cell cytoplasm, and the calcium then moves through the basolateral membrane of the cell by facilitated diffusion. The rate of calcium absorption is directly proportional to the quantity of this calcium-binding protein. Furthermore, this protein remains in the cells for several weeks after the 1,25-dihydroxycholecalciferol has been removed from the body, thus causing a prolonged effect on calcium absorption.

132. Ans. (c) Gastrocolic reflex *Ref: Ganong Review of Medical Physiology, 23rd ed. p 478*
Guyton Textbook of Medical Physiology, 11th ed. p776

- Reflexes from the gut to the prevertebral sympathetic ganglia and then back to the gastrointestinal tract. These reflexes transmit signals long distances to other areas of the gastrointestinal tract, such as signals from the

stomach to cause evacuation of the colon (the gastrocolic reflex), signals from the colon and small intestine to inhibit stomach motility and stomach secretion (the enterogastric reflexes), and reflexes from the colon to inhibit emptying of ileal contents into the colon (the colonoileal reflex).
- Distention of the stomach by food initiates contractions of the rectum and, frequently, a desire to defecate. The response is called the gastrocolic reflex, and may be amplified by an action of gastrin on the colon. Because of the response, defecation after meals is the rule in children. In adults, habit and cultural factors play a large role in determining when defecation occurs.

133. Ans. (b) Na^+ *Ref: Guyton Textbook of Medical Physiology, 11th ed. p 816*

In the absence of sodium transport through the intestinal membrane, virtually no glucose can be absorbed. The reason is that glucose absorption occurs in a cotransport mode with active transport of sodium. There are two stages in the transport of sodium through the intestinal membrane.
- First is active transport of sodium ions through the basolateral membranes of the intestinal epithelial cells into the blood, thereby depleting sodium inside the epithelial cells.
- Second, decrease of sodium inside the cells causes sodium from the intestinal lumen to move through the brush border of the epithelial cells to the cell interiors by a process of facilitated diffusion. That is, a sodium ion combines with a transport protein, but the transport protein will not transport the sodium to the interior of the cell until the protein itself also combines with some other appropriate substance such as glucose.

134. Ans. (c) Pavlov's pouch *Ref: Ganong Review of Medical Physiology, 23rd ed. p 292*
Guyton Textbook of Medical Physiology, 11th ed. p 798

The cephalic phase of gastric secretion occurs even before food enters the stomach, especially while it is being eaten. It results from the sight, smell, thought, or taste of food, and the greater the appetite, the more intense is the stimulation. Neurogenic signals that cause the cephalic phase of gastric secretion originate in the cerebral cortex and in the appetite centers of the amygdala and hypothalamus. They are transmitted through the dorsal motor nuclei of the vagi and thence through the vagus nerves to the stomach. A conditioned reflex is a reflex response to a stimulus that previously elicited little or no response, acquired by repeatedly pairing the stimulus with another stimulus that normally does produce the response. In Pavlov's classic experiments, the salivation normally induced by placing meat in the mouth of a dog was studied. A bell was rung just before the meat was placed in the dog's mouth, and this was repeated a number of times until the animal would salivate when the bell was rung even though no meat was placed in its mouth. In this experiment, the meat placed in the mouth was the unconditioned stimulus (US), the stimulus that normally produces a particular innate response. The conditioned stimulus (CS) was the bell ringing.

135. Ans. (b) Pepsinogen *Ref: Ganong Review of Medical Physiology, 23rd ed. p 437*
Guyton Textbook of Medical Physiology, 11th ed. p 799

The most important of the pancreatic enzymes for digesting proteins are trypsin, chymotrypsin, and carboxypolypeptidase.

Stomach	*Pepsins (pepsinogens)*	*HCl*	*Proteins and polypeptides*
	Gastric lipase		Triglycerides
Exocrine pancreas	Trypsin (trypsinogen)	Enteropeptidase	Proteins and polypeptides
	Chymotrypsins (chymotrypsinogens)	Trypsin	Proteins and polypeptides
	Elastase (proelastase)	Trypsin	Elastin, some other proteins
	Carboxypeptidase A (procarboxypeptidase-A)	Trypsin	Proteins and polypeptides

Contd...

Contd...

Stomach	*Pepsins (pepsinogens)*	*HCl*	*Proteins and polypeptides*
	Carboxypeptidase B (procarboxypeptidase B)	Trypsin	Proteins and polypeptides
	Colipase (procolipase)	Trypsin	Fat droplets
	Pancreatic lipase	—	Triglycerides
	Bile salt-acid lipase		Cholesteryl esters
	Cholesteryl ester hydrolase	—	Cholesteryl esters
	Pancreatic α-amylase	Cl^-	Starch
	Ribonuclease	—	RNA
	Deoxyribonuclease	—	DNA
	Phospholipase A_2 (pro-phospholipase A^2)	Trypsin	Phospholipids

136. Ans. (c) Cholecystokinin *Ref: Guyton Textbook of Medical Physiology, 11th ed. p 803*

- By far the most potent stimulus for causing the gallbladder contractions is the hormone cholecystokinin.
- Cholecystokinin (CCK) is secreted by cells in the mucosa of the upper small intestine. It has a plethora of actions in the gastrointestinal system, but the most important appear to be the stimulation of pancreatic enzyme secretion, the contraction of the gallbladder (the action for which it was named), and relaxation of the sphincter of Oddi, which allows both bile and pancreatic juice to flow into the intestinal lumen.
- All three are enzymes, cholecystokinin is a hormone.

137. Ans. (c) Food in the stomach *Ref: Guyton Textbook of Medical Physiology, 11th ed. p 798*

Acid is secreted even if food is in the stomach but if question and options appear like this then mark option C. Cephalic Phase: The cephalic phase of gastric secretion occurs even before food enters the stomach, especially while it is being eaten. It results from the sight, smell, thought, or taste of food, and the greater the appetite, the more intense is the stimulation. Neurogenic signals that cause the cephalic phase of gastric secretion originate in the cerebral cortex and in the appetite centers of the amygdala and hypothalamus. They are transmitted through the dorsal motor nuclei of the vagi and thence through the vagus nerves to the stomach. This phase of secretion normally accounts for about 20 per cent of the gastric secretion associated with eating a meal. Gastric Phase: Once food enters the stomach, it excites (1) long vagovagal reflexes from the stomach to the brain and back to the stomach, (2) local enteric reflexes, and (3) the gastrin mechanism, all of which in turn cause secretion of gastric juice during several hours while food remains in the stomach. The gastric phase of secretion accounts for about 70 percent of the total gastric secretion associated with eating a meal and therefore accounts for most of the total daily gastric secretion of about 1500 milliliters. Intestinal Phase: The presence of food in the upper portion of the small intestine, particularly in the duodenum, will continue to cause stomach secretion of small amounts of gastric juice, probably partly because of small amounts of gastrin released by the duodenal mucosa.

138. Ans. (a) 1 *Ref: Refer explanation of Chapter 5, AIPGEE Q-15*

Refer explanation of 130

139. Ans. (b) Copper *Ref: Ganong Review of Medical Physiology, 23rd ed. p 532*

Ceruloplasmin is the major copper-carrying protein in the blood, and in addition plays a role in iron metabolism.

Name	*Principal function*	*Binding characteristics*	*Serum or plasma concentration*
Albumin	Binding and carrier protein; osmotic regulator	Hormones, amino acids, steroids, vitamins, fatty acids	4500–5000 mg/dL
Orosomucoid	Uncertain; may have a role in inflammation		Trace; rises in inflammation
α_1-antiprotease	Trypsin and general protease inhibitor	Proteases in serum and tissue secretions	1.3–1.4 mg/dL
α-fetoprotein	Osmotic regulation; binding and carrier protein	Hormones, amino acids	Found normally in fetal blood
α_2-macroglobulin	Inhibitor of serum endoproteases	Proteases	150–420 mg/dL
Antithrombin-III	Protease inhibitor of intrinsic coagulation system	1:1 binding to proteases	17–30 mg/dL
Ceruloplasmin	Transport of copper	Six atoms copper/mol	15–60 mg/dL
C-reactive protein	Uncertain; has role in tissue inflammation	Complement C1q	< 1 mg/dL; rises in inflammation
Fibrinogen	Precursor to fibrin in hemostasis		200–450 mg/dL
Haptoglobin	Binding, transport of cell-free hemoglobin	Hemoglobin 1:1 binding	40–180 mg/dL
Hemopexin	Binds to porphyrins, particularly heme for heme recycling	1:1 with heme	50–100 mg/dL
Transferrin	Transport of iron	Two atoms iron/mol	3.0–6.5 mg/dL

140. Ans. (a) Enteropeptidase

141. Ans. (a) Formation of sinusoids

142. Ans. (b) Stercobilin *Ref: Guyton Textbook of Medical Physiology, 11th ed. p 817*

The feces normally are about three-fourth water and one-fourth solid matter that itself is composed of about 30 percent dead bacteria, 10 to 20 percent fat, 10 to 20 percent inorganic matter, 2 to 3 percent protein, and 30 percent undigested roughage from the food and dried constituents of digestive juices, such as bile pigment and sloughed epithelial cells. The brown color of feces is caused by stercobilin and urobilin, derivatives of bilirubin. The odor is caused principally by products of bacterial action; these products vary from one person to another, depending on each person's colonic bacterial flora and on the type of food eaten. The actual odoriferous products include indole, skatole, mercaptans, and hydrogen sulfide.

143. Ans. (a) Sustentacular cells *Ref: Guyton Textbook of Medical Physiology, 11th ed. p 664*

- A taste bud, which has a diameter of about 1/30 millimeter and a length of about 1/16 millimeter. The taste bud is composed of about 50 modified epithelial cells, some of which are supporting cells called sustentacular cells and others of which are taste cells.

144. Ans. (d) Endocrine dysfunction of the pancreas *Ref: Ganong Review of Medical Physiology, 23rd ed. p 322*
Guyton Textbook of Medical Physiology, 11th ed. p 975

A glucose tolerance test is a medical test in which glucose is given and blood samples taken afterward to determine how quickly it is cleared from the blood. The test is usually used to test for diabetes, insulin resistance, and sometimes reactive hypoglycemia and acromegaly, or rarer disorders of carbohydrate metabolism. In the most commonly performed version of the test, an oral glucose tolerance test (OGTT), a standard dose of glucose is ingested by mouth and blood levels are checked two hours later.

Procedure

- A zero time (baseline) blood sample is drawn.
- The patient is then given a measured dose (below) of glucose solution to drink within a 5 minutes timeframe.
- Blood is drawn at intervals for measurement of glucose (blood sugar), and sometimes insulin levels. The intervals and number of samples vary according to the purpose of the test. For simple diabetes screening, the most important sample is the 2 hours sample and the 0 and 2 hours samples may be the only ones collected. A laboratory may continue to collect blood for up to 6 hours depending on the protocol requested by the physician.

145. Ans. (b) Glycated hemoglobin *Ref: Refer explanation of Chapter 4 COMEDK/KCET Q-3*

Refer explanation of Ans. 101

146. Ans. (a) Oxyntic cells *Ref: Guyton Textbook of Medical Physiology, 11th ed. p 795*

The stomach mucosa has two important types of tubular glands: oxyntic glands (also called gastric glands) and pyloric glands. The oxyntic (acid-forming) glands secrete hydrochloric acid, pepsinogen, intrinsic factor, and mucus. The pyloric glands secrete mainly mucus for protection of the pyloric mucosa from the stomach acid. They also secrete the hormone gastrin.

147. Ans. (d) Ileum *Ref: Guyton Textbook of Medical Physiology, 11th ed. p 797*

Secretion of intrinsic factor: The substance intrinsic factor, essential for absorption of vitamin B12 in the ileum, is secreted by the parietal cells along with the secretion of hydrochloric acid.

148. Ans. (d) Beta cell dysfunction *Ref: Guyton Textbook of Medical Physiology, 11th ed. p 972*

Injury to the beta cells of the pancreas or diseases that impair insulin production can lead to type I diabetes. Viral infections or autoimmune disorders may be involved in the destruction of beta cells in many patients with type I diabetes, although heredity also plays a major role in determining the susceptibility of the beta cells to destruction by these insults. In some instances, there may be a hereditary tendency for beta cell degeneration even without viral infections or autoimmune disorders.

149. Ans. (b) Increase secretion of bicarbonate by pancreas

150. Ans. (b) 0.6 mg *Ref: Guyton Textbook of Medical Physiology, 11th ed. p*

Daily loss of iron: A man excretes about 0.6 milligram of iron each day, mainly into the feces. Additional quantities of iron are lost when bleeding occurs. For a woman, additional menstrual loss of blood brings long-term iron loss to an average of about 1.3 mg/day.

151. Ans. (c) HCI and intrinsic factor *Ref: Guyton Textbook of Medical Physiology, 11th ed. p 795*

In addition to mucus-secreting cells that line the entire surface of the stomach, the stomach mucosa has two important types of tubular glands: oxyntic glands (also called gastric glands) and pyloric glands. The oxyntic (acid-forming) glands secrete hydrochloric acid, pepsinogen, intrinsic factor, and mucus. The pyloric glands secrete mainly mucus for protection of the pyloric mucosa from the stomach acid. They also secrete the hormone gastrin.

- Oxyntic gland from the body of the stomach

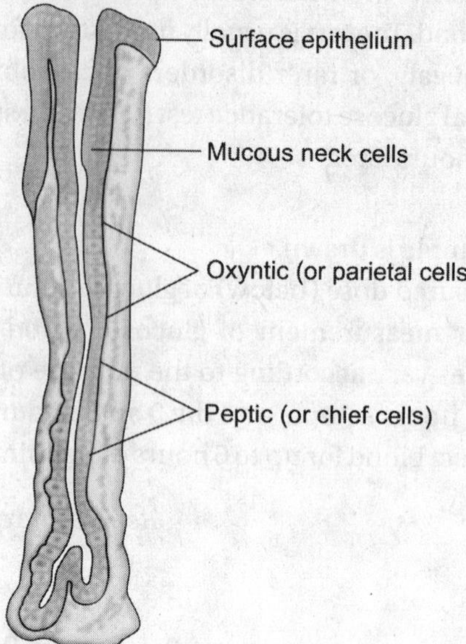

152. Ans. (d) Gloss pharyngeal nerve *Ref: http://en.wikipedia.org/wiki/pharyngeal_reflex*

In the case of the pharyngeal gag reflex:

- The sensory limb is mediated predominantly by CN IX (glossopharyngeal nerve).
- The motor limb by CN X (vagus nerve).

CARDIOVASCULAR PHYSIOLOGY

153. Ans. (a) Flat bones *Ref: Guyton Textbook of Medical Physiology, 11th ed. p 420*

In the early weeks of embryonic life, primitive, nucleated red blood cells are produced in the yolk sac. During the middle trimester of gestation, the liver is the main organ for production of red blood cells, but reasonable numbers are also produced in the spleen and lymph nodes. Then, during the last month or so of gestation and, after birth, red blood cells are produced exclusively in the bone marrow. The bone marrow of essentially all bones produces red blood cells until a person is 5 years old. The marrow of the long bones, except for the proximal portions of the humeri and tibiae, becomes quite fatty and produces no more red blood cells after about age 20 years. Beyond this age, most red cells continue to be produced in the marrow of the membranous bones, such as the vertebrae, sternum, ribs, and ilia. Even in these bones, the marrow becomes less productive as age increases.

154. Ans. (d) Liver disease *Ref: Robbins Basic Pathology, 8th ed. p 898*

Prothrombin time (PT): This assay tests the extrinsic and common coagulation pathways. The clotting of plasma after addition of an exogenous source of tissue thromboplastin (e.g. brain extract) and Ca^{++} ions is measured in seconds. A prolonged PT can result from deficiency or dysfunction of factor V, factor VII, factor X, prothrombin, or fibrinogen. The clinical features of chronic hepatitis are extremely variable and are not predictive of outcome. In some patients, the only signs of chronic disease are persistent elevations of serum transaminases. The most common symptom is fatigue; less common symptoms are malaise, loss of appetite, and occasional bouts of mild jaundice. Physical findings are few, the most common being spider angiomas, palmar erythema, mild hepatomegaly, hepatic tenderness, and mild splenomegaly. Laboratory studies may reveal prolongation of the prothrombin time and, in some instances, hyperglobulinemia, hyperbilirubinemia, and mild elevations in alkaline phosphatase levels.

155. Ans. (b) Multiple nuclei *Ref: Guyton Textbook of Medical Physiology, 11th ed. p 103*

Cardiac muscle is one of three major types of muscle, the others being skeletal and smooth muscle. These three types of muscle all form in a process known as myogenesis. The cells that constitute cardiac muscle, called cardiomyocytes or myocardiocytes, contain only one, unique nucleus. Cardiac muscle fibers arranged in a latticework, with the fibers dividing, recombining, and then spreading again. The dark areas crossing the cardiac muscle fibers are called intercalated discs; they are actually cell membranes that separate individual cardiac muscle cells from one another. At each intercalated disc, the cell membranes fuse with one another in such a way that they form permeable 'communicating' junctions (gap junctions) that allow almost totally free diffusion of ions. Therefore, from a functional point of view, ions move with ease in the intracellular fluid along the longitudinal axes of the cardiac muscle fibers, so that action potentials travel easily from one cardiac muscle cell to the next, past the intercalated discs. Cardiac muscle is a syncytium of many heart muscle cells in which the cardiac cells are so interconnected that when one of these cells becomes excited, the action potential spreads to all of them, spreading from cell to cell throughout the latticework interconnections.

156. Ans. (a) Plasmin *Ref: Guyton Textbook of Medical Physiology, 11th ed. p 464*

The plasma proteins contain a euglobulin called plasminogen (or profibrinolysin) that, when activated, becomes a substance called plasmin (or fibrinolysin). Plasmin is a proteolytic enzyme that resembles trypsin, the most important proteolytic digestive enzyme of pancreatic secretion. Plasmin digests fibrin fibers and some other protein coagulants, such as fibrinogen, Factor V, Factor VIII, prothrombin, and Factor XII. Therefore, whenever plasmin is formed, it can cause lysis of a clot by destroying many of the clotting factors, thereby sometimes even causing hypocoagulability of the blood.

157. Ans. (c) HbA *Ref: Ganong Review of Medical Physiology, 23rd ed. p 523*

In normal adult human hemoglobin (hemoglobin A), the two polypeptides are called α chains, each of which contains 141 amino acid residues, and β chains, each of which contains 146 amino acid residues. Thus, hemoglobin A is designated α2β2. Not all the hemoglobin in the blood of normal adults is hemoglobin A. About 2.5% of the hemoglobin is hemoglobin A2, in which β chains are replaced by δ chains (α2δ2).

HbA	$\alpha_2\beta_2$	95-98% of adult hemoglobin
HbF	$\alpha_2\gamma_2$	2% of adult hemoglobin
HbA_2	$\alpha_2\delta_2$	2.5% of adult hemoglobin
HbS	Sickle cell hemoglobin	α—normal; β—abnormal
HbA_c	Glycosylated hemoglobin	Glucose molely attached to valine in each β chain

158. Ans. (a) Heparin *Ref: Ganong Review of Medical Physiology, 23rd ed. p 535, 590*
Guyton Textbook of Medical Physiology, 11th ed. p 464

Heparin is another powerful anticoagulant, but its concentration in the blood is normally low, so that only under special physiologic conditions does it have significant anticoagulant effects. However, heparin is used widely as a pharmacological agent in medical practice in much higher concentrations to prevent intravascular clotting. Heparin is produced by many different cells of the body, but especially large quantities are formed by the basophilic mast cells located in the pericapillary connective tissue throughout the body. Mast cells are abundant in tissue surrounding the capillaries of the lungs and to a lesser extent capillaries of the liver. The action of heparin lasts about 1.5 to 4 hours. The injected heparin is destroyed by an enzyme in the blood known as heparinase.

159. Ans. (a) 2, 7, 9, 10 *Ref: Guyton Textbook of Medical Physiology, 11th ed. p 862*

Substances formed in the liver that are used in the coagulation process include fibrinogen, prothrombin, accelerator globulin, Factor VII, and several other important factors. Vitamin K is required by the metabolic processes of the liver for the formation of several of these substances, especially prothrombin and factors VII, IX, and X. In the absence of vitamin K, the concentrations of all these decrease markedly, and this almost prevents blood coagulation.

160. Ans. (c) Plasmin *Ref: Refer explanation of Chapter 6 AIPGEE Q-4*

Refer explanation of Ans 156.

161. Ans. (a) Large veins *Ref: Guyton Textbook of Medical Physiology, 11th ed. p 162*
Ganong Review of Medical Physiology, 23rd ed. p 549

- The velocity of blood flow is inversely proportional to vascular cross-sectional area.
- When blood flows from the venules to the large veins, its average velocity increases as the total cross-sectional area of the vessels decreases. In the great veins, the velocity of blood is about one-fourth that in the aorta, averaging about 10 cm/s.

162. Ans. (d) Eosinophilia *Ref: http://en.wikipedia.org/wiki/Eosinophilia*

- Diagnosis of eosinophilia is via a complete blood count (CBC), but diagnostic procedures directed at the underlying cause vary depending on the suspected condition(s). An absolute eosinophil count is not generally needed if the CBC shows marked eosinophilia.
- Eosinophilia can be idiopathic (primary) or, more commonly, secondary to another disease. In the Western World, allergic or atopic diseases are the most common causes, especially those of the respiratory or integumentary systems. In the developing world, parasites are the most common cause. A parasitic infection of nearly any bodily tissue can cause eosinophilia. Diseases that feature eosinophilia as a sign include the following:
  - Allergic disorders, e.g. asthma, hay fever, drug allergies
    Allergic skin diseases, e.g. pemphigus, dermatitis herpetiformis
  - Parasitic infections
  - Some forms of malignancy, e.g.Hodgkin's lymphoma, some forms of non-Hodgkin lymphoma
  - Systemic autoimmune diseases (e.g. SLE)
  - Some forms of vasculitis (e.g. Churg-Strauss syndrome)
  - Cholesterol embolism (transiently)
  - Coccidioidomycosis (Valley fever), a fungal disease prominent in the US Southwest
  - Interstitial nephropathy
  - Hyperimmunoglobulin E syndrome, an immune disorder characterized by high levels of serum IgE.

163. Ans. (a) Factor IX *Ref: Ganong Review of Medical Physiology, 23rd ed. p 535*

Examples of diseases due to deficiency of clotting factors

Deficiency of factor	*Clinical syndrome*	*Cause*
I	Afibrinogenemia	Depletion during pregnancy with premature separation of placenta; also congenital (rare)
II	Hypoprothrombinemia (hemorrhagic tendency in liver disease)	Decreased hepatic synthesis, usually secondary to vitamin K deficiency
V	Parahemophilia	Congenital
VII	Hypoconvertinemia	Congenital
VIII	Hemophilia A (classic hemophilia)	Congenital defect due to various abnormalities of the gene on X chromosome that codes for factor VIII; disease is therefore inherited as sex-linked characteristic

Deficiency of factor	*Clinical syndrome*	*Cause*
IX	Hemophilia B (Christmas disease)	Congenital
X	Stuart-Prower factor deficiency	Congenital
XI	PTA deficiency	Congenital
XII	Hageman trait	Congenital

164. Ans. (d) Thalassemia *Ref: Ganong Review of Medical Physiology, 23rd ed. p 535, 534, http://en.wikipedia.org/wiki/Ibuprofen Robbins Basic Pathology, 8th ed. p 632*

- Christmas disease—blood clotting disorder caused by a mutation of the Factor IX gene.
- Von Willebrand disease (vWD) is the most common hereditary coagulation abnormality arises from a qualitative or quantitative deficiency of von Willebrand factor (vWF), a multimeric protein that is required for platelet adhesion.
- Ibuprofen has an antiplatelet effect, though it is relatively mild and somewhat short-lived compared with aspirin or prescription antiplatelet drugs.
- Thalassemia (British English: thalassemia) are forms of inherited autosomal recessive blood disorders that originated in the Mediterranean region. In thalassemia, the disorder is caused by the weakening and destruction of red blood cells. Thalassemia is caused by variant or missing genes that affect how the body makes hemoglobin. People with thalassemia make less hemoglobin and fewer circulating red blood cells than normal, which results in mild or severe anemia.

165. Ans. (c) Self-renewal

166. Ans. (d) Louder than the first heart sound *Ref: Guyton Textbook of Medical Physiology, 11th ed. p 110*

When the ventricles contract, one first hears a sound caused by closure of the AV valves. The vibration is low in pitch and relatively long-lasting and is known as the first heart sound. When the aortic and pulmonary valves close at the end of systole, one hears a rapid snap because these valves close rapidly, and the surroundings vibrate for a short period. This sound is called the second heart sound.

167. Ans. (a) Disseminated intravascular coagulation (DIC) *Ref: Ganong Review of Medical Physiology, 23rd ed. p 534 Guyton Textbook of Medical Physiology, 11th ed. p 466*

Occasionally, the clotting mechanism becomes activated in widespread areas of the circulation, giving rise to the condition called disseminated intravascular coagulation. This often results from the presence of large amounts of traumatized or dying tissue in the body that releases great quantities of tissue factor into the blood. Frequently, the clots are small but numerous, and they plug a large share of the small peripheral blood vessels. This occurs especially in patients with widespread septicemia, in which either circulating bacteria or bacterial toxins especially endotoxins activate the clotting mechanisms. Plugging of small peripheral vessels greatly diminishes delivery of oxygen and other nutrients to the tissues, this situation can leads to or exacerbates circulatory shock. It is partly for this reason that septicemic shock is lethal in 85 percent or more of patients. A peculiar effect of disseminated intravascular coagulation is that the patient on occasion begins to bleed. The reason for this is that so many of the clotting factors are removed by the widespread clotting that too few procoagulants remain to allow normal hemostasis of the remaining blood. Disseminated intravascular coagulation is serious complication of septicemia, extensive tissue injury, and other diseases in which fibrin is deposited in the vascular system and many small- and medium-sized vessels are thrombosed. The increased consumption of platelets and coagulation factors causes bleeding to occur at the same time.

168. Ans. (b) Aggregation of platelets at damaged blood vessels

Ref: Guyton Textbook of Medical Physiology, 11th ed. p 457

Hemostasis is achieved by several mechanisms:

- Vascular constriction
- Formation of a platelet plug
- Formation of a blood clot as a result of blood coagulation
- Eventual growth of fibrous tissue into the blood clot to close the hole in the vessel permanently.

169. Ans. (b) Cyanocobalamin *Ref: Guyton Textbook of Medical Physiology, 11th ed. p 423*

Vitamin B12, also called cobalamin, is a water-soluble vitamin with a key role in the normal functioning of the brain and nervous system, and for the formation of blood. A common cause of red blood cell maturation failure is failure to absorb vitamin B12 from the gastrointestinal tract. This often occurs in the disease pernicious anemia, in which the basic abnormality is an atrophic gastric mucosa that fails to produce normal gastric secretions. The parietal cells of the gastric glands secrete a glycoprotein called intrinsic factor, which combines with vitamin B12 in food and makes the B12 available for absorption by the gut. Once vitamin B12 has been absorbed from the gastrointestinal tract, it is first stored in large quantities in the liver, then released slowly as needed by the bone marrow.The minimum amount of vitamin B12 required each day to maintain normal red cell maturation is only 1 to 3 micrograms, and the normal storage in the liver and other body tissues is about 1000 times this amount. Therefore, 3 to 4 years of defective B12 absorption are usually required to cause maturation failure anemia.

170. Ans. (d) When diameter of blood vessels increases *Ref: Ganong Review of Medical Physiology, 23rd ed. p 540*

The flow of blood in straight blood vessels, like the flow of liquids in narrow rigid tubes, is normally laminar. Laminar flow occurs at velocities up to a certain critical velocity. At or above this velocity, flow is turbulent. Laminar flow is silent, but turbulent flow creates sounds. The probability of turbulence is also related to the diameter of the vessel and the viscosity of the blood. This probability can be expressed by the ratio of inertial to viscous forces as follows:

- Where Re is the Reynolds number, named for the man who described the relationship; ρ is the density of the fluid; D is the diameter of the tube under consideration; V is the velocity of the flow; and η is the viscosity of the fluid.
- The higher the value of Re, the greater the probability of turbulence. When D is in cm, V is in cm/s1, and η is in poise; flow is usually not turbulent if Re is less than 2000. When Re is more than 3000, turbulence is almost always present.

171. Ans. (b) Pulmonary vasoconstriction in hypoxia *Ref: Ganong Review of Medical Physiology, 23rd ed. p 628*

Guyton Textbook of Medical Physiology, 11th ed. p 518

The peripheral chemoreceptor system

Special nervous chemical receptors, called chemoreceptors, are located in several areas outside the brain. They are especially important for detecting changes in oxygen in the blood. The chemoreceptors transmit nervous signals to the respiratory center in the brain to help regulate respiratory activity. Most of the chemoreceptors are in the carotid bodies. However, a few are also in the aortic bodies. There is a carotid body near the carotid bifurcation on each side, and there are usually two or more aortic bodies near the arch of the aorta. Each carotid and aortic body (glomus) contains islands of two types of cells, type I and type II cells, surrounded by fenestrated sinusoidal capillaries. Type I glomus cells have O_2-sensitive K^+ channels, whose conductance is reduced in proportion to the degree of hypoxia to which they are exposed. This reduces the K^+ efflux, depolarizing the cell and causing Ca^{2+} influx, primarily via L-type Ca^{2+} channels. The Ca^{2+} influx triggers action potentials and transmitter release, with consequent excitation of the afferent nerve endings. The smooth muscle of pulmonary arteries contains similar O2- sensitive K+ channels, which mediate the vasoconstriction caused by hypoxia. This is in contrast to systemic arteries, which contain adenosine triphosphate (ATP) dependent K^+ channels that permit more K^+ efflux with hypoxia and consequently cause vasodilation instead of vasoconstriction.

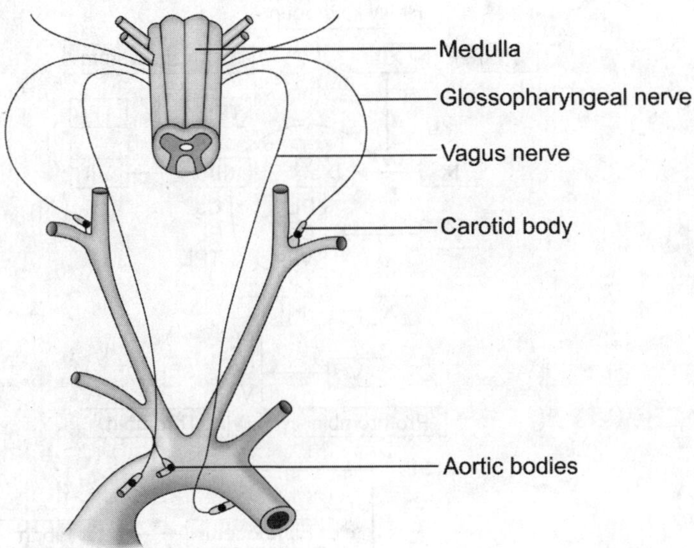

Respiratory control by peripheral chemoreceptors in the carotid and aortic bodies.

172. Ans. (c) Christmas disease *Ref: Refer explanation of Chapter 6 AIPGEE Q-11*

Refer explanation of Ans. 163.

173. Ans. (c) Flat bones *Ref:Refer explanation of Chapter 6 AIPGEE Q-1*

Refer explanation of Ans. 153.

174. Ans. (c) Ferrous form *Ref: Ganong Review of Medical Physiology, 23rd ed. p 458*
Guyton Textbook of Medical Physiology, 11th ed. p 425

Most of the iron in the diet is in the ferric (Fe^{3+}) form, whereas it is the ferrous (Fe^{2+}) form that is absorbed. Like most mineral nutrients, the majority of the iron absorbed from digested food or supplements is absorbed in the duodenum by enterocytes of the duodenal lining. These cells have special molecules that allow them to move iron into the body. To be absorbed, dietary iron can be absorbed as part of a protein, such as heme protein or must be in its ferrous Fe^{2+} form. A ferric reductase enzyme on the enterocytes brush border, reduces ferric Fe^{3+} to Fe^{2+}. A protein called divalent metal transporter 1 DMT1, which transports all kinds of divalent metals into the body, then transports the iron across the enterocyte's cell membrane and into the cell.

175. Ans. (b) Labile factor *Ref: Ganong Review of Medical Physiology, 23rd ed. p 533*

In the presence of phospholipids from aggregated platelets, Ca^{2+}, and factor V, activated factor X catalyzes the conversion of prothrombin to thrombin.

The clotting mechanism (a: active form of clotting factor, TPL: Tissue thromboplastin; TFI: Tissue factor pathway inhibitor)

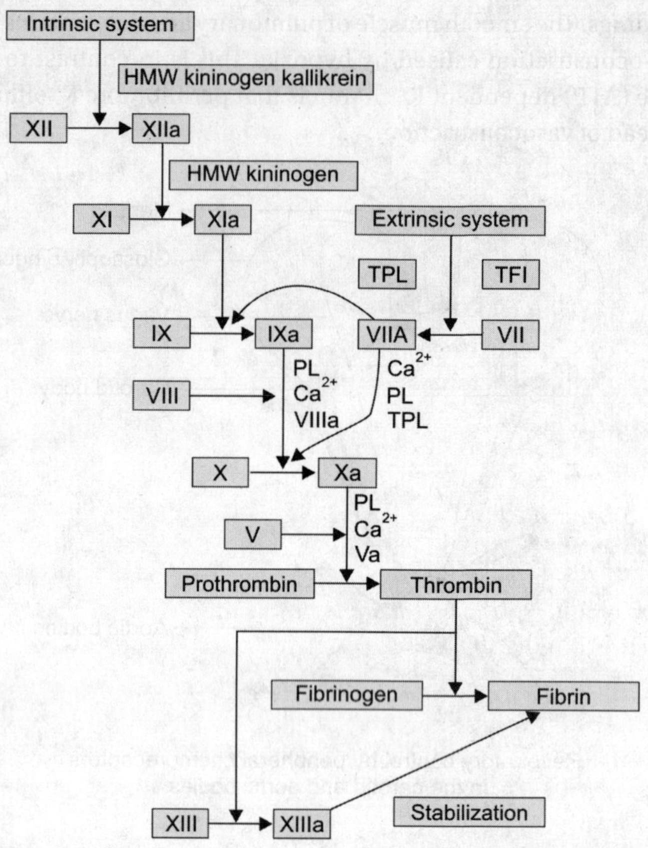

176. Ans. (b) Albumin *Ref: Ganong Review of Medical Physiology, 23rd ed. p 552*

The principal proteins synthesized by the liver are listed:

Acute-phase proteins
Albumin
Clotting factors
Steroid-binding and other hormone-binding proteins

Albumin is quantitatively the most significant, and accounts for the majority of plasma oncotic pressure. Many of the products are acute-phase proteins, proteins synthesized and secreted into the plasma on exposure to stressful stimuli. Others are proteins that transport steroids and other hormones in the plasma, and still others are clotting factors. Following blood loss, the liver replaces the plasma proteins in days to weeks. The only major class of plasma proteins not synthesized by the liver is the immunoglobulins.

177. Ans. (c) Spleen *Ref: Ganong Review of Medical Physiology, 23rd ed. p; Guyton Textbook of Medical Physiology, 11th ed. p 863, 180*

Blood cells passing through the splenic pulp before entering the sinuses undergo thorough squeezing. Therefore, it is to be expected that fragile red blood cells would not withstand the trauma. For this reason, many of the red blood cells destroyed in the body have their final demise in the spleen. After the cells rupture, the released hemoglobin and the cell stroma are digested by the reticuloendothelial cells of the spleen, and the products of digestion are mainly reused by the body. When the red blood cells have lived out their life span (on average, 120 days) and have become too fragile to exist in the circulatory system, their cell membranes rupture, and the released hemoglobin is phagocytized by tissue macrophages (also called the reticuloendothelial system) throughout the body. The hemoglobin is first split into globin and heme, and the heme ring is opened to give (1) free iron, which is transported in the blood by transferrin, and (2) a straight chain of four pyrrole nuclei, which is the substrate from which bilirubin will eventually be formed. The first substance formed is biliverdin, but this is rapidly reduced to free bilirubin, which is gradually released from the macrophages into the plasma.

178. Ans. (b) Posttranslation modifications *Ref: Faseb J. 1988 Apr;2(7):2252-61. Cofactors in and as Posttranslational Protein Modifications. Rucker RB, Wold F*

As cofactors for enzymes catalysing covalent modifications	*Examples of type of modifications*	*Related physiological phenomena*
Ascorbic acid	Reductant in prolyl and lysyl hydroxylations	Accumulation of underhydroxylated collagen and enhanced degradation of collagen when ascorbate is limiting; increased fragility of small blood vessels and capillaries; loss of extracellular matrix integrity; scurvy
Vitamin K	Putative role in carbanion formation at the γ-position of glutamyl residues in coagulation factors (e.g. prothrombin) and γ-carboxyglutamyl-enriched proteins in mineralized tissue (e.g. osteocalcin)	Hemorrhagic disorders, prolonged clotting time; impaired development and new bone formation when vitamin K is limiting
Pyrroloquinoline	Provides carbonyl function at the active site of lysyl oxidase; important to the oxidative deamination of lysyl (collagen or elastin) and hydroxylysyl (collagen) residues for eventual formation of cross-linking	Cofactor for the copper-containing amine oxidases; site of action of many dietary and pharmacological inhibitors of collagen-elastin cross-linking, such as hydrazines and aminonitriles
Copper	Cofactor for lysyl oxidase	Deficiency causes decreased collagen and elastin cross-linking; reduced tensile properties of collagen fibers and elasticity in elastic fibers
Manganese	Cofactor for many glycosyl transferases	Deficiency causes abnormal accumulation and turnover of glycoproteins in cartilaginous structures
Iron	Coordination of oxygen in numerous oxidases and hydroxylases	Effects of deficiencies in vitro, as the result of iron chelating agents (e.g. α, α-dipyridyl) are similar to those for ascorbic acid deficiency

Selected examples of cofactors and essential nutrients involved in protein posttranslalional covalent modifications

179. Ans. (d) Generates impulses at the highest rate *Ref: Guyton Textbook of Medical Physiology, 11th ed. p 120*

Why does the sinus node rather than the A-V node or the Purkinje fibers control the heart's rhythmicity? The answer derives from the fact that the discharge rate of the sinus node is considerably faster than the natural self-excitatory discharge rate of either the A-V node or the Purkinje fibers. Each time the sinus node discharges, its impulse is conducted into both the A-V node and the Purkinje fibers, also discharging their excitable membranes. But the sinus node discharges again before either the A-V node or the Purkinje fibers can reach their own thresholds for self-excitation. Therefore, the new impulse from the sinus node discharges both the A-V node and the purkinje fibers before self-excitation can occur in either of these. Thus, the sinus node controls the beat of the heart because its rate of rhythmical discharge is faster than that of any other part of the heart. Therefore, the sinus node is virtually always the pacemaker of the normal heart.

180. Ans. (b) Arterioles *Ref: Guyton Textbook of Medical Physiology, 11th ed. p 161*

The function of the arteries is to transport blood under high pressure to the tissues. For this reason, the arteries have strong vascular walls, and blood flows at a high velocity in the arteries. The arterioles are the last small branches of the arterial system; they act as control conduits through which blood is released into the capillaries. The arteriole has a strong muscular wall that can close the arteriole completely or can, by relaxing, dilate it several fold, thus having the capability of vastly altering blood flow in each tissue bed in response to the need of the tissue. The function of the capillaries is to exchange fluid, nutrients, electrolytes, hormones, and other substances between the blood and the interstitial fluid. To serve this role, the capillary walls are very thin and have numerous minute capillary pores permeable to water and other small molecular substances. The venules collect blood from the capillaries, and they gradually coalesce into progressively larger veins. The veins function as conduits for transport of blood from the venules back to the heart; equally important, they serve as a major reservoir of extra blood. Because the pressure in the venous system is very low, the venous walls are thin. Even so, they are muscular enough to contract or expand and thereby act as a controllable reservoir for the extra blood, either a small or a large amount, depending on the needs of the circulation.

181. Ans. (a) Capillary blood flow *Ref: Ganong Review of Medical Physiology, 23rd ed. p 543*

A large amount of blood can be added to the venous system before the veins become distended to the point where further increments in volume produce a large rise in venous pressure. The veins are therefore called capacitance vessels. The small arteries and arterioles are referred to as resistance vessels because they are the principal site of the peripheral resistance.

182. Ans. (c) Amount of hemoglobin in the blood *Ref: Guyton Textbook of Medical Physiology, 11th ed. p 505*

Normally, about 97 percent of the oxygen transported from the lungs to the tissues is carried in chemical combination with hemoglobin in the red blood cells. The remaining 3 percent is transported in the dissolved state in the water of the plasma and blood cells. Thus, under normal conditions, oxygen is carried to the tissues almost entirely by hemoglobin.

183. Ans. (b) 5 *Ref: Guyton Textbook of Medical Physiology, 11th ed. p 531*

The term cyanosis means blueness of the skin, and its cause is excessive amounts of deoxygenated hemoglobin in the skin blood vessels, especially in the capillaries. This deoxygenated hemoglobin has an intense dark blue-purple color that is transmitted through the skin. In general, definite cyanosis appears whenever the arterial blood contains more than 5 gm of deoxygenated hemoglobin in each 100 milliliters of blood. A person with anemia almost never becomes cyanotic because there is not enough hemoglobin for 5 grams to be deoxygenated in 100 milliliters of arterial blood. Conversely, in a person with excess red blood cells, as occurs in polycythemia vera, the great excess of available hemoglobin that can become deoxygenated leads frequently to cyanosis, even under otherwise normal conditions.

184. Ans. (a) Predominantly streamline *Ref: Refer explanation of Chapter 6, AIPGEE Q-18*

Refer explanation of Ans. 170.

185. Ans. (a) Right coronary artery and during diastole *Ref: Guyton Textbook of Medical Physiology, 11th ed. p 249-250*

The left coronary artery supplies mainly the anterior and left lateral portions of the left ventricle, whereas the right coronary artery supplies most of the right ventricle as well as the posterior part of the left ventricle in 80 to 90 percent of people. The coronary capillary blood flow in the left ventricle muscle falls to a low value during systole, which is opposite to flow in vascular beds elsewhere in the body. The reason for this is strong compression of the left ventricular muscle around the intramuscular vessels during systolic contraction. During diastole, the cardiac muscle relaxes and no longer obstructs blood flow through the left ventricular muscle capillaries, so that blood flows rapidly during all of diastole.

186. Ans. (c) Von wille brands factor *Ref: Guyton Textbook of Medical Physiology, 11th ed. p 458*

When platelets come in contact with a damaged vascular surface, especially with collagen fibers in the vascular wall, the platelets themselves immediately change their own characteristics drastically. They begin to swell; they assume irregular forms with numerous irradiating pseudopods protruding from their surfaces; their contractile proteins contract forcefully and cause the release of granules that contain multiple active factors; they become sticky so that they adhere to collagen in the tissues and to a protein called von Willebrand factor that leaks into the traumatized tissue from the plasma; they secrete large quantities of ADP; and their enzymes form thromboxane A2. The ADP and thromboxane in turn act on nearby platelets to activate them as well, and the stickiness of these additional platelets causes them to adhere to the original activated platelets.

187. Ans. (c) Monocyte *Ref: Guyton Textbook of Medical Physiology, 11th ed. p 431*

The monocytes have a short transit time, 10 to 20 hours in the blood, before wandering through the capillary membranes into the tissues. Once in the tissues, they swell to much larger sizes to become tissue macrophages, and, in this form, can live for months unless destroyed while performing phagocytic functions.

188. Ans. (c) Heme *Ref: Guyton Textbook of Medical Physiology, 11th ed. p 863*

The hemoglobin is first split into globin and heme, and the heme ring is opened to give (1) free iron, which is transported in the blood by transferrin, and (2) a straight chain of four pyrrole nuclei, which is the substrate from which bilirubin will eventually be formed. The first substance formed is biliverdin, but this is rapidly reduced to free bilirubin, which is gradually released from the macrophages into the plasma.

189. Ans. (b) Bleeding time

190. Ans. (d) O negative *Ref: http://en.wikipedia.org/wiki/Blood_type#Red_blood_cell_compatibility*

- Blood group AB individuals have both A and B antigens on the surface of their RBCs, and their blood plasma does not contain any antibodies against either A or B antigen. Therefore, an individual with type AB blood can receive blood from any group (with AB being preferable), but cannot donate blood to any group other than AB. They are known as universal recipients.
- Blood group A individuals have the A antigen on the surface of their RBCs, and blood serum containing IgM antibodies against the B antigen. Therefore, a group A individual can receive blood only from individuals of groups A or O (with A being preferable), and can donate blood to individuals with type A or AB.

Red blood cell compatibility table								
	Donor							
Recipient	O^-	O^+	A^-	A^+	B^-	B^+	AB^-	AB^+
O^-	✓	✗	✗	✗	✗	✗	✗	✗
O^+	✓	✓	✗	✗	✗	✗	✗	✗
A^-	✓	✗	✓	✗	✗	✗	✗	✗
A^+	✓	✓	✓	✓	✗	✗	✗	✗
B^-	✓	✗	✗	✗	✓	✗	✗	✗
B^+	✓	✓	✗	✗	✓	✓	✗	✗
AB^-	✓	✗	✓	✗	✓	✗	✓	✗
AB^+	✓	✓	✓	✓	✓	✓	✓	✓

- Blood group B individuals have the B antigen on the surface of their RBCs, and blood serum containing IgM antibodies against the A antigen. Therefore, a group B individual can receive blood only from individuals of groups B or O (with B being preferable), and can donate blood to individuals with type B or AB.

- Blood group O (or blood group zero in some countries) individuals do not have either A or B antigens on the surface of their RBCs, and their blood serum contains IgM anti-A and anti-B antibodies against the A and B blood group antigens. Therefore, a group O individual can receive blood only from a group O individual, but can donate blood to individuals of any ABO blood group (i.e. A, B, O or AB). If a patient in a hospital situation were to need a blood transfusion in an emergency, and if the time taken to process the recipient's blood would cause a detrimental delay, O Negative blood can be issued. They are known as universal donors.

191. Ans. (a) VIII a and V a *Ref: Ganong Review of Medical Physiology, 23rd ed. p 533*

The endothelium of the blood vessels also plays an active role in preventing the extension of clots. All endothelial cells except those in the cerebral microcirculation produce thrombomodulin, a thrombin-binding protein, on their surfaces. In circulating blood, thrombin is a procoagulant that activates factors V and VIII, but when it binds to thrombomodulin, it becomes an anticoagulant in that the thrombomodulinthrombin complex activates protein C. Activated protein C (APC), along with its cofactor protein S, inactivates factors V and VIII and inactivates an inhibitor of tissue plasminogen activator, increasing the formation of plasmin.

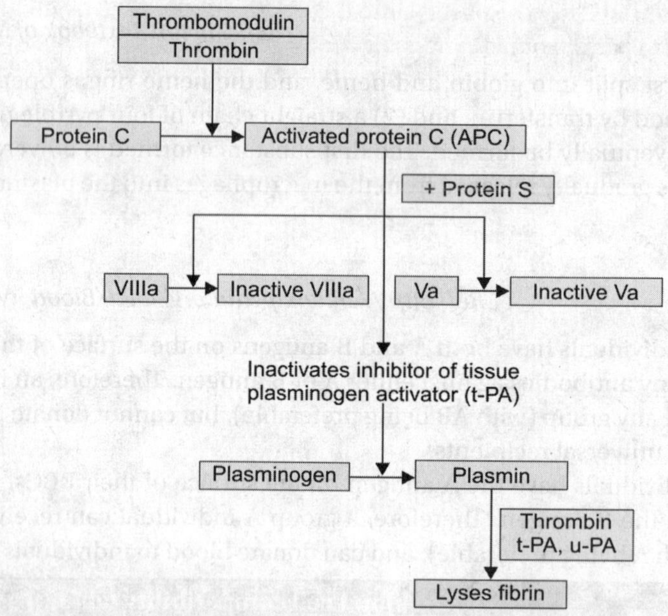

The fibrinolytic system and its regulation by protein C.

192. Ans. (a) Sudden closure of mitral and tricuspid valve

Ref: Guyton Textbook of Medical Physiology, 11th ed. p 110

When the ventricles contract, one first hears a sound caused by closure of the A-V valves. The vibration is low in pitch and relatively long-lasting and is known as the first heart sound. When the aortic and pulmonary valves close at the end of systole, one hears a rapid snap because these valves close rapidly, and the surroundings vibrate for a short period. This sound is called the second heart sound.

193. Ans. (a) Bradykinin *Ref: Guyton Textbook of Medical Physiology, 11th ed. p 202*

- Bradykinin: Several substances called kinins cause powerful vasodilation when formed in the blood and tissue fluids of some organs.
- Bradykinin causes both powerful arteriolar dilation and increased capillary permeability. For instance, injection of 1 microgram of bradykinin into the brachial artery of a person increases blood flow through the arm as much as sixfold, and even smaller amounts injected locally into tissues can cause marked local edema resulting from increase in capillary pore size.

- There is reason to believe that kinins play special roles in regulating blood flow and capillary leakage of fluids in inflamed tissues. It also is believed that bradykinin plays a normal role to help regulate blood flow in the skin as well as in the salivary and gastrointestinal glands.

194. Ans. (d) Chelate calcium *Ref: Guyton Textbook of Medical Physiology, 11th ed. p 467*

Any substance that deionizes the blood calcium will prevent coagulation. The negatively charged citrate ion is especially valuable for this purpose, mixed with blood usually in the form of sodium, ammonium, or potassium citrate. The citrate ion combines with calcium in the blood to cause an unionized calcium compound, and the lack of ionic calcium prevents coagulation. Citrate anticoagulants have an important advantage over the oxalate anticoagulants because oxalate is toxic to the body, whereas moderate quantities of citrate can be injected intravenously. After injection, the citrate ion is removed from the blood within a few minutes by the liver and is polymerized into glucose or metabolized directly for energy.

195. Ans. (d) AV node *Ref: Guyton Textbook of Medical Physiology, 11th ed. p 118-119*

The ends of the sinus nodal fibers connect directly with surrounding atrial muscle fibers. Therefore, action potentials originating in the sinus node travel outward into these atrial muscle fibers. In this way, the action potential spreads through the entire atrial muscle mass and, eventually, to the A-V node. The atrial conductive system is organized so that the cardiac impulse does not travel from the atria into the ventricles too rapidly; this delay allows time for the atria to empty their blood into the ventricles before ventricular contraction begins. It is primarily the A-V node and its adjacent conductive fibers that delay this transmission into the ventricles. The impulse reaches the A-V node about 0.03 second after its origin in the sinus node. Then there is a delay of another 0.09 second in the A-V node itself before the impulse enters the penetrating portion of the A-V bundle, where it passes into the ventricles.

196. Ans. (c) 75% *Ref: Guyton Textbook of Medical Physiology, 11th ed. p 506*

The oxygen-hemoglobin dissociation curve, which demonstrates a progressive increase in the percentage of hemoglobin bound with oxygen as blood PO_2 increases, which is called the per cent saturation of hemoglobin. Because the blood leaving the lungs and entering the systemic arteries usually has a PO_2 of about 95 mm Hg, one can see from the dissociation curve that the usual oxygen saturation of systemic arterial blood averages 97 per cent. Conversely, in normal venous blood returning from the peripheral tissues, the PO_2 is about 40 mm Hg, and the saturation of hemoglobin averages 75 percent.

197. Ans. (c) 7.35 to 7.40 *Ref: Guyton Textbook of Medical Physiology, 11th ed. p 570*
Ganong Review of Medical Physiology, 23rd ed. p 615

The pH of the arterial plasma is normally 7.40 and that of venous plasma slightly lower. Blood pH is regulated to stay within the narrow range of 7.35 to 7.45, making it slightly basic. Blood that has a pH below 7.35 is too acidic, whereas blood pH above 7.45 is too basic.

198. Ans. (b) Afterload *Ref: http://www.ncbi.nlm.nih.gov/pmc/articles/PMC2575587/pdf/cc6975.pdf*
'Understanding cardiac output' Critical Care 2008, 12:174 (doi:10.1186/cc6975)

- The heart rate is perhaps the simplest determinant of cardiac output to visualize: the faster the heart beats, the more blood can be pumped over a particular period of time.
- Increased contractility of the heart muscle results in increased cardiac output
- Preload is the degree of myocardial distension prior to shortening. As initially demonstrated by Otto Frank and Ernest Starling, an intrinsic property of myocardial cells is that the force of their contraction depends on the length to which they are stretched: the greater the stretch (within certain limits), the greater the force of contraction. An increase in the distension of the ventricle will therefore result in an increase in the force of contraction, which will increase cardiac output.
- Afterload is the force against which the ventricles must act in order to eject blood, and is largely dependent on the arterial blood pressure and vascular tone. reducing afterload can increase cardiac output.

199. Ans. (a) 3:1 *Ref: http://en.wikipedia.org/wiki/bone_marrow#examination*

The ratio between myeloid series and erythroid cells is relevant to bone marrow function, and also to diseases of the bone marrow and peripheral blood, such as leukemia and anemia. The normal myeloid-to-erythroid ratio is around 3:1; this ratio may increase in myelogenous leukemias, decrease in polycythemias, and reverse in cases of thalassemia.

200. Ans. (c) Ventricular pressure falls below atrial pressure *Ref: Ganong Review of Medical Physiology, 23rd ed. p 509.*

Once the ventricular muscle is fully contracted, the already falling ventricular pressures drop more rapidly. This is the period of protodiastole, which lasts about 0.04 s. It ends when the momentum of the ejected blood is overcome and the aortic and pulmonary valves close, setting up transient vibrations in the blood and blood vessel walls. After the valves are closed, pressure continues to drop rapidly during the period of isovolumetric ventricular relaxation. Isovolumetric relaxation ends when the ventricular pressure falls below the atrial pressure and the AV valves open, permitting the ventricles to fill. Filling is rapid at first, then slows as the next cardiac contraction approaches. Atrial pressure continues to rise after the end of ventricular systole until the AV valves open, then drops and slowly rises again until the next atrial systole.

201. Ans. (d) Factor VIII deficiency *Ref: Refer explanation of Chapter 6, AIPGEE Q-11*

Refer explanation of Ans. 163.

202. Ans. (b) Beta-thalassemia trait *Ref: http://en.wikipedia.org/wiki/hemoglobin_A2*

Hemoglobin A2 (HbA2) is a normal variant of hemoglobin A that consists of two alpha and two delta chains ($\alpha2\delta2$) and is found at low levels in normal human blood. Hemoglobin A2 may be increased in beta thalassemia or in people who are heterozygous for the beta thalassemia gene.

203. Ans. (d) Cholestatic liver disease *Ref: http://www.easl.eu/assets/application/files/b664961b2692dc2_file.pdf*

204. Ans. (c) Hemolytic anemia *Ref: http://en.wikipedia.org/wiki/Thrombocytosis*

Increase platelet counts can be due to a number of disease processes:

- Essential (primary)
  - Essential thrombocytosis (a form of myeloproliferative disease)
  - Other myeloproliferative disorders, such as chronic myelogenous leukemia, polycythemia vera, myelofibrosis
- Reactive (secondary)
  - Inflammation
  - Surgery (which leads to an inflammatory state)
  - Hyposplenism (decreased breakdown due to decreased function of the spleen)
  - Splenectomy
  - Asplenia (absence of normal spleen function)
  - Iron deficiency anemia or hemorrhage

Over-medication with drugs that treat thrombocytopenia, such as eltrombopag or romiplostim, may also result in thrombocytosis. Other causes include the following:

- Kawasaki disease
- Soft-tissue sarcoma
- Osteosarcoma
- Dermatitis (rarely)

- Inflammatory bowel disease
- Rheumatoid arthritis
- Nephritis
- Nephrotic syndrome
- Bacterial diseases, including pneumonia, sepsis, meningitis, urinary tract infections, and septic arthritis.

205. Ans. (c) Explains the increase in cardiac output that occurs when venous return is increased

Ref: Ganong Review of Medical Physiology, 23rd ed. p 109, 515

The relation between initial fiber length and total tension in cardiac muscle is similar to that in skeletal muscle; there is a resting length at which the tension developed on stimulation is maximal. In the body, the initial length of the fibers is determined by the degree of diastolic filling of the heart, and the pressure developed in the ventricle is proportionate to the volume of the ventricle at the end of the filling phase (Starling's law of the heart). The length tension relationship in cardiac muscle is similar to that in skeletal muscle as the muscle is stretched, the developed tension increases to a maximum and then declines as stretch becomes more extreme. Starling pointed this out when he stated that the 'energy of contraction is proportional to the initial length of the cardiac muscle fiber'(Starling's law of the heart or the FrankStarling law). For the heart, the length of the muscle fibers (i.e. the extent of the preload) is proportional to the end-diastolic volume. The relation between ventricular stroke volume and enddiastolic volume is called the FrankStarling curve.

206. Ans. (a) Decreased level of prothrombin

Ref: Ganong Review of Medical Physiology, 23rd ed. p 535. Refer explanation of Chapter 6 AIPGEE Q-11

Deficiency of factor:	*Clinical syndrome*	*Cause*
I	Afibrinogenemia	Depletion during pregnancy with premature separation of placenta; also congenital (rare)
II	Hypoprothrombinemia (hemorrhagic tendency in liver disease)	Decreased hepatic synthesis, usually secondary to vitamin K deficiency
V	Parahemophilia	Congenital
VII	Hypoconvertinemia	Congenital
VIII	Hemophilia A (classic hemophilia)	Congenital defect due to various abnormalities of the gene on X chromosome that codes for factor VIII; disease is therefore inherited as sex-linked characteristic
IX	Hemophilia B (Christmas disease)	Congenital
X	Stuart-Prower factor deficiency	Congenital
XI	PTA deficiency	Congenital
XII	Hageman trait	Congenital

Examples of diseases due to deficiency of clotting factors

207. Ans. (a) Correct the anemia but not the neurological symptoms

Ref: http://en.wikipedia.org/wiki/Folic_acid#cite_ref-merck.com_63-11

One way to differentiate between folate deficiency from vitamin B12 deficiency is by testing for methylmalonic acid levels. Normal MMA levels indicate folate deficiency and elevated MMA levels indicate vitamin B12 deficiency. Folate deficiency is treated with supplemental oral folate of 400 to 1000 μg per day. This treatment is very successful in replenishing tissues, even if deficiency was caused by malabsorption. Patients with megaloblastic anemia need to be tested for vitamin B12 deficiency before folate treatment, because if the patient has vitamin B12 deficiency, folate supplementation can remove the anemia, but can also worsen neurologic problems.

208. Ans. (a) 1–4 m/sec *Ref: Ganong Review of Medical Physiology, 23rd ed. p 492*

Tissue	*Conduction rate (m/s)*
SA node	0.05
Atrial pathways	1
AV node	0.05
Bundle of His	1
Purkinje system	4
Ventricular muscle	1

Conduction speeds in cardiac tissue.

209. Ans. (a) Closure of semilunar valves *Ref: Guyton Textbook of Medical Physiology, 11th ed. p 110*

When the ventricles contract, one first hears a sound caused by closure of the A-V valves. The vibration is low in pitch and relatively long-lasting and is known as the first heart sound. When the aortic and pulmonary valves close at the end of systole, one hears a rapid snap because these valves close rapidly, and the surroundings vibrate for a short period. This sound is called the second heart sound.

210. Ans. (a) XII

211. Ans. (a) Albumin *Ref: Ganong Review of Medical Physiology, 23rd ed. p 482*

Albumin is quantitatively the most significant, and accounts for the majority of plasma oncotic pressure. Many of the products are acute-phase proteins, proteins synthesized and secreted into the plasma on exposure to stressful stimuli. Others are proteins that transport steroids and other hormones in the plasma, and still others are clotting factors. Following blood loss, the liver replaces the plasma proteins in days to weeks. The only major class of plasma proteins not synthesized by the liver is the immunoglobulins.

RESPIRATORY PHYSIOLOGY

212. Ans. (d) Metabolic acidosis *Ref: Guyton Textbook of Medical Physiology, 11th ed. p 396*

Characteristics of primary acid-base disturbances

	pH	*H^+*	*PCO_2*	*HCO_3^-*
Normal	7.4	40 mEq/L	40 mm Hg	24 mEq/L
Respiratory acidosis	↓	↑	↑↑	↑
Respiratory alkalosis	↑	↓	↓↓	↓
Metabolic acidosis	↓	↑	↓	↓↓
Metabolic alkalosis	↑	↓	↑	↑↑

The primary event is indicated by the double arrows (↑↑ or ↓↓). Note that respiratory acid-base disorders are initiated by an increase or decrease in PCO_2, whereas metabolic disorders are initiated by an increase or decrease in HCO_3^-

213. Ans. (d) Reduced surface tension by surfactant *Ref: Ganong Review of Medical Physiology, 23rd ed. p 597*

The low surface tension when the alveoli are small is due to the presence in the fluid lining the alveoli of surfactant, a lipid surface-tension-lower in gagent. Surfactant is a mixture of dipalmitoylphosphatidylcholine (DPPC), other lipids, and proteins. If the surface tension is not kept low when the alveoli become smaller during expiration, they collapse in accordance with the law of Laplace. In spherical structures like the alveoli, the distending pressure equals two times the tension divided by the radius ($P = 2T/r$); if T is not reduced as r is reduced, the tension overcomes the distending pressure. Surfactant also helps to prevent pulmonary edema.

214. Ans. (a) Apneusis *Ref: Guyton Textbook of Medical Physiology, 11th ed. p 515*
Ganong Review of Medical Physiology, 23rd ed. p 627

- Apneusis is an abnormal pattern of breathing characterized by deep, gasping inspiration with a pause at full inspiration followed by a brief, insufficient release.
- It is caused by damage to the pons or upper medulla caused by strokes or trauma. Specifically, concurrent removal of input from the vagus nerve and the pneumotaxic center causes this pattern of breathing. It is an ominous sign, with a generally poor prognosis.
- It can also be temporarily caused by some drugs, such as ketamine.

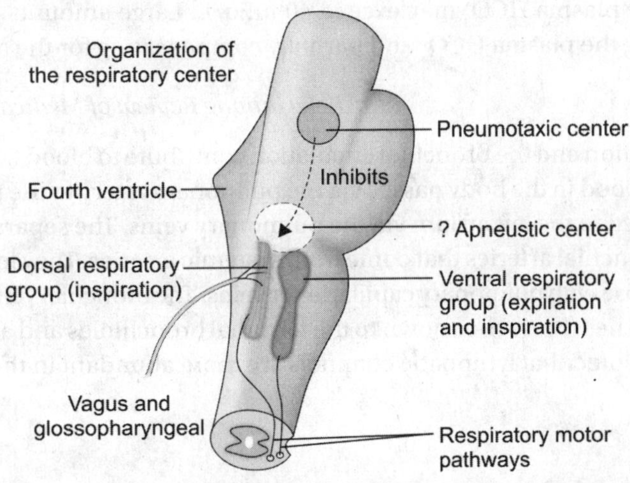

215. Ans. (a) It has high affinity for hemoglobin *Ref: Guyton Textbook of Medical Physiology, 11th ed. p 499, 509*

Carbon monoxide combines with hemoglobin at the same point on the hemoglobin molecule as does oxygen; it can therefore displace oxygen from the hemoglobin, thereby decreasing the oxygen carrying capacity of blood. Further, it binds with about 250 times as much tenacity as oxygen.

The oxygen diffusing capacity can be calculated from measurements of:

- Alveolar PO_2
- PO_2 in the pulmonary capillary blood
- The rate of oxygen uptake by the blood

However, measuring the PO_2 in the pulmonary capillary blood is so difficult and so imprecise that it is not practical to measure oxygen diffusing capacity by such a direct procedure, except on an experimental basis. To obviate the difficulties encountered in measuring oxygen diffusing capacity directly, physiologists usually measure carbon monoxide diffusing capacity instead and then calculate the oxygen diffusing capacity from this.

216. Ans. (d) Decreasing workload, decreasing duration of exercise *Ref: Ganong Review of Medical Physiology, 23rd ed. p 618 Guyton Textbook of Medical Physiology, 11th ed. p- 540*

A person remaining at high altitudes for days, weeks, or years becomes more and more acclimatized to the low PO_2, so that it causes fewer deleterious effects on the body. And, it becomes possible for the person to work harder without hypoxic effects or to ascend to still higher altitudes. The principal means by which acclimatization comes about are:

- A great increase in pulmonary ventilation
- Increased numbers of red blood cells
- Increased diffusing capacity of the lungs
- Increased vascularity of the peripheral tissues
- Increased ability of the tissue cells to use oxygen despite low PO_2.

217. Ans. (a) Shift of oxyhemoglobin curve to the right

218. Ans. (a) Low blood pH *Ref: Ganong Review of Medical Physiology, 23rd ed. p 622*
Guyton Textbook of Medical Physiology, 11th ed. p 531

Hypercapnia is a condition of abnormally elevated carbon dioxide (CO_2) levels in the blood. Retention of CO_2 in the body (hypercapnia) initially stimulates respiration. Retention of larger amounts produces symptoms due to depression of the central nervous system: confusion, diminished sensory acuity, and, eventually, coma with respiratory depression and death. In patients with these symptoms, the PCO_2 is markedly elevated, severe respiratory acidosis is present, and the plasma HCO_3 may exceed 40 mEq/L. Large amounts of HCO_3 are excreted, but more HCO_3 is reabsorbed, raising the plasma HCO_3 and partially compensating for the acidosis.

219. Ans. (a) Air conditioning *Ref: Ganong Review of Medical Physiology, 23rd ed. p 590-591*

Both the pulmonary circulation and the bronchial circulation contribute to blood flow in the lung. In the pulmonary circulation, almost all the blood in the body passes via the pulmonary artery to the pulmonary capillary bed, where it is oxygenated and returned to the left atrium via the pulmonary veins. The separate and much smaller bronchial circulation includes the bronchial arteries that come from systemic arteries. They form capillaries, which drain into bronchial veins or anastomose with pulmonary capillaries or veins. The bronchial veins drain into the azygos vein. The bronchial circulation nourishes the trachea down to the terminal bronchioles and also supplies the pleura and hilar lymph nodes. It should be noted that lymphatic channels are more abundant in the lungs than in any other organ.

220. Ans. (d) Factor X

221. Ans. (b) Shift of oxygen dissociation curve to left *Ref: Ganong Review of Medical Physiology, 23rd ed. p 621*

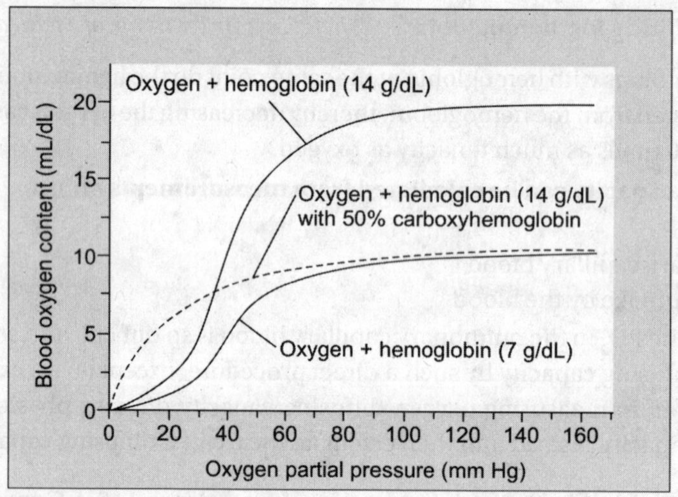

Effects of anemia and CO on hemoglobin binding of O_2.

Normal oxyhemoglobin (14 g/dL hemoglobin) dissociation curve compared with anemia (7 g/dL hemoglobin) and with oxyhemoglobin dissociation curves in CO poisoning (50% carboxyhemoglobin). Note that the CO-poisoning curve is shifted to the left of the anemia curve.

- CO is toxic because it reacts with hemoglobin to form carbon monoxyhemoglobin (carboxyhemoglobin, COHb), and COHb cannot take up O_2. Carbon monoxide poisoning is often listed as a form of anemic hypoxia because the amount of hemoglobin that can carry O_2 is reduced, but the total hemoglobin content of the blood is unaffected by CO. The affinity of hemoglobin for CO is 210 times its affinity for O_2, and COHb liberates CO very slowly. An additional difficulty is that when COHb is present the dissociation curve of the remaining HbO_2 shifts to the left, decreasing the amount of O_2 released. This is why an anemic individual who has 50% of the normal amount of HbO_2 may be able to perform moderate work, whereas an individual whose HbO_2 is reduced to the same level because of the formation of COHb is seriously incapacitated.

222. Ans. (b) Sodium balance

223. Ans. (b) Pulmonary reserve *Ref:Refer explanation of Chapter 7 AIPGEE Q-8*

Refer explanation of Ans. 219.

224. Ans. (b) ↓ pH of blood *Ref:Refer explanation of Chapter 7 AIPGEE Q-7*

Refer explanation of Ans. 218.

225. Ans. (d) Langerhans *Ref: http://en.wikipedia.org/wiki/Enterochromaffin_cell. Eur J Respir Dis. 1982 May;63(3):202-20. The Clara cell (http://www.ncbi.nlm.nih.gov/pubmed/7047186)*

All cells except langerhans are found in lung.

- The Clara cells are a group of cells, sometimes called 'nonciliated bronchiolar secretory cells,' found in the bronchiolar epithelium of mammals including man.
- 'Kulchitsky cells are a type of enteroendocrine and neuroendocrine cell occurring in the epithelia lining the lumen of the digestive tract and the respiratory tract.
- Langerhans cells are found in lungs only during diseased conditions like histiocytosis; otherwise they are usually found in lymph nodes and gastrointestinal tract epithelium.

226. Ans. (c) Thrombosis *Ref: Ganong Review of Medical Physiology, 23rd ed. p 534*

Formation of clots inside blood vessels is called thrombosis to distinguish it from the normal extravascular clotting of blood. Thromboses are a major medical problem. They are particularly prone to occur where blood flow is sluggish because the slow flow permits activated clotting factors to accumulate instead of being washed away. They also occur in vessels when the intima is damaged by atherosclerotic plaques, and over areas of damage to the endocardium. They frequently occlude the arterial supply to the organs in which they form, and bits of thrombus (emboli) sometimes break off and travel in the bloodstream to distant sites, damaging other organs. An example is obstruction of the pulmonary artery or its branches by thrombi from the leg veins (pulmonary embolism).

227. Ans. (c) Melanocytes and (d) Clara cells

228. Ans. (d) Bicarbonate *Ref: Ganong Review of Medical Physiology, 23rd ed. p 612*

The solubility of CO_2 in blood is about 20 times that of O_2; therefore, considerably more CO_2 than O_2 is present in simple solution at equal partial pressures. The CO_2 that diffuses into red blood cells is rapidly hydrated to H_2CO_3 because of the presence of carbonic anhydrase. The H_2CO_3 dissociates to H^+ and HCO_3, and the H^+ is buffered, primarily by hemoglobin, while the HCO_3 enters the plasma.

229. Ans. (d) Hypoventilation *Ref: Guyton Textbook of Medical Physiology, 11th ed. p 531*

Hypercapnia means excess carbon dioxide in the body fluids. One might suspect, on first thought, that any respiratory condition that causes hypoxia would also cause hypercapnia. However, hypercapnia usually occurs in association with hypoxia only when the hypoxia is caused by hypoventilation. Traditionally, hypoxia has been divided into four types. Numerous other classifications have been used, but the four type system still has considerable utility if the definitions of the terms are kept clearly in mind. The four categories are:

- Hypoxic hypoxia, in which the PO_2 of the arterial blood is reduced

- Anemic hypoxia, in which the arterial PO_2 is normal but the amount of hemoglobin available to carry O2 is reduced;
- Stagnant or ischemic hypoxia, in which the blood flow to a tissue is so low that adequate O_2 is not delivered to it despite a normal PO_2 and hemoglobin concentration
- Histotoxic hypoxia, in which the amount of O_2 delivered to a tissue is adequate but, because of the action of a toxic agent, the tissue cells cannot make use of the O_2 supplied to them.

230. Ans. (d) Increased concentration of oxygen *Ref: Ganong Review of Medical Physiology, 23rd ed. p 611,636*
Guyton Textbook of Medical Physiology, 11th ed. p 508

A rise in temperature or a fall in pH shifts the curve to the right. When the curve is shifted in this direction, a higher PO_2 is required for hemoglobin to bind a given amount of O_2. Conversely, a fall in temperature or a rise in pH shifts the curve to the left, and a lower PO_2 is required to bind a given amount of O_2. In addition to pH changes, several other factors are known to shift the curve. Three of these, all of which shift the curve to the right, are

- Increased carbon dioxide concentration,
- Increased blood temperature
- Increased 2,3-biphosphoglycerate (BPG), a metabolically important phosphate compound present in the blood in different concentrations under different metabolic conditions. The normal BPG in the blood keeps the oxygen-hemoglobin dissociation curve shifted slightly to the right all the time. In hypoxic conditions that last longer than a few hours, the quantity of BPG in the blood increases considerably, thus shifting the oxygen-hemoglobin dissociation curve even farther to the right. This causes oxygen to be released to the tissues at as much as 10 mm Hg higher tissue oxygen pressure than would be the case without this increased BPG. Therefore, under some conditions, the BPG mechanism can be important for adaptation to hypoxia, especially to hypoxia caused by poor tissue blood flow. A shift of the oxygenhemoglobin dissociation curve to the right in response to increases in blood carbon dioxide and hydrogen ions has a significant effect by enhancing the release of oxygen from the blood in the tissues and enhancing oxygenation of the blood in the lungs. This is called the Bohr Effect.

231. Ans. (d) 2–3 percent of the total energy spent *Ref: Ganong Review of Medical Physiology, 23rd ed. p 599*

- Estimates of the total work of quiet breathing range from 0.3 up to 0.8 kg-m/min. The value rises markedly during exercise, but the energy cost of breathing in normal individuals represents less than 3% of the total energy expenditure during exercise. The work of breathing is greatly increased in diseases such as emphysema, asthma, and congestive heart failure with dyspnea and orthopnea.

232. Ans. (c) Dipalmitoyl lecithin *Ref: Ganong Review of Medical Physiology, 23rd ed. p597*

Component	*Percentage composition*
Dipalmitoylphosphatidylcholine	62
Phosphatidylglycerol	5
Other phospholipids	10
Neutral lipids	13
Proteins	8
Carbohydrate	2

Approximate composition of surfactant. The low surface tension when the alveoli are small is due to the presence in the fluid lining the alveoli of surfactant, a lipid surface-tension-lowering agent. Surfactant is a mixture of dipalmitoylphosphatidylcholine (DPPC), other lipids, and proteins. Surfactant is important at birth. The fetus makes respiratory movements in utero, but the lungs remain collapsed until birth. After birth, the infant makes several strong inspiratory movements and the lungs expand. Surfactant keeps them from collapsing again. Surfactant deficiency is an important cause of infant respiratory distress syndrome (IRDS, also known as hyaline membrane disease), the serious pulmonary disease that develops in infants born before their surfactant system is functional. Surface tension in the lungs of these infants is high, and the alveoli are collapsed in many areas (atelectasis).

233. Ans. (a) Increased dead air space *Ref: Robbins Basic Pathology, 8th ed. p 717*

Emphysema and chronic bronchitis are often clinically grouped together and referred to as chronic obstructive pulmonary disease (COPD), since many patients have overlapping features of damage at both the acinar level (emphysema) and bronchial level (bronchitis), almost certainly because one extrinsic triggercigarette smokingis common to both.

Disorders associated with airflow obstruction: The spectrum of chronic obstructive pulmonary disease

Clinical term	*Anatomic site*	*Major pathologic changes*	*Etiology*	*Signs/symptoms*
Chronic bronchitis	Bronchus	Mucous gland hyperplasia, hypersecretion	Tobacco smoke, air pollutants	Cough, sputum production
Bronchiectasis	Bronchus	Airway dilation and scarring	Persistent or severe infections	Cough, purulent sputum, fever
Asthma	Bronchus	Smooth muscle hyperplasia, excess mucus, inflammation	Immunologic or undefined causes	Episodic wheezing, cough, dyspnea
Emphysema	Acinus	Airspace enlargement; wall destruction	Tobacco smoke	Dyspnea
Small airway disease,* bronchiolitis	Bronchiole	Inflammatory scarring/ obliteration	Tobacco smoke, air pollutants, miscellaneous	Cough, dyspnea

Emphysema is a condition of the lung characterized by abnormal permanent enlargement of the airspaces distal to the terminal bronchiole, accompanied by destruction of their walls and without obvious fibrosis.

234. Ans. (a) Minus 6 mm Hg *Ref: Ganong Review of Medical Physiology, 23rd ed. p 592*

Inspiration is an active process. The contraction of the inspiratory muscles increases intrathoracic volume. The intrapleural pressure at the base of the lungs, which is normally about 2.5 mm Hg (relative to atmospheric) at the start of inspiration, decreases to about 6 mm Hg.

235. Ans. (a) Inversely related to lung compliance *Ref: Ganong Review of Medical Physiology, 23rd ed. p 598*
Guyton Textbook of Medical Physiology, 11th ed. p 475

The work of inspiration can be divided into three fractions: (1) That required to expand the lungs against the lung and chest elastic forces, called compliance work or elastic work, (2) that required to overcome the viscosity of the lung and chest wall structures, called tissue resistance work, and (3) that required to overcome airway resistance to movement of air into the lungs, called airway resistance work.

236. Ans. (b) 4 mm *Ref: Guyton Textbook of Medical Physiology, 11th ed. p 237*

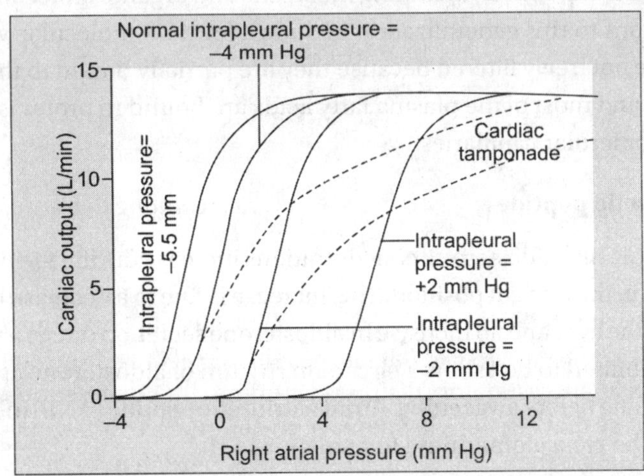

The normal external pressure is equal to the normal intrapleural pressure (the pressure in the chest cavity), which is –4 mm Hg.

237. Ans. (a) Increase in respiratory rate *Ref: Ganong Review of Medical Physiology, 23rd ed. p 617*

Dyspnea is by definition difficult or labored breathing in which the subject is conscious of shortness of breath; hyperpnea is the general term for an increase in the rate or depth of breathing regardless of the patient's subjective sensations. Tachypnea is rapid, shallow breathing.

RENAL PHYSIOLOGY

238. Ans. (c) Sensing NaCl concentration in the macula densa

Ref: Ganong Review of Medical Physiology, 23rd ed. p 651-652

- Signals from the renal tubule in each nephron feedback to affect filtration in its glomerulus. As the rate of flow through the ascending limb of the loop of Henle and first part of the distal tubule increases, glomerular filtration in the same nephron decreases, vice versa. This process, which is called tubuloglomerular feedback, tends to maintain the constancy of the load delivered to the distal tubule.
- The sensor for this response is the macula densa. The amount of fluid entering the distal tubule at the end of the thick ascending limb of the loop of Henle depends on the amount of Na^+ and Cl in it.

239. Ans. (b) Tubular excretion

240. Ans. (d) Juxtaglomerular cells *Ref: Guyton Textbook of Medical Physiology, 11th ed. p 223*

Renin is synthesized and stored in an inactive form called prorenin in the juxtaglomerular cells (JG cells) of the kidneys. The JG cells are modified smooth muscle cells located in the walls of the afferent arterioles immediately proximal to the glomeruli.When the arterial pressure falls, intrinsic reactions in the kidneys themselves cause many of the prorenin molecules in the JG cells to split and release renin.

241. Ans. (d) 125 mL/minute *Ref: Guyton Textbook of Medical Physiology, 11th ed. p 316*

In the average adult human, the GFR is about 125 ml/min, or 180 L/day. Urine formation begins with filtration of large amounts of fluid through the glomerular capillaries into Bowman's capsule. Like most capillaries, the glomerular capillaries are relatively impermeable to proteins, so that the filtered fluid (called the glomerular filtrate) is essentially protein-free and devoid of cellular elements, including red blood cells. The concentrations of other constituents of the glomerular filtrate, including most salts and organic molecules, are similar to the concentrations in the plasma. Exceptions to this generalization include a few low-molecular-weight substances, such as calcium and fatty acids, that are not freely filtered because they are partially bound to the plasma proteins. Almost one half of the plasma calcium and most of the plasma fatty acids are bound to proteins, and these bound portions are not filtered through the glomerular capillaries.

242. Ans. (b) Atrial natriuretic peptide *Ref: Ganong Review of Medical Physiology, 23rd ed. p 358*

In normal individuals, plasma aldosterone concentrations increase during the portion of the day that the individual is carrying on activities in the upright position. This increase is due to a decrease in the rate of removal of aldosterone from the circulation by the liver and an increase in aldosterone secretion due to a postural increase in renin secretion. Individuals who are confined to bed show a circadian rhythm of aldosterone and renin secretion, with the highest values in the early morning before awakening. Atrial natriuretic peptide (ANP) inhibits renin secretion and decreases the responsiveness of the zona glomerulosa to angiotensin II.

243. Ans. (d) Creatinine *Ref:BMJ. 2006 October 7;333(7571):733737. How to measure renal function in clinical practice (http://www.ncbi.nlm.nih.gov/pmc/articles/PMC1592388/)*

Creatinine is the closest to an ideal endogenous substance for measuring glomerular filtration rate. Plasma creatinine is almost exclusively a product of the metabolism of creatine and phosphocreatine in skeletal muscle, although ingestion of meat may also contribute slightly. In patients with stable renal function, serum creatinine levels are usually constant, with variability daily of about only 8%. Creatinine is freely filtered at the glomerulus and is not reabsorbed, but up to 15% is actively secreted by the tubules.

244. Ans. (b) Vasa recta *Ref: Ganong Review of Medical Physiology, 23rd ed. p 654*

The concentrating mechanism depends upon the maintenance of a gradient of increasing osmolality along the medullary pyramids. This gradient is produced by the operation of the loops of Henle as countercurrent multipliers and maintained by the operation of the vasa recta as countercurrent exchangers. A countercurrent system is a system in which the inflow runs parallel to, counter to, and in close proximity to the outflow for some distance. This occurs for both the loops of Henle and the vasa recta in the renal medulla.

245. Ans. (c) 375 mg/min *Ref: Guyton Textbook of Medical Physiology, 11th ed. p 331*

The plasma glucose of a healthy person almost never becomes high enough to cause excretion of glucose in the urine, even after eating a meal. However, in uncontrolled diabetes mellitus, plasma glucose may rise to high levels, causing the filtered load of glucose to exceed the transport maximum and resulting in urinary glucose excretion.

246. Ans. (a) 125 ml/min *Ref: Refer explanation of Chapter 8 COMEDK/KCET Q-2*

Refer explanation of Ans. 241.

247. Ans. (a) Calmodulin *Ref: Guyton Textbook of Medical Physiology, 11th ed. p 914 http://en.wikipedia.org/wiki/Calmodulin#Structure*

Calmodulin is a small, highly conserved protein approximately 148 amino acids long (16706 Daltons). It contains four EF-hand motifs, each of which binds a Ca^{2+} ion. Calcium-Calmodulin Second Messenger System Another second messenger system operates in response to the entry of calcium into the cells.Calcium entry may be initiated by:

- Changes in membrane potential that open calcium channels or
- A hormone interacting with membrane receptors that open calcium channels. On entering a cell, calcium ions bind with the protein calmodulin. This protein has four calcium sites, and when three or four of these sites have bound with calcium, the calmodulin changes its shape and initiates multiple effects inside the cell, including activation or inhibition of protein kinases.

3 Biochemistry

CARBOHYDRATE

1. Which is not monosaccharide? *(AIIMS Nov 2013)*

a. Glucose b. Galactose
c. Fructose d. Maltose

2. Oxygen-dependent killing is done through: *(AIPG 2010)*

a. NADPH oxidase
b. Superoxide dismutase
c. Catalase
d. Glutathione peroxidase

3. Acetyl CoA coverts to all *except*: *(AIPG 2013)*

a. Glucose b. Fatty acids
c. Cholesterol d. Ketone bodies

4. The most lipogenic carbohydrate is: *(AIPG 2010)*

a. Fructose b. Glucose
c. Ribose d. Sucrose

5. Regarding HMP shunt, all of the following are true, *except* that: *(AIPG 2008)*

a. It occurs in cytosol
b. Oxidative phase generates NADPH
c. Nonoxidative phase generates pyruvate
d. No ATP is produced in the cycle

6. For glucose estimation in blood, the mode of transport from a PHC to laboratory is: *(AIPG 2007)*

a. Sodium fluoride
b. EDTA
c. Citrate
d. 0.9% Saline

7. During phagocytosis, the metabolic process called respiratory burst involves the activation of: *(AIPG 2006)*

a. Oxidase
b. Hydrolase
c. Peroxidase
d. Dehydrogenase

8. What is the most sensitive indicator of cellular energy? *(AIPG 2012)*

a. ATP b. ADP
c. AMP d. Phosphocreatinine

9. Maltose, which is produced as a breakdown of starch, is a: *(AIPG 2012)*

a. Disachharide b. Monosaccharide
c. Polysaccharide d. None of above

10. Carbohydrates when taken in excessive form is stored in which form? *(AIPG 2012)*

a. Glycogen b. Fatty acid
c. Protein d. Glucose

11. The uptake of glucose by the liver increases following a carboxylate meal because: *(COMED-KCET 2009)*

a. There is increased phosphorylation of glucose by glucose by glucokinase
b. GLUT-2 is stimulated by insulin
c. Glucokinase has a low Km for glucose
d. Hexokinase in liver has a high affinity for glucose

12. Which of the following is false about starvation ketoacidosis? *(KCET 2013)*

a. Metabolic acidosis
b. Smell of acetone in breath
c. Benedict's test positive
d. Rothera's test is positive

13. Glucose transporters present in the Beta cells of the Islets of Langerhans is: *(COMED-KCET 2014)*

a. GLUT 1 b. GLUT 2
c. GLUT 3 d. GLUT 4

14. Glucose concentration in gingival cervicular fluid is: *(COMED-KCET 2014)*

a. 2 to 3 times greater than in serum
b. 2 to 3 times lesser than in serum
c. 10 times greater than in serum
d. 10 times lesser than in serum

15. Diatary fiber is rich in: *(KCET 2005)*
a. Starch b. Cellulose
c. Collagen d. Inulin

16. The following Carbohydrate is called Animal Starch: *(KCET 2006)*
a. Glucose b. Fructose
c. Sucrose d. Glycogen

17. The storage form of carbohydrates in our body is: *(KCET 2006)*
a. Starch b. Glycogen
c. Sucrose d. Cellulose

18. Glucose tolerance test is usually done to access: *(COMED 2006)*
a. Acute pancreatitis
b. Carcinoma of head and pancreas
c. Acinar function of the pancreas
d. Endocrine dysfunction of the pancreas

19. Which one of the following human tissues contains the greatest amount of body glycogen? *(COMED 2005)*
a. Liver b. Kidney
c. Skeletal muscle d. Cardiac muscle

20. The monosaccharide glucose is best described by which one of the following statements? *(COMED 2005)*
a. It usually exists in the furanose form
b. It is a ketose
c. It possesses an anomeric C-2 carbon atom
d. It forms the part of disaccharide sucrose

21. Substrate for gluconeogenesis is:
a. Glycogen b. Acetyl CoA
c. Glycerol d. Leucine

LIPIDS

22. Richest source of cholesterol is: *(AIIMS Nov 2013)*
a. Coconut oil b. Ghee
c. Hydrogenated fat d. Eggs

23. Which of the following fatty acid should be present in breast milk for normal growth of baby? *(AIIMS May 2011, Nov 2013)*
a. Palmitoleic acid
b. Arachidonic acid
c. Linolenic acid
d. Docosahexaenoic acid (DHEA)

24. N3-polyunsaturated fatty acid (PUFA) is present in least quantity in which of the following? *(AIIMS Nov 2007)*
a. Mustard oil b. Corn oil
c. Groundnut oil d. Fish oil

25. Membrane fluidity is increased by: *(AIIMS May 2005)*
a. Stearic acid b. Palmitic acid
c. Cholesterol d. Linoleic acid

26. Rothera's test is used for the detection of: *(AIPG 2011)*
a. Ketones b. Glucose
c. Fatty acid d. Proteins

27. In Niemann Pick disease, which of the following substance accumulation in CNS is in excess? *(AIPG 2011)*
a. Glycerophosphatidase
b. Phosphoinositides
c. Sphingomyelins
d. Glucocerebrosides

28. The highest percentages of polyunsaturated fatty acids (PUFAs) are present in: *(AIPG 2010)*
a. Groundnut oil b. Palm oil
c. Margarine d. Soya bean oil

29. Eicosapentaenoic acid is present in: *(AIPG 2010)*
a. Soya bean oil b. Corn oil
c. Safflower oil d. Fish oil

30. The most important source of reducing equivalents for fatty acid synthesis in the liver is: *(AIPG 2010)*
a. Glycolysis
b. TCA cycle
c. Uronic acid pathway
d. HMP pathway

31. Insulin causes lipogenesis by all, *except*: *(AIPG 2010)*
a. That it increases acetyl-CoA carboxylase activity
b. That it increases the transport of glucose into the cells
c. That it inhibits pyruvate dehydrogenase
d. That it increases intracellular CAMP level

32. N-3 PUFA is present in all of the following, *except*: *(AIPG 2008)*
a. Mustard oil b. Fish oil
c. Corn oil d. Groundnut oil

33. Which of the following has maximum cholesterol content? *(AIPG 2008)*
a. Egg b. Coconut oil
c. Hydrogenated fat d. Ghee

34. Calorific value of fat is? *(AIPG 2012)*
a. 7 b. 9
c. 5 d. 4

35. Non polar lipids act as: *(COMED 2008)*
a. Electric insulators
b. Ions
c. Non-electric insulators
d. Electrolytes

36. Lipofuscin is an insoluble endogenous pigment, also known as: *(KCET 2008)*
a. Lipochrome
b. Wear-and-tear pigment
c. Aging pigment
d. All of the above

37. Which of the following fatty acids cannot be synthesized in humans? *(KCET 2009)*
a. Palmitic acid b. Stearic acid
c. Oleic acid d. Linoleic acid

38. Under metabolic conditions associated with a high rate of fatty acid oxidation the liver produces: *(COMED 2010)*
a. Glutamate b. Aceto acetate
c. Cholesterol d. Glycine

39. The main pathway for '*De Novo*' synthesis of fatty acids occurs in: *(KCET 2010)*
a. Mitochondria b. Nucleus
c. Cytosol d. None of the above

40. In prolonged starvation the main source of energy to brain is: *(KCET 2011, COMED 2013)*
a. Glucose
b. Fruclose
c. Fatty acids
d. Ketone bodies

41. The main function of HDL is: *(KCET 2013)*
a. Transport cholesterol from liver to peripheral tissues
b. Esterification with PUFA
c. Both of the above
d. None of the above

42. Cholesterol levels in a normal person should be preferably less than: *(KCET 2013)*
a. 200 mg/dl
b. 180 mg/dl
c. 150 mg/dl
d. 120 mg/dl

43. The absorption of dietary triglycerides from the gut is mainly as: *(COMED 2014)*
a. Triglycerides
b. Mono acyl glycerol
c. Di acyl glycerol
d. Fatty acids and glycerol

PROTEIN AND AMINO ACIDS

44. Which of the following amino acid is both ketogenic and glucogenic is? *(AIIMS May 2013)*
a. Isoleucine b. Leucine
c. Arginine d. Glycine

45. Amino acid residue used in the detection of the strength of collagen is: *(AIIMS Nov 2007)*
a. Proline b. Hydroxyproline
c. Glycine d. Hydroxylysine

46. Which of the following separation techniques depends on the molecular size of proteins? *(AIIMS May 2006)*
a. Chromatography on a carboxymethyl cellulose column
b. Isoelectric focusing
c. Gel filtration chromatography
d. Chromatography on a diethylaminoethyl (DEAE) cellulose column

47. The protein rich in basic amino acids, which functions in the packaging of DNA in chromosomes, is? *(AIIMS May 2006)*
a. Histone
b. Collagen
c. Hyaluronic acid-binding protein
d. Fibrinogen

48. The primary role of chaperones is to help in: *(AIIMS May 2006)*
a. Protein synthesis
b. Protein degradation
c. Protein denaturation
d. Protein folding

49. Which of the following is the main function of serum albumin? *(AIPG 2011)*
a. Oncotic pressure maintenance
b. Toxin transport
c. Buffering action
d. Drug binding and transport

50. All are genetic amino acid deficiency diseases *except*: *(AIPG 2013)*
a. Phenylketonuria
b. Homocystinuria
c. Galactosemia
d. Alkaptonuria

51. False about denaturation of proteins is all, *except* that: *(AIPG 2009)*
a. Unfolding occurs
b. Disruption of secondary structure
c. Sequence of amino acid remains the same
d. Biological activity is retained

52. Proteins that precipitate on heating at 45°C and redissolve on boiling are: *(AIPG 2008)*
a. Albumin
b. Bence Jones proteins
c. Gamma globulin
d. Myosin

53. Folding of proteins is done by all of the following, *except*: *(AIPG 2008)*
a. Chaperons b. Zinc finger motif
c. Peroxidase d. None of these

54. Ketones cannot be taken by: *(AIPG 2008)*
a. Brain b. Heart
c. Liver d. RBCs

55. Protein purification and separation is done by all of the following, *except*: *(AIPG 2008)*
a. Chromatography
b. Centrifugation
c. Electrophoresis
d. Densitometry

56. All of the amino acids are involved in the formation of urea and ammonia in kidney, *except*:
a. Glycine b. Aspartate
c. Glutamate d. Arginine

57. The human plasma lipoprotein containing the highest percentage of triacylglycerol by weight is: *(AIPG 2006)*
a. Chylomicrons b. HDL
c. LDL d. All of the above

58. Proteins are linear polymers of amino acids. They fold into compact structures. Sometimes these folded structures associate to form homo- or heterodimers. Which one of the following refers to this associated form? *(AIPG 2006)*
a. Denatured state
b. Molecular aggregation
c. Precipitation
d. Quaternary structure

59. The amino acid residue having an imino side chain is: *(AIPG 2005)*
a. Lysine b. Histidine
c. Tyrosine d. Proline

60. Phenylketonuria is a disease due to: *(AIPG 2012)*
a. Improper metabolism of amino acids
b. Improper metabolism of carbohydrates
c. Improper metabolism of enzymes
d. Inability to convert fatty acids into carbohydrates

61. Cofactor required for lipoprotein lipase activity is: *(COMED 2008)*
a. Apo A-II b. Apo C-II
c. Apo C-III d. Apo B-II

62. The first plasma protein to be generated after severe protein deficiency: *(COMED 2008)*
a. Albumin b. Globulin
c. Fibrinogen d. Thrombin

63. Bence Jones protein found in the urine may be suggestive of: *(KCET 2008)*
a. Hyperparathyroidism
b. Hodgkin's disease
c. Multiple myeloma
d. Christian's syndrome

64. Ehrlich test is done to detect: *(COMED 2011)*
a. Bilirubin b. Urobilinogen
c. Bile salts d. Protein

65. Plasma ceruloplasmin is a: *(COMED 2011)*
a. Alpha 1 globulin b. Alpha 2 globulin
c. Beta 1 globulin d. Beta 2 globulin

66. The nitrogen content in 50 gm of a typical dietary protein is most likely to be: *(COMED 2011)*
a. 5 g
b. 8 g
c. 10 g
d. 16 g

67. Mannose 6 phosphate containing freshly synthesized proteins are directed to: *(COMED 2012)*

a. Nucleus b. Lysosomes
c. Mitochondria d. Golgi apparatus

68. In the body, metabolism of 10 g of protein would produce approximately: *(COMED 2012)*

a. 1 Kcal b. 41 Kcal
c. 410 Kcal d. 4100 kcal

69. The first plasma protein to be generated after severe protein deficiency is: *(COMED 2014)*

a. Albumin b. Globulin
c. Fibrinogen d. Thrombin

70. The amino acid which undergoes most significant hepatic oxidative deamination which is used for urea synthesis is: *(COMED 2014)*

a. Glutamine b. Glutamate
c. Aspartate d. Arginine

71. The class of amino acids that contain only non-essential amino acids is: *(COMED 2007)*

a. Acidic b. Basic
c. Aromatic d. Branded chain

72. Aspartate aminotransferase is released: *(COMED 2005*

a. By viable cells b. After cell necrosis
c. Either of the two d. None of the above

NUCLEIC ACID AND NUCLEOTIDE

73. The sigma (σ) subunit of prokaryotic RNA polymerase: *(AIPG 2006)*

a. Binds the antibiotic rifampicin
b. Is inhibited by β-amanitin
c. Specifically recognizes the promoter site
d. Is part of the core enzyme

74. RNA interference, all involved *except*: *(AIPG 2012)*

a. Drosha b. Pasha
c. mRNA d. miRNA

75. DNA replication measured by: *(AIPG 2012)*

a. Sphygmomanometer
b. Spirometer
c. Spectrophotometer
d. pH metre

76. In DNA molecule adenine always forms a linkage with: *(COMED 2013)*

a. Guanine b. Cytosine
c. Thymine d. Uracil

77. Lesch-Nyhan syndrome is due to deficiency of: *(KCET 2006)*

a. HGPRTase (Total)
b. PRPP Glutamine Amino Transferase
c. CTP synthetase
d. OMP Decarboxylase

ENZYMES

78. Which of the following liver enzymes is predominantly mitochondrion? *(AIIMS Nov 2010)*

a. SGOT (AST) b. SGPT (ALT)
c. GGT d. 5′ Nucleotidase

79. Enzyme that regulates the conversion of ethanol to acetaldehyde is: *(AIIMS Nov 2007)*

a. Alcohol dehydrogenase
b. Acetaldehyde dehydrogenase
c. Catalase
d. Xanthene oxidase

80. Which of the following enzymes at a pH of 8.6 has a function in bone mineralization and hydrolysis of phosphoric esters? *(AIIMS Nov 2007)*

a. Acid phosphatase
b. Alkaline phosphatase
c. Collagenase
d. Hyaluronidase

81. Enzyme stable at acidic pH is: *(AIPG 2008)*

a. Trypsin
b. Pepsin
c. Chymotrypsin
d. Carboxypeptidase

82. Oxidation of ethanol to aldehydes is done by which of the following enzymes? *(AIPG 2008)*

a. Alcohol dehydrogenase
b. Catalase
c. Acetaldehyde dehydrogenase
d. Xanthene oxidase

83. Coenzyme required for transamination is: *(AIPG 2008)*

a. Thiamine phosphate
b. Pyridoxine
c. Alpha-ketoglutarate
d. Cobalamine

84. Enzymes that move a molecular group from one molecule to another are known as: *(AIPG 2005)*
a. Ligases
b. Oxidoreductases
c. Transferases
d. Dipeptidases

85. The enzyme phosphofructokinase-l is strongly activated by: *(COMED 2008)*
a. Cyclic AMP
b. Adenosine triphosphate
c. Citrate
d. Fructose-2,6-bisphosphate

86. Biotin is required for the activity of: *(KCET 2009)*
a. Pyruvate carboxylase
b. Lactate dehydrogenase
c. Succinate thiokinase
d. Phosphohexose isomerase

87. Enzymes which play an important role in calcification are: *(COMED 2010)*
a. Enolase and calcitonin
b. Alkaline phosphatase and catalase
c. Alkaline phosphatase and pyrophosphatase
d. Pyrophosphatase and carbonic anhydrase

88. Which one of the following enzyme provides a link between glycolysis and the citric acid cycle? *(COMED 2010)*
a. Lactate dehydrogenase
b. Pyruvate kinase
c. Citrate synthase
d. Pyruvate dehydrogenase

89. Insulin increases the activity of: *(COMED 2010)*
a. HMG-CoA reductase
b. HMG-CoA layse
c. HMG-CoA synthase
d. Thiolase

90. LDH has following number of iso-enzymes: *(KCET 2011)*
a. 5 b. 3
c. 11 d. 2

91. Mutation in the oxidative enzymes (peroxisomes) could lead to: *(COMED 2012)*
a. Zellweger's syndrome
b. Gaucher's disease
c. Epidermolysis bullosa
d. Leber's neuropathy

92. A patient with hereditary fructose intolerance is deficient in which of the following enzymes? *(COMED 2013)*
a. Aldolase B b. Fructokinase
c. Triokinase d. All of the above

93. Which of the following is not a characteristic feature of allosteric enzymes? *(COMED 2013)*
a. They are multienzyme complexes
b. Follow Michaelis-Mentem kinetics
c. Presence of modulator site
d. Give sigmoid shaped curve

94. The level of the following enzymes are elevated in myocardial infarction *except*: *(KCET 2013)*
a. Lactate dehydrogenase
b. Alanine amino transferase
c. Creatine kinase
d. Aspartate amino transferase

95. Enzymes increase reaction rates by: *(KCET 2007)*
a. Altering the free energy of the action
b. Decreasing the energy of activation
c. Enhancing the forward reaction
d. Inhibiting the backward reaction

96. Von Gierke's Disease is associated with a deficiency of: *(KCET - 2007, COMED - 2006)*
a. Glucose-6-Phosphate dehydrogenase
b. Glucose-6-Phosphate in liver
c. Phosphorylase in muscle
d. Hexokinase

97. The enzyme known to cause spontaneous thrombosis as an adverse reaction is: *(COMED 2007)*
a. Tyrosine kinase b. Aromatase
c. Asparaginase d. Collagenase

VITAMINS

98. Which of the following factors are associated with vitamin K? *(AIIMS May 2010)*
a. II, VII, IX and X
b. III, X and XII
c. V, VIII, X and IX
d. II, VII, VII, IX and X

99. Pernicious anemia occurs due to the deficiency of: *(AIIMS May 2010)*
a. Folic acid b. Cobalamine
c. Riboflavin d. Pyridoxine

100. A patient complains of swollen joints, loose teeth, anemia and tiny bleeding points around the hair orifices. The patient is most likely suffering from the deficiency of: *(AIIMS Nov 2006)*

a. Vitamin A b. Vitamin E
c. Vitamin B1 d. Vitamin C

101. The maximum content of vitamin E is found in: *(AIIMS Nov 2006)*

a. Cod liver oil b. Fish liver oil
c. Wheat germ oil d. Shark liver oil

102. Vitamin which deficiency leads to pyurvate and lactic acid is: *(AIPG 2013)*

a. Thiamine b. Riboflavin
c. Niacin d. Pyrodoxine

103. Vitamin not involved in tooth development: *(AIPG 2013)*

a. Vit A b. Vit C
c. Vit E d. Vit D

104. Wernicke-Korsakoff psychosis is due to: *(AIPG 2010)*

a. Thiamine b. Vitamin C
c. Pyridoxine d. INH

105. Earliest sign of vitamin A deficiency is: *(AIPG 2010)*

a. Conjunctival xerosis
b. Bitot spot
c. Nyctalopia
d. Color blindness

106. Thiamine deficiency causes decreased energy production because: *(AIPG 2009)*

a. It is required for the process of transamination
b. It is a cofactor in oxidative reduction
c. It is a coenzyme for transketolase in pentose phosphate pathway
d. It is a coenzyme for pyruvate dehydrogenase

107. True about vitamin K is: *(AIPG 2008)*

a. Vitamin K2 is produced by plants
b. Vitamin K1 is produced by intestinal *Escherichia coli*
c. Bile is required for the absorption of vitamin K that is water soluble
d. Bile is required for the absorption of vitamin K that is fat soluble

108. Increase in lactate and pyruvate is seen in the deficiency of: *(AIPG 2007)*

a. Pyridoxine
b. Thiamine
c. Niacin
d. Retinoic acid

109. Vitamin B_{12} acts as a coenzyme to which one of the following enzymes?: *(AIPG 2007)*

a. Iso citrate dehydrogenase
b. Homocysteine methyltransferase
c. Glycogen synthase
d. Glucose-6-phosphate dehydrogenase

110. Lactic acidosis takes place in the deficiency of: *(AIPG 2012)*

a. Pantothenic acid b. Pyridoxine
c. Thiamine d. Riboflavin

111. Vitamin B_6 is also known as: *(AIPG 2012)*

a. Pyridoxine b. Niacin
c. Riboflavin d. Thiamine

112. Which vitamin is synthesized by intestinal bacteria? *(KCET 2008)*

a. Vitamin A b. Vitamin K
c. Vitamin D d. Vitamin E

113. One of the symptoms of vitamin A deficiency is: *(KCET 2008)*

a. Nyctalopia b. Xerophthalmia
c. Bitot's spot d. Keratomalacia

114. One molecule of beta carotene gives rise to: *(KCET 2008)*

a. One unit of vitamin A
b. Two units of vitamin A
c. Three units of vitamin A
d. Four units of vitamin A

115. Burning feet syndrome occurs due to deficiency of: *(COMED 2009)*

a. Niacin b. Pantothenic acid
c. Riboflavin d. Folic acid

116. Vitamin D: *(KCET 2009)*

a. Absorption requires bile pigments
b. Synthesis is regulated at the reaction catalyzed by 25 hydroxylase
c. Deficiency in adults leads to rickets
d. Along with PTH increases calcium resorption from bone

117. The mineral having sparing action on vitamin E: *(COMED 2013)*
a. Chromium b. Iron
c. Iodine d. Selenium

118. The Schilling test is used for detecting: *(COMED 2014)*
a. Presence of intrinsic factor
b. Deficiency of riboflavin
c. Excretion of folic acid
d. Capillary fragility

119. Figlu excretion test is used to detect:
a. Folic acid deficiency
b. Biotin deficiency
c. Pantothenic acid deficiency
d. Vit-B 12 deficiency

120. Deficiency of vitamin C causes the following *except*: *(COMED 2006)*
a. Painful swollen gums
b. Abnormal collagen
c. Anemia
d. Diarrhea

121. Which one of the following vitamin is bound to gastric intrinsic factor? *(COMED 2005)*
a. Vitamin K b. Folic acid
c. Vitamin B12 d. Vitamin D

122. Which of the following enzymatic reaction is directly related to vitamin K? *(COMED 2005)*
a. Activation of factor X
b. Regulation of blood calcium level
c. Conversion of fibrinogen to fibrin
d. Synthesis of prothrombin

123. All are Antimutagens, *except*: *(MH 2009)*
a. Vitamin A b. Aflatoxin
c. Vitamin C d. Curcumin

NUTRITION

124. Which of the following is the most important constituent of diet? *(AIIMS Nov 2006)*
a. Proteins b. Water
c. Vitamins d. Minerals

HEMOGLOBIN AND PORPHYRINS

125. Beta-oxidation of odd-chain FAs produces all *except*: *(AIIMS May 2006)*
a. Succinyl CoA b. Propionyl CoA
c. Acetyl-CoA d. Malonyl CoA

126. Hb1AC or glycohemoglobulin level of >9% indicates: *(COMED 2012)*
a. Normal
b. Mild diabetes control
c. Gestational diabetes
d. Poor diabetes control

127. The amino acid required for the sysnthesis of haem is: *(COMED 2013)*
a. Glutamine b. Glutamic acid
c. Glycine d. Lysine

MOLECULAR BIOLOGY AND BIOTECHNOLOGY

128. Number of base pairs found in human genome DNA is: *(AIIMS May 2013)*
a. 1.5 billion b. 3 billion
c. 4.5 billion d. 6.2 billion

129. Hybridization of two homologous but not identical DNA strands can be increased by: *(AIIMS May 2011)*
a. Decreasing the sodium chloride concentration in the medium
b. Increasing dimethyl-formamide in the medium
c. Ionic strengths
d. Increasing the wash temperature

130. Which of the following is not a post transcriptional modification of RNA? *(AIIMS May 2006)*
a. Splicing b. 5-Capping
c. 3-Polyadenylation d. Glycosylation

131. During which phase of the cell cycle the cellular content of DNA is doubled? *(AIIMS Nov 2005, COMED 2005)*
a. Mitotic phase b. G1 phase
c. G2 phase d. S phase

132. Denaturation of DNA means: *(AIPG 2010)*
a. Fragmentation of DNA molecules
b. Reversible separation of DNA
c. Irreversible separation of DNA
d. Coagulation of DNA

133. DNA recombination technique is possible due to: *(AIPG 2010)*
a. Restriction endonuclease
b. Cosmid
c. Polymerase chain reaction
d. Exonuclease

134. The cell component that is genetically continuous from one cell generation to the next is: *(AIPG 2005)*
a. Nuclear membrane b. Golgi complex
c. Central bodies d. Chromatin

135. Transcription is the synthesis of:: *(COMED 2008)*
a. Single-stranded complimentary copy of DNA
b. Double-stranded complimentary copy of DNA
c. Complimentary copy of RNA
d. Complimentary copy of RNA

MISCELLANEOUS

136. The process of studying chromosome shape, size and fine structure under microscope is known as: *(AIIMS May 2013)*
a. Chromosome mapping
b. Karyotyping
c. Gene mapping
d. Genotype

137. Prothrombin time is increased in: *(AIIMS Nov 2008)*
a. Von Willebrand's disease
b. Haemophilia
c. Warfarin therapy
d. Liver disease

138. A patient suffers from hypogonadism, failure to thrive, loss of taste and inability to maintain stability. This is most suggestive of deficiency of: *(AIIMS Nov 2006)*
a. Zinc b. Chromium
c. Copper d. Potassium

139. The type of collagen present in hyaline cartilage is: *(AIPG 2011)*
a. Type I b. Type II
c. Type III d. Type IV

140. Sickle-cell anemia substitution of valine in place of glutamic acid is by: *(AIPG 2010)*
a. Missense mutation
b. Nonsense mutation
c. Deletion
d. Silent mutation

141. All of following have receptors which are transcription factor *except*: *(AIPG 2010)*
a. Insulin b. Estrogen
c. Glucocorticoids d. Vitamin D

142. ATP is the store house of: *(AIPG 2010)*
a. Energy b. Phosphate
c. Protein d. Glucose

143. Ehlers Danlos syndrome (EDS) is all *except*: *(AIPG 2009)*
a. Autosomal dominant
b. Autosomal recessive
c. X-linked dominant
d. X-linked recessive

144. Calcium is primarily found in which of the following forms in blood circulation? *(AIPG 2008)*
a. Calcium phosphate
b. Ion form
c. Free calcium
d. Calcium in bound form

145. Iron is present in all of the following, *except*: *(AIPG 2006)*
a. Myoglobin b. Cytochrome
c. Catalase d. Pyruvate kinase

146. A patient presents with following parameters pH 7.6. The pCO_2 is 30 mm Hg, of 102 mm Hg and HCO_3 is 20 mEq/L. Which of the following correctly describes the compensatory mechanism? *(AIPG 2012)*
a. Respiratory alkalosis
b. Metabolic alkalosis
c. Respiratory acidosis
d. Metabolic acidosis

147. Iron absorption is least affected by: *(AIPG 2012)*
a. Milk b. Calcium
c. NaCl d. Ascorbic acid

148. The antibody produced during primary immune response is: *(COMED 2008)*
a. IgM b. IgG
c. IgA d. IgE

149. Serum creatine kinase-3 (CK-3) is elevated in: *(COMED 2009, 2007)*
a. Muscular dystrophy
b. Myocardial infarction
c. Alcoholic cirrhosis
d. Brain tumors

150. The quantity of water lost in expired air in each 24 hrs is about: *(KCET 2011)*
a. 200 ml b. 400 ml
c. 600 ml d. 800 ml

151. A relatively mobile component of the electron transporting respiratory chain is: *(COMED 2012)*
a. Flavoprotein b. Cytochrome CL
c. Ubiquinone d. Cytochrome A

152. Example of a preventive antioxidant is: *(COMED 2012)*
a. Catalase
b. Tocopherol
c. Superoxide dismutase
d. Urate

153. Stain used to make the wetted area of filter paper strip more visible is: *(COMED 2013)*
a. Eosin stain b. Haemotoxin stain
c. Ninhydrin stain d. Blue stain

154. Ammonia produces by brain is trapped as: *(KCET 2007)*
a. Urea b. Uria acid
c. Creatinine d. Glutamine

155. Thyroxine is derived from: *(KCET 2006)*
a. Tyrosine b. Tyramine
c. Taurine d. Tryptophan

156. Mucopolysaccharide which function as a lubricant and shock absorber in synovial fluid is: *(KCET 2005)*
a. Heparin
b. Hyaluronic acid
c. Keratin sulphate
d. Chondroitin-4-Sulphate

157. Electron transport chain (ETC) and ATP synthesizing structures are located in: *(KCET 2005)*
a. Outer membrane of mitochondria
b. Mitochondrial matrix
c. Inner membrane of mitochondria
d. Microsomes

158. Transport form of iron is: *(COMED 2007)*
a. Transferrin
b. Ferritin
c. Apo ferritin
d. Lactoferritin

159. Intestinal absorption of Ca^{2+} is decreased by: *(COMED 2006)*
a. Proteins
b. Lactose
c. Phytic acid
d. Acidity

160. Supporting cells of taste buds are: *(COMED 2005)*
a. Sustenticular cells
b. Taste cells
c. Von Ebner cells
d. Acini

161. Which one of the following is the precursor of both gonadal and adrenocortical hormone? *(COMED 2005)*
a. Progesterone
b. Cortisol
c. Testosterone
d. Corticosterone

Answers with Explanations

CARBOHYDRATE

1. Ans. (d) Maltose *Ref: Satyanarayan 3rd ed. p 11*

- A carbohydrate is a large biological molecule, or macromolecule, consisting of carbon (C), hydrogen (H), and oxygen (O) atoms, usually with a hydrogen: oxygen atom ratio of 2:1
- Considering the polymerization degree (PD) of carbohydrates, they can be classified in Monosaccharides, disaccharides and Polysaccharides.

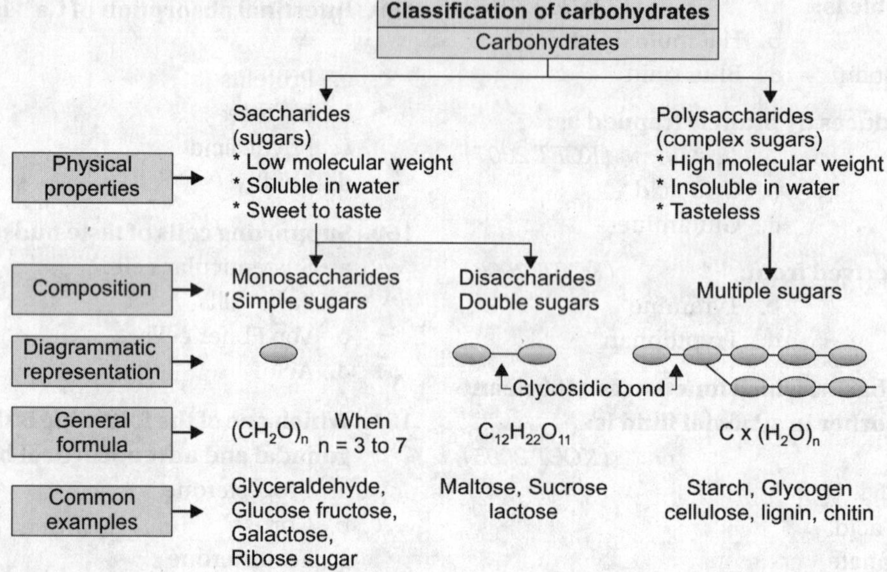

2. Ans. (a) NADPH oxidase *Ref: Lippincott's 3rd ed. p 148*

- NADPH oxidase is a membrane-associated enzyme that catalyzes the production of superoxide.
- It is considered one of the major sources of superoxide anions in humans as well as bacteria, used in oxygen-dependent killing mechanisms for invading pathogens.
- Oxygen-dependent mechanisms are the most potent and they act via respiratory burst, the basis of which is the activation of a flavoprotein oxidase, known as NADPH oxidase.

3. Ans. (a) Glucose *Ref: Satyanarayan 3rd ed. p 149*

- Acetyl coenzyme A or acetyl-CoA is an important molecule in metabolism, used in many biochemical reactions.
- Its main function is to convey the carbon atoms within the acetyl group to the citric acid cycle (Krebs cycle) to be oxidized for energy production.
- Acetyl-CoA is produced during the second step of aerobic cellular respiration, pyruvate decarboxylation, which occurs in the matrix of the mitochondria.
- Acetyl-CoA then enters the citric acid cycle.
- Acetyl-CoA is also an important component in the biogenic synthesis of the neurotransmitter acetylcholine.
- Choline, in combination with acetyl-CoA, is catalyzed by the enzyme choline acetyl transferase to produce acetylcholine and a Coenzyme A byproduct.

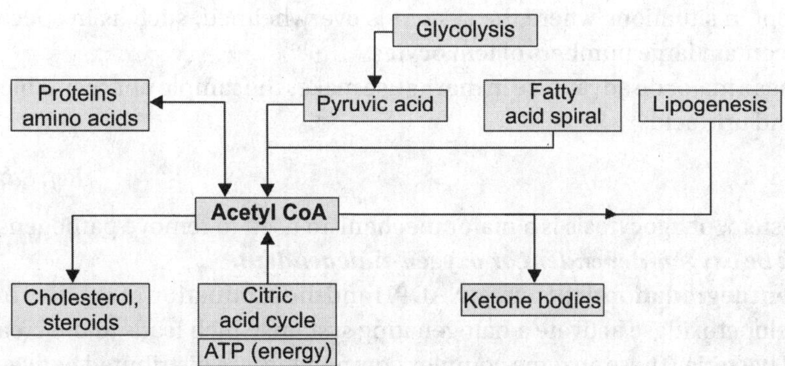

4. Ans. (a) Fructose *Ref: Modern Nutrition in Health and Disease by Maurice Edward - 7th ed. p 79*

- Fructose, a naturally occurring hexose, is a component of many fruits, vegetables, and sweeteners.
- Fructose is sweeter, more soluble, and less glucogenic than glucose or sucrose, so it has been recommended as a replacement for these sugars in the diets of diabetic and obese people.
- Fructose is absorbed primarily in the jejunum and metabolized in the liver.
- When consumed in excess of dietary glucose, it may be malabsorbed.
- Fructose is more lipogenic than glucose or starches.
- Fructose is known to increase blood pressure more than other carbohydrates.

5. Ans. (c) Nonoxidative phase generates pyruvate *Ref: Harper's 28th ed. p 174*

- The pentose phosphate pathway (also called the phosphogluconate pathway and the hexose monophosphate shunt) is a process that generates NADPH and pentoses (5-carbon sugars).
- There are two distinct phases in the pathway. The first is the oxidative phase, in which NADPH is generated, and the second is the non-oxidative synthesis of 5-carbon sugars.
- This pathway is an alternative to glycolysis.
- While it does involve oxidation of glucose, its primary role is anabolic rather than catabolic.
- For most organisms, it takes place in the cytosol; in plants, most steps take place in plastids.

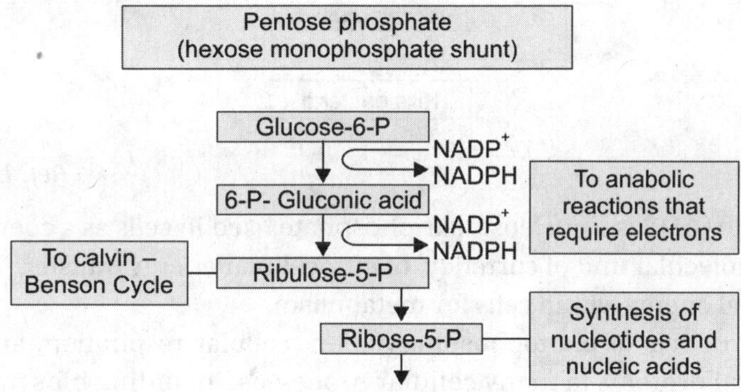

6. Ans. (a) Sodium fluoride *Ref.: www.ncbi.nlm.nih.gov › NCBI › Literature › Bookshelf*

- Both red cells and leukocytes contain glycolytic enzymes. Therefore glucose will be consumed and the concentration of glucose in a sample of whole blood will decline with time.
- The rate of loss is generally said to be approximately 5% per hour, but may be as rapid as 40% in 3 hours.
- Consumption of glucose in whole blood samples can be prevented by adding sodium fluoride to the specimen to inhibit the glycolytic enzymes.

- This approach is the generally applied method in the clinical laboratory.
- It is effective except in situations where the system is overwhelmed, such as in specimens from patients with leukemia, which contain large numbers of leukocytes.
- Sodium fluoride has a major disadvantage in that its use makes the sample unacceptable for other determinations such as sodium and uric acid.

7. Ans. (a) Oxidase *Ref: Satyanarayan 3rd ed. p 657*

- In the immune system, phagocytosis is a major mechanism used to remove pathogens and cell debris.
- ***Degradation can be oxygen-dependent or oxygen-independent.***
- **Oxygen-dependent degradation** depends on NADPH and the production of reactive oxygen species. Hydrogen peroxide and myeloperoxidase activate a halogenating system, which leads to the creation of hypochlorite and the destruction of bacteria. These enzyme complex components are distributed between cytoplasm and plasma membrane in a resting cell, but once the cell is activated, they migrate to the plasma membrane. At the plasma membrane, they associate with cytochrome components and generate active oxidase.
- Oxygen-independent degradation depends on the release of granules, containing proteolytic enzymes such as defensins, lysozyme, and cationic proteins. Other antimicrobial peptides are present in these granules, including lactoferrin, which sequesters iron to provide unfavorable growth conditions for bacteria.

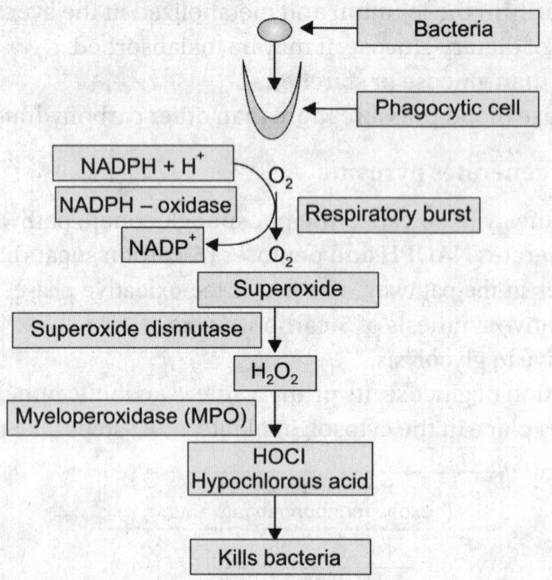

8. Ans. (a) ATP *Ref: Lippincott's 3rd ed. p 72, 78, 80*

- Adenosine triphosphate (ATP) is a nucleoside triphosphate used in cells as a coenzyme.
- It is often called the 'molecular unit of currency' of intracellular energy transfer.
- ATP transports chemical energy within cells for metabolism.
- It is one of the end products of photophosphorylation, cellular respiration, and fermentation and used by enzymes and structural proteins in many cellular processes, including biosynthetic reactions, motility, and cell division.
- ATP serves the major transducer of free energy.

9. Ans. (a) Disachharide *Ref: Satyanarayan 3rd ed. p 18, 21*

- Maltose also known as maltobiose or malt sugar, is a disaccharide formed from two units of glucose joined with an $\alpha(1\rightarrow4)$ bond, formed from a condensation reaction.
- Maltose is the disaccharide produced when amylase breaks down starch.

- Maltose is a disaccharide formed by the union of two glucose units (monosaccharide).
- It is found in beverages, beer, cereal, pasta, potatoes and in many processed products which have been sweetened.

10. Ans. (a) Glycogen *Ref: Satyanarayan 3rd ed. p 263, 382*

- Glycogen is a multibranched polysaccharide of glucose that serves as a form of energy storage in animals and fungi.
- The polysaccharide structure represents the main storage form of glucose in the body.
- In humans, glycogen is made and stored primarily in the cells of the liver and the muscles, and functions as the secondary long-term energy storage.
- Muscle glycogen is converted into glucose by muscle cells, and liver glycogen converts to glucose for use throughout the body including the central nervous system.
- Glycogen is found in the form of granules in the cytosol/cytoplasm in many cell types, and plays an important role in the glucose cycle.
- The most common disease in which glycogen metabolism becomes abnormal is diabetes.

11. Ans. (a) There is increased phosphorylation of glucose by glucose by glucokinase *Ref: Harper's, 28th ed. p 149,150*

The overall equation for glycolysis from glucose to lactate s as follows:

- Glucose + 2 ADP + 2 P1 → 2 Lactate + 2 ATP + $2H_2O$
- All of the enzymes of glycolysis are found in the cytosol. Glucose enters glycolysis by phosphorylation to glucose 6-phosphate, catalyzed by hexokinase, using ATP as the phosphate donor. Under physiologic conditions, the phosphorylation of glucose to glucose-6-phosphate can be regarded as irreversible. Hexokinase is inhibited allosterically by its product, glucose-6-phosphate.
- In tissues other than the liver (and pancreatic β-islet cells), the availability of glucose for glycolysis (or glycogen synthesis in muscle, and lipogenesis in adipose tissue controlled by transport into the cell, which in turn is regulated by insulin. Hexokinase has a high affinity (low Km) for glucose, and in the liver it is saturated under normal conditions, and so acts at a constant rate to provide glucose-6-phosphate to meet the cell's need. Liver cells also contain an isoenzyme of hexokinase, glucokinase, which has a Km very much higher than the normal intracellular concentration of glucose. The function of glucokinase in the liver is to remove glucose from the blood following a meal, providing glucose-6-phosphate in excess of requirements for glycolysis, which is used for glycogen synthesis and lipogenesis.

12. Ans. (c) Benedict's test positive *Ref: Satyanarayana 3rd ed. p 295, 386*

Ketosis is a state of elevated levels of ketone bodies in the body. There are two major cause of ketoacidosis.

- Most commonly diabetic ketoacidosis resulting from increased fat metabolism due to shortage of insulin.
- Alcoholic ketoacidosis, which can occur with acute alcohol intoxification.
- A mild acidosis may result from prolonged fasting or when following a ketogenic diet or a very low caloric diet.
- When the body is in ketosis, subjects often smell of acetone.
- Nitroprusside tube test (modified Rothera's test) is sensitive for ketones in urine. Option 'C' Benedict's test is employed for identifying reducing agent of sugars.

13. Ans. (b) GLUT 2 *Ref: Lippincott's 3rd ed. p 95*

- GLUT 2 glucose transporters are found in pancreatic β cells. These cells must have the capability to sense a higher concentration of glucose in order to release insulin when appropriate.
- GLUT 2 transporters are low affinity glucose transporters (with high Km) and only transport glucose when the concentration of circulating glucose is greater than 5 mM, the normal concentration of glucose in blood.
- In this manner, glucose is only transported into the β cells when glucose levels increase from basal levels after consumption of carbohydrates.

Glucose transporters		
	Location	*Glucose affinity*
GLUT 1	Erythrocytes other tissues	High (≅ 1 mmol/L)
GLUT 2	Liver, pancreatic B cells	Lowest (≅ 15 mmol/L)
GLUT 3	Brain, other tissues	High (≅ 1 mmol/L)
GLUT 4 tissue	Muscles, adipose translocation ↑ by insulin	Low (≅ 5 mmol/L)
GLUT 5	Small intestine	Medium

14. Ans. (a) 2 to 3 times greater than in serum *Ref: Carranza's - 10th ed. p 346*

- Glucose concentration in gingival crevicular fluid is 3-4 times greater than that in serum.
- Glucose hexosamine and hexuronic acid are the two of the compounds found in gingival fluids

15. Ans. (b) Cellulose *Ref: Satyanarayana-3rd ed. p 508*

- Cellulose is an organic compound with the formula $(C_6H_{10}O_5)n$.
- Humans can digest cellulose to some extent, but it mainly acts as a hydrophilic bulking agent for feces and is often referred to as a 'dietary fiber'.
- Cellulose has no taste, is odorless, is hydrophilic, is insoluble in water and most organic solvents, is chiral and is biodegradable.

16. Ans (d) Glycogen *Ref: Satyanarayana-3rd ed. p 21*

- Glycogen is the principal storage form of glucose in animal cells.
- In humans, the most glycogen is found in the liver (10% of the liver mass), whereas muscles only contain a relatively low amount of glycogen (1% of the muscle mass). In addition, small amounts of glycogen are found in certain glial cells in the brain.
- Glycogen is a type of carbohydrate which is reserved in animals, hence it is termed as 'animal starch' for its resemblance with starch found in plants.
- Glycogen is a highly branched glucose polymer.

17. Ans. (b) Glycogen *Ref: Satyanarayana-3rd ed. p 21*

- Glycogen is a quick storage vehicle for the body to keep large amounts of glucose when it is not needed by the body.
- It is classed as a polysaccharide.
- It is stored in both the liver and muscles, but the liver store is more readily available for energy and blood sugar level maintenance, while the muscle store is mostly used for muscle fuel.
- The major site of daily glucose consumption (75%) is the brain via aerobic pathways.
- Glycogen is considered the principal storage form of glucose and is found mainly in liver and muscle, with kidney and intestines adding minor storage sites.

18. Ans. (d) Endocrine dysfunction of the pancreas *Ref: Satyanarayana-3rd ed. p 681*

- Glucose tolerance test is usually done to access Endocrine dysfunction of the pancreas.
- The glucose tolerance test is a lab test to check how your body breaks down sugar.
- The most common glucose tolerance test is the oral glucose tolerance test (OGTT).
- The oral glucose tolerance test is used to screen pregnant women for gestational diabetes between 24 and 28 weeks of pregnancy. It may also be used when the disease is suspected, even though fasting blood glucose level is normal.

	Normal	*Impaired fasting glucose or glucose tolerance*	*Overt diabetes*
Fasting glucose	< 110 mg/dL	110–139 mg/dL	≥ 140 mg/dL
	< 6.1 mmol/L	6.1–7.8 mmol/L	≥ 7.8 mmol/L
2h after oGTT	< 140 mg/dL	140–199 mg/dL	≥ 200 mg/dL
	< 7.8 mmol/L	7.8–11.1 mmol/L	≥ 11.1 mmol/L

19. Ans. (c) Skeletal muscle *Ref: Satyanarayana-3rd ed. p 263*

- Glycogen is the storage form of glucose. It is stored in liver (68%) as well as muscle) 1-2%).
- But, as our body contains more muscle mass the storage amount of glycogen in muscle is about 250 gm where as in liver it is only 75 gm.

20. Ans. (d) It forms the part of disaccharide sucrose *Ref: Satyanarayana-3rd ed. p 18*

- Sucrose is a sugar, the organic compound commonly known as table sugar, cane sugar, beet sugar or, usually, just sugar.
- The molecule is a disaccharide composed of the monosaccharides glucose and fructose with the molecular formula $C_{12}H_{22}O_{11}$.
- In sucrose, the components glucose and fructose are linked via an ether bond between C1 on the glucosyl subunit and C2 on the fructosyl unit.
- Sucrose does not melt at high temperatures.
- Sucrose is formed by plants and cyanobacteria but not by other organisms.
- Sucrose is found naturally in many food plants along with the monosaccharide fructose.

21. Ans. (c) Glycerol *Ref: Lippincott's 3rd ed. p 115*

- Gluconeogenesis (abbreviated GNG) is a metabolic pathway that results in the generation of glucose from non-carbohydrate carbon substrates such as pyruvate, lactate, glycerol, glucogenic amino acids, and fatty acids.
- In vertebrates, gluconeogenesis takes place mainly in the liver and, to a lesser extent, in the cortex of kidneys.
- In many other animals, the process occurs during periods of fasting, starvation, low-carbohydrate diets, or intense exercise.

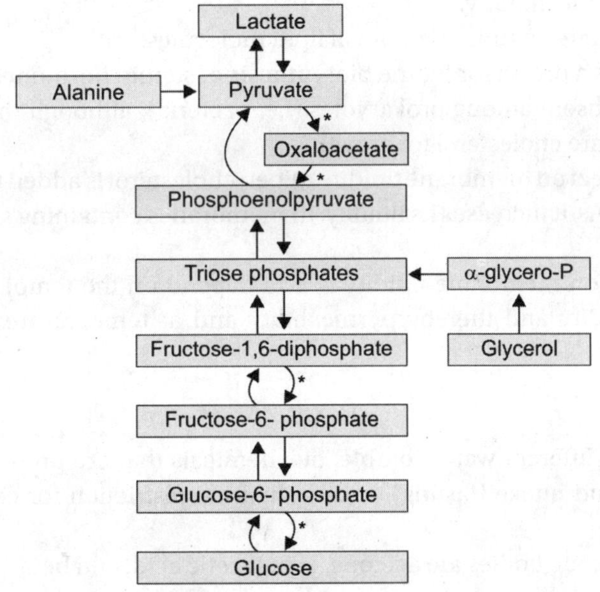

LIPIDS

22. Ans. (d) Eggs *Ref: Satyanarayan 3rd ed. p 510*

- Cholesterol is a steroid lipid (fat) found in the blood of all animals and is necessary for proper functioning of our cell membranes and production of hormones.
- While there can be negative health benefits associated with low cholesterol, cholesterol deficiency is rare.
- Our bodies already manufacture all the cholesterol we need, so it is not necessary to consume more.
- Excessive consumption of cholesterol has been shown to increase the risk of heart disease and stroke.
- Cholesterol is only found in animal food products, and thus, vegans are likely to have lower cholesterol thannon-vegans.

23. Ans. (b) Arachidonic acid and (d) Docosahexaenoic acid (DHEA) *Ref: Harper's 28th ed. p 200*

- Breast milk is the ideal food for growing infants.
- Breast milk contains the perfect balance of fat carbohydrate. Proteins, vitamins,minerals that an infant needs to thrive
- Breast milk contains tow fatty acid ie. Arachidonic acid (AA) and Docohexaenic acid (DHA). They are essential for normal growth, (DHA). They are essential for normal growth eyesight and brain development.
- Breast milk also contains digestive enzymes hormones, growth factors, antibodies.
- Breastfeeding also helps to stimulate the uterus to return to normal size and to control postpartum bleeding.

24. Ans. (b) Corn oil *Ref: Lippincott's 3rd ed. p 360*

- Plant oils, such as corn oil and sunflower seed oil, contain a high proportion of PUFAs.
- N6-PUFA: Corn oil, sunflower oil, soya bean oil, poultry, meat.
- N3-PUFA: Flax seed oil, cod liver oil, oily fish (e.g. Herrings).
- Oily fish is the richest dietary source of N3-PUFA while only a very small amount of N3 PUFA is present in corn oil.

25. Ans. (c) Cholesterol *Ref: Satyanarayan 3rd ed. p*

- Cholesterol is an organic molecule.
- It is a sterol and an essential structural component of animal cell membranes that is required to establish proper membrane permeability and fluidity.
- Cholesterol is thus considered within the class of lipid molecules.
- Cholesterol also serves as a precursor for the biosynthesis of steroid hormones, bile acids, and vitamin D.
- It is almost completely absent among prokaryotes (i.e. bacteria), although there are some exceptions such as Mycoplasma, which require cholesterol for growth.
- Cholesterol has a dual effect on membrane fluidity. When cholesterol is added to a membrane mainly composed of saturated long-chain FAs, it increases its fluidity. In membranes containing significant cis-FAs, it decreases the fluidity.
- The effect of cholesterol on membrane fluidity is also depend on the temperature at temperature below Tm cholesterol increase fluidity and thereby permeability and at temperature above Tm cholesterol decrease fluidity.

26. Ans. (a) Ketones *Ref: Satyanarayan 3rd ed. p 295*

- Ketone bodies are three different water-soluble, biochemicals that are produced by the liver from fatty acids during periods of low food intake (fasting) or carbohydrate restriction for cells of the body to use as energy instead of glucose.
- The three endogenous ketone bodies are acetone, acetoacetic acid, and beta-hydroxybutyric acid.

- Rothera's test: Positive by acetone and acetoacetic acid
- Gerhardt's test: Positive by acetoacetic acid only, not by acetone

27. Ans. (c) Sphingomyelins *Ref: Satyanarayan 3rd ed. p 307*

- Niemann-Pick disease is an inherited condition involving lipid metabolism, which is the breakdown, transport, and use of fats and cholesterol in the body.
- Mutations in the SMPD1 gene cause Niemann-Pick disease types A and B. They stop the body from making an enzyme, acid sphingomyelinase, that breaks down lipids.
- Symptoms are related to the organs in which sphingomyelin accumulates.
- Accumulation of Sphingomyelin in the central nervous system (including the cerebellum) results in unsteady gait (ataxia), slurring of speech (dysarthria) and discoordinated swallowing (dysphagia). Basal ganglia dysfunction causes abnormal posturing of the limbs, trunk, and face (dystonia).

28. Ans. (c) Margarine *Ref: Harper's 28th ed. p 122*

- Safflower oil contains the highest percentage of PUFAs and the lowest percentage of saturated fatty acids (SFAs).
- Margarine is nothing but the hydrogenated safflower yield.

29. Ans. (d) Fish oil *Ref: Lippincott's 3rd ed. p 361*

- Eicosapentaenoic acid (EPA or also icosapentaenoic acid) is an omega-3 fatty acid.
- EPA is a polyunsaturated fatty acid (PUFA) that acts as a precursor for prostaglandin-3 (which inhibits platelet aggregation), thromboxane-3, and leukotriene-5 groups (all eicosanoids).
- It is obtained in the human diet by eating oily fish or fish oil, e.g. cod liver, herring, mackerel, salmon, menhaden andsardine, and various types of edible seaweed. It is also found in human breast milk.
- However, fish does not naturally produce EPA, but obtain it from the algae they consume.
- Fish oil contains Docosahexaenoic acid (DHA) and Eicosapentaenoic acid (EPA).

30. Ans. (d) HMP pathway *Ref: Harper's 28th ed. p 177*

- The pentose phosphate pathway (also called the phosphogluconate pathway and the hexose monophosphate shunt) is a process that generates NADPH and pentoses (5-carbon sugars).
- There are two distinct phases in the pathway. The first is the oxidative phase, in which NADPH is generated, and the second is the non-oxidative synthesis of 5-carbon sugars.

The primary results of the Pathway are:

- The generation of reducing equivalents, in the form of NADPH, used in reductive biosynthesis reactions within cells. (e.g. fatty acid synthesis)
- Production of ribose-5-phosphate (R5P), used in the synthesis of nucleotides and nucleic acids.
- Production of erythrose-4-phosphate (E4P), used in the synthesis of aromatic amino acids.

31. Ans. (c) That it inhibits pyruvate dehydrogenase and (d) That it increases intracellular CAMP level
Ref: Harper's 28th ed. p 197

Insulin stimulates lipogenesis by:

- It enhances acetyl CoA carboxylase activity.
- It increases the transport of glucose into the cells (e.g. adipose tissue)
- It also increases the availability of pyruvate for fatty acid synthesis as well as glycerol 3 phosphate for esterification of fatty acid which is newly formed.
- It converts the inactive form of pyruvate dehydrogenase to the active form in adipose tissue (not in liver).
- It decreases the level of intracellular cAMP, hence it inhibits lipolysis in adipose tissue.

32. Ans. (c) Corn oil *Ref: Lippincott's 3rd ed. p 360*

Refer answer no. 3

33. Ans. (a) Egg *Ref: Satyanarayan 3rd ed. p 510*

Refer answer no. 1

34. Ans. (b) 9 *Ref: Satyanarayan 3rd ed. p 503*

	Calorific values of foodstuff Energy value (cal/g)	
Foodstuff	*In bomb calorimeter*	*In the body*
Carbohydrate	4.1	4
Fat	9.4t	9
Protein	5.4	4
Alcohol	7.1	7

35. Ans. (a) Electric insulators

- Lipids may be regarded as organic substances, relatively insoluble in water and soluble in organic solvents (alcohol, ether etc), that are related to fatty acids and utilized by the living cells.
- Lipids can be classified as follows:
  - Simple lipids:
    - Fats and oils
    - Waxes
  - Complex or Compound lipids:
    - Phospholipids (Glycerophospholipids and Sphingophospholipids)
    - Glycolipids
    - Lipoproteins
    - Other complex lipids
  - Derived lipids
  - Miscellaneous lipids
  - Neutral lipids
- Cell membrane consists mainly of phospholipid and protein molecule
- Phospholipid has two ends—Hydrophobic/Non-polar end and Hydrophilic/polar end.

36. Ans. (d) All of the above *Ref: Satyanarayan, 3rd ed. p 7*

- The lysosomal enzymes are responsible for maintaining the cellular compounds in a dynamic state, by their degradation and recycling. The degraded products leave the lysosomes, usually by diffusion, for reutilization by the cell. Sometimes, however, certain residual products, rich in lipids and proteins, collectively known as lipofusin accumulate in the cell. Lipofuscin is the age pigment or wear and tear pigment which has been implicated in ageing process.

37. Ans. (d) Linoleic acid *Ref: Biochemistry- U. Satyanarayan, 3rd ed. p 31*

- Essential fatty acids: The acids that cannot be synthesized by the body and, therefore, should be supplied in the diet are known as essential fatty acids (EFA). Chemically, they are polyunsaturated fatty acids, namely linoleic acid (18: 2; 9,12) and linolenic acid (18: 2; 9,12,15). Arachidonic acid (20: 4; 5, 8, 11, 14) becomes essential, if its precursor linoleic acid is not provided in the diet in sufficient amounts.

- Functions of EFA: Essential fatty acids are required for the membrane structure and function, transport of cholesterol, formation of lipoproteins, prevention of fatty liver etc. they are also needed for the synthesis of another important group of compounds, namely eicosanoids.
- Deficiency of EFA: The deficiency of EFA results in phrynoderma or toad skin, characterized by the presence of horny eruptions on the posterior and lateral parts of limbs, on the back and buttocks, loss of hair and poor wound healing.

38. Ans. (b) Aceto acetate *Ref: Biochemistry- U. Stayanarayana, 3rd ed. p 305*

- Regulation of ketogenesis: The ketone body formation occurs primarily due to non-availability ofcarbohydrates to the tissues. This is an outcome of excessive utilization of fatty acids to meet the energy requirements of the cells. The hormones glucagon stimulates ketogenesis whereas insulin inhibits.
- It results in an accumulation of acetyl COA and its diversion for over production of ketone bodies.

39. Ans. (c) Cytosol *Ref: Harper's illustrated Biochemistry, 28th ed*

- The main pathway for de novo synthesis of Fatty acids (Lipogenesis) occurs in the cytosol.

40. Ans. (d) Ketone bodies *Ref: Harper's 25th ed. p 124*

- Ketone bodies are three different water-soluble, biochemicals that are produced as by-products when fatty acids are broken down in the liver for energy. Two of the three are used as a source of energy in the heart and brain while the third (acetone) is a breakdown product of acetoacetic acid.
- Radioactive tracing of acetone determines that between 2% and 30% is excreted from the body, the remainder is diverted into one of two known metabolic pathways both of which lead to pyruvate.
- Pyruvate can be oxidized to acetyl-CoA or it can go through gluconeogenesis to build glucose. In the brain, ketone bodies are a vital source of energy during fasting or strenuous exercise. Although termed 'bodies', they are molecules, not particles.
- Ketone bodies can be used for energy. Ketone bodies are transported from the liver to other tissues, where acetoacetate and beta-hydroxybutyrate can be reconverted to acetyl-CoA to produce energy, via the citric acid cycle.
- Acetone in low concentrations is taken up by the liver and goes through the methylglyoxal pathway which ends with pyruvate. Acetone in high concentrations due to prolonged fasting or a ketogenic diet is absorbed by cells other than those in the liver and enters a different pathway via 1,2-propanediol. Though the pathway follows a different series of steps the end result is still pyruvate.

41. Ans. (b) Esterification with PUFA *Ref: Lippincott's 3rd ed. p 233-244*

HDLs perform a number of important functions including the following:

- HDL is a reservoir of apolipoproteins C-2 and chylomicrons and apo
- HDL uptake of unesterified cholesterol
- When cholesterol is taken up by HDL it is immediately esterified by plasma enzyme phosphatidyl choline: Cholestrol acyltransferase. This energy in synthesized by the liver.
- The selective transfer of cholesterol from peripheral cells to HDLs and from HDLs to the liver for bile and to steroidogenic cells for hormone synthesis.

42. Ans. (a) 200 mg/dl *Ref: Biochemistry- U. Stayanarayana, 3rd ed. p 315*

- Cholesterol is a waxy material found in all parts of your body.
- It helps to make cells, some hormones, and vitamin D.
- Cholesterol comes from two sources: your body and the foods you eat.
- Your liver makes all the cholesterol your body needs.

- Ideally your total cholesterol level should be less than 200. This is considered healthy.
- The higher your level of total cholesterol (240 or above), the more chance you have of getting heart disease.
- Your good cholesterol level (HDL) should be 35 or higher. Preferably around 50.
- Ideally your bad cholesterol level (LDL) should be less than 130. Preferably less than 100.

43. Ans. (b) Mono acyl glycerol *Ref: Biochemistry- U. Stayanarayana, 3rd ed. p 174*

- In the mouth, carbohydrates are broken down by amylase into maltose (disaccharide) and then move down the esophagus, which produces mucous for lubrication, but no digestive enzymes.
- In the duodenum, disaccharides are broken down into monosaccharides by enzymes called maltases, sucrases, and lactases; the monosaccharides produced are then absorbed into the bloodstream and transported to cells to be used in metabolic pathways to harness energy.
- In the stomach, proteins are broken down into peptides, which are then broken down into single amino acids that are absorbed in the bloodstream through the small intestine.
- Lipids are digested mainly in the small intestine by bile salts through the process of emulsification, which allows lipases to divide lipids into fatty acids and monoglycerides.
- Monoglycerides and fatty acids enter absorptive cells in the small intestine through micelles; they leave micelles and recombine into chylomicrons, which then enter the bloodstream.
- Fat-soluble vitamins are absorbed in the same manner as lipids; water-soluble vitamins can be directly absorbed into the bloodstream from the intestine.

PROTEIN AND AMINO ACIDS

44. Ans. (a) Isoleucine *Ref: Satyanarayan 3rd ed. p 364*

Acids are divided based

(A) Side chain (B) Ability to produce in body or not

(C) Polarity of R group (D) Catabolic pathway of the amino acid

I. Based on the structure of side chain

- Aliphatic Amino acids

Acidic amino acids—Asparate, Asparagine, Glutamate, Glutamine

- Neutral aliphatic amino acids—Glycine, Alanine, Serine, Theonine, Valine, Leucine and Isoleucine
- Basic amino acids—Arginine, Lysine, Histidine
- Branched chain—Valine, Leucine and Isoleucine
- Sulfur containing—Cysteine and Methionine
- Amide groups—Asparagine and Glutamine
- Hydroxy amino acids—serine threonine and tyrosine
- Simple amino acids—Glycine and alanine

- Aromatic amino acids—phenyl alanine and tyrosine and tryptophan and histidine
- Imino acids—proline

Nonpolar R groups	*Polar but uncharged R groups*	*Polar but charged groups*
Alanine, Serine, Valine, Leucine and Isoleucine, Methionine, phenyl alanine, proline, tryptophan and valine.	Asparagine, cysteine, glutamine, glycine serine, threonine and tyrosine	**Negatively charged (acidc amino acids)** Aspartic acid and Glutamic acid and **Positively charged (basic amino acids)** histadine, Arginine and Lysine

Based on catabolism fat II.					
Glucogenic amino acids		*Ketogenic amino acids*		*Both glucogenic and ketogenic amino acids*	
Amino acid	*Product*	*Amino acid*	*Product*	*Amino acid*	*Product*
Alanine serine	Pyruvate	Leucine	Acetoacetate	Phenylalanine	Fumarate
Glycine	Pyruvate succinate			Tyrosine	Acetoacetate
Threonine valine	Propoinate			Isoleucine	Propinyl CoA Acetyl CoA
Proline	Ketoglutarate				
Histidine					
Arginine					
Lysine (glutamic acid)					
Cystine	Pyruvate				
Hydroxy proline					
Aspartic acid	Oxaloacetate				

- Heterocycyclic Histidine and tryptophan, proline
- Dicarboxylic amino acids—Aspartic acid and Glutamic acid.
- Dibasic amino acids—Arginine and Lysine

++++ S0 tryptophan is both aromatic as well as heterocyclic.

**** proline is both heterocyclic and imino acid. It is the only DNA coded heterocyclic Alpha amino acid.

II. Based on polarity and side group (little bit confusing)

Based on whether they can be produced in body or not.

III. Essential and nonessential

- Essential amino acids are not synthesized in the food and are supplied in the diet
- Non-essential amino acids are synthesized in the body even if they are not present in the food Semi- essential synthesized in the body in small quantities and not absolutely essential in the food.

Essential	*Non-essential*	*Semi essential*
Threonine valine leucine isoleucine, methionine, phenyl alanine, tryptophan, Remember H. VITTAL LMP	Glycine, serine, cysteine, cystine, proline, hydroxyl praline, or nithine,citrulline, tyrosine	Arginine*, Histidine *

Conditionally essential (required to some degree in growing children): Glycine, cysteine, cystine, proline, hydroxyl proline, ornithine, citrulline, tyrosine.

Semi essential are synthesized in the body in small quantities and not absolutely essential in the food—arginine and histidine.

So, two statements can be made:

- All acidic amino acids (Asparate, Asparagine, Glutamate, Glutamine) are Non-essential amino acids.
- All branched chain amino acids (Valine, leucine and isoleucine) are essential amino acids.

Aromatic Amino acids which contain aromatic ring in the side chain. A closed ring structure formed by six carbon atoms, with a single hydrogen atom attached to each one is called as Aromatic ring. Also called a phenyl ring or a benzene ring.

Heterocyclic amino acids chemical compounds containing at least one heterocyclic ring, which by definition has atoms of at least two different elements, plus the compound has at least one amine (nitrogen-containing) group.

The prefix hetero means 'other.' The nitrogen atom is an 'other' atom an atom other than carbon-in the ring itself. **Only Benzene containing (purely aromatic)** phenyl alanine and tyrosine Aromatic amino acids Tryptophan, phenyl alanine and tyrosine and histidine. Heterocyclic- Tryptophan, Histidine and proline.

Tryptophan has indole substituted alanine hence it is aromatic as well as heterocyclic. Histadine is imidazole substituted alanine. This hetero cyclic ring is aromatic in nature. All the amino acids have primary amino groups. whereas Proline secondary amino group incorporated in five ringered structure (imino group).

45. Ans. (b) Hydroxyproline *Ref: Lippincott's 3rd ed. p 45*

- Amino acid present in collagen are hydroxy proline and hydroxylysine, and they are generally absence in most other protein.
- These residual amino acid result due to the hydroxylation of proline and lysine
- Hydroxyproline is one of the most important amino acid in order to stabilize the triple helical structure of collagen
- Hydroxyproline maximizes the interchain hydrogen-bond formation and helps to strengther the fibre.

46. Ans. (c) Gel filtration chromatography *Ref: Satyanarayan 3rd ed. p 724*

Gel Filtration Chromatography

The most important factors to understand about gel filtration are:

- Gel filtration separates molecules based solely on their size.
- Larger molecules elute first from the column.
- Smaller molecules elute later from the column.
- Gel filtration chromatography is used primarily to purify proteins or other molecules of interest.
- Gel filtration chromatography can be used to estimate the size of unknown proteins.

Principles of gel filtration chromatography

- In gel filtration or molecular exclusion chromatography, molecules in solution are separated by size as they pass through a column of cross-linked beads that form a three-dimensional network.
- These polymer beads (frequently made of dextran, agarose, or acrylamide) comprise the stationary phase. The liquid phase is the solvent that is found both around the beads and in the pores of the stationary phase matrix.
- Molecules that are larger than the pores will not enter the stationary phase, staying in the solution (mobile phase) surrounding the beads. Hence, they elute first from the column.
- Smaller molecules will enter the pores in the beads and so move more slowly through the column.
- Molecules of intermediate size will enter the stationary phase to some extent, but will not spend as much time there as do the smaller molecules.

To summarize, larger molecules will elute from the column first, and the smallest molecules will elute last, with intermediate molecules strung out in between.

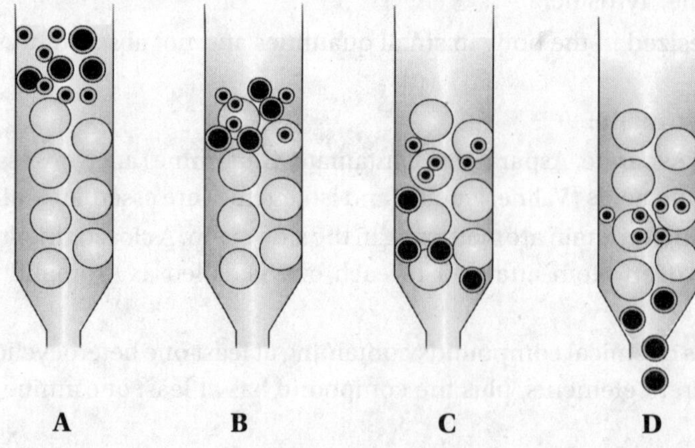

Gel filtration chromatography: Open circles represent the gel filtration beads, large filled circles are large molecules, and small filled circles are small molecules.

47. Ans. (a) Histone *Ref: Harper's 27th ed. p 322*

- In biology, histones are highly alkaline proteins found in eukaryotic cell nuclei that package and order the DNA into structural units called nucleosomes.
- They are the chief protein components of chromatin, acting as spools around which DNA winds, and play a role in gene regulation.
- Five major families of histones exist: H1/H5, H2A, H2B, H3 and H4. Histones H2A, H2B, H3 and H4 are known as the core histones, while histones H1 and H5 are known as the linker histones.

In all, histones make five types of interactions with DNA:

- Helix-dipoles from alpha-helices in H2B, H3, and H4 cause a net positive charge to accumulate at the point of interaction with negatively charged phosphate groups on DNA
- Hydrogen bonds between the DNA backbone and the amide group on the main chain of histone proteins
- Nonpolar interactions between the histone and deoxyribose sugars on DNA
- Salt bridges and hydrogen bonds between side chains of basic amino acids (especially lysine and arginine) and phosphate oxygens on DNA
- Non-specific minor groove insertions of the H3 and H2B N-terminal tails into two minor grooves each on the DNA molecule.

48. Ans. (d) Protein folding *Ref: Harper's 27th ed. p 37*

- Protein folding is a process in which a polypeptide folds into a specific, stable, functional, three-dimensional structure. It is the process by which a protein structure assumes its functional shape or conformation.
- Intramolecular chaperones are essential for protein folding, but not required for protein function. chaperones play a critical role in protein folding both in vivo and in vitro.
- Intramolecular chaperones are classified into two groups on the basis of their roles in protein folding.

The Type I intramolecular chaperones mediate the folding of proteins into their respective tertiary structures and are mostly produced as the N-terminal sequence extension.

The type II intramolecular chaperones mediate the formation of the quaternary or functional structure of proteins, and usually are located at the C-terminus of the protein.

49. Ans. (a) Oncotic pressure maintenance *Ref: Harper's 28th ed. p 569*

- Serum albumin is produced by the liver, occurs dissolved in blood plasma and is the most abundant blood protein in mammals.
- Albumin is essential for maintaining the oncotic pressure needed for proper distribution of body fluids between blood vessels and body tissues; without albumin, the high pressure in the blood vessels would force more fluids out into the tissues.
- Albumin functions primarily as a carrier protein for steroids, fatty acids, and thyroid hormones in the blood and plays a major role in stabilizing extracellular fluid volume by contributing to oncotic pressure (known also as colloid osmotic pressure) of plasma.
- Albumin is a globular, water-soluble, unglycosylated serum protein of approximate molecular weight of 65,000 Daltons.

50. Ans. (c) Galactosemia *Ref: Satyanarayan 3rd ed. p 376*

Alkaptonuria (black urine disease or alkaptonuria)

- It is a rare inherited genetic disorder of phenylalanine and tyrosine (an amino acid.) metabolism.
- This is an autosomal recessive condition that is due to a defect in the enzyme homogentisate 1,2- dioxygenase which participates in the degradation of tyrosine.

- Alkaptonuria is often asymptomatic, but the sclera of the eyes may be pigmented (often only at a later age), and the skin may be darkened in sun-exposed areas and around sweat glands; sweat may be coloured brown.

Homocystinuria

- It is also known as cystathionine beta synthase deficiency or CBS deficiency.
- It is an inherited disorder of the metabolism of the amino acid methionine.
- It is an inherited autosomal recessive trait, which means a child needs to inherit a copy of the defective gene from both parents to be affected.

Phenylketonuria (PKU)

- It is an autosomal recessive metabolic genetic disorder characterized by a mutation in the gene for the hepatic enzyme phenylalanine hydroxylase (PAH), rendering it non-functional.
- This enzyme is necessary to metabolize the amino acid phenylalanine (Phe) to the amino acid tyrosine.
- When PAH activity is reduced, phenylalanine accumulates and is converted into phenylpyruvate (also known as phenylketone), which can be detected in the urine.

51. Ans. (b) Disruption of secondary structure *Ref: Satyanarayan 3rd ed. p 61*

- Denaturation of proteins involves the disruption and possible destruction of both the secondary and tertiary structures.
- Since denaturation reactions are not strong enough to break the peptide bonds, the primary structure (sequence of amino acids) remains the same after a denaturation process.
- Denaturation disrupts the normal alpha-helix and beta sheets in a protein and uncoils it into a random shape.
- The most common observation in the denaturation process is the precipitation or coagulation of the protein.
- Heat can be used to disrupt hydrogen bonds and non-polar hydrophobic interactions.
- Medical supplies and instruments are sterilized by heating to denature proteins in bacteria and thus destroy the bacteria.

52. Ans. (b) Bence Jones proteins *Ref: Delmar's Manual of Laboratory and Diagnostic Tests, p 827*

- Bence Jones protein a low-molecular-weight, heat-sensitive urinary protein found in multiple myeloma.
- Bence Jones reaction the classic means of identifying Bence Jones protein, which precipitates when urine (from patients with this type of proteinuria) is gradually warmed to 45-70°C and redissolves when the urine is heated to near boiling; as the specimen cools, the Bence Jones protein precipitates in the indicated range of temperature and redissolves as the temperature of the specimen becomes less than 30-35°C.

53. Ans. (d) None of these *Ref: Satyanarayan 3rd ed. p 560, 573,*

- A cluster of amino acid residues having a characteristic three-dimensional folding pattern is termed as motif. It carries out a specific function, e.g. Zn finger motif.
- Chaperones are not present when the macromolecules perform their normal biological functions and have correctly completed the processes of folding and/or assembly.
- The mechanism of protein folding shown that soya bean seed coat peroxidase (SBP) is also taken part in it.

54. Ans. (c) Liver and (d) RBCs *Ref: Satyanarayan 3rd ed. p293-295, 385*

- Ketone bodies are three different water-soluble, biochemicals that are produced by the liver from fatty acids during periods of low food intake (fasting) or carbohydrate restriction for cells of the body to use as energy instead of glucose.
- The three endogenous ketone bodies are acetone, acetoacetic acid, and beta-hydroxybutyric acid.
- Two of the three are used as a source of energy in the heart and brain while the third (acetone) is a degradation breakdown product of acetoacetic acid.
- In the brain ketone bodies are also used to make Acetyl CoA into long chain fatty acids because long chain fatty acids cannot pass through the blood brain barrier.

- In the brain, ketone bodies are a vital source of energy during fasting or strenuous exercise.
- The liver breaks down protein to produce glucose during starvation for the very few glucose obligate cells that cannot use ketone bodies. Although the liver actively produces ketone bodies, it lacks thiophorase and, therefore, is unable to use ketone bodies as fuel.
- RBCs do not contain mitochondria, hence it lacks ketone bodies because mitochondria is the seat of ketone body oxidation.

55. Ans. (d) Densitometry *Ref: Biochemistry By Mary Campbell, Shawn Farrell, 7th ed. p 135*

- The basic aim of protein purification is to isolate the particular protein of interest from other contaminating proteins.
- The characteristics of proteins and other biomolecules that are utilized in different procedures are solubility size change adsorption property and specific binding site.
- The main separating methods used in protein purification and separation are:

Properties	*Methods*
Size or mass	• Centrifugation • Gel filteration • Dialysis and ultrafilteration • Gel electrophoresis
Charge	• Ion exchange chromatography • Electrophoresis • Isoelectric focusing
Solubility	• Change in PH • Change in ionic strength • Decrease in dielectric constant
Specific binding	• Affinity chromatography

56. Ans. None of the above *Ref: Medical Biochemistry by S. Ramakrishnan, 3rd ed. p 323*

- Glutamine generates ammonia in liner and kidney via glutamine deamination.
- Arginine is produced in kidney by a blood citrulline.
- In kidney catabolism of glycine takes place, here it forms serine and ammonia.
- In vitro studies, demonstrated the capacity for the formation of renal ammonia from aspartate.

57. Ans. (a) Chylomicrons *Ref: Satyanarayan 3rd ed. p 317*

- Chylomicrons are lipoprotein particles that consist of triglycerides (85-92%), phospholipids (6-12%), cholesterol (1-3%), and proteins (1-2%).
- The role of lipoprotein particles is to transport triacylglycerols and cholesterol in the blood between all the tissues of the body. The most common being the liver and the adipocytes of adipose tissue.
- Particles are synthesized in the small intestine and the liver, but interestingly not in the adipocytes.

58. Ans. (d) Quaternary structure *Ref: Satyanarayan 3rd ed. p 58*

- Proteins are polymers specifically polypeptides—sequences formed from various L-α-amino acids.
- Each unit of a protein is called an amino acid residue because it is the residue of every amino acid that forms the protein by losing a water molecule.

Primary structure

- The primary structure of a protein refers to the linear sequence of amino acids in the polypeptide chain.
- The primary structure is held together bycovalent bonds such as peptide bonds, which are made during the process of protein biosynthesis or translation.

- The two ends of the polypeptide chain are referred to as the carboxyl terminus (C-terminus) and the amino terminus (N-terminus) based on the nature of the free group on each extremity.

Secondary structure

- Secondary structure refers to highly regular local substructures. Two main types of secondary structure, the alpha helix and the beta strand or beta sheets.
- These secondary structures are defined by patterns of hydrogen bonds between the main-chain peptide groups.

Tertiary structure

- Tertiary structure refers to the three-dimensional structure of a single, double, or triple bonded protein molecule.
- The alpha-helixes and beta pleated-sheets are folded into a compact globular structure.
- The folding is driven by the non-specific hydrophobic interactions, the burial of hydrophobic residues from water, but the structure is stable only when the parts of a protein domain are locked into place by specific tertiary interactions, such as salt bridges, hydrogen bonds, and the tight packing of side chains and disulfide bonds.

Quaternary structure

- Quaternary structure is the three-dimensional structure of a multi-subunit protein.
- The quaternary structure is stabilized by the same non-covalent interactions and disulfide bonds as the tertiary structure.
- Complexes of two or more polypeptides (i.e. multiple subunits) are called multimers. Specifically it would be called a dimer if it contains two subunits, a trimer if it contains three subunits, a tetramer if it contains four subunits, and a pentamer if it contains five subunits.

59. Ans. (d) Proline *Ref: Harper's 27th ed. p 254*

- Proline is different from other amino acids in that its side chain pyrrolidine ring includes both the α-amino group and the α-carbon.
- This imino acid forces a 'bend' in a polypeptide chain, sometimes causing abrupt changes in the direction of the chain.
- Proline is an α-amino acid, one of the twenty DNA-encoded amino acids.
- Its codons are CCU, CCC, CCA, and CCG.
- It is not an essential amino acid, which means that the human body can synthesize it.
- Proline is biosynthetically derived from the amino acid L-glutamate and its immediate precursor is the imino acid (S)-1-pyrroline-5-carboxylate (P5C).

60. Ans. (a) Improper metabolism of amino acids *Ref: Satyanarayan 3rd ed. p 351*

Phenylketonuria (PKU)

- Phenylketonuria (PKU) is an autosomal recessive metabolic genetic disorder characterized by a mutation in the gene for the hepatic enzyme phenylalanine hydroxylase (PAH), rendering it non-functional.
- This enzyme is necessary to metabolize the amino acid phenylalanine (Phe) to the amino acid tyrosine
- It is a disease due to Improper metabolism of amino acids.
- Phenylketonuria is caused by lack of the enzyme needed to convert phenylalanine to tyrosine.
- Symptoms include intellectual disability, seizures, nausea, vomiting, an eczema-like rash, and a mousy body odor.
- The diagnosis is based on a blood test.
- A strict phenylalanine-restricted diet allows for normal growth and development.

61. Ans. (b) Apo C-II *Ref: Biochemistry- U. Satyanarayana, 1st ed. p 330*

- The enzyme 'lipoprotein lipase' is present in the capillary walls of adipose tissue, cardiac and skeletal muscle besides other tissues.

- It hydrolyses a portion of triacylglycerols present in chylomicrons and VLDL to liberate free fatty acids and glycerol.
- Lipoprotein lipase is activated by apo C II.

62. Ans. (c) Fibrinogen *Ref: Internet*

- Fibrinogen is a plasma protein and blood clotting factor-I. It is a soluble glycoprotein that constitutes 2–3% of plasma proteins.
- Albumin
- It is the major constituent (60%) of plasma proteins with a concentration of 3.5 to 5.0 g/dL.
- Albumin is exclusively synthesized in the liver.
- For this reason, measurement of serum albumin concentration is conveniently used to assess liver function (synthesis decreases in liver damage).
- Functions of albumin are as follows:
  - Osmotic function
  - Transport function
  - Nutritive function
  - Buffering function
- Globulins constitute several proteins that are separated into 4 distinct bands α, $\alpha 2$, β and γ globulins on electrophoresis.
- They are generally bigger in size than albumin and perform a variety of functions which include transport and immunity.
- Some of the important globulins are $\alpha 1$ antitrypsin, haptoglobin, ceruloplasmin transferring and the 5 immunoglobulins.
- **Thrombin**
- Prothrombin, which is blood clotting factor II, is converted into thrombin in presence of factors Va and Xa, besides phospholipids and Ca^{++}.
- Thrombin helps in conversion of fibrinogen to fibrin.

63. Ans. (c) Multiple myeloma *Ref: Harsh Mohan, 3rd ed. p 536*

About two-third cases of myeloma excrete Bence Jones (light chain) proteins in the urine, consisting of either kappa or lambda light chains, alongwith presence of Bence Jones paraproteins in the serum.

64. Ans. (b) Urobilinogen *Ref: Chatterijee 5th ed. p 651*

- Urobilinogen presence is checked by Ehrlich's test and Schesinger's test.
- Ehrlich's test consists of adding few ml of urine, few crystals of p-dimethyl amnion benzaldehyde and acidifying with HCL
- Cherry red color is seen in presence of normal amount of urobilinogen.

Note: Students need not go into much detailing of the test. Also note about urobilinogen:

- Urobilinogen is a colourless product of bilirubin reduction. It is formed in the intestines by bacterial action. Some urobilinogen is reabsorbed, taken up into the circulation and excreted by the kidney. This constitutes the normal 'enterohepatic urobilinogen cycle'.
- Increased amounts of bilirubin are formed in hemolysis, which generates increased urobilinogen in the gut. In liver disease (such as hepatitis), the intrahepatic urobilinogen cycle is inhibited also increasing urobilinogen levels. Urobilinogen is converted to the yellow pigmented urobilin apparent in urine.
- The urobilinogen (also known as stercobilinogen) in the intestine is then oxidized to brown stercobilin, which gives the feces their characteristic color.
- Low urine urobilinogen may result from complete obstructive jaundice or treatment with broad-spectrum antibiotics, which destroy the intestinal bacterial flora (obstruction of bilirubin passage into the gut or failure of urobilinogen production in the gut).

- Low urine urobilinogen levels may result from congenital enzymatic jaundice (hyperbilirubinemia syndromes) or from treatment with drugs that acidify urine, such as ammonium chloride or ascorbic acid.
- Elevated levels may indicate hemolytic anemia (excessive breakdown of red blood cells), overburdening of the liver, increased urobilinogen production, re-absorption—a large hematoma, restricted liver function, hepatic infection, poisoning or liver cirrhosis.

65. Ans. (b) Alpha 2 globulin *Ref: Harper's 26th ed. p 5*

- Ceruloplasmin is a $\alpha 2$ globulin.
- Ceruloplasmin is an enzyme (EC 1.16.3.1) synthesized in the liver containing 6 atoms of copper in its structure.
- Ceruloplasmin carries more than 95% of the total copper in healthy human plasma.
- The rest is accounted for by macroglobulins.
- Ceruloplasmin exhibits a copper-dependent oxidase activity, which is associated with possible oxidation of Fe2+ (ferrous iron) into Fe3+ (ferric iron), therefore assisting in its transport in the plasma in association with transferrin, which can carry iron only in the ferric state.
- The molecular weight of human ceruloplasmin is reported to be 151kDa.

66. Ans. (b) 8 g *Ref: Harper's 26th ed. p 479*

- Mg N × 6.25 = 1 mg protein, as nitrogen is 16% of most proteins.
- Now we have to calculate nitrogen content in 50 gm that is 500 mg of protein
- Therefore, 500 = 80 mg = 8 gm 6.25

67. Ans. (b) Lysosomes *Ref: Harper's 27th ed. p 515*

Targeting sequence or compound	*Organelle targeted*
Single peptide	Membrane of ER
Amino terminal KDEL sequence (Lys -Asp-Glu-Leu)	Luminal surface or ER
Amino terminal sequence (20-80 residues)	Mitochondrial matrix
NLS (e.g – Pro_2- Lys_2-Ala- Lys- Val)	Nucleus
PTS (e.g: Ser -Lys -Leu)	Peroxisome
Mannose-6 - phosphate	Lysosome

68. Ans. (b) 41 Kcal *Ref: Satyanarayan 3rd ed. p 503*

- The energy value of carbohydrates, fats and protein when metabolized in body are 4, 3, 4 kcal/g respectively so.

1 g of protein 4 k cal

10 g of protein give 10 × 4 kcal = 40 kcal.

69. Ans. (c) Fibrinogen

70. Ans. (b) Glutamate *Ref: Harper's 28th ed. p 241*

In urea cycle glutamate is the only amino acid that undergoes rapid oxidative deamination by using glutamate dehydrogenase, which uses NAD or NADP as a coenzyme.

This process leads to two distinct toxic compounds:

- Hydrogen Peroxide
- Ammonia

71. Ans. (a) Acidic *Ref: Satyanarayan 3rd ed. p 47*

Chemical Classification of amino acid

- **Neutral Amino Acid**
  - Glycine
  - Alanine
  - Valine
  - Leucine
- **Basic Amino Acid**
  - Lysine
  - Arginine
  - Histidine
- **Acidic Amino Acid**
  - Aspartic Acid
  - Glutamic Acid
  - Asparagines
  - Glutamine

  } these all are non- essential amino acids.

Essential amino acids	*Non-essential amino acids*
Histidine	Alanine
Isoleucine*	Arginine**
Leucine*	Asparagine
Lysine	Aspartic acid
Methionine	Cysteine**
Phenylalanine	Glutamic acid
Threonine	Glutamine**
Tryptophan	Glycine**
Valine*	Proline**
	Selenocysteine**
	Serine
	Taurine**
	Tyrosine**
*Branched-chain amino acid	
**Conditionally essential amino acid	

72. Ans. (b) After cell necrosis *Ref: Lippincott's 3rd ed.p 249*

Aspartate Aminotransferase (AST)

- Aspartate Aminotransferase (AST) catalyses conversion of nitrogenous portion of amino acid. It is essential to energy production in Krebs cycle.

NUCLEIC ACID AND NUCLEOTIDE

73. Ans. (c) Specifically recognizes the promoter site *Ref: Satyanarayan 3rd ed. p 544*

- A sigma factor (σ factor) is a protein needed only for initiation of RNA synthesis.
- It is a bacterial transcription initiation factor that enables specific binding of RNA polymerase to gene promoters.

- RNA polymerase (RNAP or RNApol), also known as DNA-dependent RNA polymerase, is an enzyme that produces primary transcript RNA. Incells, RNAP is necessary for constructing RNA chains using DNA genes as templates, a process called transcription.
- RNA polymerase = core RNA polymerase + sigma subunit
- Binding regions
- RNA = The sigma subunit (specifically recognizes the promoter region, binds to it and initiates transcription)
- DNA = The promoter region
- Transcription = sigma (RNA) + Promoter (DNA).

74. Ans. (c) mRNA *Ref: Harper's 28th ed. p 350*

- RNA interference (RNAi) is a biological process in which RNA molecules inhibit gene expression, typically by causing the destruction of specific mRNA molecules.
- Historically, it was known by other names, including co-suppression, post transcriptional gene silencing (PTGS), and quelling.
- Two types of small ribonucleic acid (RNA) molecules microRNA (miRNA) and small interfering RNA (siRNA) are central to RNA interference.
- Drosha is a type III RNase, which plays a critical role in miRNA biogenesis.
- Drosha and its double-stranded RNA-binding partner protein Pasha/DGCR8 likely recognize and cleave miRNA precursor RNAs or pri-miRNA hairpins cotranscriptionally.
- Both Drosha and Pasha are localized to the cell nucleus, where processing of pri-miRNA to pre- miRNA occurs.

75. Ans. (c) Spectrophotometer *Ref: Advances in Genetics by E.W. Caspari, Vol. 19, p 146*

- DNA concentration can be assessed using four different methods: absorbance (optical density), agarose gel electrophoresis, fluorescent DNA-binding dyes and a luciferase-pyrophosphorylation—coupled quantitation system.
- The two most common methods of measuring DNA purity and concentration are absorbance (measured using a spectrophotometer) and agarose gel analysis.
- Spectrophotometry is a very popular method for nucleic acid quantification as it is a simple, accurate and non-destructive method for the measurement of nucleic acid.

76. Ans. (c) Thymine *Ref: Pamela C. Champe 3rd ed. p 395*

- As DNA is a double stranded where bases of one strand of DNA are paired with the bases of the second strand, the adenine is always paired with a thymine and a cytosine is always paired with a guanine by hydrogen bonds.
- Therefore, one polynucleotide chain of the DNA double helix is always the complement of the other. Given the sequence of bases on one chain, the sequence of bases on the complementary chain can be determined. The specific base pairing in DNA the amount of adenine equals the amount of thymine; the amount of guanine equals the total amount of pyrimidines. The base pairs are held together by hydrogen bonds, two hydrogen bonds present between A and T three between G and C. These hydrogen bond stabilize the structure of the double helix.

77. Ans. (a) HGPRTase (Total) *Ref: Satyanarayan 3rd ed. p 395*

- Lesch Nyhan syndrome (LNS), also known as Nyhan's syndrome, Kelley-Seegmiller syndrome and juvenile gout, is a rare inherited disorder caused by a deficiency of the enzyme hypoxanthine- guanine phosphoribosyltransferase (HGPRT), produced by mutations in the HPRT gene located on the X chromosome.
- The HGPRT deficiency causes a build-up of uric acid in all body fluids. This results in both hyperuricemia and hyperuricosuria, associated with severe gout and kidney problems
- Neurological signs include poor muscle control and moderate intellectual disability.
- LNS is an X-linked recessive disease.
- LNS is characterized by three major hallmarks: neurologic dysfunction, cognitive and behavioral disturbances including self-mutilation, and uric acid overproduction (hyperuricemia).

ENZYMES

78. Ans. (a) SGOT (AST) *Ref: Satyanarayan 3rd ed. p 107, 455*

- AST is found in the liver, heart, skeletal muscle, kidneys, brain, and red blood cells, and it is commonly measured clinically as a marker for liver health.
- There are two general categories of 'liver enzyme' used in liver function tests.
  - Alanine aminotransferase (SGPT)
  - Aspartate aminotransferase (SGOT)
- ALT is a cytoplasmic enzyme as it presents in cytoplasm while SGOT is predominantly mitochondrial inside the liver as it is located mainly in the mitochondria (about 80%) and the remaining 20% in the cytosol.
- SGPT is more specific for the diagnosis of liver disease while SGOT is for heart disease.

Remember

Cytosolic and mitochondrial enzymes are used as evidence for hepatocellular damage. Membrane- bound enzymes are used as evidence for cholestasis.

79. Ans. (a) Alcohol dehydrogenase *Ref: Satyanarayan 3rd ed. p 327*

- Alcohol is generally absorbed by the stomach and intestine.
- Less than 2% is mainly excreted by lungs urine and sweat.
- In the liver, alcohol (ethamol) gets oxidised and forms acetaldehyde by alcohol dehydrogenase.

CH_2CHO

$CH_2CH_2 - OH$ Alcohol dehydrogenase (ethnol) → Acetaldehyde

NAD_2 → $NADH + H_2$

- In later stage, acetaldehyde oxidized by aldehyde dehydrogenase producing acetate.

80. Ans. (b) Alkaline phosphatase *Ref: Internet*

An phosphate with an optimum functioning at 8.6, it is present throughout the body. Phosphates hydrolyse organic phosphate ester.

81. Ans. (c) Chymotrypsin *Ref: Satyanarayan 3rd ed. p 170*

- Pepsin is an enzyme whose zymogen (pepsinogen) is released by the chief cells in the stomach and that degrades food proteins into peptides.
- Pepsin is a digestive protease, a member of the aspartate protease family.
- Pepsin is most active in acidic environments between 37°C and 42°C.
- Pepsin exhibits maximal activity at pH 2.0 and is inactive at pH 6.5 and above.
- The stability of pepsin at high pH has significant implications on disease attributed to laryngopharyngeal reflux.

82. Ans. (a) Alcohol dehydrogenase *Ref: Satyanarayan 3rd ed. p 327*

Refer ans no. 2

83. Ans. (b) Pyridoxine *Ref: Satyanarayan 3rd ed. p 332*

- Transamination (or aminotransfer) is a chemical reaction between two molecules. One is an amino acid, which contains an amine (NH2) group. The other is a keto acid, which contains a keto (=O) group. In transamination, the NH2 group on one molecule is exchanged with the =O group on the other molecule. The amino acid becomes a keto acid, and the keto acid becomes an amino acid.
- Pyridoxal-phosphate (PLP) is a prosthetic group of certain enzymes. PLP is also the active form of vitamin B6, which comprises three natural organic compounds, pyridoxal, pyridoxamine and pyridoxine.

- PLP acts as a coenzyme in all transamination reactions, and in certain decarboxylation, deamination, and racemization reactions of amino acids.
- PLP also is necessary for the enzymatic reaction governing the release of glucose from glycogen.

84. Ans. (c) Transferases *Ref: Satyanarayan, 3rd ed. p 86*

- Transferase is the general name for the class of enzymes that enact the transfer of specific functional groups (e.g. a methyl or glycosyl group) from one molecule (called the donor) to another (called the acceptor).
- Mechanistically, an enzyme that catalyzed the following reaction would be a transferase:

$$\text{X group} + \text{Y} \xrightarrow[\text{transerase}]{} \text{X} + \text{Y group}$$

85. Ans. (d) Fructose-2,6-bisphosphate *Ref: Biochemistry- U. Satyanarayana, 3rd ed. p 246,247*

- Phosphofructokinase (PFK) is the most important regulatory enzyme in glycolysis. This enzyme catalyzes the rate-limiting committed step. PFK is an allosteric enzyme regulated by allosteric effectors. ATP citrate and H^+ ions (low PH) are the most important allosteric inhibitors, whereas fructose-2,6-bisphosphate, AMP and Pi are the allosteric activators.

86. Ans. (a) Pyruvate carboxylase *Ref: Biochemistry- U. Satyanarayan, 3rd ed. p 147*

- Biotin (formerly known as anti-egg white injury factor, vitamin B7 or vitamin H) is a sulfur containing B-complex vitamin. It directly participates as a coenzyme in the carboxylation reactions.
- Biochemical functions: Biotin serves as a carrier of CO_2 in carboxylation reactions. The reaction catalysed by pyruvate carboxylase, converting pyruvate to oxaloacetate has been investigated in detail. This enzyme has biotin bound to the apoenzyme linked to the ε-amino group of lysine, forming the active enzyme (holoenzyme). Biotin-enzyme reacts with CO_2 in presence of ATP (provides energy) to form a carboxybiotin-enzyme complex. This high energy complex hands over the CO_2 to pyruvate (carboxylation reaction) to produce oxaloacetate.
- As a coenzyme, biotin is involved in various metabolic reactions.
  - Gluconeogenesis and citric acid cycle
  - Fatty and synthesis
  - Propionyl CoA
- It was once believed that all the carboxylation reaction in the biological system are dependent on biotin. This was tater proved to be wrong. These are a few carboxylation reactions which do not require biotin, e.g. formation of carbonyl phosphate in urea cycle. Incorporation of CO_2 in purine synthesis.

87. Ans. (c) Alkaline phosphatase and pyrophosphatase *Ref: Harper, 28th ed. p 540 and Biochemistry- U. Satyanarayana, 3rd ed. p 125 and Sembulingam, 4th ed. p 380*

- Alkaline phosphatase is concerned with the process of bone formation. There is an overproduction of alkaline phosphates related to more cellular activity of the bone.
- In rickets, plasma level of calcitrol is decreased and alkaline phosphates activity is elevated.

88. Ans. (d) Pyruvate dehydrogenase *Ref: Biochemistry- U. Stayanarayana, 3rd ed. p 135, 252*

- The enzyme pyruvate dehydrogenase catalyses (oxidative decarboxylation) the irreversible conversion of pyruvate to acetyl CoA.
- Pyruvate is converted to acetyl CoA by oxidative decarboxylation. This is an irreversible reaction, catalysed by a multienzyme complex, known as pyruvate dehydrogenase complex (PDH), which is found only in the mitochondria.
- Citric acid cycle involves the oxidation of acetyl CoA to CO_2 and H_2O. Pyruvate is end product of glycolysis.

89. Ans. (a) HMG-COA reductase *Ref: Harper, 27th ed. p 231*

Cholesterol synthesis --- is controlled by regulation of HMG CoA reductase, which is rate limiting enzyme.

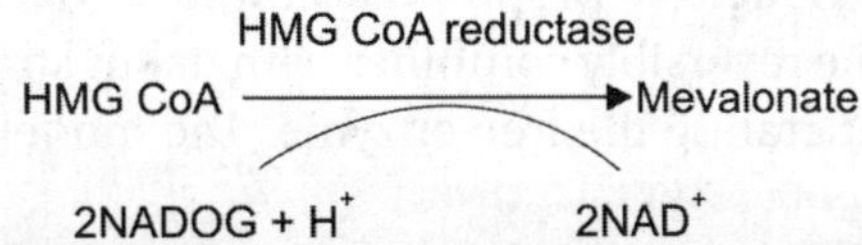

HMG CoA reductase activity	
Increased by	*Decreased by*
• Insulin	• Mevalonate, Cholesterol
• Thyroid	• Glucagon cortisol • Drugs – Atorvastatin, Lovastatin etc.

90. Ans. (b) 3 *Ref: Harper's 25th ed. p 57*

- L-Lactate dehydrogenase is a tetramic enzyme whose four subunits occur in two isoforms, designated H (for heart) and M (for muscle). The subunits can combine to yield catalytically 5 active isozymes of L-lactate dehydrogenase:

Lactate dehydrogenase	*Isozyme subunits*
L1	HHHH
L2	HHHM
L3	HHMM
L4	HMMM
L5	MMMM

91. Ans. (a) Zellweger's syndrome *Ref: Handbook of Pediatric Autopsy Pathology, p 436*

- Zellweger's syndrome: it occurs in individuals with mutation or inherited absence of peroxisomes in all tissue.
- There is also a generalized loss of proxisomal functions.
- The disease causes severe neurological symptoms and most patient may die in the first year of life.

92. Ans. (a) Aldolase B *Ref: Pamale C. Chamfer 3rd ed. p no. 136-137*

A severe disturbance of liver and kidney metabolism as a result of aldolase B deficiency (hereditary fructose intolerance, HFI), which is estimated to occur in 1: 20,000 live births

- The first symptoms appear when a baby is weaned and begins to be fed food containing sucrose or fructose.
- Fructose 1-phosphate accumulates, and ATP and inorganic phosphate levels fall significantly, with adenine being converted to uric acid, causing hyperuricemia. The decreased availability of hepatic ATP affects gluconeogenesis (causing hypoglycemia with vomiting), and protein synthesis (causing a decrease in blood clotting factors and other essential proteins).
- If fructose (and, therefore, sucrose) is not removed from the diet, liver failure and death can occur.
- Diagnosis of HFI can be made on the basis of fructose in the urine, or by a restriction fragment length polymorphism test.

Hereditary Fructose Intolerance ('Fructose Poisoning')

- Absence of aldolase B leads to intracellular trapping of fructose 1-Phosphate.
- Can cause hepatic failure and death
- Rapid detection and removal of fructose and sucrose from the diet is the only therapy.

93. Ans. (b) Follow Michaelis-Mentem kinetics *Ref: Pamale C. Chamfer 3rd ed. p 58-59, 62-63*

Michaelis mentem equation

A. Reaction model: Michaelis and Menten proposed a simple model showing features of enzyme catalyzed reactions. In this model, the enzyme reversibly combines with its substrate to form an ES complex that subsequently breaks down to product, regenerating the free enzyme. The model involving one substrate molecule is represented below:

$$E + S \underset{K-1}{\overset{K1}{\rightleftharpoons}} ES \xrightarrow{K2} E + P$$

Where S is the substrate
ES is the enzyme substrate complex
P is the product
K1, K-1 and K2 are rate constants
E is the enzyme
Allosteric enzyme show sigmoid curve whereas Michaelis and Mentem show hyperbolic curve.

94. Ans. (b) Alanine amino transferase *Ref: Davidson's 20th ed. p 594*

- Changes in plasma enzyme concentration after myocardial infarction:: Creatine kinase and troponin are first to rise, followed by aspartate aminotransferase (ASt) and then lactate (hydroxybutyrate) dehydrogenase (LDH).
- In patients treated with a thrombolytic agent, reperfusion is usually accompanied by a rapid rise in plasma creatine kinase due to a washout effect.

95. Ans. (b) Decreasing the energy of activation *Ref: Biochemistry- U. Stayanarayana, 3rd ed. p 98*

- The prime function of enzyme is catalysis.
- Enzyme increases reaction rates by decreasing the energy of activation.
- The energy required by the reactant to undergo the reaction is termed as activation energy.

96. Ans. (b) Glucose-6-Phosphate in liver *Ref: Biochemistry- U. Stayanarayana, 3rd ed. p 269*

von Gierke's disease (described by von Gierke in 1929) represents the largest group of glycogen storage disorders (GSD). There is an enzyme defect in glucose-6-phosphatase so that glucose-6- phosphate cannot be converted into free glucose but is metabolised to lactic acid or incorporated into glycogen.

- Large quantities of glycogen are formed and stored in hepatocytes, renal and intestinal mucosa cells. The liver and kidneys become enlarged.
- Abnormalities of lipids may lead to xanthoma formation.
- Uric acid is often elevated and may cause clinical gout.
- Galactose, fructose, and glycerol are metabolised to lactate. The elevated blood lactate levels cause metabolic acidosis.

97. Ans. (c) Asparaginase *Ref: Internet*

- L-asparaginase is a chemotherapeutic agent commonly used in the treatment of both adult and pediatric acute lymphoblastic leukemia (ALL).
- A major complication is thrombosis, resulting from reduced synthesis of proteins such as antithrombin III.
- Hypofibrinogenemia, also a side effect, may be a marker of thrombosis and decreased protein synthesis.

VITAMINS

98. Ans. (a) II, VII, IX and X *Ref: Satyanarayan 3rd ed. p 130*

Vitamin K play key roles in the regulation of three physiological processes:

- Blood coagulation: prothrombin (factor II), factors VII, IX, and X, and proteins C, S, and Z.

- Bone metabolism: osteocalcin, also called bone Gla protein (BGP), matrix Gla protein (MGP), periostin, and the recently discovered Gla-rich protein (GRP).
- Vascular biology: growth arrest-specific protein 6 (Gas 6) Unknown function: proline-rich g-carboxy glutamyl proteins (PRGPs) 1 and 2, and transmembrane g-carboxy glutamyl proteins (TMGs) 3 and 4.

Like other lipid-soluble vitamins (A, D, E), vitamin K is stored in the fat tissue of the human body.

Types of Vitamin K

- Vitamin K1, phylloquinone, is present in plants.
- Vitamin K2, menaquinone, is synthesized by intestinal bacteria.
- Vitamin K3, menadione, is a synthetic form.

99. Ans. (b) Cobalamine *Ref: Satyanarayan 3rd ed. p 152*

- Pernicious anemia occurs due to the deficiency of vitamin B12 (cobalamin), so vitamin B12 is also termed as antipernicious anemia vitamin.
- Pernicious anemia (also known as Biermer's anemia, Addison's anemia, or Addison Biermer anemia) is one of many types of the larger family of megaloblastic anemias.
- Vitamin B12 deficiency can result from a diet lacking in vitamin B12, which is found mainly in meat, eggs and milk. Vitamin B12 deficiency anemia can also occur if your small intestine can not absorb vitamin B12.

The characteristics of this disease are as follows:

- Less than 1 million RBC count and peripheral blood smear shows macrocytosis and poikilocytosis.
- RBC shows a characteristic 'tear-drop' or pear-shaped.
- Howell Jolly bodies and Cabot's rings are seen.
- Beefy red tongue shows glossitis, glossodynia and glossopyrosis.
- Gradual atrophy of papillae of tongue: bald tongue/Hunter's glossitis/Moeller's glossitis (similar to 'bald tongue of Sandwich,' seen in pellagra).
- Lowered alkaline phosphatase levels.

Deficiency of vitamin B12 is also associated with neuronal degeneration and demyelination of nervous system.

100. Ans. (d) Vitamin C *Ref: Satyanarayan 3rd ed. p 134*

Vitamin C is also called ascorbic acid. It cannot be made by the human body and so is an essential component of the diet. Vitamin C is needed to make a substance called collagen which is required for the health and repair of various tissues in the body, including:

Vitamins	*Major natural dietary sources*	*Deficiency-associated symptoms*	*Recommended daily allowance in healthy adults*
Vitamin A	Liver, leafy green vegetables, carrots, sweet potatoes, and pumpkins	Night blindness, xerosis, impaired immunity and changes in epithelial tissues and teeth	Adult male: 900 μg/d. Adult female: 700 μg/d
Vitamin B1 (thiamine)	Fortified breads, cereals, pastas, whole grains, dried beans, peas, and soybean	Wernicke encephalopathy, Korsakoff syndrome, and beriberi	Adult male: 1.2 mg/d. Adult female: 1.1 mg/d
Vitamin B9 (folate)	Liver, leafy green vegetables, dried beans, and cereals	Macrocytic megaloblastic anemia, diarrhea, anorexia, weight loss weakness, headaches, and behavior changes	Adults: 400 μg

Contd...

Contd...

Vitamins	*Major natural dietary sources*	*Deficiency-associated symptoms*	*Recommended daily allowance in healthy adults*
Vitamin B12 (cobalamin)	Meat, milk, shellfish, and eggs	Macrocytic megaloblastic anemia, peripheral nerve damage, coordination disorders, ataxia and cognitive impairments	Adults: 2.4 μg/d
Vitamin C (ascorbic acid)	Citrus fruits, green peppers, strawberries, tomatoes, broccoli, leafy greens, and melons	Scurvy (bleeding and bruising, hair and tooth loss, and joint pain and swelling)	Adult male, non-smoker: 90 mg/d. Adult female, non-smoker: 75 mg/d, Adult female, smoker: 110 mg/d
Vitamin D	Some fatty fish (mackerel, Salm on,and sardines), fish liver oils, and eggs, as well as fortified milk, formula, orange juice, and cereals	Increased incidence of Certain cancers, heart disease, and osteoporosis	Adults ages 19–50: 5 μg/d. Adults ages 51–70: 10 μg/d. Adults ages ≥71: 15 μg/dc
Vitamin E	Avocados, nuts and seeds, olives, green leafy vegetables, and vegetable oils	Ataxia, peripheral Neuropathy, pigmented	Adults: 15 mg/d
Vitamin K	Green leafy vegetables and in some vegetable oils, including soybean, cottonseed, canola, and olive oils	Stomach pains, bleeding, cartilage calcifi cation, malformat ion of developing bone, and atherosclerosis	Adult male: 120 μg/d. Adult female: 90 μg/dc

- Skin
- Bone
- Cartilage
- Ligaments and tendons
- Blood vessel walls
- Teeth

101. Ans. (c) Wheat germ oil *Ref: Satyanarayan 3rd ed. p 129*

- Vitamin E is a naturally occurring antioxidant.
- It is also termed as anti-sterility vitamin as it is essential for normal reproduction.
- It is absorbed from small intestine along with fat in the presence of bile salts.
- Rich sources of vitamin are:
  - Wheat germ oil
  - Cotton seed oil
  - Peanut oil
  - Corn oil
  - Sunflower oil
  - Also present in meat, milk, butter, eggs.
- Its deficiency will lead to sterility, degenerative changes in muscle, megaloblastic anemia and changes in CNS.

Liver oil of certain fish, viz. halibut, cod and shark, is very rich in vitamin A. Fish liver oil is the richest natural source of vitamin D. It is also found in liver, egg yolk and milk to a certain extent.

102. Ans. (a) Thiamine *Ref: Harper's 28th ed. p 473*

- The role of thiamin diphosphate in pyruvate dehydrogenase means that in deficiency there is impaired conversion of pyruvate to acetyl CoA.
- Metabolic acidosis can be seen in thiamine deficiency. This is due to increased lactic acid production from thiamine deficiency.
- Thiamine pyrophosphate (thiamine derivative) is the coenzyme for the conversion of pyruvate to acetyl coenzyme A. Without it, pyruvate is under used and converts to lactate.
- In vitro, thiamine deficiency produces accumulation of pyruvate and lactate, reduction of acetate, citrate and alpha-keto-glutarate and reduced acetylcholine synthesis.

103. Ans. (c) Vit E *Ref: Shafer's 7th ed. p 439*

- Play an important role in the tooth development.
- Due to the deficiency of vitamin D, there will be the developmental abnormalities of dentin and enamel
- Deficiency of vitamin D will also cause Rickets, which also affects the tooth development.
- Vitamin C deficiency will cause the severe changes in periodontal tissues as well as pulp of the teeth.

104. Ans. (a) Thiamine *Ref: Satyanarayan 3rd ed. p 137*

- Wernicke-Korsakoff syndrome (WKS) also called wet brain, Korsakoff's psychosis, and alcoholic encephalopathy.
- It is due to brain damage caused by a lack of vitamin B1 (thiamine).
- Lack of vitamin B1 is common in people with alcoholism. It is also common in persons whose bodies do not absorb food properly (malabsorption).
- The disease is characterized by apathy, loss of memory and rhythmical to and fro motion of the eyeballs.

105. Ans. (c) Nyctalopia *Ref: Lippincott's 3rd ed. p 382*

- Nyctalopia also called 'Night Blindness' is a condition making it difficult or impossible to see in relatively low light.
- Earliest sign of vitamin A deficiency is nyctalopia.
- Night blindness is due to a disorder of the cells in the retina that are responsible for vision in dim light.
- There may be several common causes of nyctalopia:
  - Lack of vitamin A, which can cause a disorder of the retina
  - Cataracts, which are cloudy areas in the lens of the eye
  - Some forms of retinal degeneration, such as retinitis pigmentosa
  - Certain medications
  - Birth defects

106. Ans. (c) It is a coenzyme for transketolase in pentose phosphate pathway *Ref: Satyanarayan 3rd ed. p 496*

- Thiamine plays a central role in energy-yielding metabolism, especially carbohydrate metabolism.
- Transketolase is an important enzyme in a biochemical pathway called the pentose phosphate pathway.
- In this set of biochemical reactions, a molecule called glucose-6-phosphate, which is derived from the sugar glucose, is modified by transketolase, yielding two productsa sugar called ribose-5-phosphate and a molecule called reduced nicotinamide adenine dinucleotide phosphate (NADPH).
- Both of these molecules are essential for the production of numerous other important molecules in the cell.
- Ribose-5-phosphate is needed for the synthesis of nucleic acids, complex sugar molecules, and other compounds.
- NADPH provides hydrogen atoms for chemical reactions that result in the production of steroids, fatty acids, amino acids, certain neurotransmitters, and other molecules.
- In addition, NADPH plays an important role in the synthesis of glutathione, a compound that is essential in the body's defense against oxidative stress.

- To function properly, all cells require certain levels of NADPH and ribose-5-phosphate, and the biochemical reaction mediated by transketolase is crucial for maintaining the appropriate levels of both molecules.

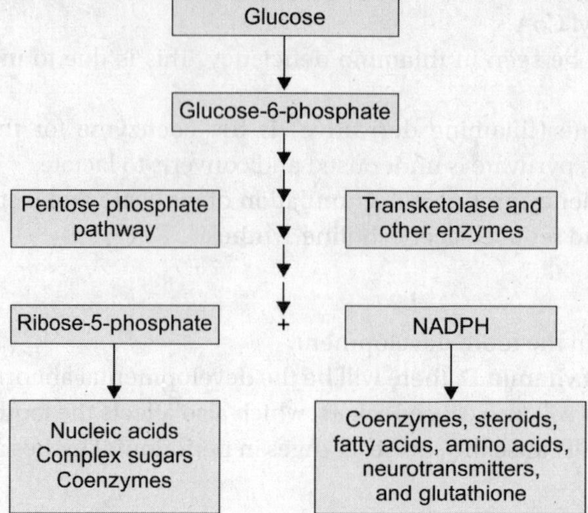

107. Ans. (d) Bile is required for the absorption of vitamin K that is fat soluble *Ref: Satyanarayan 3rd ed. p 130*

- Vitamin K is a necessary participant in synthesis of several proteins that mediate both coagulation and anticoagulation.
- Vitamin K deficiency is manifest as a tendency to bleed excessively.
- Vitamin K-dependent proteins include:
  - Coagulation proteins: factors II (prothrombin), VII, IX and X
  - Anticoagulation proteins: proteins C, S and Z
  - Others: bone proteins osteocalcin and matrix-Gla protein, and certain ribosomal proteins
- The chief source of vitamin K is synthesis by bacteria in the large intestine.
- Bile is necessary for the absorption of vitamin K.

108. Ans. (a) Pyridoxine *Ref: Harper's 28th ed. p 473*

Refer Ans no. 5

109. Ans. (b) Homocysteine methyltransferase *Ref: Satyanarayan 3rd ed. p 156*

In the cells of mammals, there are two different co-enzyme forms of vitamin B12:

- Methylcobalamin
  - Used by the enzyme methionine synthase (Homocysteine methyltransferase) to turn homocysteine (HCY) into methionine. Methionine is further converted to the important methyl donor, S- adenosylmethionine (SAM, aka SAMe) (more info at S-adenosylmethionine (SAMe)).
- 5'-deoxyadenosylcobalamin
  - Used by the enzyme methylmalonyl-CoA mutase to convert methylmalonyl-CoA to succinyl-CoA.
  - Used by the enzyme leucine aminomutase to convert B-leucine into L-leucine and vice-versa.

110. Ans. (c) Thiamine *Ref: Harper's 28th ed. p 473*

- Lactic acidosis is a form of metabolic acidosis due to the inadequate clearance of lactic acid from the blood.
- Lactate is a byproduct of anaerobic respiration and is normally cleared from the blood by the liver, kidney and skeletal muscle.
- Lactic acidosis occurs when the body's buffering systems are overloaded and tends to cause a pH of ≤7.25 with plasma lactate ≥5 mmol/L.

- It is usually caused by a state of tissue hypoperfusion and/or hypoxia. This causes pyruvic acid to be preferentially converted to lactate during anaerobic respiration.
- Hyperlactatemia is defined as plasma lactate >2 mmol/L.
- Due to increased pyruvate and lactic acid, it will lead to lactic acidosis.

111. Ans. (a) Pyridoxine *Ref: Satyanarayan 3rd ed. p 143*

List of vitamins

Vitamin A
- Chemical names (vitaminer)—retinol, retinal, and four carotenoids (including beta carotene).
- Fat soluble
- Deficiency may cause night-blindness and keratomalacia (eye disorder that results in a dry cornea)

Vitamin B1
- Chemical name (vitaminer)—thiamine
- Water soluble
- Deficiency may cause beriberi, Wernicke-Korsakoff syndrome

Vitamin B2
- Chemical name (vitaminer)—riboflavin
- Water soluble
- Deficiency may cause ariboflavinosis

Vitamin B3
- Chemical names (vitaminer)—niacin, niacinamide
- Water soluble
- Deficiency may cause pellagra

Vitamin B5
- Chemical name (vitaminer)—pantothenic acid
- Water soluble
- Deficiency may cause paresthesia

Vitamin B6
- Chemical names (vitaminer) - pyridoxine, pyridoxamine, pyridoxal
- Water soluble
- Deficiency may cause anemia, peripheral neuropathy

Vitamin B7
- Chemical name (vitaminer)—biotin
- Water soluble
- Deficiency may cause dermatitis, enteritis

Vitamin B9
- Chemical names (vitaminer)—folic acid, folinic acid
- Water soluble
- Deficiency may cause pregnancy deficiency linked to birth defects

Vitamin B12
- Chemical names (vitaminer)—cyanocobalamin, hydroxycobalamin, methylcobalamin
- Water soluble
- Deficiency may cause megaloblastic anemia.

Vitamin C
- Chemical names (vitaminer)—ascorbic acid
- Water soluble
- Deficiency may cause megaloblastic anemia

Vitamin D

- Chemical names (vitaminer)—ergocalciferol, cholecalciferol
- Fat soluble
- Deficiency may cause rickets, osteomalacia

Vitamin E

- Chemical names (vitaminer)—tocopherols, tocotrienols
- Fat soluble
- Deficiency is uncommon. May cause mild hemolytic anemia in newborns

Vitamin K

- Chemical names (vitaminer)—phylloquinone, menaquinones
- Fat soluble
- Deficiency may cause bleeding diathesis.

112. Ans. (b) Vitamin K *Ref: Satyanarayan, 3rd ed. p 130*

Vitamin K exists in different forms

- Vitamin K1 (phylloquinone) is present in plants.
- Vitamin K2 (menaquinone) is produced by the intestinal bacteria and also found in animals.
- Vitamin K3 (menadione) is a synthetic form.

113. Ans. (a) Nyctalopia *Ref: Satyanarayan, 3rd ed. p 123*

As per the answer key provided but according to the available data all options are correct

- The vitamin A deficiency manifestations are related to the eyes, skin and growth.
- Deficiency manifestations of the eyes: Night blindness (nyctalopia) is one of the earliest symptoms of vitamin A deficiency. The individuals have difficulty to see in dim light since the dark adaptation time is increased. Prolonged deficiency irreversibly damages a number of visual cells.
- Severe deficiency of vitamin A leads to xerophthalmia. This is characterized by dryness in conjunctiva and cornea, and keratinization of epithelial cells. In certain areas of conjunctiva, white triangular plaques known as Bitot's spots are seen.
- If xerophthalmia persists for a long time, corneal ulceration and degeneration occur. These results in the destruction of cornea, a condition referred to as keratomalacia, causing total blindness. Vitamin A deficiency blindness is mostly common in children of the developing countries.

114. Ans. (b) Two units of vitamin A *Ref: Richard A Harvey (Biochemistry), 3rd ed. p 380*

Plant Foods contain β-carotene, which can be oxidatively cleaved in the intestine to yield two molecules of retinol (vitamin A). In humans, the conversion is inefficient, and the vitamin A activity of β-carotene is only about one sixth that of retinol.

115. Ans. (b) Pantothenic acid *Ref: Harper's, 28th ed. p 468*

The Vitamins

Vitamin		*Functions*	*Deficiency disease*
	Lipid-soluable		
A	Retinol, β-carotene	Visual pigments in the retina; regulation of gene expression and cell differentiation (β-carotene is an antioxidant)	Night blindness, xerophthalmia; keratinization of skin
D	Calciferol	Maintenance of calcium balance; enhances intestinal absorption of Ca^{2+} and mobilizes bone mineral; regulation of gene expression and cell differentiation	Rickets = poor mineralization of bone; osteomalacia = bone demineralization

Contd...

Contd...

Vitamin		*Functions*	*Deficiency disease*
E	Tocopherols, tocotrienols	Antioxidant, especially in cell membranes; roles in cell signaling	Extremely rare—serious neurologic dysfunction
K	Phylloquinone: menaquinones	Coenzyme in formation of γ-carboxyglutamate in enzymes of blood clotting and bone matrix	Impaired blood clotting, hemorrhagic disease
	Water-Soluble		
B1	Thiamine	Coenzyme in pyruvate and α-ketoglutarate dehydrogenases, and transketolase; regulates Cl^- channel in nerve conduction	Peripheral nerve damage (beriberi) or central nervous system lesions (Wernicke-Korsakoff syndrome)
B2	Riboflavin	Coenzyme in oxidation and reduction reactions (FAD and FMN); prosthetic group of flavoproteins	Lesions of corner of mouth, lips, and tongue, seborrheic dermatitis
Niacin	Nicotinic acid, nicotinamide	Coenzyme in oxidation and reduction reactions; functional part of NAD and NADP; role in intracellular calcium regulation and cell signaling	Pellagra-photosensitive dermatitis, depressive psychosis
B6	Pyridoxine, pyridoxal, pyridoxamine	Coenzyme in transamination and decarboxylation of amino acids and glycogen phosphorylase; modulation of steroid hormone action	Disorders of amino acid metabolism, convulsions
	Folic acid	Coenzyme in transfer of one-carbon fragments	Megaloblastic anemia
B12	Cobalamin	Coenzyme in transfer of one-carbon fragments and metabolism of folic acid	Pernicious anemia = megaloblastic anemia with degeneration of the spinal cord
	Pantothenic acid	Functional part of CoA and acyl carrier protein; fatty acid synthesis and metabolism	Peripheral nerve damage (nutritional melalgia or **'burning foot syndrome'**)
H	Biotin	Coenzyme in carboxylation reactions in gluconeogenesis and fatty acid synthesis; role in regulation of cell cycle	Impaired fat and carbohydrate metabolism, dermatitis
C	Ascorbic acid	Coenzyme in hydroxylation of proline and lysine in collagen synthesis; antioxidant; enhances absorption of iron	Scurvy-impaired wound healing, loss of dental cement, subcutaneous hemorrhage

116. Ans. (a) Absorption requires bile pigments and (d) Along with PTH increases calcium resorption from bone

Ref: Biochemistry- U. Satyanarayan, 3rd ed. p 123-125,127

As per the key answer given is (4) but according to references it should be Both (1) and (4).

- Vitamin D is a fat soluble vitamin. It resembles sterols in structure and functions like a hormone.
- Absorption, transport and storage: Vitamin D is absorbed in the small intestine for which bile is essential. Through lymph, vitamin D enters the circulation bound to plasma α2-globulin and is distributed throughout the body. Liver and other tissues store small amounts of vitamin D.
- Synthesis of 1,254-DHCC: Cholecalciferol is first hydroxylated at 25th position to 25- hydroxycholecalciferol (25 OH D3) by a specific hydroxylase present in liver, 25-OH D3 is the major storage and circulatory form or vitamin D. Kidney possesses a specific enzyme. 25- hydroxycholecalciferol (calciol) 1-hydroxylase which hydroxylates

25-hydroxycholecalciferol at position 1 to produce 1,25-dihydroxycholecalciferol (1,25-DHCC). 1,25 DHCC contains 3 hydroxyl groups (1,3 and 25 carbon) hence referred to as calcitriol. Both the hydroxylase enzymes (of liver and kidney) require cytochrome P450, NADPH and molecular oxygen for the hydroxylation process.

- Acton of calcitriol on the bone: In the osteoblasts of bone, calcitriol stimulates calcium uptake for deposition as calcium phosphate. Thus, calcitriol is essential for bone formation. The bone is an important reservoir of calcium and phosphate. Calcitriol along with parathyroid hormone increases the mobilization of calcium and phosphate from the bone. This causes elevation in the plasma calcium and phosphate levels.
- Deficiency of vitamin D causes rickets in children and osteomalacia in adults.

117. Ans. (d) Selenium *Ref: Pamale C Champe 3rd ed.*

Functions	Selenium works as an antioxidant with vitamin E to protect cells from damage that may lead to cancer, heart disease, and other health problems. Selenium appears to have a sparing action on vitamin E.
Deficiencies	The effects of a deficiency of selenium are not clear, but may involve the heart muscle or thyroid functioning.
Excesses	The tolerable upper intake level is 400 micrograms for both adult males and females.
Amount needed	The recommended intake level is 55 micrograms for both adult males and females.
Food sources	The best food sources of selenium are seafood, liver, kidney and meats. Grain products and seed also contain selenium, but the amount depends on the selenium content of the soil in which they are grown.

118. Ans. (a) Presence of intrinsic factor *Ref: Pamale C Champe 3rd ed.*

The Schilling test has multiple stages:

- Stage 1: Oral vitamin B12 plus intramuscular vitamin B12
- Stage 2: Vitamin B12 and intrinsic factor
- Stage 3: Vitamin B12 and antibiotics
- Stage 4: Vitamin B12 and pancreatic enzymes
- Combined stage 1 and stage 2

119. Ans. (a) Folic acid deficiency *Ref: Biochemistry- U. Satyanarayan, 3rd ed. p 152*

- The amino acid histidine is metabolized to glutamic acid in mammalian tissue. Formiminoglutamic acid (FIGLU) is an intermediary in this reaction, and tetrahydrofolic acid is the coenzyme that converts it to glutamic acid.
- A test for folate deficiency concerns the measurement of urinary FIGLU excretion after a histidine load.
- Actually in folic acid deficiency, FIGLU accumulates and excreted in urine.

120. Ans. (d) Diarrhea *Ref: Biochemistry- U. Satyanarayan, 3rd ed. p 134*

The first symptoms of vitamin C deficiency tend to be:

- Tiredness and weakness
- Muscle and joint pains
- Easy bruising
- Spots that look like tiny, red-blue bruises on the skin.

Other symptoms can include:

- Dry skin
- Splitting hair

- Painfull swelling and discoloration of the gums
- Spontaneous bleeding from the gums.
- Ancmia
- Nosebleeds.
- Poor healing of wounds.
- Abnormal collagen
- Problems fighting infections.
- Bleeding into joints, causing severe joint pains.
- Changes in the bones.
- Tooth loss.
- Weight loss.

121. Ans. (c) Vitamin B12 *Ref: Biochemistry- U. Satyanarayan, 3rd ed. p 153*

- Intrinsic factor (IF), also known as gastric intrinsic factor (GIF), is a glycoprotein produced by the parietal cells of the stomach.
- It is necessary for the absorption of vitamin B12 (cobalamin) later on in the small intestine.
- In humans, the gastric intrinsic factor protein is encoded by the GIF gene.
- The intrinsic factor is secreted by the stomach. It is present in the gastric juice as well as in the gastric mucous membrane.
- The optimum pH for its action is 7 and it is inactivated at temperatures above 45°C.

122. Ans. (d) Synthesis of prothrombin *Ref: Lippincott's 3rd ed. p 387*

Function of Vitamin K

- Formation of γ carboxyglutamate.
- Interaction of prothrombin with platelets.
- Role of γ carboxyglutamate residues in other proteins.

123. Ans. (b) Aflatoxin *Ref: Satyanarayana, 3rd ed. p 122, 133, 667, 658-660*

Cancer: Free radicals can damage DNA, and cause mutagenicity and cytotoxicity, and thus play a key role in carcinogenesis. It is believed that Reactive Oxygen Species (ROS) can induce mutations, and inhibit DNA repair process, that results in the inactivation of certain tumor suppressor genes leading to cancer.

Further, free radicals promote biochemical and molecular changes for rapid growth of tumor cells.

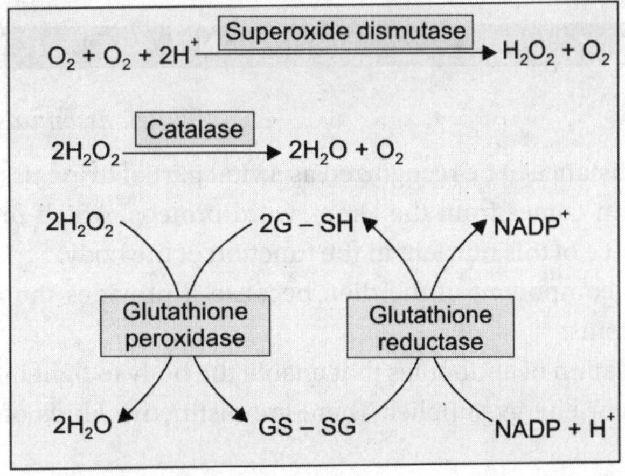

Nutrient antioxidants:

- Tocopherols (vitamin E): Vitamin E is fat soluble, and among the tocopherols, α-tocopherol present in all cellular membranes, and products against lipid peroxidation α-Tocopherol can directly act on oxyradicals (e.g. O_2, OH, singlet oxygen), thus serves as an important chain breaking antioxidant.

The antioxidant enzyme system (G-SH-reduced glutathione; GS-SG-oxidized glutathione)

- Ascorbic acid (vitamin C): It is a vitamin that participants in many normal metabolic reactions of the body. Ascorbic acid is an important water-soluble antioxidant in biological fluids. Vitamin C efficiently scavenges free radicals, and inhibits lipid peroxidation. It also promotes the regeneration of α-tocopherol (from α-tocopheroxyl radical produced during scavenging of ROS). As an antioxidant, vitamin C reduces the risk of cancer, contract, and coronary heart disease.
- Carotenoids: These are the natural compounds with lipohilic properties. About 500 different carotenoids have been identified, among them β-carotene is most important. It can act as an antioxidant under low partial pressure of O_2. β-Carotene usually functions in association with vitamin C and E. Carotenoids (most important β-carotene) function as antioxidants and reduce the risk of cancer initiated by free radicals and strong oxidants. β-Carotene is found to be beneficial to prevent heart attacks. This is also attributed to the antioxidant property. Lycopene, a fat soluble pigment is a carotenoid. It is responsible for colour of certain fruits and vegetables (e.g. tomato). Lycopene possesses antioxidant property. Lutein and zeaxanthin are also carotenoid pigments that impart yellow or green colour to fruits and vegetables. These pigments can also serve as antioxidants.
- Selenuim: It is an essential trace element, and is proved to be a significant antioxidant. Selenium works with vitamin E in fighting free radicals. It is also required for the required for the function of an important antioxidant enzyme, namely glutathione peroxidase.
- α-Lipoic acid: It is vitamin-like compound, produced in the body, besides the supply from plant and animal sources. α-Lipoic acid plays a key role in recycling other important antioxidants such as ascorbic acid, α-tocopherol and glutathione.

Besides the above, there is many other important nutrient antioxidants, some of them are listed below:

- Coenzyme Q10 of ubiquinone family
- Proanthocyanidins of grape seeds
- Catechins of green tea
- Curcuminoids of turmeric
- Quercetin of onions
- Aflatoxins are produced by Aspergillus favus when groundnuts or coconuts are stored in moist conditions. Aflatoxins are hepatotoxic and carcinogenic.

NUTRITION

124. Ans. (a) Proteins *Ref: Essentials of Biochemistry By Naik 1st ed.p 147*

- Protein was the first substance to be recognized as a vital part of living tissue.
- In fact, the word protein comes from the Greek word proteos, which means 'primary' or 'taking first place,' indicating the importance of this nutrient in the function of the body.
- Protein is an essential component of the diet, because it provides the amino acids that the body needs to synthesize its own proteins.
- Proteins aid in the formation of antibodies that enable the body to fight infection.
- Proteins serve as a major energy supplier. There are distinctive kinds of proteins, each performing a unique function in the body.

- Proteins form a major part of human body, next to water.
- The composition of proteins in the body is like that muscle contains about 1/3 protein, bone about 1/5 part and skin consists of 1/10 portion. The rest part of proteins is in the other body tissues and fluids. Even blood contains loads of proteins. In fact, the hemoglobin molecule is composed of proteins.

HEMOGLOBIN AND PORPHYRINS

125. Ans. (d) Malonyl CoA *Ref: Harper's 27th ed. p 189*

Beta-oxidation is the process by which fatty acid molecules are broken down in the mitochondria to generate acetyl-coA, which enters the citric acid cycle, and NADH and FADH2, which are used by the electron transport chain.

β-oxidation of odd chain fatty acids

- In general, fatty acids with an odd number of carbons are found in the lipids of plants and some marine organisms.
- Many ruminant animals form a large amount of 3-carbon propionate during the fermentation of carbohydrates in the rumen.
- Chains with an odd-number of carbons are oxidized in the same manner as even-numbered chains, but the final products are propionyl-CoA and acetyl-CoA.
- Propionyl-CoA is first carboxylated using a bicarbonate ion into D-stereoisomer of methylmalonyl-CoA, in a reaction that involves a biotin co-factor, ATP, and the enzyme propionyl-CoA carboxylase.
- The bicarbonate ion's carbon is added to the middle carbon of propionyl-CoA, forming a D-methylmalonyl-CoA. However, the D conformation is enzymatically converted into the L conformation by methylmalonyl-CoA epimerase, then it undergoes intramolecular rearrangement, which is catalyzed by methylmalonyl-CoA mutase (requiring B12 as a coenzyme) to form succinyl- CoA.
- The succinyl-CoA formed can then enter the citric acid cycle

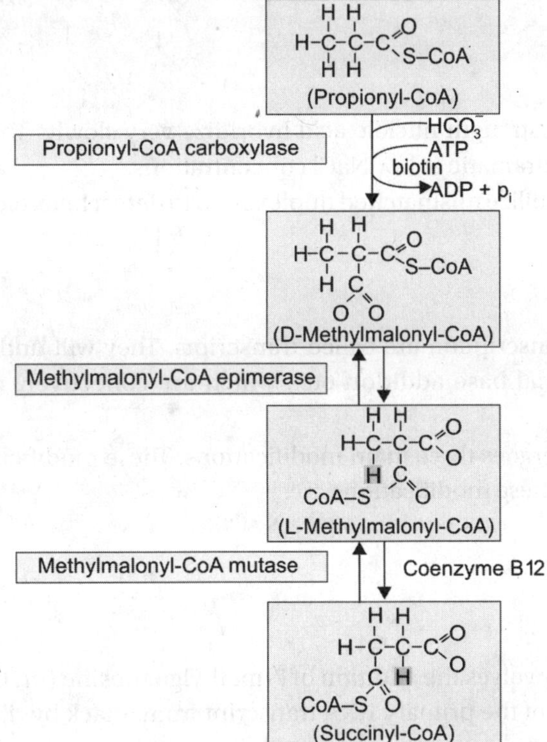

126. Ans. (d) Poor diabetes control *Ref: Pamela C. Champe 3rd ed. p 34*

- Increased amount of glycohemoglobin level in RBC indicates Diabetes mellitus
- The rate of formation of HbA_{1c} is directly proportional to the average blood glucose concentration over the previous several month:

Means blood glucose level	*HbA_{1c}*
110 mg/dl	6%
150 mg/dl	7%
225-275 mg/dl	8-9%

- So, when AhA_{1c} concentration is > 9% it indicates poor diabetes control.

127. Ans. (c) Glycine *Ref: Pamela C. Chamfer 3rd ed. p 276-277*

- Liver is the major sites of heme biosynthesis which synthesizes a number of heme proteins.

MOLECULAR BIOLOGY AND BIOTECHNOLOGY

128. Ans. (b) 3 billion *Ref: Harper's 28th ed.p 317*

- The human genome is the complete set of genetic information for humans (Homo sapiens).
- This information is encoded as DNA sequences within the 23 chromosome pairs in cell nuclei and in a small DNA molecule found within individual mitochondria.
- Human genomes include both protein-coding DNA genes and noncoding DNA.
- The total length of the human genome is over 3 billion base pairs.
- The genome is organized into 22 paired chromosomes, the X chromosome (one in males, two in females) and, in males only, one Y chromosome, all being large linear DNA molecules contained within the cell nucleus.
- The haploid human genome contains approximately 20,000 protein-coding genes, significantly fewer than had been anticipated.

129. Ans. (c) Ionic strengths *Ref: Harper's 28th ed.p 317*

- Ionic strength: at low ionic strength nucleic acid hybridize very slowly. The effect of higher ionic strength on reassociation rates is more dramatic at low NaCl concentrations.
- High salt concentrations stabilize mismatched duplexes, so to detect heterologous probes, the salt concentration must be kept high.

130. Ans. (d) Glycosylation *Ref: Lippincott's 3rd ed. p 422, 423*

The RNA produced during transcription are called transcripts. They will undergo many alteration such as base modification, splicing, terminal base addition etc., which are collectively referred to as post-transcriptional modification.

The pre-mRNA molecule undergoes three main modifications. These modifications are occurs in the cell nucleus before the RNA is translated. These modifications are:

- 5′ capping,
- 3′ polyadenylation, and
- RNA splicing

5′ capping:

- Capping of the pre-mRNA involves the addition of 7-methylguanosine (m7G) to the 5′ end.
- The cap protects the 5′ end of the primary RNA transcript from attack by ribonucleases that have specificity to the 3′5′ phosphodiester bonds.

3′ polyadenylation:

- The pre-mRNA processing at the 3′ end of the RNA molecule involves cleavage of its 3′ end and then the addition of about 250 adenine residues to form a poly(A) tail.
- The cleavage and adenylation reactions occur if a polyadenylation signal sequence (5′- AAUAAA-3′) is located near the 3′ end of the pre-mRNA molecule, which is followed by another sequence, which is usually (5′-CA-3′). The second signal is the site of cleavage.
- The poly (A) tail is synthesized, it binds multiple copies of poly(A) binding protein, which protects the 3′end from ribonuclease digestion.

RNA splicing:

- RNA splicing is the process by which introns, regions of RNA that do not code for protein, are removed from the pre-mRNA and the remaining exons connected to re-form a single continuous molecule.
- Although most RNA splicing occurs after the complete synthesis and end-capping of the pre-mRNA, transcripts with many exons can be spliced co-transcriptionally.
- The splicing reaction is catalyzed by a large protein complex called the spliceosome assembled from proteins and small nuclear RNA molecules that recognize splice sites in the pre-mRNA sequence.

131. Ans. (d) S phase *Ref: Lippincott's 3rd ed. p 404*

The cell cycle, or cell-division cycle, is the series of events that take place in a cell leading to its division and duplication (replication) that produces two daughter cells.

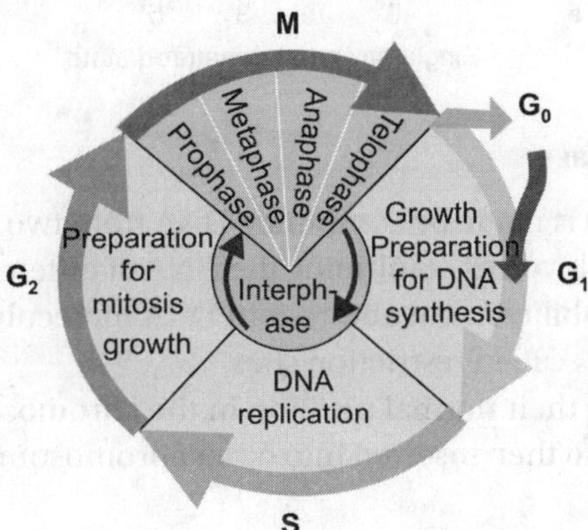

State	*Description*	*Abbreviation*	
Quiescent/senescent	Gap 0	G_0	A resting phase where the cell has left the cycle and has stopped dividing.
Interphase	Gap 1	G_1	Cells increase in size in Gap 1. The G_1 control mechanism ensures that everything is ready for DNA synthesis.
	Synthesis	S	DNA replication occurs during this phase.
	Gap 2	G_2	During the gap between DNA synthesis and mitosis, the cell will continue to grow. The G_2 control mechanism ensures that everything is ready to enter the M (mitosis) phase and divide.
Cell division	Mitosis	M	Cell growth stops at this stage and cellular energy is focused on the orderly division into two daughter cells. A checkpoint in the middle of mitosis ensures that the cell is ready to complete cell division.

132. Ans. (b) Reversible separation of DNA *Ref: Satyanarayan 3rd ed. p 78*

- DNA denaturation, also called DNA melting, is the process by which double-stranded deoxyribonucleic acid unwinds and separates into single-stranded strands through the breaking of hydrophobic stacking attractions between the bases.
- Although 'denaturation' can also refer to the separation of DNA strands.
- DNA is heated and denatured into single-stranded state, and the mixture is cooled to allow strands to rehybridize.
- Hybrid molecules are formed between similar sequences and any differences between those sequences will result in a disruption of the base-pairing.

The process of DNA melting is also used in molecular biology techniques, notably in the polymerase chain reaction.

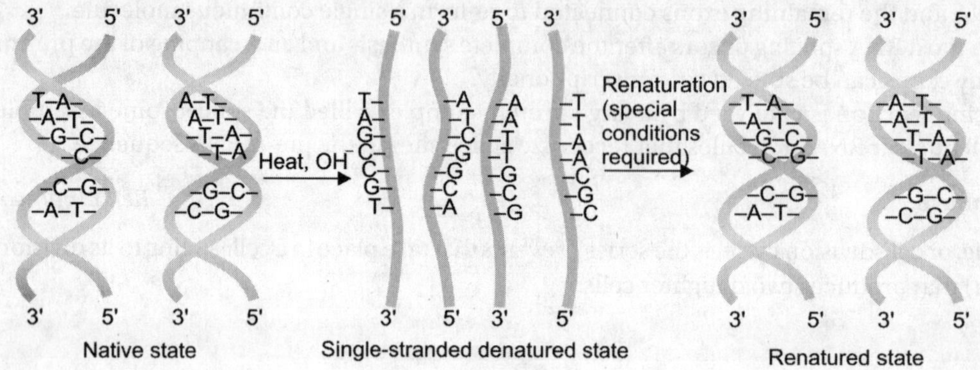

133. Ans. (a) Restriction endonuclease *Ref: Satyanarayan 3rd ed. p 578, 579*

- Recombinant DNA (or rDNA) is made by combining DNA from two or more sources.
- In practice, the process often involves combining the DNA of different organisms.
- The process depends on the ability to cut and re-join DNA molecules at points which are identified by specific sequences of nucleotide bases called restriction sites.
- DNA fragments are cut out of their normal position in the chromosome using restriction enzymes (also called restriction endonucleases) and then inserted into other chromosomes or DNA molecules using enzymes called ligases.

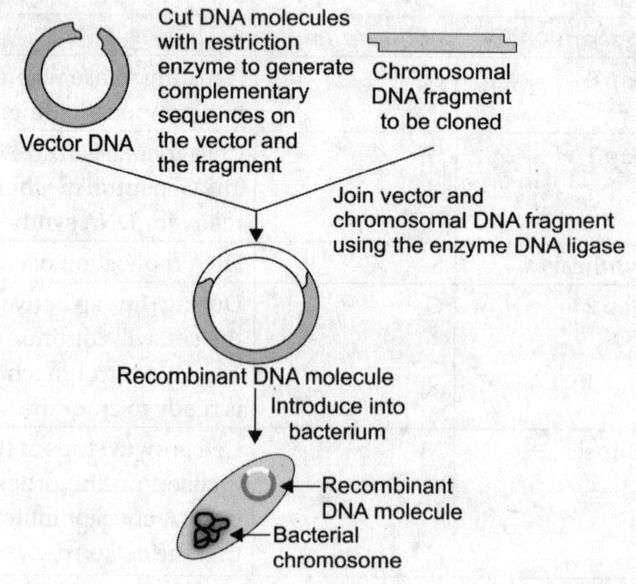

134. Ans. (d) Chromatin *Ref: Clinical Hematology: Theory and Procedures, Volume 936, p 45 by Mary Louise Turgeon*

- Chromatin is the combination or complex of DNA and proteins that make up the contents of the nucleus of a cell.
- The primary functions of chromatin are:
  - To package DNA into a smaller volume to fit in the cell,
  - To strengthen the DNA to allow mitosis
  - To prevent DNA damage, and
  - To control gene expression and DNA replication.
  - The chromatin is continuous from one cell generation to the next and also from one generation of multicellular organism to the next.

135. Ans. (c) Complimentary copy of RNA *Ref: Biochemistry- U. Satyanarayana, 3rd ed. p 543*

Transcription is a process in which ribonucleic acid (RNA) is synthesized from DNA. The word gene refers to the functional unit of the DNA that can be transcribed. Thus, the genetic information stored in DNA is expressed through RNA. For this purpose, one of the two strands of DNA serves as a template (non-coding strand or sense strand) and produces working copies of RNA molecules. The other DNA strand which does not participate in transcription is referred to as coding strand or antisense strand (frequently referred to as coding strand since with the exception of T for U, primary mRNA contains codons with the same base sequence).

MISCELLANEOUS

136. Ans. (b) Karyotyping *Ref: Lippincott's 3rd ed. p 456*

- A karyotype is the number and appearance of chromosomes in the nucleus of a eukaryotic cell. The term is also used for the complete set of chromosomes in a species, or an individual organism.
- Karyotypes describe the number of chromosomes, and what they look like under a light microscope.
- The study of karyotypes is important for cell biology and genetics, and the results may be used in evolutionary biology and medicine.
- Karyotypes can be used for many purposes; such as to study chromosomal aberrations, cellular function, taxonomic relationships, and to gather information about past evolutionary events.

137. Ans. (d) Liver disease *Ref: Satyanarayan 3rd ed. p 458*

- A prothrombin time (PT) test measures how long it takes for a clot to form in a blood sample.
- A clot is a thick lump of blood that the body produces to seal leaks, wounds, cuts, and scratches and prevent excessive bleeding.
- The blood's ability to clot is a complex process involving platelets (also called thrombocytes) and proteins called clotting factors.
- PT is the first one to be prolonged in vitamin K deficiency.
- Platelets are oval-shaped cells made in the bone marrow.
- Most clotting factors are made in the liver.
- When a blood vessel breaks, platelets are first to the area to help seal the leak and temporarily stop or slow the bleeding. But for the clot to become strong and stable, the action of clotting factors is required.
- The PT test can be used to evaluate the action of five different clotting factors (I, II, V, VII, and X). If any factor is missing, deficient, or defective, clotting time may be delayed. Blood that takes too long to clot in a PT test may be a sign of:
  - A hereditary deficiency in clotting factors (such as in the bleeding disorders hemophilia and von Willebrand disease)
  - Liver disease (because most clotting factors are made in the liver)

- Vitamin K deficiency (because vitamin K is a necessary component of several clotting factors)
- Therapy using warfarin, a blood-thinning medication
- Certain medical conditions in which the body uses up or destroys clotting factors too rapidly.

138. Ans. (a) Zinc *Ref: Satyanarayan 3rd ed. p 420*

- 2 gram is the total amount of Zn present in an adult body.
- Daily requirement of Zn is 10-15 mg/day, it is increased during pregnancy and lactation.
- Dietary sources is milk, beans, nuts, eggs, meat, fish.
- Erythrocytes contains higher amount of Zn.

Severe zinc deficiency: Bullous-pustular dermatitis, alopecia, diarrhea, emotional disorder, weight loss, intercurrent infections, hypogonadism in males; it is fatal if unrecognized and untreated.

Moderate zinc deficiency: Growth retardation and delayed puberty in adolescents, hypogonadism in males, rough skin, poor appetite, mental lethargy, delayed wound healing, taste abnormalities and abnormal dark adaptation.

Mild zinc deficiency: Oligospermia, slight weight loss and hyperammonemia.

139. Ans. (b) Type II *Ref: Harper's 28th ed. p 542*

- Hyaline cartilage is a type of cartilage found on many joint surfaces.
- It is pearly bluish in color with firm consistency and has a considerable amount of collagen.
- It contains no nerves or blood vessels.
- Hyaline cartilage matrix is mostly made up of type II collagen and chondroitin sulfate, both of which are also found in elastic cartilage.
- Hyaline cartilage exists on the ventral ends of ribs; in the larynx, trachea, and bronchi; and on the articular surface of bones.
- Hyaline cartilage matrix is produced by chondrocytes and contains three major classes of molecules, i.e. Collagen molecules, Proteoglycans, and Multiadhesive glycoproteins.
- Hyaline cartilage provides a model for the developing skeleton of the fetus.
- Hyaline cartilage of articular joint surfaces do not possess a perichondrium.

140. Ans. (a) Missense mutation *Ref: Harper's 28th ed. p 356,357*

- In genetics, a missense mutation (a type of nonsynonymous mutation) is a point mutation in which a single nucleotide change results in a codon that codes for a different amino acid.
- Missense mutations can render the resulting protein nonfunctional. and such mutations are responsible for diseases such as Epidermolysis bullosa, sickle-cell disease.
- The most common variant of sickle-cell disease, the 20th nucleotide of the gene for the beta chain of hemoglobin is altered from the codon GAG to GUG. Thus, the 6th amino acid glutamic acid is substituted for valine notated as an 'E6V' mutation and the protein is sufficiently altered to cause the sickle-cell disease.

141. Ans. (a) Insulin *Ref: Harper's 28th ed. p 455*

- In the field of molecular biology, nuclear receptors are a class of proteins found within cells that are responsible for sensing steroid and thyroid hormones and certain other molecules.
- Nuclear receptors have the ability to directly bind to DNA and regulate the expression of adjacent genes, hence these receptors are classified as transcription factors.
- Nuclear receptors play key roles in both embryonic development and adult homeostasis.
- Ligands that bind to and activate nuclear receptors include lipophilic substances such as endogenous hormones, vitamins A and D, and xenobiotic endocrine disruptors.
- Nuclear receptors are the androgen receptor, estrogen receptors, glucocorticoid receptor, and progesterone receptor.

142. Ans. (a) Energy *Ref: Satyanarayan 3rd ed. p 223*

- Adenosine triphosphate (ATP) is considered by biologists to be the energy currency of life.
- It is the high-energy molecule that stores the energy.
- The ATP is synthesized in the tiny energy factories called mitochondria by a process called glycolysis.
- It is used to transport energy to cells for biochemical processes, including muscle contraction and enzymatic metabolism, through its hydrolysis to ADP.
- ATP is hydrolyzed to AMP when it is incorporated into DNA or RNA.
- ATP is an energy-rich molecule, which releases free energy when it is broken down to either ADP (adenosine diphosphate) or AMP (adenosine monophosphate).
- It is sometimes called 'the spark of life.

143. Ans. (c) X-linked dominant *Ref: Satyanarayan 3rd ed. p 223*

- Ehlers-Danlos syndrome (EDS) is an inherited connective tissue disorder with different presentations that have been classified into several primary types.
- EDS is caused by a defect in the structure, production, or processing of collagen or proteins that interact with collagen, such as mutations in the COL5A or COL3A genes.
- The collagen in connective tissue helps tissues resist deformation.
- Collagen is an important contributor to the physical strength of skin, joints, muscles, ligaments, blood vessels and visceral organs; abnormal collagen renders these structures more elastic.
- Depending on the individual, the severity of the mutation can vary from mild to life-threatening.
- Inheritance patterns within this group include:
  - X-linked recessive
  - autosomal dominant, and
  - autosomal recessive

144. Ans. (b) Ion form *Ref: Satyanarayan 3rd ed. p 406*

- Calcium is one of the most abundant mineral present in our body.
- Milk and its products are the best sources of calcium
- 800 mg/day is the daily requirement of Calcium in adult men and women, while its requirement will be increased during pregnancy and lactation in females.
- Calcium is present in blood plasma in ionic form and its normal concentration in plasma is 9-11 mg/dl.
- It plays an important role in the development of bones and teeth, muscle contraction, blood coagulation, nerve transmission, membrane integrity and permeability, activation of enzyme release of harmone, calmodulin mediated action. Action on heart etc.

145. Ans. (d) Pyruvate kinase *Ref: Satyanarayan 3rd ed. p 250*

Myoglobin

- It is an iron- and oxygen-binding protein found in the muscle tissue of vertebrates in general and in almost all mammals.
- It is related to hemoglobin, which is the iron- and oxygen-binding protein in blood, specifically in the red blood cells.
- Myoglobin is only found in the bloodstream after muscle injury. It is an abnormal finding, and can be diagnostically relevant when found in blood.

Cytochromes

- Cytochromes are, in general, membrane-bound (i.e. inner mitochondrial membrane) hemeproteins containing heme groups and are primarily responsible for the generation of ATP via electron transport.
- The heme group is a highly-conjugated ring system (which allows its electrons to be very mobile) surrounding a metal ion, which readily interconverts between the oxidation states.

- For many cytochromes, the metal ion present is that of iron, which interconverts between Fe2+ (reduced) and Fe3+ (oxidized) states (electron-transfer processes) or between Fe2+ (reduced) and Fe3+(formal, oxidized) states (oxidative processes).

Catalase

- It is a common enzyme found in nearly all living organisms exposed to oxygen (such as vegetables, fruit or animals).
- It catalyzes the decomposition of hydrogen peroxide to water and oxygen.
- It is a very important enzyme in protecting the cell from oxidative damage by reactive oxygen species (ROS).
- Catalase is a tetramer of four polypeptide chains, each over 500 amino acids long.
- It contains four porphyrin heme (iron) groups that allow the enzyme to react with the hydrogen peroxide.

Pyruvate kinase

- It is an enzyme involved in glycolysis.
- It catalyzes the transfer of a phosphate group from phosphoenolpyruvate(PEP) to ADP, yielding one molecule of pyruvate and one molecule of ATP.

146. Ans. (d) Metabolic acidosis *Ref: Internet*

- If the patient has primary respiratory alkalosis with compensatory metabolic acidosis

PH	*Primary disorder and parameter*	*Compensatory mechanisms*	*Compensatory mechanism and parameter*
Decrease	Metabolic acidosis (↓HCO_3)	Hyperventilation	Respiratory alkalos (↓PCO_2)
Decrease	Respiratory acidosis (↑PCO_2)	Increased HCO_3 reabsorption by kidney	Metabolic alkalosis (↑HCO_3)
Increase	Metabolic alkalosis (↑HCO_3)	Hypoventilation	Respiratory acidosis (↑PCO_2)
Increase	Respiratory alkalosis (↓PCO_2)	Decreased HCO_3 reabsorption by kidney	Metabolic acidosis (↓HCO_3)

147. Ans. (c) NaCl *Ref: Harper's 28th ed. p 463*

Factor affecting iron absorption are:

- Phosphate content in a diet is inversely proportional to the Ee absorption, i.e. if the phosphate content in a diet is more. The iron absorption will be decreased and vice versa.
- In malabsorption syndrome like steatorrhea, iron absorption was impaired
- Ascorbic acid (vitamin C) increases the absorption of iron (Acidity and cysteine also doing the same)
- Fe absorption increases by 2-10 times in iron deficiency anemia
- However, calcium and a glass of milk also reduce the availability of iron significantly.
- Phytate and oxalate interfere iron absorption.

148. Ans. (a) IgM *Ref: Biochemistry- U. Satyanarayana, 3rd ed. p 188,189*

IgM is the largest immunoglobulin composed of 5 Y-shaped units (IgG type) held together by a J polypeptide chain. Thus, IgM is a pentamer. Due to its large size, IgM cannot traverse blood vessels, hence it is restricted to the blood stream, IgM is the first antibody to be produced in response to an antigen and is the most effective against invading microorganisms. It may be noted that IgM can simultaneously combine with 5 antigenic sites due to its pentameric structure.

149. Ans. (a) Muscular dystrophy *Ref: Satyanarayana, 3rd ed. p 111*

Isoenzymes of creatine phosphokinase

Creatine kinase (CK) or creatine phosphatase (CPK) catalyses the inter-conversion of phosphocreatine (or creatine phosphate) to creatine.

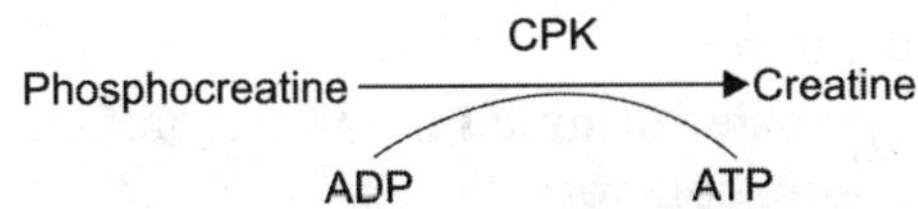

CPK exists as three isoenzymes. Each isoenzyme is a dimer composed of two subunits-M (muscle) or B (brain) or both.

Isoenzyme	*Subunit*	*Tissue of origin*
CPK1	BB	Brain
CPK2	MB	Heart
CPK3	MM	Skeletal muscle

In healthy individuals, the isoenzyme CPK2 (MB) is almost undetectable in serum with less than 2% of total CPK. After the myocardial infarction (MI), within the first 6-18 hours, CPK2 increases in the serum to as high as 20% (against 2% normal). CPK2 isoenzyme is not elevated in skeletal muscle disorders. Therefore, estimation of the enzyme CPK2 (MB) is the earliest reliable indication of myocardial infarction.

150. Ans. (b) 400 ml *Ref: Harper's 25th ed. p 57*

Distribution of water

- Average 60% of body weight, Men 55-70%, Women 45-60%
- Average 70 kg normal man contains 24 lit of water

Water intake

- Exogenous water 0.5–5 lit controlled by thirst center and hypothalamus
- Endogenous water 300–350 ml/day

Water output

- Urine 1-2 l/day
- Skin 450 ml/day
- Lungs 400 ml/day
- Feces - 150 ml/day

The loss of water by via skin and lungs is called as insensible water loss.

151. Ans. (c) Ubiquinone *Ref: Pamila Champe 3rd ed. p 74*

- All the members of the respirating chain are protein except coenzyme Q.
- Coenzyme Q is a quinine dominative with along isopremoid tail. It is also called ubiquinone because it is ubiquitous in biologic system.
- It plays an active role as election transport respiratory chain.

152. Ans. (a) Catalase *Ref: U. Satyanarayans 7th ed. p 658-659*

Antioxidants in relation to lipid peroxidation:

- Preventive antioxidants that will block the initial production of free radicals, e.g. catalase, glutathione peroxidase.
- Chain breaking antioxidants that inhibit the propagative phase of lipid peroxidation, e.g. superoxide dismutase, vitamin E, uric acid.

Antioxidants according to their nature and action

- Nonenzymatic antioxidants
  - Nutrient antioxidants, e.g. carotenoids (β carotene), α tocopherol, ascorbic acid selenium.
  - Metabolic antioxidants, e.g. gluthione, ceruloplasmin, albumin, bilirubin, transferrin, uric acid.
- Enzymatic antioxidants, e.g. superoxide dismutase, catalase, glutathione peroxidase, glutathione reductase.

Antioxidatns according to their location
- Intracellular antioxidants, e.g. superoxide dismutase, catalase, glutathione peroxidase.
- Cell membrane antioxidants, e.g. α tocopherol
- Plasma antioxidants, e.g. β carotene, ascorbic acid, bilrubin, uric acid, ceruloplasmin, transferring.

153. Ans. (c) Ninhydrin stain *Ref: Pamale C. Chamfer 3rd ed. p 14, 15*

- Ninhydrin can also be used to monitor deprotection in solid phase peptide synthesis (Kaiser test). The chain is linked via its C-terminus to the solid support, with the N-terminus extending off it. When that nitrogen is deprotected, a ninhydrin test yields blue. Amino-acid residues are attached with their N-terminus protected, so if the next residue has been successfully coupled onto the chain, the test gives a colorless or yellow result.
- Ninhydrin is also used in amino acid analysis of proteins. Most of the amino acids, except proline, are hydrolyzed and react with ninhydrin. Also, certain amino acid chains are degraded. Therefore, separate analysis is required for identifying such amino acids that either react differently or do not react at all with ninhydrin. The rest of the amino acids are then quantified colorimetrically after separation by chromatography.
- A solution suspected of containing the ammonium ion can be tested by ninhydrin by dotting it onto a solid support (such as silica gel); treatment with ninhydrin should result in a dramatic purple color if the solution contains this species. In the analysis of a chemical reaction by thin layer chromatography (TLC), the reagent can also be used (usually 0.2 % solution in either n-butanol or in ethanol). It will detect, on the TLC plate, virtually all amines, carbamates and also, after vigorous heating, amides.
- When ninhydrin reacts with amino acids, the reaction also releases CO_2. The carbon in this CO_2 originates from the carboxyl carbon of the amino acid. This reaction has been used to release the carboxyl carbons of bone collagen from ancient bones for stable isotope analysis in order to help reconstruct the palaeodiet of cave bears. Release of the carboxyl carbon (via ninhydrin) from amino acids recovered from soil that has been treated with a labeled substrate demonstrates assimilation of that substrate into microbial protein. This approach was successfully used to reveal that some ammonium oxidizing bacteria, also called nitrifying bacteria use urea as a carbon source in soil.
- A stain obtained after a thumbprint is treated with ninhydrin.
- A ninhydrin solution is commonly used by forensic investigators in the analysis of latent fingerprints on porous surfaces such as paper. Amino acid containing fingermarks, formed by minute sweat secretions which gather on the finger's unique ridges, are treated with the ninhydrin solution which turns the amino acid finger ridge patterns purple and therefore visible.
- The first step in determining the primary structure of a polypeptide is to identify and quantitate its constituent amino acids. A purified sample of the polypeptide is to identify and quantitate its constituent amino acids. A purified sample of the polypeptide to be analyzed is first hydrolyzed by strong acid at 1100C for 24 hours. This treatment cleaves the peptide bonds, and releases the individual amino acids, which can be separated by cation-exchange chromatography.
- The amino acids bind to the column with different affinities, depending on their charges, hydrophobicity, and other characteristics. Each amino acid is sequentially released from the chromatography column by eluting with solutions of increasing ionic strength and pH. The separated amino acids contained in the eluate from the column are quantitated by heating them with ninhydrin a reagent that forms a purple compound with most amino acids, ammonia, and amines. The amount of each amino acid is determined spectrophotometrically by measuring the amount of light absorbed by the ninhydrin derivative. The analysis described above is performed using an amino acid analyzer.

154. Ans. (d) Glutamine *Ref: Biochemistry- U. Satyanarayana, 3rd ed. p 336*

- Ammonia produces by brain is trapped as glutamine.
- G lutamine synthetase is present predominantly in the brain, kidneys, and liver.
- GS in the brain participates in
  - The metabolic regulation of glutamate,

- The detoxification of brain ammonia,
- The assimilation of ammonia,
- Recyclization of neurotransmitters, and
- Termination of neurotransmitter signals.

155. Ans. (a) Tyrosine *Ref: Satyanarayan 3rd ed. p 349*

- Thyroxine is a derivative of tyrosine.
- It is formed by the iodination and joining of peptide-linked tyrosyl residues of thyroglobulin.
- Proteolysis of thyroglobulin yields thyroxine.
- Thyroxine is also called tetraiodothyronine, or T4, because of the four iodine atoms of the thyroid hormone.

156. Ans. (b) Hyaluronic acid *Ref: Satyanarayan 3rd ed. p 23*

- Hyaluronic acid (HA) is a biopolymer found naturally in the body.
- It is a linear polysaccharide ('many sugars') with unique physical and biochemical properties such as visco-elasticity and water-binding ability.
- Hyaluronic acid gives the synovial fluid its characteristic viscoelastic properties. It enables the fluid to act as a lubricant, shock absorber and a filter controlling the movement of cells and large molecules within the joint.
- Hyaluronic acid forms a coating over the entire inner surface of the joint, which acts as a viscoelastic shield over the articular cartilage and protects it from mechanical damage. This coating also protects the cartilage and synovium from free radicals and other inflammatory factors. In addition, hyaluronic acid protects from pain by masking the local nociceptors.
- Hyaluronic acid forms the backbone of the proteoglycan aggregates that are essential for the structural and functional integrity of the articular cartilage.

157. Ans. (c) Inner membrane of mitochondria *Ref: Satyanarayan 3rd ed. p 226*

- The electron transport chain is present in the inner mitochondrial membrane and is the final common pathway by which electrons derived from different fuels of the body flow to oxygen.
- Electron transport and ATP synthesis by oxidative phosphorylation proceed continuously in all tissues that contain mitochondria.
- The components of the electron transport chain are located in the inner membrane.
- The inner mitochondrial membrane is unusually rich in protein, half of which is directly involved in electron transport and oxidative phosphorylation.
- The inner mitochondrial membrane is highly convoluted. The convolutions, called cristae, serve to greatly increase the surface area of the membrane.
- The matrix contains mitochondrial RNA and DNA (mtRNA and mtDNA) and mitochondrial ribosomes.

158. Ans. (a) Transferrin *Ref: Biochemistry- U. Satyanarayana, 3rd ed. p 415*

- The iron (Fe^{2+}) entering the mucosal cells by absorption are oxidized to ferric form (Fe^{3}) with the help of enzyme ferroxidase.
- Iron is stored in liver, spleen and bone marrow in the form of ferritin.
- Transport form of iron is transferrin.
- Hemosiderin is another form of iron storage protein. It holds about 35% of iron by weight.

159. Ans. (c) Phytic acid *Ref: Biochemistry- U. Satyanarayana, 3rd ed. p 406*

- Phytic acid a saturated cyclic acid, is the principal storage form of phosphorus in many plant tissues, especially bran and seeds.

- Phytate is not digestible to humans or nonruminant animals, so it is not a source of either inositol or phosphate if eaten directly.
- Moreover, phytic acid chelates and thus makes unabsorbable certain important minor minerals such as zinc and iron, and to a lesser extent, also macro minerals such as calcium and magnesium.

160. Ans. (a) Sustenticular cells *Ref: Guyton 11th ed. p 664*

- The taste bud is composed of about 50 modified epithelial cells, some of which are supporting cells called 'Sustenticular cells'and others of which are 'Taste Cells.
- Taste buds are the cells or group of cell which help in taste perception
- Taste buds are absent on the filliform papillae.

161. Ans. (a) Progesterone *Ref: Lippincott's 3rd ed. p 235*

- Progesterone is the precursor of both gonadal and adrenocortical hormone.

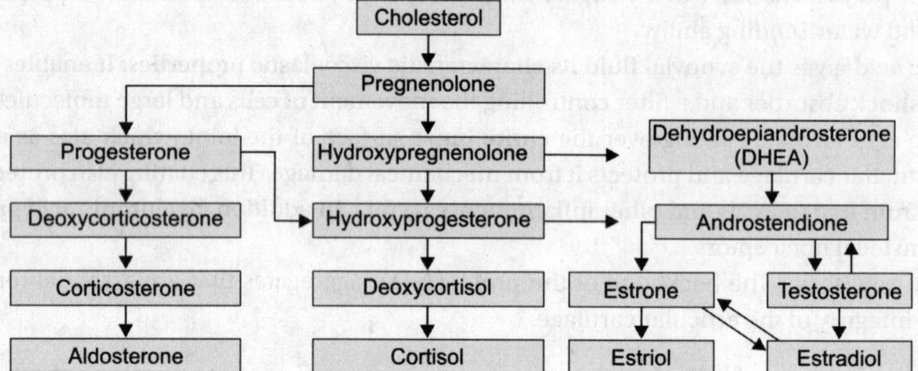

4 Dental Material

GENERAL CLASSES AND PROPERTIES OF DENTAL MATERIAL

1. Munsell's system is used to: *(AIIMS May 2010)*
   a. Define and measure color qualitatively
   b. Define and measure the physical properties of gold alloys
   c. Evaluate the brittleness of different alloys
   d. Measure different colors quantitatively

2. Which of the following tests is classified as micro hardness test? *(AIIMS Nov 2010, May 2007)*
   a. Brinell hardness
   b. Knoop hardness
   c. Rockwell hardness
   d. None of the above

3. If the rate of loading is increased, the mechanical properties of a material: *(AIIMS Nov 2010)*
   a. Increases
   b. Decreases
   c. Constant
   d. Becomes unpredictable

4. Which is correct regarding setting of condensation silicone? *(AIPGEE 2011)*
   a. Polymerization occurs with repeated elimination of small molecules
   b. Polymerization occurs with elimination of a single by-product
   c. Polymerization occurs by addition of molecules of monomers
   d. Condensation does not occur at all

5. Torsional force is: *(AIPGEE 2005, COMED 2012)*
   a. Compression
   b. Tensile force
   c. Shear
   d. Transverse bending force

6. In acrylic resin denture. True is: *(AIPGEE 2013)*
   a. For each 1% increase in weight by water absorption, produces 0.23% linear expansion
   b. For each 10% increase in weight by water absorption, produce 0.23 linear expansion
   c. There is total 2.3% expansion in a year
   d. There is 2.3 increase in weight of the denture in 5 years

7. For complete wetting, angle should be: *(AIIMS Nov 2013)*
   a. Minimum in hard tissues
   b. Maximum in both dentin and enamel
   c. Minimum in dentin and maximum in enamel
   d. Minimum in enamel and maximum in dentin

8. What is used for d measurement of d setting time? *(AIIMS Nov 2013)*
   a. Viket's needle test
   b. Vicker's test
   c. Brinell test
   d. Cold bend test

9. The term used for a material with high compressive strength but low tensile strength is: *(AIIMS Nov 2008)*
   a. Ductile
   b. Malleable
   c. Brittle
   d. Resilient

10. The angle between adhesive and adherent is 0°. This indicates: *(AIIMS Nov 2007)*
   a. Rough surface between the adhesive and adherent
   b. Presence of irregularities between the adherent surfaces
   c. Complete wetting of the surfaces
   d. That molecules of adhesive and adherent are at a tangent to each other

11. Like the eutectic transformation, the peritectic reaction is an invariant reaction (i.e. it occurs at a particular composition and temperature). The reaction can be written as: *(AIIMS May 2006)*
a. Liquid + b → a
b. Liquid + b → Liquid + a
c. Liquid → a-solid solution + b-solid solution
d. a+b → Liquid

12. Poisson's ratio is: *(AIIMS Nov 2007)*
a. Lateral strain by axial strain within elastic limit
b. Equal to flexural strength
c. More in amalgam
d. Low for gold alloy

13. Strain is: *(AIIMS Nov 2007)*
a. The new length upon original length after a load is applied
b. The original length upon new length after a load is applied
c. The force applied to change the length
d. The difference between the two lengths upon original length

14. The chroma in color is: *(KCET 2008)*
a. Dominant color of an object
b. Degree of saturation
c. Type of color
d. Lightness or darkness of color

15. Which of the following are the microhardness tests done to check the hardness? *(KCET 2009)*
a. Brinell and Rockwell tests
b. Knoop and Vickers tests
c. Shore and Barcol tests
d. Knoop and Brinell test

16. Direct coupling or by the exchange of a hydrogen atom from one growing chain to another in a polymerization chain reaction is termed as: *(KCET 2009)*
a. Introduction
b. Propagation
c. Termination
d. Chain transfer

17. A true eutectic alloy has melting point: *(KCET 2011)*
a. Above that of low fusing metal
b. Above the melting point of either metal
c. Below that of high fusion metal
d. Below the melting point of either metal

18. Modern dental noble metal casting alloys generally have equiaxed fine grain structures because of the incorporation of small amounts of: *(KCET 2012)*
a. Chromium
b. Indium
c. Iridium
d. Palladium

19. Relative lightness or darkness of the color is known as: *(KCET 2013)*
a. Hue
b. Chroma
c. Value
d. Saturation

20. A good adhesive should possess all of the following, *except*: *(KCET 2013)*
a. High adherend wetting
b. High contact angle
c. Low contact angle
d. High flow

21. Deformation that is recovered up on removal of an externally applied force or pressure is known as: *(KCET 2013)*
a. Young's modulus
b. Plastic strain
c. Elastic strain
d. Flexural strain

22. Which of the following is not true of polymethyl methacrylate? *(KCET 2013)*
a. Knoop hardness number 18 to 20
b. Tensile strength of 60 MPa
c. Density of 1.13 gm/cm^2
d. Modulus of elasticity of 3.4 GPa

23. On the stress strain curve the area below the curve showing the energy required to fracture the material is known as: *(KCET 2013)*
a. Ultimate tensile strength
b. Resilience
c. Toughness
d. Yield strength

24. Brazilian test is used to determine the ultimate tensile strength of: *(COMED 2008)*
a. Ductile materials
b. Flexible materials
c. Brittle materials
d. Malleable materials

25. **The relative hardness of elastomers is determined by using:** (*COMED 2008*)
a. Rockwell tester
b. Barcol indenter
c. Noop pyramid
d. Shore durometer

26. **Resistance of a material to permanent deformation is known as:** (*COMED 2008*)
a. Elongation
b. Resiliency
c. Ductility
d. Fracture strength

27. **A test for mutagenesis of a material done on mammalian cells is:** (*COMED 2008*)
a. Styles test
b. Ame's test
c. MTT test
d. Cytotoxicity test

28. **Similarity in the chemical structure of estrogen is seen with:** (*COMED 2008*)
a. HEMA
b. Polyether
c. Bisphenol A
d. Gutta-percha

29. **The melting point of titanium is______degrees in celsius:** (*COMED 2009*)
a. 1056 b. 1560
c. 1668 d. 1886

30. **The most toxic form of mercury is:** (*COMED 2009*)
a. Methyl and ethyl mercury
b. Mercury vapour
c. Inogranic mercury forms
d. Mercury sulfide

31. **Hardness test used for elastic materials:**
a. Brinnel hardness test (*COMED 2009*)
b. Rockwell hardness test
c. Vicker's hardness test
d. Knoop's hardness test

32. **Which of the following hardness tests is independent of the ductility of the material?** (*COMED 2006*)
a. Rockwell hardness test
b. Vicker's hardness test
c. Knoop's hardness test
d. Brinnel hardness test

33. **Space lattice refers to:** (*COMED 2006*)
a. Inter atomic movement
b. Inter atomic imbalance
c. Arrangement of atoms
d. Arrangement of molecules

34. **The modulus of elasticity of an alloy refers to its:** (*COMED 2006*)
a. Flexibility b. Ductility
c. Stiffness d. Malleability

35. **Which of the following causes allergic reactions commonly?** (*MH 2009*)
a. Mercury b. Beryllium
c. Nickel d. Cobalt

36. **Relative inability of a material to sustain plastic deformation before fracture of a material occurs is:** (*MH 2011*)
a. Brittleness b. Toughness
c. Resiliency d. Ductility

37. **The dentin desensitizing agents that acts by precipitating proteins in dentinal tubular fluid is:** (*MH 2014*)
a. Strontium chloride
b. Potassium oxalate
c. Fluoride
d. Hydroxy ethyl methacrylate

AUXILIARY DENTAL MATERIALS

38. **Which of the following is the correct glass transition temperature of impression compound?** (*AIIMS May 2010, 2008*)
a. 39°C b. 43.5°C
c. 65°C d. 100°C

39. **Which of the following is used as a surface hardener in impression material?** (*AIIMS Nov 2010*)
a. 2% K_2SO_4
b. 0.2% K_2SO_4
c. 2% sodium sulphate
d. 0.2% sodium sulphate

40. **Addition of 2% potassium sulphate and 0.5% borax to agar agar helps in:** (*AIIMS Nov 2010*)
a. Regulating setting time and expansion of plaster
b. Imparting color and taste
c. Regulating strength and consistency of gel
d. Minimized shrinkage of impression

41. Hardening solution is used with which of the following impression materials? *(AIIMS Nov 2010, 2008)*

a. Zinc oxide eugenol b. Alginate
c. Agar agar d. Polysulfide

42. Alginate is made dust free by which one of the following methods? *(AIIMS Nov 2010)*

a. Adding metallic compounds
b. Coating particles with dihydric alcohol (diglycerol)
c. Removing diatomaceous earth particles
d. Changing the matrix

43. Fins or spines on casting are produced due to: *(AIPGEE 2011)*

a. Prolonged heating
b. Rapid heating rate
c. High powder/liquid ratio
d. Thin investment materials

44. Which is described as the best working time of elastomeric impression material? *(AIPGEE 2011)*

a. From the beginning of mixing to just after the appearance of elastic properties
b. From the beginning of mixing to a stage when the impression can be removed from the mouth with minimum of distortion
c. From the beginning of mixing to just before the appearance of elastic properties
d. From the beginning of mixing to the loss of lustre of impression material

45. Polysulfide materials are not used routinely, because of: *(AIPGEE 2011)*

a. Unpleasant odour and taste
b. Low accuracy
c. Least permanent deformation
d. Highest curing shrinkage

46. Rough irregular surface on elastomeric impression material is due to: *(AIPGEE 2011)*

a. Improper application of pressure
b. Air incorporated during mixing
c. Improper ratio of polymer and monomer
d. Presence of saliva in impression area

47. The method to reduce back pressure porosity is: *(AIPGEE 2009)*

a. To use a rounded casting
b. By decreasing the flare
c. By adjusting space to 1/4 inch from casting
d. By decreasing melting pressure

48. Which one of the following is true about an agar hydrocolloid impression material? *(AIPGEE 2008)*

a. It liquefies at a temperature of 71100°C
b. It solidifies at a temperature of 5070°C
c. It cannot register fi ne surfaces
d. It facilitates fabrication of metal dies

49. Difference between gelation and liquefaction temperature is called: *(AIPGEE 2007)*

a. Imbibition b. Syneresis
c. Hysteresis d. Adsorption

50. The function of 2% potassium sulphate in a gypsum product is: *(AIPGEE 2007)*

a. To regulate the setting expansion
b. To regulate the setting time
c. To act as a retarder
d. To act as an accelerator

51. The use of quartz in gypsum-bonded investments is: *(AIPGEE 2007)*

a. To counteract expansion
b. To provide strength
c. To act as a retarder
d. To counteract contraction

52. The flow of impression compound at 37°C is: *(AIPGEE 2007)*

a. 2% b. 4%
c. 6% d. 10%

53. In the investment for gold, the strength is provided by: *(AIPGEE 2007)*

a. Silica b. Gypsum
c. Cristobalite d. Carbon

54. Which of the following is not true about elastomeric impression? *(AIPGEE 2006)*

a. Single-mix materials have higher viscosity
b. Shear thinning is related to the viscosity of monophase impression materials
c. Improper mixing of material can cause permanent deformation of impression
d. Putty-wash technique of impression reduces the dimensional change on setting

55. Which one of the following agents is used as a die hardener? *(AIPGEE 2005)*

a. Cynoacrylate
b. Nail polish
c. Volatile relief agents
d. Composite resin

56. Addition of surface active agent like gum Arabic with lime to hemihydrates: *(AIPGEE 2013)*
a. Would increase water requirement
b. Would decrease water requirement
c. Would not affect water requirement
d. Increases surface activity

57. Which material is not used to make special tray in children: *(AIPGEE 2013)*
a. Vacuum cure Thermoplastic resin
b. Light cure acrylic resin
c. Cold cure acrylic resin
d. Vacuum cure polyurethane

58. Which wax is used for arrangement of teeth in India during summer season in try in stage? *(AIPGEE 2013)*
a. Utility wax
b. Type 1 modelling wax
c. Type 3 modelling wax
d. Base plate

59. Composition of Cold mold seal is: *(AIPGEE 2013)*
a. Sodium alginate
b. Isopropyl alcohol
c. Glycerine
d. Calcium Alginate

60. Gypsum bonded investments should not be heated above: *(AIPGEE 2013)*
a. 250°C b. 200°C
c. 700°C d. 450°C

61. Pickling solution for gypsum bonded casting is: *(AIPGEE 2013, COMED 2005)*
a. 50% HCl
b. 50% phosphoric acid
c. 50% HF
d. 37% phosphoric acid

62. Incomplete casting is the result of: *(AIPGEE 2012)*
a. More porous investment in the mould
b. Narrow sprue diameter
c. Hallow sprue pin
d. Larger reservoir

63. What is a c-factor in dental material? *(AIPGEE 2012)*
a. Condensation of Amalgam
b. Carving of amalgam
c. Polymerization shrinkage of composite resins
d. Cement strength

64. Denture cleansers main component is: *(AIIMS May 2012)*
a. H_2O_2 b. Sodium perborate
c. Alkali agents d. Detergents

65. Which of the following is not used as an abrasive in dentifrices? *(AIIMS May 2012)*
a. Calcium carbonate
b. Sodium chloride
c. Silicate
d. Amylose

66. Chemically activated resin P/L ratio: *(AIIMS May 2012)*
a. 3:1 by vol, 2:1 by wt
b. 2:1 by vol, 3:1 by wt
c. 1:3 by vol, 1:2 by wt
d. 2:1 by vol, 1:3 by wt

67. In cold cure resin activator is: *(AIIMS May 2012)*
a. Dibutyl phthalate
b. Dimethyl-p-toluidine
c. Glycol dimethacrylate
d. Benzoyl peroxide

68. w/p ratio of type iv dental stone: *(AIIMS Nov 2013)*
a. 6 to .7
b. 4 to .5
c. 22 to .24
d. 28 to .30

69. In impression compound filler in 'alginate' is: *(AIIMS Nov 2013)*
a. Potassium alginate
b. Calcium sulphate
c. Diatomaceous earth
d. Sodium phosphate

70. Addition silicone what is done for better cast: *(AIIMS Nov 2013)*
a. Apply chloroform
b. Apply ketone
c. Delay pouring
d. All of the above

71. Which of the following is true regarding corrosion of amalgam restoration? *(AIIMS Nov 2007)*
a. It can extend up to a depth of 100-500 μm
b. It decreases if the tin content of alloy decreases
c. It is promoted by g2 phase of alloy particles
d. It is resisted most by CuSn phase in high-copper amalgam

72. Which of the following components acts as an accelerator in ZOE impression paste? *(AIIMS May 2007)*

a. Zinc sulphate and zinc chloride
b. Zinc chloride and eugenol
c. Zinc sulphate and eugenol
d. Glycerine

73. The impression material of choice to be used in oral submucous fibrosis is: *(AIIMS Nov 2006)*

a. Addition silicone
b. Condensation silicone
c. Zinc oxide eugenol
d. Impression compound

74. Which of the following is not a true wax? *(AIIMS May 2006)*

a. Paraffin
b. Ozokerite
c. Cocoa butter
d. Candelilla

75. Which of the following is not true about casting gypsum-bonded investment material? *(AIIMS May 2006)*

a. It is used for cast metal alloys
b. 50-65% of gypsum changes to form a-hemihydrate
c. The investment material is not heated above 700°C temperature
d. Heating above 700°C causes formation of sulphur dioxide from copper sulphate

76. In the air abrasive technique, the abrasive particles used are: *(AIIMS May 2009)*

a. 27 μm aluminium oxide
b. 50 μm aluminium oxide
c. Iron oxide
d. HCl

77. Advantage of acid etching that led to its widespread use is reduction in: *(AIIMS Nov 2008)*

a. Microleakage
b. Porosity of restorative material
c. Polymerization shrinkage of restoration
d. Coefficient of thermal expansion of restoration

78. Which of the following is a mucostatic impression material? *(AIIMS Nov 2008)*

a. Agar
b. Alginate
c. ZOE paste
d. Side effect

79. Which of the following is used as a gypsum hardening agent? *(AIIMS Nov 2008)*

a. 0.2% potassium sulphate
b. 2% potassium sulphate
c. 0.2% sodium sulphate
d. 2% sodium sulphate

80. Difference between the gelation and liquefaction temperature is called: *(AIIMS Nov 2008)*

a. Imbibition b. Syneresis
c. Hysteresis d. Adsorption

81. Which of the following impression materials requires a hardener? *(AIIMS Nov 2008)*

a. Agar b. Alginate
c. Elastomers d. Side effect

82. The working time of an elastomeric impression material is defined as: *(AIIMS Nov 2008)*

a. The time from the start of the mixing till the material is fully set
b. The time elapsed from the beginning of mixing until curing has advanced
c. The time from the start of mixing till just before the elastic properties have fully developed
d. None of the above

83. The function of 2% potassium sulphate in a gypsum product is: *(AIIMS Nov 2008)*

a. To regulate the setting expansion
b. To regulate the setting time
c. To act as a retarder
d. None of the above

84. Tg of an impression material is: *(AIIMS Nov 2008)*

a. 39°C b. 43.5°C
c. 65°C d. 100°C

85. The major disadvantage of polysulfide impression material in clinical practice is: *(AIIMS Nov 2008)*

a. Poor biocompatibility
b. Poor tear strength
c. That it is radiolucent
d. That it stains clothes and has unacceptable odour

86. Dimensional stability of an elastomeric impression material can be given in descending order as: *(AIIMS Nov 2008)*

a. Polysulfide > polyether > condensation silicone > addition silicone
b. Polyether > condensation silicone > polysulfide > addition silicone

c. Addition silicone > polyether > polysulfide > condensation silicone
d. Addition silicone > condensation silicone > polysulfide > polyether

87. Rough surface of elastomeric impression results from: *(AIIMS Nov 2008)*
a. Inadequate mixing
b. Nonrinsing of the oral cavity by patient before the impression
c. Too rapid polymerization
d. Incomplete polymerization caused by premature removal from the mouth

88. The diameter of sprue and subsurface porosity will have: *(AIIMS Nov 2006)*
a. Direct relationship
b. Inverse relationship
c. Inverse square relationship
d. No relationship

89. The length of sprue and subsurface porosity will have: *(AIIMS Nov 2006)*
a. Direct relationship
b. Inverse relationship
c. Inverse square relationship
d. No relationship at all

90. Carnauba wax: *(AIIMS May 2006)*
a. Increases smoothness
b. Decreases flow
c. Is 30-40%
d. Increases hardness

91. Which of the following impression material is most biocompatible? *(KCET 2005)*
a. Polysulfide b. Condensation silicone
c. Addition Silicone d. Polyether

92. According to ADA specification No. 3 Type I Impression Compound, at 45°C, should have a minimum flow: *(KCET 2005)*
a. More than 65% b. More than 75%
c. More than 85% d. More than 95%

93. Loss of gloss test in gypsum product is an indication for: *(KCET 2005)*
a. Adequate mixing time
b. Adequate working time
c. Initial set
d. Final set

94. Rouge, used as dental abrasive, is chemically known as: *(KCET 2005)*
a. Tin oxide b. Iron oxide
c. Ethyl silicate d. Zirconium silicate

95. Type IV gold alloy contains: *(KCET 2006)*
a. 2% gold b. 13% gold
c. 75% gold d. 80% gold

96. Non-gamma 2 alloy is: *(KCET 2006)*
a. Resistant to marginal leakage
b. Resistant to discoloration
c. Resistant to sensitization
d. Resistant to corrosion

97. The irreversible hydrocolloid impression material used in removal partial denture prosthesis construction: *(KCET 2006)*
a. Agar Agar b. Alginate
c. Silicone d. Thiobal

98. The average particle size of powered gold is: *(KCET 2006)*
a. 10 um b. 15 um
c. 30 um d. 0.1 mm

99. The best method to control gelation time while mixing alginate material is: *(KCET 2006)*
a. Alter the temperature of water
b. Alter the water/powder ratio
c. Increase the mixing time
d. Reduce the percentage of retarder

100. The modulus of elasticity of an alloy refers to The best method to control gelation time: *(KCET 2006)*
a. Flexibility
b. Ductility
c. Stiffness
d. Malleability

101. The percentage of free monomer in a heat-cured acrylic resin is: *(KCET 2007)*
a. 3% to 5%
b. 8% to 10%
c. 0.2% to 0.5%
d. 0.600 to 0.8%

102. For Dental Amalgam, the elastic modulus and tensile strength is: *(KCET 2007)*
a. 40 Gpa and 60–100 Mpa
b. 21 Gpa and 27–55 Mpa
c. 350 Gpa and 110–120 Mpa
d. 360 Gpa and 125–130 Mpa

103. The inability of the air in the mould to escape through the pores in the investment leads to: *(KCET 2008)*
a. Localized shrinkage porosity
b. Back pressure porosity
c. Subsurface porosity
d. Suck back porosity

104. The premature termination of the flow of molten metal during solidification is termed: *(KCET 2008)*
a. Gas inclusion porosity
b. Subsurface porosity
c. Localized shrinkage porosity
d. Back pressure porosity

105. Which one of the following is a superabrasive? *(KCET 2008)*
a. Sand
b. Silicon carbide
c. Diamond
d. Aluminum oxide

106. Class II stone, densite or improved stone is: *(KCET 2008)*
a. Type III b. Type IV
c. Type V d. None of the above

107. Crocus cloth is: *(KCET 2008)*
a. Emery b. Garnet
c. Pumice d. Rouge

108. Which one of the following impression materials is elastic, sets by a chemical reaction and is catalyzed by chloroplatinic acid? *(KCET 2009)*
a. Condensation silicone
b. Poly ethers
b. Poly sulfides
d. Poly vinyl siloxane

109. With indirect spruing, which one of the following porosities can be minimized? *(KCET 2009)*
a. Back pressure porosity
b. Localized shrinkage porosity
c. Pin hole porosity
d. Micro porosity

110. The main difference between powders of dental plaster and dental stone is: *(KCET 2009)*
a. Chemical composition
b. Solubility in water
c. Particle shape and size
d. Shelf life

111. The ranking of tear strength from the lowest to highest of all impression materials generally is as follows: *(KCET 2010)*
a. Hydrocolloids, silicones, polyether, polysulfide
b. Silicones, hydrocolloids, polyether, polysulfide
c. Polysulfide, hydrocolloids, silicones, polyether
d. Hydrocolloids, polyether, silicones, polysulfide

112. The strength of gypsum products is generally expressed in terms of: *(KCET 2010)*
a. Tensile strength
b. Wet strength
c. Green strength
d. Compressive strength

113. Which of the following impression materials is easy to pour and difficult to remove the stone caste from the impressions? *(KCET 2011)*
a. Addition polysilicone
b. Condensation polysilicone
c. Polyether
d. Polysulfide

114. As per ADA No. 25 minimum amount of setting expansion required for type V gypsum product is: *(KCET 2011)*
a. 0.05 b. 0.10
c. 0.15 d. 0.20

115. Which one of the following waxes can be added to the paraffin wax to partially or entirely replace the carnauba wax? *(KCET 2012)*
a. Bee wax
b. Candelilla wax
c. Ceresin
d. Microcrystalline wax

116. Clogging of an abrasive wheel with debris, causing reduction of abrasive action is called: *(KCET 2012)*
a. Blinding
b. Buffing
c. Dressing
d. Truing

117. Which of the following detergent used in dentifrice? *(KCET 2012)*
a. Carrageenan
b. Disodium pyrophosphate
c. Sodium lauryl sulphate
d. Sorbitol

118. By-product of condensation reaction between silicone base and alkyl silicate in presence of tin octate: *(KCET 2012)*
a. Ethyl alcohol b. Glycol
c. Acetate d. Propanolol

119. Attachment of the sprue at right angle to the broad flat surface of the pattern will cause: *(KCET 2012)*
a. Micro porosity
b. Pinhole porosity
c. Subsurface porosity
d. Suck back porosity

120. The chief difference between model plaster powder and dental stone powder is: *(KCET 2012)*
a. Chemical formula
b. Particle size and shape
c. Shelf life
d. Solubility in water

121. Which of the following impression material is not hydrophobic? *(KCET 2013)*
a. Polyethers
b. Reversible hydrocolloid
c. Polysulfide polymer
d. Condensation silicone

122. The length of the sprue former should be adjusted for gypsum-bonded investment so that the top of the wax pattern is within: *(COMED 2008)*
a. 6 mm of the open end of the ring
b. 10 mm of the open end of the ring
c. 1 mm of the open end of the ring
d. 2 mm of the open end of the ring

123. Component of inlay wax which makes it flake resistant is: *(COMED 2008)*
a. Paraffin
b. Carnauba
c. Gum dammar
d. Candellila

124. A technique of combining reversible and irreversible hydrocolloid that could bond to irreversible hydrocolloid is known as:
(COMED 2009)
a. Injecting technique
b. Laminate technique
c. Immersion technique
d. Tempering technique

125. Sprue former direction should be at:
(COMED 2010, 2007)
a. 45 degree b. 90 degree
c. 95 degree d. 180 degree

126. Binder in phosphate bonded investment is:
(COMED 2010)
a. Magnesium oxide and phosphate
b. Magnesium oxide and phosphate acid
c. Magnesium oxide and monoammonium phosphate
d. Magnesium oxide and orthophosphoric acid

127. Gypsum bonded investment should not be heated above: *(COMED 2010)*
a. 700°C
b. 750°C
c. 800°C
d. 900°C

128. Which one of the following is not added in small amount to be used as grain refiners?
(COMED 2010)
a. Iridium b. Ruthenium
c. Indium d. Platinum

129. The purpose of investment setting expansion is to compensate for: *(COMED 2010)*
a. Casting shrinkage
b. Casting expansion
c. Wax elimination
d. Alloy melting

130. Placing a ring liner approximately 3.25 mm short of the ends of the ring tends to: *(COMED 2010)*
a. Produce a more uniform expansion and the expansion will not be in a vertical direction hence no distortion
b. Produce a more uniform contraction
c. Produce to change
d. Produce distortion

131. ADA specification number for gypsum products are described under: *(COMED 2011)*
a. 4 b. 1
c. 12 d. 25

132. A materials that facilitate removal of impression from cast is: *(COMED 2011)*
a. Rosin b. Starch
c. Sodium chloride d. Borates

133. For accurate inter-occlusal records the material of choice is: *(COMED 2011)*
a. 28 gauge casting wax
b. ZOE bite registration paste
c. Elastomeric bite registration material
d. Base plate wax

134. The best pickling solution for gypsum bonded investment is: *(COMED 2011)*
a. Hydrochloric acid
b. Nitric acid
c. Sulphuric acid
d. Phosphoric acid

135. The safest method for soaking dental cast is: *(COMED 2011)*
a. Placing in saturated solution of calcium sulphate
b. Placing in water
c. Placing in saturated solution of sodium chloride
d. Placing in solution of gypsum slurry

136. The most practical method for avoiding any possible distortion of the wax pattern is: *(COMED 2011)*
a. Use of heated instruments during carving of the wax pattern
b. Invest the wax pattern immediately
c. Swaging the wax pattern in a closed vessel
d. Applying finger pressure during cooling of the wax

137. Overheating of impression compound during softening will lead to reaching out of more soluble constituents such as: *(COMED 2012)*
a. Rosin b. Talc
c. Waxes d. Stearlic acid

138. Condenstion reaction of silicones occur in presence of: *(COMED 2012)*
a. Lead dioxide b. Titanium dioxide
c. Stannous octate d. Platinum salt

139. Dimension stability of hydrocolloids may be achieved by: *(COMED 2012, 2005)*
a. Optimizing
b. Using cold water
c. Prolonged manipulation
d. Using humidor

140. The length of the sprue former should be adjusted for gypsum bonded investment so that the top of the wax pattern is: *(COMED 2012)*
a. Within 6 mm of the open end of the ring
b. Within 10 mm of the open end of the ring
c. Within the 1 mm of the one end of the ring
d. Within 2 mm of opened of the ring

141. Increased spatulation of gypsum products: *(COMED 2012)*
a. Increase setting time
b. Decrease setting time
c. Does not interfere with setting time
d. Only produces more exothermic heat

142. The laminate impression technique utilizes a combination of 2 impression materials: *(COMED 2012)*
a. Light body and heavy body
b. PVS and polyether
c. Polyether and polysulfide
d. Alginate and agar

143. Gypsum bonded investments are used for: *(COMED 2012)*
a. Gold alloy
b. Bank metal alloy
c. Silver palladium alloy
d. Porcelain casting

144. The most successful Materials for soft liner applications have been: *(COMED 2013)*
a. Impression of plaster
b. Silicone rubbers
c. Waxes
d. Irreversible hydrocolloids

145. Rough surface and uneven surface of elastomeric impression results from: *(COMED 2013)*
a. Inadequate mixing
b. Air bubbles
c. Too rapid polymerization
d. Incomplete polymerization caused by premature removal from mouth

146. Which of the following is not a mouth temperature wax? *(COMED 2013)*
a. Adaptol
b. Korrecta type 1
c. HL physiologic paste
d. Lowa wax

147. An ideal location to attach a sprue for a posterior cast restoration is: *(COMED 2013)*
a. Central fossa b. Cusp tips
c. Marginal ridge d. Contact point

148. Identify the material used in maxillo-facial prosthesis: *(COMED 2013)*
a. Polyurethane elastomers
b. Polycarbonate
c. Autopolymerizing acrylic resin
d. Polyvinyl chloride

149. Antibiotic prophylaxis is not recommended in: *(COMED 2014)*
a. Making of impressions
b. Dental extraction
c. Replantation of a tooth
d. Gingivectomy

150. The monophase elastomeric material can be used as both tray and syringe material because it has: *(COMED 2014)*
a. A long setting time
b. It is economical
c. Pseudoplastic properties
d. Better recording of tissues

151. In air-abrasive technology the abrasive particles used are *(KCET 2007)*
a. Iron oxide
b. Tin oxide
c. Aluminium oxide
d. Solicon oxide

152. Finer particle size of silica: *(KCET 2007)*
a. Slower the hygroscopic expansion
b. Greater the hygroscopic expansion
c. Normal setting expansion
d. No setting expansion

153. Putty wash technique (two-stage): *(KCET 2007)*
a. Light body and putty used at the same time
b. Putty used first and light body used second
c. Light body first and putty later
d. None of the above

154. Back pressure porosity in casting is due to: *(COMED 2005)*
a. High casting pressure
b. Low investment permeability
c. Small size and improper direction of sprue
d. Sprue

155. Type I gypsum product is: *(COMED 2005)*
a. Impression plaster
b. Class I stone/hydrocal
c. Class II stone/densite
d. Modelplaster

156. The setting expansion of gypsum products can be reduced by: *(COMED 2005)*
a. Increased spatulation
b. Adding potassium sulphate
c. Less water/powder ratio
d. Allowing setting under water

157. Gases dissolved in molten metals are liberated when cooled, giving rise to: *(COMED 2005)*
a. Suck back porosity
b. Gas inclusion porosity
c. Localized shrinkage porosity
d. Microporosity

158. The water/powder ratio of alginate is: *(COMED 2005)*
a. 100 ml of water + 60 gm of powder
b. 40 ml of water + 40 gm of powder
c. 40 ml of water + 15 gm of powder
d. 15 ml of water + 40 gm of powder

159. To make vinyl polysiloxane hydrophilic, the following is added: *(COMED 2005)*
a. Mineral oil
b. Surfactant
c. Water
d. Plasticizer

160. Which die material has a hazardous potential during fabrication? *(COMED 2006)*
a. Improve stone
b. Silver amalgam
c. Electrodeposited silver
d. Epoxy resin

161. The role of magnesium chloride in ZnOE impression paste is: *(COMED 2006)*
a. Retarder
b. Modifier
c. Plasticizer
d. Accelerator

162. Impression material that does not harden by chemical reaction: *(COMED 2007)*
a. Zinc oxide eugenol
b. Impression compound
c. Alginate
d. Plaster of Paris

163. Desensitizing agent used in dentrifice: *(COMED 2007)*
a. Sodium chloride
b. Potassium nitrate
c. Ammonium sulphate
d. Glycerine

164. A laminate technique impression utilizes: *(COMED 2007)*
a. Syringe agar and chilled tray alginate
b. Syringe agar and tray agar
c. Syringe agar and impression compound
d. Chilled alginate and impression compound

165. The polishing agent which can be used to polish amalgam restorations is: *(COMED 2007)*
a. Garner b. Emery
c. Silex d. Alumina

166. Gum Dammar helps to: *(MH 2009)*
a. Lower the melting point
b. Decrease flow at mouth temperature
c. Improves smoothness
d. Harden the wax

167. Maximum elastic recovery is seen with: *(MH 2010)*
a. Condensation silicon
b. Addition silicon
c. Polysulfide
d. Polyether

168. Working and setting time of elastomers can be measured by: *(MH 2010)*
a. Rheometer
b. Reciprocating rheometer
c. Odontometer
d. Gnathodynometer

169. Hot spot is another name for: *(MH 2010)*
a. Localized shrinkage porosity
b. Gas inclusion porosity
c. Microporosity
d. Suck-back porosity

170. Mucostatic impression material is: *(MH 2010)*
a. Impression compound
b. Impression wax
c. ZnOE impression paste
d. Bite registration paste

171. The principle material by weight in set agar is: *(MH 2011)*
a. Water b. Soluble borate
c. Agar d. Sulphate

172. A two component system in the form of two pastes contains alginate sol in one and______as reactor: *(MH 2011)*
a. Calcium b. Silica
c. Silicone d. Sodium

173. Polyether should be stored in_____environment: *(MH 2011)*
a. Dry b. Wet
c. Humid d. Warm

174. The fusion temperature of the imp compound indicates a definite________during cooling: *(MH 2011)*
a. High coefficient of thermal expansion
b. Increase in plasticity
c. Reduction in plasticity
d. Leaching of plasticizer

175. Which type of porosity is generally associated with fine grained alloy? *(MH 2011)*
a. Suckback porosity
b. Microporosity
c. Localized shrinkage
d. Pinhole porosity

176. ____ is a potassium-aluminium-silicate mineral with a large coefficient of thermal expansion: *(MH 2011)*
a. Leucite b. Potash
c. Feldspar d. Lithia disilicate

177. A dentist can best control the setting time of Alginate impression material without altering its properties by: *(MH 2014)*
a. Using perforated tray
b. Altering water : powder ratio
c. Reducing the rate of mixing
d. Altering the temperature of water

178. Time dependent deformation produced in a completely set solid subjected to a constant stress is termed as: *(MH 2014)*
a. Static creep
b. Elongation
c. Dynamic creep
d. Flexibility

DIRECT RESTORATIVE MATERIALS

179. The mechanism of adhesion of glass ionomer cement (GIC) restoration with tooth surface is by means of: *(AIIMS May 2011)*
a. Carboxyl group of polymer chains
b. Chelates with metal ions
c. C = C double bond
d. Hydroxyl group

180. Which of the following is the most stable restoration for a GV Black class V unstable erosive lesion? *(AIIMS May 2011)*
a. Acid etch composite
b. RM GIC
c. GIC
d. Compomer

181. After amalgam polishing, the outermost surface has crystals arranged flattened to tooth surface. This is known as: *(AIIMS May 2011)*
a. Beelby's layer b. Weetby's layer
c. Sealb's layer d. Deltoid layer

182. Fluoride released from GIC restoration is replaced by: *(AIIMS May 2011)*
a. Hydroxyl ion b. Aluminium ion
c. Silicate ion d. Carboxylate ion

183. In acid etching, the gel form is preferred to the solution form because: *(AIIMS Nov 2010, 2008)*
a. Of more concentrated action of acid
b. It can be easily washed off
c. Of the ease of placement over the area to be acid etched, without getting spread
d. All of the above

184. A dentin primer: *(AIIMS Nov 2010)*
a. Etches the dentin
b. Increases the surface energy and wets the dentin surface
c. Removes the smear layer
d. Conditions the dentin

185. In etching of enamel, the depth achieved (in micrometer) is: *(AIIMS Nov 2010)*
a. 0 to 0.5 b. 0.5 to 5
c. 5 to 50 d. 50 to 100

186. Which dental cement is the most kind to the pulp? *(AIIMS Nov 2010)*
a. Silicate b. Polycarboxylate
c. Composite d. GIC

187. Regarding the setting reaction of ZnO and eugenol, the incorrect statement is: *(AIIMS Nov 2010)*
a. ZnO forms hydroxide with H_2O
b. Dehydrated ZnO acts with dehydrated eugenol
c. Reaction is autocatalytic
d. Water is a by-product

188. The corrosion that does not take place in high copper amalgam is: *(AIIMS Nov 2010)*
a. Electrical b. Electrochemical
c. Penetrating d. No corrosion

189. Best root-end-filling material is: *(AIPGEE 2010)*
a. MTA b. ZOE
c. Amalgam d. $Ca(OH)_2$

190. Which of the following is used as moisture active adhesive? *(AIPGEE 2010)*
a. Cyanoacrylate b. Methyl methacrylate
c. BISGMA d. Composite resin

191. Polymerization shrinkage of composite causes compression stress of: *(AIPGEE 2009)*
a. 1 MPa b. 2.5 MPa
c. 5 MPa d. 30 MPa

192. Which is the best material for treatment of noncarious class V cavities in unstable acid erosion cases? *(AIPGEE 2009)*
a. GIC b. RM-GIC
c. Compomer d. Composite

193. Bonding of GIC to tooth structure is brought about by: *(AIPGEE 2009)*
a. Metal ions b. Hydroxyl bond
c. Carboxyl bond d. Ionic bond

194. Before restoring a tooth with composite, the area is etched. Accidental contamination occurs with saliva. Therefore: *(AIPGEE 2009)*
a. The area is re-etched before restoration
b. The area is air-dried using an air spray and continue with restoring
c. Wipe the saliva with cotton and continue to restore
d. Add excess composite material and cure it

195. Order of setting of GIC is: *(AIPGEE 2009)*
a. Gelation, migration and post-setting contraction
b. Migration, gelation and setting contraction
c. Concentration, gelation and migration
d. None of the above

196. The purpose of indium in amalgam is to: *(AIPGEE 2009)*
a. Eliminate Hg phase
b. Increase the surface free energy of dentin
c. Decrease Hg release on mastication
d. Decrease Hg release on abrasion

197. Action of primer is: *(AIPGEE 2009)*
a. To remove the smear layer
b. To increase the surface free energy of dentin
c. To form a thin layer between collagen and resin
d. To bond with composite

198. For zinc oxide eugenol, all of following are true *except* that: *(AIPGEE 2008)*
a. Eugenol is the plasticizer
b. Methyl methacrylate is added for strength
c. EBA is added for strength as 37.5% for liquid and 62.5% for eugenol
d. Rosin decreases the brittleness of set cement

199. Which of the following is true for hybrid ionomers? *(AIPGEE 2008)*
a. Surface conditioning of tooth is required
b. Similar translucency as compared to conventional GIC
c. Lesser diametric tensile strength than conventional GIC
d. Dentin bonding agent has to be applied

200. Which of the following is a characteristic feature of high-copper amalgam alloy? *(AIPGEE 2007)*
a. Low compressive strength
b. High marginal breakdown
c. Less marginal breakdown
d. High creep

201. Water-resistant sealant among the following is: *(AIPGEE 2007)*
a. Cyanoacralates
b. Bis-GMA
c. Methylmethacrylate
d. None

202. Which of the following restorative materials demonstrate maximum water solubility? *(AIPGEE 2007)*
a. Light cure GIC
b. Microfilled composite
c. Conventional composites
d. Hybrid composites

203. How much fraction of methyl mercury is absorbed from the gut? *(AIPGEE 2006, KCET 2006)*
a. 20% b. 50%
c. 80% d. 100%

204. What fraction of inhaled mercury vapour is retained in the body? *(AIPGEE 2006)*
a. 45–55% b. 55–65%
c. 65–85% d. >85%

205. Which of the following has the highest creep value? *(AIPGEE 2006)*
a. Low-copper amalgam alloy
b. Admix alloy
c. Single-composition alloy
d. Creep value of all the above alloys is the mentioned same

206. Which of the following cements that bond to tooth structure has an anticarcinogenic effect, has a degree of translucency and does not irritate the pulp? *(AIPGEE 2006)*
a. Polycarboxylate cement
b. Resin cement
c. Silicate cement
d. Glass ionomer cement

207. How soon after contamination by moisture does zinc-containing amalgam restoration starts expanding? *(AIPGEE 2006)*
a. 12 h b. 12 days
c. 35 days d. 1 week

208. Amalgam achieves 70% of the strength by: *(AIPGEE 2006)*
a. 2 hours b. 4 hours
c. 8 hours d. 16 hours

209. Nano fillers are in the range of: *(AIPGEE 2006)*
a. 10–100 µm
b. 0.1–1 µm
c. 0.01–0.1 µm
d. 0.005–0.01 µm

210. Ormocers are: *(AIPGEE 2005)*
a. Organically modified composites
b. Inorganically modified composites
c. Organically modified glass ionomer cement
d. Inorganically modified glass ionomer cement

211. Zinc phosphate compared to GIC has: *(AIPGEE 2013, COMED 2006)*
a. Higher compressive strength
b. Higher tensile strength
c. Higher modulus of elasticity
d. Greater film thickness

212. Important property of pit and fissure sealant is: *(AIPGEE 2013)*
a. Low viscosity
b. Color
c. High Filler content
d. Fluoride release

213. Which of the following cement provides maximum resistance to enamel decalcification when used with orthodontic bands? *(AIPGEE 2013)*
a. GIC
b. Silicate
c. $ZnPO_4$
d. Zinc polycarboxylate

214. Working time of plaster influenced by: *(AIPGEE 2013)*
a. W/P ratio
b. Rapid mixing
c. Addition of warm water
d. Gypsum particles present in the mix

215. Fluoride release from GIC restoration: *(AIPGEE 2012)*
a. Initially more than gradually decreases
b. Remain constant
c. Increases few months after placement
d. It is less in the beginning after that it is increased

216. During normal acid etching, enamel rods have been etched up to 15 μm. What depth of enamel is etched? *(AIIMS Nov 2012)*
a. 510 μm b. 25 μm
c. 1015 μm d. >15 μm

217. In mechanical trituration of amalgam, what is adversely affected? *(AIIMS Nov 2012)*
a. Hardness of d filling
b. Tarnish resistance
c. Final gloss of filling
d. Working time

218. Dentin conditioner: *(AIIMS Nov 2008)*
a. Removes the smear layer
b. Increases the surface free energy of dentin
c. Forms a thin layer between collagen and resin
d. Bonds with composite

219. ZOE-based sealer is all, *except*: *(AIIMS May 2005)*
a. AH26 b. Grossman cement
c. Endomethasone d. Wach's cement

220. A radiopaque area is observed under a 3-month-old class II silver amalgam filling. The base used most probably was: *(AIIMS Nov 2008)*
a. Calcium hydroxide
b. ZOE
c. Zinc phosphate
d. Zinc oxide with formocresol

221. After amalgam is polished, the metal surface is flattened. This layer is called: *(AIIMS Nov 2008)*
a. Deilby's layer b. Beelby's layer
c. Teelby's layer d. Whitby's layer

222. Which one of the following cements is truly adherent to the tooth structure? *(AIIMS Nov 2008)*
a. Glass ionomer cement
b. Zinc oxide eugenol
c. Calcium hydroxide
d. Zinc phosphate

223. Which of the following cements has obtundent property? *(AIIMS Nov 2008)*
a. GIC b. ZOE
c. Calcium hydroxide d. Zinc phosphate

224. Overtrituration of silver and mercury: *(AIIMS Nov 2008)*
a. Causes reduction in contraction
b. Increases strength in lathe cut but reduces strength in spherical alloy
c. Gives a dull and crumbly amalgam mix
d. Decreases the creep

225. Which one of the following is a characteristic feature of high-copper amalgam alloy? *(AIIMS Nov 2008)*
a. Low compressive strength
b. High marginal breakdown
c. Less marginal fracture
d. High creep

226. Decrease in creep: *(AIIMS May 2007)*
a. Occurs with undertrituration or overtrituration of amalgam
b. Occurs with decrease in condensation pressure
c. Occurs with increase in condensation pressure
d. Cannot be predicted

227. The percentage of copper present in a high-copper amalgam is: *(AIIMS May 2007)*
a. 5–12% b. 12–32%
c. 32–52% d. More than 62%

228. All of the following are true about polymerization shrinkage of composite resin except that: *(AIIMS Nov 2006)*
a. More surface area of the bonded surface causes less polymerization shrinkage compared to the surface area of an unbonded restoration
b. Class V composite restorations cause more amount of contraction than gold restoration
c. Etching and priming reduce polymerization shrinkage
d. Amount of shrinkage is less in all enamel margins

229. All of the following are disadvantages of composite resin restorations, *except*: *(AIIMS Nov 2006)*
a. Greater localized occlusal wear
b. Recurrent secondary caries
c. Technique sensitive
d. More time consuming

230. Diametral tensile strength of glass ionomer cement is: *(AIIMS Nov 2006)*
a. Greater than zinc phosphate
b. Same as zinc phosphate
c. Lower than zinc phosphate
d. None of the above

231. Which of the following bonds is present in completely set polyalkanoate (or GI) cement? *(AIIMS Nov 2006)*
a. Chemical bond b. Ionic bond
c. Covalent bond d. Hydrogen bond

232. Etching of dentin does not include:
a. Removal of smear layer *(AIIMS Nov 2006)*
b. Exposure of collagen fibres
c. Opening of dentinal tubules
d. Increase in surface energy

233. Which of the following is true about glass ionomer cement? *(AIIMS Nov 2005)*
a. There is no crosslinking between sodium and fluorine ions
b. The liquid should not be refrigerated
c. It is strongly contraindicated in mouth breathers
d. Its strength is more than that of silicate

234. Delayed contraction of amalgam: *(AIIMS Nov 2005)*
a. Increases with increase in tin content
b. Is seen as the last stage of reaction between mercury and alloy
c. Increases with increase in the mercury: alloy ratio
d. Increases with increase in the alloy particle size

235. The blue light used to polymerize composite resin is harmful to eye if one looks at it, which portion of the eye is affected? *(KCET 2005)*
a. Cornea
b. Retina
c. Lens
d. None of the above

236. Once triturated, the Dental amalgam should be condensed with in: *(KCET 2005)*
a. 5 minutes b. 6 Minutes
c. 3 minutes d. 15 minutes

237. Which of the following is not a direct restorative material ? *(KCET 2005)*
a. Dentin bonding agent
b. Composite resin
c. Dental amalgam
d. Dental ceramic

238. Particle size of Micro filled composite Restorative Resin. Is in the following range: *(KCET 2005)*
a. 0.04-0.4 micrometer
b. 0.4-1 micro meter
c. 0.5-3 micrometer
d. 8-12 micro meter

239. Liquid used in ploycarboxylate cement is:
a. Poly acrylic acid *(KCET 2007)*
b. Phosphoric acid
c. Eugenol
d. Methacrylic acid

240. The filler size (silica) in homogeneous microfilled composites is: *(KCET 2008)*
a. 1–2 μm b. 4 μm
c. 0.04 μm d. 0.5–3 μm

241. Of the various glass ionomer products, the highest cumulative release of fluoride after 30 days is from: *(KCET 2008)*
a. Type I glass ionomer
b. Type II glass ionomer
c. Glass ionomer liner (conventional)
d. Glass ionomer liner (light cure)

242. Coefficient of thermal expansion of amalgam is:
a. 6.6 alpha (ppm/K) *(KCET 2008)*
b. 11.4 alpha (ppm/K)
c. 14.0 alpha (ppm/K)
d. 25.0 alpha (ppm/K)

243. Photosensitizer used in light-activated composite resins is: *(KCET 2008)*
a. Organosilane b. Benzoyl peroxide
c. Colloidal silica d. Camphorquinone

244. Eames technique for proportioning alloy and mercury is: *(KCET 2008)*
a. 1:1 by volume b. 8:5 by weight
c. 5:8 by volume d. 1:1 by weight

245. Degassing means: *(KCET 2008)*
a. Removal of residual surface contamination
b. Removal of grease
c. Addition of gasses
d. Disinfecting

246. The effects associated with cold working can be eliminated by a heat treatment called: *(KCET 2009)*
a. Age hardening heat treatment
b. Annealing heat treatment
c. Homogenization heat treatment
d. Solution heat treatment

247. The effect of trituration on the strength in an amalgam restoration depends on: *(KCET 2009)*
a. Amalgam alloy
b. Trituration time
c. Speed of amalgamator
d. All of the above

248. The commonly used acid for etching enamel and dentine is: *(KCET 2009)*
a. Dilute sulphuric acid
b. Phosphoric acid
c. Concentrated acetic acid
d. 37% hydrochloric acid

249. Which one of the following restorative materials is having coefficient of thermal expansion close to that of tooth enamel and dentin? *(KCET 2010)*
a. Microfilled composite resins
b. Pure gold
c. Silver amalgam
d. Type II glass ionomer cement

250. Polyacid modified composites are designated as: *(KCET 2011)*
a. Compomers b. Giomers
c. Hybrid ionomere d. Ormocers

251. Direct filling gold formed by electrolytic precipitation is called by all the terms, *except*: *(KCET 2011)*
a. Crystalline gold b. Granular gold
c. Mat gold d. Sponge gold

252. The dominant phase in well condensed, low copper dental amalgam is: *(KCET 2011)*
a. Ag_2Hg_3
b. Ag3Sn
c. CuSn
d. Sn8Hg8

253. Which glass ionomer cement develops early resistance to water intake on setting? *(KCET 2011)*
a. Reinforced auto cure glass ionomer cement
b. Compomer
c. Resin modified glass ionomer cement
d. Ceramic reinforced glass ionomer cement

254. The components of fourth generation dentin bonding systems are described as: *(KCET 2012)*
a. Self-etching adhesive
b. Self-etching primer/adhesive
c. Total etching multiple bottle
d. Total etching single bottle

255. Which one of the following dental cements does not contain water as part of the composition of the liquid component? *(KCET 2012)*
a. Zinc phosphate cement
b. Zinc oxide eugenol cement
c. Zinc silicophosphate cement
d. Zinc polycarboxylate cement

256. The first generation and second generation flowable composites are intended to be used for: *(KCET 2012)*
a. Class V and class II restorations, respectively
b. Pit and fissure sealants and small anterior restorations respectively
c. Class I and class II restorations, respectively
d. Pit and fissure sealants and class I restorations, respectively

257. Which of the following materials has the coefficient of the thermal expansion closer to that of the tooth enamel? *(KCET 2013)*
a. Porcelain
b. Gold
c. Composite
d. Glass ionomer cement

258. The pure form of gold in dentistry is known as: *(KCET 2013)*
a. Cohesive gold
b. Non-cohesive gold
c. Class I casting gold
d. Class IV casting gold

259. Higher the mercury alloy ratio in amalgam leads to: *(KCET 2013)*
a. Increased strength
b. Increased matrix material formation
c. Decreased creep
d. All of the above

260. All forms of direct filling Gold are degassed by heating in the blue inner core of ethanol flame *except*: *(COMED 2009)*
a. Platinized gold foil
b. Electrolytic precipitate
c. Powdered gold
d. Alloyed electrolytic precipitate

261. Powdered gold is marketed is: *(COMED 2009)*
a. William's E-Z gold
b. Morgan's E-Z gold
c. Robert's E-Z gold
d. Taggart's E-Z gold

262. The total copper content in admixed alloy ranges from approximately: *(KCET 2007)*

a. 1 to 6 weight precent
b. 9 to 20 weight precent
c. 30 to 40 weight precent
d. 360 Gpa and 125–130 Mpa

263. Frozen Slab technique is applicable to: *(COMED 2011, 2005)*

a. Zinc phosphate cement
b. Glass ionomer cement
c. Zinc oxide eugenol cement
d. Resin cement

264. pH of which cement remains below 7 even after 1 month after insertion into the cavity? *(COMED 2011)*

a. GIC b. Zinc phosphate
c. Resin cement d. Silicate cement

265. Electralloy RV is alloy of Gold and? *(COMED 2011)*

a. Carbon b. Platinum
c. Calcium d. Palladium

266. Which lasers can be used to cure composite resins? *(COMED 2011, 2005)*

a. Argon b. NdYAG
c. ErYAG d. CO_2

267. Mode of failure during dislodgement of prosthesis cemented with zinc poly carboxyl ate cement is usually seen at the: *(COMED 2011)*

a. Cement tooth interface
b. Cement prosthesis interface
c. Cleavage through the cement layer
d. Fracture of tooth or prosthesis

268. Desorbtion is a term which is used to describe: *(COMED 2012)*

a. Strain hardening
b. Process of removing the absorbed impurities
c. Recrystallization
d. Grain growth

269. All of the following statements are true for zinc oxide eugenol cements, *except*: *(COMED 2012)*

a. Equal lengths of base paste and accelerator paste are mixed together until the mix has a uniform color
b. Increase in temperature and humidity shorten the setting time
c. The mix appears thick at the start of mixing but after 30 seconds of additional spatulation it becomes more fluid
d. Water accelerates but heat retards the setting of zinc oxide eugenol cements

270. Which of the following agents is used to prevent the formation of deleterious oxides on gold foil? *(COMED 2012)*

a. Methane b. Ammonia
c. Hydrogen peroxide d. Carbon monoxide

271. Mode of failure during dislodgement of prosthesis cemented with zinc polycarboxylate cement is usually seen at the: *(COMED 2012)*

a. Cement tooth interface
b. Cement prosthesis interface
c. Cleavage through the cement layer
d. Fracture of tooth or prosthesis

272. The cement filling material which has the most server injurious effect on pulp is: *(COMED 2013)*

a. Copper cement
b. Zine oxyphosphate cement
c. Silicate cement
d. Calcium hydroxide

273. The Knoop Hardness Number of Microfilled Compossible Restorative material ranges from: *(KCET 2007)*

a. 50–60 KHN b. 25–35 KHN
c. 15–20 KHN d. 40–48 KHN

274. The minimum film thickness for luting a single crown: *(KCET 2007)*

a. 20 pm b. 25 pm
c. 35 pm d. 45 pm

275. The cements which adhere to the tooth are: *(COMED 2005)*

a. Silicate and GIC
b. ZnO eugenol and GIC
c. GIC and Zn polycarboxylate
d. GIC and Zn phosphate

276. For esthetic areas where high luster is required the restoration used usually: *(COMED 2005)*

a. Glass ionomer restoratives
b. Hybrid resin composites
c. Microfilled resin composites
d. Macrofilled resin composites

277. The solid solution of silver and mercury is called: *(COMED 2005)*
a. β-phase of amalgam
b. γ1-phase of amalgam
c. ε-phase of amalgam
d. Silver copper eutectic

278. Minimum thickness for type I zinc phosphate cement should be: *(COMED 2006)*
a. 15 micron b. 25 micron
c. 50 micron d. None of the above

279. Which cement base has the highest modulus of elasticity? *(COMED 2006)*
a. Zn polycarboxylate
b. Polymer reinforced ZnOE
c. Zn phosphate
d. GIC

280. Ammonia treated gold foil is called: *(COMED 2006)*
a. Cohesive foil b. Non-cohesive foil
c. Corrugated foil d. Non-corrugated foil

281. The deoxidizing agent added to dental alloy is: *(COMED 2006)*
a. Palladium b. Silver
c. Copper d. Zinc

282. Which of the following materials should not be used as liners or bases under composite restorations? *(COMED 2006)*
a. Resin modified GIC
b. Flowable composite
c. Zinc oxide eugenol
d. Compomer

283. The polyacid modified composites are known as: *(COMED 2006)*
a. Compomers b. Hybrid ionomers
c. Polycarboxylates d. Polyacrylates

284. If the Hg:alloy ratio is 6:5 then percentage of mercury in amalgam restoration is: *(MH 2009)*
a. 42.5% b. 45.6%
c. 52.4% d. 54.5%

285. The size of amalgam particle is: *(MH 2009)*
a. 15–35 micrometer b. 25–40 micrometer
c. 40–60 micrometer d. 80–100 micrometer

286. pH of liquid polycarboxylate cement is: *(MH 2009)*
a. 3.5 b. 1.7
c. 7 d. 11

287. Delayed expansion of amalgam can be up to: *(MH 2009)*
a. 400 micrometer b. 150 micrometer
c. 200 micrometer d. 50 micrometer

288. Most important mechanical property of dental cement is: *(MH 2012)*
a. Compressive strength
b. Tensile strength
c. Coefficient of thermal conductivity
d. Adhesiveness

289. An acidic agent that dissolves the inorganic structure in dentin that allows infiltration of adhesive resin is: *(MH 2014)*
a. Dentin bonding agent
b. Dentin conditioner
c. Primer
d. None of the above

290. Minimum solubility of dental cements to oral fluids is seen in: *(MH 2014)*
a. GIC
b. Zinc polycarboxylate
c. Zinc phosphate
d. Resin cement

291. Eames technique is otherwise known as: *(MH 2014)*
a. No squeeze cloth technique
b. Increasing dryness technique
c. Bloting mix
d. Mortar and pestle mix

292. The acid used in etching ceramic during repair of ceramic restorations is: *(MH 2014)*
a. Hydrochloric acid
b. Hydrofluoric acid
c. Sulphuric acid
d. Orthophosphoric acid

INDIRECT RESTORATIVE AND PROSTHETIC MATERIALS

293. Condensation shrinkage of porcelain during firing depends on: *(AIIMS May 2010)*
a. Rate of firing temperature
b. Shape and size of particle
c. Uniformity of particle size
d. Type of investment used

294. Addition of fluoride flux during soldering of cobalt-chromium alloy or joint of two stainless steel wires: *(AIIMS Nov 2010)*
a. Lowers the melting range of solder
b. Prevents the formation of copper oxide
c. Prevents the formation of chromium oxide.
d. Prevents the flow of material if undesirable

295. Nickel added to wrought gold alloy acts as: *(AIIMS Nov 2010)*
a. A strengthener
b. A scavenger
c. A whitener
d. A hardener

296. Back pressure porosity can be reduced by: *(AIPGEE 2011)*
a. Vacuum investing
b. Proper or increased burnout temperature
c. Reduced firing temperature
d. All of the above

297. Zone of flame used for melting metal alloys is: *(AIPGEE 2010)*
a. Combustion zone b. Reducing zone
c. Oxidizing zones d. Central zone

298. Which of the following is not a noble metal? *(AIPGEE 2008)*
a. Gold b. Ruthenium
c. Silver d. Osmium

299. Which part of flame has the maximum heat content? *(AIPGEE 2007)*
a. Reducing zone
b. Combustion zone
c. Oxidizing zone
d. Central zone

300. Which of the following is not a function of flux? *(AIPGEE 2013)*
a. To remove any oxide coating on parent metal
b. To restrict the flow of solder over the parent metal
c. To protect metal surface from oxidation during soldering procedures
d. To permit the flow of solder over parent metal

301. Addition of chromium to casting base metal alloy doesn't cause: *(AIPGEE 2013)*
a. Decrease in modulus of elasticity
b. Increase in corrosion resistance
c. Increase in hardness
d. Increase in tensile strength

302. The main purpose of chromium in stainless steel is: *(AIPGEE 2013)*
a. Corrosion resistance
b. Strength
c. Rigidity
d. Scavenger

303. Cold bend test is used to measure: *(AIPGEE 2013)*
a. Ductility
b. Malleability
c. Compressive strength
d. Tensile strength

304. Which of the following cannot be completely burn-out while casting? *(AIPGEE 2013)*
a. Pattern wax b. Inlay wax
c. Acrylic d. Composite

305. Annealing is: *(AIIMS May 2012)*
a. Hardening heat treatment
b. Softening heat treatment
c. Precipitating heat treatment
d. Stress relieving heat treatment

306. At what temperature is benzoyl peroxide activated? *(AIIMS Nov 2012)*
a. 37°C b. 25°C
c. 50°C d. 60°C

307. Twinning is seen with: *(AIIMS Nov 2012)*
a. SS b. NiTi
c. CoCr d. All

308. Antiflux material all, *except*: *(AIIMS Nov 2012)*
a. Graphite
b. Iron oxide
c. Calcium carbonate in alcohol
d. Fluoride

309. In CoCr base metal alloy what is d function of chromium? *(AIIMS Nov 2013)*
a. Responsible for surface irregularities
b. Increases corrosion n tarnish resistance
c. Act as a scavenger
d. Increase the strength

310. During which stage does maximum shrinkage on firing of ceramic occur: *(AIIMS Nov 2008, May 2007)*
a. High bisque
b. Low bisque
c. During condensation
d. All of the above

311. The function of the fluoride flux in soldering of cobalt-chromium alloy is: *(AIIMS Nov 2008)*
a. To decrease the melting point of the solder
b. To decrease the formation of copper oxide
c. To decrease the formation of chromium oxide
d. To stop the flow of molten solder in undercut areas

312. Insufficient closure of flasks during packing of denture base resin results in: *(AIIMS Nov 2008)*
a. Poor color stability
b. Increase in vertical dimension
c. Less polymerization shrinkage
d. Localized porosities

313. Porosity in porcelain at condensation is determined by: *(AIIMS Nov 2008, May 2007)*
a. The shape and size of particles
b. The uniform distribution of particle size
c. The number of particles
d. None of the above

314. Stainless steel is:
a. Iron chromium cobalt
b. Iron nickel chromium
c. Iron copper cobalt
d. Iron

315. Casting porosity, which is caused by the inability of air to escape through the pores in the investment, is: *(KCET 2005)*
a. Localized shrinkage porosity
b. Suck-back porosity
c. Back pressure porosity
d. Micro porosity

316. Which of the following is a castable dental ceramic? *(KCET 2005)*
a. Aluminous porcelain
b. IPS Empress 2
c. In-Cream
d. Dicor

317. Invisible light cured denture base resin, Camphor-quinone serves as the: *(KCET 2005)*
a. Activator b. Initiator
c. Retarded d. Filler

318. The process of heating a cast alloy to eliminate composition difference is: *(KCET 2006)*
a. Hardening heat treatment
b. Softening heat treatment
c. Homogenization
d. Crystallization

319. Galvanism is: *(KCET 2006)*
a. Tarnishing
b. Electrolytic corrosion
c. Chemical corrosion
d. Annealing

320. Shape memory exhibited by: *(KCET 2006)*
a. Beta titanium
b. Nickel titanium
c. Cobalt chromium
d. Nickel Chromium

321. How much minimum amount of alloy percentage by weight of noble element in high noble metals? *(KCET 2006)*
a. 60% by weight of noble elements
b. 30% gold
c. 40% by weight of noble elements
d. Less than 40% by weight of noble elements

322. Stabilization of stainless steel is achieved by addition of: *(KCET 2006)*
a. Carbon b. Chromium
c. Nickel d. Titanium

323. Steel is an alloy of iron in which the carbon content is: *(KCET 2007)*
a. Less than 18% b. Less than 2%
c. More than 8% d. None of the above

324. Helium-neon (He-Ne) lasers are examples for: *(KCET 2008)*
a. Excimer lasers b. Gas lasers
c. Diode lasers d. Solid state lasers

325. Compared with porcelain teeth, acrylic teeth have all of the following, *except*: *(KCET 2009)*
a. Chemical bond to denture
b. Hard and brittle
c. Minimal abrasion of opposing dentition
d. Silent on contact

326. Most commonly used initiator for the polymerization of methyl methacrylate is: *(KCET 2009)*
a. Hydrogen peroxide b. Benzoyl peroxide
c. Isopropyl alcohol d. Hydroquinone

327. Which of the following cast gold alloys is used for fabricating partial denture frameworks? *(KCET 2009)*
a. Type I-soft b. Type II-hard
c. Type III-hard d. Type IV-extra hard

328. Which of the following increases castability of base metal alloys? *(KCET 2009)*
a. Tin b. Beryllium
c. Molybdenum d. Carbon

329. Purpose of adding indium to metal alloy in porcelain fused to metal is: *(KCET 2009)*
a. To improve bonding
b. To increase strength
c. To decrease porosity
d. To match the thermal expansion of metal and porcelain

330. Wax addition instrument is: *(KCET 2009)*
a. PKT No-2 b. PKT No-5
c. PKT No-4 d. PKT No-3

331. In brazing, the filler metal has a melting point of: *(KCET 2009)*
a. 250°C
b. Below 452°C
c. 80–100°C
d. Above 450°C

332. Which form of stainless steel is used for the manufacturing of orthodontics wire? *(KCET 2010)*
a. Austenitic
b. Martenstic
c. Ferritic
d. All the three form can be used

333. Solder and flux used for joining elgiloy wires are: *(KCET 2011)*
a. Gold solder and borax flux
b. Gold solder and fluoride flux
c. Silver solder and borax flux
d. Silver solder and fluoride flux

334. Ceramics fired to metals are processed by: *(KCET 2011)*
a. Heat pressing
b. Machining
c. Sintering
d. Slip casting

335. All of the following components are present in the liquid composition of the heat cure acrylic resins, *except*: *(KCET 2011)*
a. Glycol dimethacrylate
b. Hydroquinone
c. Methyl methacrylate
d. N. N-dihydroxyethyl para toludine

336. The term ordered hardening heat treatments used in which of the following dental alloys? *(KCET 2012)*
a. Gold copper b. Nickel chromium
c. Nickel titanium d. Sliver palladium

337. Distorted grains observed in the microstructure of a wrought metal indicates that it has been: *(KCET 2012)*
a. Cold worked b. Heat hardened
c. Recrystalized d. Stress relief annealed

338. Transformation between the austenitic and martensitic forms of NiTi can be induced by: *(KCET 2013)*
a. Temperature b. Stress
c. Both of the above d. None of the above

339. The first layer of porcelain applied on a metal ppm crown would be: *(KCET 2013)*
a. Opaque b. Body
c. Incisal d. Both A and C

340. Passivation effect in any alloy is imparted due which of the following? *(KCET 2013)*
a. Zinc b. Copper
c. Chromium d. Nickel

341. A metal which has been cold worked would exhibit: *(KCET 2013)*
a. Decreased strength b. Increased strength
c. Decreased hardness d. Increased ductility

342. Which of the following listed below is the best source of heat to carry out a soldering process? *(KCET 2013)*
a. Hydrogen b. Natural gas
c. Acetylene d. Propane

343. Which of the following types of stainless steel has the best corrosion resistance? *(KCET 2013)*
a. Carbon b. Ferrite
c. Austenitic d. Martensitic

344. High fusing porcelains are used: *(COMED 2008)*
a. For crowns
b. In denture teeth
c. With titanium alloys
d. Over aluminous core porcelain

345. Laser welding: *(COMED 2008)*
a. Involves high heat generation
b. Can be done with pure titanium
c. Is not used in dentistry
d. Can be done with pure gold

346. Feldspathic porcelain: *(COMED 2008)*
a. Shows reliable chemical bonding with metals
b. Has high tensile strength
c. Is no longer used
d. Shows insignificant firing shrinkage

347. Which one of the following may not be used during the flasking of dentures? *(COMED 2008)*
a. Petroleum b. Tin foil
c. Tin foil substitute d. Silicone lubricant

348. The commonest type of porosity that results in fluid resin technique is: *(COMED 2008)*
a. Polymerization shrinkage porosity
b. Porosity due to inadequate pressure
c. Air inclusion porosity
d. Porosity due to increased heat

349. The first porcelain tooth material was introduced by: *(COMED 2008)*
a. DeChemant
b. Ash
c. Plateau
d. McClean

350. During soldering the solidus temperature of the filler metal should be: *(COMED 2009)*
a. Greater than the substrate metal
b. Lesser than the substrate metal
c. Equal to the substrate metal
d. Temperature not relevant

351. To prevent sensitization of austenitic stainless steel at elevated temperature the element used is: *(COMED 2009)*
a. Chlorine b. Titanium
c. Nickel d. Carbon

352. The accepted polymer to monomer ratio for packing of polymethyl methacrylate resin is: *(COMED 2009)*
a. 3:1 b. 4:1
c. 10:1 d. 5:1

353. Which of the following fuel gases used for soldering has the highest heat content? *(COMED 2009)*
a. Hydrogen b. Natural gas
c. Acetylene d. Propane

354. The calcium content in alloyed electrolytic precipitate is: *(COMED 2009)*
a. 0.10% b. 0.20%
c. 0.50% d. 0.80%

355. The linear solidification shrinkage of Type IV Ni-Cr-based casting alloys is: *(COMED 2009)*
a. 2.30% b. 1.56%
c. 1.37% d. 3%

356. The solvent flux used for base metal soldering is: *(COMED 2009)*
a. Boric acid b. Borax
c. Fluoride d. Rouge

357. Residual monomer content of chemically activated resins is: *(COMED 2009)*
a. 0.2% to 0.5%
b. 2% to 5%
c. 0.3% to 0.5%
d. 3% to 5%

358. The most heat producing and efficient burning zone in a soldering flame is: *(COMED 2009)*
a. Cold mixing zone
b. Partial combustion zone
c. Reducing zone
d. Oxidizing zone

359. The stainless steel having LEAST corrosion resistance is: *(COMED 2009)*
a. Ferritic
b. Austenitic
c. Martensitic
d. Duplex

360. Nickel titanium alloy was first introduced as an orthodontic wire by: *(COMED 2009)*
a. Andreasen b. Buehler
c. Burrstone d. Bishara

361. NiTi instruments are flexible because of is: *(COMED 2009)*
a. Plasticity b. Rigidity
c. Super elasticity d. Hardness

362. VLC Resins are also called as: *(COMED 2009)*
a. Microwave-activated resins
b. Tertiary amine-activated resins
c. Light activated resins
d. Heat activated resins

363. Which is the only nearly pure metal used for dental casting process? *(COMED 2010)*
a. Pure gold
b. Palladium
c. Pure silver
d. Pure titanium (CPTi)

364. Compared with noble metals, base metals show: *(COMED 2010)*

a. Increased hardness
b. Increased ductility
c. Better biocompatibility
d. Increased density

365. The deoxidizing agent added to dental alloys is: *(COMED 2010)*

a. Palladium b. Silver
c. Copper d. Zinc

366. Compared with dental alloys ceramics show: *(COMED 2010)*

a. High ductility
b. High hardness
c. Low esthetic value
d. Susceptibility to brittle fracture

367. The advantage of resin teeth over porcelain teeth is: *(COMED 2010)*

a. Greater wear resistance
b. Increased hardness
c. Better dimensional stability
d. Greater impact resistance

368. Compared with cast alloys wrought alloys have: *(COMED 2010)*

a. High strength b. Low hardness
c. High ductility d. Crystalline structure

369. The preferred material for repair of fractured denture base is: *(COMED 2010)*

a. Chemically cure resin
b. Heat cure resin
c. Light cure resin
d. Vinyl resin

370. The materials used to outline the area to be soldered in order to restrict the flow of solder are called: *(COMED 2011)*

a. Antiflux b. Flux
c. Soldering d. Welding

371. Dr Taggart is associated with: *(COMED 2012)*

a. Discovery of ceramics
b. Lost wax technique
c. Acid etch technique
d. Bleaching procedures

372. Which is the best choice of heat source for soldering, from the following fuel gases? *(COMED 2012)*

a. Propane b. Acetylene
c. Natural gas d. Hydrogen

373. The best fuel gas when used with oxygen is: *(COMED 2012)*

a. Hydrogen b. Natural gas
c. Propane d. Acetylene

374. What is incorporated in porcelain during firing? *(COMED 2013)*

a. Argon b. Helium
c. Hydrogen d. Oxygen

375. The volumetric shrinkage exhibited by heat polymerized denture resin polymerized mass is: *(COMED 2013)*

a. 0.07% b. 0.7%
c. 7% d. 70%

376. Tissue conditioning materials are: *(COMED 2013)*

a. Elastomers b. Elastopolymers
c. Polymers d. Impression plaster

377. Linear coefficient of thermal expansion of metal used metal ceramic restoration range from: *(COMED 2013)*

a. $11.5–12.5 \times 10^{-6}/°C$
b. $10.5–11.5 \times 10^{-6}/°C$
c. $13.5–14.5 \times 10^{-6}/°C$
d. $16.5–17.5 \times 10^{-6}/°C$

378. During casting procedures creation of a "Hot spot" means: *(COMED 2013)*

a. The presence of reservoir resulting in delayed solidification of metal
b. Sprue former is attached at right angle creating a localized lingering of molten metal after casting has solidified
c. The length of sprue is too long resulting in ready flow of molten metal
d. Use of too high temperature resulting in localized disintegration of metal

379. The alloy that possesses 'Super elasticity' is: *(COMED 2005)*

a. Nitinol
b. Stainless steel
c. Cobalt-chromium-nickel
d. Gold-palladium

380. Casting flux is used to: *(COMED 2005)*

a. Prevent the oxidation of material during melting
b. Increase the melting point of the flux
c. Prevent the contamination of the metal and the liner
d. All of the above

381. Percentage of gold in a high noble gold alloy is: *(COMED 2005)*
a. <25% b. 25%
c. >40% d. 00%

382. The main form of iron carbide in 18/8 stainless steel is: *(COMED 2005)*
a. Martensite b. Austenite
c. Ferrite d. Pearlite

383. Cross linking in denture base resin is contributed by: *(COMED 2006)*
a. Benzoyl peroxide b. Glycol DMA
c. N-paratoludine d. Methyl methacry

384. In metal ceramic crowns, the function of indium and tin is: *(COMED 2006)*
a. Improve bonding
b. Decrease porosity
c. React with porcelain to form an opaque layer
d. Improve thermal expansion

385. Quartz in dental porcelain is: *(COMED 2006)*
a. Strengthener
b. Binder
c. Pigmeny
d. Crackminimizer

386. Advantage of titanium over other base metal alloy is: *(COMED 2007)*
a. Low weight
b. Low cost
c. Low strength
d. Low melting point

387. Function of wetting agents used in casting procedures is: *(COMED 2007)*
a. To facilitate wetting of ring liner
b. To facilitate mixing investment
c. To reduce contact angle of a liquid with wax surface
d. For better wax elimination

388. Solvent flux used for base metal alloy is: *(COMED 2007)*
a. Fluoride b. Boric acid
c. Borax d. Graphite

389. Ceramic fusion is an example of: *(COMED 2007)*
a. Liquid phase sintering
b. Solid-phase sintering
c. Sintering
d. Oxidation reduction reaction

390. Delayed ceramic fracture of ceramic crown in molar is due to cyclic loading of: or the crown contours of molars are subjected to: *(MH 2010)*
a. Dynamic stress/fatigue failure
b. Static stress/fatigue failure
c. Both a and b
d. None of the above

391. Purest form of metal used in dental casting: *(MH 2010)*
a. CpTi b. NiTi
c. Gold d. Co-Cr

392. Non-traumatic gingival retraction is seen with: *(MH 2010)*
a. Cord b. Expansyl
c. Electrocautery d. Copper band

393. Alternate to gallium-indium is: *(MH 2010)*
a. Gold b. Mercury
c. Chromium d. Titanium

394. Inhibitor used in monomer: *(MH 2010)*
a. Methyl methacrylate
b. Hydroquinone
c. N, N dimethyl paratoulidine
d. Dibutylpthalate

395. Stress relaxation in denture base resins generally produces: *(MH 2011)*
a. Sagging b. Crazing
c. Creeping d. Fracture lines

396. Long curing cycle for acrylic dentures is: *(MH 2012)*
a. 9 hrs 100°C
b. 9 hrs 70°C
c. 10 hrs 100°C
d. 10 hrs 70°C

397. Boiling point and melting point of methyl methacrylate: *(MH 2012)*
a. 100.8°C and -48°C
b. 100°C and -48°C
c. 100°C and -40°C
d. 100.8°C and -40°C

398. In acrylic restorative materials, the pumping action of alternately imbibing and exuding fluids is termed as: *(MH 2014)*
a. Imbibition
b. Percolation
c. Syneresis
d. Evaporation

Answers with Explanations

GENERAL CLASSES AND PROPERTIES OF DENTAL MATERIAL

1. Ans. (d) Measure different colors quantitatively *Ref: Craig's 12th ed. p 30, 31*

- In colorimetry, the Munsell color system is a color space that specifies colors based on three color dimensions: hue, value (lightness), and chroma (color purity).
- It was created by Professor Albert H. Munsell in the first decade of the 20th century.

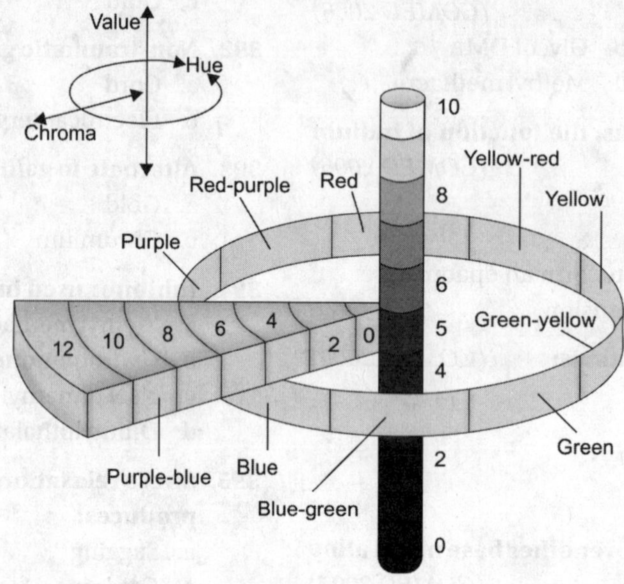

Munsell color system

- Munsell's system is used to measure different colors quantitatively.
- It is one of the most commonly used method in order to define and measure the color quantitively.

Things to remember

Today's aesthetic dentistry is based on value of the tooth; hence it is the most important component.

- Hue-based shade guide Vitapan Classical
- Value-based shade guide Vita 3D Master
- Chroma-based shade guide Ivoclar Chromoscope

2. Ans. (b) Knoop hardness *Ref: Phillips, 11th ed. p 968*

- Two microhardness test methods are the Knoop hardness test and Vickers hardness test.
- Both the Knoop hardness test and Vickers hardness test methods use specific measurements from the indent, in conjunction with formulas, to calculate material hardness.
- The Knoop hardness test is performed by applying controlled force of 1000 grams or less for a specific amount of time to an indenter in a rhombus-shape (elongated four-sided pyramid).
- The hardness of the material is determined by the depth to which the Knoop indenter penetrates.
- The impression is measured microscopically and, when combined with the amount of the test load, can be used to calculate the hardness value on the Knoop scale.
- Brinell and Rockwell are macrohardness tests.

3. Ans. (b) Decreases *Ref: Arthur Morley. Strength of Materials, 1916 ed. p 52*

- Factors affecting the mechanical properties of s dental cement.
- On increasing the temperature, the mechanical properties of a material decrease and the opposite is true for cooling.
- Rate of loading is directly proportional to the material property, i.e. when rate of loading increases, the material property increases and vice versa.

4. Ans. (a) Polymerization occurs with repeated elimination of small molecules *Ref: Phillips, 11th ed. p 162*

- When the primary molecule react with the formation of by-product such as water, ammonia, alcohol and halogen acid. The process is termed as step growth polymerization.
- Due to the formation of these by-product, the step growth polymerization is termed as condensation polymerization.
- When the polymerization of monomers is done by an addition reaction, addition polymerization takes place.

5. Ans. (c) Shear *Ref: Phillips, 11th ed. p 78*

- When a force acts on a constrained body, to this external force application, a resistance is developed. To the applied external force an equal intensity force is developed internally which acts on opposite direction and whole procedure is termed as stress.
- Stress is denoted by S or σ.
- When a force is applied to a body from any angle or direction, and after several forces are combined to develop complex stress in a structure.
- In general applied force may be axial, shear, bending or torsional.
- Shear stress is produced by a twisting or torsional action on a material.

6. Ans. (a) For each 1% increase in weight by water absorption, produces 0.23% linear expansion
Ref: Phillips, 12th ed. p 489

- When polymethyl methacrylate placed in aqueous environment, it absorbs small amount of water.
- A water molecule occupy its position between the polymer chain after penetrating the methyl methacrylate molecules.
- Water sorption value of polymethyl methacrylate is 0.69 mg/cm^2.
- It is seen that, in acrylic resin denture for each 1% increase in weight by water absorption, it produces about 0.23% linear expansion.
- The linear expansion, which occurs due to water absorption is equal to the thermal shrinkage during polymerization.

7. Ans. (a) Min in hard tissues *Ref: Phillips, 11th ed. p 37*

Wetting:

- Relative interfacial tension between a liquid and a solid substrate that results in a contact angle of less than 90 degree.
- Contact angle measured the extend to which an adhesive wets the surface of an adherend.
- At 00 contact angle for complete wetting.
- At 180 degree contact angle no wetting occurs.

8. Ans. (a) Viket's needle test *Ref: Phillips, 11th ed. p 262*

Vicat tesy for setting time:

- The initial and final setting time can be determined accurately by using a penetrometer with a needle.
- The needle is applied to the surface of the impression material for 10 seconds and a reading is taken.

- The initial set is the time at which the needle no longer completely penetrates the specimen to the bottom of the ring.
- The final set is the time of the first of three identical non maximum penetration reading.

9. Ans. (c) Brittle *Ref: Phillips, 11th ed. p 73*

- Brittleness: Relative inability of a material in order to cause plastic deformation before the material fractures. This means tensile strength is less.
- Ductility: Ability of a material to sustain large permanent deformation under tensile load before it fractures.
- Malleability: Ability of a material to sustain considerable permanent deformation without rupture under compression.
- Resilience: Amount of energy absorbed within a unit volume of structure when it is stressed to its proportional limit.

10. Ans. (c) Complete wetting of the surfaces *Phillips, 11th ed. p 37-8.*

- Wetting is the ability of a liquid to maintain contact with a solid surface, resulting from intermolecular interactions when the two are brought together.
- The degree of wetting (wettability) is determined by a force balance between adhesive and cohesive forces.
- Wetting deals with the three phases of materials: gas, liquid and solid.
- The contact angle (θ), is the angle at which the liquid vapour interface meets the solid liquid interface. The contact angle is determined by the resultant between adhesive and cohesive forces.

		Strength of:	
Contact angle	*Degree of wetting*	*Solid/liquid interactions*	*Liquid/liquid interactions*
θ = 0	Perfect wetting	Strong	Weak
0 < θ < 90°	High wettability	Strong	Strong
		Weak	Weak
90° = θ < 180°	Low wettability	Weak	Strong
θ = 180°	Perfectly non-wetting	Weak	Strong

11. Ans. (a) Liquid + b → a *Ref: Phillips. 11th ed. p. 134-135*

Like the eutectic transformation true peritectic reaction is an invariant reaction (i.e. it occurs at a particular composition and temperature)

- The reaction can be represented by: Liquid + beta phase alpha phase?
- The alpha phase is a silver rich a phase.
- The beta phase is platinum rich.
- α + β is the two phase region resulting from limited solid solubility.
- The peritectic transformation occurs at the point P at which the liquid plus the platinum rich β phase transforms into the silver rich α phase.

12. Ans. (a) Lateral strain by axial strain within elastic limit *Ref: Craig's 12th ed. p 61*

Poisson's ratio

- Poisson's ratio is defined as the ratio of lateral strain to the axial strain within elastic limit. It is a unitless value as it is a ratio of same unit (two strains).

Material	*Poisson's ratio*
Resin composite	0.30
Enamel	0.33
Amalgam	0.33

13. Ans. (d) The difference between the two lengths upon original length *Ref: Phillips 11th ed. p 74*

Strain:

- It is defined as the change in length (?L= L-L0) per original length (Lo) of the body when it is subjected to a load.
- Strain (E) Deformation/original length = (L-Lo)/Lo or ?L/L.
- It can also be defined as change in length per unit initial length.
- When stress is applied on a body. Strain is induced.

14. Ans. (b) Degree of saturation *Ref: Phillips, 11th ed. p 41*

- Chroma-Degree of saturation of a particular hue

15. Ans. (b) Knoop and Vickers tests *Ref: Phillips, 11th ed. p 97-98, 360-361*

In metallurgy, the concept of hardness is 'resistance to indentation'. Most of the surface hardness tests are based on the ability of the surface of a material to resist penetration by a diamond point - steel ball under a specified load. Barcol, Brinell, Rockwell, Shore, Vickers and Knoop hardness tests are used m t frequently. The Knoop and Vickers tests are classified as microhardness tests and the Brinell's and Rockwell tests are macrohardness tests. This is because Knoop and Vickers employ loads which are much less in force and have a less area of indentation. The load commonly employed is 9.8 N and the resulting indentation will be small and will have a limited depth of only around 19 μm. On the other hand, Brinell and Rockwell give indentations over much larger areas. The Shore and the Barcol tests measure the hardness of rubber and plastic type of materials.

16. Ans. (c) Termination *Ref: Phillips, 11th ed. p 158*

Termination: Although chain termination can result from chain transfer, addition polymerization reactions are most often terminated either by direct coupling of two free radical chain ends or by the exchange of a hydrogen atom from one growing chain to another.

17. Ans. (d) Below the melting point of either metal *Ref: Craig's 11th ed. p 172*

- A eutectic system is a mixture of chemical compounds or elements that have a single chemical composition that solidifies at a lower temperature than any other composition made up of the same ingredients. This composition is known as the eutectic composition and the temperature at which it solidifies is known as the eutectic temperature.
- On a phase diagram the intersection of the eutectic temperature and the eutectic composition gives the eutectic point. Non-eutectic mixtures will display solidification of one component of the mixture before the other. Not all binary alloys have a eutectic point; for example, in the silver-gold system the melt temperature (liquidus) and freeze temperature (solidus) both increase monotonically as the mix changes from pure silver to pure gold.
- Eutectic alloys have two or more materials and have a eutectic composition. When a non-eutectic alloy solidifies, its components solidify at different temperatures, exhibiting a plastic melting range. Conversely, when a well-mixed, eutectic alloy melts, it does so at a single, sharp temperature.
- Some uses include:
  - Eutectic alloys for soldering, composed of tin (Sn), lead (Pb) and sometimes silver (Ag) or gold (Au) especially $Sn_{63}Pb_{37}$ alloy formula for electronics.
  - Casting alloys, such as aluminium-silicon and cast iron (at the composition of 4.3% carbon in iron producing an austenite-cementite eutectic).
  - Silicon chips are bonded to gold-plated substrates through a silicon-gold eutectic by the application of ultrasonic energy to the chip. See eutectic bonding.
  - Brazing, where diffusion can remove alloying elements from the joint, so that eutectic melting is only possible early in the brazing process.

18. Ans. (c) Iridium *Ref: Phillip's 11th ed. p 117*

Modern dental noble metal casting alloys generally have equiaxed five gram structure because of the incorporation of small amounts of iridium ruthenium or rhenium as grain refinement elements (generally less than about 1 wt% for palladium alloy and much smaller quantity for gold alloy.

19. Ans. (c) Value *Ref: Philips 11th ed. p 49*

Hue—describes the dominant color of an object, e.g. Red, Green, Blue.

Chroma—represents degree of saturation of a particular hue.

Value identifies the lightness or darkness of color.

20. Ans. (b) High contact angle *Ref: Philips 11th ed. p 38*

The property of adhesion by adhesive agent depends on the wetting surface

- When contact angle completely is Oº, the liquid contacts it's the surface completely and spread freely.
- Small contact angle on slightly contaminated surface.
- Large angle formed by poor wetting.

21. Ans. (c) Elastic strain *Ref: Philips 11th ed. p 73*

Elastic strain is reversible in nature. It is defined as the deformation which is recovered up on removal of an externally applied force on pressure.

22. Ans. (d) Modulus of elasticity of 3.4 GPa *Ref: Philips 11th ed. p 166*

Properties of polymethyl methacrylate:

- Knoop hardness number 18.20
- Tensile strength approx. 60 MPa
- Density 1.19 g/cm^3
- Modulous of elasticity 2.4 Gpa (approx.)

23. Ans. (c) Toughness *Ref: Philip's 11th ed. p 74*

Toughness is the ability of material to absorb elastic energy and to deform plastically before fracture. It is measured as the total area under a plot of tensile stress versus tensile strains.

24. Ans. (c) Brittle materials *Ref: Phillips, 11th ed. p 85,86*

- Ultimate tensile strength, shear strength, compressive strength, and flexural strength, each of which is a measure of stress required to fracture a material.
- Brittle materials have a tensile strength that is markedly lower than the corresponding compressive strength, because of their inability to plastically deform and reduce the tensile stress at flaw tips. This is true of all brittle dental materials, such as amalgams, composites, cements, and ceramics. The failure of these materials in clinical usage is most often associated with their low tensile strengths and the presence of flaws within the tensile stress region.
- Due to their brittleness, assembling of ceramics pieces is generally achieved through brazing but thermal stresses during cooling frequently induce cracking of the material used for brazing. In order to check if such damage is avoidable, it is necessary to characterize the brittle to ductile transition (BDT) of the material. Simple compression is not suited for crack studies, because of mixed loading (mode II + compressive mode I cracking). Another type of test, the cylinder splitting test, known as the Brazilian test, can be carried out by applying compressive forces on two opposite generatrix of a cylinder: this causes a uniform tensile stress on the plane containing the axis of the cylinder and the generatrix, leading to mode I cracking. The advantage of this test is to avoid expensive and random machining of brittle samples. This study shows that the Brazilian test is well adapted for the measurement of toughness and the characterization of the BDT of materials whose room temperature behavior is brittle.

25. Ans. (d) Shore durometer *Ref: Phillips, 11th ed. p 97,98*

Hardness is the ability to resist scratching. In elastomers, the indentation disappears after removal of load which is normally seen with Brinell and Vickers, etc. Shore durometer is used in such cases. This test can also be used to evaluate soft denture liners, mouth protectors and maxillofacial elastomers.

26. Ans. (b) Resiliency *Ref: Phillips, 11th ed. p 75,74*

- Mechanical properties of any material are expressed most often in units of stress and/or strain. They can represent measurements of:
  - Elastic or reversible deformation (i.e. proportional limit, resilience, and modulus of elasticity);
  - Plastic or irreversible deformation (e.g. percent elongation and hardness); or
  - A combination of elastic and plastic deformation, such as toughness and yield strength.
- Resilience the relative amount of elastic energy per unit volume released on unloading of a test specimen.

27. Ans. (a) Styles test *Ref: Craig, 12th ed. p 30*

- Mutagenesis assays assess the effect of a biomaterial on a cell's genetic material.
- **AME's Test**
  - It is the most widely used short term mutagenesis test.
  - It uses mutant stocks of Salmonella typhimurium that require exogenous histidine.
- **Style's Cell Transformation Test**
  - This test on mammalian cells was developed to offer an alternative to bacterial tests (AME's Test) which may not be relevant to mammalian systems.
  - This assay quantities the ability of potential carcinogens to transform standardized cell lines so they will grow in soft agar.
- **Cytotoxicity Tests**
  - These tests assess cell death caused by a material by measuring cell number of growth before and after exposure to that material.
- **MTT Test**
  - It is a commonly used enzymatic test for Cytotoxicity.
  - This test measures the activity of cellular dehydrogenases which convert a chemical called MTT, via several cellular reducing agents, to a blue, insoluble formazan compound.

28. Ans. (c) Bisphenol A *Ref: Phillips, 11th ed. p 199*

- Estrogenecity is the ability of a chemical to act as the hormone estrogen does in the body.
- If these chemicals are not indigenous to the body, the substance is called 'xenoestrogen'.
- The concern about estrogen in dentistry center around a chemical called Bisphenol A (BPA), which is a synthetic starting point for all Bis-GMA composites.
- E-Screen Assay test is commonly used to assess xenoestrogenic activity.
- This in vitro test relies on the growth response of breast cancer cells that are estrogen sensitive to purposed estrogenic compounds.

29. Ans. (c) 1668 *Ref: Phillips, 11th ed. p 108*

Titanium	
Atomic weight	47.9
Melting point	1668°C
Boiling point	3260°C
Density	4.51 g/cm^3
Linear coefficient	0.085×10^{-4}/°C
Of thermal expansion	

30. Ans. (a) Methyl and ethyl mercury *Ref: Phillips, 11th ed. p 198*

- Mercury occurs in three forms:
  - Metal (HgO)
  - Inorganic mercury (Hg^{2+})
  - Organic form (Methyl or ethyl mercury)
- Methyl mercury is the most toxic form of mercury and is very efficiently absorbed from the gut (90% to 95%).
- The primary source of methyl in the diet, with fish (shark, sword fish and tuna) contributing a significant portion.
- The half life ranges from 20 to 90 days depending on the form with methyl mercury exhibiting the longest half life and inorganic forms having the shortest half life.

31. Ans. None *Ref: Dental Materials at a Glance by J. Anthony, 1st ed. p 5*

- Shore hardness test measures penetration of a blunt indenter into a soft or elastic materials, which is not given in the option in the above question.
- The other options are used for brittle and ductile materials and not for elastic materials.
- Hence, the answer was none of the above according to the key.

32. Ans. (c) Knoop's hardness test *Ref: Phillips, 11th ed. p 98*

Knoop hardness number

- It is consider as a micro hardness test.
- It is used to measure the value for hard as well as soft material.
- It is independent of the ductility of the material.
- It employs a diamond-tipped tool that is cut in the geometrical configuration.

33. Ans. (c) Arrangement of atoms

Space Lattice

- Atomic arrangements in crystalline solids can be described with respect to a network of lines in three dimensions.
- The intersections of the lines are called "lattice sites" (or lattice points). Each lattice site has the same environment in the same direction.
- Space lattice may be result of primary and secondary bonds.
- A particular arrangement of atoms in a crystal structure can be described by specifying the atom positions in a repeating "unit cell".

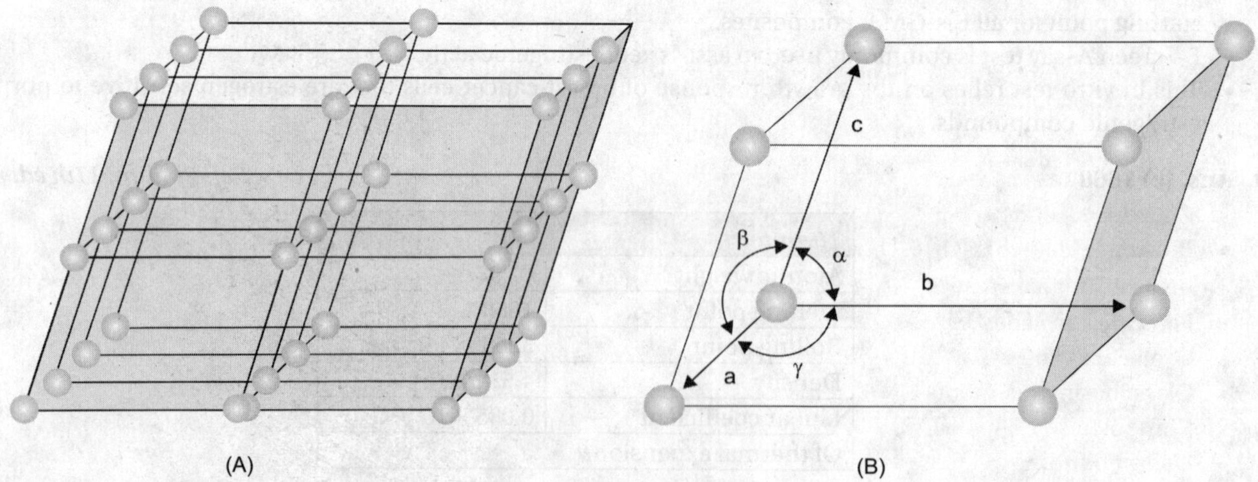

34. Ans. (c) Stiffness *Ref: Phillips, 11th ed. p 80*

- Youngs modulus is the measure of stiffness of an isotropic elastic material and that of mild steel is 210000 MPa.
- The SI unit is known as Pascal, though the practical units that are used are megapascals or gigapascals.
- Mild steel has a tensile strength that is relatively low, is less expensive and malleable making it the most common form of steel.

35. Ans. (c) Nickel *Ref: Phillip, 11th ed. p 176*

- Nickel is the most allergic among all the material with incidence of 10–20% and most common in women.

36. Ans. (a) Brittleness *Ref: Philips, 11th ed. p 94, 95, 74*

- Brittleness: The relative inability of a material to sustain plastic deformation before fracture.
- A material is brittle if, when subjected to stress, it breaks without significant deformation (strain). Brittle materials absorb relatively little energy prior to fracture, even those of high strength.
- Breaking is often accompanied by a snapping sound. Brittle materials include most ceramics and glasses (which do not deform plastically) and some polymers, such as PMMA and polystyrene.
- Many steels become brittle at low temperatures (see ductile-brittle transition temperature), depending on their composition and processing.
- When used in materials science, it is generally applied to materials that fail when there is little or no evidence of plastic deformation before failure.

37. Ans. (a) Strontium chloride *Ref: Philips, 11th ed. p 374*

CLASIFICATION OF DESENSITIZING AGENTS

- Mode of Administration
  - At home desensitizing agents
  - In-office treatment
- On the basis of mechanism of action

Nerve desensitization

- Potassium nitrate

Protein precipitation

- Gluteraldehyde
- Silver nitrate
- Strontium chloride hexahydrate
- Zinc chloride

Plugging dentinal tubules

- Sodium fluoride
- Stannous fluoride
- Strontium chloride
- Potassium oxalate
- Calcium phosphate
- Calcium carbonate
- Bio active glasses (SiO_2, P_2O_5, CaO, Na_2O)

Dentine adhesive sealers

- Fluoride varnishes
- Oxalic acid and resin
- Glass ionomer cements
- Composites
- Dentin bonding agents

Lasers
- Neodymium:yttrium aluminum garnet (Nd:YAG) laser
- GaAlAs (galium-aluminium-arsenide laser)
- Erbium-YAG laser

Homeopathic medication
- Propolis

AUXILIARY DENTAL MATERIALS

38. Ans. (a) 39°C *Ref: Phillips, 11th ed. p 33.*

- Glass transition temperature, at which the material losses its hardness or brittleness on heating or forms a rigid mass.
- Approx 39°C is the glass transition temperature and 43.5°C is the fusion temperature of impression compound.
- Material removed from the mouth after glass transition temperature is reached.
- Fusion temperature is the temperature at which the impression compound becomes plastic.

39. Ans. (a) 2% K_2SO_4 *Ref: Phillips 11th ed. p 265, 269*

The following material can be added to the impression material in order to increase the surface hardness:
- 2% K_2SO_4 (most widely used)
- $ZnSO_4$
- Magnesium sulphate
- Potash alum.

40. Ans. (a) Regulating setting time and expansion of plaster *Ref: Phillips, 11th ed. p 235*

41. Ans. (c) Agar agar *Ref: Phillips. 11th ed. p. 247*

Reversible hydrocolloid
- Based on thermoreversible gelation of natural polysaccharide agar (isolated from red algae/seaweeds)
- Agar sols form gels upon cooling of a hot solution to (30–40)°C
- Agar gels melt to sols upon heating to (90–95)°C
- Composition:
  - Agar
  - Borax to increase the gel strength
  - Potassium sulphate as a gypsum hardener
  - Water dispersion medium
- Advantages:
  - Very good biological properties
  - Excellent surface detail reproduction
- Disadvantages:
  - Need special equipment (water bath) and special technique
  - Dimensionally instable—evaporation or imbibition
  - Low strength and poor tear resistance
  - Slow setting time

42. Ans. (b) Coating particles with dihydric alcohol (diglycerol) *Ref: Phillips 11th ed. p 240*

- In order to make dustless alginate, manufactures add glycerine to the alginate powder.
- Addition of glycerine, agglomerates the particles due to this the powder become denser and not releasing the dust particle after tumbling.

43. Ans. (b) Rapid heating rate *Ref: Phillip's. 11th ed. p 339*

- Rapid heating rate is one of the cause of casting.
- Because of flaking of the investment when water or steam pours into the mould, it will results the surface roughness. In order to avoid it, investment filled ring should be heated for at least 60 min from room temperature to 700°C.
- When the bulk of the investment is more, it requires more time for heating.

44. Ans. (c) From the beginning of mixing to just before the appearance of elastic properties *Ref: Phillip's 11th ed. p 216*

- Working time is measured at room temperature.
- Setting time is measured at mouth temperature.
- Working and setting times can be assesses with the help of penetrometer.
- Working times of elastomeric impression material is starting from the beginning of mixing to just before the appearance of elastic property.
- Working and setting time decreases when the velocity increases.

	Mean working time (min)		*Mean setting time (min)*	
Impression material	23°C	37°C	23°C	37°C
Polyether	3.3	2.3	9.0	8.3
Condensation silicone	3.3	2.5	11.0	8.9
Addition silicone	3.1	1.8	8.9	5.9
Polysulfide	6.0	4.3	16.0	12.5

45. Ans. (a) Unpleasant odour and taste *Ref: Phillip's 11th ed. p 232*

Polysulfide

- Also known as mercaptan or thiokol
- Supplied in the form of two pastes—a base and a catalyst

Examples: Permlastic (SDS/Kerr), Coe-Flex, Omniflex (GC America)

The base paste consists of:

- Polysulfide polymer
- Suitable filler (titanium dioxide or lithopone)
- Plasticizer (e.g. dibutyl phthalate)
- Sulphur small amount that enhances reaction (catalyst)

The catalyst paste:

- Lead dioxide
- Plasticizer—chlorinated paraffin
- Approx same amount of filler as in base paste
- Oleic or stearic acid—retarders—control the rate of setting

Advantages	*Disadvantages*
Good tear strength	Poor dimension stability
Good elasticity	Offensive odor
Low cost	Stains clothing
	Long setting time

46. Ans. (c) Improper ratio of polymer and monomer *Ref: Phillip's 11th ed. p 230*

Effects of mishandling that occur with the use of nonaqueous elastomeric impression materials

Type of failure	*Causes*
Bubbles	• Too rapid polymerization from high humidity or temperature • Excessively high accelerator/base ratio with condensation silicone • Too rapid polymerization, preventing flow • Air incorporated during mixing
Distortion	• Resin tray not aged sufficiently, still undergoing polymerization shrinkage • Lack of adhesion of rubber to the tray caused by not applying enough coats of adhesive, filling tray with material too soon after applying adhesive or using the wrong adhesive • Lack of mechanical retention for those materials where adhesive is ineffective • Development of elastic properties in the material before tray is seated • Excessive bulk of material (if such technique is used) • Continued pressure against impression material that has developed elastic properties • Movement of tray during polymerization • Premature removal from mouth • Improper removal from mouth • Delayed pouring of the polysulfide or condensation silicone impression
Rough or uneven surface of impression material	• Incomplete polymerization caused by premature removal from the mouth • Improper ratio or mixing of components • Presence of oil or other organic material on the teeth • For addition silicone, agents that contaminate the material and inhibit polymerization
Irregularly shaped voids	• Moisture or debris on surface of teeth

47. Ans. (c) By adjusting space to 1/4 inch from casting *Ref: Phillip's 11th ed. p 346*

Strickland and Sturdevant (1959) reported on ways to eliminate back pressure porosity. They found that 3 to 5 winds on a centrifugal casting machine or 20 PSI minimum pressure for air pressure casting machines produced a 'high enough' casting pressure to eliminate back pressure porosity. In order to more easily vent gases, they recommended placing the pattern 1/4" from the end of the ring. Phillips (1982) stated that 'proper burnout, an adequate mold and casting temperature, and a sufficiently high water/powder ratio will help to eliminate this phenomena.'

48. Ans. (a) It liquefies at a temperature of 71100°C *Ref: Phillip's 11th ed. p 234-239*

Refer Ans no. 47.

49. Ans. (c) Hysteresis *Ref: www.slideshare.net/SaranshMalot/elastic-impression-materials*

Refer Ans no. 47.

50. Ans. (d) To act as an accelerator *Ref: Phillip's 11th ed. p 269*

The function of 2% potassium sulphate in a gypsum product is to act as an accelerator.

51. Ans. (d) To counteract contraction *Ref: Phillip's 11th ed. p 297*

Gypsum bonded investment is composed of:

- α $CaSO_4$.1/2 H_2O- 30 to 35%
- Quarrtz- 60 to 65%.
- Cristobalite- 5%.
- Quartz and cristobalite are the two allotropic forms of silica that are commonly employed for the formulation of dental investments.
- There is an a-to b-phase transformation for cristobalite and quartz from 220 to 275 8°C and at 573 8°C, respectively, and these lead to volumetric expansion on heating. Such expansion has been utilized to compensate for much of the alloy thermal contraction, but it must lead to a slightly less dense mass which may therefore weaken it.
- In the case of cristobalite, the expansion is isotropic and the change is rapid, this would create a differential shearing movement between the refractory material and the binder, creating stress and therefore potentially crack nucleation sites.
- In the case of quartz the expansion is anisotropic and may exaggerate the differential shear and thus the localized cracking and disruption of contact points within the mass.

52. Ans. (a) 2% and (c) 6% *Ref: http://virtual.usc.ed.u.co/uscvirtual/courses/CODBIOMAT/document/norma_3.pdf*

Dental impression compound shall be of the flowing types:

- Type I: Impression compound is the material shall be suitable for taking impressions in the oral cavity
- Type II: Tray compound is the material shall be suitable for forming trays to be used in the oral cavity.

Flow. Type I compound

The flow at 37°C, shall be no more than 6%

The flow at 45°C, shall be not less than 85%

Flow. Type II compound

The flow at 37°C, shall be not more than 2%

The flow at 45°C, shall be not less than 70% nor more than 85%

- Type I compound shall record accurately the surface detail of the test block.

53. Ans. (b) Gypsum *Ref: Phillip's 11th ed. p 296, 267*

- The essential ingredients of the casting gold alloys are α-hemihydrates of gypsum, quartz or cristobalite.
- A-hemihydrates of gypsum provide strength to the gold investment.
- Gypsum product act as a binder in order to provide the rigidity to the investment.
- Amount of binder will decide how the strength of the investment.
- Quartz is meant to counteract the contraction.

54. Ans. (a) Single-mix materials have higher viscosity *Ref: Phillip's 11th ed. p 217-22*

- When a single mix monophase material is used medium viscosity material is used.
- Monophase technique (e.g. polyether)—the same mix of medium viscosity metrial is used for both a stock tray and syringe.

- Medium body polyether and addition silicone are often used for monophase or single viscosity technique.
- The material in the tray retains its medium viscosity and when seated, it can force the syringe material to flow past critical area of tooth preparation.

55. Ans. (a) Cynoacrylate *Ref: Phillip's 11th ed. p 317*

- In order to increase the abrasive resistance, silver plating, die hardner, and coating the surface with cyanoacrylate is done.
- All these method play an important role to increase the die dimension slightly and thus reducing its accuracy.

56. Ans. (c) Would not affect water requirement *Ref: Phillip's 11th ed. p 258*

- Calcium sulphate hemihydrate is the principal constituent of dental plaster as well as dental stone.
- Small amount of addition of surface active agent like gum Arabic with calcium carbonate to the hemihydrates would decrease the water requirement of dental plaster as well as stone.

57. Ans. (d) Vacuum cure polyurethane *Ref: Delmar's Dental Assisting by Donna, 2nd ed. p 636*

Customs Tray's:

- Acrylic tray resins self-curing customer tray
- Acrylic tray resins light curing customer tray
- Vacuum forced custom tray
- Thermoplastic tray material custom trays

58. Ans (c) Type 3 modelling wax *Ref: Phillip's 11th ed. p 292*

Modelling wax

It is of three types:

- Type 1: Soft wax used for building veneers.
- Type 2: Medium wax pattern trial in the mouth during normal climatic condition
- Type 3: Hard wax used for arrangement of teeth in India during summer season in try in stage

59. Ans. (a) Sodium alginate *Ref: Nallaswamy 1st ed. p 213*

Cold mould seal is widely used separating media because of its effective and easy manipulation.

Composition

- Sodium alginate solution –2% in H_2O.
- Sodium phosphate.
- Glycerine.
- Alcohol.
- Preservative.

Option a is the answer because sodium alginate is the chief components of cold mould seal.

60. Ans. (c) 700°C *Ref: Phillips 11th ed. p 297*

- After dehydration all forms of gypsum shrink between 200-400°C.
- Between 400 and 700°C, a slight expansion is noted.
- Lateral shrinkage in gypsum is caused due to the decomposition and the release of sulphur dioxide.
- It is imperative, that gypsum investment should not be heated above 700°C.

61. Ans. (a) 50% HCl *Ref: Phillips 11th ed. p 335*

- When the surface oxides from the casting are removed from the surface termed as pickling.
- In this procedure the gypsum bonded investment should be heated with 50% HCl.

- 50% HCl removes all the oxide coating and residual investment.
- Sometime the fumes of HCl also corrode laboratory metal furnishing.

62. Ans. (b) Narrow sprue diameter *Ref: Phillips 11th ed. p 347*

- Sometimes incomplete casting or no casting occurs when the molten alloy is not properly filled into the mould.
- It occurs due to two factors:
  - Insufficient venting of mould.
  - High viscosity of the fused metal.
- If there is insufficient venting, i.e. air does not escape from the mold, the molten alloy does not enters properly into the mold and solidify and results incomplete casting.
- Due to the high viscosity of the fused metal, it is not able to flow timely and same thing will occur when the narrow sprue diameter, is present. So it is also a responsible factor of incomplete casting.

63. Ans. (c) Polymerization shrinkage of composite resins *Ref: Phillips 11th ed. p 416*

Polymerization Shrinkage:

- Composite materials shrinks during curing.
- It can lead to failure of interfacial bonding.
- It is usually more significant when the cavity preparation extends up to the root surface causing 'V' shaped gap formation between the composite and the root surface due to polymerization shrinkage.
- The configuration factor (C factor) is the ratio of bonded surface of the restoration to the unbounded surfaces.
- The highest the value of 'C' factor, the greater is the potential for bond disruption due to polymerization shrinkage.
- C factor = Bonded surface/unbounded surface
  - For class I restoration = C=5.
  - For class II restoration = C=1/4
  - For class III restoration = C= 2
- Therefore, class I restoration are at more risk to the effects of polymerization shrinkage.

64. Ans. (b) Sodium perborate *Ref: Nallaswamy 1st ed. p 222*

- A denture should be cleaned with the help of brush and paste. It can be cleaned by using the following two types of cleaning agent.

Chemical cleanser:

- It involves the use of chemical agent such as sodium perborate, chlorhexidine, or nystatin in order to cleans the denture.
- Denture should be kept in the dilute solution of these chemicals.

Ultrasonic cleaner:

- In this method, small bubble are formed sonically which bombarded against the denture and in this way it cleans the denture thoroughly.
- Denture is also cleans by soaking and brushing with a denture brush.

65. Ans. (d) Amylose *Ref: Craig's 12th ed. p 162*

- Abrasives constitute at least 50% of a typical toothpaste.
- These insoluble particles help remove plaque from the teeth.
- The removal of plaque and calculus helps minimize cavities and periodontal disease.
- Representative abrasives include particles of aluminum hydroxide ($Al(OH)_3$), calcium carbonate ($CaCO_3$), Sodium chloride, various calcium hydrogen phosphates, various silicates and zeolites, and hydroxyapatite ($Ca_5(PO_4)_3OH$).

66. Ans. (a) 3:1 by vol, 2:1 by wt *Ref: Phillips 11th ed. p 727*

- Heat activated resin and chemically activated resin are different from one another in the sense by which benzoyl peroxide is divided to yield free radicals.
- Powder, liquid ratio (P:L) is 3:1 by volume and 2:1 by weight. In this ratio all the powder particle is thoroughly wet in the liquid molecule.
- Volumetric shrinkage is 6% and linear shrinkage is 0.5% at this ratio.

67. Ans. (b) Dimethyl-p-toluidine *Ref: Phillips 11th ed. p 734*

Chemically activated denture base resins:

- Denture polymerization is induced by chemical activator.
- Polymerization is completed at room temperature.
- It is also termed as cold-cure, resin, self-cure resin or autopolymerizing resin.
- Tertiary amine such as dimethyl para-toluidine is used as activator.

68. Ans. (c) 22 to .24 *Ref: Craig's 12th ed. p 316*

69. Ans. (c) Diatomaceous earth *Ref: Craig's 12th ed. p 275*

Component	*Function*	*Weight percentage*
Potassium alginate	Soluble alginate	15
Calcium sulphate	Reactor	16
Zinc oxide	Filler particle	4
Potassium titanium fluoride	Accelerator	3
Diatomaceous earth	Filler particle	60
Sodium phosphate	Retarder	2

70. Ans. (c) Delay pouring *Ref: Applied Dental Materials by John F p 170*

- Addition reaction of addition silicone gives cross linking between two types of siloxane pre polymer.
- Pouring should be delayed in order to the evolution of hydrogen so that the cast surface will be free from pits.

71. Ans. (d) It is resisted most by CuSn phase in high-copper amalgam *Ref: Phillips 11th ed. p 5178*

General Setting Reaction of high copper alloy:

Ag-Sn-Cu	+	Hg	→	Ag_3 Sn	+	Ag_2Hg_3	+	Cu_6Sn_5
silver-tin-copper		mercury		silver-tin gamma		silver-mercury gamma 1		copper-tin eta

Note that NO gamma 2 is formed.

72. Ans. (b) Zinc chloride and eugenol *Ref: Phillips 11th ed. p. 208, 252*

Components Percentage

Tube no. 1 (Base)

Zinc oxide (French-processed or U.S.P.)	87
Fixed vegetable or mineral oil	13

Tube no. 2 (Accelerator)

Oil of cloves or eugenol	12
Gum or polymerized rosin	50
Filler (silica type)	20
Lanolin	3
Resinous balsam	10
Accelerator solution ($CaCl_2$) and color	5

Phillips mentions $CaCl_2$ as an accelerator and eugenol is the component of accelerator paste and hence the most probable answer is (b).

73. Ans. (a) Addition silicone *Ref:http://www.ijdr.in/article.asp?issn=09709290;year=2012; volume=23;issue=3;spage=407;epage=41 0;aulast=Afroz*

- Oral submucous fibrosis is a premalignant condition in which rigidity of the lip, tongue, and palate results in reduced mouth opening and tongue movement.
- Limited mouth opening, mucosal rigidity, and reduced salivary flow makes prosthodontic procedures difficult in these patients and affects the stability, retention, and the support of removable prostheses.
- The burning sensation in the mouth that these patients experience reduces the tolerance to prostheses.
- Light-body additional silicones are materials of choice for OSMF patients in closed-mouth technique as it has excellent flow, good production of details and tear strength, causing no irritation to soft tissues.

74. Ans. (c) Cocoa butter *Ref: Craig 12th ed. p. 339*

Natural waxes	*Synthetic*	*Additives*
Mineral	Acrawax	Stearic acid
• Paraffin	Aerosol OT	Glyceryl
• Microcrystalline	Castorwax	Tristearate
• Barnsdahl	Flexo-wax C	Oils
• Ozokerite	Epolene N-10	Turpentine
• Ceresin	Albacer	Colorants
• Montan	Aldo 33	Natural resins
Plant	Durawax 1032	**Rosin**
• Carnauba		• Copal
• Ouricury		• Dammar
• Candelilla		• Sanarac
• Japan wax		• Mastic
• Cocoa butter		• Shellac
Insect		• Kauri
• Beeswax		**Synthetic resin**
Animal		• Elvax
• Spermaceti		• Polyethylene
		• Polystyrene

- Cocoa butter and Japan wax is not a true wax.
- They are mainly fats composed of glycerides of stearic, palmitic, oleic, lauric and lower fatty acids.
- Cocoa butter is a brittle substance at the room temperature.
- Japan wax is a tough, malleable, and sticky material.

75. Ans. (a) It is used for cast metal alloys *Ref: Phillips. 11th ed., p 2967*

Types of Investments:

Gypsum-bonded investments

- Used for casting gold alloys.

Phosphate-bonded investments

- Used for alloys used in ceramometal restorations.

Ethyl silica-bonded investments

- Used for casting base metal alloy partial dentures.

Gypsum-bonded investments

- The mold materials most commonly used in the casting of dental gold alloys.
- Decomposes at high temperatures; not suitable for casting high-melting gold alloys, or base metal alloys.
- The main ingredients of the dental inlay investment employed with the conventional gold casting alloys are: a-hemihydrate of gypsum, quartz or cristobalite, which are allotropic forms of silica. a-hemihydrate of gypsum, in investments, provides greater strength. a-hemihydrate of gypsum serves as a binder to hold other ingredients together and provide rigidity. The strength of the investment is dependent on the amount of binder present.
- A slight expansion takes place between 400°C and approximately 700°C (1292°F), and then a large contraction occurs.
- This later shrinkage is most likely caused by the decomposition and release of sulphur gases, such as sulphur dioxide.
- Gypsum investments should not be heated above 700°C (1292°F).

76. Ans. (a) 27 µm aluminium oxide *Ref: Vimal Sikri 2nd ed. p 453*

- Air abrasive technique is a non rotary hard tissue cutting method.
- In place of rotary method, it uses pseudomechanical kinetic energy.
- Aluminium oxide is the most widely used abrasive particle with an average particle, i.e. 25 to 30 micron.
- The normal exit pressure is about 60–120 pounds per square inch is used in this technique.

Uses of air abrasive technique:

- Detecting early carious lesions.
- As an adjunct to acid etching.
- As a repair modality in ceramic, composite.
- As preventive measure in pit and fissure sealant.

77. Ans. (a) Microleakage *Ref: Phillips 11th ed. p 383*

Acid etching:

- Etching of dental surface with an acid in order to remove the smear layer and open enamel tubules, increased retention of resin sealant and promote mechanical retention.
- A concept of etching, with phosphoric acid, first proposed by Buonocore in 1955 to increase the bond strength between the composite resin and etched enamel.
- It improves mechanical bonding and also sealed interfacial gaps.
- It is known to reduce the problem of microleakage in the restoration.

78. Ans. (c) ZOE paste *Ref: Phillips 11th ed. p 208*

Mucostatic impression material: An impression material which records without distorting the tissues and these are used to record the impression of patient with excessively mobile soft tissue.

For example: Impression plaster and ZOE.

- These impression materials do not compress the tissue while taking the impression.
- These are generally used to make impression of edentulous patient.

79. Ans. (b) 2% potassium sulphate *Ref: Phillips 11th ed. p 235*

Reversible hydrocolloid: Agar

- Agar is an organic hydrophilic colloid (polysaccharide) extracted from certain types of seaweed.
- Agar is a sulphuric ester of a liver polymer of galactose.
- Borax is used to strengthen the gel, and it also retard the setting time.
- Potassium sulphate is used as a gypsum hardening agent.
- As a bactericidal and plasticizer we add thymol and glycerine in it.

80. Ans. (c) Hysteresis *Ref: Internet*

Hysteresis

- The temperature lag between the liquefaction temperature and the gelation temperature and the gelation temperature.
- Liquefaction temperature is the temperature at which gel changes to sol (70 to 100°C)
- Gelation temperature is the temperature at which sol changes to gel (37 to 50°C)

Imbibition

- It is the water sorption, i.e. the gel swells when placed in water.

Syneresis

- It is the expression of fluid on to the surface of gel structure.

81. Ans. (a) Agar *Ref: Phillips 11th ed. p 235*

Agar reversible hydrocolloids require a gypsum hardener.

82. Ans. (b) The time elapsed from the beginning of mixing until curing has advanced *Ref: Phillips 11th ed. p 210*

There are four types of elastomeric impression material:

- Polysulfide
- Condensation silicone.
- Addition silicone.
- Polyethers.
  - The working time of an elastomeric impression material is defined as the time elapsed from the beginning of mixing and ends just before the elastic properties have fully developed.
  - Setting time can be defined as the time elapsed from the beginning of mixing until curing has advanced.
  - Three types of mixing system are available to mix the catalyst and base thoroughly i.e.
    - Hand mixing
    - Static automixing
    - Dynamic mechanical mixing.

83. Ans. (d) None of the above *Ref: Phillips 11th ed. p 265*

- In gypsum, potassium sulphate is the most commonly used accelerator. It is effective in higher than 2% concentration.
- Sodium chloride also act as an accelerator in gypsum but in higher concentration (>2%) it act as a retarder.
- At concentration 3.4% sodium sulphate acts as a good accelerator.
- Borates, citrates and acetates act as a retarder in gypsum product.

84. Ans. (a) 39°C *Ref: Phillips 11th ed. p 33*

- Tg of an impression material is the glass transition temperature, i.e. 39°C. Also refer ans no. 10.

85. Ans. (d) That it stains clothes and has unacceptable odour *Ref: Phillips 11th ed. p 232*

Polysulfide:

- The main component of polysulfide material is a multifunctional mercaptan or polymer of polysulfide.
- Its characteristic brown color is due to the presence of lead dioxide, which is catalyst or accelerator.
- Hot and humid condition accelerate the setting of reaction.
- Water is a by-product of the reaction.

Advantage of polysulfide:

- Working time is longer.
- Modest cost.
- High tear resistance.
- Margins are easily seen.

Disadvantages of polysulfide:

- Custom tray is required
- Stretching will cause distortion.
- Stains clothing.
- Has unacceptable odour.
- Pour within 1 hour.

86. Ans. (c) Addition silicone > polyether > polysulfide > condensation silicone *Ref: Phillips 11th ed. p 224*

- Dimensional stability of an elastomeric impression material can be given in descending order as Addition silicone > polyether > Polysulfide > Condenstaion silicone.

87. Ans. (d) Incomplete polymerization caused by premature removal from the mouth *Ref: Phillips 11th ed. p 230*

Rough surface of elastomeric impression result from:

- Incomplete polymerization caused by premature removal from the mouth.
- Presence of oil or other organic material on the teeth.
- Improper ratio or mixing of components.
- For addition silicone, agents that contaminate the material and inhibit polymerization.
- Too rapid polymerization from high humidity.
- Excessively high accelerator/base ratio with condensation silicone.

88. Ans. (a) Direct relationship *Ref: Phillips 11th ed. p 342*

- Subsurface porosity occurs due to the simultaneous nucleation of solid grain and gas bubble at the first moment that the metal freezes at the mould walls.
- It can be diminished by controlling the rate at which the molten metal enters the mould.
- In order to control the rate of entry of molten metal there is a direct relationship with the diameter of sprue. i.e. subsurface porosite α Diameter of sprue.

89. Ans. (b) Inverse relationship *Ref: Phillips 11th ed. p 346*

- The length of sprue and subsurface porosity have inverse relationship, i.e. on increasing the length of sprue the molten metal enters into the mould slowly and it will leads to less chances of sub-surface porosity.

90. Ans. (b) Decreases flow and (d) Increases hardness *Ref: Phillips 11th ed. p 286*

Carnauba wax

- It has a high melting point.
- It increases the hardness.
- It decreases the flow at mouth temperature.
- It gives glossiness to the surface.
- It has an agreeable odour.
- It is used in 25%.

Candellila wax

- It can be used instead of carnauba wax.
- Low melting temperature.
- Not as hard as carnauba wax.

91. Ans. (a) Polysulfide *Ref: Phillips 11th ed. p 229 (A)*

- Polysulfide is one of the most biocompatible impression material because it shows least cell death and high viable cell in an in vivo study.

92. Ans. (c) More than 85% *Ref: Applied Dental Materials by John F 149 9th ed*

- According to ADA specification No. 3 Impression compound are of:
- **Type I:**
  - Low fusing compound green stick compound.
  - Medium fusing compound- impression compound.
- **Type II:**
  - High fusing compound- Tray compound.
- **Flow:**
  - High fusing compound have a flow less than 2% at 37°C and less than 70 to 85% at 45°C.
  - Low fusing compound have a flow less than 3% at 37°C and less than 80 to 85% at 45°C.

93. Ans. (c) Initial set *Ref: Phillips 11th ed. p 261*

Setting time can be divided into:

- Working time:
  - The mixture is in semi fluid condition and it can be manipulated as one wishes. It is approximately 5 to 7 minutes.
- Initial setting time:
  - The mix has become semi-hard and firm.
  - All manipulation must be completed before this stage.
  - In other words end of working time is the initial setting time.
  - At this time material losses its surface shine and smoothness (loss of gloss) due to the surface water of the mix.
  - Initial setting time varies with different type of gypsum products.
- Final setting time:
  - It is the time when the mix is completely set and hard.
  - At this stage cast can be separated from the impression without causing any damage.

94. Ans. (b) Iron oxide *Ref: Phillips 11th ed. p 370*

Rouge

- It is an iron oxide in fine form.
- It is blended with various soft binders into a cake or bar form.

- When impregnated in cloth it is called crocus cloth.
- It is used to polish high noble metal alloys.
- It is contraindicated for polishing stainless steel and Co-Cr alloys as iron contaminates the surface and facilitate corrosion.
- It is used as a coloring agent in impression compound.
- Rouge is mixed with chloroform and can be used as antiflux.

95. Ans. (c) 75% gold *Ref: Phillips 11th ed. p 575*

Typical composition of casting gold alloys:

Type	*Au (%)*	*Ag (%)*	*Cu (%)*	*Pu/Pd (%)*	*Zn (%)*
Low strength	85	11	03	—	1
Medium strength	75	12	10	2	1
High strength	70	14	10	5	1
Extra strength	65	09	15	10	1

96. Ans. (d) Resistant to corrosion *Ref: Phillips 11th ed. p 517*

- Gamma 2 phase is highly susceptible to corrosion.
- As soon as the corrosion products are formed, they initially seal the gap between the set amalgam and surface of the tooth and lessen the microleakage.
- Gamma 2 phase is absent in high copper amalgam that's why it is highly resistant to corrosion.
- Gamma 2 phase is also possess more susceptibility to creep.

97. Ans. (b) Alginate *Ref: Phillips 11th ed. p 244*

- The primary impression for removable partial denture should be made by irreversible hydrocolloid (alginate) impression material.
- Alginate is chosen because it is economical, elastic, and easy to manipulate.
- The alginate impression is poured using dental plaster and the resulting primary cast is used to design the prosthesis.
- The secondary impression is made after prosthetic mouth preparation and the material of choice for it is also alginate.

98. Ans. (b) 15 um *Ref: Phiilips 11th ed. p 551*

- Gold powder is formed by electrolytic precipitation. It is formed into shapes by sintering, which cause self-diffusion between particles, so the crystals actually grow together.
- Granular (powdered) gold is formed by chemical precipitation or by atomizing the metal.
- Blend of varying particle sizes average-15 microns and maximum-74 microns.
- Pellets mixed with soft wax and then wrapped with gold foil no. 3
- Ratio of gold foil to powder - 1:3 small pellets. 1:9 large pellets.
- It is used to build up bulk of restoration. Surface pits may occur.

99. Ans. (a) Alter the temperature of water *Ref: Phillips 11th ed. p 242*

Gelation time: Normal gelation time is 3 to 4 minutes at room temperature. But at mouth temperature which is 37°C the material will set little quicker.

According to ADA:

- Type I- Fast setting- 1 to 2 minutes.
- Type II- Normal setting- 2 to 4 minutes.

Control of gelation time:

By altering the temperature of the mixing water. Higher the temperature of water quicker setting. Cool water as well as pre cooled mixing bowl and spatula needed in hot, temperature climates.

- Gelation is tested by fingertip the material should not be sticky or tacky, but feel stiff.

Note: Control of setting should be done by changing the water powder ratio and mixing time.

100. Ans. (c) Stiffness *Ref: Phillips 11th ed. p 80*

Elastic modulus or modulus of elasticity or Young's modulus:

- It represents the relative stiffness or rigidity of the material within the elastic range.
- Young's modulus is ratio of stress to strain.
- Higher the modulus, stiffer or rigid is the material.
- It is difficult to compress, pull or twist or even to cause a small amount of strain in a rigid material.
- The dental structure must exhibit high elastic limit and high modulus of elasticity.

101. Ans. (c) 0.2% to 0.5% *Ref: Phillips 11th ed. p 736*

The amount of free monomer in:

- Polymerization by chemical activation 3% to 5%.
- Polymerization by heat activation 0.2% to 0.5%.

102. Ans. (b) 21 Gpa and 27–55 Mpa *Ref: Phillips 11th ed. p 512*

Physical property of amalgam:

- Maximum allowable creep = 1%
- Minimum compressive strength after 1 hour = 80 MPa.
- Minimum compressive strength after 24 hr = 300 MPa.
- Tensile strength = 48 65 MPa.
- Modulus of elasticity- Approx 21 GPa.
- Dimensional change within 24 hour = -15 to + 20 µm/cm.

103. Ans. (b) Back pressure porosity *Ref: Phillips 11th ed. p 346*

Entrapped-air porosity on the inner surface of the casting sometimes referred to as back-pressure porosity, can produce large concave depressions. This is caused by the inability of the air in the mold to escape through the pores in the investment of by the pressure gradient that displaces the air pocket toward the end of the investment via the molten sprue and button.

104. Ans. (c) Localized shrinkage porosity *Ref: Phillips, 11th ed. p 342*

Localized shrinkage porosity is generally caused by premature termination of the flow of molten metal during solidification.

105. Ans. (c) Diamond *Ref: Phillips, 11th ed. p 368*

Diamond is a transparent, colorless mineral composed of carbon. It is the hardest known substance. Diamond is called a supera brasive because of its ability to abrade any other known substance. Diamond abrasives are supplied in several forms, including bonded abrasive rotary instruments, flexible metal-backed abrasive strips, and diamond polishing pastes. They are mostly used on ceramic and resin-based composite materials.

106. Ans. (b) Type IV *Ref: Phillips, 11th ed. p 275*

High strength type IV gypsum products are:

- Densite
- Dental stone

107. Ans. (d) Rouge *Ref: Phillips, 11th ed. p 368, 372*

- Crocus cloth is an abrasive sheet similar to sand paper or emery cloth but covered with a layer of very fine loose iron oxide particles rather than with bound grains of abrasive. "For final metal and gemstone finishing."
- This cloth comes in various grits, including fine, course and medium.
- One process in which a crocus cloth is often used is metal cleaning. After the metal has been treated with aluminum oxide, the sandpaper is used to smooth and polish the surface of the metal. The cloth can do this because of the fine grains it has, which also make it possible for it to bring out a deep shine in metals. It also can be used to repair scratches in surfaces by buffing them out.

108. Ans. (d) Poly vinyl siloxane *Ref: Phillips, 11th ed. p 214-216*

- Addition Silicone: The addition silicones are frequently called polyvinyl siloxane or vinyl polysiloxane impression materials. In contrast to the condensation silicones, the addition reaction polymer is terminated with vinyl groups and is cross-linked with hydride groups activated by a platinum salt catalyst.
- The base paste contains polymethyl hydrogen siloxane, as well as other siloxane prepolymers. The catalyst paste contains divinyl polydimethyl siloxane and other siloxane prepolymers. If the "catalyst" paste contains the platinum salt activator, then the paste labeled "base" must contain the hybrid silicone. Retarder may also be present in the paste that contains the platinum catalyst. Both pastes contain fillers.
- One of the disadvantages of the silicone impression materials is their inherent hydrophobic nature.
- A nonionic surfactant is added to the paste to render the surface of the impression hydrophilic. This surfactant migrates towards the surface of the impression material and has its hydrophilic segment oriented toward the surface. This phenomenon allows the impression material to more readily wet soft tissue and enhance the ability or gypsum products to capture maximum detail when poured into an impression.

109. Ans. (b) Localized shrinkage porosity *Ref: Phillips, 11th ed. p 345 and Science of Dental Material (Clinical Application) Prof. V. Shama Bhat and Prof B,T, Nandish, p 464*

Effects of technical factors on the porosity resulting from metal solidification

Type of porosity	*Increase in sprue thickness*	*Increase in sprue length*	*Increase in melt temperature*	*Increases in mold temperature*
Localized shrinkage	Reduced	Increased	Reduced	Reduced
Subsurface porosity	Increased	Reduced	Increased	Increased
Microporosity	No effect	No effects	Reduced	Reduced

With permission from Ryge G. Rozak SF and Fairhurst CW, J Am Dent Assoc 54:746, 1957.

Indirect spruing, the reservoir bar provides extra liquid to compensate solidification shrinkage (localized shrinkage porosity). In this method, 3 or 4 patterns can be invested as shown, with a common bar (reservoir). This method also saves expensive phosphate bonded investment and also casting time.

110. Ans. (c) Particle shape and size *Ref: Phillips, 11th ed. p 257*

The principal constituent of gypsum based products such as dental plasters and stones is calcium sulphate hemihydrates, that is $(CaSO_4)$ H_2O or $CaSO_4$ ½ H_2O. Depending on the method of calcinations, different forms of the hemihydrates can be obtained. These forms are referred to as α-hemihydrates, α-modified hemihydrates and β-hemihydrates. The use of α and β prefixes seem to suggest two phase from the point of view of the phase rule, but this is not the case. The α and β designations are retained because of tradition and convenience. It should not be inferred that there are mineralogical differences between them. The differences between α and β-hemihydrates are a result of difference in crystal size, surface area, and degree of lattice perfection. The β from, which is known as dental plaster, consists for large irregularly shaped orthorhombic crystal particles with capillary pores, whereas the α form consists of smaller, regularly shaped crystalline particles in the form of rods or prisms. The α-modified hemihydrates are made by boiling gypsum in a 30% aqueous solution of calcium chloride and magnesium chloride. This process yields the smoothest, most dense powder particles of the three types and the powder is used primarily for dies. The α-hemihydrates is called artificial stone, die stone, or improved stone.

111. Ans. (a) Hydrocolloids, silicones, polyether, polysulfide *Ref: Phillip's 11th ed. p 227-228*

Tear Strength: A tear strength test measures the resistance to fracture of an elastomeric material subjected to a tensile force acting perpendicular to a surface flaw. The ranking of tear strength from the lowest to highest of all impression materials generally is as follows: hydrocolloids (agar and alginate), silicones (addition and condensation), polyether, and polysulfide.

112. Ans. (d) Compressive strength *Ref: Phillip's, 11th ed. p 271*

The strength of gypsum products is generally expressed in terms of compressive strength, although tensile strength should also be considered in order to secure a satisfactory guide to the total strength characteristics.

113. Ans. (c) Polyether *Ref: Phillip's 11th ed. p 227*

- The stiffness increases as following order: polysulfides, condensation silicones, addition silicone and polyether.
- The polyether is difficult to remove from the undercut areas because of very high modulus of elasticity.

114. Ans. (b) 0.10 *Ref: Phillip's 11th ed. p 273; Craig's 12th ed. p 397*

- As per ADA No. 25 minimum amount of setting expansion required for type V gypsum product is 0.10.

115. Ans. (b) Candelilla wax *Ref: Phillip's 11th ed. p 286*

- Candililla and paraffin wax can be added to, partially or entirely replace the carnauba wax.
- The candililla wax having same general qualities as the carnauba wax, but its melting is low so it is not as hard as carnauba wax.

116. Ans. (a) Blinding *Ref: Philip's 12th ed. p 241*

- The clogging of the abrasive instrument with debris is called abrasive blinding.
- Abrasive blinding occurs when the debris generated from grinding or polishing occludes the small spaces between the abrasive particles on the tools and reduces the depth that particles can penetrate into the substrate.

117. Ans. (c) Sodium lauryl sulphate *Ref: Phillip's 11th ed. p 374*

- Toothpastes contain sodium lauryl sulphate (SLS) or related surfactants (detergents). SLS is found in many other personal care products, as well, such as shampoo, and is mainly a foaming agent, which enables uniform distribution of toothpaste, improving its cleansing power.

118. Ans. (a) Ethyl alcohol *Ref: Phillip's 11th ed. p 213*

- Ethyl alcohol is the by-product of condensation reaction between silicone base and alkyl silicate in presence of tin octate.
- Cross linking of a hydroxy-terminated polydimethyl siloxane by an alkyl silicate catalyzed by tin or stannous octoate. Ethyl alcohol is a byproduct which volatilizes leading to dimensional change.

119. Ans. (d) Suck back porosity *Ref: Phillip's 11th ed. p 343*

- Attachment of the sprue at right angle to the broad flat surface of the pattern will cause suck back porosity.
- Suck back porosity often occurs at an occulo-axial or incisal-axial line angle.

120. Ans. (b) Particle size and shape *Ref: Phillip's 11th ed. p 257*

- Dental plaster possess beta hemihydrates particle while stone have alpha hemihydrates crystal.
- Alpha and beta particle of plaster and stone are differ in their size, shape and porosity

121. Ans. (b) Reversible hydrocolloid *Ref: Phillip's 11th ed. p 237*

- A hydrocolloid has hydrophilic colloid particles spread throughout water and can be either irreversible or reversible. Examples of a hydrocolloid are agar gel and proteins.
- Agar hydrocolloid materials are derived from reversible agar gels.
- Reversible hydrocolloids offer the following advantages:
  - A custom tray is not required;
  - No separate components are mixed, thus the chance for error is reduced;
  - They are relatively hydrophilic and inexpensive;
  - They are pleasant tasting and clean to use;
  - Casts are easily removed from the impression;
  - and compatibility with stone allows the creation of bubble-free casts.
- The disadvantages are
  - The initial start-up cost of the conditioning unit,
  - Casts must be poured immediately,
  - and the material has a low tear strength when impressing narrow, deep sulci.

122. Ans. (a) 6 mm of the open end of the ring *Ref: Phillips, 11th ed. p 322*

The length of the sprue former depends on the length of the casting ring. If the sprue is too short, the wax pattern may be so far removed from the end of the casting ring that gases cannot be adequately vented to permit the molten alloy to fill the ring completely. When these gases are not completely eliminated, porosity may result. Therefore the sprue length should be adjusted so that the top of the wax pattern is within 6 mm of the open end of the ring for gypsum bonded investments. With the higher-strength phosphate-bonded investments, it may be possible to position the wax pattern within 3 to 4 m of the top of the investment.

123. Ans. (c) Gum dammar *Ref: Phillips, 11th ed. p 285*

- Inlay wax is a specialized dental wax that can be applied to dies to form direct or indirect patterns for the lost-wax technique used for casting metals or hot pressing of ceramics.

Paraffin wax	40 to 60 wt%
Gum dammar	• Added to paraffin to improve its smoothness in molding and to render it more resistant to cracking and flaking • It also increases toughness of the wax • Enhances smoothness and luster of the surface
Carnauba wax	• Added to decrease the flow at mouth temperature
	• Contributes to the glossiness of the wax surface
Candellila wax	• It can be added to partially or entirely replace carnauba wax
	• Its melting point is lower and it is not as hard as carnauba
Cerasin	• May replace part of the paraffin to modify the toughness and carving characteristics of the wax

- In modern inlay waxes, carnauba wax is often replaced in part with certain synthetic waxes. Because of their high melting point, more paraffin can be incorporated and the general working qualities of the product are improved.

124. Ans. (b) Laminate technique *Ref: Phillips 11th ed. p 245*

Laminate technique

- A recent modification to the traditional agar procedure is the combined agar procedure is the combined agar alginate technique. The hydrocolloid in the tray is replaced with a mix of chilled alginate that bonds with the agar expressed from a syringe. The alginate gels by a chemical reaction, whereas the agar gels by means of contact with the cool alginate rather than with the water circulating through the tray.

- Laminate technique is the most cost-effective way of producing an impression with adequate detail.
- The main disadvantage to this technique are
  - The bond between the agar and the alginate is not always sound
  - The higher viscosity of the alginate material displaces the agar hydrocolloid during seating
  - The dimensional inaccuracy of the alginate limits its use to single units.

125. Ans. (a) 45 degree *Ref: Phillips, 11th ed. p 321*

The sprue former should not be attached at a right angle to a broad flat surface. Such an orientation leads to turbulence within the mold cavity and sever porosity in this region. When this same pattern is sprued at a 45-degree angle to the proximal area, a satisfactory casting is obtained.

126. Ans. (c) Magnesium oxide and monoammonium phosphate *Ref: Phillips, 11th ed. p 310*

The binder consists of magnesium oxide (basic) and a phosphate that is acid in nature. Originally phosphoric acid was used, but monoammonium phosphate has replaced it, because it can be incorporated into the investment powder.

127. Ans. (a) 700°C *Ref: Phillips, 11th ed. p 297*

A slight expansion takes place between 400°C and approximately 700°C (1292°F), and a large contraction then occurs. This later shrinkage is most likely caused by decomposition and the release of sulfur gases, such as sulfur dioxide. This decomposition not only causes shrinkage but also contaminates the castings with the sulfides of the non nobles alloying elements, such as silver and copper. Thus it is imperative that gypsum investments not be heated above 700°C (1292°F). However, for gypsum products containing carbon, the maximum temperature should be 650°C (1202°F). In this way, proper fit and uncontaminated alloys are obtained.

128. Ans. (d) Platinum *Ref: Phillips, 11th ed. p 652*

Platinum has high fusion temperature and is one of the eight noble metals. It whitens the alloy and is resistant to tarnish and corrosion. On the other hand, addition of large amounts of copper decreases fusion temperature. Iridium, Ruthenium, Rhenium—help to decrease the grain size, they are added in small quantities (about 100 to 150 ppm). Platinum—also helps to reduce grain size but it is added in large amount, i.e. 3%.

129. Ans. (a) Casting shrinkage *Ref: Phillips, 11th ed. p 316*

The compensation for the shrinkage inherent in the dental casting procedure may be obtained by either one or both of the following two methods.

- Setting or hygroscopic expansion of the investment.
- Thermal expansion of the investment.

Both of these techniques are currently in use and are commonly termed the hygroscopic expansion (low-heat) method and the thermal expansion (high heat) method, respectively. As their names alone might indicate, the high heat method requires thermal expansion of the investment to occur between room temperature and a high temperature (650°C–700°C for gypsum-bonded investments and up to 1050°C for phosphate-bonded investment).

130. Ans. (a) Produce a more uniform expansion and the expansion will not be in a vertical direction hence no distortion *Ref: Phillips, 11th ed. p 323-324*

- The most commonly used technique to provide investment expansion is to line the walls of the ring with a ring liner.
- The use of one liner (C) increases the normal setting expansions compared with no liner. Using a thicker liner material or two layers of liner (D) provides even greater semi hygroscopic expansion and also affords a more unrestricted normal setting expansion of the investment.

- The expansion of the investment is always greater in the unrestricted longitudinal direction than in the radical direction, that is toward the ring. Therefore it is desirable to reduce the expansions in the longitudinal direction. Placing the liner somewhat short (3.25 mm) of the ends of the ring tends to produce a more uniform expansion; thus there is less chance for distortion of the wax pattern and the mold.

131. Ans. (d) 25 *Ref: Phillips 11th ed. p 273*

According to ADA specification number 25 gypsum products are classified as:

Type I: impression plaster

Type II: dental plaster

Type III: dental stone

Type IV: die stone, low expansion

Type V: die stone, high expansion

132. Ans. (b) Starch *Ref: Mannapallil's, 2nd ed. p 92*

- Starch swells up when placed under water and expands and helps to separate the impression from cast.

133. Ans. (b) ZOE bite registration paste *Ref: Philips 11th ed. p 253*

- ZOE impression paste does not give any resistance for closing of mandible and are more stable than wax. Hence are more accurate.

134. Ans. (a) Hydrochloric acid *Ref: Philips 11th ed. p 336*

- Pickling is the process of removing oxide and tarnish of casting made with gold based or palladium based alloys which uses gypsum bonded investment for casting.
- Best picking solution for gypsum bonded investment is 50% hydrochloric acid.

135. Ans. (a) Placing in saturated solution of calcium sulphate *Ref: Phillips 11th ed. p 94*

- Immersion in water leads to dissolution of gypsum, hence not indicated.
- Best method is to soak it into water containing plaster debris

136. Ans. (b) Invest the wax pattern immediately *Ref: Philips 11th ed. p 289-290*

- Distortion of wax pattern can occur during the formation or removal from the die or mouth.
- Waxes have elastic memory and tend to return to their original shape after their manipulation.
- Wax pattern should be retained in the die for many hours so that distortion is avoided and equilibrium is reached.
- Casting have best fit when the wax pattern in invested soon after its removal from the preparation.

137. Ans. (d) Stearlic acid *Ref: Phillips 11th ed. p 250*

Impression compound shellac, stearic acid and gutta-percha are added to improve plasticity and workability. Prolonged immersion or over heading of impression compound will lead to its brittle and growing as the material will lead out having low molecular weight as stearic acid.

138. Ans. (c) Stannous octate *Ref: Phillips 11th ed. p 213*

- The curving of condensation silicone involves a reaction of tri and tetra functional alkyl silicates in presence of stannous octate.
- Ethyl alcohol is a by-product of the condensation setting reaction.

139. Ans. (d) Using humidor *Ref: Phillips 11th ed. p 247*

If pouring of the impression was delayed it should be rinsed in tap water, disinfected, wrapped in a surgical paper towel, saturated with water and placed in a sealed plastic bag or a humidor.

140. Ans. (a) Within 6 mm of the open end of the ring *Ref: Philips 11th ed. p. 322*

The length of the sprue former depends on the length of the casting ring. If the sprue is too short the wax pattern may be so far removed from the end of the casting ring that gases cannot be adequately vented to permit the molten alloy to fill the ring completely. When these gases are not completely eliminated, porosity may result. Therefore the sprue length should be adjusted so that the top of the wax pattern is within 6 mm of the open end of the ring for gypsum bonded investments with the higher-strength phosphate bonded investment. It may be possible to position the wax pattern within 3–4 mm of the top of the investment.

141. Ans. (b) Decrease setting time *Ref: Philips 11th ed. p 265*

Setting time is decreased by
- Gypsum particle as impurities
- Finer particle size of hemihydrates
- Decreased water power ratio
- Faster mixing breaks the particles which in turn act as crystals and hence increases the speed of setting. Hence, the setting time decrease.
- Temperature above 50 degree retards the reaction.

142. Ans. (d) Alginate and agar *Ref: Philips 11th ed. p 245*

Laminate Technique: It is a recent modification to the traditional agar procedure. It consists of combined agar-alginate technique.
- The hydrocolloid in the tray is replaced with a mix of chilled alginate that bonds with the agar.
- Nevertheless, it is the most cost-effective way of producing an impression with adequate detail.

143. Ans. (a) Gold alloy *Ref: Philips 11th ed. p 296*

Generally there are two types of investment:
- Gypsum bonded investment
- Phosphate bonded investment

The Gypsum-based investment is used for gold alloy inlays, onlays crowns and FPD's.

The phosphate based investment used to produce frameworks for metal-ceramic prostheses and for some base metal alloys.

ADA specification No. 2 for casting investment for dental gold alloys encompasses 3 types of investment, i.e.
- Type I for casting of inlays or crowns
- Type II for casting of inlays, onlays or crowns
- Type III for construction of partial dentures with gold alloys.

144. Ans. (b) Silicone rubbers *Ref: Craig's 12th ed. p 541-543*

- Soft or plasticized acrylic, vinyl polymers, and copolymers, as well as natural and silicone rubber products, are used as denture liners for patients having irritation of the denture bearing mucosa, area of severe undercuts, or congenital or acquired defects of the palate. Some products have an inhibitory effect on the growth of candida albicans while others appear to support the growth of microorganism. Desirable properties are (a) high bond strength to the denture base, (b) dimensional stability of the liner during and after processing, (c) long term resilience, (d) low water sorption, (e) color stability, (f) biocompatibility.

- The silicones were more stable.
- Soft liners have an important place in denture prosthetics but require improved strength, improved adhesion to the denture base.

145. Ans. (c) Too rapid polymerization and (d) Incomplete polymerization caused by premature removal from mouth *Ref: Philips 11th ed. p 244*

Causes of rough or uneven surface of elastomeric impression:

- Too rapid polymerization due to high ambient temperatures.
- Incomplete polymerization caused by premature removal from mouth.
- Inhibitory of polymerization by accidental incorporation of impurities as in case of addition silicone.
- Improper proportioning of case of catalyst particularly condensation silicones.

146. Ans. (b) Korrecta type 1 *Ref: Stewart Rudd Kuebker 2nd ed. p 385*

- The fluid wax impression is used either to make a reline impression for existing partial denture or to correct the distal extension edentulous ridge portion of the original master cast.
- The term fluid wax is used to the waxes that have the ability to flow at mouth temperature. The most frequently used fluid waxes are Iowa Wax, developed by Dr Smith.
- Korrecta Wax no 1 was used to support the softer no 4 wax if extension beyond that length. The no 1 wax, however neither available nor is an example of fluid wax.

147. Ans. (b) Cusp tips *Ref: Shillnburg 3rd ed. p 368*

- The sprue former is a small diameter tube made of wax, plastic or metal. One end of the sprue former is attached to the wax pattern and the other end to the crucial former.
- The sprue former should be attached to the wax pattern at its point of greatest bulk, amending centre occlusal contact if possible.
- To a flat wall of the mold, a "hot spot" may be created at the point If the sprue is directed at a right angle.
- Hence the most correct answer from the given option is "CUSP TIPS".

148. Ans. (d) Polyvinyl chloride *Ref: Nallasawamy p 714*

Here according to the exam paper key answer is Polyvinyl chloride but all references studies shows that it is used in maxillo-facial prosthesis.

149. Ans. (a) Making of impressions *Ref: www.sahealth.sa.gov.au/.../Prevention+of+Endo+or+Infection+of+Prosth.*

Prophylaxis always required Dental Procedures

- Extractions
- Periodontal procedures including surgery, subgingival scaling and root planning
- Replanting avulsed teeth
- Other surgical procedures (e.g. implant placement, apicoectomy)

Prophylaxis is not required for Dental Procedures:

- Oral examination
- Infiltration and block local anaesthetic injection
- Restorative dentistry
- Supragingival rubber dam clamping and placement of rubber dam
- Intracanal endodontic procedures
- Removal of sutures

- Impressions and construction of dentures
- Orthodontic bracket placement and adjustment of fixed appliances
- Application of gels
- Intraoral radiographs
- Supragingival plaque removal

150. Ans. (c) Pseudoplastic properties *Ref: Philips 11th ed. p 220*

Pseudoplastic liquid:
- It is observed in monophase elastomeric impression material which is also termed as single mix.
- Here, the viscosity changes according to the shear exerted.
- It can be used for both as a tray as well as syringe material.
- When mixed on a paper pad the viscosity is more and so can be used as tray material.
- When loaded in a syringe the amount of force exerted increases the viscosity. This is called shear thinning pseudoplastic behavior. It has greater flow as a syringe material.

151. Ans. (c) Aluminium oxide *Ref: Phillips 11th ed. p 373*

- In air abrasive technology the abrasive particles used is 25 to 30 µm aluminium oxide.
- These are used to remove enamel, dentin, and restorative material.
- It is beneficial due to its following advantage:
  - Minimal heat generation.
  - Minimal vibration.
  - Minimum microfracture.
- **Uses of air abrasive:**
  - Cavity preparation.
  - Removal of defective composite fillings.
  - Endodontic access through porcelain crown.
  - Superficial removal of stains.
  - Cleaning of tooth surface before adhesive bonding.
  - Roughening of internal surfaces of indirect porcelain.
  - Composite restoration.

152. Ans. (b) Greater the hygroscopic expansion *Ref: Phillips 11th ed. p 302*

- The fineness of silica particle is directly proportional to the hygroscopic expansion.
- Finer the particle size, more will be hygroscopic expansion.
- Normal setting expansion is 0.4 to 0.6%.
- Normal hygroscopic expansion is 1.2 to 2.2%.

153. Ans. (b) Putty used first and light body used second *Ref: Phillips 11th ed. p 221*

- In a putty wash technique putty is used first and the light body is used second.
- It is used to take impression by heavy filled elastomers such as condensation silicone. There are 3 ways of putty wash technique, i.e.
  1. One stage impression
     - Also known as twin mix or laminate technique.
     - Here, putty and wash are recorded simultaneously.
  2. Two stage unspace—Here, putty is recorded first and relieved by a thin layer of wash after setting.
  3. Two stage spaced—Here, a space is created for the wash by the use of polythene.

154. Ans. (b) Low investment permeability *Ref: Phillips 11th ed. p 346*

- Back pressure porosity is a void in a casting due to the inability of the air inside the mold to be adequately displaced by the incoming molten metal.
- It can be seen as a concave depression on the surface of the casting.
- Dense investment will prevent air venting.

155. Ans. (a) Impression plaster *Ref: Phillips 11th ed. p 273*

- Gypsum products used in dentistry are based on calcium sulphate hemihydrates ($CaSO_4 . 2H_2O$).
- According to ANS1/ADA specification number 25. The types of gypsum products are:
  - Type I- dental plaster. Impression plaster.
  - Type II- Dental plaster (Model plaster).
  - Type III Dental stone- Die.
  - Type IV- Dental stone, die, high strength, low expansion.
  - Type V- Dental stone, Die, High strength, high expansion.

156. Ans. (c) Less water/powder ratio *Ref: Phillip's 11th ed. p 265, 270*

- Potassium sulphate is added to the mixture in order to increase accelerate the setting as well as to reduces the expansion.
- Sodium chloride and borax can also be used to reduce the expansion.

157. Ans. (b) Gas inclusion porosity *Ref: Phillip's 11th ed. p 344*

Gas inclusion porosity

- It is due to gas which is mechanically entrapped by molten metal in a mold or carried during casting procedure.
- Voids are spherical and larger in size in compare to pin hole porosity.

158. Ans. (c) 40 ml of water + 15 gm of powder *Ref: Phillip's 11th ed. p 241*

- According to the most of the manufacturer's the water/powder ratio of alginate is 3:1. So the option c is more appropriate from all the given option. As:
  - When water is 3 ml the powder will be 1 gm.
  - So, when powder = 15 gm.
  - Water will be 3 × 15 = 45 gm or 45 ml.
  - Hence, Water:Powder = 45:15 or 3:1.

159. Ans. (b) Surfactant *Ref: Phillip's 11th ed. p 215*

A-silicone impression materials (addition silicones, poly vinyl siloxane, vinyl siloxane). Supplied as a two-component 1:1 system

Composition:

Base paste:

- Vinyl terminated polysiloxane polymer
- Pt catalyst
- Filler (cristobalite, talc)
- Surfactant (hydrophilic agent)

Catalyst:

- Vinyl terminated polysiloxane polymer
- Cross-linking agent
- Filler, silicone oil (adjust viscosity of duplicating materials)

160. Ans. (c) Electrodeposited silver *Ref: Phillip's 12th ed. p 213, 434*

- During fabrication, electrodeposited silver has a hazardous potential.
- During plating procedure, silver cyanide is used as a electrolyte and hydrogen cyanide gas is given off.
- Polysulfide impression electroplated easily while hydrocolloid impressions electroplated with difficulty.

161. Ans. (d) Accelerator *Ref: Phillip's 12th ed., p. 252*

Composition of Zinc Oxide Eugenol:

I Base (Tube no. 1)

- Zinc oxide- 80 to 87%.
- Magnesium chloride- 1%.
- Innert vegetable or mineral oil- 12 to 19%.

II Accelerator or catalyst (Tube no. 2)

- Eugenol- 12 to 15%.
- Gum- 50 to 58%.
- Filler 16 to 20%.
- Lanolin- 3%.
- Resinous balsam- 5 to 10%.
- Accelerator ($MgCl_2$, $CaCl_2$ or moisture)- 4 to 5%.

162. Ans. (c) Alginate *Ref: Phillip's 12th ed. p 234*

- It is a thermoplastic compound, i.e. it softens when heated and hardens when cooled.
- This process does not involve a chemical reaction.

Impression compound is available in 2 forms:

- Stick form: used for modifying impression trays. Softening temperature is 700°C
- Sheet form: used to take impressions of the mouth. Softening temperature is 55-600°C.

Properties

- Poor surface detail
- High coefficient of thermal expansion (contraction of up to 0.3% when removed from mouth to room temperature)
- Distorts wen removed over undercut areas
- Mucocodisplacive
- Poor dimensional stability
- Can be modified by re-heating
- Non-toxic and non-irritant
- Good shelf life

Advantages

- Non-irritant and non-toxic
- Reusable (but with re-use the constituents are leached out)
- Can be reheated and readapted
- Can support other materials for wash impressions
- Mucocompressive

Disadvantages

- Poor dimensional stability
- Poor surface detail
- Expansion coefficient
- Will distort if removed from undercuts

163. Ans. (b) Potassium nitrate *Ref: Phillip's 12th ed. p 374*

- Dentinal Hypersensitivity (DH) is characterized by short sharp pain arising from exposed dentin in response to stimuli typically thermal, evaporative, tactile, osmotic or chemical—that cannot be ascribed to any other dental defect or disease.
- Potassium nitrate has been used as a desensitizing agent to treat dentinal hypersensitivity.
- The effectiveness of a potassium nitrate is evaluated both in the form of a toothpaste and a mouthwash in a clinical study.

164. Ans. (a) Syringe agar and chilled tray alginate *Ref: Phillip's 12th ed. p 245*

Laminate technique/alginate agar method:

- In this technique agar in the syringe is injected on to the area to be recorded, an impression tray containing chilled alginate is placed over it.
- The alginate sets by chemical reaction whereas agar gel by means of contact with cool alginate. Since agar is in contact with teeth maximum detail care be obtained.

165. Ans. (c) Silex *Ref: Restorative Dental Material by Floyd Avery, 1st ed. p 411*

- The purpose of polishing is to create a smoother finish on the restoration or the tooth surface.
- Once a restoration has been placed in the mouth, recontouring, finishing, and polishing the surface are all necessary.
- By restoring normal contours, smoothing margins, and creating a high luster shine, the overall appearance and longevity of the restoration itself are increased.
- When polishing an amalgam restoration, light, intermittent strokes with a fine pumice or fine silex in a slurry mix can be used but it is important not to overpolish.
- To avoid overpolishing, rinse and evaluate the restoration frequently.
- Most amalgam restorations can be polished at least 24 hours after placement. This allows sufficient time for the amalgam to set.
- However, the current use of high copper amalgams can be polished about 8–12 minutes after placement because they set much faster.

166. Ans. (c) Improves smoothness *Ref: Phillip, 11th ed. p 286*

- Gum Dammar or Dammar Resin is natural resin added to paraffin to improve its smoothness in molding to render it more resistant to cracking and flaking.
- It increases the toughness of the wax and enhances smoothness and luster of the surface.

167. Ans. (b) Addition silicon *Ref: Phillips, 11th ed. p 227*

- Addition silicons are also known as "vinyl poly-siloxane"
- Addition silicons are the most ideally elastic of current available material
- These materials exhibit the lowest permanent distortion after strain in compression
- Relative amount of permanent deformation following strain in compression increases in the order
- Polysulfide, condensation silicon, addition silicon, polyether

168. Ans. (b) Reciprocating rheometer *Ref: Phillips, 11th ed. p 223*

- In the British standard test, a reciprocating rheometer is used to measure the working and setting time of elastomers
- Penetrometer tests have been used to assess both

169. Ans. (d) Suck-back porosity *Ref: Phillips, 11th ed. p 343-344*

- Hot spot is created by the hot metal impinging from the sprue channel on a point of the mold wall
- This hot spot causes the local region to freeze last and results in what is known as 'suck back porosity'
- Often occurs at occlusoaxial or incisoaxial line angle that is not well rounded
- It can be eliminated by flaring the point of sprue attachment and reducing the mold-melt temperature differential, that is lowering the casting temperature by 300°C.

170. Ans. (b) Impression wax *Ref: Phillips, 11th ed. p 208*

- ZnOE impression paste and impression plaster are called mucostatic impression materials
- This is because they do not compress the tissues during seating of the impression tray
- They are ideal for making impression of edentulous jaws

171. Ans. (a) Water *Ref: Philips 11th ed. p 235*

Composition of Agar:

- Agar Basic constituent composing 13–17% for tray material and 6–8% for syringe material form the dispersed phase
- Borates 0.2–0.5% - Improves the strength of the gel
- Potassium sulphate 1–2%. It counters retarding effect of borates, allows proper setting of the cast or die
- Wax, hard 0.5–1% acts as a filler
- Thixotropic material 0.3–0.5% - as plasticizer, e.g. Glycerine and Thymol. Thymol acts as a bactericide too.
- Alkyl benzoates 0.1% acts as a preservative and prevents growth of molds
- Traces of coloring and flavoring agents for patients comfort, to improve appearance and tests and differentiate various phases of setting in chromatic materials
- Water 84–85% the major compartment while acts as the dispersion or continuous phase.

172. Ans. (a) Calcium *Ref: Philips 11th ed. p 245*

- 2 paste system, one containing the alginate sol, other contains calcium reactor.
- These are said to contain silicone and have superior tear resistance.

173. Ans. (a) Dry *Ref: Philips 11th ed. p 225-226*

- Addition silicon and Polyether impression can be stored up to 24 hours to a week without distortion
- But Polyether absorbs water and might also leach its plasticizer. Hence it should be kept in dry, cool environment to retain its accuracy.

174. Ans. (c) Reduction in plasticity *Ref: Philips 11th ed. p 250*

- The compound disc is completely immersed in a water bath at 55-60°C for about 4–5 minutes to ensure complete softening. Gauze is placed at the bottom of the water bath to prevent adherence. However if it is left in too long some of the constituents may be leached out into the water bath, altering the properties of the material (it is often the plasticizer stearic acid that is leached out).
- If the compound is kneaded water will become incorporated and act as a plasticizer. The compound is loaded on to the tray and firm pressure is used to seat the tray home in the mouth.
- After the impression has been taken it is carefully examined, a common mistake is not softening the compound enough. In this is the case the impression can be reheated in a separate bowl of water (cross infection control) and the impression is repeated.
- The fusion temperature of compound is 43°C.
- The fusion temperature of the imp compound indicates a definite reduction in plasticity during cooling
- Poor surface detail

- High coefficient of thermal expansion (contraction of up to 0.3% when removed from mouth to room temperature)
- Distorts when removed over undercut areas
- Mucocodisplacive
- Poor dimensional stability
- Can be modified by re-heating
- Non-toxic and non-irritant
- Good shelf life

175. Ans. (b) Microporosity *Ref: Philips 11th ed. p 343,344*

Microporosity:

- That part of the pore space that has a characteristic dimension less than 1 micron.
- In general, this includes not only very small pores but also the porosity associated with surface roughness.
- The water in this pore space is part of the capillary-bound water and the small-pore water. Water in micropores is not expected to flow on production.
- The term is also defined as porosity that cannot be seen at magnifications less than 50x.
- Occurs due to solidification shrinkage
- Mostly found in fine grain alloy castings when the solidification is too rapid for the micro-voids to segregate to the liquid pool
- Commonly not detectable unless the casting is sectioned

176. Ans. (a) Leucite *Ref: Philips 11th ed. p 668*

Leucite [$K(AlSi_2O_6)$]

- Leucite is a potassium-aluminium-silicate
- Formed by Feldspar at 1150°C to 1530°C by incongruent melting
- Leucite is a major crystalline component of dental porcelains.
- The presence of tetragonal leucite in dental porcelains increases their coefficients of thermal expansion due to its high coefficient of thermal expansion (2025 × 10^{-6}/°C).
- This is particularly useful for those porcelains designed for bonding to precious metals and nickel alloys.
- Feldspar glasses have only (< 10 ppm/°C)
- Mainly used in Leucite enriched porcelain

177. Ans. (d) Altering the temperature of water *Ref: Philips 11th ed. p 242*

Controlling setting time of alginate

- The best method of controlling the gelation time of alginate-type hydrocolloid materials is to alter the temperature of the water used in the mix.
- The higher the temperature of the water, the faster gelation will occur.
- Higher temperatures accelerate the chemical reaction.
- The temperature of the water must be regulated carefully within a few degrees of that recommended by the manufacturer to obtain a constant and reliable gelation time.
- The average recommended temperature of water is 70°F (21°C).
- Changing the water-powder ratio and the mixing time will alter the gelation time, but these methods of control also impair certain properties of the material.
- The amount of the retarder in the material can be regulated only by the manufacturer since the action of the retarder changes the nature of the material.

178. Ans. (a) Static creep *Ref: Philips 11th ed. p 495*

- Creep is defined as the time dependent plastic strain of a material under a static load or constant stress near its melting point.
- Static creep—It is a time dependent deformation produced in a completely set solid subjected to a constant stress.
- Dynamic creep—It produced when the applied stress is fluctuating, such as in fatigue type test.
- Sag resistance is the ability of metal to resist creep under its own weight.

DIRECT RESTORATIVE MATERIALS

179. Ans. (a) Carboxyl group of polymer chains *Ref: Phillips 11th ed. p 475*

- Glass ionomer cement is a tooth colored material, introduced by Wilson and Kent in 1972.
- GIC bond chemically to tooth structure and release fluoride for relatively long period.
- Bonding occurs due to the reaction occurs between carboxyl group of poly acid and calcium of hydroxyl apatite.
- Bonding with enamel is higher than that of dentin, due to greater inorganic content.

180. Ans. (c) GIC *Ref: Phillips 11th ed. p 482*

- When the tooth surface is loss due to the chemomechanical wear is termed as erosion.

Uses of GIC:

- Anterior esthetic restoration material for class III and V restoration.
- For luting.
- For core build up.
- For eroded area.
- For ART.
- As an orthodontic brackets adhesive.
- As restoration for deciduous teeth.
- Used in lamination/sandwich technique.

181. Ans. (a) Beelby layer *Ref: Vimal Sikri 2nd ed. p 302*

- The polishing agent remove material from the surface molecule and thus provide a very smooth surface. This microcrystalline layer is referred to as a polish layer or Beilby layer.
- Polishing can be done by rubber abrasive points, fine particle discs, stripes, flexible paper, backed discs, finishing burs, and polishing paste used with rotary instruments.

182. Ans. (a) Hydroxyl ion *Ref: Internet*

- As soon as the fluoride ion is released, it is replaced by hydroxyl and phosphate ion in order to maintain the electrolyte balance in the cement matrix.

183. Ans. (c) Of the ease of placement over the area to be acid etched, without getting spread

Ref: Phillips 11th ed. p 384,385

- The etchant is supplied in the form of aqueous gel in order to allow its precise placement over a specific area which is not possible, if it is used in solution form.
- The gel form of phosphoric acid is made by adding colloidal silica or polymer beads to the acid.
- Solution form is also useful in the region where larger area is needed to be etched. For example, composite veneer.

184. Ans. (b) Increases the surface energy and wets the dentin surface *Ref: Sturdevant. 4th ed. p 245; 5th ed. p 210 or Vimal Sikri 2nd ed. p 361*

- Primers are the monomers dissolved in solvents like water, acetone or alcohol.
- The primer is used to displace residual moisture, thus creating a surface upon which the hydrophobic bonding resin can adhere.
- The primer assists the adhesive to flow into and penetrate the etched tooth surface.
- The primer often contains a hydrophilic portion that interacts with the moisture present in the tooth structure, as well as a hydrophobic end that provides bonding sites for the methacrylate monomers in the bonding resin.
- A dentin primer increases the surface energy and wets the dentin surface.

185. Ans. (c) 5 to 50 *Ref: en.wikipedia.org/wiki/Tooth_*

Enamel

- Invented in 1955, acid-etching employs dental etchants and is used frequently when bonding dental restoration to teeth.
- This is important for long-term use of some materials, such as composites and sealants.
- By dissolving minerals in enamel, etchants remove the outer 10 micrometers on the enamel surface and make a porous layer 550 micrometers deep.
- This roughens the enamel microscopically and results in a greater surface area on which to bond.
- Use of 30–40% of phosphoric acids caused a dissolution of about 10 μm of organic component of enamel.

186. Ans. (b) Polycarboxylate *Ref: Phillips 11th ed. p 469*

Zinc polycarboxylate cement:

- According to biocompatibility with pulp cements arranging in decreasing order.
- ZOE and polycarboxylate <GIC < $ZnPO_4$ < resin cement and silicate cements.

Reaction of different cements towards pulp

Most pulpally kind	*Moderately pulpally kind cement*	*Least pulpally kind cement*
• Polycarboxylate. • Hydrous GIC • ZOE	Semihydrous GIC $ZnPO_4$ with a protective varnish	Semihydrous GIC and $ZnPO_4$ without a varnish and resin cements

187. Ans. (b) Dehydrated ZnO acts with dehydrated eugenol *Ref: Vimal Sikri 2nd ed. p 214*

Setting reaction of zinc oxide and eugenol:

- Eugenol is colorless liquid which is slightly soluble in water, ethanol and chloroform.
- Eugenol is not react with anhydrous zinc oxide.
- Water plays an important role in the setting of ZnO and eugenol and, it is also a byproduct of the reaction. It acts as an initiator of the setting reaction, i.e. $ZnO + H_2O$?Zn $(OH)_2$ Zn $(OH)_2$ + 2E (eugenol) ?ZnE_2 (Zinc eugenolate) + $2H_2O$
- Here, when zinc oxide react with water forms a hydroxide of zinc.
- Reaction is autocatalytic in nature.

188. Ans. (c) Penetrating *Ref: Phillips 11th ed. p 517, 519*

- High copper amalgam is less susceptible to corrosion due to the reduced amount or absence of tin mercury phase.
- It does not possess gamma 2 phase in the final set mass.
- It is the material of choice with improved mechanical properties, corrosion characteristics better marginal integrity

- Low copper and high copper amalgams undergo two kinds of corrosion, i.e. chemical and electrochemical corrosion.
- Chemical corrosion is generally found on the occlusal surface and produce a black Ag-S tarnish film.
- Electrochemical corrosion is occurs when amalgamcomes in direct contact with the adjacent metallic restoration such as gold crown.

189. Ans. (a) MTA *Ref: Grossman's 12th ed. p 317-319*

Mineral trioxide aggregate (MTA) was developed at Loma Linda University in the 1990s as a root-end filling material.

- Introduced by Mahmoud torabinejad.
- It is used in surgical as well as in non-surgical procedure such as:
  - Root end fillings.
  - Direct pulp caping.
  - Apexification
  - Perforation repair in roots.
- MTA may be ideal material for use against bone.
- MTA when hydrated becomes a colloidal gel that solidify to form a strong and impermeable barrier.
- Excellent sealing properties.
- Least cytotoxic compared to other materials.
- Facilities regeneration of periodontal ligament.
- It is insoluble in tissue fluids.
- It is an ideal root end filling materials as it adhere and adapt to the dentinal walls of the root end, preparation, it also prevent the leakage of microorganisms and their byproduct into the periradicular tissues.

190. Ans. (a) Cyanoacrylate *Ref: Dental Hard Tissue and Bonding by George Eliades, 1st ed. p 76*

- In general, cyanoacrylate is an acrylic resin that rapidly polymerises in the presence of water (specifically hydroxide ions), forming long, strong chains, joining the bonded surfaces together.
- Majorly used as a die hardener.
- Cyanoacrylate is used as a forensic tool to capture latent fingerprints on non-porous surfaces like glass, plastic, etc. Cyanoacrylate is warmed to produce fumes that react with the invisible fingerprint residues and atmospheric moisture to form a white polymer (polycyanoacrylate) on the fingerprint ridges.
- Low-viscosity resin used as moisture-active adhesive

191. Ans. (c) 5 MPa *Ref: Phillips 11th ed. p. 402*

- As we all know that, composite resin is set by polymerization.
- Shrinkage occurs during polymerization, because when we cure monomer, it is converted from an aggregate of free flowing molecule to a rigid assembly of cross linked polymer chain.
- Generally monomer molecules are held together by Van der Wall forces, but after polymerization, the monomers are held together by the strong covalent bond having potential energy space of 20% less in compare to unreacted monomer.
- It result the volume contraction and shrinkage stress.
- 7 MPa is the magnitude of stress in this condition.

192. Ans. (a) GIC *Ref: V Sikri 2nd ed. p 433*

Erosion is defined as the loss of the surface of tooth due to chemomechanical wear. It is generally cause by exogeneous and endogeneous acid. Regurgitation of stomach acid can cause erosion in the maxillary anteriors.

Resin modified GIC is widely used in class V, erosion, abrasion cavities and in rampant caries also.

193. Ans. (c) Carboxyl bond *Ref: Phillips 11th ed. p 475*

- One of the most important characteristic of GIC is to adhere chemically to mineralized tooth tissues by the carboxyl group.
- It exhibit the chelation of carboxyl group of the polyacid with the calcium of enamel and dentin.
- It requires, the tooth surface to be cleaned of debris and smear layer and have proper conditioning prior to the placement of GIC.

194. Ans. (a) The area is re-etched before restoration *Ref: V Sikri 2nd ed. p 402*

- Etching should be done with 37% phosphoric acid which creates the microporosite on the surface of etched enamel or dentin.
- Etchant should be applied just for 10 to 15 seconds.
- Etchant timing is increased in case of deciduous tooth.
- Gel etchant is preferred over liquid etchant.
- After etching the surface energy of enamel is increased.
- During etching the field of work should be free from debris and moisture.
- After etching the field should be dried, it appear clean, white and frosted.
- If it is contaminated with saliva it should be re-etched. Until we gain completely etched isolated surface for the application of dentin bonding agent.

195. Ans. (b) Migration, gelation and setting contraction *Ref: Sikri S 2nd ed. p 430*

Setting reaction: Stages based on the work of crisp and Wilson 1972–1974

- Decomposition: Of glass and release of cement forming metal ions (Al^{3+} and Ca^{+})
- Migration: Of these metal ions into the aqueous phase of the cement.
- Gelation: Of the polyacid by metal ions leading to set.
- Post set hardening: When metal ions become increasingly bound to the polyacid chain (continues for 24 hours).
- Further Slow maturation: Take place even after 24 hours. Translucency develops further as does resistance of desiccation and acid attack.

196. Ans. (c) Decrease Hg release on mastication *Ref: Craig 12th ed. p 238*

Function of some ingredients of amalgam:

- Selenium—Improves the biocompatibility of amalgam.
- Indium—Decrease the mercury vapour release during mastication.
- Platinum—Hardens alloy and corrosion resistant.
- Palladium—Hardens and whitens alloy.
- Mercury—Gives plasticity and softness. Essential for setting reaction.
- Zinc—Quickens the setting time, increases ultimate strength, de oxidizes.
- Copper—Decreases flow, increases strength and hardness, quick setting.
- Tin—Decreases expansion, helps in amalgamation.
- Silver—Increases strength and setting expansion, decreases flow and setting time, resist tarnish and corrosion, improves color.

197. Ans. (b) To increase the surface free energy of dentin *Ref: Phillips. 11th ed. p. 402*

Primer

The primer is a resin-based liquid with highly hydrophilic properties, which makes it very effective on dentin. The application of a primer increases the surface energy of the dentin. It infiltrates the exposed collagen weave, surrounds the fibres and displaces the water content.

- The special properties of the primer or bonding agent allow it to infiltrate deep inside the dentinal tubules and bond with the collagen fibres.

- The moistness of the dentin prevents infiltration of the hydrophobic adhesive after conditioning. This is why hydrophobic conditioning of the dentin is required beforehand with a primer that contains amphiphilic monomers, e.g. HEMA, PENTA, or 4-META, in organic solvents.
- By using solvents such as ethanol or acetones/H_2O, the monomers are able to infiltrate inside the organic structure. This displaces the water content inside the dentine tubules and replaces it with the monomers.
- As aqueous solvents evaporate more slowly than organic solvents, it is important to know the solvent content of the primer and take this into account during application.
- Great care should be taken during clinical application of the primer, which should be allowed to react for a minimum of 30 s. At the end of the reaction time the volatile components (solvents) are evaporated with an indirect jet of air (pointed towards the dental mirror).
- A thin monomer film remains after the solvent has been completely evaporated. The primer in the dentine renders it hydrophobic and compatible with the adhesive.

198. Ans. (a) Eugenol is the plasticizer *Ref: Phillips. 11th ed. p. 489*

The chemical composition of ZOE is typically:[3]

- Zinc oxide, ~69.0%
- White rosin, ~29.3%
- Zinc acetate, ~1.0% (improves strength)
- Zinc stearate, ~0.7% (acts as accelerator)
- Liquid (Eugenol, ~85%, Olive oil ~15%)
- ZOE impression pastes are dispensed as two separate pastes. One tube contains zinc oxide and vegetable or mineral oil; the other contains eugenol and rosin.
- The vegetable or mineral oil acts as a plasticizer and aids in offsetting the action of the eugenol as an irritant.
- Oil of cloves, which contains 70% to 85% eugenol, is sometimes used in preference to eugenol because it produces less burning sensation for patients when it contacts the soft tissues.
- The addition of rosin to the paste in the second tube facilitates the speed of the reaction and yields a smoother, more homogenous product.
- Canada balsam and Peru balsam are often used to increase flow and improve mixing properties.
- If the mixed paste is too thin or lacks body before it sets, a filler (such as a wax) or an inert powder (such as kaolin, talc, or diatomaceous earth) may be added to one or both of the original pastes.

199. Ans. (a) Surface conditioning of tooth is required *Ref: Phillips 12th ed. p. 326*

- Surface conditioning of tooth with mild acid is necessary for proper bond formation between the tooth and restoration.
- Hybrid ionomer containing non-reactive filler particle less carb0xylic acid is available for bonding to tooth structure and dentin bonding system is needed.

200. Ans. (c) Less marginal breakdown *Ref: Phillips. 11th ed. p. 504*

On the basis of copper content, amalgam is of two types i.e.

- Low copper amalgam (<6%)
- High copper amalgam (13 to 30% of copper)
  - High copper amalgam have improved mechanical property like resistance to corrosion, less marginal breakdown, low creep, good compressive strength and better marginal integrity.
  - This all, improved quality of high copper amalgam is due to elimination of g2 phase (SnHg)

201. Ans. (a) Cyanoacralates *Ref: Adhesives and Sealants by David J Dunn p 22*

- Cyanoacrylate adhesives are known for their fast adhesion and ability to bond a wide variety of substrates.
- Cyanoacrylate provide good moisture resistance

202. Ans. (b) Microfilled composite *Ref: Phillips. 11th ed. p. 419*

The values of water sorption for each are as follows:

- Conventional GIC 0.5 to 0.7 mg/cm^2;
- Resin-modified ionomer 0.5 to 0.6 mg/cm^2;
- Light-cured GIC less than conventional GIC, which is 1.25 mg/cm^2;
- Traditional composite 0.5 0.7 mg/cm^2
- Microfilled composite 1.4 to 1.7 mg/cm^2,
- Hybrid composite 0.5 to 0.7 mg/m^2

Hence, the highest solubility is shown by one that absorbs most water.

203. Ans. (d) 100% *Ref: Phillips 11th ed. p 198*

- Approximately 90 to 95% methyl mercury is absorbed from the gut and it is one of the most toxic form of mercury.
- 50 µg of Hg/mm^3 is considered safe and it is the maximum level of occupational exposure.
- Mercury is fourteen times denser than H_2O.
- Half life of Hg is 55 days.
- 15 µg/l of Hg in urine and 4 µg/ml of Hg in blood is the acceptable normal level.

204. Ans. (c) 65–85% *Ref: Advances in Mercury Technology p 9*

- Elemental mercury (Hg0)—Approximately 80% of inhaled mercury vapour is absorbed vapour is absorbed via the lungs and retained in the body.
- The amount remain the same whether the inhalation in the body.
- The amount remain the same whether the inhalation is done from nose or mouth.
- Elemental mercury is poorly absorbed in the gastrointestinal tract.
- Skin absorption is insignificant in relation to human exposure to mercury vapour.
- Alkyl mercurials are absorbed completely in GIT and retained in the body.

205. Ans. (a) Low-copper amalgam alloy *Ref: Craig 12th ed. p 243*

	Compressive strength (MPa)			*Tensile strength 24 hr*
Amalgam	*1 hour*	*7 days*	*Creep (%)*	*(MPa)*
Low copper	145	343	2.0	60
Admix	137	431	0.4	48
Single composition	262	510	0.13	64

206. Ans. (d) Glass ionomer cement *Ref: Craig. 12th ed. p. 485*

- Resin cement does not have anticarcinogenic properties.
- Silicate has an irritant effect on pulp and does not bond to the tooth.
- Polycarboxylate bonds to the tooth but is not translucent.
- Hence, the best option is (d).

207. Ans. (c) 35 days *Ref: Phillips 11th ed. p 510 (C)*

- A large expansion can be seen, when zinc containing low and high copper alloy is contaminated by moisture at the time of trituration and condensation.
- Expansion will starts after 3 to 5 days of restoration and may be continuous for a long time (up to a month) until and unless it reaches to it maximum value (400 µm or 4%). The whole procedure is known as delayed expansion.
- Delayed expansion is seen only in zinc containing alloy and it is absent in zinc free alloy.
- It is due to the reaction occurs between the zinc and water.

208. Ans. (c) 8 hours *Ref: Phillips 11th ed. p 515*

- Amalgam gain strength slowly.
- Amalgam gain only 6% compressive strength at the end of 20-min in compare to strength after 1 week.
- Amalgam achieves 70% of the strength by 8 hours.
- Sometime amalgam gain its strength even at the end of a 6-month period.

209. Ans. (d) 0.005–0.01 μm *Ref: Phillips 12th ed. p 281*

Classification of reinforcing filler particles by size	
Class of filler	*Particle size*
Macrofiller	10 to 100 μm
Small/fine filler	0.1 to 10 μm
Midfiller	1 to 10 μm
Minifiller	0.1 to 1 μm
Microfiller	0.01 to 0.1 μm
Nanofiller	0.005 to 0.1 μm

210. Ans. (a) Organically modified composites *Ref: Sikri 2nd ed. p 423*

Ormocer:

- The acronym of organically modified ceramic is ormocer.
- It can be used for anterior as well as posterior restoration.
- Ormocer possess inorganic organic network matrix.
- It is very rigid, high molecular weight, possess performed structure, exhibit low shrinkage during polymerization.
- Ormocer matrix is composed of ceramic polysiloxane (silicone-oxygen chain).

Physical properties:

Fluoride release	Present
Water sorption	10.4 mg/mm^3
Vicker's hardness	80
Compressive strength	420 MPa
Polymerization shrinkage	1.88%

211. Ans. (c) Higher modulus of elasticity *Ref: Phillips- 11th ed. p 463*

Material	*Tensile strength*	*Modulus of elasticity*	*Compressive strength*
Zinc phosphate	5.5 MPa	13.7 GPa	104 MPa
GIC	6.6 MPa	13 GPa	150 MPa

212. Ans. (a) Low viscosity *Ref: Phillips 11th ed. p 397*

- Pit and fissure sealant is a non-invasive procedure.
- If includes the placement of resin sealant onto the deep pits and fissure without out tooth structure.
- It includes several type of resin such as cyanoacrylate polyurethanes, bis GMA.
- Sealant possess low viscosity so that it flow easily into the depth of pit and fissure and wet the surface.
- In order to increase wetting, the surface should be conditioned by acid etching.

213. Ans. (a) GIC *Ref.: http://www.jaypeejournals.com/eJournals/ShowText.aspx?ID=3607&Type=FREE&TYP=*

TOP & IN = eJournals/images/JPLOGO.gif&IID=284&isPDF=YES

- Enamel Decalcification can occur whenever bacterial plaque is retained on the enamel surface for prolonged period.
- Fluoride releasing cements can be used to prevent the demineralization but at the same time cement should to firmly adhere to the tooth under the bands.
- Conventional GIC and resin modified GIC had the least amount of demineralization compared to zinc phosphate and zinc polycarboxylate.
- Conventional GIC showed 6.61 μ while RMGIC showed 6.90 μ demineralization.

214. Ans. (a) W/P ratio *Ref: Craig 12th ed. p 318*

Working time of dental plaster:

- Working time is defined as the time available to use a workable mix.
- It is measured from the moment when the powder is mixed with the water.
- The freshly mixed mass possess a semifluid consistency.
- It can be poured into a mould.
- The viscosity of the mixed mass increases, and mass can no longer flow easily and in this way it was unable to produce the fine details.
- In this way working time of plaster is influenced by W/P ratio.

215. Ans. (a) Initially more than gradually decreases *Ref: V. Sikri 2nd ed. p 434*

- The release of fluoride is one of the main advantages of glass ionomer cements.
- Glass ionomer cements is a filling material with anticariogenic effects.
- However, fluoride release can be influenced by factors such as solubility, fluoride content of the material, nature of the dissolving medium and temperature.
- Although the pattern of fluoride release changes a lot according to the methodology used, researchers agree that greater quantities of fluoride are released during the first days and after that the level of fluoride released falls to a constant level.
- Glass ionomer cements also take up fluoride from the oral environment.
- Glass ionomer cements take up the fluoride from fluoride dentifrice and release it, which means that this material might be looked upon as a "rechargeable slow release fluoride system".

216. Ans. (d) >15 µm *Ref: V Sikri 2nd ed. p 402*

- Invented in 1955, acid-etching employs dental etchants and is used frequently when bonding dental restoration to teeth.
- This is important for long-term use of some materials, such as composites and sealants.
- By dissolving minerals in enamel, etchants remove the outer 10 micrometers on the enamel surface and make a porous layer 550 micrometers deep.
- This roughens the enamel microscopically and results in a greater surface area on which to bond.
- There are three types of patterns formed by acid-etching.
- Type 1 is a pattern where predominantly the enamel rods are dissolved;
- Type 2 is a pattern where predominantly the area around the enamel rods are dissolved; and
- Type 3 is a pattern where there is no evidence left of any enamel rods.
- Besides concluding that type 1 is the most favorable pattern and type 3 the least.

217. Ans. (d) Working time *Ref: Phillips 11th ed. p 526*

Following changes can be noted due to mechanical Trituration

- Increase in strength.
- Smooth carved surface is achieve.
- Luster will retain longer after polishing.
- Physical property remain same but only it shorten the working time.
- Mix may be warm when removed from capsule.

218. Ans. (a) Removes the smear layer *Ref: Vimal Sikri 2nd ed. p 365*

Outstanding features of the material

- Removes smear layer and impurities from the dentin surface without opening dentin tubulae.
- Enhances bonding strength of glass ionomer, resin, and zinc phosphate cements to dentin; helps prevent marginal leakage.
- Fast and economical to use.
- Dentin conditioning can be performed by chemical, thermal or mechanical means
- Dentin Conditioning Gel is a high molecular weight, polyacrylic acid dentin bond conditioner for removing the smear layer from dentin prior to bonding and cementation.
- It is applied to dentin for only 20 seconds prior to placement of glass ionomer cements or other dentin bonding materials.
- The product is thixotropic, stays where placed and washes off easily.

219. Ans. (a) AH26 *Ref: Grossman's 12th ed. p 301*

Sealers are materials used along with a solid core material for observation of the cleared root canal space. They can be divided into four main types:

- Silicone based: Lee Endofill, Roekoseal, Guttaflow.
- Urethane methocrylate: Endoroz, EZ fill.
- Paraformaldehyde containing: Reibler's paste. Abturahon
- ZOE based Wach's, Grossman's, Tubliseal, Kerr's, Endomethasone and Nogenol.
- Resin based AH26, AH plus, Epiphany.
- GIC based Ketac Endo.
- Ca(OH)2 based Sealapex, Apexit, CRCS, Vitapex.
- Solvent based Chlorosin, chlorpercha, klorpercha N-Ø

220. Ans. (c) Zinc phosphate *Ref: Craig 12th ed. p 491*

- 'Bases' are the materials, which are placed over the pulpal/axial wall and act as a substitute for most dentin.
- Thickness of bases is depends upon the amount of dentin lost. It should be at least 2 mm.
- It protects the pulp.
- Zinc phosphate, polycarboxylate, GIC, $Ca(OH)_2$ and zinc oxide eugenol are used as bases.
- Zinc phosphate is the most commonly used base applied under class II amalgam.

221. Ans. (b) Beelby's layer *Ref: Vimal Sikri 2nd ed. p 302*

- During finishing, some scratches are left on the casting.
- These scratches are reduced or eliminate during the procedure of final polishing.
- After final polishing, a microcrystalline surface layer will remains on the surface which is termed as "Beilby layer".

222. Ans. (a) Glass ionomer cement *Ref: Phillips 11th ed. p 475*

GIC:

- Developed by Wilson and Kent in England in 1972.
- It is a potential replacement for silicate cement.
- It adheres to enamel as well as dentin by chelation of carboxyl group of polyacid with calcium.
- There is a continuous leach of fluoride throughout the lifetime of the cement.
- Polycarboxylate cement is adhering to tooth by chemical bonding.
- Due to the greater inorganic content of enamel, the bond strength of cement to enamel is greater than that of dentin.

223. Ans. (b) ZOE *Ref: Craig 12th ed. p 504*

- The set cement of zinc oxide eugenol has a pH of 6.6 to 8.0 has little or no effect on pulp when placed in deep cavities. The presence of free eugenol has an obtundent effect on the pulp and reduce the pain that may be associated with the antibacterial properties of the cement.
- Eugenol is a parasubstituted phenolic compound, used as a liner.

224. Ans. (b) Increases strength in lathe cut but reduces strength in spherical alloy *Ref: Craig 12th ed. p 251*

Over trituration	*Tensile strength*	*Compressive strength*	*Creep*
Lathe alloy spherical alloy admixed	Increase Decrease Decrease	Increase Decrease Decrease	Increase Increase Increase
Under trituration	TS	CS	Creep
Lathe alloy Spherical alloy Admixed	Increase Decrease Decrease	Increase Decrease Decrease	Decrease Decrease Decrease

225. Ans. (a) Low compressive strength *Ref: Phillips 11th ed. p 512, 504, 540*

High copper alloy:

- It has high early strength.
- Low creep.
- Good corrosion resistance.
- Good resistance to marginal fracture.

226. Ans. (c) Occurs with increase in condensation pressure *Ref: Phillips 11th ed. p 516*

Creep:

- It is defined as the time dependent plastic deformation.
- Creep of dental amalgam is a slow progressive permanent deformation of set amalgam which occur under constant stress or intermittent stress.
- Creep values for low and high copper amalgam is 0.8 to 8.0 and less than 0.17% respectively.

Factors affecting creep:

- Microstructure.
- Effect of manipulative variables.
- Mercury alloy ratio.
- Condensation pressure.
- Timing of trituration.

Over trituration increases creep, and under trituration decrease creep.

- Higher condensation pressure will express excess mercury from the mix and it reduces deleterious effect of mercury like increased creep. Hence, option c is the answer of choice.

227. Ans. (b) 12–32% *Ref: Craig 12th ed. p 237*

Dental amalgam

It is an alloy of mercury with silver tin, copper, zinc and other minor ingredients.

Classification of dental amalgam alloy:

- According to the presence of number of alloy metal.
  - Binary alloy contains silver and tin.
  - Ternary alloys HV silver, tin and copper.
  - Quaternary alloys contain silver, tin, copper and zinc or indium.
- According to shape of particle.
  - Irregular.
  - Spherical.
  - Spheroidal.
- According to copper content of alloy.
  - Low copper alloy contains copper- 2 to 6%
  - High copper alloy contains copper- 12 to 30%.
- According to zinc content.
  - Zinc containing alloy- Zinc-0.01 to 1%.
  - Zinc free alloy contain less than 0.01% zinc.
- According to presence of Nobel metal.
  - Noble metal alloy contain gold or palladium.
  - Non-noble metal alloy does not contain any noble metal.

228. Ans. (a) More surface area of the bonded surface causes less polymerization shrinkage compared to the surface area of an unbonded restoration *Ref: Studervants 5th ed. p 504/Phillips 11th ed. p 416*

- Polymerization shrinkage is a term used to composite shrink while hardening.
- Configuration factor = $\frac{\text{Bonded surface area (C-factor)}}{\text{Unbounded surface area}}$
- **The higher the C-factor, the greater is for bond disruption from polymerization effects.**

Preparation	*C-factor*
Class IV	1/4 = 0.25
Class II	2/1 = 2
Class I	5/1 = 5

229. Ans. (b) Recurrent secondary caries *Ref: Vimal Sikri- 2nd ed. p 409*

Failure of composite restoration

- Marginal discoloration due to long exposure of tea and coffee.
- Polymerization shrinkage leads to microleakage due to which secondary caries will occur.
- Marginal fracture.
- Greater occlusal wear.
- Technique sensitive.

Advantages of composite

- Esthetic.
- Conservative.
- Repairable.
- Low thermal conductivity.

230. Ans. (a) Greater than zinc phosphate *Ref: Phillips-11th ed. p 451*

Cement type	*24-hr-diametral tensile strength*	*Compressive strength (MPa)*	*Pulp response*	*Setting time (minutes)*	*Film thickness (mm)*
Zinc phosphate	5.5	104	Moderate	5.5	20
GIC	6.2	86	Mild to moderate	7	21
ZOE type I	—	6–28	Mild	4–10	25
Resin	—	70–172	Moderate	2–4	< 25
Polycarboxylate	6.2	55	Mild to Moderate	6	21

231. Ans. (b) Ionic bond *Ref: Phillips 11th ed. p 473*

- During setting reaction of glass ionomer cement, various ions are released such as sodium, fluorine, aluminium and calcium.
- These all ions can be seen during the phase of dissolution.
- During gelation phase, the setting occurs by the cross linking of Ca ions.
- On further stage these Ca ions are replaced with Al ions and this indicate that it is an ionic bond.

232. Ans. (d) Increase in surface energy *Ref: Vimal Sikri 2nd ed. p 364,365*

Acid etching of dentin will leads to:

- Removal of smear layer.
- Demineralized the superficial dentin of 3 to 7 micrometer.
- Expose microporous collagen.
- It will open the tubules for the penetration of a primer to form resin tags.
- Reduce surface energy due to heterogeneous composition.

233. Ans. (a) There is no crosslinking between sodium and fluorine ions *Ref: Phillips 11th ed. p 473, 474*

GIC:

- The polyacrylic chain is crosslinked by calcium ions that are replaced by aluminium ion within 24 hours.
- There is no crosslinking between sodium and fluoride ions.
- Sodium ions are replaced by the hydrogen ions of carboxyl group.
- All the remaining ions are displaced within the set cement.

234. Ans. (b) Is seen as the last stage of reaction between mercury and alloy *Ref: Phillips 11th ed. p 509*

Dimensional change:

- ADA specification No 1 requires that amalgam should neither contract nor expand more than 20 micrometer/cm measured at 37°C, between 5 minutes and 24 hours after the beginning of trituration, with a device that is accurate to at least 0.5 micrometer.
- Amalgam can expand or contract depending on its manipulation.

- Ideally the dimensional change should be small.
- Severe contraction will leads to microleakage and secondary caries.
- Contraction occurs, when the particle begins to dissolve in Hg and AgHg grow.
- Excess mercury will cause expansion.
- Delayed contraction of amalgam has no relation with tin content.

235. Ans. (c) Lens *Ref: Phillips 11th ed. p. 47*

- Dental curing lights have many applications in dentistry, including photopolymerization of resins for pit and fissure sealants, cavity restorations, bonding of indirect restorations, orthodontic bonding and tooth bleaching.
- Most of these lights emit intense blue light in the 400- to 500-nm wavelength range, and some also emit in the ultraviolet A (UVA) range (315–400 nm).
- Although blue light (and, for some resins, UVA light) is essential for the polymerization reaction to occur in light-cured resins, prolonged exposure to blue and UVA light has adverse health effects, especially ocular damage.
- The greatest ocular hazard related to blue light occurs at about 440 nm (close to the peak wavelength of many light-emitting diode curing lights), whereas the maximum UV hazard peaks at 270 nm.
- Blue light is transmitted through the ocular media and absorbed by the retina.
- At chronic low levels of exposure, the blue light amplifies retinal aging and degeneration by causing photochemical injury to the pigmented epithelium and choroid of the retina.
- The clinical manifestations of retinal damage include acute photo retinitis and, in severe cases, premature age-related macular degeneration.
- In contrast, UV light is primarily absorbed by the conjunctiva, cornea and lens before it reaches the retina.
- Therefore, UVA radiation causes corneal injury or photokeratitis, as well as cataractogenesis, the transient or permanent opacification of the lens, and personnel who use curing lights on a daily basis may be at risk for ocular damage.

236. Ans. (c) 3 minutes *Ref: Phillips 11th ed. p 527*

- In order to compact the alloy in the prepared cavity condensation is done.
- After trituration, condensation is done, condensation of partially mixed material may fracture and break up the matrix.
- Condensation should be as rapid as possible and a fresh mix of amalgam should be condensed for 3 to 4 minutes.
- The field of operation should be dry before application.

237. Ans. (d) Dental ceramic *Ref: Phillips 11th ed.*

- **Direct restorative materials includes:**
  - Dentin bonding agents.
  - Restorative resins.
  - Dental cements.
  - Dental amalgam.
  - Direct filling gold.
- **Indirect restorative and prosthetic material:**
  - Dental casting and soldering.
  - Wrought alloys.
  - Dental ceramics.
  - Denture base resins.
  - Dental implants.

238. Ans. (a) 0.04–0.4 micrometer *Ref: Phillips 11th ed. p 419*

Refer: Ans-31

239. Ans. (a) Poly acrylic acid *Ref: Phillips 11th ed. p 466*

- Liquid used in polycarboxylate cement is an aqueous solution of polyacrylic acid or a copolymer of acrylic acid with other carboxylic acids such as itaconic acid.
- 30,000 to 50,000 is the molecular weight of polyacids.
- 32% to 42% by weight is acid concentration of liquid in polycarboxylate cement.
- Small fraction of fluoride release is also present.
- Powder composition is very much similar to zinc phosphate cement.
- Powder particle of cement consist of oxide of zinc, magnesium, bismuth, aluminium.
- It is bonded to the tooth surface chemically by carboxyl bond (-COOH).

240. Ans. (c) 0.04 μm *Ref: Phillips, 11th ed. p 404*

Filler particles are most commonly produced by grinding or milling quartz or glasses to produce particles ranging in size from 0.1 to 100 μm. Submicron silica particles of colloidal size (~0.04 μm), referred to collectively as microfiller or individually as microfillers, are obtained by a pyrolytic or precipitation process.

241. Ans. (d) Glass ionomer liner (light cure) *Ref: Philips, 11th ed. p 481*

Cumulative Fluoride Release from Various Glass Ionomer Products

Cement type	*Fluoride released (μg)*	
	14 days	*30 days*
Type II glass ionomer	440	650
Cermet	200	300
Alloy admix glass ionomer (silver alloy admix)	3350	4040
Type I glass ionomer	470	700
Glass ionomer liner (conventional)	1000	1300
Glass ionomer liner (light-cured)	1200	1600

242. Ans. (d) 25.0 alpha (ppm/K) *Ref: Phillips, 11th ed. p 55*

Coefficient of Thermal Expansion (α) of Dental Materials Relative to that of Tooth Enamel and Dentin

Material	A *(ppm K^{1})*	*α material/α tooth enamel*
Aluminous porcelain	6.6	0.58
Dentin	8.3	0.75
Commercially pure titanium	8.5	0.77
Type II glass ionomer	11.0	0.96
Tooth enamel	11.4	1.00
Gold-palladium alloy	13.5	1.18
Gold (pure)	14.0	1.23
Palladium-silver alloy	14.8	1.30
Amalgam	25.0	2.19

Material	A *(ppm K^{-1})*	*α material/α tooth enamel*
Composite	14–50	1.2–4.4
Denture resin	81.0	1.77
Pit and Fissure sealant	85.0	7.46
Inlay wax	400.0	35.1

243. Ans. (d) Camphorquinone *Ref: Phillips, 11th ed. p 400,408*

- Light-cured composite-A particle-filled resin consisting of a single paste that becomes polymerized through the use of a photosensitive initiator system (CO and an amine initiator) and a light source activator (visible blue light)
- Camphorquinone (CQ) is a commonly used photosensitizer that absorbs blue light with wavelengths between 400 and 500 nm. Only small quantities of CQ are required (0.2 wt% or less in the paste). A number of amine initiators are suitable for interaction with CQ, such as dimethylaminoetheyl methacrylate (DMAEMA), which is also present at low levels, that is, approximately 0.15 wt%.

244. Ans. (d) 1:1 by weight *Ref: Phillips, 11th ed. p 521-522*

- The method for reducing the mercury content of the restoration is to reduce the original mercury/alloy ratio.
- The present-day alloys are designed for manipulation with reduced mercury/alloy ratios.
- This method is known as the minimal mercury technique or the Eames technique, in recognition of the dentist who developed the concept.
- Sufficient mercury must be present in the original mix to provide a coherent and plastic mass after trituration; however, the amount of mercury present must also be low enough so that the mercury content of the restoration is at an acceptable level without the need to remove an appreciable amount during condensation.
- The mercury content of the finished restoration should be comparable to that of the original mercury/alloy ratio, usually about 50 wt% with lesser amounts (~42 wt %) being used with spherical alloys.

245. Ans. (a) Removal of residual surface contamination *Ref: Phillips, 11th ed. p 545*

Degassing Process of removing gases (or other impurities) from a solid (or a liquid).

246. Ans. (b) Annealing heat treatment *Ref: Phillips, 11th ed. p 551-552*

- Heating (sometimes called annealing) to remove the volatile protective coating is accomplished by holding individual pellets over an flame of pure alcohol or by placing a group of pellets or other gold form on a so-called annealing plate that is heated by electricity, gas or a burning alcohol flame. The annealing temperature range from 6500 to 7000°C, depending on the selected method and the heating time.
- The gold form is heated until it exhibits a dull red color. It is important not to under heat or overheat the gold segment. If the protective adsorbed layer is not driven off, the gold remains noncohesive and it will not bond to other desorbed segments.
- With the exception of noncohesive golds, the DFGs are received by the dentists in a cohesive condition. During manufacture and packaging, these products are never handled manually, and there are various heating stages that remove gaseous surface contamination. However, during storage and packaging they are exposed to the atmosphere. Because gas can absorb on the surface of the gold, it is necessary for the dentist or dental assistant to heat the foil or pellet immediately before it is carried into the prepared cavity. This step is commonly called annealing, heat treatment, or degassing. Although it is possible that a certain amount of recrystallization or stress relief may occur, these are unintentional because the primary purpose is to produce an atomically clean surface.

247. Ans. (d) All of the above *Ref: Phillips, 11th ed. p 513*

Effect of trituration: The effect of trituration on strength depends on the type of amalgam alloy, the trituration time and the speed of the amalgamator. Either under trituration or over trituration decreases the strength in both traditional and high-copper amalgams.

248. Ans. (b) Phosphoric acid *Ref: Phillips, 11th ed. p 383-385*

- The first meaningful proof of intraoral adhesion was reported in 1955 by Michael Buonocore. He etched the enamel surface with acids and then placed an acrylic restorative material on the micromechanically roughened surface. The monomers of the acrylic resin wet the etched surface, flowed into the etch pits, and generated retentive resin tags. One of the surface conditioning agents he used phosphoric acid, is still the most widely used etchant today for bonding in enamel and dentin.
- A number of acidic agents have been used to produce the required microporosity. However, phosphoric acid at a concentration between 30% and 50% typically 37% is the preferred etching agent. Concentrations greater than 50% result in the deposition of an adherent layer of monocalcium phosphate monohydrate on the etched surface, which inhibits further dissolution.
- The etching time for most etching gels is approximately 25 second. The advantage of such short etching times is that they yield acceptable bond strength in most instances, while conserving enamel and reducing treatment time.
- When the enamel is dry, it should have a white, frosted appearance, indicative of the proper etching treatment.

249. Ans. (d) Type II glass ionomer cement *Ref: Phillip's 11th ed. p 55; Craig's 11th ed. p 53*

Linear coefficient of thermal expansion of various materials

Material	*Coefficient × 10^{-6}/C*
Inlay waxes	350–450
Silicone impression material	210
Polysulfide impression material	140
Pit and fissure sealants	71–94
Acrylic resin	76.0
Mercury	60.6
Resin composites	14–50
Zinc oxide-eugenol cement	3 5
Amalgam	22-28
Silver	19.2
Copper	16.8
Gold	14.4
Porcelain	12.0
Tooth (crown portion)	**11.4**
Glass ionomer (type 2)	**10.2–11.4**

So it is clear from the above table that it is GIC with coefficient of thermal expansion close to that of tooth enamel and dentin.

250. Ans. (a) Compomers *Ref: Phillip's 11th ed. p 472; Craig's 12th ed. p 244*

They are the hybrids of dental composites and glass ionomer cement. They are also known as polyacid-modified resin composites.

Compomers

- Compomers or poly acid-modified composites are used for restorations in low stress-bearing areas.
- Compomers are recommended for patients at medium risk of developing caries.

Composition and setting reaction

- Compomers contain poly acid-modified monomers with fluoride-releasing silicate glasses and are formulated without water.
- The volume percent filler ranges from 42% to 67% and the average filler particle size ranges from 0.8 to 5.0 micrometer.
- Setting occurs primarily by light-cured polymerization, but an acid-base reaction also occurs as the compomer absorbs water after placement and upon contact with saliva.

251. Ans. (b) Granular gold *Ref: Phillip's 11th ed. p 547*

DFGs that are currently available are divided into 3 categories

- Foil (also known as fibrous gold)
- Electrolytic precipitate (also called crystalline gold, sponge gold or mat gold)
- Granular gold (also called powdered gold)

252. Ans. (a) Ag_2Hg_3 *Ref: Marzouk, p 106*

PHASES OF AMALGAM

- **Ag_3Sn (gamma)**
  - Mechanically it is the strongest
- **Ag_2Hg_3 (gamma 1)**
  - Noblest phase, most resistant to tarnish and corrosion every effort should be made to keep this in maximum available space in the bonding matrix of final products.
- **Sn_8Hg (gamma 2)**
  - Least resistant to tarnish and corrosion
  - Responsible for failure of restoration
- **Hg phase (Mercury phase) remember this point**
  - Mechanically the weakest phase Ag_2Hg_3 dominant phase in well condensed, low copper dental amalgam

253. Ans. (c) Resin modified glass ionomer cement *Ref: Phillip's 11th ed. p 482*

Resin modified GIC (Hybrid Ionomer)

- Powder contains
- Ion leachable fluoroaluminosilicate glass particle and initiator for curing
- Liquid contains
- Polyacid with methacrylate and hydroxyethyl methacrylate
- Setting reaction
- Initial setting by polymerization
- Final set of conventional acid base setting
- Advantages
- Less moisture sensitivity
- Greater early strength
- Improved translucency
- Higher dimetrile strength

- Lower elastic modulus
- Greater plastic deformation
- Greater bond strength when used with composite
- Disadvantage
- More polymerization shrinkage and micro leakage
- Lesser wetting capacity
- Transient temperature increase while setting

254. Ans. (c) Total etching multiple bottle *Ref: Sikri, 2nd ed. p 376*

Evolution of dentin bonding systems

- 1st generation Cavity primers with low bond strength
- 2nd generation Dentin enamel bonding agents with improved bond strength to etch enamel.
- 3rd generation Etching of dentin and partially removal of smear layer
- 4th generation Total etch technique and formation of hybrid layer and resin tags (multi bottle, i.e. 3)
- 5th generation One bottle system and self-etch primers
- 6th generation One step bonding system with proper bond to enamel and dentin; type I are compatible with self-cured composites and type II are not.
- 7th generation Single bottle no mix self-etching adhesive, not compatible with self-cured composite.

255. Ans. (b) Zinc oxide eugenol cement *Ref: Phillip's 11th ed. p 490*

The chemical composition of ZOE is typically:

- Zinc oxide, ~ 69.0%
- White rosin, ~ 29.3%
- Zinc acetate, ~ 1.0% (improves strength)
- Zinc stearate, ~ 0.7% (acts as accelerator)
- Liquid (Eugenol, ~ 85%, Olive oil ~15%)
- ZOE impression pastes are dispensed as two separate pastes. One tube contains zinc oxide and vegetable or mineral oil; the other contains eugenol and rosin. The vegetable or mineral oil acts as a plasticizer and aids in offsetting the action of the eugenol as an irritant.

256. Ans. (d) Pit and fissure sealants and class I restorations, respectively *Ref: Phillip's 11th ed. p 362*

- First generation: Flowable composite have low filler levels and should be used as pit and fissure sealant and also used as liner under class I and Class II Composite Restoration. It is introduced in 1996
- Second generation: Introduced from 2000 promise. It has gigher filler and improved properties. These can be used to restore small Class I and II restoration

257. Ans. (d) Glass ionomer cement *Ref: Phillip's 11th ed. p 55; Craig's 11th ed. p 53*

Refer Ans 54

258. Ans. (a) Cohesive gold *Ref: Philips- 11th ed. p 547*

- Cohesive gold is nearly pure gold so treated as to be free of adsorbed surface gases and impurities so that it will weld under pressure at room temperature; in dentistry, used as a restorative material placed directly into a prepared cavity and welded by pressure.
- Non-cohesive gold should be annealed to remove the surface contaminants before using it as restorative material.

259. Ans. (b) Increased matrix material formation *Ref: Philips- 11th ed. p 513*

- Alloy-mercury ratios vary between 5:8 and 10:8.

- Those mixes containing greater quantities of mercury are wetter and increased matrix material formation and are generally used with hand mixing which requires the removal of excess mercury following trituration and during condensation.
- For optimum properties, the final set amalgam should contain less than 50% mercury. Require the removal of excess mercury following trituration and during condensation.
- This ratio depends on: alloy type, particles size, and shape; therefore manufacturer instruction should be followed.

260. Ans. (c) Powdered gold *Ref: Phillips 11th ed. p 551-553*

Powdered gold—This form is supplied as irregularly shaped, pre-condensed pellets or clumps of particles that can be produced by comminution, chemical precipitation or atomization from the molten state. The atomized and chemically precipitated powders are first mixed with a soft wax to form pellets. These wax-gold pellets are wrapped with foil.

- During degassing, powdered gold must be heated in a flame to ensure the complete burning away of wax proper description is a matter of heating long enough at a temperature that removes gases, and in the case of powdered gold, burns away the wax, e.g. it takes 15 to 20 sec.
- Completing burning away of wax is not possible in the blue inner core of ethanol frame, because it takes more temperature and prolonged heating for its elimination. Therefore, powdered gold degassing is not performed in blue inner core.

261. Ans. (b) Morgan's E-Z gold *Ref: Phillips, 11th ed. p 551*

A type of powdered gold, Golden (originally by Morgan, Hastings Co. later by Williams Gold refining Co, Inc, Buffalo, NY) was introduced in the easily 1960s. The individual particles or granules, averaging 15 µm, are gathered into masses of irregular shape ranging in size from 1 to 3 mm.

262. Ans. (b) 9 to 20 weight precent *Ref: Phillips, 11th ed. p 505*

Admixed Alloys

This is the oldest type of high-copper alloy. The alloy powder purchased from the manufacturer is a mixture of powders of 2 alloys. One is traditional low-copper alloy. The other is a powder often a silver-copper eutectic. Addition of these two increases the overall copper content. The total copper content of commercial admixed alloys ranges from about 9–20%. The alloy particles are either spheres or lathe-cut.

263. Ans. (a) Zinc phosphate cement *Ref: Craig's 11th ed. p 598*

- The technique for handling zinc phosphate cement can be altered to achieve enhanced properties of the cement. The compressive strength of the material can be decreased. The film thickness can be maintained within acceptable limits, and the possibility of pulpal damage can be kept low by maintaining temperature changes in the cement similar to those obtained from a room temperature-slab technique.
- The technique advocated by this report is as follows: 1. Store the aluminum slab with vinyl covering in a freezer at –15°C to –20°C in a plastic bag to prevent ice formation on the surface. 2. Remove the slab when ready to mix. 3. Quickly wipe the slab clean. 4. Dispense twice as much powder and liquid as recommended on the slab. 5. Start timer. 6. Slowly incorporate the powder into the liquid over a large area of the slab for 2 minutes. 7. Allow the mix to remain on the slab. 8. The instrument for placing the cement can be placed under the slab. The casting can be placed on a corner of the slab. 9. At 10 minutes, place the cement into the casting(s) and seat. 10. Remove excess cement. 11. Clean the slab by rinsing in water and gently wiping. 12. Dry the slab, place it in the plastic bag, and return it to the freezer.
- Zinc phosphate setting reaction is exothermic in nature and this heat can reduce the working time drastically.
- The glass lab can be cooled to about 180°C to 240°C but not below the dew point. This reduced temperature facilitates the longer working time and is names as frozen slab technique.

264. Ans. (d) Silicate cement *Ref: Philips 11th ed. p 487*

pH of silicate cement

- Less than 3—at time of insertion
- Below 7—even after month
- More acidic than zinc phosphate and silicophosphate
- Classified as severe irritant
- Considered as standard to compare severity reaction of pulp with other cement.

265. Ans. (c) Calcium *Ref: http://www.scribd.com/doc/42500701/Direct-Filling-Gold*

- It was a newest form of electroytically precipitated direct filling gold than alloyed with calcium and was named electralloy RV.
- Contains 0.1% calcium.
- Increased strength by dispersion strengthening.

266. Ans. (a) Argon *Ref: Philips 11th ed. p 412*

Argon laser lamps

- Highest intensity
- Single wavelength—490 micron

267. Ans. (b) Cement prosthesis interface *Ref: Philips 11th ed. p 112*

- Failure of zinc poly carboxylate cement occurs usually at cement metal (prosthesis) interface.

268. Ans. (b) Process of removing the absorbed impurities *Ref: Philips 11th ed. p 550*

- Desorption is a process of removing the absorbed impurity in order to provide a totally clean surface by physical or chemical action.
- Desorption is essential to the achievement of cohesive mass.
- This process is generally used to clean the direct filling gold.

269. Ans. (d) Water accelerates but heat retards the setting of zinc oxide eugenol cements *Ref: Craig's 12th ed. p 498*

ZOE cements ADA specification No 30

- The setting reaction of ZOE is accelerated by increase in temperature and humidity.

270. Ans. (b) Ammonia *Ref: Phillips 11th ed. p 549*

- The manufacture can supply the fat to the dentist essentially free of surface contaminants termed as cohesive but some adsorption of gases may occur during storage. So most gold sheets are provided with an adsorbed protective gas film such as ammonia because it will reduce the adsorption of gas and termed as non-cohesive foil.
- This volatile film is removed by heating to restore the cohesive charterer.

271. Ans. (b) Cement prosthesis interface *Ref: Philips - 11th ed. p. 470*

- Zinc polycarboxylate and zinc phosphate cement is generally used to cements the fixed prosthesis.
- The adhesion of the cement to tooth structure is better with zinc phosphate than in zinc polycarboxylate.
- In zinc polycaboxylate cement, the failure occurs usually at the cement metal interface.
- In zinc phosphate cement, the failure occurs at the cement tooth interface due to which dislodgement of the prosthesis occurs.

272. Ans. (c) Silicate cement *Ref: Sturtevant 5th ed. p 499, 857 & Vimal Sikkri 2nd ed. p 220*

- Silicate cement is the first fluoride releasing cement. It has anti cariogenic property but at the same time it cause pulpal irritation and solubility.
- Calcium hydroxide help to promotes the formation of a dentin bridge, which would close the exposure. The preripheral 0.5 to 1 mm of the dentin excavation should be left available for bonding the light cured glass ionomer cement base subsequently applied.

273. Ans. (b) 25-35 KHN *Ref: Phillips 11th ed. p 419*

Material	*KHN (Knoop hardness)*
Unfilled acrylic	15
Traditional composite	55
Hybrid composite	50-60
Microfilled composite	25-35
Enamel	360-430
Dentin	68

274. Ans. (b) 25 pm *Ref: Craig 12th ed. p 482*

- According ANS1/ADA specification 8 (type I), the film thickness of luting cement should be 25 μm.

Cement	*Film thickness (μm)*
Zinc Phosphate	20
ZOE (type I)	25
Silicophosphate	25
Glass ionomer	24
Zinc polycarboxylate	25

275. Ans. (b) ZnO eugenol and GIC *Ref: Philips - 11th ed. p. 470, 475*

- Zinc polycarboxylate cements have the ability to adhere to enamel and dentin.
- GIC adhere to the tooth by a chemical bond. It involves chelation of COOH group of polyacid in the liquid with Ca^{2+}.
- Most of dental cements possess mechanical means of retention to the tooth.

276. Ans. (c) Microfilled resin composites *Ref: Philips - 11th ed. p 425*

- Advantage of microfilled composite-
  - Highly polishable.
  - Smooth surface finish.
  - Easy to repair.
- The quality of lusture depends on the filler particle size. The finer is the size of particle the better will be its finish and hence it gives high lusture.
- Microfilled composite contains the particle size of 0.04 to 0.4 μm to provide excellent luster in aesthetic areas.

277. Ans. (a) β-phase of amalgam *Ref: Phillips-11th ed. p 502*

The solid solution of silver and amalgam is known as β_1 phase of amalgam.

During amalgamation, the following various phases are formed:

γ1 - Ag2 Hg3

γ2 - Sn7-8Hg

ε Cu3Sn

?- Cu6Sn5

Silver copper eutectic Ag-Cu

278. Ans. (b) 25 micron *Ref: Phillips-11th ed. p 458*

- For type I zinc phosphate cement, the film thickness is about 25 microns as it consist of fine grained particle for luting.
- For type II zinc phosphate cement, the film thickness is about 40 microns. As it consist of medium grained particle for luting as well as restoration (filling).
- In literature, the film thickness value ranges from 25 to 150 μm.

279. Ans. (c) Zn phosphate *Ref: Phillips-11th ed. p 451*

Zinc phosphate cement

- It is a popular luting and basing agent.
- It possess highest modulus of elasticity from all given option.
- It is commonly used as a base beneath amalgam restoration.
- The phosphoric acid is thought to injure the pulp.

Cement	*Modulus of elasticity*
Zinc polycarboxylate	5.1
Polymer reinforced ZOE	2.5
GIC	7.3
Zinc phosphate	13.5

280. Ans. (b) Non-cohesive foil *Ref: Philips - 11th ed. p 549*

Non-cohesive gold:

Manufacturer can subject the foil to a volatile agent such as ammonia, which is adsorbed on surface of gold. This volatile substance acts as a protective film to prevent adsorption of non-volatile materials and premature cohesion of pellets in their container. This ammonia treated foil is called as non cohesive gold.

281. Ans. (d) Zinc *Ref: Vimal Sikri-2nd ed. p 228*

- Zinc is added to the alloy in order to suppress the oxidation of the key elements of the alloys.
- It is also responsible for delayed expansion.
- When zinc is contaminated with moisture prior to the setting will leads to the formation of ZnO and H_2 gas that expands the amalgam excessively and results pain.

282. Ans. (c) Zinc oxide eugenol *Ref: Textbook of Operative Dentistry by Satish Chandra, 1st ed., p 163*

Zinc oxide eugenol

- Excellent sealing qualities.
- Bacteriostatic in nature.
- Used for temporary restoration and as sealers.
- It should not be used as liner or bases under composite restoration because ZOE inhibits the polymerization of the resin.
- Actually ZOE are mostly used as liner.

283. Ans. (d) Polyacrylates *Ref: Philips - 11th ed. p 485*

- Dental compomers are materials which are used in dentistry as restorative material.
- They were introduced in the early 1990s as a hybrid of two other dental materials: dental composites and glass ionomer cement.
- They are also known as polyacid-modified resin composites.
- They are used for restorations in low stressbearing areas.
- Compomer contains poly acidmodified monomers and fluoride-releasing silicate glasses. An acid-base reaction occurs as the compomer absorbs water after contact with saliva, which facilitats cross-linking structure and fluoride release.
- Compomers do show a fluoride ion release, like a glass ionomer cement. The level of this fluoride release however is only around 10% of that released by a glass ionomer, and therefore its usefulness in preventing recurrent caries on primary tooth is questionable.

284. Ans. (d) 54.5% *Ref: Phillip, 11th ed. p 522*

- Mercury/alloy ratio of 6/5 (6:5) indicates that 6 parts of mercury are to be used with 5 parts of alloy by weight.
- A mix of amalgam prepared with a mercury/alloy ratio of 6:5 contain 54.5% mercury.
- The recommended mercury/alloy ratio for most modern lathe-cut alloy is approximately 1:1 or 50% mercury (Eames tech).
- With spherical alloy, the recommended amount of mercury is closer to 42% because spherical particles have lower surface/volume ratio.

285. Ans. (a) 15–35 micrometer *Ref: Phillip, 11th ed. p 501*

- The size of the powder particle is controlled by the manufacturer.
- The average particle sizes of modern powders range between 15 and 35 μm.
- A very small particle greatly increases the surface area per unit volume of the powder. A powder containing tiny particles requires a greater amount of mercury to form an acceptable amalgam.

286. Ans. (b) 1.7 *Ref: Phillip, 11th ed. p 469*

The pH of the cement liquid is approximately 1.7. However the liquid is rapidly neutralized by the powder

- This is the first cement developed with potential for adhesion to tooth structure

COMPOSITION

Powder:

- ZnO Basic ingredient
- Mg oxide Modifier
- Bismuth and Al oxide—Improves smoothness of mix
- Stannous fluoride Anti-cariogenic property

Liquid:

Polyacrylic acid } decrease viscosity
Itaconic acid }

Maleic acid

Tricarboxcyllic acid

287. Ans. (a) 400 micrometer *Ref: Phillip, 11th ed. p 510*

- If zinc containing low copper amalgam is contaminated by moisture during trituration or condensation, large expansion can take place.

- The expansion usually starts after 3 to 5 days and may continue for a month, reaching value greater than 400 µm (4%). This type of expansion is known as delayed expansion or secondary expansion.
- This is due to formation of H_2 gas in the restorations leading to pain, sensitivity and protrusion of the restoration.

288. Ans. (a) Compressive strength *Ref: Still searching*

289. Ans. (b) Dentin conditioner *Ref: Phillip, 11th ed. p 381*

Dentin conditioner	An acidic agent that dissolves the inorganic structure in dentin, resulting in a collagen mesh that allows infiltration of an adhesive resin
Dentin bonding agent	A thin layer of resin between conditioned dentin and the resin matrix of a composite
Primer	A hydrophilic, low-viscosity resin that promotes bonding to a substrate, such as dentin.
Hybrid layer	An intermediate layer of resin, collagen, and dentin produced by acid etching of dentin and resin infiltration into the conditioned dentin
Preventive-resin restoration (PRR)	A conservative, sealed, resin-based composite restoration, usually placed in a minimally prepared occlusal fissure area, with the sealant extending into contiguous uncut fissures

290. Ans. (d) Resin cement *Ref: Phillip, 11th ed. p 482-489*

Resins

- Methyl methyacrylate based resin of the 1950s did not adhere to tooth, underwent polymerization shrinkage, had a high coefficient of thermal expansion, underwent microleakage, and excess removal was difficult.
- Today resin cements are a popular choice due to their high compressive and tensile strengths, low solubility and aesthetic qualities. They do have limitations like technique sensitivity and high cost.

291. Ans. (a) No squeeze cloth technique *Ref: Sturdevant's Art and Science of Operative Dentistry, 4th ed. p 150*

Types of trituration

- Eames or no squeeze cloth or minimal mercury technique: the mercury alloy ratio according to this is 1:1 or 50% mercury.
- Increased dryness or squeeze cloth technique.

292. Ans. (b) Hydrofluoric acid *Ref: Operative Dentistry by Dr Moiz Khan p 57*

- Fractured PFM and all ceramic are repaired by etching the fractured surface with the 9.6% hydrofluoric acid for 2 minutes.
- It provides microretentive porosities and to facilitate mechanical retention.
- Due to etching with hydrofluoric acid there is increase in surface area and it enhances the micromechanical bonding of cement between ceramics and tooth surfaces.

INDIRECT RESTORATIVE AND PROSTHETIC MATERIALS

293. Ans. (b) Shape and size of particle *Ref: Phillips 11th ed. p 671*

- Condensation is the process of packing the porcelain powder particles together and of removing the liquid binder. The term also includes any process by which an unfired dental porcelain paste is compacted.

Firing shrinkage

- Firing shrinkage of porcelain usually reaches an approximate volume of 40%.
- Densely condensed porcelain built up structure undergoes less firing shrinkage.

- Condensation shrinkage of porcelain during firing depends on distribution or particles size in a mass of fritted powder.
- 25.95% if they are most densely packed volumetric shrinkage.

294. Ans. (c) Prevents the formation of chromium oxide *Ref: Phillips 11th ed. p 609*

- Flux is a compound, applied to metal surface in order to prevent the formation of oxides as well as other undesirable substances which reduce the quality of soldered area.
- Soldering flux is used to wet and melt the ends of the metal from where we want to joined them together.
- Compound such as boric acid borax or boric anhydride are used as flux for noble metal alloys.
- Fluoride flux is used to dissolve the oxide of chromium, nickel and cobalt.

Fluxes may be divided according to their primary purpose:

- Type I—surface protectioncovers the metal surface and prevents access to oxygen.
- Type II—reducing agentreduces any oxides present, exposing the clean metal.
- Type III—solventdissolves any oxide present and carries them away.

295. Ans. (a) Astrengthener *Ref: Phillips 10th ed. p 652*

- Wrought alloy are plastically deformed.
- Nickel provides additional strengthening to the gold alloy and whiten the alloy as well.
- Nickel may decrease the alloys tarnish resistance if we used it in large quantity.

296. Ans. (b) Proper or increased burnout temperature

297. Ans. (b) Reducing zone *Ref: Phillips 11th ed. p 615*

The flame can be divided into four zones:

- Cold mixing zone.
- Partial combustion zone.
- Reducing zone.
- Oxidizing zone.

Mixing zone

- The first long cone like zone emanating directly from the nozzle of the torch in which air and gas are mixed.
- It is dark in color.
- No heat is present in this zone.

Combustion zone

- This surrounds the inner zone.
- It is green in color.
- It is a zone of partial combustion.
- It has an oxidizing nature.

Reducing zone

- Lies beyond the combustion zone.
- It is blue in color.
- It is the hottest part of the flame.
- It is used for fusion of casting alloy.

Oxidizing zone

- Outermost zone.
- Not used for fusion.

298. Ans. (c) Silver *Ref: Craig 12th ed. p 360*

Metallic elements used in dental alloy

- **Noble metal:**
  - Ruthenium.
  - Rhodium.
  - Palladium.
  - Osmium.
  - Iridium.
  - Platinum.
  - Gold.
- **Base**
  - Nickel
  - Copper
  - Zinc.
  - Gallium.
  - Silver.
  - Tin.
  - Indium

299. Ans. (a) Reducing zone *Ref: Phillips 11th ed. p 615*

Zone of flame	*Nature of flame*	*Use*
Cold mixing zone	Unburned gas	Not used
Combustion zone (Green)	Oxidizing	Not used
Reducing zone (Blue)	Hottest zone	Used for soldering and melting alloy
Oxidizing zone	Burned gas	Not used

300. Ans. (b) To restrict the flow of solder over the parent metal *Ref: Phillips 11th ed. p 609*

Functions of flux:

- Eliminate any oxide coating a parent metal.
- It is designed for presoldering.
- It possess optimum activity in breaking down oxides.
- To protect metal surface from oxidation during soldering procedures.
- To permit the flow of solder over parent metal.

301. Ans. (a) Decrease in modulus of elasticity *Ref: Phillips 11th ed. p 637*

Chromium

- It increases the corrosion resistance.
- Increases hardness.
- Increases in tensile strength.
- It reduces the melting point.
- 30% of Cr is considered the upper limit for attaining maximum mechanical properties.

Physical property

- Melting point 18–75°C
- Boiling point 26–65°C
- Density 7.19 gm/cm^3

302. Ans. (a) Corrosion resistance *Ref: Philips 11th ed. p 637*

- Chromium is added to iron, carbon and other elements to form stainless steel.
- Stainless steel is highly resistance to corrosion and this property is achieved due to presence of chromium.
- Chromium is also known to impart corrosion resistance to cobalt and nickel alloy. It comprises two of the major groups of base metal alloy used in dentistry.
- It provide this corrosion resistance by forming a very thin, adherent surface oxide that prevent the diffusion of oxygen or other coroding species to the underlying bulk metal.

303. Ans. (a) Ductility *Ref: Phillips 11th ed. p 96*

Ductility:

- It is a property of metal, which may be drawn readily into a wire, by subjecting a tensile force.
- Higher the tensile strength, higher will be its ductility and thinner will be its ductility and thinner will be the wire.
- Method of measurement of ductility:
  - By percentage elongation.
  - By measuring the reduction in area.
- Cold bend test.
- The bend test is essentially measuring a metal's ductility.
- Ductility defines how easily a metal can bend without breaking.
- The higher the ductility of a metal, the more it can bend without breaking or becoming deformed from its original shape.
- This is important because certain metals must handle pressure without snapping yet still be ductile enough to bend slightly and not lose their support or shape.
- Copper and steel are two metals that have a high ductility and do well under pressure.

304. Ans. (d) Composite *Ref: V Sikri 2nd ed. p 297*

- During casting, all the wax pattern and acrylic is completely burnout.
- The purpose of burnout is to make room for the liquid metal.

305. Ans. (b) Softening heat treatment *Ref: Phillip's 11th ed. p 621*

- Annealing, in metallurgy and materials science, is a heat treatment that alters a material to increase its ductility and to make it more workable.
- It involves heating a material to above its critical temperature, maintaining a suitable temperature, and then cooling.
- Annealing can induce ductility, soften material, relieve internal stresses, refine the structure by making it homogeneous, and improve cold working properties.
- The three stages of the annealing process that proceed as the temperature of the material is increased are:
  - recovery,
  - recrystallization, and
  - grain growth.
- The first stage is recovery, and it results in softening of the metal through removal of primarily linear defects called dislocations and the internal stresses they cause. Recovery occurs at the lower temperature stage of all annealing processes and before the appearance of new strain-free grains. The grain size and shape do not change.
- The second stage is recrystallization, where new strain-free grains nucleate and grow to replace those deformed by internal stresses. If annealing is allowed to continue once recrystallization has completed, then grain growth (the third stage) occurs.

- In grain growth, the microstructure starts to coarsen and may cause the metal to lose a substantial part of its original strength. This can however be regained with hardening.

306. Ans. (c) 50°C *Ref: Phillips 11th ed. p 730*

- Benzoyl peroxide acts as an initiator, which is present in the polymer powder.
- It initiates polymerization reaction.
- When it is heated at 60°C. Its molecule begins to decompose to yield electrically neutral species possess unpaired electron.
- This free radical react with the monomer molecule to initiate the polymerization.
- The reaction is terminated by the coupling of two growing chains (transfer of H+ from one chain to other).

307. Ans. (b) NiTi *Ref: Phillips 11th ed. p 630*

- Transformation of custenite NiTi to martensite NiTi is done by the process of twinning.
- Deformation of α titanium alloy is significantly done by twinning.
- It achieves great importance in dental implants as well as some cast restoration.

308. Ans. (d) Fluoride *Ref: Craig's 12th ed. p 436*

Antiflux

- Antiflux is material that confines solder attachment or flow.

Significance

- Helps to confine the solder to required area.
- Maintain the connector shape and thickness.
- Limits flow of solder.
- Applied before application of flux.

Types of antiflux

- Graphite in lead pencil.
- Iron oxide in chloroform.
- Calcium carbonate in alcohol and water.

309. Ans. (b) Increases corrosion n tarnish resistance *Ref: Phillip's 11th ed. p 637*

Refer Ans no. 10.

310. Ans. (a) High bisque *Ref: Vimal Sikri 2nd ed. p 465*

Bisque is defined as the surface appearance of an unglazed porcelain.

- **Low bisque**
  - Porous surface
  - Shrinkage in minimal
  - Little fusion
  - Extremely week fired body
- **Medium bisque**
  - Pores are present on the surface
  - A lot of shrinkage
- **High bisque**
  - Minimum porosity
  - Maximum shrinkage
  - Strong fired body

311. Ans. (c) To decrease the formation of chromium oxide *Ref: Phillips 11th ed. p 609*

Flux:

- It is a compound used to dissolve or prevents the formation of oxides and other undesirable material from the surface of the part to be soldered or brazed.
- It is applied to the metal surface.
- It increases the quality or strength of a soldered metal.
- Fluxes can be divided into 3 types:
  - Type I—Surface protection
  - Type II—Reducing agent.
  - Type III—Solvent.
- Fluoride fluxes are used to dissolve cobalt, nickel and chromium oxides.
- Fluorides fluxes may also be used in post soldering

312. Ans. (b) Increase in vertical dimension *Ref: Phillips 11th ed. p 728*

Packing:

- Packing is defined as the adaptation and the placement of denture base resin within the mold cavity.
- Overpacking—It is a condition when the excess of material is placed in mold cavity, it will cause the malpositioning of prosthetic teeth.
- Under packing—It is a condition when small quantity of material is placed within mold cavity. It will leads to porosity in denture base.
- Insufficient closure of flask during packing of denture base resin will results in increase in vertical dimension while closure of flask, the excess resin will be found and termed as flash.

313. Ans. (a) The shape and size of particles *Ref: Phillips- 11th ed. p 671*

Porcelain condensation

- Porcelain is supplied in powder form for ceramic, metal-ceramic and for some other application. These powder particles are mixed either with water or in other vehicle.
- Cu-Sn phase is least susceptible to corrosion in compare to gamma 2 phase.

314. Ans. (b) Iron-nickel-chromium *Ref: Phillips 11th ed. p 638*

- Stainless steel is formed when 12% to 30% chromium is added to iron.
- They are of 3 types:
  - Austentic stainless steel.
  - Martensitic stainless steel.
  - Ferritic stainless steel.
- Composition of stainless steel:

Type of steel	*Chromium (wt%)*	*Nickel (wt%)*	*Carbon (wt%)*
Austentic	16 to 26	7 to 22	0.25
Martensitic	11.5 to 17	2.5	0.15 to 1.20
Ferritic	11.5 to 27	0	0.20

315. Ans. (c) Back pressure porosity *Ref: Phillips 11th ed. p 346*

Back pressure porosity:

- It is caused by inability of the air in the mould to escape through the pores in the investment.
- The entrapment is frequently found in the pocket at the fitting surface of crown or mesio occlusal distal casting.

- It is occasionally found even on the outside surface of casting.
- It occurs when the casting temperature or mould temperature is so low that the solidification of alloy occurs before the entrapped air can escape.

316. Ans. (d) Dicor *Ref: Phillips- 11th ed. p 681*

Castable glass ceramic (DICOR), was developed by corning glass works.

Composition:

- Tetra- silica fluoro mica glass ceramic 55%.
- Glass 45% (SiO_2, MgF_2, and MgO)
- Small amount of aluminium oxide, zirconia oxide and cerium oxide.
- The ceramics are cast into the mold prepared by phosphate investment material.
- The crown is cast by heating a ceramic ingot in zirconia crucible at 1380°C with motorized centrifugal casting machine using fluoride mica glass.
- The machine remains spinning for 4½ minutes. Followed by removal of investment.
- Dicor crown should be loaded on the occlusal surface, within marginal ridge area.

317. Ans. (b) Initiator *Ref: Phillips- 11th ed. p 737*

- As organic filler particle, acrylic resin is present.
- As a activator, visible light is present.
- As a initiator, Camphorquinone is present.

318. Ans. (c) Homogenization *Ref: Phillips- 11th ed. p 129*

- Homogenization is a process in which the alloy is held at a temperature near its solidus, to cause atomic diffusion to relieve coring and thereby resulting in uniformity of composition in the alloy.
- Duration of heating is at least six hours.
- Homogenized alloy is more resistant to corrosion and has more ductility.

319. Ans. (b) Electrolytic corrosion *Ref: Phillips 11th ed. p 61*

Galvanism:

- Presence of dissimilar metallic restoration in opposing or adjacent teeth causes galvanism.
- These restorations in conjunction with saliva or gingival crevicular fluid which act as an electrolyte make up an electrical cell.
- When two restorations contact each other the electrical cell is short-circuited.
- This result in flow of current through the pulp and the patient may experience pain.
- This is called galvanic corrosion or electrolyte corrosion.

320. Ans. (b) Nickel titanium *Ref: Phillips 11th ed. p 648*

- In the oral environment nickel titanium orthodontic wires possessing true shape memory characteristics.
- Widely used in dentistry in the form of orthodontic wires for clinical uses.
- It possesses superior springback to non superelastic as well as super elastic NiTi wire.

321. Ans. (b) 30% gold *Ref: Phillips- 11th ed. p 570*

Alloy type	*Total noble metal content*
High noble	≥ 40 wt% A_4
	≥ 40 wt% noble metal elements
Noble	≥ 25 wt% noble metal elements
Predominantly base metal (PB)	≤ 25 wt% nobel metal elements

322. Ans. (d) Titanium *Ref: Phillips- 11th ed. p 640*

- Stabilization is essentially concerned with the removal of the deleterious effect of carbon by the addition of alloying elements such as niobium, titanium or vanadium which form carbides that are more stable than chromium carbides.
- Stabilization in austenitic and ferritic stainless steel was achieved by using titanium.
- In a titanium-stabilized steel, welding usually results in reoxidation of titanium.

323. Ans. (b) Less than 2% *Ref: Phillips- 11th ed. p 636 (B)*

Type of steel	*Carbon content (wt%)*
A. Stainless steel	
• Ferritic	0.20 max
• Austentic	0.25 max
• Martensitic	0.15 to 1.20
B. Carbon steel	>2.1

324. Ans. (b) Gas lasers *Ref: Carranza, 10th ed. p 1036*

Current and Potential Applications of Lasers in Dentistry

Type	*Active medium*	*Dental applications*
Gas lasers	Argon (Ar)	Curing of composite materials, tooth whitening, intraoral soft tissue surgery, sulcular debridement (subgingival curettage in perioontitis and periimplantitis)
	Helium-neon (HeNe)	Analgesia, treatment of dentin hypersensitivity, aphthous ulcer treatment
	Carbon dioxide (CO_2)	Intraoral soft tissue and soft tissue surgery, aphthous ulcer treatment, removal of gingival melanin pigmentation, treatment of dentin hypersensitivity, analgesia

325. Ans. (b) Hard and brittle *Ref: Deepak Nallaswamy, p 7*

- Acrylic and porcelain teeth

Property	*Acrylic*	*Porcelain*
Abrasion resistance	**Low**	**High**
Adjustability	Easy to adjust	Difficult to trim
Bonding	Chemical	Mechanical
Staining	Easily stained	Does not stain
Percolation	Absent if acrylic denture base is used	Present when acrylic denture bas is used
Clicking sound	Absent	Present
Ease of fabrication	Easy	Difficult
Ease of rebasing	Difficult to remove acrylic teeth	Easy to remove porcelain teeth
Trauma to denture bearing area	Less	More

- Resin teeth display greater impact resistance and ductility than porcelain teeth. As a result, resin teeth are less likely to chip or fracture on impact, such as when denture is dropped. Furthermore, resin teeth are easier to adjust and display greater resistance to shock (temperature). Ceramic teeth have better dimensional stability and wear resistance, but they cause significant wear of opposing teeth and gold surface. Hence, ceramic teeth should not oppose such surface, if out of option they are used; they should be polished regularly to reduce abrasive damage.

- Very commonly consideration with resin teeth is that they are capable of chemical bonding with commonly used denture base resins, ceramic teeth are also retained by other means such as mechanical undercuts, silanization, etc.

326. Ans. (b) Benzoyl peroxide *Ref: Phillips, 11th ed. p 165, 731*

- Most poly (methyl methacrylate) resin systems include powder and liquid components. The powder consists of prepolymerized spheres of poly (methyl methacrylate) and a small amount of benzoyl peroxide. The benzoyl peroxide is responsible for starting the polymerization process and is termed as the initator. The liquid is predominantly nonpolymerized methyl methacrylate with small amounts of hydroquinone. Hydroquinone is added as an inhibitor and it prevents undesirable polymerization or setting of the liquid during storage.
- Glycol dimethacrylate, crosslinking agent in poly (methyl methacrylate) denture base resins is chemically and structurally similar to methyl methacrylate and therefore may be incorporate into growing polymer chains.

327. Ans. (d) Type IV-extra hard *Ref: Phillips, 11th ed. p 571-572*

- Type 1: Low strength for castings subjected to very slight stress (e.g. inlays), the minimum yield strength (0.2% offset) is 80 MPa, and the minimum percent elongation is 18%.
- Type 2: Medium strength for castings subjected to moderate stress (e.g. inlays, onlays, and full crowns), the minimum yield strength (0.2% offset) is 180 MPa, and the minimum percent elongation is 10%.
- Type 3: High strength for casting subjected to high stress (e.g. onlays, thin copings, pontics, crowns and saddles), the minimum yield strength (0.2% offset) is 270 MPa, and the minimum percent elongation is 5%.
- Type 4: Extra-high strength for castings subjected to very high stress (e.g. saddles, bars, clasps, thimbles, certain single units, and partial denture frameworks), the minimum yield strength (0.2%) offset) os 360 MPa, and the minimum percent elongation is 3%.

Alloy type	*Minimum yield strength (0.2%) or proof stress of nonproportional elongation (MPa)*	*Minimum elongation after fracture (%)*
Type 1	80	18
Type 2	180	10
Type 3	270	5
Type 4	360	3

Types 1 and 2 alloys are often referred to as inlay alloys. The development of modern direct and indirect tooth colored filling materials has virtually eliminated the use of types 1 and 2 gold alloys. Traditional types 3 and 4 alloys are generally called crown and bridge alloys, although type 4 alloys also are used occasionally for high stress application such as removable partial denture frameworks.

328. Ans. (b) Beryllium *Ref: Phillips, 11th ed. p 600*

The beryllium containing alloys as a group did not demonstrate overall superiority to the non-beryllium containing alloys, although the highest castability value of the 14 alloys rested was exhibited by a nickel chroimium beryllium alloy.

329. Ans. (a) To improve bonding *Ref: Phillips, 11th ed. p 582*

- Oxidizable elements such as Sn, In or Fe are included in each alloy to promote adherence to porcelain. However, because of their sag potential, the use of these alloys must be limited to crowns and three unit FPDs.
- Indium and/or tin can be added to improve bonding with the porcelain veneer. Gallium contributes to a homogenous microstructure.
- Ruthenium is used primarily as a grain refiner. Palladium-based alloys absorb small amounts of carbon that increase the brittleness of the alloy.

330. Ans. (a) PKT No-2 *Ref: Contemporary Fixed Prosthodontics By Stephen F. Rosenstiel, 4th ed. p 562*

Waxing instruments can be categorized by the intent of their design: wax addition, carving, or burnishing of the popular PKTs (designed by Dr Peter K. Thomas).

Specifically for the additive waxing instrument

- No. 1 and no. 2 are wax addition instruments,
- No. 3 is a burnisher for refining occlusal anatomy, and
- No. 4 and 5 are wax carvers
- The PKT no. 1 instrument is used for large increments he smaller no. 2 is used for lesser additions.

331. Ans. (d) Above 450°C *Ref: Phillips, 11th ed. p 608*

Metal joining operations are generally divided into these categories.

- Brazing
- Soldering
- Welding

The definitions of all three look exactly the same but there is minute difference in each. Difference between soldering and brazing is that brazing requires heating temperature above 4500°C but below the solidus temperature of substrate metals. The difference between these two processes and welding is that welding may not require a filler metal and metal surfaces to be joined will fuse locally. For dental application, the term soldering is commonly used to describe the buildup of the contact area or the joining of two metal parts, such as component of fix partial dentures or intraoral appliances.

332. Ans. (a) Austenitic *Ref: Phillip's 11th ed. p 639*

Austenitic steel is used for dental application because of the following excellent properties:

- Greater ductility and ability to undergo, more cold workable without fracturing.
- Substantial strengthening during cold working (some transformation to martensitic phase).
- Greater ease of welding.
- Ability to overcome sensitization.
- Less critical grain growth.
- Ease of formation.

333. Ans. (d) Silver solder and fluoride flux *Ref: Phillip's 11th ed. p 609, 611, 612*

- Use of gold solder with Elgiloy a type of nickel titanium derivative will form a layer of an alloy which will melt at 900°. Hence use of silver solder is indicated.
- The oxide layer on this highly reactive metal is more stable and borax flux is not able to dissolve this layer as they are just protective flux.

334. Ans. (c) Sintering *Ref: Phillip's 11th ed. p 665*

- Sintering is a method for creating objects from powders, including metal and ceramic powders. It is based on atomic diffusion.

- Diffusion occurs in any material above absolute zero, but it occurs much faster at higher temperatures.
- In most sintering processes, the powdered material is held in a mold and then heated to a temperature below the melting point.
- The atoms in the powder particles diffuse across the boundaries of the particles, fusing the particles together and creating one solid piece.
- Because the sintering temperature does not have to reach the melting point of the material, sintering is often chosen as the shaping process for materials with extremely high melting points such as tungsten and molybdenum.
- Sintering is traditionally used for manufacturing ceramic objects but finds applications in almost all fields of industry.
- The study of sintering and of powder-related processes is known as powder metallurgy. A simple, intuitive example of sintering can be observed when ice cubes in a glass of water adhere to each other.

335. Ans. (d) N. N-dihydroxyethyl para toludine *Ref: Phillip's 11th ed. p 723*

Most (poly) methyl methacrylate resin systems include powder and liquid components.

Powder	*Liquid*
Prepolymerized spheres of polymethylmethacrylate	Nonpolymerized methyl methacrylate
Benzoylperoxide (initiator)	Hydroquinone (inhibitor)
	Glycol dimethacrylate (cross linking agent)

336. Ans. (a) Gold copper *Ref: Hussain's 11th ed. p 234*

- Gold copper alloy is heated to a temperature within the ordering range for a period of time as recommended by the manufacturer and then it is quenched.

337. Ans. (a) Cold worked *Ref: Craig's 11th ed. p 178*

- Distorted grains observed in the microstructure in the wrought metal indicates that it has been cold worked.
- The deformation of the metal mass occurs by slippage of one portion past another along definite crystallization planes.
- The greater the degree of cold working, the greater the degree of grain boundary deformation.
- It can be reversed by stress relieving, annealing, and recrystallization.

338. Ans. (c) Both of the above *Ref: Phillip's 11th ed. p 646*

- Nickel titanium, also known as nitinol, is a metal alloy of nickel and titanium, where the two elements are present in roughly equal atomic percentages e.g. Nitinol 55, Nitinol 60.
- Nitinol alloys exhibit two closely related and unique properties: shape memory and superelasticity (also called pseudoelasticity).
- Shape memory is the ability of nitinol to undergo deformation at one temperature, then recover its original, undeformed shape upon heating above its "transformation temperature". Superelasticity occurs at a narrow temperature range just above its transformation temperature.
- Nitinol's unusual properties are derived from a reversible solid-state phase transformation known as a martensitic transformation, between two different martensite crystal phases, requiring 10,00020,000 psi (69138 MPa) of mechanical stress.
- Hence, transformation is induced by temperature as well as stress.

339. Ans. (a) Opaque *Ref: Shillinburg 3th ed. p 471*

Opaque porcelain is a special type of porcelain is a special type of porcelain which is used to conceal metal core in PFM. It contains a high concentration of opacifiers. It is first layer applied before the application of regular porcelain.

340. Ans. (c) Chromium *Ref: Craig 12th ed. p 397*

Chromium resists corrosion well because of the formation of a strongly adherent coating of oxide on the surface, which prevents further reaction with the metal below the surface. The formation of such an oxide layer is called passivation. The surface coating is not visible, even at high magnification, but the film adds to the metallic luster of the metal. The degree of passivity is influenced by a number of factors, such as alloy composition, heat treatment, surface condition, stress in the appliance and the environment in which the appliance is placed.

341. Ans. (b) Increased strength *Ref: Phillip's 11th ed. p 633, 634*

- The cold working of the metal increasing the hardness, yield strength, and tensile strength.
- The effects of cold working may be reversed by annealing the material at high temperatures where recovery and recrystallization reduce the dislocation density.

342. Ans. (d) Propane *Ref: Philips 11th ed. p 613*

Propane gas:

- Best choice of fuel gas.
- Highest heat content.
- Butane also has the same characteristics.

Acetylene gas:

- Highest flame temperature
- Chemically unstable gas
- Temperature varies in one part of the flame to another.

343. Ans. (c) Austenitic *Ref: Philip's 11th ed. p 638*

The austentic stainless steels are the most corrosion resistant alloys of the three major type and are the stainless steels used for orthodontic wires, endodontic instruments, and crowns in pediatric dentistry.

344. Ans. (b) In denture teeth *Ref: Phillips 11th ed. p 711*

The manufacture of denture teeth constitutes virtually the sole current use for high-fusing or medium-fusing dental porcelains. Denture teeth are made by packing two or more porcelains of differing translucencies for each tooth into metal molds. They are fired on large trays in high-temperature ovens.

345. Ans. (b) Can be done with pure titanium *Ref: Phillips, 11th ed. p 616,617*

- Commercially pure titanium (CP Ti) that is used in dentistry for crowns, FPDs, and partial denture frameworks is a highly reactive metal in air. The thin oxide film that forms instantaneously on a cleaned surface converts this metal from an active to a passive state. At temperatures used for soldering procedures, the thickness of the titanium oxide layer increases and may spontaneously debond from the parent metal surface at temperatures exceeding 8500°C. Thus the process of soldering this metal using traditional torch-soldering or oven-soldering procedures is technique- sensitive, and the quality of the soldered joint is quire variable
- To effectively join titanium components of dental crowns, FPDs, and partial denture frameworks, the technician can perform laser welding and plasma welding in an argon gas atmosphere. Since laser welding is associated with a lower thermal influence on the parts being joined than is plasma welding, it is the preferred method for dental applications. An advantage of welding is that the joint will be composed of the same pure titanium as the substrate components, thereby preserving the excellent biocompatibility potential of CP Ti and avoiding the risk for galvanic corrosion effects within the prosthesis.

346. Ans. (a) Shows reliable chemical bonding with metals *Ref: Phillips, 11th ed. p 656-660*

Potassium and sodium feldspar are naturally occurring elements. They are used for preparation of many dental porcelains designed for metal ceramic crowns and many other dental glasses and ceramics. This forms the crystalline mineral leucite when melted. This is used for manufacturing porcelain for metal bonding.

347. Ans. (a) Petroleum *Ref: Phillips, 11th ed. p 725-726*

Following materials are used as separating medium:

- Tin foil
- Cellulose lacquers
- Water soluble alginate solutions
- Silicone lubricants

Petroleum cannot be used as a separating medium as:

- It would allow water diffusion from mold surface to denture base;
- A portion of base would fuse with mould;
- It does not form thin uniform coat. Currently, most popular separating agents alginate and produce thin insoluble calcium alginate films on the mould surface.

348. Ans. (c) Air inclusion porosity *Ref: Phillips, 11th ed. p 736-737*

- **The fluid resin technique employs a pourable, chemically activated resin for the fabrication of denture bases.**
- **Advantages claimed for the fluid resin technique include**
  - Improved adaptation to underlying soft tissues,
  - Decreased probability of damage to prosthetic teeth and denture bases during deflasking,
  - Reduced material costs
  - And simplification of the flasking, deflasking, and finishing procedures
- **Potential disadvantages of the fluid resin technique include**
  - Noticeable shifting of prosthetic teeth during processing
  - Air entrapment within the denture base material (air inclusion porosity)
  - Poor bonding between the denture base material and acrylic resin teeth, and
  - Technique sensitivity

349. Ans. (a) DeChemant *Ref: Phillips, 11th ed. p 660*

The first porcelain tooth material was patented in 1789 by a French dentist (DeChemant) in collaboration with a French pharmacist (Duchateau).

350. Ans. (b) Lesser than the substrate metal *Ref: Phillips, 11th ed. p 608,609*

Soldering is commonly done to build up of a contact area or the joining of two metal parts such as components of a fixed partial denture. It involves the substrate metal to be joined, a filler metal, a flux and a heat source:

- The primary difference between soldering and brazing is that brazing requires a heating temp above 4500°C but below the solidus temperature of the substrate metal.

Ideal requirements of a dental solder

- It should melt at low temperature. The fusion temperature of the solder should be at least 500°C lower than the parent metal Gold solders 690 to 8700°C, Silver solders 620 to 7000°C
- When melted, it should be wet and flow freely over the parent metal
- Its color should match that of metal being joined

- It should be resistant to tarnish and corrosion
- It should resist pitting during heating and application

Application of soldering

- For soldering various types of wires in orthodontics
- In pedodontics, to construct various types of space maintainers
- In RPD for soldering of clasps
- In FPD for
  - Joining various components of fixed partial denture
  - For repair of perforation in crown and bridges
  - To develop contact points in crowns
  - For cutting and rejoining an ill-fitting distorted bridge.

351. Ans. (b) Titanium *Ref: Phillips, 11th ed. p 579, 640*

- Stainless steel is resistant to tarnish and corrosion due to chromium oxide layer formation but when 18-8 stainless steels are heated to 400–900°C chromium combines with carbon and forms chromium carbide as a result, the corrosion resistance of steel is reduced. This is called sensitization.
- To prevent this, titanium is added to stainless steel as titanium carbide in preference to chromium this is called stabilization of stainless steel.

352. Ans. (a) 3:1 *Ref: Deepak Nallaswamy, 1st ed. p 213,214*

Mixing of Powder and Liquid (Acrylic)

This Polymer monomer monomer proportion:

- 3:1 by volume
- 2:1 by weight

If too much monomer is used (low polymer monomer ratio) then:

- There will be greater curing or polymerization shrinkage.
- More time is needed to reach the packing consistency.
- Porosity can occur in the denture.

If too little monomer is used (high polymer monomer ratio).

- Not all the polymer beads will be wetted by monomer and the cured acrylic will be granular.
- Dough will be difficult to manage and it may not form a continuous plastic mass during processing.

353. Ans. (d) Propane *Ref: Phillips, 11th ed. p 612, 613*

Fuel gas characteristics	*Flame temperature*		*Heat content*	
Fuel (with oxygen)	°C	°F	*Kcal/m³*	*(BTU/ft³)*
Hydrogen	2660	4820	2362	275
Natural gas	2680	4855	8898	1000
Propane	2850	5160	21221	2385
Acetylene	3140	5685	12884	1448

Various gases used are

- Hydrogen has lowest heat content (275 Btu)
- Natural gas temperature 2680°C and heat content is four time that of H_2 (1000 Btu)
- Acetylene highest flame temperature (3140°C) and higher heat content than H_2 or natural gas (1448 Btu)
- Propane best choice, has the highest heat content (2385 Btu) and good flame temp (2850°C)

Hence remember
Highest heat content → Propane
Lowest heat content → Hydrogen
Highest flame temperature → Acetylene
Lowest flame temperature → Hydrogen

354. Ans. (a) 0.10% *Ref: Phillips 11th ed. p 550*

Alloyed Electrolytic Precipitate one form of electrolytic precipitate is alloyed with calcium. The alloy is converted to a mat form by sintering at an elevated temperature. The calcium content of the finished product is about 0.1%. In this product, the granular gold, alloyed with a trace of calcium, is manufactured electrolytically. Its purpose is to produce stronger restorations by dispersion strengthening.

355. Ans. (a) 2.30% *Ref: Phillips, 11th ed. p 577*

Base metal alloys (Ni-Cr,Co-Cr) have high hardness, modules of elasticity, sag resistance, yield strength, high fusion temp, and casting shrinkage (2.25%).

Linear solidification Shrinkage of casting alloys

Alloy type	*Casting shrinkage (%)*
• Type I (Au-based)	1.56
• Type II (Au-based)	1.37
• Type III (Au-based)	1.42
• Type IV (Ni-Cr based)	2.30

Comparative Properties of High noble alloys and Base metals for Metal Ceramic Prostheses

Properly	*High noble alloy*	*Co-Cr*	*Ni-Cr*	*CP–Ti*
1. Biocompatibility	Excellent	Excellent	Fair	Excellent
2. Density	14 g/cm^3	7.5 g/cm^3	8.7 g/cm^3	4.5 g/cm^3
3. Elastic Modulus	90 GPa	145–220 GPa	207 GPa	103 GPa
4. Sag Resistance	Poor to excellent	Excellent	Excellent	Good
5. Technique	Minimal	Moderately high	Moderately high	Extremely high
6. Bond to porcelain	Excellent	Fair	Good to Excellent	Fair
7. Metal cost	High	Low	Low	Low

356. Ans. (c) Fluoride *Ref: Phillips, 11th ed. p 609 and Deepak Nallaswamy, 1st ed. p 667*

Soldering Flux

- The purpose of a flux is to eliminate any oxide coating on the substrate metal surface when the filler metal is molten and ready to flow into place
- Fluxes may be divided into the following three types, according to their primary purpose

Type I Surface protection covers the metal surface and prevents access to oxygen so that no oxides can form.

Type II Reducing agent reduces any oxides present and exposes clean metal

Type III Solvent dissolves any oxides present and carries them away

- Fluxes for use with noble metal alloys are based on boric or borate compounds such as boric acid, boric and hydride and borax. They act as protective fluxes (Type II) for low stability oxides such as CuO.

- In base metal alloys, fluoride fluxes (Type III) are used to dissolve chromium, nickel and cobalt oxides. They usually contain borates as glass formers (protective) and the fluoride dissolves any metal oxide with which it comes in contact, acting as a solvent.

Disadvantages of flux

- Excess flux may become entrapped within the filler metal and cause a weakened joint
- Residual flux that is covered with porcelain can cause discoloration and bubbling of the porcelain
- Flux, when combined with metal oxides, forms a glass during the soldering process that is difficult to remove completely.

357. Ans. (d) 3% to 5% *Ref: Phillips, 11th ed. p 736*

- Resins polymerized via chemical activation generally display 3–5% free monomer whereas heat activated resins exhibit 0.2% to 0.5% free monomer.

358. Ans. (c) Reducing zone *Ref: Phillips, 11th ed. p 615*

The flame can be divided into four zones and the portion of the flame used to heat the soldering assembly is at the tip of the reducing zone, because this produces the most efficient burning process and the most heat. An improperly adjusted torch or improperly positioned flame can lead to oxidation of the substrate or filler metal and may result in a poor solder joint. It is also possible to introduce carbon into substrate and filler metal by using the unburned gas portion of the flame. To prevent oxide formation, the technician should not remove the flame once it has been applied to the joint area until the soldering process has been completed. The flame provides protection from oxidation, especially at the soldering temperature.

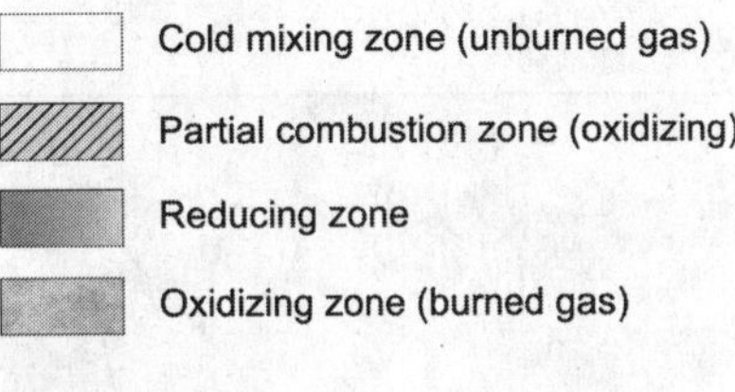

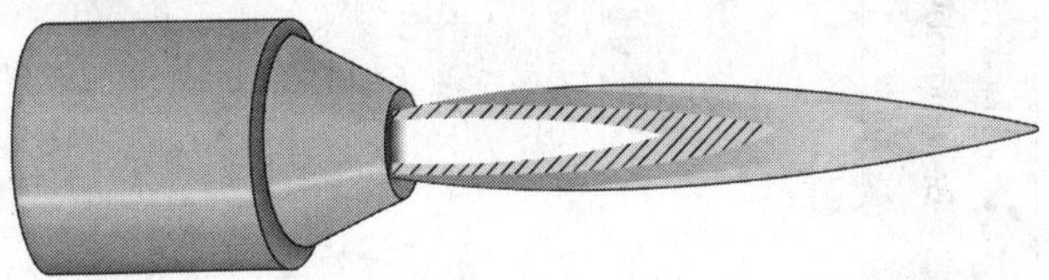

Mixing, combustion, reducing, and unburned gas zones in a propane-oxygen torch flame

359. Ans. (c) Martensitic *Ref: Phillips, 11th ed. p 637-639*

Three major types of stainless steels		
I. Ferritic	*II. Martensitic*	*III. Austenitic*
• AISI series 400 stainless steel • Provide good corrosion resistance • No readily work—herdenable • Little application in dentistry	• Share AISI series 400 designation • Least corrosion resistance • Can be heat treated • Can be used for surgical and cutting instruments	• AISI series 300 stainless steels • Most corrosion resistant alloys • Used for orthodontic wires Endodontic instruments and crowns in pediatric dentistry • Greater ductility and ability to undergo more cold work without fracturing

360. Ans. (a) Andreasen *Ref: Phillips, 11th ed. p 646*

Nickel-titanium Alloys

- A Nickel-titanium orthodontic wire alloy was first introduced commercially (Nitinol, 3M Unitek, Monrovia, CA) during the 1970s, following research by Andreasen and his colleagues.
- The alloy name "Nitinol" originally came from the two elements nickel and titanium, and the Naval Ordinance Laboratory where these alloys were first developed by Buehler and associates.

361. Ans. (c) Super elasticity *Ref: Phillips, 11th ed. p 647*

Nitinol wire	
→ Elastic modulus	40 GPa
→ Yield strength	430 MPa
→ Tensile strength	1500 MPa

Nitinol wire

- The NiTi inter metallic compound can exist in different crystal structures
  - Austenitic NiTi phase has complex ordered bcc (Cesium chloride) structure
  - Mertensitic NiTi phase distorted monoclinic, triclinic or hexagonal structure
  - R-phase or Rhombohedral crystals structure intermediate phase during transformation between martensitic, and austenitic NiTi
- Transformation between the austenitic and martensitic forms of NiTi can be induced by both temperature and stress Austenitic NiTi is the high temperature low stress form whereas martensitic NiTi is the low temperature, high stress form.

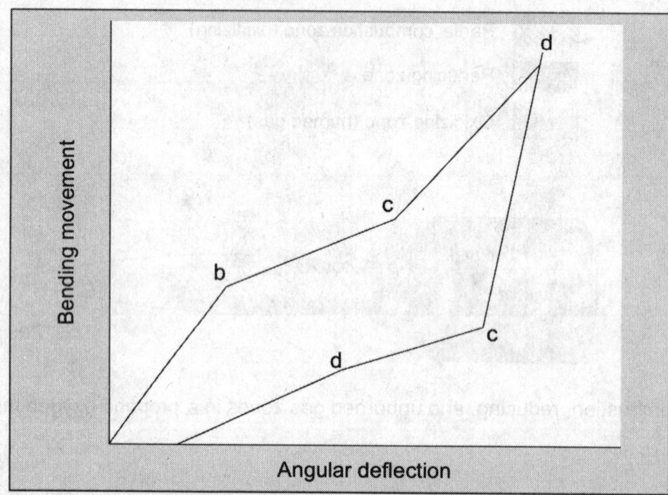

Schematic bending movement V.S angular deflection curve for a NiTi wire, showing regions of super elasticity

- Segment a-b - Initial deformation (elastic) of the wire
- Segment b-c - Where austenitic NiTi structure transforms to martensitic NiTi structure (responsible for superelastic behavior)
- Segment c-d - Further elastic deformation occurs with increasing stress
- Segment d-e - Loss of elastic strain in martensitic structure
- Segment e-f - Transformation back to austenific structure and finally loss of elastic strain, as the stress or bonding moment decreases to zero
- Superelastic behaviour is due to transition from austenitic NiTi form to Mastensitic NiTi structure. It is desired clinically, because very low and nearly constant forces for tooth movement are provided by the wire during unloading (deactivation).

362. Ans. (c) Light activated resins *Ref: Phillips, 11th ed. p 737*

A visible light-activated denture base resin has been available to the dental community for several years. This material has been described as a composite having a matrix of urethane dimethacrylate, microfine silica, and high molecular weight acrylic resin monomers. Acrylic resin beads are included as organic filler. Visible light is the activator, whereas camphorquinone serves as the initiator for polymerization.

363. Ans. (d) Pure titanium (CPTi) *Ref: Phillip's, 11th ed. p 579*

The use of commercially pure titanium (CPTi) and titanium alloys increased significantly over the last two decades of the twentieth century. These metals can be used for all metal and metal ceramic prostheses, as well as for implants and removable partial denture frameworks. Titanium is considered the most biocompatible metal used for dental prostheses. Because of the unique properties of titanium, and especially its biocompatibility, it does not fall within the classification of base metals. It is worthy of a separate class of metals.

364. Ans. (a) Increased hardness *Ref: Phillip's, 11th ed. p 604*

- Base metal alloys (Ni-Cr, Co-Cr) have high hardness, modulus of elasticity, sag resistance, yield strength, high fusion temperature and casting shrinkage (2–2.5%).
- They have lower proportional limit and ductility than gold alloys.
- Pure gold is most ductile and most malleable of all metals.
- Mechanical properties of removable partial denture alloys.

Metal type	*Yield strength (MPa)*	*Tensile strength (MPa)*	*Elongation (%)*	*Hardness (Hv)*	*Elastic modulus (GPa)*
Co-Cr	710	870	1.6	432	224
Ni-Cr	690	800	3.8	300	182
Co-Cr-Ni	470	685	8.0	264	198
Fe-Cr	703	841	9	309	202
Type IV Gold	493	776	7	264	90
CPTi	344	345	13	210	103
Ti-6V-4Al	870	925	5	320	117

365. Ans. (a) Palladium *Ref: Phillips, 10th ed. p 652, 653*

Effects of constituents of Gold alloys:

1. Palladium and platinum - Fine grain structure.
2. Copper - Age hardening.
3. Silver - To balance color, if Cu is present.
4. Nickel - To strength the alloy.
5. Zinc - Scavenger.

366. Ans. (d) Susceptibility to brittle fracture *Ref: Phillips, 11th ed. p 698*

The brittle fracture behavior of ceramics and their low tensile strengths compared with those predicted from bond between atoms can be understood by considering stress concentrations around surface flaws. As ceramics tend to have no mechanism for plastically deforming without fracture as do metals, cracks may propagate through a ceramic material at low average stress levels. As a result, ceramics and glasses have tensile strengths that are much lower than their compressive strengths.

367. Ans. (d) Greater impact resistance *Ref: Phillips, 11th ed. p 755*

- Resin teeth display greater impact resistance and ductility than porcelain teeth. As a result, resin teeth are less likely to chip or fracture on impact, such as when a denture is dropped. Furthermore, resin teeth are easier to adjust and display greater resistance to thermal shock. In comparison, porcelain teeth display better dimensional stability and increased wear resistance. Unfortunately, porcelain teeth often cause significant wear of opposing enamel and gold surfaces, especially when contacting surfaces have been roughened. As a result, porcelain teeth should not oppose such surfaces, and if they are used they should be polished periodically to reduce abrasive damage.
- Resin teeth are capable of chemical bonding with commonly used denture base resins. Porcelain teeth do not form chemical bonds with denture resins and must be retained by other means, for example, mechanical undercuts and silanization.

368. Ans. (a) High strength *Ref: Phillips, 11th ed. p 633-634*

Wrought alloy's have high strength as compared to casting alloys.

369. Ans. (a) Chemically cure resin *Ref: Phillip's, 11th ed. p 747-748*

- Despite the favorable physical characteristics of denture base resins, denture bases sometimes fracture. In most instance, these fractures may be repaired using compatible resins. Repair resins may be light, heat, or chemically activated.
- Chemically activated resins generally are preferred over heat and light-activated resins, despite the fact that chemically activated resins display lower transverse strengths. The principal advantage of chemically activated resins is that they may be polymerized at room temperature. Heat and light activated repair materials must be placed in water baths and light chambers, respectively. Heat generated by water baths and light chambers often cause stress release and distortion of previously polymerized denture base segments.

370. Ans. (a) Antiflux *Ref: Phillips 11th ed. p 608*

Antiflux: substance that prevents the flow of molten solder on areas of coated substance. For example, graphite, rouge mixed with chloroform.

371. Ans. (b) Lost wax technique *Ref: Phillips 11th ed. p 565*

- Lost wax technique: In 1907 Taggart's presents the fabrication of cast inlay restorations to New York odontological group which was developed in 1905.
- It was his instant success.

372. Ans. (a) Propane *Ref: Phillips 11th ed. p 613*

Propane

- Best choice
- Have good flame temperature
- Highest heat content

Acetylene

- Highest flame temperature
- Variation in temperature may be > 1000°C

Natural gas

- Four times the heat content of hydrogen

Hydrogen

- Low heat content

373. Ans. (c) Propane *Ref: Philips 11th ed. p. 613*

- The best heat source for soldering is propane. Actually both propane and butane have the advantage of being relatively pure compounds. Hence there is the best fuel gas when used with oxygen.
- It has a good flame temperature.

374. Ans. (b) Helium *Ref: Craig's p 450 449*

- An alternate method uses the principle of diffusion to secure improved density in fused porcelain. A diffusible gas such as helium may be introduced to the furnace at low pressure during the sintering (densification) stage.
  - The helium gas (instead of air) is entrapped in the interstitial spaces, due to its molecular diameter is smaller than the porcelain lattice.
  - It diffuses outward under the pressure of the shrinking porcelain.

375. Ans. (c) 7% *Ref: Philip's 12th ed. p 739*

Usually the accepted polymer to monomer ratio is 3:1 by volume, using this ratio the volumetric shrinkage may be limited to approximately 6% and linear shrinkage is 0.5%. The volumetric shrinkage exhibited by polymerized mass is 7%.

376. Ans. (c) Polymers *Ref: Deepka Nallaswamy 1st ed. p 224*

- Tissue lining materials are those which aid to decrease the force per unit area transmitted to the supporting tissue.

Composition

- Tissue conditioners are composed of polyethylmethacrylate and a mixture of aromatic ester and ethyl alcohol. Tissue conditioners are available as three component systems.
- Polymer (powder)
- Monomer (liquid)
- Liquid plasticizer (flow control)
- A gel is formed when these materials are mixed, with the ethyl alcohol having a greater affinity for the polymer.

Uses of tissue conditioners

The major uses of these tissue conditioning materials include:

- Baseplate stabilization
- To diagnose the outcome of resilient liners
- Liners in surgical splints
- Temporary obturator
- Trial denture base
- Tissue treatment
- Functional impression material.

377. Ans. (c) 13.5–14.5 × 10^{-6}/°C

Liner coefficient of thermal expansion	
Biomaterials/structures LCTE (ppm/C)	*LCTE (ppm/C)*
Aluminous dental porcelain	4
Alumina	6.5–8
In -Ceram	8–10
Cp-titanium	8–9
Traditional dental cements	8–10
Tooth structure	9–11

Contd...

Contd...

Biomaterials/structures LCTE (ppm/C)	*LCTE (ppm/C)*
Stainless steel	11
PFM ceramics	14
PFM alloys	14
Gold foil	14–15
Gold casting alloys	16–18
Co-Cr alloys	18–20
Hybrid glass -ionomers	20–25
Dental amalgam	25
Packable composites	28–35
Anterior and flowable composites	35–50
Composite cements	40
PMMA direct filling resins	72–83
Dental wax	60–600

378. Ans. (b) Sprue former is attached at right angle creating a localized lingering of molten metal after casting has solidified *Ref: Vimal Sikri 2nd ed. p 291*

Angulation of the sprue former

- It should not be attached at right angle to a broad surface because the melt may impinge the mold surface and produce a so called 'Hot-spot' producing suck back porosity.
- An angle of 45° is usually preferably. The sprue former should be directed away from any thin or delicate parts of the pattern, since molten metal may abrade or fracture investment in this area and result in casting failure.
- When molten metal strikes against the mold wall at 90 degree angle and if the mold metal temperature differential is more, it creates a hot spot, the molten metal in this area will solidify last, leading to localized shrinkage porosity, if there is no continuous supply of molten metal.

379. Ans. (a) Nitinol *Ref: Philip's 11th ed. p 622*

- Nickel titanium, also known as nitinol, is a metal alloy of nickel and titanium, where the two elements are present in roughly equal atomic percentages, e.g. Nitinol 55, Nitinol 60.
- Nitinol alloys exhibit two closely related and unique properties: shape memory and superelasticity (also called pseudoelasticity).
- Shape memory is the ability of nitinol to undergo deformation at one temperature, then recover its original, undeformed shape upon heating above its "transformation temperature".
- Superelasticity occurs at a narrow temperature range just above its transformation temperature; in this case, no heating is necessary to cause the undeformed shape to recover, and the material exhibits enormous elasticity, some 10–30 times that of ordinary metal.

380. Ans. (a) Prevent the oxidation of material during melting *Ref: Philip's 11th ed. p 602, 609*

Fluxes are specifically used

- To remove gas or prevent its absorption into the melt,
- To reduce metal loss,
- To remove specific impurities and nonmetallic inclusions,
- To refine metallic constituents, or to lubricate and control surface structure in the semicontinuous casting of mill alloys.

381. Ans. (c) >40% *Ref: Phillips-11th ed. p 570*

Contents of high noble gold alloy is:

- > 40 wt% gold.
- > 60 wt% of (Au, Pt, Pd, Rh, Ru, Ir, Os)

382. Ans. (b) Austenite *Ref: Phillips 11th ed. p 638*

18: 8 Stainless steel.

- It is a type of austenite stainless steel, consist of:
- Chromium-18%
- Nickel-8%.
- Carbon- Less than 0.25%
- Both 302 and 304 stainless steel are termed as 18 : 8 Stainless steel based on the percentage of chromium and nickel in their composition.
- This steel is used for making orthodontic bands, wires, brackets and other appliances.
- On heating between 400 and 9000°C this steel becomes prone to corrosion.
- Austenite is the main form of iron carbide and provides resistance to corrosion.

383. Ans. (b) Glycol DMA *Ref: Phillips 11th ed. p 722 -724*

- **Heat-activated resins:**
  - Polymethyl methacrylate powder.
  - Methylmethacrylate- liquid monomer.
  - Benzoyl peroxide- Initiator.
  - Glycol dimethacrylate- crosslinking agent 1–2% by volume.
- **Light activated resins:**
  - Camphorquinone activator.
- **Self-cured resin:**
  - Dimethyl para toludine activator.

384. Ans. (a) Improve bonding *Ref: Skinner's 10th ed. p 435*

- In PFM alloys, silver may discolor porcelain veneers.
- Copper strengthens gold-based alloys ($AuCu_3$).
- Both palladium and platinum increase casting temperature, strength, and corrosion resistance of the alloy.
- Palladium lowers cost and improves rigidity and sag resistance of PFM alloys.
- Zinc (traces) increases castability and forms intermetallic (gold) compounds to harden the alloy.
- Iron improves mechanical properties and, in PFM alloys, increases sag resistance and bond strength with porcelain.
- Tin acts as a bonding element in PFM alloys and a hardening agent in palladium-gold alloy.
- Iridium acts as a grain refiner in gold-based PFM alloy.
- Indium serves as a bonding agent in PFM alloys.

385. Ans. (a) Strengthener *Ref: Vimal Sikri 2nd ed. p 459*

- Quartz (i.e. silica) 15% is used in dental porcelain.
- It provides a crystalline phase in a dental porcelain.
- It acts as a strengthner.
- It imparts more strength, firmness and translucency.
- Small quantity of iron in quartz will discolor the porcelain so it should be removed.
- It is insoluble in water and acid.
- It helps in retaining the shape during fusing.

386. Ans. (a) Low weight *Ref: Phillips 11th ed. p 579*

Titanium

- Titanium is a light weight metal with a low density and thus the only metal that may be used in an almost pure.
- It has a very high melting point (1668°C) in comparison with the alloy used in dentistry. It has relatively low elastic modulus and a very low coefficient of thermal expansion.
- It is highly corrosion resistant at mouth temperature and is regarded as biocompatible.
- It is frequently used for the construction of implants.
- The most frequently used titanium alloy in medical and dental consist of titanium 90%, aluminium 6% and vanadium 4%.

387. Ans. (c) To reduce contact angle of a liquid with wax surface *Ref: Restorative Dental Material by Robert George Criag 11th ed. p 524*

- The surface of a wax pattern that is not completely wetted with investment results in surface irregularities in the casting that destroy its accuracy.
- These irregularities can be minimized by applying a surface-active wetting agent on the wax.
- The function of the wetting agent is to reduce the contact angle of a liquid with the wax surface.
- Wetting agents also remove any oily film that is left on the wax pattern from the separating medium.
- The contact angles are 98° for the plain wax surface and 61° for the treated wax surface.
- The lower contact angle indicates that the treated wax surface has an affinity for water, which results in the investment being able to spread more easily over the wax.
- Because the surface-active agents are quite soluble, rinsing the wax pattern with water after the application defeats the purpose of their use.

388. Ans. (a) Fluoride *Ref: Phillip, 11th ed. p 609*

- **Flux:** Compound applied to metal surfaces that dissolve or prevents the formation of oxides and other undesirable substance that may reduce the quality or strength of soldered or brazed area.
- They are classified according to their primary purpose.
- **Type I:** (surface protection) covers the metal surface and prevents access to oxygen so that no oxide can form.
- **Type II:** Reducing agent Reduces any oxides present and expose clean metal.
- **Type III:** Solvent dissolves any oxides present and carries them away.
- Fluxes for use with noble metal alloys are generally based on boric or boric compounds such as boric acid, boric anhydride and borax.
- They act as protective fluxes (type I) by forming low-temperature glass. They are also reducing fluxes (type II) for low stability oxides such as copper oxides.
- Oxides that are formed a base metal alloy are more stable. Fluoride fluxes (type III) are used to dissolve chromium, nickel and cobalt oxides.

389. Ans. (b) Solid-phase sintering *Ref: Phillip, 11th ed. p 671-672*

- The purpose of firing is simply to sinter the particle of powder together properly to form the prosthesis.
- Melting temperature of newer alumina ceramic is too high: Hence, liquid phase sintering does not happen. Particles fuse in solid phase sintering alone

Stages in firing	*Changes in porcelain*
Low Bisque	Less shrinkage, very porous
Medium Bisque	More shrinkage
High Bisque	Shrinkage complete

390. Ans. (a) Dynamic stress/fatigue failure *Ref: Phillips, 11th ed. p 91*

- Ceramic orthodontic brackets and activated wires within the brackets represent a clinical system that can exhibit static fatigue failure.
- The delayed fracture of molar ceramic crowns that are subjected to periodic cycle forces may be caused by dynamic fatigue failure.
- The failure begins as a flaw that propagates until catastrophic fracture occurs.

391. Ans. (a) CpTi *Ref: http://monographs.iarc.Fr/ENG/monographs/vol174/mono74-6.pdf*

- At room temperature, it has hexagonal close-packed structure (α form) at 882°C it transforms to a BCC (β form).
- Alloys with all α structure develops good strength and toughness and have superior resistance to oxygen contamination at elevated temperatures, but poor forming characteristics.
- Therefore, for dental casting, the purest form of metal is commercially pure (unalloyed) titanium (CpTi) available in 4 grades.
- Titanium is very resistant to electro chemical corrosion and it suffers from abrasive wear.

392. Ans. (b) Expansyl *Ref: http://www.promed.ie/dental#66772*

- It is a viscous paste placed directly into the sulcus
- Presence of aluminium chloride washes away with water
- It is a cartilage delivery system
- It causes no damage to tissue and preserves the epithelial attachment it is painless and ergonomic
- It is a paste used for atraumatic gingival retraction that opens the sulcus, displacing the tissue and leaving the field dry, ready for impression and cementation
- Expansyl guarantees a regular, reversible retraction of the gum.

393. Ans. (b) Mercury *Ref: ATB of Dental Material by Chandra 2nd ed. p 219*

- The use of mercury in dental amalgam restorations has become the subject of political controversy despite its long history of safe clinical use and alternative materials based on gallium and indium rather than mercury have been developed.
- The cytotoxicities of mercury nitrate, gallium nitrate and Indium were assessed.

394. Ans. (b) Hydroquinone *Ref: Phillips, 11th ed. p 722-723*

- Liquid (monomer): Major component of liquid
- Inhibitor: Hydroquinone 0.003% to 0.1%
- Accelerator: Tertiary amines, sulfinic acids or more stable salts of sulfinic acid. Amines such as N, Ndimethyl-p-toulidine increase the peroxide decomposition and causes the polymerization of the monomer at room temperature
- Plasticizers: They are low molecular weight esters like dibutyl phthalate. Result in softer and more resilient polymer
- Cross-linking agent 2 to 14% they help resistance against crazing. Glycoldimethacrylate.

395. Ans. (b) Crazing *Ref: Philips- 11th ed. p 744*

Crazing

- A network of fine cracks on or under the surface of a material such as enamel, glaze, metal, or plastic.
- Caused by stress relaxation of processing stresses in acrylic denture base
- Affect clinically specially aesthetics and physical properties
- Are the flaws or micro cracks in denture base
- Seen as small linear crack, and gives hazy or foggy appearance to denture

- May also be due to partial dissolution of resin by solvent like ethyl alcohol
- Mainly due to tensile stress
- Starts on surface of resin and perpendicular to the tensile force.

396. Ans. (b) 9 hrs 70°C *Ref: Phillip's 11th ed. p 733*

At 740°C (1650 F) for 8 hours or longer, with no terminal boiling treatment. A second technique is consist of processing in a 740°C water bath for 8 hours and then increasing the temperature to 1000°C for 1 hour a third technique involves processing the resin at 740°C for approximately 2 hours and increasing the temperature of the water bath to 1000°C and processing for 1 hour.

397. Ans. (a) 100.8°C and -48°C *Ref: Phillips 11th ed. p 165*

Methyl methacrylate is a transparent liquid at room temperature with the following physical properties:

- Molecular weight 100
- Melting point = –480°C
- Boiling point = 100.80°C (note: how close this is to the boiling point of water)
- Density = 0.945 g/mL at 200°C
- Heat of polymerization = 12.9 kcal/mol

398. Ans (b) Percolation *Ref: http://www.cram.com/flashcards/orpr-midterm-669917*

Percolation:

The pumping action of alternately pumping out the imbibing fluids at the tooth-restoration interface caused by temperature changes when the restorative material and tooth tissues have greatly differing coefficients of thermal change.

5 General Pathology

CELLULAR ADAPTATIONS, CELL INJURY, AND CELL DEATH

1. Which of the following statements is not true regarding its association with increased aging? *(AIIMS May 2011)*
a. Damage to the tissues due to free radical injury
b. Increased superoxide dismutase
c. Increased accumulation of free radicals
d. Increased cross-linkages in collagen

2. The fading of nuclear chromatin of a necrotic cell is called: *(AIIMS May 2010) (AIIMS May 2007) (AIPGEE 2007)*
a. Karyolysis
b. Karyorrhexis
c. Pyknosis
d. Hyperchromatism

3. Apoptosis is suggestive of: *(AIIMS Nov 2007) (AIPGEE 2006)*
a. Coagulative necrosis
b. Liquefactive degeneration
c. Neoangiogenesis
d. Epithelial dysplasia

4. Internucleosomal cleavage of DNA is a characteristic of: *(AIIMS Nov 2005)*
a. Reversible cell injury
b. Irreversible cell injury
c. Necrosis
d. Apoptosis

5. Chemotherapeutic drugs can cause: *(AIIMS May 2005)*
a. Only necrosis
b. Only apoptosis
c. Both necrosis and apoptosis
d. None of the above

6. Caspases are involved in: *(AIPGEE 2008)*
a. Cell necrosis
b. Atherosclerosis
c. Cell apoptosis
d. Inflammation

7. Cytoplasmic cytochrome C is associated with:
a. Glycolysis
b. Apoptosis
c. Drug metabolisation
d. All of the above

8. All of the following statements are true regarding reversible cell injury, *except*: *(AIPGEE 2005)*
a. Formation of amorphous densities in the mitochondrial matrix
b. Diminished generation of adenosine triphosphate (ATP)
c. Formation of blebs in the plasma membrane
d. Detachment of ribosomes from the granular endoplasmic reticulum

9. Enzymatic digestion is the predominant event in the following type of necrosis: *(KCET 2005)*
a. Coagulative necrosis
b. Caseous necrosis
c. Liquefactive necrosis
d. Fibrinoid necrosis

10. An increase in the number of cells in an organ or tissue is: *(KCET 2007) (AIPGEE 2005)*
a. Hypertrophy b. Hyperplasia
c. Aplasia d. Metaplasia

11. The process of 'phagocytosis' was discovered by: *(KCET 2008)*
a. Celsus b. Elie Metchnikoff
c. Virchow d. None of the above

12. Inactive precursors of enzymes are known as: *(KCET 2008)*
a. Apoenzymes b. Coenzymes
c. Proenzymes d. Holoenzymes

13. The dominant histologic feature of infarction is: *(KCET 2009)*
a. Liquefactive necrosis
b. Coagulative necrosis
c. Chronic inflammation
d. Scar tissue

14. Free radicals can be inactivated by the following enzymes *except*: *(KCET 2009)*
a. Glutathione peroxidase
b. Catalase
c. Superoxide dismutase
d. Myeloperoxidase

15. The necrotic tissue and deposits of immune complexes complement and plasma protein produce a smudgy eosinophilic deposit is termed as: *(KCET 2010)*
a. Coagulative necrosis
b. Fibrinoid necrosis
c. Caseous necrosis
d. Fatty necrosis

16. Tigered effect of heart is seen in: *(KCET 2011)*
a. Fatty change b. Hyaline change
c. Amyloidosis d. Atrophy

17. Which of the following is not true of distrophic calcification? *(KCET 2013)*
a. Occurs in damaged tissue
b. Tuberculous lesions
c. Atherosclerotic lesions
d. Serum calcium levels are high

18. Generation of free radicals occurs by all of the following mechanisms *except*: *(KCET 2013)*
a. Normal metabolism
b. Oxygen toxicity
c. Reperfusion after ischemic injury
d. All of the above

19. Mercury is toxic because it: *(COMEDK 2005)*
a. Complexes with haemoglobin to form methaemoglobin
b. Inhibits haemoglobin synthesis, producing anemia
c. Inhibits anaerobic glycolysis
d. Binds to sulfydryl groups

20. Caseation necrosis is suggestive of: *(COMEDK 2007) (COMEDK 2008)*
a. Tuberculosis
b. Sarcoidosis
c. Leprosy
d. Midline lethal granuloma

21. Through which mechanism do phagocytes kill bacteria? *(COMEDK 2008)*
a. Membrane attach complex killing
b. Oxidative and non-oxidative killing
c. Zipper killing
d. Chemotaxis

22. Pathologic calcification is seen in: *(COMEDK 2009)*
a. Scleroderma
b. Lichen planus
c. Dystrophic epidermolysis bullosa
d. Lupus erythematosis

23. The activation of caspases is likely to lead to: *(COMEDK 2012)*
a. Apoptotic cell death
b. Blood coagulation
c. Mitotic cell division
d. GI to S phase of cell cycle

24. Non-caseating granulomas are characteristic of: *(COMEDK 2012)*
a. Tuberculosis
b. Syphilis
c. Sarcoidosis
d. Actinomycosis

25.______is defined as a programmed cell death: *(MHPGDCET 2011)*
a. Apoptosis b. Gangrene
c. Necrosis d. Neoplasia

26. All of the following are nonapoptotic bodies *expect*: *(MHPGDCET 2012)*
a. Chromatin bodies
b. Cell membrane with organelles
c. Nuclear fragmentation
d. Pyknotic nucleus

ACUTE AND CHRONIC INFLAMMATION

27. All of the following is true about cerebral oedema *except*: *(AIIMS Nov 2007)*
a. It can result in herniation of the brain from foramen magnum
b. It results from increased lymphatic drainage
c. It results in an increase in intracranial pressure
d. It can result from an increase in plasma protein concentration

28. All of the following are mediators of inflammation, *except*: *(AIIMS May 2005)*
a. Tumour necrosis factor
b. Interleukin-1
c. Myeloperoxidase
d. Prostaglandins

29. Interleukin and leukotrienes are: *(AIPGEE 2008)*
a. Cytokines
b. Hormones
c. Enzymes
d. Liposyn

30. Immediate transient permeability in cells is increased by: *(AIPGEE 2007)*
a. Direct injury and necrosis
b. Endothelial gaps by histamine
c. Endothelial gaps by serotonin
d. Leucocyta mediated endothelial injury

31. All of the following vascular changes are observed in acute inflammation, *except*: *(AIPGEE 2005)*
a. Vasodilation
b. Stasis of blood
c. Increased vascular permeability
d. Decreased hydrostatic pressure

32. Langhans type of giant. Cell is found in: *(KCET 2005)*
a. Fat necrosis b. Malignancy
c. Tuberculosis d. Acute inflammation

33. Transudate differs from exudates in having the following *except*: *(KCET 2005)*
a. Few inflammatory cells
b. Glucose content
c. Low protein content
d. Low specific gravity

34. The commonly used fluorescent dye in the detection of tubercle bacilli is: *(KCET 2008)*
a. Acridine orange
b. Thioflavin
c. Congo red
d. Auramine and rhodamine

35. Which of the following cell types contains a vasoactive amine that is released in the inflammatory process? *(KCET 2009)*
a. Plasma cells b. Mast cells
c. T-lymphocytes d. B-lymphocytes

36. Coating of bacteria particles with host proteins to facilitate phagocytosis is known as: *(COMEDK 2012)*
a. Chemotaxis
b. Chemokine
c. Opsonisation
d. Membrane attack complex

37. Histamine and serotonin are secreted from: *(MHPGDCET 2011)*
a. Macrophages b. Platelets
c. B cells d. RBC

38. All of the following are antioxidants *except*: *(MHPGDCET 2012)*
a. NADPH oxidase
b. Glutathione peroxidase
c. Catalase
d. Superoxide dismutase

39. Mediators of inflammation are all *except*: *(AIPG/NEET 2013)*
a. TNF b. IFN
c. PG d. Myeloperoxidase

40. Oxygen dependent respiratory burst killing is done through: *(AIPG/NEET 2013)* *(AIPG 2006 and kar 2010)*
a. Nadph oxidase
b. Myeloperoxidase
c. Superoxide dismutase
d. Glutathione dismutase

41. Immediate transient permeability is caused by: *(AIPG/NEET 2013)*
a. Endothelial injury by histamine
b. Direct cell injury
c. Endothelial retraction
d. Gap between cells

TISSUE RENEWAL AND REPAIR: REGENERATION, HEALING AND FIBROSIS

42. Which of the following hormones have greatest effect on granulation tissue in wound healing? *(AIIMS May 2010)*
a. ADH
b. Oestrogen
c. Cortisol
d. Parathormone

43. Earliest transient changes following tissue injury: *(AIPGEE 2011)*
a. Neutropenia b. Neutrophilia
c. Monocytosis d. Lymphocytosis

44. Healing of wounds is retarded by: *(AIPGEE 2007)*
a. Proteins b. Cortisol
c. UV light d. Vitamin C

45. Collagen seen in the basement membrane is: *(AIPGEE 2007)*
a. Type IV b. Type VI
c. Type VIII d. Type IX

46. Wound contraction involves in: *(MHPGDCET 2012)*
a. Primary healing
b. Secondary healing
c. Tertiary healing
d. All of the above

HEMODYNAMIC DISORDERS, THROMBOEMBOLIC DISEASE AND SHOCK

47. Which of the following is the first sign that appeared in haemorrhagic shock? *(AIIMS May 2010)*
a. Hypotension b. Tachycardia
c. Vasoconstriction d. Syncope

48. The cardiopulmonary resuscitation should be: *(AIIMS May 2010)*
a. 2 inches per second
b. 1 inch per second
c. 2 inches per 5 seconds
d. 2 inches per 10 seconds

49. The first manifestation of shock is: *(AIIMSMay2008)* *(AIIMS May 2007)(AIPGEE 2007)*
a. Tachycardia
b. Vasoconstriction
c. Constriction of pupil
d. Bradycardia

50. Most common causes of pulmonary embolism are: *(AIPGEE 2009)*
a. Lymphangitis b. Endarteritis
c. Thrombosis d. Buerger's disease

51. Nutmeg liver is seen in: *(KCET 2005)*
a. Thrombosis b. Embolism
c. CVC liver d. Alcoholism

52. Severe generalized edema is called as: *(KCET 2005)*
a. Myxoedema b. Pitting edema
c. Anasarca d. Dependent edema

53. Transfusion transmitted diseases are all *except*: *(KCET 2007)*
a. HIV b. Hepatitis C
c. CMV d. Tuberculosis

54. The most common site of origin for venous thrombi leading to pulmonary embolism is: *(KCET 2009)*
a. Ascending aorta b. Portal vein
c. Deep leg veins d. Right atrium

55. Secondary hemorrhage occurs: *(KCET 2010)*
a. Within 6 hours after surgery
b. 7 to 14 days after surgery
c. As a result of violent recovery after operation
d. Due to blood transfusion line being discontinued

56. Which of the following is not a constituent of Virchow's triad? *(KCET 2011)*
a. Damage to endothelium due to injury or inflammation
b. Diminished rate of blood flow
c. Increased coagulability of blood
d. Increased venous blood pressure

57. Ivy technique is a test done to measure the: *(KCET 2011)*
a. Bleeding time
b. Capillary fragility
c. Prothrombin time
d. Platelet survival time

58. Which type of necrosis is most characteristic of ischemia of heart and kidney? *(KCET 2013)*
a. Coagulative
b. Liquefactive
c. Caseous
d. Fibrinoid

59. Which of the following organ is the characteristic site for haemorrhagic infarction? *(KCET 2013)*
a. Heart b. Intestine
c. Kidney d. Spleen

60. Saddle embolus causes sudden death by blocking: *(COMEDK 2008)*
a. Coronary arteries
b. Cerebral arteries
c. Pulmonary arteries
d. Renal arteries

61. Venous emboli are most often lodged in: *(COMEDK 2009)*

a. Intestines b. Lungs
c. Kidneys d. Heart

62. The infarct of the following organ is invariably hemorrhagic: *(COMEDK 2010)*

a. Kidney b. Lung
c. Spleen d. Heart

63. Endotoxic shock initiated by: *(AIPG/NEET 2013)*

a. Endothelial injury
b. Peripheral vasodilation
c. Inadequate blood volume
d. Cytokine action

GENETIC DISORDERS

64. Which of the following gene is responsible for hereditary nonpolyposis colon carcinoma? *(AIIMS May 2011)*

a. P53 b. Apc
c. Bcra2/1 d. MLH1

65. Which of the following is categorized in the list of obligate carriers having disease with recessive trait? *(AIIMS Nov 2010)*

a. Phenotypically normal woman with affected brother and son but normal daughter
b. Phenotypically diseased woman with affected husband and daughter but normal son
c. Phenotypically normal woman with diseased husband and son but normal daughter
d. Phenotypically diseased woman with diseased husband and affected son and daughter

66. A male patient with hypogonadism has at least two X chromosomes and one or more than one Y chromosome. He is suffering from: *(AIIMS Nov 2008)*

a. Klinefelter's syndrome
b. Turner's syndrome
c. Down's syndrome
d. Nursing bottle syndrome

67. Which of the following procedures is a routine technique for karyotyping using light microscopy? *(AIIMS May 2006)*

a. C-banding
b. G-banding
c. Q-banding
d. Brd V-staining

68. Albino girl gets married to a normal boy. What are the chances of their having an affected child and what are the chances of their children being carriers? *(AIIMS May 2006)*

a. None affected, all carriers
b. All normal
c. 50% carriers
d. 50% affected, 50% carriers

69. A 25-year-old male presented with pigmentation of nose and pinna. After voiding, his urine becomes dark. His spine is most likely to show: *(AIIMS Nov 2005)*

a. Atlantoaxial subluxation
b. Spondyloptosis
c. Basilar invagination
d. Calcification of disc

70. Which of the following is known as the guardian of the genome? *(AIIMS May 2005)*

a. P53 b. Mdm2
c. P14 d. ATM

71. A 25-year-old male had pigmented macules over the palm, sole and oral mucosa. He also had anaemia and pain in abdomen. The most probable diagnosis is: *(AIIMS May 2005)*

a. Albright's syndrome
b. Cushing's syndrome
c. Peutz-Jeghers syndrome
d. Incontinentia pigmenti

72. Down syndrome translocation occurs as which of the following? *(AIPGEE 2011)*

a. 46XY-141[14,21]
b. 47XY+21 t[14,21]
c. 47XY ,14 t[14,21]
d. 46XY t[14,21]

73. ORF stands for: *(AIPGEE 2011)*

a. Open reading frame
b. Oncogene removing factor
c. Oncogenic removing frequency
d. Open reduction fracture

74. Which of the following tests is not used for the detection of specific aneuploidy? *(AIPGEE 2011)*

a. FISH
b. RT-PCR
c. QF-PCR
d. Microarray

75. Ehlers-Danlos syndrome is: *(AIPGEE 2009)*
a. Autosomal dominant
b. Recessive
c. X-linked dominant
d. X-linked recessive

76. All the following methods are used to detect mutations, *except*: *(AIPGEE 2007)*
a. Single-stranded conformational polymorphism
b. Denaturating gradient gel electrophoresis
c. Gel electrophoresis
d. Northern blot analysis

77. All the following are functions of mRNA, *except*: *(AIPGEE 2007)*
a. Posttranscriptional modification
b. Posttranslational modification
c. Gene silencing
d. DNA replication

78. Differential expression of the same gene depending on the parent of origin is referred to as: *(AIPGEE 2005)*
a. Genomic imprinting
b. Mosaicism
c. Anticipation
d. Nonpenetrance

79. DiGeorge's syndrome is due to: *(COMEDK 2012)*
a. Congenital thymic aplasia
b. Deficiency of complement factors
c. Inborn error of metabolism
d. Chromosomal anomaly

80. A male is haemophillic, his wife is normal, which is true (refer to AIMS nov. 2010 and AIPG 2006 for same pattern of question). *(AIPG/NEET 2013)*
a. His sons are affected
b. All the daughters are carrier
c. 50% of his daughters are carriers
d. 50% sons are carrier

81. Primary amenorrhoea, sterility, short height is all these features are NOT seen in all except (In other words the features are seen in):*(AIPG/NEET 2013)*
a. 47XXX b. 46XY
c. 45X0 d d. 46xxx

82. Medical ethics in genetic counselling involve all *except*: *(AIPG/NEET 2013)*
a. Beneficence b. Confidentiality
c. Informed consent d. Direct guidance

DISEASES OF IMMUNITY

83. Which of the following investigations should be done immediately to best confirm a nonmatched blood transfusion reaction? *(AIIMS Nov 2010)*
a. Indirect Coombs' test
b. Direct Coombs' test
c. Antibody in patient's serum
d. Antibody in donor's serum

84. All are true about Widal test, *except*: *(AIIMS Nov 2010)*
a. Baseline differs depending on the endemicity of disease
b. O antibodies last longer and hence are not an indicator of recent infection
c. H antigen cannot differentiate between subtypes
d. High titre value in a single Widal test is not confirmative

85. Toll-like receptors on the NK cells recognize bacterial products and stimulate immune response by: *(AIIMS May 2008)*
a. Perforin and granzyme-mediated apoptosis
b. FADD ligand-mediated cell death
c. Transcription of nuclear factor mediated by (NF-_B) which recruits cytokines
d. Release of lipoxins

86. The average number of CD4 cells in body fluid is: *(AIIMS May 2006)*
a. 8001000/mm^3
b. 8001200/mm^3
c. 500800/mm^3
d. 400600/mm^3

87. Cell type which lacks HLA antigen is: *(AIIMS May 2005)*
a. Monocyte
b. Thrombocytes
c. Neutrophil
d. Red blood cells

88. The following methods of diagnosis utilize labelled antibodies, *except*: *(AIIMS May 2005)*
a. Enzyme linked immunosorbent assay (ELISA)
b. Haemagglutination inhibition test
c. Radioimmunoassay
d. Immunofluorescence

89. All of the following are a part of the innate immunity, *except*: *(AIIMS May 2005)*
a. Complement
b. NK cells
c. Macrophages
d. T cells

90. Autoimmunity can be caused due to all of the following, *except*: *(AIIMS May 2005)*
a. The presence of forbidden clones
b. Expression of cryptic antigens
c. Negative selection of T cells in the thymus
d. Inappropriate expression of the MHC proteins

91. Bence Jones proteins are derived from: *(AIPGEE 2011)*
a. Alpha globulin
b. Beta globulin
c. Gamma globulin
d. Delta globulin

92. Regarding myasthenia gravis which of the following is not true? *(AIPGEE 2011)*
a. Antibody formed to ACh receptors
b. Accumulation of ACh at cleft
c. Antibody binds to ACh
d. Anticholinesterases are used in the management

93. Number of CD4 cells in a drop of blood in a normal person is: *(AIPGEE 2011)*
a. 500700
b. 400800
c. 7001000
d. 8001200

94. A child on administration of penicillin for sore throat develops rashes, urticaria. This reaction is mediated by: *(AIPGEE 2008)*
a. IgE
b. IgM
c. IgG
d. IgD

95. Complement deposition in kidney, skin, joints and choroid plexus is seen in: *(AIPGEE 2008)*
a. Systemic lupus erythematosus
b. Myasthenia gravis
c. Goodpasture's syndrome
d. Scleroderma

96. Cross β-pleated sheet conformation to amyloidosis is determined by: *(AIPGEE 2007)*
a. Electron microscopy
b. X-ray crystallography
c. Light microscopy
d. Congo red stain

97. Flow cytometry analysis is done for: *(AIPGEE 2007)*
a. Blood glucose estimation
b. LDL fraction estimation
c. CD4/CD8 counts
d. None

98. Acid phosphatase positivity is shown by: *(AIPGEE 2007)*
a. T lymphocytes
b. B lymphocytes
c. Myelocytes
d. Monocytes

99. Which of the following immunoglobulins mediates type I hypersensitivity? *(AIPGEE 2005)*
a. IgA
b. IgG
c. IgM
d. IgE

100. The most lethal of complications due to blood transfusion is: *(AIPGEE 2005)*
a. Jaundice
b. Antigen antibody reaction
c. Hepatitis B transmission
d. HIV transmission

101. Sago spleen is found in: *(KCET 2005) (COMEDK 2005)*
a. Chronic inflammation
b. Amyloidosis
c. Tuberculosis
d. Syphilis

102. Poststreptococcal acute glomerulonephritis is an example for: *(KCET 2009)*
a. Type I hypersensitivity
b. Type II hypersensitivity
c. Type III hypersensitivity
d. Type IV hypersensitivity

103. Mast cells: *(COMEDK 2005)*
a. Possess receptors for complement components
b. Can synthesize TNF-alpha
c. Release histamine
d. Antigen recognized by IgA

104. Secondary amyloidosis is seen most commonly in: *(COMEDK 2009) (COMEDK 2012)*
a. Actinomycosis
b. Tuberculosis
c. Rabies
d. Secondary lues

105. HLA B27 histocompatibility antigen is seen in: *(COMEDK 2012)*
a. Sjogren's disease
b. Ankylosing spondylitis
c. Felty's syndrome
d. Scleroderma

106. The antibody indicative of acute hepatitis: *(MHPGDCET 2010)*
a. IgM anti-HBc
b. HBsAb/anti-HBs
c. IgG anti-HBc
d. HBeAb/anti-HBe

107. Long standing T cell activation leads to? *(MHPGDCET 2011)*
a. Acute anaphylactic reaction
b. Granuloma formation
c. Delayed response
d. Acute inflammatory reaction

108. Type 1 hypersensitivity is mediated by: *(AIPG/NEET 2013) (AIPG 2005)*
a. IgA b. IgD
c. IgE d. IgM

109. CD4 is not important for which of the following: *(AIPG/NEET 2013) (AIIMS May 10 medical paper)*
a. Antibody production
b. Cytotoxicity of T Cells
c. Memory B cells
d. Opsonisation

NEOPLASIA

110. When malignant cells resemble more primitive undifferentiated cells than those from which they arose, they are said to be: *(AIIMS May 2010)*
a. Anaplastic b. Metaplastic
c. Hypoplastic d. Desmoplastic

111. Which of the following is not a tumour suppressor gene? *(AIIMS May 2008)*
a. NF-1 b. WT-1
c. PTEN d. RAS

112. Myogenin, an immunohistochemical marker, is used in: *(AIIMS May 2008)*
a. Rhabdomyosarcoma
b. Malignant hyperthermia
c. Retinoblastoma
d. Osteogenic sarcoma

113. The most common bone tumour that occurs in children is: *(AIIMS Nov 2006)*
a. Osteosarcoma
b. Ewing's sarcoma
c. Metastatic carcinoma
d. Multiple myeloma

114. The most common histological type of thyroid cancer is: *(AIIMS May 2006)*
a. Medullary type b. Papillary type
c. Follicular type d. Anaplastic type

115. The inheritance pattern of familial retinoblastomas is: *(AIIMS Nov 2005)*
a. Autosomal recessive
b. Autosomal dominant
c. X-linked dominant
d. X-linked recessive

116. The tumour suppressor gene p53 induces cell cycle arrest at: *(AIIMS Nov 2005)*
a. G2M phase b. SG2 phase
c. G1S phase d. G0 phase

117. Which is the most common site of metastatic disease? *(AIIMS May 2005)*
a. Lung b. Bone
c. Liver d. Brain

118. Occupational cancers are common in: *(AIPGEE 2011)*
a. Liver b. Lung
c. Skin d. Leukaemia

119. Which of the following is least form of occupational cancers (another version of the above question)? *(AIPGEE 2011)*
a. Lungs b. Liver
c. Skin d. Leukaemia

120. Prostate specific antigen is used as: *(AIPGEE 2010, 2011)*
a. Tumour marker
b. Proto oncogene
c. Oncogene
d. Bacterial antigen

121. Leukaemia is not common in which of the following syndromes? *(AIPGEE 2011)*
a. Downs syndrome
b. Blooms syndrome
c. Turners syndrome
d. Immunedeficiency syndrome

122. Plasmocytoma of B cell origin is: *(AIPGEE 2009)*
a. Hodgkin's lymphoma
b. Plasmocytoma
c. Multiple myeloma
d. Lymph node metastatic tumour

123. All of the following immunohistochemical markers are positive in the neoplastic cells of granulocytic sarcoma, *except*: *(AIPGEE 2006)*
a. CD45Ro
b. CD43
c. Myeloperoxidase
d. Lysozyme

124. A simple bacterial test for mutagenic carcinogens is: *(AIPGEE 2005)*
a. Ames test b. Redox test
c. Bacteriophage d. Gene splicing

125. Features of a benign tumour are all *except*: *(KCET 2008)*
a. Absence of hyperchromasia of nucleus
b. Retained basal polarity
c. Slow growth
d. Presence of local invasion

126. Somatic mutation of PTEN is seen in: *(KCET 2011)*
a. Retinoblastoma
b. Osteosarcoma
c. Carcinoma breast
d. Endometrial carcinoma

127. Carcinoembryonic antigen is associated with: *(KCET 2011)*
a. Hepatocellular carcinoma
b. Medullary carcinoma of thyroid
c. Seminoma
d. Carcinoma of colon

128. A patient presents with jaundice, physical examination reveals an enlarged nodular liver, CT of the abdomen shows a cirrhotic liver with a large mass CT-guided biopsy of the mass demonstrates a malignant tumor derived from hepatic parenchymal cells. Infection with which of the following viruses would most directly related to the development of this tumor? *(KCET 2011)*
a. Epstein barr virus
b. Human herpes virus type A
c. Human T lymphocyte virus
d. Hepatitis B virus

129. Which of the following is known to arise from the sunlight? *(COMEDK 2008) (COMEDK 2012)*
a. Basal cell carcinoma
b. Ewing's sarcoma
c. Kaposi sarcoma
d. Verruca vulgaris

130. A hamartoma is: *(COMEDK 2008)*
a. Any collection of blood clot
b. A haemorrhagic cyst of the thigh
c. A developmental malformation
d. A tumour of soft tissue

131. Most common salivary gland tumour that arises in jaws is: *(COMEDK 2008)*
a. Pleomorphic adenoma
b. Adenoid cystic carcinoma
c. Mucoepidermoid carcinoma
d. Acinic cell carcinoma

132. Malignant ulcer is differentiated from benign by? *(COMEDK 2011)*
a. Heaping up of margins
b. Fibrous scars radiating from crater
c. Induration of base
d. Clean base

133. Which of the following arises from totipotent cells? *(MHPGDCET 2009)*
a. Hamartoma
b. Teratoma
c. Embryoma
d. Chloriostoma

134. Reversible conversion of one type of adult cell to another type of adult cell is known as: *(MHPGDCET 2009)*
a. Metaplasia
b. Dysplasia
c. Anaplasia
d. Hyperplasia

135. Chromosome responsible for Breast carcinoma: *(MHPGDCET 2010)*
a. 5 b. 11
c. 17 d. 21

136. Carotid body tumour diagnosis is: *(MHPGDCET 2010)*
a. Chemodectoma
b. Carotid body paraganglioma
c. Both 1 and 2
d. None of the above

137. Philadelphia chromosome is associated with which Leukaemia: *(MHPGDCET 2010)*
a. Chronic myeloblastic leukaemia
b. Acute myeloblastic leukaemia
c. Chronic lymphoid leukaemia
d. Acute lymphoblastic leukaemia

138. Which bone tumour occurs in epiphysis: *(AIPG/NEET 2013)*
a. Osteoclastoma
b. Ewing's sarcoma
c. Chondromyxoid fibroma
d. Osteosarcoma

139. Haemopoietic stem cell are differentiated from committed progenitor cell by (reconstitution of all bone marrow cells not in option as what is mention in medical paper): *(AIPG/NEET 2013)*
a. Are multipotent stem cells that give rise to all haemotogenous cell lineages
b. Cant differentiate further and less differenciating capacity than progenitor cell
c. Only present in bone and absent extra medullary
d. Stem cells can replicate only a specific number of time (limited self renewal) whereas progenitor cells can replicate indefinitely
e. Meiosis is seen (alternative option)

INFECTIOUS DISEASES

140. Cardiovascular complications of HIV infection include all of the following, *except*: *(AIIMS May 2011)*
a. Pericardial effusion
b. Cardiac tamponade
c. Congestive cardiac failure
d. Aortic aneurysm

141. All of the following are symptoms seen in systemic inflammatory response syndrome (SIRS) except (Options were slightly different in the exam): *(AIIMS May 2011)*
a. Oral temperature >38°C in the mouth
b. Infectious or noninfectious aetiology
c. Leukocytosis
d. Thrombocytopenia

142. All of the following statements about Staphylococcus aureus are true, *except*: *(AIIMS Nov 2010)*
a. Most common source of infection is cross-infection from infected people
b. About 30% of population is healthy nasal carriers
c. Epidermolysis and TSS toxins are superantigens
d. Methicillin resistance is chromosomally mediated

143. Which stage of Plasmodium vivax is infective to mosquito? *(AIIMS Nov 2010)*
a. Sporozoite
b. Gametocyte
c. Merozoite
d. Zygote

144. About pseudomonas, all are true, *except*: *(AIIMS Nov 2010)*
a. Strict aerobe
b. Can grow in disinfectant in hospital
c. Infection is mostly due to endogenous source
d. Most common organism in burn patient

145. Monocytes are seen in tuberculosis, monocytic leukaemia, typhoid and *(AIIMS Nov 2010)*
a. Pernicious anaemia
b. Hodgkin's disease
c. Parasitic infection
d. Subacute bacterial endocarditis

146. Infectious mononucleosis is caused by: *(AIIMS Nov 2010)*
a. EBV
b. HSV
c. CMV
d. VZV

147. The vector of Lyme's disease is: *(AIIMS May 2008)*
a. Ticks
b. Mites
c. Fleas
d. Aedes mosquito

148. Thirty-eight children consumed eatables procured form a single source at a picnic party. Twenty children developed abdominal cramps followed by vomiting and watery diarrhoea 610 hours after the party. The most likely aetiology for the outbreak is: *(AIIMS May 2006)*
a. Rotavirus infection
b. Enterotoxigenic E. coli infection
c. Staphylococcal toxin
d. Clostridium perfringens infection
e. Coli infection

149. In a postoperative intensive care unit, five patients develop postoperative wound infection in the same ward. The best method to prevent cross infection in other patients in the same ward is to: *(AIIMS May 2006)*
a. Give antibiotics to all other patients in the ward
b. Fumigate the ward
c. Disinfect the ward with sodium hypochlorite
d. Practice proper handwashing

150. A 5-year-old boy passed 18 loose stools in last 24 hours and vomited twice in last 4 hours. He is irritable but drinking fluids. The optional therapy for this child is: *(AIIMS May 2006)*

a. Intravenous fluids
b. Oral rehydration fluids
c. Intravenous fluid initially for 4 hours followed by oral fluids
d. Plain water ad libitum

151. All of the following can be a cause of resurgent malaria *except*: *(AIPGEE 2011)*

a. Genetic alterations in the host
b. Drug resistance in parasite
c. Resistance of the vector to DDT
d. Antigenic variation in parasites

152. Phlegmon is: *(AIPGEE 2011)*

a. STD
b. Types of cellulitis
c. Types of osteomyelitis
d. Veneral disease

153. Heterozygous sickle cell anaemia gives protection against: *(AIPGEE 2011)*

a. G6PD b. Malaria
c. Thalassaemia d. Dengue fever

154. What is seen in acute infection? *(AIPGEE 2011)*

a. Leukocytosis
b. Leukopenia
c. Lymphocytosis
d. Neutropenia

155. The most common malignancy seen in AIDS is: *(AIPGEE 2011) (AIPGEE 2009)*

a. Kaposi's sarcoma
b. Hodgkin's tumour
c. SCC
d. Osteosarcoma

156. CSF glucose levels are normal in which type of meningitis? *(AIPGEE 2011)*

a. Viral b. Pyogenic
c. Tubercular d. Carcinomatous

157. Which of following is not transmitted by lice? *(AIPGEE 2010)*

a. Q fever
b. Trench fever
c. Relapsing fever
d. Epidemic typhus

158. Chronic carrier state is seen in all, *except*: *(AIPGEE 2010)*

a. Measles b. Diphtheria
c. Typhoid d. Gonorrhoea

159. Risus sardonicus is seen in: *(AIPGEE 2010)*

a. Tetanus b. Tetany
c. Leprosy d. Actinomycosis

160. Which exposure caries maximum risk of transmission of HIV? *(AIPGEE 2010)*

a. Sexual intercourse
b. Blood transfusion
c. Transplacental
d. Needle prick

161. True about CSF changes in bacterial meningitis is: *(AIPGEE 2010)*

a. Increased protein
b. Increased glucose
c. Normal glucose level
d. Decreased protein level

162. Reactive arthritis is caused by: *(AIPGEE 2009)*

a. Staphylococcus aureus
b. H. influenza
c. Shigella sp
d. E. coli

163. Which one of the following clinical findings excludes the diagnosis of polymyositis? *(AIPGEE 2006)*

a. Neck muscle involvement
b. Extraocular muscle involvement
c. Abdominal muscle involvement
d. None of the above

164. In patients infected with HIV have: *(AIPGEE 2005)*

a. Elevated blastogenesis
b. Depressed serum globulin levels
c. High T4T8 ratio
d. Thrombocytopenia

165. Lepra cells seen in leprosy are: *(COMEDK 2005)*

a. Lymphocytes
b. Plasma cells
c. Vacuolated histiocytes
d. Neutrophils

166. Virchow's lepra cells are seen in: *(COMEDK 2005)*

a. Tuberculoid leprosy
b. Indeterminate leprosy
c. Borderline tuberculoid leprosy
d. Lepromatousleprosy

167. Human immunodeficiency virus binds to macrophages having: *(COMEDK 2008)*
a. CD4 molecule
b. CD4 and CCR5 molecules
c. CD4 and CCR5 molecules
d. CXCR and CCR5 molecules

168. Ghon complex of the lung usually: *(COMEDK 2009) (COMEDK 2012)*
a. Undergoes cavitation
b. Undergoes calcification
c. Progresses to tuberculous pneumonia
d. Progresses to military tuberculosis

169. Which one of the following developmental stages of plasmodium is transmitted from humans to anopheles mosquito? *(COMEDK 2012)*
a. Sporozoite
b. Gametocyte
c. Merozoite
d. Hlpnozoite

ENVIRONMENTAL AND NUTRITIONAL PATHOLOGY

170. All of the following lead to severe adverse effects *except*: *(AIIMS Nov 2007)*
a. Death
b. Diabetes
c. Prolonged hospitalization
d. Immobility

171. A 2-year-old boy presents with fever for 3 days, which responded to administration of paracetamol. Three days later, he developed acute renal failure, marked acidosis and encephalopathy. His urine showed plenty of oxalate crystals. The blood anion gap and osmolal gap were increased. Which of the following is the most likely diagnosis? *(AIIMS Nov 2005)*
a. Paracetamol poisoning
b. Diethyl glycol poisoning
c. Severe malaria
d. Hanta virus infection

172. Which of the following is not given in transparenteral nutrition? *(AIPGEE 2010)*
a. Carbohydrate
b. Fat
c. Fibre
d. Micronutrient

173. In iron deficiency anaemia, which of the following are seen in peripheral blood smear? *(AIPGEE 2007)*
a. ↑TIBC, ↑Ferritin
b. ↓TIBC, ↑Ferritin
c. ↑TIBC, ↓Ferritin
d. ↓TIBC, ↓Ferritin

174. A young girl has consumed barium carbonate with suicidal intent. She complains of generalized muscle weakness. The most likely electrolyte abnormality is: *(AIPGEE 2006)*
a. Hyponatremia
b. Hypocalcaemia
c. Hypokalaemia
d. Hypomagnesaemia

175. A child is below the third percentile for height. Growth velocity is normal, but chronological age is more than the skeletal age. The most likely diagnosis is: *(AIPGEE 2006)*
a. Constitutional delay in growth
b. Genetic short stature
c. Primordial dwarfism
d. Hypopituitarism

176. Vitamin B12 deficiency can give rise to all of the following, *except*: *(AIPGEE 2005)*
a. Myelopathy
b. Optic atrophy
c. Peripheral neuropathy
d. Myopathy

177. All of the following are true about manifestations of vitamin E deficiency, *except*: *(AIPGEE 2005)*
a. Haemolytic anaemia
b. Posterior column abnormalities
c. Cerebellar ataxia
d. Autonomic dysfunction

178. What fraction of inhaled mercury vapours is retained in the body? *(COMEDK 2006)*
a. 45 to 55%
b. 55 to 65%
c. 65 to 85%
d. >85%

179. Which of the following is not a pigment disorder? *(COMEDK 2005)*
a. Vitiligo
b. Melasma
c. Freckle
d. Seborrheic keratosis

180. Squamous metaplasia in the respiratory epithelium is induced by deficiency of: *(COMEDK 2010) (COMEDK 2011)*
a. Vitamin D
b. Vitamin B
c. Vitamin A
d. Vitamin C

181. Primary defect in scurvy is: *(AIPG/NEET 2013)*
a. Decrease mineralization
b. Decrease osteoid matrix formation
c. Increase bone resorption
d. Decrease bone mass with normal

DISEASES OF INFANCY AND CHILDHOOD

182. A malignant tumour of children that metastasizes to bones often is: *(AIPGEE 2006)*
a. Wilms' tumour
b. Neuroblastoma
c. Adrenal gland tumour
d. Granulosa cell tumour of ovary

183. Abnormal function of epithelial chloride channel protein is the cause of: *(KCET 2009)*
a. Ehlers-Danlos syndrome
b. Marfan syndrome
c. Cystic fibrosis
d. Diabetes insipidus

BLOOD VESSELS

184. Raynaud's disease, rashes on the face and fever are included in the spectrum of: *(AIIMS May 2008)*
a. Scleroderma
b. SLE
c. Erythema multiforme
d. Pemphigus

185. Bedsore is an example of: *(AIIMS May 2006)*
a. Typical ulcer
b. Trophic ulcer
c. Venous ulcer
d. Postthrombotic ulcer

186. The tissue of the origin of the Kaposi's sarcoma is: *(AIIMS May 2005)*
a. Lymphoid
b. Vascular
c. Neural
d. Muscular

187. All of following cause headache of vascular origin, *except*: *(AIPGEE 2011) (AIPGEE 2010)*
a. Giant cell arteritis
b. Anaesthesia dolorosa
c. Cluster headache
d. Hemicrania

188. CANCA is associated with: *(AIPGEE 2007)*
a. Proteinases 3
b. Myeloperoxidase
c. Alkaline phosphatase
d. Lactate dehydrogenase

189. All of the following are risk factors for atherosclerosis, *except*: *(AIPGEE 2006)*
a. Increased waist hip ratio
b. Hyperhomocysteinaemia
c. Decreased fibrinogen levels
d. Decreased HDL levels

190. Cystic hygroma is a: *(KCET 2009)*
a. Hemangioma
b. Lymphangioma
c. Lung abscess
d. Liver cirrhosis manifestation

THE HEART

191. Best marker for dyslipidaemia: *(AIIMS Nov 2010)*
a. LDL/HDL ratio
b. Cholesterol level
c. Cholesterol/triglycerides level
d. APO-1 level

192. A cell that contains hemosiderin, derived from RBCs that have been extravasated into the tissues, is: *(COMEDK 2005)*
a. Siderophage b. Melanophage
c. Plasma cell d. Lymphocyte

RED BLOOD CELL AND BLEEDING DISORDERS

193. A 9-year-old girl after tonsillectomy presents with uncontrolled bleeding with laboratory findings of prolonged aPTT, normal PT and a normal platelet count. What could be the deficiency? *(AIIMS Nov 2009)*
a. Factor IX
b. Factor VIII
c. Factor VII
d. Von Willebrand disease

194. Which of the following is true about haemophilia A? *(AIIMS May 2010) (AIPGEE 2007)*
a. Increased BT
b. Increased PT
c. Increased PTT
d. Increased platelet count

195. Cooley's anaemia is commonly known as: *(AIIMS Nov 2009)*
a. Beta thalassaemia major
b. Beta thalassaemia minor
c. Beta thalassaemia intermedia
d. Alpha thalassaemia

196. Haemophilia A is due to defective gene for which one of the following factors? *(AIIMS Nov 2009)*
a. Factor VII b. Factor VIII
c. Fibrinogen d. Platelets

197. Prothrombin time is increased in:
a. Von Willebrand's disease *(AIIMS Nov 2008)*
b. Haemophilia
c. Warfarin therapy
d. Liver disease

198. Hair-on-end appearance is seen in:
a. Thalassaemia *(AIIMS Nov 2008)*
b. Sickle cell anaemia
c. Aplastic anaemia
d. Megaloblastic anaemia

199. Bart's hydrops fetalis is lethal because: *(AIIMS May 2008)*
a. Hb Bart's cannot bind oxygen
b. The excess alpha globin insoluble precipitates
c. Hb Bar's cannot release oxygen to fetal tissues
d. Microcytic red cells become trapped in the placenta

200. Which of the following is not true about thalassaemia? *(AIIMS May 2008)*
a. Increase in number of globin chain
b. There is erythrocyte fragility and haemolysis
c. Hypochromic, microcytic anaemia is present
d. There is severe anaemia and thrombocytopenia

201. Which one of the following can be used in the management of a haemophilic patient?
a. Ascorbic acid *(AIIMS Nov 2007)*
b. Tranexamic acid
c. Acetic acid
d. Palmitic acid

202. In a blood sample, antiserum A and antiserum B and Rh positive factor are added. No agglutination is seen. The blood group is: *(AIIMS Nov 2006)*
a. O group and Rh^+
b. O group and Rh
c. AB group and Rh
d. AB group and Rh^+

203. All cause secondary polycythaemia *except*:
a. High altitude *(AIPGEE 2011)*
b. Hemangioblastoma
c. Myeloproliferative disorder
d. Pheochromocytoma

204. Fibrin degradation product help in detection of: *(AIPGEE 2011)*
a. Haemophilia b. DIC
c. Purpura d. Thrombasthenia

205. All are true about hereditary spherocytosis, *except*: *(AIPGEE 2011)*
a. Increased osmotic fragility
b. Increase in surface:volume ratio
c. MCHC is increased but MCV is normal
d. They tolerate less osmotic swelling than normal cells

206. Reticulocytosis is seen in all, *except*:
a. Blood transfusion *(AIPGEE 2007)*
b. Acute blood loss
c. Polycythaemia vera
d. Thrombocytopenic purpura

207. Increased number of reticulocytes are seen in all, *except*: *(AIPGEE 2007)*
a. Acute blood loss
b. Hereditary spherocytosis
c. PNH
d. Iron deficiency anaemia

208. Deficiency of all the three components of coagulation factor VIII results in:
a. Von Willebrand's disease
b. Hemophilia A
c. Parahemophilia
d. Haemophilia B

209. Heparin overdose is treated by: *(AIPGEE 2005)*
a. Copper sulphate
b. Protamine sulphate
c. Dextran sulphate
d. Cellulose sulphate

210. Hemophilia A is due to deficiency of: *(KCET 2009)*
a. Factor II
b. Factor V
c. Factor VIII
d. Factor IX

211. In haemolytic anaemias, the urobilinogen level in the blood would: *(COMEDK 2008)*
a. Increase
b. Be absent
c. Decrease
d. Mildly decrease

212. Transport form of iron is: *(COMEDK 2008)* *(MHPGDCET 2010)*
a. Transferrin
b. Ferritin
c. Apoferritin
d. Lactoferrin

213. Increased levels of hemoglobin A2 is characteristic of? *(COMEDK 2011)*
a. Sickle cell trait
b. Thalassaemia minor
c. Glucose-6-phosphate dehydrogenase deficiency
d. Thalassaemia

214. In fanconi anemia there is a: *(COMEDK 2012)*
a. Deficiency of copper
b. Mutation in DNA repair gene
c. No increased risk of sq cell cover
d. Purely, a nutritional disorder etiology

215. In disease of which of the following organs, there is prolonged bleeding: *(MHPGDCET 2009)*
a. Liver
b. Heart
c. Lungs
d. Kidney

216. Classical haemophilia is caused due to deficiency of: *(MHPGDCET 2009)*
a. Factor VIII
b. Factor IX
c. Factor V
d. Factor XI

217. Increased clotting time is seen in: *(MHPGDCET 2010)*
a. DVT
b. Vit. C deficiency
c. Von-Willebrand's disease
d. Haemophilia

218. Which of the following is/are responsible for Microcytic hypochromic anemia? *(MHPGDCET 2011)*
a. Lead poisoning
b. Iron deficiency anemia
c. Sideroblastic anemia
d. All of the above

DISEASES OF WHITE BLOOD CELLS, LYMPH NODES, SPLEEN, AND THYMUS

219. Increased monocytic count is seen in typhoid and: *(AIIMS May 2007)*
a. Parasitic infections
b. Subacute bacterial endocarditis
c. Hodgkin's lymphoma
d. None of the above

220. Bacteria are most commonly engulfed by: *(AIIMS Nov 2006)*
a. Neutrophilic leucocytes
b. Large granular lymphocytes
c. Small lymphocytes
d. Killer cells

221. In a leukaemic patient, gingival bleeding occurs during oral prophylaxis because of: *(AIIMS May 2006)*
a. Increased leukocytes count
b. Increased calcium level in blood
c. Platelet disorder
d. Deficiency of clotting factor

222. Raised LAP score is seen in: *(AIPGEE 2007)*
a. PNH
b. CML
c. Megaloblastic anaemia
d. Myelofibrosis

223. All the following are primary granules, *except*: *(AIPGEE 2007)*
a. Lysozyme
b. Myeloperoxidase
c. Lactoferrin
d. BPI

224. Leucocytosis is seen in: *(AIPGEE 2007)*
a. Megaloblastic anaemia
b. Blood transfusion
c. Steroids
d. Dengue

225. Lymphocytes are located in each of the following tissues or organs *except*: *(KCET 2009)*

a. Brain b. Spleen
c. Lymph nodes d. Thymus gland

226. The type of acute myelogenous leukemia associated with a high incidence of disseminated intravascular coagulation is: *(KCET 2009)*

a. Acute erythroleukemia
b. Acute promyelocytic leukemia
c. Acute megakaryocytic leukemia
d. Acute myelomonocytic leukemia

227. The most striking haematological finding in agranulocytosis is: *(COMEDK 2005)*

a. Decreased absolute neutrophil count
b. Increased absolute neutrophil count
c. Decreased absolute basophil count
d. Increased absolute basophil count

228. Leukocyte alkaline phosphatase (LAP) is elevated in: *(COMEDK 2007)*

a. Pernicious anemia
b. Sickle cell anemia
c. Polycythemia vera
d. Plummer-Vinson syndrome

229. Acute pyogenic infection produces: *(COMEDK 2008)*

a. Leukopenia b. Leukocytosis
c. Neutropenia d. Lymphopenia

230. "AUER RODS" are seen in: *(COMEDK 2010)*

a. Lymphoblast b. Myeloblast
c. Neurophils d. Basophils

231. In Troisier's sign, the lymph nodes involved are? *(COMEDK 2011)*

a. Right axillary nodes
b. Left axillary nodes
c. Right supra-clavicular nodes
d. Left supra-clavicular nodes

232. A 20 years old male complains of recurrent attacks of sore throat since 2 years. The total leucocyte count was 1000/ul. A differential count revealed severe neutropenia. The diagnosis is: *(COMEDK 2012)*

a. Subleukemic leukemia
b. Infectious mononucleosis
c. Agranulocytosis
d. Leukoerythroblastic anemia

LUNG

233. The physiologic dead space is decreased by: *(AIIMS May 2005)*

a. Upright position
b. Positive pressure ventilation
c. Neck flexion
d. Emphysema

234. If pneumothorax occurs in a patient: *(AIPGEE 2011)*

a. The surfactant will be reduced
b. The intrapleural pressure becomes more negative
c. Deep breathing is noticed
d. Exaggerated breath sounds

235. During ABG chances of median nerve damage is maximum with: *(AIPGEE 2010)*

a. Radial artery
b. Brachial artery
c. Femoral artery
d. Internal carotid artery

236. The proper rate of rescue breathing in an adult is: *(AIPGEE 2005)*

a. 4 times per minute
b. 12 times per minute
c. 20 times per minute
d. 28 times per minute

237. In cardiopulmonary resuscitation, chest compression is done on the: *(AIPGEE 2005)*

a. Upper part of sternum
b. Xiphisternum
c. Middle of the lower part of the sternum
d. Left side of the chest

238. In lobar pneumonia, the presence of fibrin support exudates with disintegration of red cell is seen to the stage of: *(COMEDK 2010)*

a. Congestion
b. Red hepatisation
c. Grey hepatisation
d. Resolution

HEAD AND NECK

239. Fordyce disease is a condition resulting from: *(AIIMS May 2009)*

a. Aberrant sebaceous glands
b. Cholesterol deposits
c. Capillary fragility
d. Hyperkeratosis

240. Most common site of occurrence of sialolith is in: *(AIPGEE 2009)*

a. Parotid
b. Sublingual
c. Submandibular
d. All of the above

241. Most common tumour of the parotid gland is: *(AIPGEE 2009)*

a. Pleomorphic adenoma
b. Warthin's tumour
c. Adenocarcinoma
d. Sialometaplasia

242. Saw tooth rete pegs are seen in which of the following oral lesions? *(AIPGEE 2009)*

a. Lichen planus
b. Leukoplakia
c. Leukoedema
d. Lichenoid reaction

243. True about ranula is: *(AIPGEE 2005)*

a. Also known as epulis
b. Cyst in floor of mouth
c. Thyroglossal cyst
d. Type of mucous retention cyst

244. Mucin in mucous cells is usually demonstrated by: *(KCET 2008)*

a. PAP stain
b. H and E stain
c. Mucicarmine stain
d. Mallory stain

GASTROINTESTINAL TRACT

245. All of the following statements about Wilson's disease are true, *except*: *(AIPGEE 2010)*

a. It is an autosomal recessive disorder
b. Serum ceruloplasmin level less than 20 mg/dL
c. Urinary copper excretion is less than 100 μg/day
d. Zinc acetate is effective as maintenance therapy

246. In hepatolenticular disease which one is true? *(AIPGEE 2010)*

a. Increased ceruloplasmin level in blood
b. Increased urinary excretion of copper
c. Reduced hepatic copper level
d. Presence of Kayser-Fleischer rings in the retina of eyes

247. The Histologic criterion for diagnosis of acute appendicitis is neutrophilic infiltration of: *(COMEDK 2009)*

a. Mucosa
b. Submucosa
c. Muscularis propria
d. Serosa

LIVER AND BILIARY TRACT

248. Pain due to gallstones can be perceived in all areas *except*: *(AIIMS May 2011)*

a. Right shoulder
b. Right hypochondrium
c. Right iliac fossa
d. Epigastrium

249. Recent HBV infection is determined by the presence of HBsAg and: *(AIPGEE 2008)*

a. HbeAg
b. HbcAg
c. HbeAb
d. HbsAb

250. Which of the following is the first marker of hepatitis B infection? *(AIPGEE 2007)*

a. Anti-HBsAg
b. HBeAg
c. HBcAg
d. HBsAg

251. Extrahepatic cholestasis is seen in: *(AIPGEE 2007)*

a. Haemolytic anaemia
b. Obstructive jaundice
c. Pancreatic carcinoma
d. Viral hepatitis

252. An extrahepatic cholestasis is association with: *(AIPGEE 2007)*

a. Increased bilirubin in urine
b. Increased urobilinogen in urine
c. Increased bilirubin and urobilinogen in serum
d. Increased bilirubin in serum

253. Dark-coloured urine and clay-coloured stools are seen in: *(AIPGEE 2007)*

a. Neonatal jaundice
b. Haemolytic anaemia
c. Hepatocellular jaundice
d. Severe dehydration

254. Unconjugated hyperbilirubinaemia in jaundice is most likely due to: *(AIPGEE 2005)*

a. Hepatitis
b. Cirrhosis
c. Obstruction of bile canaliculi
d. Increased breakdown of red cells

255. 5′-nucleotidase activity is increased in: *(AIPGEE 2005)*

a. Bone diseases
b. Prostate cancer
c. Chronic rental failure
d. Cholestatic disorders

256. Which one of the following serum levels would help in distinguishing an acute liver disease from chronic liver disease? *(AIPGEE 2005)*
a. Aminotransaminase
b. Alkaline phosphatase
c. Bilirubin
d. Albumin

257. In a patient suffering from liver disease, the main complication encountered during extraction is: *(KCET 2009)*
a. Syncope
b. Postoperative infection
c. Prolonged bleeding
d. Convulsions

258. A diagnosis of chronic hepatitis is made if liver disease is present for a minimum of: *(COMEDK 2007)*
a. 3 weeks b. 6 weeks
c. 6 months d. 3 months

PANCREAS

259. In type II diabetes, patients are advised to increase intake of: *(AIPGEE 2010)*
a. Protein b. Fat
c. Carbohydrate d. Fibre

KIDNEY

260. Which of the following is associated with thiazide diuretics? *(AIIMS Nov 2010)*
a. Hyperkalaemic paralysis
b. Hypouricaemia
c. Hypolipidaemia
d. Impotence

261. Hyponatraemia with increased Na^+ concentration in the body is seen with: *(AIIMS Nov 2010)*
a. Renal tubular acidosis
b. Diuretic therapy
c. Nephrotic syndrome
d. Vomiting

262. Bence Jones proteinuria may be seen in: *(AIPGEE 2011)*
a. Alpha heavy chain disease
b. Gamma heavy chain disease
c. Mu heavy chain disease
d. Epsilon heavy chain disease

263. Urine VMA is associated with: *(AIPGEE 2008)*
a. Diabetes mellitus
b. Neurofibroma
c. Schwannoma
d. Neuroectodermal disease

264. Which of the following is the hallmark of chronic renal failure? *(AIPGEE 2007)*
a. Metabolic acidosis
b. Hypercalcemia
c. Hypokalaemia
d. Increased proneness to hypoxia

265. Urine analysis of a patient associated with haematuria and glomerulonephritis shows: *(AIPGEE 2007)*
a. Isomorphic red cells
b. Red cell casts
c. WBC casts
d. Hyaline cast

266. Bence Jones proteins found in the urine may be suggestive of: *(AIPGEE 2006)*
a. Hyperparathyroidism
b. Hodgkin's disease
c. Multiple myeloma
d. Christian syndrome

267. Expansile lytic osseous metastases are characteristic of primary malignancy of: *(AIPGEE 2006)*
a. Kidney b. Bronchial
c. Breast d. Prostate

268. Kimmelstiel Wilson disease is: *(COMEDK 2009)*
a. Diffuse glomerulosclerosis
b. Capillary basement membrane thickening
c. Nodular glomerulosclerosis
d. Increase in mesangial matrix

269. Nephrotic syndrome true is? *(MHPGDCET 2011)*
a. Hyperfibrinogenemia
b. Hyperlipidemia
c. Hypercoagulability
d. All of the above

270. During a routine urine examination of an adult, precipitation occurs at 60C and on increasing the temperature further, it dissolves completely. It is indicative of: *(AIPG/NEET 2013)*
a. Ketosis
b. Bence jones proteins
c. Uremia
d. Nephrotic syndrome

LOWER URINARY TRACT AND MALE GENITAL SYSTEM

No question was asked from this chapter.

FEMALE GENITAL TRACT

271. Which of the following method is used for the assessment of female fertility during menstrual cycle and the best predict time of ovulation? *(AIPGEE 2011)*
a. Basal body temperature
b. Fern test
c. Spinnbarkeit phenomenon
d. Hormonal study

BREAST

No question was asked from this chapter.

ENDOCRINE SYSTEM

272. A patient is wide eyed, very nervous with an increased systolic pressure (with widening of pulse pressure), increased pulse rate, fine skin and hair, and loss of body weight. He is probably suffering from: *(AIIMS Nov 2010)*
a. Hypothyroidism
b. Hyperthyroidism
c. Hyperpituitarism
d. Hyperparathyroidism

273. Obesity is associated with all *except*: *(AIIMS Nov 2009)*
a. Growth hormone deficiency
b. Hypothyroidism
c. Diabetes mellitus
d. Oestrogen deficiency

274. Exophthalmos, nervousness, tachycardia, heat intolerance and hypertension are indicative of: *(AIIMS May 2009)*
a. Hypothyroidism
b. Hyperthyroidism
c. Hypoparathyroidism
d. Hyperparathyroidism

275. Phaeochromocytoma is a disorder primarily occurring due to a defect in: *(AIIMS Nov 2006)*
a. Adrenal medulla
b. Kidney
c. Thyroid
d. Parathyroid

276. Obesity is not caused by: *(AIPGEE 2011)*
a. Diabetes mellitus
b. Oestrogen deficiency
c. Hypothyroidism
d. Cortisol

277. Pigmentation of skin is seen in: *(AIPGEE 2010)*
a. Addison's disease
b. Haemochromatosis
c. Cushing disease
d. Wilson's disease

278. Human chorionic gonadotropin detection is done by: *(AIPGEE 2010)*
a. ELISA
b. BIOASSAY
c. RIA
d. PCR

279. Which of the following is seen in acromegaly? *(AIPGEE 2009)*
a. Large tongue
b. Hypoglycaemia
c. Crowding of teeth
d. All of the above

280. A middle-aged female patient has eyes widely placed, sparse hair, increased systolic blood pressure, increased pulse pressure, weight loss and nervousness. She may be suffering from: *(AIPGEE 2009)*
a. Hyperthyroidism
b. Hypothyroidism
c. Hyperparathyroidism
d. Hypopituitarism

281. Brown tumour is seen in: *(AIPGEE 2006)*
a. Hyperparathyroidism
b. Pigmented villonodular synovitis
c. Osteomalacia
d. Neurofibromatosis

282. Hypercalcaemia associated with malignancy is most often mediated by: *(AIPGEE 2005)*
a. Parathyroid hormone (PTH)
b. Parathyroid hormone related protein (PTHrP)
c. Interleukin-6 (IL-6)
d. Calcitonin

283. Which of the following statements is true regarding thyroglobulin? *(COMEDK 2011)*
a. It is a specific marker for anaplastic carcinoma
b. Elevation after complete therapy suggests recurrence in well differentiated thyroid malignancies
c. Pre-operation elevation from thyroid veins is very useful for prognosis
d. Intraoperative estimation from thyroid veins is very useful for prognosis

284. Hyperthyroidism causes all, *except*: *(MHPGDCET 2010)*
a. Restlessness (emotional)
b. Weight loss
c. Anxiety
d. Sleep

285. Parry's disease is known are: *(MHPGDCET 2010)*
a. Thyrotoxicosis
b. Thyroid strom
c. Thyroid crisis
d. Exophthalmic goiter

286. Ace test is used for: *(MHPGDCET 2010)*
a. Ketosis b. Acidosis
c. Alkalosis d. None of the above

287. Calcitonin increases in which of the following conditions? *(MHPGDCET 2012)*
a. Medullary carcinoma of thyroid
b. Hepatocellular carcinoma
c. Carcinoma of colon
d. Neural tumor

SKIN

288. The type of ultraviolet radiation (UV) that is known to induce skin cancer is: *(COMEDK 2012)*
a. UVA b. UVB
c. UVC d. UVD

BONES, JOINTS, AND SOFT-TISSUE TUMORS

289. Protein that precipitates on heating at 46°C and redissolves on boiling is: *(AIIMS May 2009)*
a. Bence Jones proteins
b. Gamma globulin
c. Albumin
d. Myosin

290. Fibrous dysplasia is associated with: *(AIIMS May 2009)*
a. Ground-glass density
b. Soap-bubble appearance
c. Hair-on-end appearance
d. Sunburst appearance

291. With what type of collagen does cartilage not have any association? *(AIIMS May 2008)*
a. Type 4 b. Type 2
c. Type 6 d. Type 9

292. Osteomalacia is associated with: *(AIIMS May 2006)*
a. Decrease in osteoid volume
b. Decrease in osteoid surface
c. Increase in osteoid maturation time
d. Increase in mineral deposition rate

293. A 50-year-old man presented with multiple pathological fractures. His serum calcium was 11.5 mg/dL, phosphate was 2.5 mg/dL and alkaline phosphatase was 940 IU/dL. The most probable diagnosis is: *(AIIMS Nov 2005)*
a. Osteoporosis
b. Osteomalacia
c. Multiple myeloma
d. Hyperparathyroidism

294. Gout is disorder of: *(AIPGEE 2011)*
a. Purine metabolism
b. Pyrimidine metabolism
c. Ketone metabolism
d. Protein metabolism

295. Rhabdomyosarcoma is a disorder of: *(AIPGEE 2009)*
a. Smooth muscle
b. Striated muscle
c. Both
d. None

296. Mosaic pattern of bone is seen in: *(AIPGEE 2009)*
a. Fibrous dysplasia
b. Osteitis deformans
c. Osteomyelitis
d. Ewing's sarcoma

297. Which of the following is not a major criterion for diagnosis of multiple myeloma? *(AIPGEE 2006)*
a. Lytic bone lesions
b. Plasmacytoma on tissue biopsy
c. Bone marrow plasma cytosis > 30%
d. 'M' spike > 3 g% for IgG > 2% for IgA

298. All the statements are true about exostosis *except* that: *(AIPGEE 2006)*
a. It occurs at the growing end of bone
b. Growth continues after skeletal maturity
c. It is covered by a cartilaginous cap
d. Malignant transformation may occur

299. Bisphosphonates act by: *(AIPGEE 2006)*
a. Increasing the osteoid formation
b. Increasing the mineralization of osteoid
c. Decreasing the osteoclast mediated resorption of bone
d. All of the above

300. All of the following are known causes of osteoporosis, *except*: *(AIPGEE 2006) (AIPGEE 2005)*
a. Fluorosis
b. Hypogonadism
c. Hyperthyroidism
d. Hyperparathyroidism

301. Fine needle aspiration cytology is not suitable for diagnosing: *(AIPGEE 2006)*
a. Tubercular lymphadenitis
b. Papillary carcinoma of thyroid
c. Plasmacytoma
d. Aneurysmal bone cyst

302. Which of the following conditions is least likely to present as an eccentric osteolytic lesion?
a. Aneurysmal bone cyst *(AIPGEE 2006)*
b. Giant cell tumour
c. Fibrous cortical defect
d. Simple bone cyst

303. Rugger jersey spine is seen in: *(AIPGEE 2006)*
a. Fluorosis
b. Achondroplasia
c. Renal osteodystrophy
d. Marfan's syndrome

304. Joint erosions are not a feature of: *(AIPGEE 2006)*
a. Rheumatoid arthritis
b. Psoriasis
c. Multicentric reticulohistiocytosis
d. Systemic lupus erythematosus

305. Which is not a marker of new bone formation: *(AIPG/NEET 2013)*
a. Osteocalcin b. Alkaline phosphate
c. Procollagen d. Hydroxyproline

PERIPHERAL NERVE AND SKELETAL MUSCLE

306. One of the following is not capable of replication: *(KCET 2006)*
a. Neuron b. Liver
c. Kidney d. None of above

CENTRAL NERVOUS SYSTEM

307. In Glasgow Coma Scale, a patient with V4E5M6 (a total score of 15) indicates: *(AIIMS May 2010)*
a. A normal patient with normal verbal and eye response and obeys full commands
b. Patients withdraws to painful response with disoriented conversation
c. Atient withdraws to painful response and opens his eye to voice
d. An unconscious patient showing no verbal response

308. Increased intracranial tension can cause all *except*: *(AIIMS May 2009)*
a. Nausea and vomiting
b. Headache
c. Muscle twitching
d. Somnolence

309. Which one of the following is a benzodiazepine antagonist? *(AIIMS May 2009)*
a. Flumazenil
b. Naloxone
c. Furazolidone
d. Naltrexone

310. A person is fully conscious with regard to time, place and person; shows normal speech and responds to verbal commands. In this case, the Glasgow coma scale would be: *(AIIMS May 2007) (AIPGEE 2007)*
a. 3
b. 19
c. 14
d. 15

311. The seizures with no aura, no tonic or clonic phase that occurs asymptomatic in children with several times in a day is: *(AIPGEE 2010)*
a. Grand mal epilepsy
b. Petit mal epilepsy
c. Infantile
d. Tonicclonic

312. A 25-year-old female presents with 2-year history of repetitive, irresistible thoughts of contamination with dirt associated with repetitive hand washing. She reports these thoughts to be her own and distressing, but is not able to overcome them along with medications. She is most likely to benefit from which of the following therapies?
a. Exposure and response prevention
b. Systematic desensitization
c. Assertiveness training
d. Sensate focusing

313. Who proposed the operant conditioning theory of child psychology? *(AIPGEE 2005)*
a. Pavlov
b. Skinner
c. Jean Piaget
d. Sigmund Freud

314. Which is not true about cerebellar lesions? *(AIPGEE 2005)*
a. In ventral lesion of pons, ipsilateral facial palsy is present
b. In lower dorsal lesion of pons, contralateral hemiplegia is present
c. In upper dorsal lesion of pons, ipsilateral sensory loss of face is present
d. In lower dorsal lesion of pons, ipsilateral facial palsy is present

EYE

315. The most common retrobulbar orbital mass in adults is: *(AIPGEE 2006)*
a. Neurofibroma
b. Meningioma
c. Cavernous haemangioma
d. Schwannoma

Answers with Explanations

CELLULAR ADAPTATIONS, CELL INJURY, AND CELL DEATH

1. Ans. (b) Increased superoxide dismutase *Ref: Robbins Pathologic Basis of Disease 7th ed. p 16-17, 43*

Cell ageing occurs because of following reasons:

- As time passes cells become old.
- In addition, there is a genetic clock which is mainly determined by telomeres.
- Also presence of the free radicals causes cell aging. Cells generate energy by reducing molecular oxygen to water. During this process, small amounts of partially reduced reactive oxygen forms are produced as an unavoidable by product of mitochondrial respiration. Some of these forms are free radicals that can damage lipids, proteins, and nucleic acids. They are referred to as reactive oxygen species. A series of enzymes acts as free radical-scavenging systems and break down hydrogen peroxide and superoxide anion, these enzymes are located near the sites of generation of these oxidants and include the following:
  - Catalase, present in peroxisomes
  - Superoxide dismutases are found in many cell types and convert superoxide to H_2O.' This group includes both manganese superoxide dismutase, which is localized in mitochondria, and copper-zinc-superoxide dismutase, which is found in the cytosol.
  - Glutathione peroxidase also protects against injury by catalyzing free radical breakdown. The amount of oxidative damage, which increases as an organism ages, may be an important component of senescence. And it has been found out that as presence of superoxide dismutase scavenges free radicals it actually prevents ageing.

2. Ans. (a) Karyolysis *Ref: Robbins Pathologic Basis of Disease 7th ed. p 21*

Necrosis refers to a spectrum of morphologic changes that follow cell death in living tissue, largely resulting from the progressive degradative action of enzymes on the lethally injured cell (cells placed immediately in fixative are dead but not necrotic). As commonly used, necrosis is the gross and histologic correlate of cell death occurring in the setting of irreversible exogenous injury. Necrotic cells are unable to maintain membrane integrity and their contents often leak out. This may elicit inflammation in the surrounding tissue.

Nuclear changes appear in the form of one of three patterns, all due to nonspecific breakdown of DNA.

- The basophilia of the chromatin may fade (karyolysis), a change that presumably reflects DNase activity.
- A second pattern (also seen in apoptotic cell death) is pyknosis, characterized by nuclear shrinkage and increased basophilia. Here, the DNA apparently condenses into a solid, shrunken basophilic mass.
- In the third pattern, known as karyorrhexis, the pyknotic or partially pyknotic nucleus undergoes fragmentation. With the passage of time (a day or two), the nucleus in the necrotic cell totally disappears.

3. Ans. (a) Coagulative necrosis *Ref: Pathology by Earl Brown p 103.*

- Apoptosis is a pathway of cell death that is induced by a tightly regulated suicide program in which cells destined to die activate enzymes that degrade the cells' own nuclear DNA and nuclear and cytoplasmic proteins. Apoptotic cells break up into fragments, called apoptotic bodies, which contain portions of the cytoplasm and nucleus. The plasma membrane of the apoptotic cell and bodies remains intact, but its structure is altered in such a way that these become 'tasty' targets for phagocytes. The dead cell and its fragments are rapidly devoured, before the contents have leaked out, and therefore cell death by this pathway does not elicit an inflammatory reaction in the host. Apoptosis is a unique mechanism of cell death, distinct from necrosis, which is characterized by loss of membrane integrity, enzymatic digestion of cells, leakage of cellular contents, and frequently a host reaction.

- Coagulative necrosis implies preservation of the basic outline of the coagulated cell for a span of at least some days. The affected tissues exhibit a firm texture.
- Liquefactive necrosis is characteristic of focal bacterial or, occasionally, fungal infections, because microbes stimulate the accumulation of inflammatory cells. For obscure reasons, hypoxic death of cells within the central nervous system often evokes liquefactive necrosis. Whatever the pathogenesis, liquefaction completely digests the dead cells.
- Dysplasia, the term that literally means disordered growth. Dysplasia is encountered principally in epithelia, and it is characterized by a constellation of changes that include a loss in the uniformity of the individual cells as well as a loss in their architectural orientation.
- Neoangiogenesis literally means new blood vessel formation. It usually seen in tumors and healing tissues. Among all the options if one has to choose then by exclusion method we may choose Dysplasia.

4. Ans. (d) Apoptosis *Ref: Robbins Pathologic Basis of Disease 7th ed. p 27*

BIOCHEMICAL FEATURES OF APOPTOSIS

Many biochemical changes are noted during apoptosis which can also be seen in necrosis but following features are unique to apoptosis.

- **Protein cleavage**- is mainly carried out by cysteine proteases namely caspases. Many caspases are inactively present in cells as proenzymes and when required they cleave proteins, e.g. lamins which break up the nuclear scaffold and cytoskeleton, and thus determine the shape of the apoptotic bodies. Another example is DNAse which cleavenuclear DNA.
- **DNA breakdown**-Apoptotic cells exhibit a characteristic breakdown of DNA into large 50- to 300-kilobase pieces. Subsequently, there is internucleosomal cleavage of DNA into oligonucleosomes.
- **Phagocytic Recognition**-Apoptotic cells express phosphatidylserine in the outer layers of their plasma membranes, the phospholipid having flipped out from the inner layers. In some types of apoptosis, thrombospondin, an adhesive glycoprotein, is also expressed on the surfaces of apoptotic bodies, and other proteins secreted by phagocytes may bind to apoptotic cells and opsonize the cells for phagocytosis.' These alterations permit the early recognition of dead cells by macrophages, resulting in phagocytosis without the release of proinflammatory cellular components.

5. Ans. (c) Both necrosis and apoptosis *Ref: http://www.ncbi.nlm.nih.gov/pmc/articles/PMC3132471/ [Chemotherapeutic Approaches for Targeting Cell Death Pathways- Oncologist. Apr 2006;11(4): 342357]*

For several decades, apoptosis has taken center stage as the principal mechanism of programmed cell death in mammalian tissues. It also has been increasingly noted that conventional chemotherapeutic agents not only elicit apoptosis but other forms of nonapoptotic death, such as necrosis, autophagy, mitotic catastrophe, and senescence.

6. Ans. (c) Cell apoptosis

Refer explanation of Chapter 1 Q 4

7. Ans. (b) Apoptosis *Ref: Metal Ions in Neurological system by wolfgang Linert p 149*

Cytochrome C in the cytoplasm triggers the activation of capase. 9, which triggers the capase cascades and leads to apoptosis.

8. Ans. (b) Diminished generation of adenosine triphosphate (ATP)

Ref: Robbins Pathologic Basis of Disease 7th ed. p 20

Ultrastructural changes in reversible cell injury include:

- Plasma membrane alterations, such as blebbing, blunting, and loss of microvilli
- Mitochondrial changes, including swelling and the appearance of small amorphous densities
- Dilation of the ER, with detachment of polysomes; intracytoplasmic myelin figures may be present
- Nuclear alterations, with disaggregation of granular and fibrillar elements

9. Ans. (c) Liquefactive necrosis *Ref: Robbins Pathologic Basis of Disease 7th ed. p 21*

Once the necrotic cells undergo early altercations such as increased eosinophilia, nuclear changes (karyolysis, pyknosis, and karyorrhexis) the mass of necrotic cells have several morphologic patterns. When denaturation is the primary pattern, coagulative necrosis develops. In the presence of dominant enzyme digestion the result is liquefactive degeneration. In special circumstances caseous necrosis and fat necrosis may occur.

10. Ans. (b) Hyperplasia *Ref: Robbins Pathologic Basis of Disease 7th ed. p 6, 7, 10*

Hyperplasia is an increase in the number of cells in an organ or tissue, usually resulting in increased volume of the organ or tissue. Although hyperplasia and hypertrophy are two distinct processes, frequently both occur together, and they may be triggered by the same external stimulus. For instance, hormone-induced growth in the uterus involves both increased numbers of smooth muscle and epithelial cells and the enlargement of these cells. Hyperplasia takes place if the cellular population is capable of synthesizing DNA, thus permitting mitotic division; by contrast, hypertrophy involves cell enlargement without cell division. Hyperplasia can be physiologic or pathologic.

Metaplasia is a reversible change in which one adult cell type (epithelial or mesenchymal) is replaced by another adult cell type.'

Aplasia is defined in general as 'defective development or congenital absence of an organ or tissue'.

11. Ans. (b) Elie Metchnikoff

Ref: Harsh Mohan Textbook of Pathology 6th ed. p 4; http://en.wikipedia.org/wiki/Phagocytosis

In cell biology, phagocytosis is the process by which a cell often a phagocyte engulfs a solid particle to form an internal vesicle known as a phagosome. Phagocytosis was revealed by Élie Metchnikoff in 1882.

12. Ans. (c) Proenzymes *Ref: http://en.wikipedia.org/wiki/Zymogen http://en.wikibooks.org/wiki/Structural_Biochemistry/Enzyme/Apoenzyme_and_Holoenzyme*

Many enzymes require an additional small molecule, known as a cofactor to aid with catalytic activity. A cofactor is a non-protein molecule that carries out chemical reactions that cannot be performed by the standard 20 amino acids. Cofactors can be either inorganic molecules (metals) or small organic molecules (coenzymes).

- **Apoenzyme**- An enzyme that requires a cofactor but does not have one bound. An apoenzyme is an inactive enzyme, activation of the enzyme occurs upon binding of an organic or inorganic cofactor.
- **Holoenzyme**- An apoenzyme together with its cofactor. A holoenzyme is complete and catalytically active.
- **Proenzyme**- The inactive or nearly inactive precursor of an enzyme, converted into an active enzyme by proteolysis. Also called zymogen.
- **A zymogen (or proenzyme)** is an inactive enzyme precursor. A zymogen requires a biochemical change (such as a hydrolysis reaction revealing the active site, or changing the configuration to reveal the active site) for it to become an active enzyme. The biochemical change usually occurs in a lysosome where a specific part of the precursor enzyme is cleaved in order to activate it.

13. Ans. (b) Coagulative necrosis *Ref: Robbins Pathologic Basis of Disease 7th ed. p 21*

Coagulative necrosis implies preservation of the basic outline of the coagulated cell for a span of at least some days. The affected tissues exhibit a firm texture. Presumably, the injury or the subsequent increasing intracellular acidosis denatures not only structural proteins but also enzymes and so blocks the proteolysis of the cell. The myocardial infarct is an excellent example in which acidophilic, coagulated, anucleate cells may persist for weeks.

14. Ans. (d) Myeloperoxidase

Refer explanation of Chapter 1 Q 1

Myeloperoxidase (MPO) is a peroxidase enzyme that in humans is encoded by the MPO gene. Myeloperoxidase is most abundantly expressed in neutrophil. It is a lysosomal protein stored in azurophilic granules of the neutrophil. MPO has a heme pigment, which causes its green color in secretions rich in neutrophils, such as pus and some forms of mucus.

15. Ans. (b) Fibrinoid necrosis *Ref: Robbins Pathologic Basis of Disease 7th ed. p 213-214*

The pathogenesis of systemic immune complex disease can be divided into three phases:

- Formation of antigen-antibody complexes in the circulation
- Deposition of the immune complexes in various tissues, thus initiating, and
- An inflammatory reaction at the sites of immune complex deposition

The morphologic consequences of immune complex injury are dominated by acute necrotizing vasculitis, with necrosis of the vessel wall and intense neutrophilic infiltration. The necrotic tissue and deposits of immune complexes, complement, and plasma protein produce a smudgy eosinophilic deposit that obscures the underlying cellular detail, an appearance termed fibrinoid necrosis.

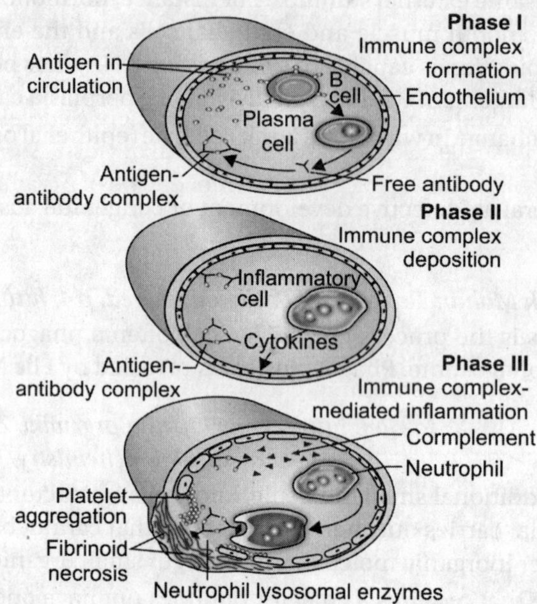

Schematic illustration of the 3 sequential phases in the induction of systemic immune complex-mediated disease (type III hypersensitivity).

16. Ans. (a) Fatty change *Ref: Robbins Pathologic Basis of Disease 7th ed. p36*

The terms steatosis and fatty change describe abnormal accumulations of triglycerides within parenchymal cells. Fatty change is often seen in the liver because it is the major organ involved in fat metabolism, but it also occurs in heart, muscle and kidney. The causes of steatosis include toxins, protein malnutrition, diabetes mellitus, obesity, and anoxia.

- Heart. lipid is found in cardiac muscle in the form of small droplets, occurring in two patterns. In one, prolonged moderate hypoxia, such as that produced by profound anemia, causes intracellular deposits of fat, which create grossly apparent bands of yellowed myocardium alternating with bands of darker, redbrown, uninvolved myocardium (tigered effect). The other pattern of hypoxia is produced by more profound hypoxia or by some forms of myocarditis (e.g. diphtheria) and shows more uniformly affected myocytes.

17. Ans. (d) Serum calcium levels are high *Ref: Robbins Pathologic Basis of Disease 7th ed. p 41*

Pathologic calcification is the abnormal tissue deposition of calcium salts, together with smaller amounts of iron, magnesium, and other mineral salts. It is a common process occurring in a variety of pathologic conditions. There are two forms of pathologic calcification. When the deposition occurs locally in dying tissues, it is known as dystrophic calcification; it occurs despite normal serum levels of calcium and in the absence of derangements in calcium metabolism. In contrast, the deposition of calcium salts in otherwise normal tissues is known as metastatic calcification, and it almost always results from hypercalcemia secondary to some disturbance in calcium metabolism. Dystrophic calcification is encountered in areas of necrosis, whether they are of coagulative, caseous, or liquefactive type, and in foci of enzymatic necrosis of fat. Calcification is almost inevitable in the atheromas of advanced atherosclerosis. It also commonly develops in aging or damaged heart valves, further hampering their function.

18. Ans. (d) All of the above *Ref: Robbins Pathologic Basis of Disease 7th ed. p 482, 24,*

- Cells generate energy by reducing molecular oxygen to water. During this process, small amounts of partially reduced reactive oxygen forms are produced as an unavoidable byproduct of mitochondrial respiration. Some of these forms are free radicals that can damage lipids, proteins, and nucleic acids. They are referred to as reactive oxygen species.
- Restoration of blood flow to ischemic tissues can result in recovery of cells if they are reversibly injured, or not affect the outcome if irreversible cell damage has occurred. However, depending on the intensity and duration of the ischemic insult, variable numbers of cells may proceed to die after blood flow resumes, by necrosis as well as by apoptosis.") The affected tissues often show neutrophilic infiltrates. As noted earlier, this ischemia-reperfusion injury is a clinically important process in such conditions as myocardial infarction and stroke. Damage may be initiated during reoxygenation by increased generation of oxygen free radicals from parenchymal and endothelial cells and from infiltrating leukocytes.
- Oxygen toxicity is a condition resulting from the harmful effects of breathing molecular oxygen (O_2) at elevated partial pressures. The biochemical basis for the toxicity of oxygen is the partial reduction of oxygen by one or two electrons to form reactive oxygen species, which are natural by-products of the normal metabolism of oxygen and have important roles in cell signalling.

19. Ans. (d) Binds to sulfydryl groups *Ref: Robbins Pathologic Basis of Disease 7th ed. p 25*

Some chemicals can act directly by combining with some critical molecular component or cellular organelle. For example, in mercuric chloride poisoning, mercury binds to the sulfhydryl groups of the cell membrane and other proteins, causing increased membrane permeability and inhibition of ATPase-dependent transport. In such instances, the greatest damage is usually to the cells that use, absorb, excrete, or concentrate the chemicals in the case of mercuric chloride, the cells of the gastrointestinal tract and kidney.

20. Ans. (a) Tuberculosis *Ref: Robbins Pathologic Basis of Disease 7th ed. p 22*

Caseous necrosis, a distinctive form of coagulative necrosis, is encountered most often in foci of tuberculous infection. The term caseous is derived from the cheesy white gross appearance of the area of necrosis. On microscopic examination, the necrotic focus appears as amorphous granular debris seemingly composed of fragmented, coagulated cells and amorphous granular debris enclosed within a distinctive inflammatory border known as a granulomatous reaction. Unlike coagulative necrosis, the tissue architecture is completely obliterated.

21. Ans. (c) Zipper killing *Ref: Robbins Pathologic Basis of Disease 7th ed. p 60*

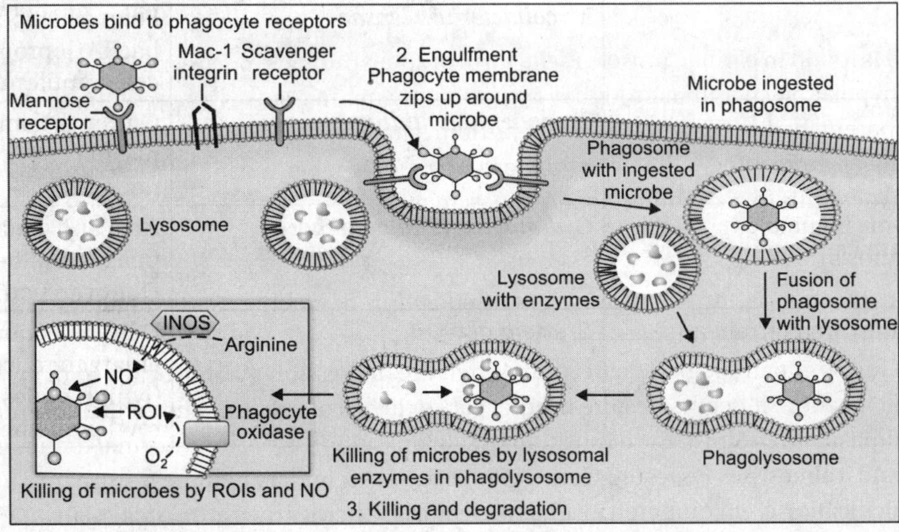

- Phagocytosis of a particle (e.g. bacterium) involves attachment and binding of Fc and C3b to receptors on the leukocyte membrane, engulfment, and fusion of lysosomes with phagocytic vacuoles, followed by destruction of ingested particles within the phagolysosomes.

22. Ans. (a) Scleroderma *Ref: Robbins Pathologic Basis of Disease 7th ed. p 237*

Systemic sclerosis is a chronic disease of unknown etiology characterized by abnormal accumulation of fibrous tissue in the skin and multiple organs. Although the term scleroderma is ingrained in the literature through common usage, this disease is better named systemic sclerosis because it is characterized by excessive fibrosis throughout the body. Virtually all organs may be involved in systemic sclerosis. Prominent changes occur in the skin, alimentary tract, musculoskeletal system, and kidney, but lesions also are often present in the blood vessels, heart, lungs, and peripheral nerves. Skin—A great majority of patients have diffuse, sclerotic atrophy of the skin, which usually begins in the fingers and distal regions of the upper extremities and extends proximally to involve the upper arms, shoulders, neck, and face. There is marked increase of compact collagen in the dermis along with thinning of the epidermis, loss of rete pegs, atrophy of the dermal appendages, and hyaline thickening of the walls of dermal arterioles and capillaries. Focal and sometimes diffuse subcutaneous calcifications may develop, especially in patients with the CREST syndrome (calcinosis, Raynaud phenomenon, esophageal dysmotility, sclerodactyly, and telangiectasia).

23. Ans. (a) Apoptotic cell death *Ref: Robbins Pathologic Basis of Disease 7th ed. p 27*

Caspases, or cysteine-aspartic proteases or cysteine-dependent aspartate-directed proteases are a family of cysteine proteases that play essential roles in apoptosis (programmed cell death), necrosis, and inflammation. Caspases are essential in cells for apoptosis, or programmed cell death, in development and most other stages of adult life, and have been termed 'executioner' proteins for their roles in the cell. A specific feature of apoptosis is protein hydrolysis involving the activation of several members of a family of cysteine proteases named caspases.` Many caspases are present in normal cells as inactive pro-enzymes, and they need to be activated to induce apoptosis. Active caspases cleave many vital cellular proteins, such as lamins, and thus break up the nuclear scaffold and cytoskeleton; in addition, caspases activate DNAses, which degrade nuclear DNA. These changes underlie the nuclear and cytoplasmic structural alterations seen in apoptotic cells.

24. Ans. (c) Sarcoidosis *Ref: Harsh Mohan Textbook of Pathology 6th ed. p 150*

Conditions	*Etiologic agent*	*Special characteristics*
I. Bacterial		
• Tuberculosis	*Mycobacterium tuberculosis*	Tuberculous granulomas with central caseation necrosis; acid-fast bacilli
• Leprosy	*Mycobacterium leprae*	Foamy histiocytes with acid-fast bacilli (lepromatous); epithelioid cell granulomas (tuberculoid)
• Syphilis	*Treponema pallidum*	Gummas composed of histiocytes: plasma cell infiltration; central necrosis
• Granuloma inguinale (Donovanosis)	*C. donovani (Donovan body)*	Anal and genital lesions; macrophages and neutrophils show Donovan bodies
• Brucellosis (Mediterranean fever)	*Brucella abortus*	Dairy infection to humans; enlarged reticuloendothelial organs (lymph nodes, spleen, bone marrow); non-specific granulomas

Contd...

Contd...

Conditions	*Etiologic agent*	*Special characteristics*
• Cat scratch disease	Coccobacillus	Lymphadenitis; reticuloendothelial hyperplasia; granulomas with central necrosis and neutrophils
• Tularaemia (Rabbit fever)	Francisella (Pasteurella) tularensis	Necrosis and suppuration (acute); tubercles hard or with minute central necrosis (chronic)
• Glanders	Actinobacillus mallei	Infection from horses and mutes; subcutaneous lesions and lymphadenitis; infective granulomas
II. Fungal		
• Actinomycosis (bacterial)	Actinomycetes israelii	Cervicofacial, abdominal and thoracic lesions; granulomas and abscesses with draining sinuses; sulphur granules
• Blastomycosis	Blastomyces dermatitidis	Cutaneous, systemic and lung lesions, suppuration, ulceration and granulomas
• Cryptococcosis	Cryptococcus neoformans	Meninges, lungs and systemic distribution; organism yeast-like with clear capsule
• Coccidioidomycosis	Coccidioides immitis	Meninges, lung and systemic distribution; granulomas and abscesses; organism cyst containing endospores
III. Parasitic		
• Schistosomiasis (Bilharziasis)	Schistosoma mansoni, haematobium, japonicium	Eggs and granulomas in gut, liver, lung; schistosome pigment; eosinophilis in bood and tissue
IV. Miscellaneous		
• Sarcoidosis	Unknown	Non-caseating granulomas (hard tubercles); asteroid and Schaumann bodies in giant cells
• Crohn's disease (regional enteritis)	Unknown ? Bacteria, ?? Viruses	Transmural chronic inflammatory infiltrates, non-caseating sarcoid-like granulomas
• Silicosis	Silica dust	Lung lesions, fibrocollagenous nodules
• Berylliosis	Metallic beryllium	Sarcoid-like granulomas in lungs, fibrosis; inclusions in giant cells (asteroids, Schaumann bodies, crystals)
• Foreign body granulomas	Talc, suture, oils, wood splinter, etc.	Non-caseating granulomas with foreign body giant cells; demonstration of foreign body

25. Ans. (a) Apoptosis *Ref: Harsh Mohan Textbook of Pathblogy 6th ed. p 34*

Classification of Morphologic Forms of Cell Injury.

Mechanism of cell injury	*Nomenclature*
Reversible cell injury	Retrogressive changes (older term: degenerations)
Irreversible cell injury	Cell death—necrosis
Programmed cell death	Apoptosis
Residual effects of cell injury	Subcellular alterations
Deranged cell metabolism	Intracellular accumulation of lipid, protein, carbohydrate
After-effects of necrosis	Gangrene, pathologic calcification

26. Ans. (b) Cell membrane with organelles *Ref: Robbins Pathologic Basis of Disease 7th ed. p 27*

Formation of cytoplasmic blebs and apoptotic bodies—The apoptotic cell first shows extensive surface blebbing, then undergoes fragmentation into membrane-bound apoptotic bodies composed of cytoplasm and tightly packed organelles, with or without nuclear fragments. The apoptotic bodies are rapidly degraded within lysosomes, Usually by macrophages and the adjacent healthy cells migrate or proliferate to replace the space occupied by the now deleted apoptotic cell (Apoptotic body will always appear as membrane bound. In question, all other options represent non-apoptotic bodies, i.e. those are not apoptotic bodies). There is any term available as nonapoptotic bodies.

ACUTE AND CHRONIC INFLAMMATION

27. Ans. (b) It results from increased lymphatic drainage *Ref: Harsh Mohan Textbook of Pathology 6th ed. p 96-97*

Oedema is caused by mechanisms that interfere with normal fluid balance of plasma, interstitial fluid and lymph flow.

The following mechanisms may be operating singly or in combination to produce oedema:

- Decreased plasma oncotic pressure
- Increased capillary hydrostatic pressure
- Lymphatic obstruction
- Tissue factors (increased oncotic pressure of interstitial fluid, and decreased tissue tension)
- Increased capillary permeability
- Sodium and water retention.

Lymphatic obstruction: Normally, the interstitial fluid in the tissue spaces escapes by way of lymphatics. Obstruction to outflow of these channels causes localised oedema, known as lymphoedema. In contrast if there is more lymphatic drainage then there are less chances of accumulation of oedematous fluid (excess fluid will be eliminated by lymphatic drainage).

28. Ans. (c) Myeloperoxidase *Ref: Harsh Mohan Textbook of Pathology 6th ed. p 136*

- Myeloperoxidase is most abundantly expressed in neutrophil granulocytes. It is a lysosomal protein stored in azurophilic granules of the neutrophil. Myeloperoxidase causes oxidative lysis by generation of oxygen free radicals, acid hydrolases act within the cell to cause destruction of bacteria in phagolysosome.

1. Cell-derived mediators
   - Vasoactive amines (Histamine, 5-hydroxytryptamine, neuropeptides)
   - Arachidonic acid metabolites (Eicosanoids)
     - Metabolites via cyclo-oxygenase pathway (prostaglandins, thromboxane A_2, prostacyclin, resolvins)
     - Metabolites via lipo-oxygenase pathway (5-HETE, leukotrienes, lipoxins)
   - Lysosomal components (from PMNs, macrophages)
   - Platelet activating factor
   - Cytokines (IL-1, TNF-α, TNF-β, IFN-γ, chemokines)
   - Free radicals (oxygen metabolites, nitric oxide)
- Plasma-derived mediators (plasma proteases)
  Products of:
   - The kinin system
   - The clotting system
   - The fibrinolytic system
   - The complement system

Chemical Mediators of Inflammation.

29. Ans. (a) Cytokines *Ref: Robbins Pathologic Basis of Disease 7th ed. p 70 Refer explanation of Chapter 2 Q 2*

Cytokines are proteins produced by many cell types (principally activated lymphocytes and macrophages, but also endothelium, epithelium, and connective tissue cells) that modulate the functions of other cell types. Long known to be involved in cellular immune responses, these products have additional effects that play important roles in both acute and chronic inflammation. Cytokines include chemokines, interferons, interleukins, lymphokines, tumour necrosis factor but generally not hormones or growth factors.

30. Ans. (b) Endothelial gaps by histamine *Ref: Robbins Pathologic Basis of Disease 7th ed. p 50*

Normal fluid exchange and microvascular permeability are critically dependent on an intact endothelium. How then does the endothelium become leaky in inflammation? The following mechanisms have been proposed: Formation of endothelial gaps in venules. This is the most common mechanism of vascular leakage and is elicited by histamine, bradykinin, leukotrienes, the neuropeptide substance P, and many other classes of chemical mediators. It occurs rapidly after exposure to the mediator and is usually reversible and short-lived (15 to 30 minutes); it is thus known as the immediate transient response.

31. Ans. (d) Decreased hydrostatic pressure
Ref: Harsh Mohan Textbook of Pathology 6th ed. p 131; Robbins Pathologic Basis of Disease 7th ed. p 50

Vasodilation is one of the earliest manifestations of acute inflammation; sometimes, it follows a transient constriction of arterioles, lasting a few seconds. Vasodilatation results in increased blood volume in microvascular bed of the area, which is responsible for redness and warmth at the site of acute inflammation. Progressive vasodilatation, in turn, may elevate the local hydrostatic pressure resulting in transudation of fluid into the extracellular space. This is responsible for swelling at the local site of acute inflammation. Vasodilation is quickly followed by increased permeability, of the microvasculature, with the outpouring of protein-rich fluid into the extravascular tissues. The loss of fluid results in concentration of red cells in small vessels and increased viscosity of the blood, reflected by the presence of dilated small vessels packed with red cells and slower blood flow, a condition termed stasis. As stasis develops, leukocytes, principally neutrophils, accumulate along the vascular endothelium. Leukocytes then stick to the endothelium, and soon afterward they migrate through the vascular wall into the interstitial tissue.

32. Ans. (c) Tuberculosis *Ref: Robbins Pathologic Basis of Disease 7th ed. p 83*

Langhans giant cells are large cells found in granulomatous conditions. They are formed by the fusion of epithelioid cells (macrophages), and contain nuclei arranged in a horseshoe-shaped pattern in the cell periphery. Although traditionally their presence was associated with tuberculosis, they are not specific for tuberculosis or even for mycobacterial disease. In fact, they are found in nearly every form of granulomatous disease, regardless of etiology. They should not be confused with Langerhans cells, which are mononuclear epidermal dendritic cells derived from monocytes.

33. Ans. (b) Glucose content *Ref: Harsh Mohan Textbook of Pathology 6th ed. p 96*

Feature	*Transudate*	*Exudate*
Definition	Filtrate of blood plasma without changes in endothelial permeability	Oedema of inflamed tissue associated with increased vascular permeability
Character	Non-inflammatory oedema	Inflammatory oedema
Protein content	Low (less than 1 gm/dl); mainly albumin, low fibrinogen: hence no tendency to coagulate	High (2.5-3.5 gm/dl), readily coagulates due to high content of fibrinogen and other coagulation factors
Glucose content	Same as in plasma	Low (less than 60 mg/dl)
Specific gravity	Low (less than 1.015)	High (more than 1.018)
pH	> 7.3	< 7.3
LDH	Low	High
Effusion LDH/serum LDH ratio	< 0.6	> 0.6
Cells	Few cells, mainly mesothelial cells and cellular debris	Many cells, inflammatory as well as parenchymal
Examples	Oedema in congestive cardiac failure	Purulent exudate such as pus

34. Ans. (d) Auramine and rhodamine *Ref: http://en.wikipedia.org/wiki/Auramine-rhodamine_stain*

The auramine-rhodamine stain (AR), also known as the Truant auramine-rhodamine stain, is a histological technique used to visualize acid-fast bacilli using fluorescence microscopy, notably species in the Mycobacterium genus Acid-fast organisms display a reddish-yellow fluorescence. Although the auramine- rhodamine stain is not as specific for acid-fast organisms (i.e. Mycobacterium tuberculosis or Nocardia) as the Ziehl-Neelsen stain, it is more affordable and more sensitive, therefore it is often utilized as a screening tool.

35. Ans. (b) Mast cells *Ref: Immunology at a Glance by BM Chain p 23*

- The two amines, histamine and serotonin, are especially important because they are present in preformed stores in cells and are therefore among the first mediators to be released during inflammation.

Histamine

Histamine is widely distributed in tissues, the richest source being the mast cells that are normally present in the connective tissue adjacent to blood vessels. It is also found in blood basophils and platelets.

Serotonin

Serotonin (5-hydroxytryptamine) is a preformed vasoactive mediator with actions similar to those of histamine. It is present in platelets and enterochromaffin cells, and in mast cells in rodents but not humans. Release of serotonin (and histamine) from platelets is stimulated when platelets aggregate after contact with collagen, thrombin, adenosine diphosphate (ADP), and antigen-antibody complexes. Platelet aggregation and release are also stimulated by platelet activating factors (PAF) derived from mast cells during IgE-mediated reactions.

36. Ans. (c) Opsonisation *Ref: Robbins Pathologic Basis of Disease 7th ed. p 59*

Phagocytosis is initiated by the expression of surface receptors on macrophages which recognise microorganisms.

- The process of coating a particle, such as a microbe, to target it for phagocytosis is called opsonization, and substances that do this are opsonins. These substances include antibodies, complement proteins, and lectins. One of the most efficient systems for opsonizing particles is coating the particles with IgG antibodies, which are termed specific opsonins.

Section C Maharahstra/Manipal/PGI

37. Ans. (b) Platelets

Refer explanation of Chapter 2 Q 35

38. Ans. (a) NADPH oxidase

Refer explanation of Chapter 1 Q 1

The NADPH oxidase (nicotinamide adenine dinucleotide phosphate-oxidase) is a membrane-bound enzyme complex. It can be found in the plasma membrane as well as in the membranes of phagosomes used by neutrophil white blood cells to engulf microorganisms.

39. Ans. (d) Myeloperoxidase

Refer explanation of Chapter 2 Q 28

40. Ans. (a) Nadph oxidase *Ref: http://en.wikipedia.org/wiki/NADPH_oxidase#Function*

Respiratory burst (sometimes called oxidative burst) is the rapid release of reactive oxygen species (superoxide radical and hydrogen peroxide) from different types of cells. Usually it denotes the release of these chemicals from immune cells, e.g. neutrophils and monocytes, as they come into contact with different bacteria or fungi.

NADPH oxidase-Under normal circumstances, the complex is latent in neutrophils and is activated to assemble in the membranes during respiratory burst. NADPH oxidase generates superoxide by transferring electrons from NADPH inside the cell across the membrane and coupling these to molecular oxygen to produce superoxide anion, a reactive free-radical. Superoxide can be produced in phagosomes, which contain ingested bacteria and fungi, or it can be produced outside of the cell. In a phagosome, superoxide can spontaneously form hydrogen peroxide that will undergo further reactions to generate reactive oxygen species (ROS).

41. Ans. (a) Endothelial injury by histamine

Refer explanation of Chapter 2 Q 30

TISSUE RENEWAL AND REPAIR: REGENERATION, HEALING AND FIBROSIS

42. Ans. (c) Cortisol *Ref: Robbins Pathologic Basis of Disease 7th ed. p114*

Healing is modified by a number of known influences and some unknown ones, frequently impairing the quality and adequacy of both inflammation and repair. These influences include both systemic and local host factors.

Systemic factors include the following:

- Nutrition-vitamin C deficiency, inhibit collagen synthesis and retard healing.
- Metabolic status Diabetes mellitus, for example, is associated with delayed healing,
- Circulatory status—can modulate wound healing. Inadequate blood supply, usually caused by arteriosclerosis or venous abnormalities (e.g. varicose veins)
- Hormones, such as glucocorticoids, have well-documented anti-inflammatory effects that influence various components of inflammation. These agents also inhibit collagen synthesis and subsequently wound healing.

Local factors that influence healing include the following:

- Infection
- Mechanical factors, such as early motion of wounds
- Foreign bodies, such as unnecessary sutures or fragments of steel, glass, or even bone, constitute impediments to healing.
- Size, location, and type of wound influence healing

43. Ans. (b) Neutrophilia *Ref: Harsh Mohan Textbook of Pathology 6th ed. p 134-135*

The escape of leucocytes from the lumen of microvasculature to the interstitial tissue is the most important feature of inflammatory response. In acute inflammation, polymorphonuclear neutrophils (PMNs) comprise the first line of body defense, followed later by monocytes and macrophages. Neutrophils are the dominant cells in acute inflammatory exudate in the first 24 hours, and monocyte- macrophages appear in the next 24-48 hours. However, neutrophils are short-lived (24-48 hours) while monocyte-macrophages survive much longer.

44. Ans. (b) Cortisol

Refer explanation of Chapter 3 Q 42

45. Ans. (a) Type IV *Ref: Robbins Pathologic Basis of Disease 7th ed. p 1198. http://en.wikipedia.org/wiki/Collagen#Types_and_associated_disorders*

Genetic Defects of Collagen Genes

Type	*Notes*	*Gene (s)*	*Disorders*
I	This is the most abundant collagen of the human body. It is present in scar tissue, the end product when tissue heals by repair. It is found in tendons, skin, artery walls, cornea, the endomysium of myofibrils, fibrocartilage, and the organic part of bones and teeth	COL1A1, COL1A2	Osteogenesis imperfecta, Ehlers-Danlos syndrome, Infantile cortical hyperostosis aka Caffey's disease
II	Hyaline cartilage, makes up 50% of all cartilage protein. Vitreous humour of the eye.	COL2A1	Collagenopathy, types II and XI
III	This is the collagen of granulation tissue, and is produced quickly by young fibroblasts before the tougher type I collagen is synthesized. Reticular fiber. Also found in artery walls, skin, intestines and the uterus	COL3A1	Ehlers-Danlos syndrome, Dupuytren's contracture
IV	Basal lamina; eye lens. Also serves as part of the filtration system in capillaries and the glomeruli of nephron in the kidney	COL4A1, COL4A2, COL4A3, COL4A4, COL4A5, COL4A6	Alport syndrome, Goodpasture's syndrome
V	Most interstitial tissue, assoc. with type I, associated with placenta	COL5A1, COL5A2, COL5A3	Ehlers-Danlos syndrome (Classical)
VI	Most interstitial tissue, assoc. with type I	COL6A1, COL6A2, COL6A3, COL6A5	Ulrich myopathy, Bethlem myopathy, Atopic dermatitis
VII	Forms anchoring fibrils in dermoepidermal junctions	COL7A1	Epidermolysis bullosa dystrophica
VIII	Some endothelial cells	COL8A1, COL8A1	Posterior polymorphous corneal dystrophy 2

Contd...

Contd...

Type	*Notes*	*Gene (s)*	*Disorders*
IX	FACIT collagen, cartilage, assoc. with type II and XI fibrils	COL9A1, COL9A2, COL9A3	EDM2 and EDM3
X	Hypertrophic and mineralizing cartilage	COL10A1	Schmid metaphyseal dysplasia
XI	Cartilage	COL11A1, COL11A2	Collagenopathy, types II and XI
XII	FACIT collagen, interacts with type I containing fibrils, decorin and glycosaminoglycans	COL12A1	
XIII	Transmembrane collagen, interacts with integrin a1b1, fibronectin and components of basement membranes like nidogen and perlecan	COL13A1	
XIV	FACIT collagen, also known as undulin	COL14A1	
XV		COL15A1	
XVI		COL16A1	
XVII	Transmembrane collagen, also known as BP180, a 180 kDa protein	COL17A1	Bullous pemphigoid and certain forms of junctional epidermolysis bullosa
XVIII	Source of endostatin	COL18A1	
XIX	FACIT collagen	COL19A1	
XX	—	COL20A1	
XXI	FACIT collagen	COL21A1	
XXII	—	COL22A1	
XXIII	MACIT collagen	COL23A1	
XXIV	—	COL24A1	
XXV	—	COL25A1	
XXVI	—	EMID2	
XXVII	—	COL27A1	
XXVIII	—	COL28A1	

46. Ans. (b) Secondary healing *Ref: Robbins Pathologic Basis of Disease 7th ed. p 113*

The feature that most clearly differentiates primary from secondary healing is the phenomenon of wound contraction, which occurs in large surface wounds. Large defects in the skin of a rabbit are reduced in approximately 6 weeks, to 5% to 10% of their original size, largely by contraction. The initial steps of wound contraction involve the formation of a network of actin-containing fibroblasts at the edge of the wound. Permanent wound contraction requires the action of myofibroblasts altered fibroblasts that have the ultrastructural characteristics of smooth muscle cells." Contraction of these cells at the wound site decreases the gap between the dermal edges of the wound.

HEMODYNAMIC DISORDERS, THROMBOEMBOLIC DISEASE AND SHOCK

47. Ans. (b) Tachycardia *Ref: Robbins Pathologic Basis of Disease 7th ed. p 139-141*

Shock, or cardiovascular collapse, is the final common pathway for a number of potentially lethal clinical events, including severe hemorrhage, extensive trauma or burns, large myocardial infarction, massive pulmonary embolism, and microbial sepsis. Regardless of the underlying pathology, shock gives rise to systemic hypoperfusion caused by reduction either in cardiac output or in the effective circulating blood volume. The end results are hypotension, followed by impaired tissue perfusion and cellular hypoxia. Shock is a progressive disorder that, if uncorrected, leads to death. Sequential pathophysiologic and clinical events in the progression of shock:

- An initial nonprogressive phase during which reflex compensatory mechanisms are activated and perfusion of vital organs is maintained.
- A progressive stage characterized by tissue hypoperfusion and onset of worsening circulatory and metabolic imbalances, including acidosis
- An irreversible stage that sets in after the body has incurred cellular and tissue injury so severe that even if the hemodynamic defects are corrected, survival is not possible. In the early nonprogressive phase of shock, a variety of neurohumoral mechanisms help maintain cardiac output and blood pressure. These include baroreceptor reflexes, release of catecholamines, activation of the renin-angiotensin axis, antidiuretic hormone release, and generalized sympathetic stimulation. The net effect is tachycardia, peripheral vasoconstriction, and renal conservation of fluid.

48. Ans. (a) 2 inches per second *Ref: http://www.heart.org/idc/groups/heart-public/@wcm/@ecc/documents/downloadable/ucm_317350.pdf*

A compression depth of at least 2 inches (5 cm) in adults and a compression depth of at least one-third of the anterior-posterior diameter of the chest in infants and children (approximately 1.5 inches [4 cm] in infants and 2 inches [5 cm] in children). Note that the range of 1½ to 2 inches is no longer used for adults, and the absolute depth specified for children and infants is deeper than in previous versions of the AHA Guidelines for CPR.

49. Ans. (a) Tachycardia

Refer explanation of Chapter4 Q 47

50. Ans. (c) Thrombosis *Ref: Robbins Pathologic Basis of Disease 7th ed. p 544*

Thrombi in the legs tend to produce few, if any, signs or symptoms in the early stages. Indeed, local manifestations, including edema distal to the occluded vein, dusky cyanosis, dilatation of superficial veins, heat, tenderness, redness, swelling, and pain may be absent in a bedridden patient. In some cases, however, pain can be elicited by pressure over affected veins, squeezing the calf muscles or forced dorsi flexion of the foot (Homans' sign). Pulmonary embolism is a common and serious clinical sequel to deep leg vein thrombosis. The contraction of surrounding muscles tends to 'milk' the contents loose from their attachments to the vein walls. Not infrequently, the first manifestation of thrombophlebitis is the development of an embolic episode; in a very ill patient pulmonary embolization often constitutes the final blow.

51. Ans. (c) CVC liver *Ref: Harsh Mohan Textbook of Pathology 6th ed. p 106*

Chronic venous congestion of the liver occurs in right heart failure and sometimes due to occlusion of inferior vena cava and hepatic vein. Grossly, the liver is enlarged and tender and the capsule is tense. Cut surface shows characteristic nutmeg appearance due to red and yellow mottled appearance, corresponding to congested centre of lobules and fatty peripheral zone respectively of deoxygenated hemoglobin in the affected tissues.

52. Ans. (c) Anasarca *Ref: Robbins Pathologic Basis of Disease 7th ed. p C*

Edema is most easily recognized grossly; microscopically, edema fluid generally manifests only as subtle cell swelling, with clearing and separation of the extracellular matrix elements. Although any organ or tissue in the body may be involved, edema is most commonly encountered in subcutaneous tissues, the lungs, and the brain. Severe, generalized edema is called anasarca.

53. Ans. (d) Tuberculosis *Ref: http://emedicine.medscape.com/article/1389957-overview*

Viral agents that are capable of being transmitted through blood transfusion include the following:

- Human immunodeficiency virus (HIV)
- Hepatitis viruses
- West Nile virus (WNV)
- Cytomegalovirus (CMV)
- Human T-cell lymphotropic viruses (HTLVs)
- Parvovirus B19

Protozoal organisms that can be passed on through transfusion include species of the genus Plasmodium, which cause malaria. Prions, which cause Creutzfeldt-Jakob disease, are also transmissible through transfusion; they cannot be destroyed using current techniques for inactivating pathogens in the blood supply.

54. Ans. (c) Deep leg veins

Refer explanation of Chapter 4 Q 50

55. Ans. (b) 7 to 14 days after surgery *Ref: http://hpathy.com/cause-symptoms-treatment/haemorrhages-bleeding/*

Classification of the hemorrhage

Depending upon the nature of vessel involved:

- Arterial hemorrhage bright red in color, jets out. Pulsation of the artery can be seen. It can be easily controlled as it is visible.
- Venous hemorrhage—dark red in color, never jets out but oozes out, difficult to control because veins get retracted, nonpulsatile
- Capillary hemorrhage red color, never jets out, slowly oozes out. It becomes significant if there are bleeding tendencies.

Depending on the timing of the hemorrhage:

- Primary hemorrhage: Occurs at the time of surgery
- Reactionary hemorrhage: Occurs after 6-12 hours of surgery. Hypertension in postoperative period, violent sneezing, coughing or retching, are the usual cause.
- Secondary hemorrhage: Occurs after 5-7 days after surgery. It is due to infection which eats away the suture material, causing sloughing of vessels wall.

Depending on the duration of hemorrhage:

- Acute hemorrhage: Occurs suddenly, e.g. esophageal variceal bleeding due to portal hypertension.
- Chronic hemorrhage: Occurs over a period of time, e.g. hemorrhoids/piles or chronic duodenal ulcers. Tuberculous ulcer of the ileum, diverticular disease of the colon.

Depending on the nature of bleeding:

- External hemorrhage: Revealed haemorrhage, e.g. epis taxis haematemesis.
- Internal hemorrhage: Concealed hemorrhage, e.g. splenic rupture following injury, ruptured ectopic gestation, liver laceration following injury.

56. Ans. (d) Increased venous blood pressure *Ref: Robbins Pathologic Basis of Disease 7th ed. p 130*

Three primary influences predispose to thrombus formation, the so-called Virchow triad:

- Endothelial injury
- Stasis or turbulence of blood flow
- Blood hypercoagulability

57. Ans. (a) Bleeding time *Ref: http://en.wikipedia.org/wiki/Bleeding_time#Ivy_method*

- **Ivy method**

The Ivy method is the traditional format for this test. While both the Ivy and the Duke method require the use of a sphygmomanometer, or blood pressure cuff, the Ivy method is more invasive than the Duke method, utilizing an incision on the ventral side of the forearm, whereas the Duke method involves puncture with a lancet or special needle. In the Ivy method, the blood pressure cuff is placed on the upper arm and inflated to 40 mmHg. A lancet or scalpel blade is used to make a shallow incision that is 1 millimeter deep on the underside of the forearm. A standard-sized incision is made around 10 mm long and 1 mm deep. The time from when the incision is made until all bleeding has stopped is measured and is called the bleeding time. Every 30 seconds, filter paper or a paper towel is used to draw off the blood. The test is finished when bleeding has stopped completely.

A normal value is less than 9 and a half minutes. A prolonged bleeding time may be a result from decreased number of thrombocytes or impaired blood vessels. However, it should also be noted that the depth of the puncture or incision may be the source of error. Normal values fall between 3 to 10 minutes depending on the method used.

- **Duke method**

With the Duke method, the patient is pricked with a special needle or lancet, preferably on the earlobe or fingertip, after having been swabbed with alcohol. The prick is about 34 mm deep. The patient then wipes the blood every 30 seconds with a filter paper. The test ceases when bleeding ceases. The usual time is about 25 minutes.

58. Ans. (a) Coagulative *Ref: Robbins Pathologic Basis of Disease 7th ed. p 21*

Coagulative necrosis implies preservation of the basic outline of the coagulated cell for a span of at least some days. The affected tissues exhibit a firm texture. Presumably, the injury or the subsequent increasing intracellular acidosis denatures not only structural proteins but also enzymes and so blocks the proteolysis of the cell. The myocardial infarct is an excellent example in which acidophilic, coagulated, anucleate cells may persist for weeks.

59. Ans. (a) Heart *Ref: Robbins Pathologic Basis of Disease 7th ed. p 134*

Thrombi are significant because they cause obstruction of arteries and veins, and they are possible sources of emboli. The significance of each depends on where the thrombus occurs. Thus, while venous thrombi may cause congestion and edema in vascular beds distal to an obstruction, a far graver consequence is that they may embolize to the lungs, causing death. Conversely, although arterial thrombi can embolize, their role in vascular obstruction at critical sites (e.g. coronary arteries resulting in myocardial infarction) is much more important.

60. Ans. (c) Pulmonary arteries *Ref: Robbins Pathologic Basis of Disease 7th ed. p 742*

PULMONARY THROMBOEMBOLISM

The morphologic consequences of embolic occlusion of the pulmonary arteries depend on the size of the embolic mass and the general state of the circulation. Large emboli may impact in the main pulmonary artery or its major branches or lodge at the bifurcation as a saddle embolus. Sudden death often ensues, owing largely to the blockage of blood flow through the lungs. Death may also be caused by acute failure of the right side of the heart (acute cor pulmonale).

61. Ans. (b) Lungs *Ref: Refer explanation of Chapter 4 Q 54*

Refer explanation of Chapter 4 Q 54

62. Ans. (d) Heart *Ref: Refer explanation of Chapter 4 Q 54*

Refer explanation of Chapter 4 Q 54
Section C Maharahstra/Manipal/PGI

63. Ans. (d) Cytokine action *Ref: Internet*

- The receptor for the endotoxin in humans is TLR-4 located on the surface of antigen presenting cells. Binding to the receptor which finally leads to the activation of the genes for the proinflammatory cytokines.

GENETIC DISORDERS

64. Ans. (d) MLH1 *Ref: Robbins Pathologic Basis of Disease 7th ed. p 287*

Inherited cancer syndromes (autosomal dominant)	
Gene	*Inherited predisposition*
RB	Retinoblastoma
p53	Li-Fraumeni syndrome (various tumours)
p16INK4A	Melanoma
APC	Familial adenomatous polyposis/colon cancer
NF1, NF2	Neurofibromatosis 1 and 2
BRCA1, BRCA2	Breast and ovarian tumors
MEN1, RET	Multiple endocrine neoplasia 1 and 2
MSH2, MLH1, MSH6	Hereditary nonpolyposis colon cancer
PATCH	Nevoid basal cell carcinoma syndrome
Familial cancers	
Familial clustering of cases, but role of inherited predisposition not clear for each individual	
• Breast cancer	
• Ovarian cancer	
• Pancreatic cancer	
Inherited autosomal recessive syndromes of defective DNA repair	
• Xeroderma pigmentosum	
• Ataxia-telangiectasia	
• Bloom syndrome	
• Fanconi anemia	

65. Ans. (a) Phenotypically normal woman with affected brother and son but normal daughter

Ref: http://en.wikipedia.org/wiki/Genetic_disorder#Single_gene_disorder

Option A represents: X-linked recessive trait
Option B represents: X-linked dominant trait
Option C represents: Y-linked or holandric trait
Option D represents: Autosomal dominant trait

66. Ans. (a) Klinefelter's syndrome *Ref: Harsh Mohan Textbook of Pathology 6th ed. p 258*

Down's syndrome: There is trisomy 21 in about 95% cases of Down's syndrome due to nondisjunction during meiosis in one of the parents. Down's syndrome is the most common chromosomal disorder and is the commonest cause of mental retardation. The incidence of producing offspring with Down's syndrome rises in mothers over 35 years of age. Klinefelter's syndrome: Klinefelter's syndrome is the most important example of sex chromosome trisomy. About 80% cases have 47, XXY karyotype while others are mosaics. Typically, these patients have testicular dysgenesis. In general, sex chromosome trisomies are more common than trisomies of autosomes. Turner's syndrome: Turner's syndrome is an example of monosomy (45, X0) most often due to loss of X chromosome in paternal meiosis.

67. Ans. (b) G-banding *Ref: Harsh Mohan Textbook of Pathology 6th ed. p 17*

When stained, chromosomes have the property of forming alternating dark and light bands. For this purpose, fixed metaphase preparation is stained by one of the following banding techniques:

- Giemsa banding or G-banding, the most commonly used.
- Quinacrine banding or Q-banding used to demonstrate bands along chromosomes.
- Constitutive banding or C-banding is used to demonstrate constitutive heterochromatin.
- Reverse staining Giemsa banding (or R-banding) gives pattern opposite to those obtained by G- banding.

Chromosomes are then photographed by examining the preparation under the microscope. From the photograph, chromosomes are cut and then arranged according to their size, centromeric location and banding patterns. The pairs of chromosomes are identified by the arm length of chromosomes. The centromere divides the chromosome into a short upper arm called p arm (p for petit in French meaning 'short') and a long lower arm called q arm (letter q next to p).

68. Ans. (a) None affected, all carriers *Ref: Internet*

- Albinism has an autosomal recessive inheritance pattern.

(Unaffected male) AA aa (affected female)

⇩

Aa Aa Aa Aa

Since all offspring carry only one recessive gene each from the affected female none of them will manifest albinism but they all are carriers.

69. Ans. (d) Calcification of disc *Ref: Robbins Pathologic Basis of Disease 7th ed. p 168*

Alkaptonuria

It is an autosomal recessive disorder in which the lack of homogentisic oxidase blocks the metabolism of phenylalanine-tyrosine at the level of homogentisic acid. Thus, homogentisic acid accumulates in the body. A large amount is excreted, imparting a black color to the urine if allowed to stand and undergo oxidation.' 'The retained homogentisic acid selectively binds to collagen in connective tissues, tendons, and cartilage, imparting to these tissues a blue-black pigmentation (ochronosis) most evident in the ears, nose, and cheeks. The most serious consequences of ochronosis, however, stem from deposits of the pigment in the articular cartilages of the joints. In some obscure manner, the pigmentation causes the cartilage to lose its normal resiliency and become brittle and fibrillated. Wear-and-tear erosion of this abnormal cartilage leads to denudation of the subchondral bone, and often tiny fragments of the fibrillated cartilage are driven into the underlying bone, worsening the damage. The vertebral column, particularly the intervertebral disc, is the prime site of attack, but later the knees, shoulders, and hips may be affected. The small joints of the hands and feet are usually spared.

70. Ans. (a) P53 *Ref: Robbins Pathologic Basis of Disease 7th ed. p 302*

p53: Guardian of the Genome

The p53 gene is located on chromosome 17p13.1, and it is the most common target for genetic alteration in human tumors.' A little over 50% of human tumors contain mutations in this gene. The fact that p53 mutations are common in a variety of human tumors suggests that the p53 protein functions as a critical gatekeeper against the formation of cancer. Indeed, it is evident that p53 acts as a 'molecular policeman' that prevents the propagation of genetically damaged cells.

71. Ans. (c) Peutz-Jeghers syndrome *Ref: Robbins Pathologic Basis of Disease 7th ed. p 859*

Peutz-Jeghers polyps are hamartomatous polyps that involve the mucosal epithelium, lamina propria, and muscularis mucosa. These hamartomatous lesions may also occur singly or multiply in the Peutz-Jeghers syndrome. This rare autosomal dominant syndrome is characterized by multiple hamartomatous polyps scattered throughout the entire gastrointestinal tract and melanotic mucosal and cutaneous pigmentation around the lips, oral mucosa, face, genitalia, and palmar surfaces of the hands. Patients with this syndrome are at risk for intussusception, which is a common cause of mortality.

72. Ans. (d) 46XY t{14,21] *Ref: Robbins Pathologic Basis of Disease 7th ed. p 175*

Down syndrome also known as trisomy 21, is a genetic disorder caused by the presence of all or part of a third copy of chromosome 21. It is typically associated with physical growth delays, characteristic facial features and mild to moderate intellectual disability. The extra chromosome content can arise through several different ways. The most common cause is a complete extra copy of chromosome 21, resulting in trisomy 21. In 1 to 2.5% of cases, some of the cells in the body are normal and others have trisomy 21, known as mosaic Down syndrome. The other common mechanisms that can give rise to Down syndrome include: a Robertsonian translocation, isochromosome, or ring chromosome. These contain additional material from chromosome 21 and occur in approximately 2.5% of cases.

- Trisomy 21 (also known by the karyotype 47,XX,+21 for females and 47,XY,+21 for males) is caused by a failure of the 21st chromosome to separate during egg or sperm development. As a result, a sperm or egg cell is produced with an extra copy of chromosome 21; this cell thus has 24 chromosomes. When combined with a normal cell from the other parent, the embryo and baby has 47 chromosomes, with three copies of chromosome 21.
- The extra chromosome 21 material may also occur due to a Robertsonian translocation in 24% cases. In this situation, the long arm of chromosome 21 is attached to another chromosome, often chromosome 14. In a male affected with down syndrome it results in a karyotype of 46XY,t(14q21q). This may be a new mutation or previously present in one of the parents. The parent with such a translocation is usually normal physically and mentally; however, during production of egg or sperm cells there is a higher chance of creating reproductive cells with extra chromosome 21 material. This results in a 15% chance of having a child with Down syndrome when the mother is affected and a less than 5% risk if the father is affected. The risk of this type of Down syndrome is not related to the mother's age. Hence in Robertsonian translocation, chromosome number is normal but still there is translocation of genetic material between chromosome number 14 and 21. This type of translocation takes place in acrocentric type of chromosomes only.

73. Ans. (a) Open reading frame *Ref: http://en.wikipedia.org/wiki/Open_reading_frame*

In molecular genetics, an open reading frame (ORF) is the part of a reading frame that contains no stop codons. The transcription termination pause site is located after the ORF, beyond the translation stop codon, because if transcription were to cease before the stop codon, an incomplete protein would be made during translation. A reading frame is a way of dividing the sequence of nucleotides in a nucleic acid (DNA or RNA) molecule into a set of consecutive, non-overlapping triplets. Where these triplets equate to amino acids or start/stop signals during translation, they are called codons.

74. Ans. (d) Microarray *Ref: http://en.wikipedia.org/wiki/Aneuploidy#Diagnosis*

Aneuploidy is typically detected through karyotyping, a process in which a sample of cells is fixed and stained to create the typical light and dark chromosomal banding pattern and a picture of the chromosomes is analyzed. Other techniques include Fluorescence in situ Hybridization (FISH), quantitative PCR of Short Tandem Repeats, quantitative fluorescence PCR (QF-PCR), quantitative PCR dosage analysis, Quantitative Mass Spectrometry of Single Nucleotide Polymorphisms, and Comparative Genomic Hybridization (CGH). A DNA microarray is a collection of microscopic DNA spots attached to a solid surface. Scientists use DNA microarrays to measure the expression levels of large numbers of genes simultaneously or to genotype multiple regions of a genome.

- Microarray is used to analyze large number of genes at one time. For single or specific gene, above-mentioned techniques are used.

75. Ans. (a) Autosomal dominant *Ref: Robbins Pathologic Basis of Disease 7th ed. p155*

Ehlers-Danlos syndromes (EDS) comprise a clinically and genetically heterogeneous group of disorders that result from some defect in the synthesis or structure of fibrillar collagen.' Other disorders resulting from mutations affecting collagen synthesis include osteogenesis imperfect, Alport syndrome, and epidermolysis bullosa.

Classification of Ehlers-Danlos syndromes			
EDS type	*Clinical findings*	*Inheritance*	*Gene defects*
Classical (VII)	Skin and joint hypermobility, atrophic scars, easy bruising	Autosomal dominant	COL5A1, COL5A2
Hypermobility (III)	Joint hypermobility, pain, dislocations	Autosomal dominant	Unknown
Vascular (IV)	Thin skin, arterial or uterine rupture, bruising, small joint hyperextensibility	Autosomal dominant	COL3A1
Kyphoscoliosis (VI)	Hypotonia, joint laxity, congenital scoliosis, ocular fragility	Autosomal recessive	Lysyl-hydroxylase
Arthrochalasia (VIIa, b)	Severe joint hypermobility, skin changes mild, scoliosis, bruising	Autosomal dominant	COL1A1, COL1A2
Dermatosparaxis (VIIc)	Severe skin fragility, cutis laxa, bruising	Autosomal recessive	Procollagen *N*-peptidase

76. Ans. (d) Northern blot analysis *Ref: http://en.wikipedia.org/wiki/Northern_blot*

The northern blot is a technique used in molecular biology research to study gene expression by detection of RNA (or isolated mRNA) in a sample. With northern blotting it is possible to observe cellular control over structure and function by determining the particular gene expression levels during differentiation, morphogenesis, as well as abnormal or diseased conditions.

- Single-stranded conformational polymorphism, denaturating gradient gel electrophoresis and gel electrophoresis: These all 3 techniques are minute variations of the gel electrophoresis technique.
- BY using these techniques, change of even single nucleotide can be detected and pointed out on that individual DNA strand.
- While Northern blot technique will only display indirect effect of the mutation in the form of mRNA.

77. Ans. (d) DNA replication *Ref: Wikipedia*

Transcription is the first step of gene expression, in which a particular segment of DNA is copied into RNA by the enzyme RNA polymerase. Post-transcriptional modification is a process in primary transcript RNA is converted into mature RNA. A notable example is the conversion of precursor messenger RNA into mature messenger RNA (mRNA), which includes splicing and occurs prior to protein synthesis.

Translation is the process in which cellular ribosomes create proteins. It is part of the process of gene expression. In translation, messenger RNA (mRNA) produced by transcription is decoded by a ribosome complex to produce a specific amino acid chain, or polypeptide, that will later fold into an active protein. Posttranslational modification (PTM) is a step in protein biosynthesis. Proteins are created by ribosomes translating mRNA into polypeptide chains. These polypeptide chains undergo PTM, (such as folding, cutting and other processes), before becoming the mature protein product. Gene silencing is a general term used to describe the epigenetic regulation of gene expression. In particular, this term refers to the ability of a cell to prevent the expression of a certain gene. Gene silencing can occur during either transcription or translation and is often used in research. In particular, methods used to silence genes are being increasingly used to produce therapeutics to combat cancer and diseases, such as infectious diseases and neurodegenerative disorders. DNA replication is the process of producing two identical replicas from one original DNA molecule. In a cell, DNA replication begins at specific locations, or origins of replication, in the genome. Unwinding of DNA at the origin and synthesis of new strands results in replication forks growing bidirectionally from the origin. A number of proteins are associated with the replication fork which helps in terms of the initiation and continuation of DNA synthesis. Most prominently, DNA polymerase synthesizes the new DNA by adding complementary nucleotides to the template strand.

78. Ans. (a) Genomic imprinting *Ref: Robbins Pathologic Basis of Disease 7th ed. p 185*

GENOMIC IMPRINTING

We all inherit two copies of each gene, carried on homologous maternal and paternal chromosomes. It is generally assumed that there is no functional difference between the genes derived from the mother or the father. Recent studies have challenged this notion, and there is accumulating evidence that, at least with respect to some genes, there are functional differences between the paternal gene and the maternal gene. These differences result from an epigenetic process, called imprinting. In most cases, imprinting selectively inactivates either the maternal or paternal allele. Thus, maternal imprinting refers to transcriptional silencing of the maternal allele, whereas paternal imprinting implies that the paternal allele is inactivated. Imprinting occurs in the ovum or the sperm, before fertilization, and then is stably transmitted to all somatic cells through mitosis.' As is often the case in medicine, genomic imprinting is best illustrated by considering two uncommon genetic disorders: Prader-Willi syndrome and Angelman syndrome.

79. Ans. (d) Chromosomal anomaly *Ref: http://en.wikipedia.org/wiki/DiGeorge_syndrome*

DiGeorge syndrome is a syndrome caused by the deletion of a small piece of chromosome 22. The features of this syndrome vary widely, even among members of the same family, and affect many parts of the body. Characteristic signs and symptoms may include birth defects such as congenital heart disease, defects in the palate, most commonly related to neuromuscular problems with closure (velopharyngeal insufficiency), learning disabilities, mild differences in facial features, and recurrent infections.

80. Ans. (b) All the daughters are carrier *Ref: Robbins Pathologic Basis of Disease 7th ed. p 655*

Like most recessive sex-linked, X chromosome disorders, haemophilia is more likely to occur in males than females. This is because females have two X chromosomes while males have only one, so the defective gene is guaranteed to manifest in any male who carries it. Because females have two X chromosomes and haemophilia is rare, the chance of a female having two defective copies of the gene is very remote, so females are almost exclusively asymptomatic carriers of the disorder. Female carriers can inherit the defective gene from either their mother or father, or it may be a new mutation.

(Affected male) XY XX (Unaffected female)

⇩

XX XX XY XY

- Female will always be carrier for hemophilia. Very rarely they will manifest the disease.

81. Ans. (c) 45X0 d *Ref: http://en.wikipedia.org/wiki/Turner_syndrome*

Turner syndrome or Ullrich-Turner syndrome (also known as 'Gonadal dysgenesis'), 45, X, encompasses several conditions in human females, of which monosomy X (absence of an entire sex chromosome, the Barr body) is most common. There are characteristic physical abnormalities which affect many but not all people with Turner syndrome, such as short stature, swelling, broad chest, low hairline, low-set ears, and webbed necks. Girls with Turner syndrome typically experience gonadal dysfunction (non-working ovaries), which results in amenorrhea (absence of menstrual cycle) and sterility. Concurrent health concerns may also be present, including congenital heart disease, hypothyroidism (reduced hormone secretion by the thyroid), diabetes, vision problems, hearing concerns, and many autoimmune diseases.

82. Ans. (c) Informed consent *Ref: http://icmr.nic.in/ijmr/2011/october/1020.pdf*

Genetic counselling is provided in places where genetic tests are carried out. The process involves pre-test counselling as well as post-test counselling to enable the individuals to face the situation and take appropriate decisions with the right frame of mind. Major ethical principles which govern the attitudes and actions of counsellors include: respect for patient autonomy, non-maleficence, beneficence, or taking action to help benefit others and prevent harm, both physical and mental, and justice, which requires that services be distributed fairly to those in need. Other moral issues include veracity, the duty to disclose information or to be truthful, and respect for patient confidentiality. Nondirective counselling, a hallmark of this profession, is in accordance with the principle of individual autonomy. High prevalence of haemoglobinopathies with availability of good and sensitive carrier detection tests and prenatal diagnostic techniques makes these good candidates for population screening of carriers along with genetic counselling for primary prevention of the disease. Screening of the extended family members of the affected child, high-risk communities and general population screening including antenatal women are the main target groups for planning a Haemoglobinopathy control programme.

DISEASES OF IMMUNITY

83. Ans. (b) Direct Coombs' test *Ref: http://en.wikipedia.org/wiki/Coombs_test*

The Direct Coombs test is used to test for autoimmune hemolytic anemia, i.e. a condition of a low count of red blood cells caused by immune system lysis or breaking of red blood cells (RBC) membranes causing RBC destruction. In certain diseases or conditions, an individual's blood may contain IgG antibodies that can specifically bind to antigens on the RBC surface membrane, and their circulating RBCs can become coated with IgG alloantibodies and/or IgG autoantibodies. Complement proteins may subsequently bind to the bound antibodies and cause RBC destruction. The direct Coombs test is used to detect these antibodies or complement proteins that are bound to the surface of red blood cells; a blood sample is taken and the RBCs are washed (removing the patient's own plasma) and then incubated with antihuman globulin (also known as 'Coombs reagent'). If this produces agglutination of RBCs, the direct Coombs test is positive, a visual indication that antibodies (and/or complement proteins) are bound to the surface of red blood cells. The indirect Coombs test is used in prenatal testing of pregnant women, and in testing blood prior to a blood transfusion. It detects antibodies against RBCs that are present unbound in the patient's serum. In this case, serum is extracted from the blood sample taken from the patient. Then, the serum is incubated with RBCs of known antigenicity; that is, RBCs with known reference values from other patient blood samples. If agglutination occurs, the indirect Coombs test is positive.

84. Ans. (b) O antibodies last longer and hence are not an indicator of recent infection *Ref: Parya p 289*

O antibodies disappear earlier within 6 months

85. Ans. (c) Transcription of nuclear factor mediated by (NF-_B) which recruits cytokines

Ref: Robbins Pathologic Basis of Disease 7th ed. p 194.

Phagocytes are recruited to sites of infection, resulting in inflammation, and here the cells ingest the microbes and are then activated to destroy the ingested pathogens. Phagocytes recognize microbes by several membrane receptors.

These include receptors for mannose residues and N-formyl methionine-containing peptides, which are produced by microbes but not by host cells, and a family of receptors that are homologous to a Drosophila protein called Toll.' Different Toll-like receptors (TLRs) are involved in responses to different microbial products. Upon recognition of the relevant microbial structure, the TLRs signal by a common pathway that leads to the activation of transcription factors, notably NF-KB (nuclear factor KB). NF-KB stimulates production of cytokines and several proteins that are responsible for the microbicidal activities of the phagocytes. Phagocytes internalize microbes into vesicles, where the microbes are destroyed by reactive oxygen and nitrogen intermediates and hydrolytic enzymes.

86. Ans. (b) 8001200/mm³ *Ref: http://www.webmd.com/hiv-aids/cd4-count-what-does-it-mean*

A review on peripheral blood CD4+ T lymphocyte counts in healthy adult Indians. Indian J Med Res 132, December 2010, pp 667-675.

CD4 cells are a type of white blood cell that fights infection. Another name for them is T-helper cells. CD4 cells are made in the spleen, lymph nodes, and thymus gland, which are part of the lymph or infection-fighting system. CD4 cells move throughout your body, helping to identify and destroy germs such as bacteria and viruses. CD4 counts are reported as the number of cells in a cubic millimeter of blood. A normal CD4 count is from 500 to 1,500 cells per cubic millimeter of blood. It is more important to pay attention to the pattern of results than to any one test result. In general, HIV disease is progressing.

If the CD4 count is going down. This means the immune system is getting weaker and you are more likely to get sick. In some people, CD4 counts can drop dramatically, even going down to zero. Public health guidelines recommend starting on preventive antiretroviral therapy if CD4 counts are under 200, whether or not you have symptoms. This is a later stage of HIV infection called AIDS (acquired immunodeficiency syndrome). Some doctors start therapy earlier, when the CD4 count reaches 350 to 500 or if you have a newly acquired infection. If therapy is effective, your CD4 count should go up or become stable.

Most doctors recommend starting medication for opportunistic infections at these levels:

- Less than 200: Pneumocystis pneumonia (PCP).
- Less than 75: Mycobacterium avium complex (MAC).
- The mean CD4+ T cell counts in the north India varied from as low as 703 to 818 cells/μl, in south India from 799 to 1048 cells/μl, 743 to 965 cells/μl in western India and 848 cells/μl in eastern India.

87. Ans. (d) Red blood cells *Ref: Harsh Mohan Textbook of Pathology 6th ed. p 64*

HLA system is considered important in the regulation of the immune system. HLA stands for Human Leucocyte Antigens because these antigens or genetic proteins in the body which determine one's own tissue from non-self (histocompatibility) were first discovered on the surface of leucocytes. Subsequently, it was found that HLA are actually gene complexes of proteins on the surface of all nucleated cells of the body and platelets. Since these complexes are of immense importance in matching donor and recipient for organ transplant, they are called major histocompatibility complex (MHC) or HLA complex. Out of various genes for histocompatibility, most of the transplantation antigens or MHC are located on a portion of chromosome 6 of all nucleated cells of the body and platelets. These genes occupy four regions or loci A, B, C and D, on the short (p) arm of chromosome 6 and exhibit marked variation in allelic genes at each locus. Depending upon the characteristics of MHC, they have been divided into 3 classes: Class I MHC antigens have loci as HLA-A, HLA-B and HLA-C. CD8+ (i.e. T suppressor) lymphocytes carry receptors for class I MHC and these cells are used to identify class I antigen on them. Class II MHC antigens have single locus as HLA-D. These antigens have further 3 loci: DR, DQ and DP. Class II MHC is identified by B cells and CD4+ (i.e. T helper) cells. Class III MHC antigens are some components of the complement system (C2 and C4) coded on HLA complex but are not associated with HLA expression and are not used in antigen identification.

88. Ans. (b) Haemagglutination inhibition test *Ref: http://virology-online.com/general/Test4.htm*
Ref: Wikipedia

Haemagglutination-inhibition test: A wide variety of different viruses possess the ability to agglutinate the erythrocytes of mammalian or avian species. The actual animal species whose erythrocytes could be agglutinated depends on the actual virus. Examples of viruses which could haemagglutinate include influenza, parainfluenza, adenoviruses, rubella, alphaviruses, bunyaviruses, flaviviruses and some strains of picornaviruses. Antibodies against the viral protein responsible for haemagglutination can prevent haemagglutination; this is the basis behind the haemagglutination-inhibition test (HAI). The specificity of the HAI test varies with different viruses. With some viruses such as influenza A, the haemagglutination antigen is the same as the antigen responsible for virus adsorption and thus virus neutralization, and therefore the HAI test is highly specific for the different strains of the virus. With other viruses, the HAI test is less specific, e.g. flaviviruses, where HAI antibodies against one flavivirus may cross-react with other related flaviviruses. HAI tests are more sensitive than complement-fixation tests but are less sensitive than EIAs and RIAs. Immunofluorescence is a technique used for light microscopy with a fluorescence microscope and is used primarily on microbiological samples. This technique uses the specificity of antibodies to their antigen to target fluorescent dyes to specific biomolecule targets within a cell, and therefore allows visualisation of the distribution of the target molecule through the sample. Immunofluorescence is a widely used example of immunostaining and is a specific example of immunohistochemistry that makes use of fluorophores to visualise the location of the antibodies Radioimmunoassay (RIA) is a very sensitive in vitro assay technique used to measure concentrations of antigens (for example, hormone levels in the blood) by use of antibodies. As such, it can be seen as the inverse of a radiobinding assay, which quantifies an antibody by use of corresponding antigens. The enzyme-linked immunosorbent assay (ELISA) is a test that uses antibodies and color change to identify a substance.

89. Ans. (d) T cells *Ref: Harsh Mohan Textbook of Pathology 6th ed. p 61*

- **Types of immunity:** Broadly speaking, immunity or body defence mechanism is divided into 2 types, each with humoral and cellular components:

  Natural or innate immunity is non-specific and is considered as the first line of defense without antigenic specificity. It has 2 major components:
  - Humoral: Comprised by complement.
  - Cellular: Consists of neutrophils, macrophages, and natural killer (NK) cells.

Specific or adaptive immunity: is specific and is characterised by antigenic specificity. It too has 2 main components:

- Humoral: Consisting of antibodies formed by B cells.
- Cellular: Mediated by T cells.

The various components of both types of immunity are interdependent and interlinked for their functions.

90. Ans. (c) Negative selection of T cells in the thymus *Ref: Internet*

In immunology, cryptic self epitopes are a source of autoimmunity.

Self epitopes, which are found in high concentration on the surface of Antigen-presenting cells (APCs) in association with its major histocompatibility complex (MHC) are known as dominant epitopes. These are stimulants of negative selection mechanisms to remove potentially self destructing autoreactive T cells. Their 'self' antigens are displayed to a developing T-cell and signal those 'self-reactive' T-cells to die via programed cell death (apoptosis) and thereby deletion from the T cell repertoire, preventing autoimmunity. However, self epitopes which appear in very low concentration on APC are termed cryptic in the sense that they do not delete autoreactive T-cells which will then join the peripheral adult T cell repertoire. This causes autoimmunity in the body.

91. Ans. (c) Gamma globulin *Ref: Robbins Pathologic Basis of Disease 7th ed. p 678*

Globulins, albumin, and fibrinogen are the major blood proteins. The normal concentration of globulins in the blood is about 2.6-4.6 g/dL. Gamma globulins are a class of globulins, identified by their position after serum protein electrophoresis. The most significant gamma globulins are immunoglobulins ('Igs'), a subclass of which is antibodies. Plasma cell neoplasms and related disorders. The common feature of this collection of entities is the proliferation of a B-cell clone that synthesizes and secretes a single homogeneous immunoglobulin or its fragments. The monoclonal immunoglobulin identified in the blood is referred to as an M component, in reference to myeloma. Since complete M components have molecular weights of 160,000 or higher, they are restricted to the plasma and extracellular fluid and are excluded from the urine in the absence of glomerular damage. However, unlike normal plasma cells, in which the production and coupling of heavy (H) and light (L) chains are tightly balanced, neoplastic plasma cells often synthesize excess L or H chains along with complete immunoglobulins. Occasionally, only L chains or H chains are produced. The free L chains, known as Bence Jones proteins, are small enough to be rapidly excreted in the urine. Designations applied to disorders associated with abnormal immunoglobulins include gammopathy, monoclonal gammopathy, dysproteinemia, and paraproteinemia. A variety of clinicopathologic entities are associated with monoclonal gammopathies.

- Multiple myeloma (plasma cell myeloma) is the most important and most common symptomatic monoclonal gammopathy. It is characterized by multiple timorous masses of neoplastic plasma cells scattered throughout the skeletal system. Solitary myeloma, or solitary plasmacytoma, is an infrequent variant consisting of a solitary neoplastic mass of plasma cells found in bone or some soft-tissue site.

92. Ans. (b) Accumulation of ACh at cleft *Ref: Robbins Pathologic Basis of Disease 7th ed. p 1344*

Now recognized as one of the best-defined forms of autoimmune disease, myasthenia gravis is a muscle disease caused by immune-mediated loss of acetylcholine receptors and having characteristic temporal and anatomic patterns as well as drug responses. When arising before age 40 years, it is most commonly seen in women, but there is equal occurrence between the sexes in older patients. Thymic hyperplasia is found in 65% and thymoma in 15% of patients. Analysis of neuromuscular transmission in myasthenia gravis shows a decrease in the number of muscle acetylcholine receptors (AChRs), and circulating antibodies to the AChR are present in nearly all patients with myasthenia gravis. In most cases, the autoantibodies against the AChR lead to loss of functional AChRs at the neuromuscular junction by: (1) Fixing complement and causing direct injury to the post-synaptic membrane, (2) increasing the internalization and degradation of the receptors, and (3) inhibiting binding and function of ACh. An acetylcholinesterase inhibitor (often abbreviated AChEI) or anti-cholinesterase is a chemical that inhibits the acetylcholinesterase enzyme from breaking down acetylcholine, thereby increasing both the level and duration of action of the neurotransmitter acetylcholine. Anti-cholinesterase are used medicinally to treat myasthenia gravis. In myasthenia gravis, they are used to increase neuromuscular transmission.

93. Ans. (d) 8001200

Refer explanation of Chapter 6 Q 86

94. Ans. (a) IgE *Ref: Harsh Mohan Textbook of Pathology 6th ed. p 75. Robbins; Pathologic Basis of Disease 7th ed. p 209*

Systemic anaphylaxis is characterized by vascular shock, widespread edema, and difficulty in breathing. In humans, systemic anaphylaxis may occur after administration of foreign proteins (e.g. antisera), hormones, enzymes, polysaccharides, and drugs (such as the antibiotic penicillin).' In the immunologic mechanism, immunoglobulin E (IgE) binds to the antigen (the foreign material that provokes the allergic reaction). Antigen-bound IgE then activates FcεRI receptors on mast cells and basophils. This leads to the release of inflammatory mediators such as histamine. These mediators subsequently increase the contraction of bronchial smooth muscles, trigger vasodilation, increase the leakage of fluid from blood vessels, and cause heart muscle depression.

- **Schematic representation of pathogenesis of 4 types of immunological tissue injury.**

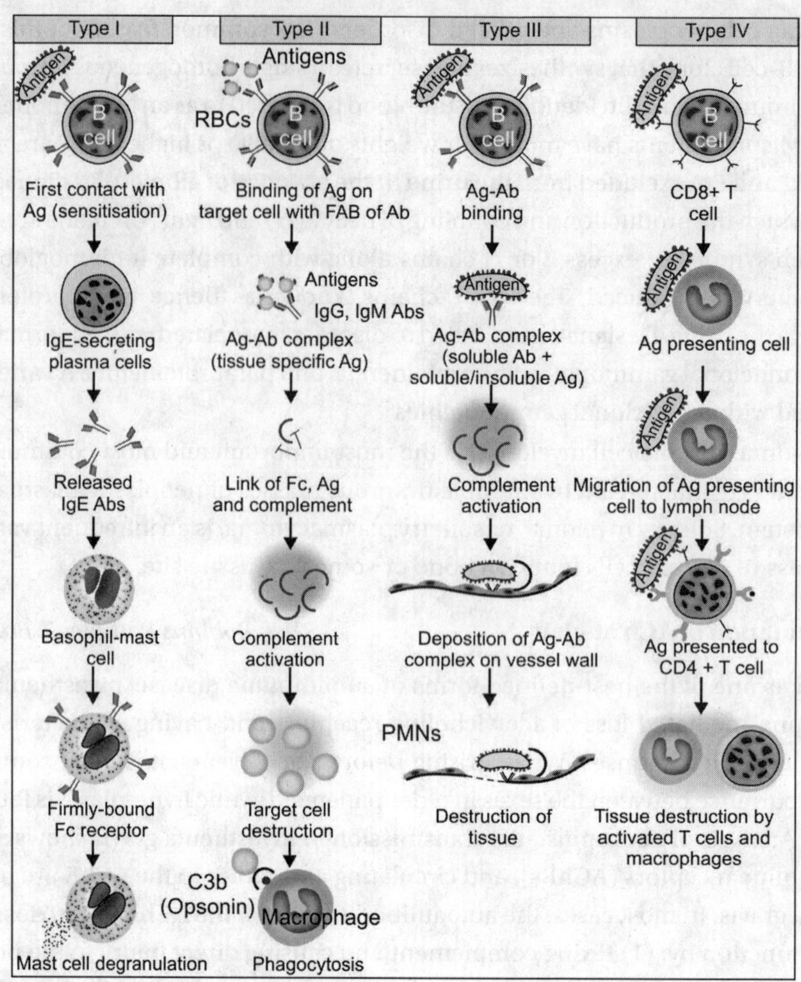

95. Ans. (a) Systemic lupus erythematosus *Ref: Harsh Mohan Textbook of Pathology 6th ed. p 78; Robbins Pathologic Basis of Disease 7th ed. p 227*

Systemic Lupus Erythematosus

SLE is the prototype of a multisystem disease of autoimmune origin, characterized by a bewildering array of autoantibodies, particularly antinuclear antibodies (ANAs). Acute or insidious in its onset, it is a chronic, remitting and relapsing, often febrile illness characterized principally by injury to the skin, joints, kidney, and serosal membranes. The exact etiology of SLE is not known. However, autoantibodies against nuclear and cytoplasmic components of the cells are demonstrable in plasma by immunofluorescence tests in almost all cases of SLE. Some of the important antinuclear antibodies (ANAs) or antinuclear factors (ANFs) against different nuclear antigens are as under:

- Antinuclear antibodies (ANA)
- Antibodies to double-stranded (anti-dsDNA)
- Anti-Smith antibodies (anti-Sm)
- Other non-specific antibodies. Besides above, there are several other antibody tests which lack specificity for SLE. These are as follows: Anti-ribonucleoproteins (anti-RNP), anti-histone antibody, antiphospholipid antibodies or lupus anticoagulant antiribosomal P antibody is antibody against the source of these autoantibodies as well as hypergammaglobulinaemia seen in SLE is the polyclonal activation of B cells brought about by following derangements:
  - Immunologic factors.
  - Genetic factors.

- Other factors.
  - Certain drugs, e.g. penicillamine D
  - Certain viral infections, e.g. EBV infection and
  - Certain hormones, e.g. oestrogen.

PATHOGENESIS: The autoantibodies formed by any of the above mechanisms are the mediators of tissue injury in SLE.

Two types of immunologic tissue injury can occur in SLE:

- Type II hypersensitivity is characterised by formation of autoantibodies against blood cells (red blood cells, platelets, leucocytes) and results in haematologic derangement in SLE.
- Type III hypersensitivity is characterised by antigen-antibody complex (commonly DNA-anti-DNA antibody; sometimes Ig-anti-Ig antibody complex) which is deposited at sites such as renal glomeruli, walls of small blood vessels, etc.

MORPHOLOGIC FEATURES: The manifestations of SLE are widespread in different visceral organs as well as show erythematous cutaneous eruptions. The principal lesions are renal, vascular, cutaneous and cardiac; other organs and tissues involved are serosal linings (pleuritis, pericarditis); joints (synovitis); spleen (vasculitis); liver (portal triaditis); lungs (interstitial pneumonitis, fibrosing alveolitis), CNS (vasculitis) and in blood (autoimmune haemolytic anaemia, thrombocytopaenia).

TREATMENT of SLE involves preventing flares and reducing their severity and duration when they occur. Treatment can include corticosteroids and anti-malarial drugs. Certain types of lupus nephritis such as diffuse proliferative glomerulonephritis require bouts of cytotoxic drugs. These drugs include cyclophosphamide and mycophenolate.

96. Ans. (b) X-ray crystallography *Ref: Harsh Mohan Textbook of Pathology 6th ed. p 82*

Ultrastructural examination and chemical analysis reveal the complex nature of amyloid. It emerges that on the basis of morphology and physical characteristics, all forms of amyloid are similar in appearance, but they are chemically heterogeneous. Based on these analysis, amyloid is composed of 2 main types of complex proteins:

- Fibril proteins comprise about 95% of amyloid.
- Non-fibrillar components which include P-component predominantly; there are several different proteins which together constitute the remaining 5% of amyloid. By electron microscopy, it became apparent that major component of all forms of amyloid (about 95%) consists of meshwork of fibril proteins. The fibrils are delicate, randomly dispersed, non-branching, each measuring 7.5-10 nm in diameter and having indefinite length. Each fibril is further composed of double helix of two pleated sheets in the form of twin filaments separated by a clear space. By X-ray crystallography and infra-red spectroscopy, the fibrils are shown to have cross-β-pleated sheet configuration which produces 1000 A° periodicity that gives the characteristic staining properties of amyloid with Congo red and birefringence under polarising microscopy. Based on these features, amyloid is also referred to as β-fibrillosis. Chemical analysis of fibril proteins of amyloid reveals heterogeneous nature of amyloid. Chemically two major forms of amyloid fibril proteins were first identified in 1970s while currently 20 biochemically different proteins are known to form amyloid fibrils in humans in different clinicopathologic settings. Thus, these proteins can be categorised as under:
  - AL (amyloid light chain) protein
  - AA (amyloid associated) protein
  - Other proteins

97. Ans. (c) CD4/CD8 counts *Ref: Journal of Clinical Virology Volume 17, Issue 2, August 2000, Ps 101108*

Flow cytometry is the standard method for the estimation of CD4/CD8 counts. In biotechnology, flow cytometry is a laser-based, biophysical technology employed in cell counting, cell sorting, biomarker detection and protein engineering, by suspending cells in a stream of fluid and passing them by an electronic detection apparatus. It allows simultaneous multiparametric analysis of the physical and chemical characteristics of up to thousands of particles per second. Flow cytometry is routinely used in the diagnosis of health disorders, especially blood cancers, but has many other applications in basic research, clinical practice and clinical trials. A common variation is to physically sort particles based on their properties, so as to purify populations of interest.

98. Ans. (a) T lymphocytes *Ref: Acid phosphatase staining pattern as an indicator of T-cell acute leukemia. Am J Clin Pathol. 1981 Dec;76(6):760-4. http://www.pathologyoutlines.com/topic/stainsacidphosphatase.html*

Acid phosphatase (staining)

- Class of enzymes that releases phosphate groups, optimally at acid pH (Mol Pathol 2002;55:65)
- Usually detected with enzyme histochemistry technique
- Examples include PAP (prostatic acid phosphatase) and TRAP (tartrate resistant acid phosphatase)
- Also useful for examining skeletal muscle pathology

It is useful in diagnosing following malignancies:

- Osteoclastic giant cells in tumors
- Acute basophilic leukemia, T-ALL (focal paranuclear), AML-M6b, T cell large granular lymphocytic leukemia, T cell prolymphocytic leukemia
- Epulis, granular cell tumor, histiocytic sarcoma

99. Ans. (d) IgE

Refer explanation of Chapter 6 Q 94

100. Ans. (b) Antigen antibody reaction *Ref: http://www.pathology.med.umich.edu/bloodbank/manual/bbch_7/*

Reaction type	*Symptoms*	*Cause*	*Prevention*
Acute hemolytic reaction	Fever, chills and fever, the feeling of heat along the vein in which the blood is being transfused, pain in the lumbar region, constricting pain in the chest, tachycardia, hypotension, and hemoglobinemia with subsequent hemoglobinuria and hyperbilirubinemia. A 'feeling of impending doom' is frequently reported by the patient as an early sign of this reaction. In an unconscious or anesthetized patient: Uncontrollable bleeding due to disseminated intravascular coagulation may be the only sign of a hemolytic transfusion reaction	Human error such as mislabeled pretransfusion specimen; the transfusion of properly labeled blood to the wrong person, or clerical errors occurring within the Blood Bank transfused red cells react with circulating antibody in the recipient with resultant intravascular hemolysis Most likely to occur when a group O patient is mistakenly transfused with group A, B, or AB blood. Patients receiving a major ABO-incompatible marrow or stem cell transplant with sufficient red cell content will likely develop an acute hemolytic reaction	Proper identification of patients, pretransfusion blood samples and blood components at the time of transfusion

Contd...

Contd...

Reaction type	*Symptoms*	*Cause*	*Prevention*
Delayed hemolytic reaction Notify the Blood Bank at the time the reaction is suspected, to allow prompt investigation. Care must be taken that subsequently transfused red cells lack the antigen corresponding to the patient's antibody.	The most common signs are a falling hematocrit (due to extravascular destruction of the transfused red blood cells) and a positive direct antiglobulin (Coombs) test (DAT). 'Delayed' hemolytic reactions commonly occurs about 4-8 days after blood transfusion, but may develop up to one month later. There may also be hemoglobinuria and a mild elevation of the serum bilirubin. Symptomatic patients may manifest fever and leukocytosis thus appearing to have an occult infection.	Many delayed hemolytic reactions will go undetected because the red cell destruction occurs slowly Delayed hemolytic reactions occur in patients who have developed antibodies from previous transfusion or pregnancy but, at the time of pretransfusion testing, the antibody in question is too weak to be detected by standard procedures. Subsequent transfusion with red cells having the corresponding antigen results in an anamnestic antibody response and hemolysis of transfused red cells.	
Febrile	Fever or chill fever A temperature rise of 1.8 F or 1.0 C from the baseline	Cytokines and antibodies to leukocyte antigens reacting with leukocytes or leukocyte fragments	
Allergic - urticaria	Allergic reactions may be associated with laryngeal edema and bronchospasm. If coupled with another sign, such as fever, evaluation for a hemolytic reaction may be indicated.	This reaction is caused by foreign plasma proteins	
Allergic - Anaphylaxis	Anaphylactic or anaphylactoid Respiratory involvement with dyspnea or stridor may be more pronounced than is usually seen in typical allergic reactions. Reactions manifest cardiovascular instability that includes hypotension, tachycardia, loss of consciousness, cardiac arrhythmia, shock and cardiac arrest.	May be due to anti-IgA	

Contd...

Contd...

Reaction type	*Symptoms*	*Cause*	*Prevention*
TRALI	Abrupt onset of noncardiogenic pulmonary edema. Severe cases may require assisted ventilation with high FIO2...	TRALI has been associated with the presence of antibodies in the donor plasma reactive to recipient leukocyte antigens or with the production of inflammatory mediators during storage of cellular blood components	Most cases of TRALI resolve within 72 hours although fatalities may occur in approximately 10 percent of cases.
Volume overlead		Transfusion-related volume overload	Infuse smaller volumes more slowly
Bacterial contamination	Hypotension, shock, fever and chills, nausea and vomiting, and respiratory distress. Diagnosis is established by Gram stain and blood culture of both the blood component and the recipient.distress	Bacterial contamination occurs when a small number of bacteria enter a blood component during collection or processing. During storage, bacteria may proliferate, resulting in a large number of organisms, and possible endotoxin, being given with the transfusion	
Hypotension	A drop of at least 10 mm Hg in systolic or diastolic arterial blood pressure in the absence of signs or symptoms of other transfusion reactions If the immediate pretransfusion blood pressure is elevated from the patient's typical blood pressure, and the arterial pressure does not fall below the patient's usual blood pressure, it should not be considered a hypotensive reaction. The onset of hypotension is during the transfusion, and resolves quickly with discontinuation of the transfusion. If hypotension persists beyond 30 minutes after discontinuing the transfusion, another diagnosis should be strongly considered.	Some reactions have been associated with angiotensin converting enzyme (ACE) inhibitor drugs or the use of leukocyte reduction filters. Hypotensive reactions have been associated with red cell and platelet transfusions.	

Contd...

Contd...

Reaction type	*Symptoms*	*Cause*	*Prevention*
Graft-vs-Host disease (GVHD)	Rash, fever, diarrhea, cytopenia and liver dysfunction 3-4 weeks after transfusion	Viable T lymphocytes in blood components are transfused, engraft and react against the recipient's tissues and the recipient is unable to reject the donor lymphocytes because of immunodeficiency, severe immunosuppression, or shared HLA antigens associated with bone marrow transplantation. Transfusion associated GVHD carries a very poor prognosis.	Irradiation of cellular components The Blood Bank must be apprised of the immune status, or diagnosis, of the patient so that cellular components intended for transfusion of immunocompromised patients and blood components from directed (designated) donors will be irradiated. Irradiation of blood red cell containing components decreases the red cell survival and increases the potassium of the component. There is no apparent effect on platelet survival. Fresh Frozen Plasma (FFP) and cryoprecipitated AHG (CRYO) need not be irradiated because these components do not contain enough viable lymphocytes to cause GVHD.

Contd...

Contd...

Reaction type	*Symptoms*	*Cause*	*Prevention*
Non-immune hemolysis	hemoglobinemia and hemoglobinuria transient hemodynamic, pulmonary and renal impairment may occur. Cardiac arrhythmia due to hyperkalemia may occur, particularly in patients with renal failure.	Lysis of red cells can occur due to improper storage, handling, or transfusion conditions. Mishandling or storage of blood components. The contents of the blood bags are available for study. The blood bag together with attached tubing and intravenous fluids should be saved for further investigations.	
Post-transfusion purpura (PTP)	Thrombocytopenia that is frequently profound, purpura, or bleeding Febrile reactions have been reported retrospectively with the implicated transfusion thrombocytopenia typically 7–48 days after transfusion PTP must be differentiated from the far more common alloimmunization to platelet antigens. Consultation with a Blood Bank physician is recommended in evaluating such patients.	The patient makes an alloantibody in response to platelet antigens in the transfused blood that for a period of time causes destruction of autologous antigen negative platelets	Platelet transfusion is of very little value in PTP; however, therapeutic plasma exchange may be beneficial. Since autologous platelets do not survive in circulation, there is no expectation that transfused platelets regardless of antigen matching will do any better. Reserved platelet transfusion for patients with active bleeding.

101. Ans. (b) Amyloidosis *Ref: Harsh Mohan Textbook of Pathology 6th ed. p 90*

Amyloid deposition in the spleen, for some unknown reasons, may have one of the following two patterns:

- **SAGO SPLEEN:** The splenomegaly is not marked and cut surface shows characteristic translucent pale and waxy nodules resembling sago grains and hence the name. Microscopically, the amyloid deposits begin in the walls of the arterioles of the white pulp and may subsequently replace the follicles.

- **LARDACEOUS SPLEEN:** There is generally moderate to marked splenomegaly (weight up to 1 kg). Cut surface of the spleen shows map-like areas of amyloid (lardaceous lard-like; lard means fat of pigs). Microscopically, the deposits involve the walls of splenic sinuses and the small arteries and in the connective tissue of the red pulp. Confirmation is by seeing Congophilia in Congo Red staining and demonstration of apple-green birefringence under polarising microscopy in the corresponding positive areas.

102. Ans. (c) Type III hypersensitivity *Ref: Robbins Pathologic Basis of Disease 7th ed. p 210* *http://en.wikipedia.org/wiki/Type_III_hypersensitivity*

(Type III) Hypersensitivity: Type III hypersensitivity occurs when antigen-antibody complexes that are not adequately cleared by innate immune cells accumulate, giving rise to an inflammatory response and attraction of leukocytes.

Some clinical examples:

Disease	*Target antigen*	*Main effects*
Systemic lupus erythematosus	Nuclear antigens	• Nephritis • Skin lesions • Arthritis
Post-streptococcal glomerulonephritis	Streptococcal cell wall antigens	• Nephritis
Polyarteritis nodosa	Hepatitis B virus surface antigen	• Systemic vasculitis
Reactive arthritis	Several bacterial antigens	• Acute arthritis
Serum sickness	Various	• Arthritis • Vasculitis • Nephritis
Arthus reaction	Various	• Cutaneous vasculitis
Farmer's Lung	Inhaled antigens (often mould or hay dust)	• Alveolar inflammation
Henoch-Schönlein purpura	Unknown, likely respiratory pathogen	• Purpura • Glomerulonephritis

103. Ans. (b) Can synthesize TNF-alpha

Tumor necrosis factor (TNF, cachexin, or cachectin, and formerly known as tumor necrosis factor alpha or TNFα) is an adipokine involved in systemic inflammation and is a member of a group of cytokines that stimulate the acute phase reaction. It is produced chiefly by activated macrophages (M1) Mast cell release histamine upon binding to immunoglobulin E.

104. Ans. (b) Tuberculosis *Ref: Robbins Pathologic Basis of Disease 7th ed. p 261*

Reactive systemic/secondry amyloidosis—The amyloid deposits in this pattern is systemic in distribution and are composed of AA protein. This category was previously referred to as secondary amyloidosis because it is secondary to an associated inflammatory condition. The feature common to most of the conditions associated with reactive systemic amyloidosis is protracted breakdown of cells resulting from a wide variety of infectious and noninfectious chronic inflammatory conditions. At one time, tuberculosis, bronchiectasis, and chronic osteomyelitis were the most important underlying conditions, but with the advent of effective antimicrobial chemotherapy, the importance of these conditions has diminished. More commonly now, reactive systemic amyloidosis complicates rheumatoid arthritis, other connective tissue disorders such as ankylosing spondylitis, and inflammatory bowel disease, particularly Crohn disease and ulcerative colitis. Among these, the most frequent associated condition is rheumatoid arthritis.

105. Ans. (b) Ankylosing spondylitis *Ref: Harsh Mohan Textbook of Pathology 6th ed. p 853*

Ankylosing spondylitis or rheumatoid spondylitis is rheumatoid involvement of the spine, particularly sacroiliac joints, in young male patients. The condition has a strong HLA-B27 association and may have associated inflammatory diseases such as inflammatory bowel disease, anterior uveitis and Reiter's syndrome.

106. Ans. (a) IgM anti-HBc *Ref: Robbins Pathologic Basis of Disease 7th ed. p 893*

Serologic Diagnosis of HBV: After exposure to HBV, the long asymptomatic 4- to 26-week incubation period (mean: 6 to 8 weeks) is followed by acute disease lasting many weeks to months. Most patients experience a self-limited illness:

- HBsAg appears before the onset of symptoms, peaks during overt disease, and then declines to undetectable levels in 3 to 6 months.
- HBeAg, HBV-DNA, and DNA polymerase appear in the serum soon after HBsAg, and all signify active viral replication.
- IgM anti-HBc becomes detectable in serum shortly before the onset of symptoms, concurrent with the onset of elevation of serum aminotransferases. Over months, the IgM antibody is replaced by IgG anti-HBc.
- Anti-HBe is detectable shortly after the disappearance of HBeAg, implying that the acute infection has peaked and the disease is on the wane
- IgG anti-HBs does not rise until the acute disease is over and is usually not detectable for a few weeks to several months after the disappearance of HBsAg. Anti-HBs may persist for life, conferring protection; this is the basis for current vaccination strategies using noninfectious HBsAg. The carrier state is defined by the presence of HBsAg in serum for 6 months or longer after initial detection. The presence of HBsAg alone does not necessarily indicate replication of complete virions, and patients may be asymptomatic and without liver damage. In contrast, chronic replication of HBV virions is characterized by persistence of circulating HBsAg, HBeAg, and HBV DNA, usually with anti-HBc and occasionally with anti-HBs. In these patients, progressive liver damage may occur.

107. Ans. (b) Granuloma formation *Ref: The Granulomatous disease by D. Geraint James p-491.*

T cell interaction leads to the formation of organised lymphoid organ structure such as granuloma.

108. Ans. (c) IgE

Refer explanation of Chapter 6 Q 94

109. Ans. (d) Opsonisation

Ref: Robbins Pathologic Basis of Disease 7th ed. p 59; http://www.ncbi.nlm.nih.gov/gene/920

Receptors for opsonins promote phagocytosis of microbes coated with various proteins and deliver signals that activate the phagocytes. The process of coating a particle, such as a microbe, to target it for phagocytosis is called opsonization, substances that do this are opsonins. These substances include antibodies, complement proteins, and lectins. One of the most efficient systems for opsonizing particles is coating the particles with IgG antibodies, which are termed specific opsonins and are recognized by the high-affinity Fry receptor of phagocytes, called FcyRI. Components of the complement system, especially fragments of the complement protein C3, are also potent opsonins, because these fragments bind to microbes and phagocytes express a receptor, called the type I complement receptor (CR1), that recognizes breakdown products of C3. CD4. This gene encodes a membrane glycoprotein of T lymphocytes that interacts with major histocompatibility complex class II antigens and is also a receptor for the human immunodeficiency virus. This gene is expressed not only in T lymphocytes, but also in B cells, macrophages, and granulocytes. It is also expressed in specific regions of the brain. The protein functions to initiate or augment the early phase of T-cell activation, and may function as an important mediator of indirect neuronal damage in infectious and immune-mediated diseases of the central nervous system.

NEOPLASIA

110. Ans. (a) Anaplastic *Ref: Robbins Pathologic Basis of Disease 7th ed. p 272*

Differentiation refers to the extent to which neoplastic cells resemble comparable normal cells, both morphologically and functionally; lack of differentiation is called anaplasia.

- Anaplasia (structural differentiation loss within cell or group of cells)
- Aplasia (organ or part of organ missing)
- Hypoplasia (below-average number of cells, especially when inadequate)
- Hyperplasia (proliferation of cells)
- Neoplasia (abnormal proliferation)
- Dysplasia (change in cell or tissue phenotype)
- Metaplasia (conversion in cell type)
- Prosoplasia (development of new cell function)
- Desmoplasia (connective tissue growth)

111. Ans. (d) RAS *Ref: Harsh Mohan Textbook of Pathology 6th ed. p 212*
Robbins Pathologic Basis of Disease 7th ed. p 300

Mutated RAS gene: This is the most common form of oncogene in human tumours, the abnormality being induced by point mutation in RAS gene. About a third of all human tumours, carry mutated RAS gene (RAS for Rat Sarcoma gene where it was first described), seen particularly in carcinoma colon, lung and pancreas. Normally, the inactive form of RAS protein is GDP (guanosine diphosphate)—bound while the activated form is bound to guanosine triphosphate (GTP). GDP/GTP are homologous to G proteins and take part in signal transduction in a similar way just as G proteins act as 'on-off switch' for signal transduction. Normally, active RAS protein is inactivated by GTPase activity, while mutated RAS gene remains unaffected by GTPase, and therefore, continues to signal the cell proliferation.

Tumor suppressor genes in human neoplasm.

Subcellular location	*Gene*	*Function*	*Tumors associated with somatic mutations*	*Tumors associated with inherited mutations*
Cell surface	TGF-β receptor E-cadherin	Growth inhibition Cell adhesion	Carcinomas of colon Carcinoma of stomach	Unknown Familial gastric cancer
Inner aspect of plasma membrane	NF-1	Inhibition of RAS signal transduction and of p21 cell-cycle inhibitor	Neuroblastomas	Neurofibromatosis type 1 and sarcomas
Cytoskeleton	NF-2	Cytoskeletal stability	Schwannomas and meningiomas	Neurofibromatosis type 2, acoustic schwannomas and meningiomas
Cytosol	APC/β-catenin	Inhibition of signal transduction	Carcinomas of stomach, colon, pancreas; melanoma	Familial adenomatous polyposis coli/colon cancer

Contd...

Contd...

Subcellular location	*Gene*	*Function*	*Tumors associated with somatic mutations*	*Tumors associated with inherited mutations*
	PTEN	Pl-3 kinase signal transduction	Endometrial and prostate cancers	Unknown
	SMAD 2 and SMAD 4	TGF-β signal transduction	Colon, pancreas tumors	Unknown
Nucleus	RB	Regulation of cell cycle	Retinoblastoma; osteosarcoma carcinomas of breast, colon, lung	Retinoblastomas, osteosarcoma
	p53	Cell-cycle arrest and apoptosis in response to DNA damage	Most human cancers	Li-Fraumeni syndrome; multiple carcinomas and sarcomas
	WT-1 p16 (INK4a)	Nuclear transcription Regulation of cell cycle by inhibition of cyclin-dependent kinases	Wilms tumor Pancreatic, breast, and esophageal cancers	Wilms tumor Malignant melanoma
	BRCA-1 and BRCA-2	DNA repair	Unknown	Carcinomas of female breast and ovary; carcinomas of male breast
	KLF6	Transcription factor	Prostate	Unknown

112. Ans. (a) Rhabdomyosarcoma *Ref: Robbins Pathologic Basis of Disease 7th ed. p 1321*

Rhabdomyosarcoma is histologically subclassified into the embryonal, alveolar, and pleomorphic variants.' The rhabdomyoblast the diagnostic cell in all types contains eccentric eosinophilic granular cytoplasm rich in thick and thin filaments. The rhabdomyoblasts may be round or elongate; the latter are known as tadpole or strap cells and may contain cross-striations visible by light microscopy. Ultrastructurally, rhabdomyoblasts contain sarcomeres, and immunohistochemically they stain with antibodies to the myogenic markers desmin, MYOD1, and myogenin.

113. Ans. (a) Osteosarcoma *Ref: Robbins Pathologic Basis of Disease 7th ed. p 1301; http://www.mdanderson.org/patient-and-cancer-information/cancer-information/cancer- types/childhood-osteosarcoma/index.html*

Ewing sarcoma and PNET account for approximately 6% to 10% of primary malignant bone tumors and follow osteosarcoma as the second most common group of bone sarcomas in children. Osteosarcoma is a bone tumor that consists of malignant cells that produce immature bone. It is the most common type of bone cancer in children and adolescents and affects more males than females. Nearly, 80% of osteosarcomas appear in the distal femur, the portion of the thigh bone closest to the knee, or the proximal tibia, the lower leg bone near the knee. Osteosarcoma may also develop in the proximal humerus, the upper arm bone connected to the shoulder. Of all childhood cancers, osteosarcoma is rare, but it is the most common bone tumor in children; it affects approximately 400 children under age 20 every year. Osteosarcomas are classified as low, intermediate or high-grade tumors. A low-grade osteosarcoma has few dividing cells in the tumor, while a high-grade osteosarcoma is filled with dead tumor cells. Most tumors that occur in children are high-grade.

114. Ans. (b) Papillary type *Ref: Robbins Pathologic Basis of Disease 7th ed. p 1177*

Most thyroid carcinomas are well-differentiated lesions. The major subtypes of thyroid carcinoma and their relative frequencies include the following:

- Papillary carcinoma (75% to 85% of cases)
- Follicular carcinoma (10% to 20% of cases)
- Medullary carcinoma (5% of cases)
- Anaplastic carcinoma (<5% of cases). Most thyroid carcinomas are derived from the follicular epithelium, except for medullary carcinomas; the latter are derived from the parafollicular or C cells.

115. Ans. (b) Autosomal dominant *Ref: http://link.springer.com/article/10.1007%2FBF00284597*

Human Genetics November (1) 1979, Volume 52, Issue 1, pp 1-54

Genetics of retinoblastoma

The genetic basis of retinoblastoma is reviewed and the following conclusions are drawn:

- The mode of inheritance of the hereditary variety of retinoblastoma (R) is autosomal dominant with about 90% penetrance. Retinoblastoma is a rare type of eye cancer that usually develops in early childhood, typically before the age of 5. This form of cancer develops in the retina, which is the specialized light-sensitive tissue at the back of the eye that detects light and color. In most children with retinoblastoma, the disease affects only one eye. However, one out of three children with retinoblastoma develops cancer in both eyes. The most common first sign of retinoblastoma is a visible whiteness in the pupil called 'cat's eye reflex' or leukocoria. This unusual whiteness is particularly noticeable in photographs taken with a flash. Other signs and symptoms of retinoblastoma include crossed eyes or eyes that do not point in the same direction (strabismus); persistent eye pain, redness, or irritation; and blindness or poor vision in the affected eye(s).

116. Ans. (c) G1S phase *Ref: http://en.wikipedia.org/wiki/P53#Function*

p53 has many mechanisms of anticancer function, and plays a role in apoptosis, genomic stability, and inhibition of angiogenesis. In its anti-cancer role, p53 works through several mechanisms:

- It can activate DNA repair proteins when DNA has sustained damage. Thus, it may be an important factor in aging.
- It can arrest growth by holding the cell cycle at the G1/S regulation point on DNA damage recognition (if it holds the cell here for long enough, the DNA repair proteins will have time to fix the damage and the cell will be allowed to continue the cell cycle).
- It can initiate apoptosis, the programmed cell death, if DNA damage proves to be irreparable.

117. Ans. (c) Liver *Ref: Kelleys Essential of Internal Medicine p 445*

Liver is the most common site of metastasis

118. Ans. (b) Lung *Ref: http://www.ccohs.ca/oshanswers/diseases/occupational_cancer.html*

Research shows that the amount of cancer related to occupational exposure varies with the type of cancer. The most common types of occupational cancer are lung cancer, bladder cancer and mesothelioma.

Type of cancer	*Related to occupational exposure estimated % (USA)*
Lung	6.3-13%
Bladder	3-19%
Mesothelioma	85-90% (men) 23-90% (women)
Leukemia	0.8-2.8%
Laryngeal	1-20% (men)
Skin cancer (non-melanoma)	1.5-6% (men)
Sinonasal and nasopharyngeal	31-43% (men)
Kidney	0-2.3%
Liver	0.4-1.1 (vinyl chloride only; men)

Mesothelioma (or, more precisely, malignant mesothelioma) is a rare form of cancer that develops from cells of the mesothelium, the protective lining that covers many of the internal organs of the body. Mesothelioma is most commonly caused by exposure to asbestos. The most common anatomical site for mesothelioma is the pleura (the outer lining of the lungs and internal chest wall), but it can also arise in the peritoneum (the lining of the abdominal cavity), the pericardium (the sac that surrounds the heart), or the tunica vaginalis (a sac that surrounds the testis).

119. Ans. (b) Liver

Refer explanation of Chapter 7 Q 118

120. Ans. (a) Tumour marker *Ref: Essential of Pathophysiology by Carol Porth p 149*

PSA is used as a tumor marker in prostate cancer and CA-125 is used as a marker in ovarian cancer.

121. Ans. (c) Turners syndrome *Ref: Science. 1984 Dec 7;226(4679):1165-71. Molecular characterization of human T-cell leukemia (lymphotropic) virus type III in the acquired immune deficiency syndrome. http://www.mayomedicallaboratories.com/test-catalog/Clinical+and+Interpretive/926 http://www.cancer.gov/cancertopics/pdq/treatment/childAML/HealthProfessional/p8*

The human T-cell leukemia (lymphotropic) virus type III (HTLV-III) appears to be central to the causation of the acquired immune deficiency syndrome (AIDS). Bloom syndrome is a genetic disorder associated with various congenital defects and predisposition to acute leukemia, pulmonary fibrosis, and Hodgkin lymphomas. Carcinoma also is commonly seen in these patients. Approximately one fourth to one half of patients develop some type of cancer with a mean age of 25 years at onset. The severity and age of onset of cancer varies among patients. Children with Down syndrome have a tenfold to twentyfold increased risk of leukemia compared with children without Down syndrome.

122. Ans. (c) Multiple myeloma *Ref: http://en.wikipedia.org/wiki/Multiple_myeloma#Pathophysiology*

B lymphocytes start in the bone marrow and move to the lymph nodes. As they progress, they mature and display different proteins on their cell surface. When they are activated to secrete antibodies, they are known as plasma cells. Multiple myeloma develops in B lymphocytes after they have left the part of the lymph node known as the germinal center. The normal cell line most closely associated with MM cells is generally taken to be either an activated memory B cell or the precursor to plasma cells, the plasmablast. The immune system keeps the proliferation of B cells and the secretion of antibodies under tight control. When chromosomes and genes are damaged, often through rearrangement, this control is lost. Often, a promoter gene moves (or translocates) to a chromosome where it stimulates an antibody gene to overproduction. A chromosomal translocation between the immunoglobulin heavy chain gene (on chromosome 14, locus q32) and an oncogene (often 11q13, 4p16.3, 6p21, 16q23 and 20q1) is frequently observed in patients with multiple myeloma. This mutation results in dysregulation of the oncogene which is thought to be an important initiating event in the pathogenesis of myeloma. The result is proliferation of a plasma cell clone and genomic instability that leads to further mutations and translocations. The chromosome 14 abnormality is observed in about 50% of all cases of myeloma. Deletion of (parts of) chromosome 13 is also observed in about 50% of cases. Production of cytokines (especially IL-6) by the plasma cells causes much of their localised damage, such as osteoporosis, and creates a microenvironment in which the malignant cells thrive. Angiogenesis (the attraction of new blood vessels) is increased. The produced antibodies are deposited in various organs, leading to renal failure, polyneuropathy and various other myeloma-associated symptoms.

123. Ans. (a) CD45Ro *Ref: Myeloid Sarcomas: A Histologic, Immunohistochemical, and Cytogenetic Study Diagnostic Pathology 2007;2:42*

A myeloid sarcoma (chloroma, granulocytic sarcoma extramedullary myeloid tumor), is a solid tumor composed of immature white blood cells called myeloblasts. A chloroma is an extramedullary manifestation of acute myeloid leukemia; in other words, it is a solid collection of leukemic cells occurring outside of the bone marrow. An immunohistochemical panel including CD43, lysozyme, myeloperoxidase (MPO), CD68 (or CD163), CD117, CD3 and CD20 can successfully identify the vast majority of MS variants in formalin-fixed paraffin-embedded tissue sections.

124. Ans. (a) Ames test *Ref: Robbins Pathologic Basis of Disease 7th ed. p 320*

Because malignant transformation results from mutations that affect oncogenes, tumor suppressor genes, genes that regulate apoptosis, and genes involved in DNA repair, it comes as no surprise that the majority of initiating chemicals are mutagenic. Their mutagenic potential has been investigated, most commonly using the Ames test, which uses the ability of a chemical to induce mutations in the bacterium Salmonella typhinrurium. The vast majority (70% to 90%) of known chemical carcinogens score positive in the Ames test." Conversely, most but not all chemicals that are mutagenic in vitro are carcinogenic in vivo.

125. Ans. (d) Presence of local invasion *Ref: Robbins Pathologic Basis of Disease 7th ed. p 281*

Comparison between benign and malignant tumors		
Characteristics	*Benign*	*Malignant*
Differentiation/anaplasia	Well differentiated; structure may be typical of tissue of origin	Some lack of differentiation with anaplasia; structure is often atypical
Rate of growth	Usually progressive and slow; may come to a standstill or regress; mitotic figures are rare and normal	Erratic and may be slow to rapid; mitotic figures may be numerous and abnormal
Local invasion	Usually cohesive and expansile well-demarcated masses that do not invade or infiltrate surrounding normal tissues	Locally invasive, infiltrating the surrounding normal tissues; sometimes may be seemingly cohesive and expansile
Metastasis	Absent	Frequently present; the larger and more undifferentiated the primary, the more likely are metastases

126. Ans. (d) Endometrial carcinoma *Ref: Robbins Pathologic Basis of Disease 7th ed. p 305*

PTEN: Phosphatase and tensin homologue, deleted on chromosome 10 (PTEN) gene, mapped on chromosome 10q23, is frequently deleted in many human cancers but at particularly high frequency in endometrial carcinomas and glioblastomas. "PTEN activity causes cell-cycle arrest and apoptosis as well as inhibition of cell motility. It has been proposed that PTEN blocks the cell cycle by increasing the transcription of the p27 Cip/Kip cell-cycle inhibitor and stabilizing the protein." With loss of PTEN, therefore, cells are released into the cell cycle.

127. Ans. (d) Carcinoma of colon

Ref: http://en.wikipedia.org/wiki/Carcinoembryonic_antigen#Diagnostic_significance

Carcinoembryonic antigen (CEA) is a glycoprotein involved in cell adhesion. It is normally produced in gastrointestinal tissue during fetal development, but the production of CEA stops before birth. Therefore, it is usually present only at very low levels in the blood of healthy adults. However, the serum levels are raised in some types of cancer, which means that it can be used as a tumor marker in clinical tests. Serum levels can also be elevated in heavy smokers. CEA is a glycosylphosphatidylinositol (GPI) cell surface anchored glycoprotein whose specialized sialofucosylated glycoforms serve as functional colon carcinoma L-selectin and E-selectin ligands, which may be critical to the metastatic dissemination of colon carcinoma cells.

128. Ans. (d) Hepatitis B virus *Ref: http://en.wikipedia.org/wiki/Hepatitis_B#Signs_and_symptoms*

Acute infection with hepatitis B virus is associated with acute viral hepatitis an illness that begins with general ill-health, loss of appetite, nausea, vomiting, bodyaches, mild fever, and dark urine, and then progresses to development of jaundice. It has been noted that itchy skin has been an indication as a possible symptom of all hepatitis virus types. The illness lasts for a few weeks and then gradually improves in most affected people. A few people may have more severe liver disease (fulminant hepatic failure), and may die as a result. The infection may be entirely asymptomatic and may go unrecognized. Chronic infection with hepatitis B virus either may be asymptomatic or may be associated with a chronic inflammation of the liver (chronic hepatitis), leading to cirrhosis over a period of several years. This type of infection dramatically increases the incidence of hepatocellular carcinoma (liver cancer).

129. Ans. (a) Basal cell carcinoma *Ref: Robbins Pathologic Basis of Disease 7th ed. p 1242*

Basal cell carcinomas are common, slow-growing tumors that rarely metastasize. They have a tendency to occur at sites subject to chronic sun exposure and in lightly pigmented people. As with squamous cell carcinoma, the incidence of basal cell carcinoma rises sharply with immunosuppression and in patients with inherited defects in DNA repair.

130. Ans. (c) A developmental malformation *Ref: Harsh Mohan Textbook of Pathology 6th ed. p 193*

Mixed tumours: When two types of tumours are combined in the same tumour, it is called a mixed tumour. Teratomas: These tumours are made up of a mixture of various tissue types arising from totipotent cells derived from the three germ cell layers ectoderm, mesoderm and endoderm. Most common sites for teratomas are ovaries and testis (gonadal teratomas) Blastomas (Embryomas). Blastomas or embryomas are a group of malignant tumours which arise from embryonal or partially differentiated cells which would normally form blastema of the organs and tissue during embryogenesis. Hamartoma: Hamartoma is benign tumour which is made of mature but disorganised cells of tissues indigenous to the particular organ, e.g. hamartoma of the lung consists of mature cartilage, mature smooth muscle and epithelium. Thus, all mature differentiated tissue elements which comprise the bronchus are present in it but are jumbled up as a mass. Choristoma: Choristoma is the name given to the ectopic islands of normal tissue. Thus, choristoma is heterotopia but is not a true tumour, though it sounds like one.

131. Ans. (c) Mucoepidermoid carcinoma *Ref: Diagn Cytopathol. 2004 Oct;31(4):271-5.Primary Intraosseous (Central) Salivary Gland Neoplasms in Jaw Bones: Report of a Mucoepidermoid Carcinoma of the Mandible Diagnosed by Fine- Needle Aspiration Cytology.*

Mucoepidermoid carcinoma is the most common histotype of malignant and benign salivary gland tumors, which occasionally arise within the facial bones of mandible and maxilla, besides their ordinary derivation from the major and minor salivary glands of the head and neck regions.

132. Ans. (a) Heaping up of margins *Ref: Robbins Pathologic Basis of Disease 7th ed. p 818*

Although over 50% of peptic ulcers have a diameter less than 2 cm, about 10% of benign ulcers are greater than 4 cm. Since carcinomatous ulcers may be less than 4 cm in diameter and may be located anywhere in the stomach, size and location do not differentiate a benign from a malignant ulcer. The classic peptic ulcer is a round to oval, sharply punched-out defect with relatively straight walls. The mucosal margin may overhang the base slightly, particularly on the upstream portion of the circumference. The margins are usually level with the surrounding mucosa or only slightly elevated. Heaping-up of these margins is rare in the benign ulcer but is characteristic of the malignant lesion. The depth of these ulcers varies, from superficial lesions involving only the mucosa and muscularis mucosa.

133. Ans. (b) Teratoma

Refer explanation of Chapter 7 Q 130

134. Ans. (a) Metaplasia

Refer explanation of Chapter 1 Q 119

135. Ans. (c) 17 *Ref: Breast Cancer Genes and Inheritance-Viviana Rivera-Varas -Copyright 1998*

Breast cancer is the most common cancer that affects women in the United States. There are at least two majors genes (BRCA1 and BRCA2) that when they mutate can cause breast cancer. These genes can be passed from parent to child, increasing the risk of developing cancer in that child that have parent carrying these genes. BRCA1 and BRCA2 genes are located on chromosome 17 and chromosome 13 respectively. There is a 90% chance of developing breast cancer for a woman that has these mutated genes. In contrast, men carrying BRCA1 have no risk to develop breast cancer, but those carrying BRCA2 genes have high risk. It is important to note that mutations in these genes can be passed on to children by either parent. A man with a mutation is just as likely to pass this gene to his children as a woman with a mutation. Hereditary cancer occurs at young age, for instance a woman in her 20s with breast cancer is more likely to have hereditary type of cancer that a woman in her 50s.

136. Ans. (c) Both 1 and 2 *Ref: Robbins Pathologic Basis of Disease 7th ed. p 789*

Two carotid arteries (one on each side of the neck) supply blood to the large, front part of the brain, where thinking, speech, personality and sensory and motor functions reside. A carotid body tumor (also called a chemodectoma or paraganglioma) is a tumor found in the upper neck at the branching of the carotid artery. Paraganglia are clusters of neuroendocrine cells dispersed throughout the body, some connected with the sympathetic nervous system and others with the parasympathetic nervous system. The largest collection of these cells is found in the adrenal medulla, where they give rise to pheochromocytomas. Tumors arising in extra-adrenal paraganglia are not surprisingly referred to as paragangliomas. Paraganglia related to the great vessels of the head and neck, the so-called aorticopulmonary chain, including the carotid bodies; aortic bodies; jugulotympanic ganglia; ganglion nodosum of the vagus nerve; and clusters located about the oral cavity, nose, nasopharynx, larynx, and orbit. These are innervated by the parasympathetic nervous system, and their tumors are referred to as nonchromaffin paragangliomas. These tumors infrequently release catecholamines, but because the neuroendocrine cells that make up these lesions sense oxygen and carbon dioxide tensions within adjacent vessels, the tumors are also sometimes referred to as chemodectomas.

137. Ans. (a) Chronic myeloblastic leukaemia *Ref: Robbins Pathologic Basis of Disease 7th ed. p 314*

The Philadelphia chromosome, characteristic of chronic myeloid leukemia and a subset of acute lymphoblastic leukemias, provides the prototypic example of an oncogene formed by fusion of two separate genes. In these cases, a reciprocal translocation between chromosomes 9 and 22.

138. Ans. (a) Osteoclastoma *Ref: Robbins Pathologic Basis of Disease 7th ed. p 1302*

Giant cell tumor is so named because it contains a profusion of multinucleated osteoclast-type giant cells, giving rise to the synonym osteoclastoma. Giant cell tumor is a relatively uncommon benign but locally aggressive neoplasm. It usually arises in patients in their twenties to forties. Giant cell tumors are believed to have a monocyte-macrophage lineage,' and the giant cells are believed to form via fusion of the mononuclear cells. Giant cell tumor is so named because it contains a profusion of multinucleated osteoclast-type giant cells, giving rise to the synonym osteoclastoma. Giant cell tumor is a relatively uncommon benign but locally aggressive neoplasm. It usually arises in patients in their twenties to forties. Giant cell tumors are believed to have a monocyte-macrophage lineage,' and the giant cells are believed to form via fusion of the mononuclear cells. Giant cell tumors in adults involve both the epiphyses and the metaphyses, but in adolescents they are confined proximally by the growth plate and are limited to the metaphysis. The majority of giant cell tumors arise around the knee (distal femur and proximal tibia), but virtually any bone may be involved. The location of these tumors in the ends of bones near joints frequently causes patients to complain of arthritic symptoms. Osteosarcoma: The tumors usually arise in the metaphyseal region of the long bones of the extremities, and almost 60% occur about the knee.

139. Ans. (a) Are multipotent stem cells that give rise to all haemotogenous cell lineages

Ref: Robbins Pathologic Basis of Disease 7th ed. p 620

Haemopoietic stem cell potential to develop all blood cells hence called as pluripotential cells while committed progenitor cells have ability to form only individual type of the cell groups, e.g. granulocytes lymphocytes, etc.

INFECTIOUS DISEASES

140. Ans. (d) Aortic aneurysm *Ref: Harrisons Principles of Internal Medicine, 18th ed. p 1549*

The heart and great vessels are not the sites most frequently affected by opportunistic infections and neoplastic processes in patients with acquired immune deficiency syndrome (AIDS). However, cardiovascular complications occur in a significant number of such patients and are the immediate cause of death in some. The spectrum of cardiovascular complications of AIDS that may be depicted at imaging includes dilated cardiomyopathy, pericardial effusion, human immunodeficiency virus-associated pulmonary hypertension, endocarditis, thrombosis, embolism, vasculitis, coronary artery disease, aneurysm, and cardiac involvement in AIDS-related tumors.

141. Ans. (d) Thrombocytopenia *Ref: Robbins Pathologic Basis of Disease 7th ed. p 84*

Systemic inflammatory response syndrome (SIRS) is an inflammatory state affecting the whole body, frequently a response of the immune system to infection, but not necessarily so. It is related to sepsis, a condition in which individuals meet criteria for SIRS and have a known infection. Criteria for SIRS were established in 1992 as part of the American College of Chest Physicians/Society of Critical Care Medicine Consensus Conference. The conference concluded that the manifestations of SIRS include, but are not limited to:

- Body temperature less than 36°C (96.8°F) or greater than 38°C (100.4°F)
- Heart rate greater than 90 beats per minute
- Tachypnea (high respiratory rate), with greater than 20 breaths per minute; or, an arterial partial pressure of carbon dioxide less than 4.3 kPa (32 mmHg)
- Leukocytosis: Leukocytes less than 4000 cells/mm^3 (4 × 109 cells/L) or greater than 12,000 cells/mm^3 (12 × 109 cells/L); or the presence of greater than 10% immature neutrophils (band forms) band forms greater than 3% is called bandemia or a 'left-shift.' SIRS can be diagnosed when two or more of these criteria are present. The causes of SIRS are broadly classified as infectious or noninfectious. As above, when SIRS is due to an infection, it is considered sepsis. Noninfectious causes of SIRS include trauma, burns, pancreatitis, ischemia, and hemorrhage

142. Ans. (a) Most common source of infection is cross-infection from infected people

Exp: No need to explain *Ref: Microbiology by Medpgnotes*

143. Ans. (b) Gametocyte *Ref: Robbins Pathologic Basis of Disease 7th ed. p 401*

The infectious stage of malaria, the sporozoites, is found in the salivary glands of female mosquitoes. When the mosquito takes a blood meal, sporozoites are released into the human's blood and within minutes attach to and invade liver cells by binding to the hepatocyte receptor for the serum proteins thrombospondin and properdin. Within liver cells, malaria parasites multiply rapidly, so as many as 30,000 merozoites (asexual, haploid forms) are released when each infected hepatocyte ruptures. P.vivax and P.ovale form latent hypnozoites in hepatocytes, which cause relapses of malaria long after initial infection. Once released from the liver, Plasmodium merozoites bind by a parasite lectinlike molecule to sialic residues on glycophorin molecules on the surface of red blood cells. Within the red blood cells, the parasites grow in a membrane-bound digestive vacuole, hydrolyzing hemoglobin through secreted enzymes. The trophozoite is the first stage of the parasite in the red blood cell and is defined by the presence of a single chromatin mass. The next stage, the schizont, has multiple chromatin masses, each of which develops into a merozoite. On lysis of the red blood cell, the new merozoites infect additional red blood cells. Although most malaria parasites within the red blood cells develop into merozoites, some parasites develop into sexual forms called gametocytes that infect the mosquito when it takes its blood meal.

144. Ans. (a) Strict aerobe *Ref: http://www.webmd.com/a-to-z-guides/pseudomonas-infection-topic-overview*

A pseudomonas infection is caused by a very common type of bacteria called Pseudomonas aeruginosa. Pseudomonas aeruginosa: It is small, nonsporulating, motile, aerobic Gram-negative rod bacteria. It produces blue green pigment pyocyanin. It is an obligate aerobe, but can also grow aerobically in the presence of nitrates and arginine. It can even grow in antiseptic solutions. Healthy people often carry these bacteria around without knowing it and without having any problems. Sometimes these germs cause minor problems like swimmer's ear and hot tub rash. But for people who are weak or ill, these germs can cause very serious even deadly infections in any part of the body. People in the hospital may get this infection. In hospitals, the bacteria can spread through medical equipment, cleaning solutions, and other equipment. They can even spread through food. When they spread to patients who are weak because of illness, surgery, or treatment, they can cause very serious infections. For example, pseudomonas is one of the main causes of pneumonia in patients who are on breathing machines. Burn victims and people with puncture wounds may get dangerous pseudomonas infections of the blood, bone, or urinary tract. The bacteria can also get into the body through IV needles or catheters. These bacteria like moist environments, such as hot tubs and swimming pools, where they can cause a skin rash or swimmer's ear. People who wear contact lenses can get serious eye infections if the bacteria get into their contact lens solutions. This can happen if you aren't careful about keeping your contact lenses and equipment sterile.

145. Ans. (d) Subacute bacterial endocarditis *Ref: http://en.wikipedia.org/wiki/Monocytosis*

Monocytosis often occurs during chronic inflammation. Diseases that produce this state:

- Infections: Tuberculosis, brucellosis, listeriosis, subacute bacterial endocarditis, syphilis, and other viral infections and many protozoal and rickettsial infections (e.g. kala azar, malaria, Rocky Mountain spotted fever).
- Blood and immune causes: Chronic neutropenia and myeloproliferative disorders.
- Autoimmune diseases and vasculitis: Systemic lupus erythematosus, rheumatoid arthritis and inflammatory bowel disease.
- Malignancies: Hodgkin's disease and certain leukaemias, such as chronic myelomonocytic leukaemia (CMML) and monocytic leukemia.
- Recovery phase of neutropenia or an acute infection.
- Miscellaneous causes: Sarcoidosis and lipid storage disease.

146. Ans. (a) EBV *Ref: Robbins Pathologic Basis of Disease 7th ed. p 369*

EBV causes infectious mononucleosis, a benign, self-limited lymphoproliferative disorder, and is associated with the development of hairy leukoplakia and a number of neoplasms, most notably certain lymphomas and nasopharyngeal carcinoma. Infectious mononucleosis is characterized by fever generalized lymphadenopathy, splenomegaly, sore throat, and the appearance in the blood of atypical activated T lymphocytes (mononucleosis cells). Some patients develop hepatitis, meningoencephalitis, and pneumonitis. Infectious mononucleosis occurs principally in late adolescents or young adults among upper socioeconomic classes in developed nations. In the rest of the world, primary infection with EBV occurs in childhood and is usually asymptomatic.

147. Ans. (a) Ticks *Ref: Robbins Pathologic Basis of Disease 7th ed. p 392*

Lyme disease, named for the Connecticut town where, in the mid-1970s, there was an epidemic of arthritis associated with skin erythema, is caused by several subspecies of the spirochete Borrelia burgdorferi." The disease, transmitted from rodents to people by Erodes deer ticks.

148. Ans. (d) Clostridium perfringens infection *Ref: Robbins Pathologic Basis of Disease 7th ed. p 393*

Ingestion of food contaminated with C. perfringens causes a brief diarrhea. Spores, usually in contaminated meat, survive cooking, and the organism proliferates in cooling food. C. perfringens enterotoxin forms pores in the epithelial cell membranes, lysing the cells and disrupting tight junctions between epithelial cells.'

149. Ans. (d) Practice proper handwashing *Ref: http://www.medscape.com/viewarticle/750224*

All surgical wounds are likely to become contaminated, usually by resident bacterial flora from skin or viscera. This may not be of clinical significance and contaminated wounds may go unnoticed. However, progression from wound contamination to clinical infection is largely determined by the adequacy of host defence, the most important immune mechanism of which is neutrophil phagocytosis which occurs during a crucial few hours intraoperatively and after operation. When a neutrophil ingests bacteria (or any foreign debris), it undergoes a 'respiratory burst', temporarily increasing its oxygen consumption which results in the production of anti-microbial oxygen free radicals. Oxygen free radicals such as superoxide ions and hydrogen peroxide are produced by the enzymes superoxide dismutase and myeloperoxidase. Variables that affect tissue oxygen delivery or enzyme function can impair the production of oxygen free radicals and allow bacteria to survive and infection to become established. Well-known variables that influence surgical site infection include surgical factors (e.g. haematoma, anastomotic leak, poor surgical technique, choice of antiseptic, prolonged or technically difficult procedure) and patient factors (immunosuppression, age, ASA status, comorbidities, colonization by S. aureus).

Factors that can be optimized in the perioperative period can be divided into:

- **Well-established interventions (supported by good evidence)**
  - Antibiotic prophylaxis
  - Proper hand hygiene
  - Aseptic technique during invasive procedures
  - Perioperative thermoregulation
- **Less certain interventions (some supporting evidence)**
  - Face masks and theatre traffic
  - Regional anaesthesia techniques
  - Inspired oxygen
  - Glycaemic control
- **Speculative interventions (no supportive evidence as yet)**
  - Goal-directed fluid management
  - Minimizing blood transfusions
  - Enhanced recovery after surgery (ERAS)
  - Avoidance of selected opioids

150. Ans. (b) Oral rehydration fluids *Ref: http://en.wikipedia.org/wiki/Dehydration#Signs_and_symptoms*

Symptoms of mild dehydration include thirst, decreased urine volume, abnormally dark urine, unexplained tiredness, lack of tears when crying, headache, dry mouth, dizziness when standing due to orthostatic hypotension, and in some cases insomnia. Other possible symptoms include cloudy urine and stinging during urination. In moderate to severe dehydration, there may be no urine output at all. Other symptoms in these states include irritability, lethargy or extreme sleepiness, seizures, sunken fontanel (soft spot) in infants, fainting, and sunken eyes. Irritability is classic sign of the moderate to severe dehydration. The treatment for minor dehydration, often considered the most effective, is drinking water and stopping fluid loss. Plain water restores only the volume of the blood plasma, inhibiting the thirst mechanism before solute levels can be replenished. Solid foods can contribute to fluid loss from vomiting and diarrhea. In more severe cases, correction of a dehydrated state is accomplished by the replenishment of necessary water and electrolytes (through oral rehydration therapy or fluid replacement by intravenous therapy).

151. Ans. (a) Genetic alterations in the host *Ref: Malaria Resurgence: a Systematic Review and Assessment of its causes. Malaria Journal 2012;11:122*

Resurgence of malaria

Malaria is returning to areas from which it had been eradicated, and spreading in to new areas, such as Central Asia, and Eastern Europe. More people are now dying of malaria than thirty years ago.

Factors contributing to resurgence are:

- Drug resistance is a problem, chloroquine is an extremely safe and cheap drug, but in Asia and an increasing area of Africa and South America the resistance levels are high. In some areas of Asia there is resistance to all the major drugs.
- Mosquitos are developing resistance to the major classes of insecticide which have been used to control the disease.

152. Ans. (b) Types of cellulitis *Ref: http://www.vetmed.vt.edu/education/Curriculum/VM8304/vet%20pathology/CASES/INFPATT/P 3-2.htm*

An abscess is a localized collection of pus caused by suppurative inflammation in a tissue, usually in response to pyogenic bacteria. As the island of necrotic tissue and neutrophils grows, a a wall of fibrous tissue is formed around it in an endeavor to confine it. A good blood supply in the tissue ensures a nutrient supply for neutrophils which cross the barrier. This fibrous wall with an active blood supply that surrounds an abscess is called a pyogenic membrane. Phlegmon refers to spreading diffuse suppurative inflammation present in the loose connective tissue. Its margins are poorly defined. Phlegmon is a rapidly progressive suppurative inflammation. Examples of phlegmon are cellulitis and acute appendicitis. Empyema is an accumulation of pus within a body cavity, especially pleura.

153. Ans. (b) Malaria *Ref: Harsh Mohan Textbook of Pathology 6th ed. p 318*

The most important and widely prevalent type of haemoglobinopathy is due to the presence of sickle haemoglobin (HbS) in the red blood cells. The red cells with HbS develop 'sickling' when they are exposed to low oxygen tension. Sickle syndromes have the highest frequency in black race and in Central Africa where falciparum malaria is endemic. Patients with HbS are relatively protected against falciparum malaria.

154. Ans. (a) Leukocytosis *Ref: Harsh Mohan Textbook of Pathology 6th ed. p 348*

Neutrophil leucocytosis. An increase in circulating neutrophils above 7,500/μl is the commonest type of leucocytosis and occurs most commonly as a response to acute bacterial infections. Some common causes of neutrophilia are as under:

- Acute infections, local or generalised, especially by cocci but also by certain bacilli, fungi, spirochaetes, parasites and some viruses. For example: pneumonia, cholecystitis, salpingitis, meningitis, diphtheria, plague, peritonitis, appendicitis, actinomycosis, poliomyelitis, abscesses, furuncles, carbuncles, tonsillitis, otitis media, osteomyelitis, etc.
- Other inflammations, e.g. tissue damage resulting from burns, operations, ischaemic necrosis (such as in MI), gout, collagen-vascular diseases, hypersensitivity reactions, etc.
- Intoxication, e.g. uraemia, diabetic ketosis, eclampsia, poisonings by chemicals and drugs.
- Acute haemorrhage, internal or external.
- Acute haemolysis.
- Disseminated malignancies.
- Myeloproliferative disorders, e.g. myeloid leukaemia, polycythaemia vera, myeloid metaplasia.
- Miscellaneous, e.g. following corticosteroid therapy, idiopathic neutrophilia.

155. Ans. (a) Kaposi's sarcoma

Kaposi's sarcoma is a malignant angiomatous tumour, first described by Kaposi, Hungarian dermatologist, in 1872. However, the tumour has attracted greater attention in thelast two decades due to its frequent occurrence in patients with HIV/AIDS. Kaposi's sarcoma (KS) is a systemic disease that can present with cutaneous lesions with or without internal involvement. Four subtypes have been described: Classic KS, affecting middle aged men of Mediterranean descent; African endemic KS; KS in iatrogenically immunosuppressed patients; and AIDS-related KS. The erythematous to violaceous cutaneous lesions seen in KS have several morphologies: macular, patch, plaque, nodular, and exophytic. The cutaneous lesions can be solitary, localized or disseminated. KS can involve the oral cavity, lymph nodes, and viscera. Classic KS tends to be indolent, presenting with erythematous or violaceous patches on the lower extremities. African endemic KS and AIDS-related KS tend to be more aggressive. The AIDS-related KS lesions often rapidly progress to plaques and nodules affecting the upper trunk, face, and oral mucosa. The diagnosis can be made with a tissue biopsy and, if clinically indicated, internal imaging should be done.

156. Ans. (a) Viral *Ref: http://en.wikipedia.org/wiki/CSF_glucose#Low_CSF_glucose_levels*

CSF glucose levels can be useful in distinguishing among causes of meningitis as more than 50% of patients with bacterial meningitis have decreased CSF glucose levels while patients with viral meningitis usually have normal

CSF glucose levels. Contrary to common belief, decrease in glucose levels during a CNS infection is not caused by increased glucose consumption by leukocytes and bacteria in the CNS, but is thought to be the result of altered glucose transport through the blood-brain barrier.

157. Ans. (a) Q fever *Ref: http://en.wikipedia.org/wiki/Q_fever*

Q fever is a disease caused by infection with Coxiella burnetii, a bacterium that affects humans and other animals. This organism is uncommon, but may be found in cattle, sheep, goats and other domestic mammals, including cats and dogs. The infection results from inhalation of a spore-like small cell variant, and from contact with the milk, urine, feces, vaginal mucus, or semen of infected animals. Rarely, the disease is tick borne.

158. Ans. (a) Measles *Ref: Robbins Pathologic Basis of Disease 7th ed. p 363*

Measles, also known as morbilli, English measles, or rubeola (and not to be confused with rubella or roseola) is an infection of the respiratory system caused by a virus, specifically a paramyxovirus of the genus Morbillivirus. Morbilliviruses, like other paramyxoviruses, are enveloped, single-stranded, negative-sense RNA viruses. Symptoms include fever, cough, runny nose, red eyes and a generalized, maculopapular, erythematous skin rash, the symptom for which measles is best known. Measles is spread through respiration (contact with fluids from an infected person's nose and mouth, either directly or through aerosol transmission), and is highly contagious 90% of people without immunity sharing living space with an infected person will catch it. An asymptomatic incubation period occurs nine to twelve days from initial exposure. The period of infectivity has not been definitively established, some saying it lasts from two to four days prior, until two to five days following the onset of the rash (i.e. four to nine days infectivity in total), whereas others say it lasts from two to four days prior until the complete disappearance of the rash. The rash usually appears between 2 and 3 days after the onset of illness. It doesn't have carrier state.

159. Ans. (a) Tetanus *Ref: Harsh Mohan Textbook of Pathology 6th ed. p 180*

Risus sardonicus or rictus grin is a highly characteristic, abnormal, sustained spasm of the facial muscles that appears to produce grinning. It is most often observed as a sign of tetanus. Tetanus: Tetanus or 'lock jaw' is a severe acute neurologic syndrome caused by tetanus toxin, tetanospasmin, which is a neurotoxic exotoxin elaborated by C. tetani. The spores of the microorganism present in the soil enter the body through a penetrating wound. In underdeveloped countries, tetanus in neonates is seen due to application of soil or dung on the umbilical stump. The degenerated microorganisms liberate the tetanus neurotoxin which causes neuronal stimulation and spasm of muscles. The incubation period of the disease is 1-3 weeks. The earliest manifestation is lockjaw or trismus. Rigidity of muscles of the back causes backward arching or opisthotonos. Death occurs due to spasm of respiratory and laryngeal muscles.

160. Ans. (b) Blood transfusion *Ref: http://hivinsite.ucsf.edu/InSite?p=kb-00&doc=kb-07-02-09*

The risk of HIV transfusion through infected blood products exceeds that of any other risk exposure. Ninety percent of recipients transfused with HIV antibody-positive blood are found to be HIV infected at follow-up.

161. Ans. (a) Increased protein *Ref: http://en.wikipedia.org/wiki/Meningitis#Blood_tests_and_imaging*

CSF findings in different forms of meningitis			
Type of meningitis	*Glucose*	*Protein*	*Cells*
Acute bacterial	Low	High	PMNs Often > $300/mm^3$
Acute viral	Normal	Normal or high	Mononuclear, < $300/mm^3$
Tuberculous	Low	High	Mononuclear and PMNs, < $300/mm^3$
Fungal	Low	High	< $300/mm^3$
Malignant	Low	High	Usually mononuclear

162. Ans. (c) Shigella sp *Ref: Robbins Pathologic Basis of Disease 7th ed. p 1309*

Reactive arthritis is defined as an episode of noninfectious arthritis of the appendicular skeleton that occurs within one month of a primary infection localized elsewhere in the body. Most of the infections are centered in the genitourinary system (Chlamydia) and the gastrointestinal tract (Shigella, Salmonella, Yersinia, Campylobacter). The triad of arthritis, nongonococcal urethritis or cervicitis, and conjunctivitis is called Reiter syndrome, but most patients with reactive arthritis do not have these defining symptoms.

163. Ans. (b) Extraocular muscle involvement *Ref: Neuromuscular diseases by Michael Swash p 286*

Polymyositis should be considered in adults and rarely in children who do not have any of the followings.

- Rash
- I movement of extraocular and facial muscles.
- History of exposure to myotoxic drugs of foxins
- Endocrinopathy
- Neurogenic disease
- Muscular dystrophy

164. Ans. (d) Thrombocytopenia *Ref: Blood Rev 2002 Mar;16(1):73-6.*

HIV-related thrombocytopenia.

Chronic thrombocytopenia is a common hematologic disorder in patients infected with the human immunodeficiency virus (HIV). Although often asymptomatic, the thrombocytopenia may be associated with a variety of bleeding abnormalities. The underlying pathophysiology includes accelerated peripheral platelet destruction and decreased ('ineffective') production of platelets from the infected megakaryocytes. HIV-related thrombocytopenia (HIV-TP) responds to antiretroviral therapy. Most studies have evaluated the use of AZT (zidovudine) and have shown increased platelet production. Combination therapy (HAART) also resulted in sustained platelet increases. When antiretroviral agents fail to improve the platelet count or cannot be used, other therapies, similar to those used in 'classic' immune thrombocytopenia (ITP), can be employed, including steroids, intravenous immunoglobulin (i.v.intravenous anti-D or splenectomy. Anti-D treatment offers advantages for HIV-TP because the duration of effect appears to be significantly longer than the response duration after i.v. therapy (initial results of our open-arm study were confirmed by our randomized trial).

165. Ans. (c) Vacuolated histiocytes *Ref: Robbins Pathologic Basis of Disease 7th ed. p 387*

Lepromatous leprosy involves the skin, peripheral nerves, anterior chamber of the eye, upper airways (down to the larynx), testes, hands, and feet. The vital organs and central nervous system are rarely affected, presumably because the core temperature is too high for growth of M. leprae. Lepromatous lesions contain large aggregates of lipid-laden macrophages (lepra cells), often filled with masses of acid- fast bacilli. Histiocyte is tissue macrophage.

166. Ans. (d) Lepromatousleprosy *Ref: Refer Explanation of Chapter 8 Q 26.*

A hallmark of LL is the accumulation of Virchow's foamy macrophages. However, the origin and nature of these lipids, as well as their function and contribution to leprosy disease, remain unclear.

167. Ans. (c) CD4 and CCR5 molecules *Ref: Robbins Pathologic Basis of Disease 7th ed. p 248*

There is abundant evidence that the CD4 molecule is a high-affinity receptor for HIV. This explains the selective tropism of the virus for CD4+ T cells and other CD4+ cells, particularly monocytes/macrophages and dendritic cells. Binding to CD4 is not sufficient for infection, however. HIV gp120 must also bind to other cell surface molecules (coreceptors) for entry into the cell. Two chemokine receptors, CCR5 and CXCR4 serve this role.

168. Ans. (b) Undergoes calcification *Ref: Robbins Pathologic Basis of Disease 7th ed. p 384; Harsh Mohan Textbook of Pathology 6th ed. p 154*

Primary Tuberculosis. In countries where bovine tuberculosis and infected milk have been eliminated, primary tuberculosis almost always begins in the lungs. Typically, the inhaled bacilli implant in the distal airspaces of the lower part of the upper lobe or the upper part of the lower lobe, usually close to the pleura. As sensitization develops, a 1 to 1.5 cm area of gray-white inflammatory consolidation emerges, known as the Ghon focus. In most cases, the center of this focus undergoes caseous necrosis. Tubercle bacilli, either free or within phagocytes, drain to the regional nodes, which also often caseate. This combination of parenchymal lung lesion and nodal involvement is referred to as the Ghon complex.

- **Fate of primary tuberculosis.**

Primary complex may have one of the following sequelae:

- The lesions of primary tuberculosis of lung commonly do not progress but instead heal by fibrosis, and in time undergo calcification and even ossification.

169. Ans. (b) Gametocyte *Ref: Refer explanation of Chapter 8 Q 143*

Refer explanation of Chapter 8 Q 143.

ENVIRONMENTAL AND NUTRITIONAL PATHOLOGY

170. Ans. (a) Death

What adverse effect does death have? Its an quite obvious answer does not need any reference or exclamation.

171. Ans. (b) Diethyl glycol poisoning *Ref: Clinical Biochemistry by Allan Gaw p 121*

Ethylene glycol poisoning occurs due to the ingestion of ethylene glycol, paracetamol or theophylline. The diagnosis may be suspected when calcium oxalate crystal are seen in the crine or when acidosis or an increased osmol gap is present in the blood. Patient may unclucle renal failure and brain damage.

172. Ans. (c) Fibre *Ref: Pediatric Surgery by Prem Puri p 78*

The parenteral formulation includes carbohydrates, fat, protein, electrolytes, vitamins, trace element and water.

173. Ans. (c) ↑TIBC, ↓Ferritin *Ref: Robbins Pathologic Basis of Disease 7th ed. p 643*

Iron-deficiency anemia (or iron-deficiency anaemia) is a common anemia (low red blood cell or hemoglobin levels) caused by insufficient dietary intake and absorption of iron, and/or iron loss from bleeding which can originate from a range of sources such as the intestinal, uterine or urinary tract. Iron deficiency causes approximately half of all anemia cases worldwide, and affects women more often than men. World estimates of iron deficiency occurrence are somewhat vague, but the true number probably exceeds one billion people. This can result if:

- The body does not make enough red blood cells
- Bleeding causes loss of red blood cells more quickly than they can be replaced. The most significant cause of iron-deficiency anemia in developing world children is parasitic worms: Hookworms, whipworms, and roundworms. Worms cause intestinal bleeding, which is not always noticeable in faeces, and is especially damaging to growing children Malaria, hookworms and vitamin A deficiency contribute to anemia during pregnancy in most underdeveloped countries. In women over 50 years old, the most common cause of iron-deficiency anemia is chronic gastrointestinal bleeding from nonparasitic causes, such as gastric ulcers, duodenal ulcers or gastrointestinal cancer. Anemia is one result of advanced-stage iron deficiency. When the body has sufficient iron to meet its needs (functional iron), the remainder is stored for later use in all cells, but mostly in the bone marrow, liver, and spleen. These stores are called ferritin complexes and are part of the human (and

other animals) iron metabolism systems. Ferritin complexes in humans carry about 4500 iron atoms and form into 24 protein subunits of two different types:

Change in lab values in iron deficiency anemia	
Change	*Parameter*
Decrease	Ferritin, hemoglobin, MCV
Increase	TIBC, transferrin, RDW

174. Ans. (c) Hypokalaemia *Ref: JIACM 2008; 9(2):133-5*

Acute severe poisoning by barium sulphate (rat poison)

Barium carbonate is a highly toxic substance used as a rodenticide. Barium is a muscle poison. Most of the toxic effects of barium result from its direct stimulation of all types of muscles, including cardiac muscle, and from its ability to cause a profound reduction in serum potassium together with an increase in intracellular potassium.

175. Ans. (a) Constitutional delay in growth *Ref: http://en.wikipedia.org/wiki/Constitutional_growth_delay*

Constitutional growth delay (CGD) is a term describing a temporary delay in the skeletal growth and thus height of a child with no other physical abnormalities causing the delay. Short stature may be the result of a growth pattern inherited from a parent (familial) or occur for no apparent reason (idiopathic). Typically at some point during childhood, growth slows down, eventually resuming at a normal rate. CGD is the most common cause of short stature and delayed puberty.

176. Ans. (d) Myopathy *Ref: Harsh Mohan Textbook of Pathology 6th ed. p 306*

Deficiency of vitamin B12 and folate may cause following clinical manifestations which may be present singly or in combination and in varying severity:

- Anaemia. Macrocytic megaloblastic anaemia is the cardinal feature of deficiency of vitamin B12 and/or folate. The onset of anaemia is usually insidious and gradually progressive.
- Glossitis. Typically, the patient has a smooth, beefy, red tongue.
- Neurologic manifestations. Vitamin B12 deficiency, particularly in patients of pernicious anaemia, is associated with significant neurological manifestations in the form of subacute combined, degeneration of the spinal cord and peripheral neuropathy, while folate deficiency may occasionally develop neuropathy only. The underlying pathologic process consists of demyelination of the peripheral nerves, the spinal cord and the cerebrum. Signs and symptoms include numbness, paraesthesia, weakness, ataxia, poor finger coordination and diminished reflexes.
- Others: In addition to the cardinal features mentioned above, patients may have various other symptoms. These include: mild jaundice, angular stomatitis, purpura, melanin pigmentation, symptoms of malabsorption, weight loss and anorexia. Vitamin B12 deficiency cause all except myopathy (All other options are correct).

177. Ans. (d) Autonomic dysfunction *Ref: Robbins Pathologic Basis of Disease 7th ed. p 455-456*

Signs of vitamin E deficiency include neuromuscular problems such as spinocerebellar ataxia and myopathies. Other neurological signs may include dysarthria, absence of deep tendon reflexes, loss of vibratory sensation and proprioception, and positive Babinski sign. Deficiency can also cause anemia due to oxidative damage to red blood cells, retinopathy and impairment of the immune response. There is also some laboratory evidence that vitamin E deficiency can cause male infertility.

178. Ans. (c) 65 to 85%

Ref: http://www.euro.who.int/_data/assets/pdf_file/0004/123079/AQG2ndEd_6_9Mercury.PDF

- WHO Regional Office for Europe, Copenhagen, Denmark, 2000
- Mercury. Geneva, World Health Organization, 1976 (Environmental Health Criteria, No.1).

Approximately, 80% of inhaled mercury vapour is absorbed via the lungs and retained in the body. The amount retained is the same whether inhalation takes place through the nose or the mouth. Elemental mercury is poorly absorbed in the gastrointestinal tract (less than 0.01% in rats), although increased blood levels of mercury have been measured in humans following accidental ingestion of several grams of metallic mercury. Skin absorption is insignificant in relation to human exposure to mercury vapour.

179. Ans. (d) Seborrheic keratosis *Ref: Robbins Pathologic Basis of Disease 7th ed. p 1237*

Seborrheic keratoses (benign epithelial tumor): These common epidermal tumors occur most frequently in middle-aged or older individuals. They arise spontaneously and may become particularly numerous on the trunk, although the extremities, head, and neck may also be involved. In people of color, multiple small lesions on the face are termed dermatosis papulosa nigra. Seborrheic keratoses have characteristic clinical features. They appear as round, flat, coinlike, waxy plaques that vary in diameter from millimeters to several centimeters. They are uniformly tan to dark brown and usually show a velvety to granular surface. Lesions may give the impression that they are 'stuck on' and may be easily peeled off. Inspection with a hand lens will usually reveal small, round, porelike ostia impacted with keratin, a feature helpful in differentiating these pigmented lesions from melanomas.

180. Ans. (c) Vitamin A *Ref: Robbins Pathologic Basis of Disease 7th ed. p 451*

Vitamin A plays an important role in the orderly differentiation of mucus-secreting epithelium; when a deficiency state exists, the epithelium undergoes squamous metaplasia and differentiation to a keratinizing epithelium. The mechanism is not precisely understood; but in cell culture systems, retinoic acid (retinol is much less potent) regulates the expression of genes encoding a number of cell receptors and secreted proteins, including receptors for growth factors.

181. Ans. (b) Decrease osteoid matrix formation *Ref: Robbins Pathologic Basis of Disease 7th ed. p 459*

Scurvy in a growing child is far more dramatic than in an adult. Hemorrhages constitute one of the most striking features. Because the defect in collagen synthesis results in inadequate support of the walls of capillaries and venules, purpura and ecchymoses often appear in the skin and in the gingival mucosa. Furthermore, the loose attachment of the periosteum to bone, together with the vascular wall defects, leads to extensive subperiosteal hematomas and bleeding into joint spaces after minimal trauma. Retrobulbar, subarachnoid, and intracerebral hemorrhages may prove fatal. Skeletal changes may also develop in infants and children. The primary disturbance is in the formation of osteoid matrix, rather than in mineralization or calcification, such as occurs in rickets. In scurvy, the palisade of cartilage cells is formed as usual and is provisionally calcified. However, there is insufficient production of osteoid matrix by osteoblasts. Resorption of the cartilaginous matrix then fails or slows; as a consequence, there is cartilaginous overgrowth, with long spicules and plates projecting into the metaphyseal region of the marrow cavity, and sometimes widening of the epiphysis.

DISEASES OF INFANCY AND CHILDHOOD

182. Ans. (b) Neuroblastoma *Ref: Robbins Pathologic Basis of Disease 7th ed. p 502*

In young children, under age 2 years, neuroblastomas generally present with large abdominal masses, fever, and possibly weight loss. In older children, they may not come to attention until metastases produce manifestations, such as bone pain, respiratory symptoms, or gastrointestinal complaints. Neuroblastomas may metastasize widely through the hematogenous and lymphatic systems, particularly to liver, lungs, and bones, in addition to the bone marrow. Proptosis and ecchymosis may also be present because the periorbital region is a common metastatic site.

183. Ans. (c) Cystic fibrosis *Ref: Robbins Pathologic Basis of Disease 7th ed. p 490*

The cystic fibrosis gene: In normal duct epithelia, chloride is transported by plasma membrane channels (chloride channels). The primary defect in cystic fibrosis results from abnormal function of an epithelial chloride channel protein encoded by the cystic fibrosis transmembrane conductance regulator (CFTR) gene on chromosome band 7g31.2.

BLOOD VESSELS

184. Ans. (b) SLE *Ref: Robbins Pathologic Basis of Disease 7th ed. p 227*

- Revised criteria for diagnosis of systemic lupus erythematosus (1997)

Criteria	*Definition*
1. Malar rash	Fixed erythema, flat or raised, over the malar eminences
2. Discoid rash	Erythematous raised patches with adherent keratotic scaling and follicular plugging; atrophic scarring may occur
3. Photosensitivity	Skin rash as a result of exposure to UV light
4. Oral ulcers	Oral or nasopharyngeal ulceration, usually painless, observed by a physician
5. Arthritis	Nonerosive arthritis involving two or more peripheral joints, characterized by tenderness, swelling, or effusion
6. Serositis	Pleuritis—convincing history of pleuritic pain or rub heard by a physician or evidence of pleural effusion, or pericarditis—documented by electrocardiogram or rub or evidence of pericardial effusion
7. Renal disorder	Persistent proteinuria > 0.5 g/dl or >3+ if quantitation not performed, or cellular casts—may be red blood cell, hemoglobin, granular, tubular, or mixed
8. Neurologic disorder	• Seizures—in the absence of offending drugs or known metabolic derangements, e.g., uremia, ketoacidosis, or electrolyte imbalance, or
	• Psychosis—in the absence of offending drugs or known metabolic derangements, e.g. uremia, ketoacidosis, or electrolyte imbalance
9. Hematologic disorder	• Hemolytic anemia—with reticulocytosis, or
	• Leukopenia—< 4.0×10^9/L (4000/μl) total on two or more occasions, or
	• Lymphopenia—< 1.5×10^9/L (1500/μl) on two or more occasions, or
	• Thrombocytopenia—< 100×10^9/L (100×10^3/μl) in the absence of offending drugs
10. Immunologic disorder	Anti-ds DNA, anti-Sm, and/or antiphospholipid
11. Antinuclear antibody	An abnormal titer of antinuclear antibody by immunofluorescence or an equivalent assay at any point in time and in the absence of drugs known to be associated with drug-induced lupus syndrome

- Clinical and pathological manifestation of systemic lupus erythematosus

Clinical manifestation	*Prevalence in patients (%)*	*Central nervous system*	50
Hematologic	100	Pleuritis	46
Arthritis	90	Myalgia	33
Skin	85	Pericarditis	25
Fever	83	Gastrointestinal	21
Fatigue	81	Raynaud phenomenon	20
Weight loss	63	Ocular	15
Renal	50	Peripheral neuropathy	14

185. Ans. (b) Trophic ulcer *Ref: http://en.wikipedia.org/wiki/Malum_perforans*

Neurotrophic ulcer or trophic ulcer is a cutaneous condition of chronic, trophic, ulcerative disease seen on the dependent parts of body in denervating diseases. Causes. This condition results from denervation of areas exposed to day-to-day friction of bony prominences. The denervation may be result of any of the following diseases:

- Spinal injuries
- Leprosy
- Peripheral nerve injury
- Diabetic neuropathy
- Tabes dorsalis
- Transverse myelitis
- Meningomyelocele

186. Ans. (b) Vascular *Ref: Robbins Pathologic Basis of Disease 7th ed. p 548*

Despite its name, in general it is not considered a true sarcoma, which is a tumor arising from mesenchymal tissue. KS, in fact, arises as a cancer of lymphatic endothelium and forms vascular channels that fill with blood cells, giving the tumor its characteristic bruise-like appearance. KSHV proteins are uniformly detected in KS cancer cells. KS lesions contain tumor cells with a characteristic abnormal elongated shape, called spindle cells. The tumor is highly vascular, containing abnormally dense and irregular blood vessels, which leak red blood cells into the surrounding tissue and give the tumor its dark color. Inflammation around the tumor may produce swelling and pain. Although KS may be suspected from the appearance of lesions and the patient's risk factors, definite diagnosis can be made only by biopsy and microscopic examination, which will show the presence of spindle cells. Detection of the KSHV protein LANA in tumor cells confirms the diagnosis.

187. Ans. (b) Anaesthesia dolorosa *Ref: Wikipedia*

Giant-cell arteritis (GCA or temporal arteritis or cranial arteritis) or Horton disease is an inflammatory disease of blood vessels most commonly involving large and medium arteries of the head, predominantly the branches of the external carotid artery. It is a form of vasculitis. The most serious complication of GCA is permanent blindness, though this can be prevented by prompt treatment with corticosteroids. Cluster headache has been historically classified as vascular headaches; for decades, it has been proposed that intense pain was caused by dilation of blood vessels which was thought to create pressure on the trigeminal nerve. While this theory was thought to be the immediate cause of the pain, the etiology (underlying cause or causes) is not fully understood and CH pathogenesis is the subject of ongoing debate. Investigations into the vascular theory of headache disorders are helping to identify the role of other possible causative mechanisms in CH. Anesthesia dolorosa or anaesthesia dolorosa is pain felt in an area (usually of the face) which is completely numb to touch. The pain is described as constant, burning, aching or severe. It can be a side effect of surgery involving any part of the trigeminal system, and occurs after 14% of peripheral surgery for trigeminal neuralgia. Hemicrania continua (HC) is a persistent unilateral headache that responds to indomethacin. It is usually unremitting, but rare cases of remission have been documented. Hemicrania continua is considered a primary headache disorder, meaning that it is not caused by another condition.(Cause of this entity is unknown and only known thing is that it responds to indomethacin).

- Definite non-association of vascular origin is seen in an anaesthesia dolorosa. Hence, correct answer is B.

188. Ans. (a) Proteinases 3 *Ref: Robbins Pathologic Basis of Disease 7th ed. p 535*

Antineutrophil Cytoplasmic Antibodies: Serum from many patients with vasculitis reacts with cytoplasmic antigens in neutrophils, indicating the presence of antineutrophil cytoplasmic antibodies (ANCAs). ANCAs are a heterogeneous group of autoantibodies directed against enzymes mainly found within the azurophil or primary granules in neutrophils, in the lysosomes of monocytes, and in ECs. The description of these autoantibodies is based on the immunofluorescent patterns of staining of ethanol-fixed neutrophils. Two main patterns are recognized: one shows cytoplasmic localization of the staining (c- ANCA), and the most common target antigen is proteinase-3 (PR3), a neutrophil granule constituent. The second shows perinuclear staining (p-ANCA) and is usually specific for myeloperoxidase (MPO).

189. Ans. (c) Decreased fibrinogen levels *Ref: http://en.wikipedia.org/wiki/Atherosclerosis#Risk_factors*

Risk factors for atherosclerosis

Modifiable

- Diabetes or impaired glucose tolerance (IGT)
- Dyslipoproteinemia (unhealthy patterns of serum proteins carrying fats & cholesterol):
  - High serum concentration of low-density lipoprotein (LDL, 'bad if elevated concentrations and small'), and/or very low density lipoprotein (VLDL) particles, i.e., 'lipoprotein subclass analysis'
  - Low serum concentration of functioning high density lipoprotein (HDL 'protective if large and high enough' particles), i.e. 'lipoprotein subclass analysis'
  - An LDL:HDL ratio greater than 3:1
- Tobacco smoking, increases risk by 200% after several pack years
- Elevated serum C-reactive protein concentrations
- Vitamin B6 deficiency
- Dietary iodine deficiency and hypothyroidism, which cause elevated serum cholesterol and of lipid peroxidation

Nonmodifiable

- Advanced age
- Male sex
- Having close relatives who have had some complication of atherosclerosis (e.g. coronary heart disease or stroke)
- Genetic abnormalities, e.g. familial hypercholesterolemia

Lesser or uncertain

The following factors are of relatively lesser importance, are uncertain or unquantified:

- Obesity (in particular central obesity, also referred to as abdominal or male-type obesity)
- Hypercoagulability
- Postmenopausal estrogen deficiency
- High intake of saturated fat (may raise total and LDL cholesterol)
- Intake of trans fat (may raise total and LDL cholesterol while lowering HDL cholesterol)
- High carbohydrate intake
- Elevated serum levels of triglycerides
- Elevated serum levels of homocysteine
- Elevated serum levels of uric acid (also responsible for gout)
- Elevated serum fibrinogen concentrations
- Elevated serum lipoprotein(a) concentrations
- Chronic systemic inflammation as reflected by upper normal WBC concentrations, elevated hs-CRP and many other blood chemistry markers, most only research level at present, not clinically done.
- Hyperthyroidism (an over-active thyroid)
- Elevated serum insulin levels
- Short sleep duration
- Chlamydia pneumoniae infection

190. Ans. (b) Lymphangioma *Ref: Robbins Pathologic Basis of Disease 7th ed. p 547*

Analogous to the cavernous hemangioma, cavernous lymphangioma (cystic hygroma) occurs in children in the neck or axilla, and only rarely, retroperitoneally. They occasionally achieve considerable size, up to 15 cm in diameter, and may fill the axilla or produce gross deformities in and about the neck. The tumors are made up of massively dilated, cystic lymphatic spaces lined by endothelial cells and separated by a scant intervening connective tissue stroma that often contains lymphoid aggregates. Because the margins of the tumor are not discrete and these lesions are not encapsulated, removal can be difficult. Cystic hygromas of the neck occur in Turner syndrome.

THE HEART

191. Ans. (a) LDL/HDL ratio *Ref: Robbins Pathologic Basis of Disease 7th ed. p 1204*

Dyslipidemias include both increased triglycerides and LDL levels and decreased levels of the 'protective' lipoprotein, HDL.

192. Ans. (b) Melanophage *Ref: Robbins Pathologic Basis of Disease 7th ed. p 562*

Heart failure cells are siderophages (hemosiderin-containing macrophages) generated in the alveoli of patients with left heart failure or chronic pulmonary edema, when the high pulmonary blood pressure causes red cells to pass through the vascular wall. Siderophages are not specific of heart failure. They are present wherever red blood cells encounter macrophages. In left heart failure, the left ventricle can not keep pace with the incoming blood from the pulmonary veins. The resulting backup causes increased pressure on the alveolar capillaries, and red blood cells leak out. Alveolar macrophages (dust cells) ingest the red blood cells, and become engorged with brownish hemosiderin. In chronic pulmonary edema, alveolar septa become thick and fibrous, again increasing pressure on alveolar capillaries and resulting in leakage of red blood cells which undergo phagocytosis by alveolar macrophages.

RED BLOOD CELL AND BLEEDING DISORDERS

193. Ans. (d) Von Willebrand disease *Ref: http://en.wikipedia.org/wiki/Von_Willebrand_disease#Diagnosis*

Laboratory findings in various platelet and coagulation disorders

Condition	*Prothrombin time*	*Partial thromboplastin time*	*Bleeding time*	*Platelet count*
Vitamin K deficiency or warfarin	Prolonged	Normal or mildly prolonged	Unaffected	Unaffected
Disseminated intravascular coagulation	Prolonged	Prolonged	Prolonged	Decreased
Von Willebrand disease	Unaffected	Prolonged or unaffected	Prolonged	Unaffected
Hemophilia	Unaffected	Prolonged	Unaffected	Unaffected
Aspirin	Unaffected	Unaffected	Prolonged	Unaffected
Thrombocytopenia	Unaffected	Unaffected	Prolonged	Decreased
Liver failure early	Prolonged	Unaffected	Unaffected	Unaffected
Liver failure, end-stage	Prolonged	Prolonged	Prolonged	Decreased
Uremia	Unaffected	Unaffected	Prolonged	Unaffected
Congenital afibrinogenemia	Prolonged	Prolonged	Prolonged	Unaffected
Factor V deficiency	Prolonged	Prolonged	Unaffected	Unaffected
Factor X deficiency as seen in amyloid purpura	Prolonged	Prolonged	Unaffected	Unaffected
Glanzmann's thrombasthenia	Unaffected	Unaffected	Prolonged	Unaffected
Bernard-Soulier syndrome	Unaffected	Unaffected	Prolonged	Decreased or unaffected
Factor XII deficiency	Unaffected	Prolonged	Unaffected	Unaffected
C1INH deficiency	Unaffected	Shortened	Unaffected	Unaffected

194. Ans. (c) Increased PTT *Ref: Refer explanation of Chapter 13 Q 193*

Refer explanation of Chapter 13 Q 193

195. Ans. (a) Beta thalassaemia major *Ref: Harsh Mohan Textbook of Pathology 6th ed. p 323*

- β-thalassaemia major, also termed Mediterranean or Cooley's anaemia is the most common form of congenital haemolytic anaemia. β-thalassaemia major is a homozygous state with either complete absence of β-chain synthesis (β° thalassaemia major) or only small amounts of β-chains are formed (β+ thalassaemia major). These result in excessive formation of alternate haemoglobins, HbF ($\alpha 2\gamma 2$) and HbA2 ($\alpha 2\delta 2$).

CLINICAL FEATURES: Clinical manifestations appear insidiously and are as under:

- Anaemia starts appearing within the first 4-6 months of life when the switch over from γ-chain to β-chain production occurs.
- Marked hepatosplenomegaly occurs due to excessive red cell destruction, extramedullary haematopoiesis and iron overload.
- Expansion of bones occurs due to marked erythroid hyperplasia leading to thalassaemic facies and malocclusion of the jaw.
- Iron overload due to repeated blood transfusions causes damage to the endocrine organs resulting in slow rate of growth and development, delayed puberty, diabetes mellitus and damage to the liver and heart.

196. Ans. (b) Factor VIII *Ref: Harsh Mohan Textbook of Pathology 6th ed. p 335*

Most of the inherited plasma coagulation disorders are due to qualitative or quantitative defect in a single coagulation factor. Out of defects in various coagulation factors, two of the most common inherited coagulation disorders are the sex-(X)- linked disorders classic haemophilia or haemophilia A (due to inherited deficiency of factor VIII), and Christmas disease or haemophilia B (due to inherited deficiency of factor IX).

197. Ans. (c) Warfarin therapy

Refer explanation of Chapter 13 Q 193

198. Ans. (a) Thalassaemia *Ref: Haironend Appearance Arch DIS Child. Sep 2006;91(9):735*

More than 80 years ago, Cooley and Lee described skeletal changes associated with haemolytic anaemias. Haironend appearance of the skull is a characteristic feature of chronic haemolysis usually seen in patients with thalassaemia and sickle cell anaemia. It results from accentuated vertical trabeculae between the inner and outer tables of the skull because of excessive bone marrow hyperplasia. An incidence of 8.3% of haironend appearance in thalassaemic patients has been reported. Though, rare, these appearances have been described in iron deficiency anaemia and cyanotic congenital heart disease.

199. Ans. (c) Hb Bar's cannot release oxygen to fetal tissues *Ref: http://en.wikipedia.org/wiki/Hemoglobin_Barts*

Hemoglobin Barts consists of four gamma chains. It is moderately insoluble, and therefore accumulates in the red blood cells. It has an extremely high affinity for oxygen, resulting in almost no oxygen delivery to the tissues. It is produced in the disease alpha-thalassemia and, in the most severe of cases, it is the only form of haemoglobin in circulation. In this situation, a fetus will develop hydrops fetalis and normally die before or shortly after birth, unless intrauterine blood transfusion is performed.

200. Ans. (a) Increase in number of globin chain *Ref: Robbins Pathologic Basis of Disease 7th ed. p 632*

The thalassemia syndromes are a heterogeneous group of inherited disorders caused by genetic lesions leading to decreased synthesis of either the a- or R-globin chain of HhA (a2 B2). B-Thalassemia is caused by deficient synthesis of the B chain, whereas a-thalassemia is caused by deficient synthesis of the a chain. All other options are correct.

201. Ans. (a) Ascorbic acid *Ref: Blood. 1983 Sep;62(3):532-7.Ascorbic acid, vitamin A, folic acid, and amino acids in blood of patients with hemophilia.*

It has been observed that plasma ascorbic acid level in hemophiliac patients is lower than normal individual hence ascorbic acid administration is definitely helpful in management of these patients.

202. Ans. (b) O group and Rh *Ref: http://en.wikipedia.org/wiki/File:ABO_blood_type.svg*

	Group A	Group B	Group AB	Group O
Red blood cell type	A	B	AB	O
Antibodies in plasma	Anti-B	Anti-A	None	Anti-A and Anti-B
Antigens in red blood cell	A antigen	B antigen	A and B antigen	None

In the blood sample, antiserum A and antiserum B are added still agglutination is not seen that means there are no antigen present in the blood sample this occurs in O negative blood with Rh negativity. If Rh+ factor is added to Rh- person → No agglutination reaction will be seen. But if Rh+ factor is added to Rh+ person → Agglutination is seen (because of presence of RH+ antibody).

203. Ans. (c) Myeloproliferative disorder *Ref: Robbins Pathologic Basis of Disease 7th ed. p 649; http://en.wikipedia.org/wiki/Polycythemia#Secondary_polycythemia*

Polycythemia, or erythrocytosis, denotes an abnormally high concentration of red cells, usually with a corresponding increase in hemoglobin level. The increase in red cells can be relative, when there is hemoconcentration due to decreased plasma volume, or absolute, when there is an increase in total red cell mass. Relative polycythemia results from any cause of dehydration, such as deprivation of water, prolonged vomiting, diarrhea, or excessive use of diuretics. It is also associated with an obscure condition of unknown etiology called stress polycythemia, or Gaisbock syndrome. Affected individuals are usually hypertensive, obese, and anxious ('stressed'). Absolute polycythemia is primary when it results from an intrinsic abnormality of the myeloid stem cells and secondary when the red cell progenitors are responding to increased levels of erythropoietin.

Conditions which may result in a physiologically appropriate secondary polycythemia include:

- Altitude related: This physiologic polycythemia is a normal adaptation to living at high altitudes
- Hypoxic disease-associated - for example in cyanotic heart disease where blood oxygen levels are reduced significantly. May also occur as a result of hypoxic lung disease such as COPD and as a result of chronic obstructive sleep apnea.
- Iatrogenic - Secondary polycythemia can be induced directly by phlebotomy (blood letting) to withdraw some blood, concentrate the erythrocytes, and return them to the body.
- Genetic conditions where the secondary polycythemia is not as a result of physiologic adaptation and occurs irrespective of body needs include:
- Neoplasms - Hemangioblastoma, Renal-cell carcinoma or liver tumors, von Hippel-Lindau disease, and endocrine abnormalities including pheochromocytoma and adrenal adenoma with Cushing's syndrome.
- People whose testosterone levels are high because of the use of anabolic steroids, including athletes who abuse steroids, or people on testosterone replacement for hypogonadism, as well as people who take erythropoietin may develop secondary polycythemia.

204. Ans. (b) DIC *Ref: Robbins Pathologic Basis of Disease 7th ed. p 657*

The consequences of disseminated intravascular coagulation (DIC) are two-fold. First, there is widespread deposition of fibrin within the microcirculation. This can lead to ischemia of the more severely affected or more vulnerable organs and to a hemolytic anemia resulting from fragmentation of red cells as they squeeze through the narrowed microvasculature (microangiopathic hemolytic anemia). Second, a hemorrhagic diathesis can dominate the clinical picture. This results from consumption of platelets and clotting factors as well as activation of plasminogen. Plasmin can not only cleave fibrin, but also digest factors V and VIII, thereby reducing their concentration further. In addition, fibrinolysis leads to the formation of fibrin degradation products, which inhibit platelet aggregation and fibrin polymerization and have antithrombin activity. All these influences lead to the hemostatic failure seen in DIC.

205. Ans. (b) Increase in surface:volume ratio *Ref: Robbins Pathologic Basis of Disease 7th ed. p 625*

Hereditary spherocytosis

This inherited disorder is caused by intrinsic defects in the red cell membrane that render red cells spheroid, less deformable, and vulnerable to splenic sequestration and destruction.

- **Model of the pathophysiology of hereditary spherocytosis.**

All other options are correct.

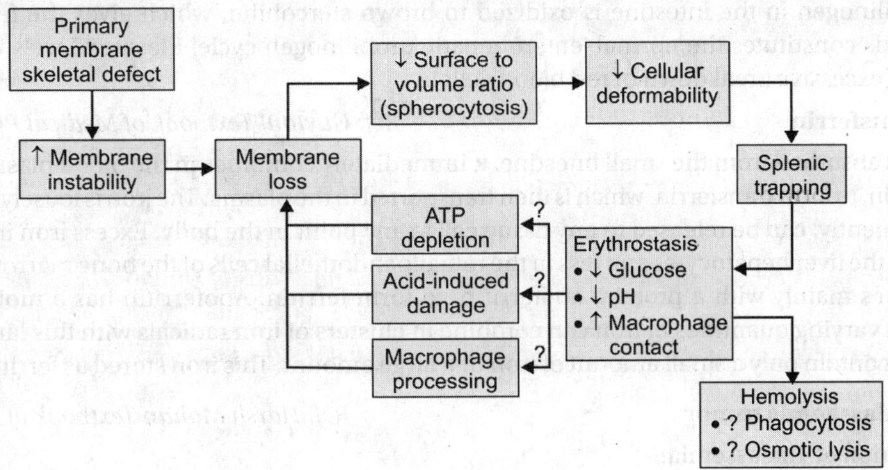

206. Ans. (b) Acute blood loss *Ref: Harrisons Principles of Internal Medicine, 18th ed. p 455, 872*

Acute blood loss is not associated with increased reticulocyte production index

207. Ans. (a) Acute blood loss

Refer answer 206.

208. Ans. (b) Hemophilia A

Ref: Text book of Oral Medicine, Oral Diagnosis and Oral Radiology by Ongole and BN Praveen

Hemophilia A is due to defective factor VIII (antihemophilic factor, AHF). This is a glycoprotein of several components, including factor VIIIc (procoagulant which participates in clotting cascade, VIIIk: Ag (Von Willebrand factor which bind to platelet and is the carrier for factor VIIIc) and VIII R: R Co (Ristocetin cofactor, which supports platelet aggregation.

209. Ans. (b) Protamine sulphate *Ref: http://en.wikipedia.org/wiki/Heparin#Antidote_to_heparin_overdose*

Protamine sulfate (1 mg per 100 units of heparin that had been given over the past four hours) has been given to counteract the anticoagulant effect of heparin. Protamine sulfate is usually administered to reverse the large dose of heparin administered during certain surgeries, especially heart surgery. It is also used in gene transfer, protein purification and in tissue cultures as a crosslinker for viral transduction. In gene therapy, protamine sulfate has been studied as a means to increase transduction rates by both viral and nonviral (e.g. utilizing cationic lipids mediated delivery mechanisms.

210. Ans. (c) Factor VIII

Refer explanation of Chapter 13 Q 208

211. Ans. (a) Increase *Ref: Robbins Pathologic Basis of Disease 7th ed. p 624, 886*

Hemolytic anemias share the following features:

- A shortened red cell life span (normal = 120 days); that is, premature destruction of red cells
- Elevated erythropoietin levels and increased erythropoiesis in the marrow and other sites, to compensate for the loss of red cells
- Accumulation of the products of hemoglobin catabolism, due to an increased rate of red cell destruction Urobilinogen is a colourless by-product of bilirubin reduction. It is formed in the intestines by bacterial action on bilirubin. About half urobilinogen is reabsorbed, taken up, via the bile duct, into circulation through the liver and excreted by the kidney. Increased amounts of bilirubin are formed in hemolysis, which generates increased urobilinogen in the gut. In liver disease (such as hepatitis), the intrahepatic urobilinogen cycle is inhibited also increasing urobilinogen levels. Urobilinogen is converted to the yellow pigmented urobilin apparent in urine. The urobilinogen in the intestine is oxidized to brown stercobilin, which gives the feces their characteristic colour. This constitutes the normal 'enterohepatic urobilinogen cycle'. Elevated levels may indicate hemolytic anaemia (excessive breakdown of red blood cells).

212. Ans. (a) Transferrin *Ref: Guyton, Textbook of Medical Physiology 11th ed. p 425*

When iron is absorbed from the small intestine, it immediately combines in the blood plasma with a beta globulin, apotransferrin, to form transferrin, which is then transported in the plasma. The iron is loosely bound in the transferrin and, consequently, can be released to any tissue cell at any point in the body. Excess iron in the blood is deposited especially in the liver hepatocytes and less in the reticuloendothelial cells of the bone marrow. In the cell cytoplasm, iron combines mainly with a protein, apoferritin, to form ferritin. Apoferritin has a molecular weight of about 460,000, and varying quantities of iron can combine in clusters of iron radicals with this large molecule; therefore, ferritin may contain only a small amount of iron or a large amount. This iron stored as ferritin is called storage iron.

213. Ans. (b) Thalassaemia minor *Ref: Harsh Mohan Textbook of Pathology 6th ed. p 321*

- Classification of Thalassemia:

Type	*Hb*	*Hb-electrophoresis*	*Genotype*	*Clinical syndrome*
α-thalassaemias				
1. Hydrops foetalis	3-10 gm/dl	Hb Barts (g_2) (100%)	Deletion of four α-genes	Fatal in utero or in early infancy
2. Hb-H disease	2-12 gm/dl	HbF (10%), HbH (2-4%)	Deletion of three α-genes	Haemolytic anaemia
3. α-thalassaemia trait	10-14 gm/dl	Almost normal	Deletion of two α-genes	Microcytic hypochromic blood picture but no anaemia
β-thalassaemias				
1. β-thalassaemia major	< 5 gm/dl	HbA (0-50%) HbF (50-98%)	$\beta^{thal}/\beta^{thal}$	Severe congenital haemolytic anaemia, requires blood transfusions
2. β-thalassaemia intermedia	5-10 gm/dl	Variable	Multiple mechanisms	Severe anaemia, but regular blood transfusions not required
3. β-thalassaemia minor	10-12 gm/dl	HbA_2 (4-9%) HbF (1-5%)	β^{A}/β^{thal}	Usually asymptomatic

214. Ans. (b) Mutation in DNA repair gene *Ref: Robbins Pathologic Basis of Disease 7th ed. p 647*

Fanconi anemia is a rare autosomal recessive disorder caused by defects in a component of a multiprotein complex required for DNA repair. Marrow hypofunction in Fanconi anemia becomes evident early in life and is accompanied by multiple congenital anomalies, such as hypoplasia of the kidney and spleen and hypoplastic anomalies of bone, often involving the thumbs or radii.

215. Ans. (a) Liver *Ref: Hematology by Ronald Hoffman p 1880*

Most of the proteins required for the coagulation cascade are produced by the liver as inactive precursors (zymogens) which are then modified into clotting factors. There are two routes for activation of the coagulation system. The intrinsic pathway is activated by contact with collagen from damaged blood vessels (or indeed any negatively charged surface). The extrinsic pathway is activated by contact with tissue factor from the surface of extravascular cells. Both routes end in a final common pathway—the proteolytic activation of thrombin and the cleaving of fibrinogen to form a fibrin clot. The intrinsic pathway is the main 'player' in this scenario, with the extrinsic pathway acting as an enhancer. Some bleeding disorders are present at birth and are passed through families (inherited). Others develop from:

- Illnesses such as vitamin K deficiency or severe liver disease
- Treatments such as the use of drugs to stop blood clots (anticoagulants) or the long-term use of antibiotics. Bleeding disorders can also result from having poorly working or too few of the blood cells that promote blood clotting (platelets). These disorders can also be either inherited or picked up (acquired). The side effects of certain drugs often lead to the acquired forms.

216. Ans. (a) Factor VIII

Refer explanation of Chapter 13 Q 196

Clotting factors in blood and their synonyms	
Clotting factor	*Synonyms*
Fibrinogen	Factor I
Prothrombin	Factor II
Tissue factor	Factor III; tissue thromboplastin
Calcium	Factor IV
Factor V	Proaccelerin; labile factor; Ac-globulin (Ac-G)
Factor VII	Serum prothrombin conversion accelerator (SPCA); proconvertin; stable factor
Factor VIII	Antihemophilic factor (AHF); antihemophilic globulin (AHG); antihemophilic factor A
Factor IX	Plasma thromboplastin component (PTC); Christmas factor; antihemophilic factor B
Factor X	Stuart factor; Stuart-Prower factor
Factor XI	Plasma thromboplastin antecedent (PTA); antihemophilic factor C
Factor XII	Hageman factor
Factor XIII	Fibrin-stabilizing factor
Prekallikrein	Fletcher factor
High-molecular-weight kininogen	Fitzgerald factor; HMWK (high-molecular-weight) kininogen
Platelets	

217. Ans. (d) Haemophilia *Ref: Shafers 6th/ed p 786*

Hemophilia

Clinical Features: Patients of haemophilia suffer from bleeding for hours or days after the injury. The clinical severity of the disease correlates well with plasma level of factor VIII activity. Haemophilic bleeding can involve any organ but occurs most commonly as recurrent painful haemarthroses and muscle haematomas, and sometimes as haematuria. Spontaneous intracranial haemorrhage and oropharyngeal bleeding are rare, but when they occur they are the most feared complications.

- Whole blood coagulation time is prolonged in severe cases only.
- Prothrombin time is usually normal.
- Activated partial thromboplastin time (APTT or PTTK) is typically prolonged.
- Specific assay for factor VIII shows lowered activity. The diagnosis of female carriers is made by the findings of about half the activity of factor VIII, while the manifest disease is associated with factor VIII activity below 25%.

218. Ans. (d) All of the above *Ref: Harsh Mohan Textbook of Pathology 6th ed. p 295*

Hypochromic anaemia due to iron deficiency is the commonest cause of anaemia the world over. It is estimated that about 20% of women in child-bearing age group are iron deficient, while the overall prevalence in adult males is about 2%. It is the most important, though not the sole, cause of microcytic hypochromic anaemia in which all the three red cell indices (MCV, MCH and MCHC) are reduced and occurs due to defective haemoglobin synthesis. Hypochromic anaemias, therefore, are classified into 2 groups:

- Hypochromic anaemia due to iron deficiency.
- Hypochromic anaemias other than iron deficiency. The latter category includes 3 groups of disorders sideroblastic anaemia, thalassaemia and anaemia of chronic disorders. In microcytic anemia, the red blood cells (erythrocytes) are usually also hypochromic, meaning that the red blood cells appear paler than usual. This is reflected by a lower-than-normal mean corpuscular haemoglobin concentration (MCHC), a measure representing the amount of haemoglobin per unit volume of fluid inside the cell; normally about 320-360 g/L or 32-36 g/dL. Typically, therefore, anemia of this category is described as 'microcytic, hypochromic anaemia'.

Causes of microcytic (hypochromic) anemia

- **Childhood**
- Iron deficiency anemia, by far the most common cause of anemia in general and of microcytic anemia in particular
- Thalassemia
- **Adulthood**
- Blood loss
- Iron deficiency anemia
- Sideroblastic anemia, congenital or acquired
- Anemia of chronic disease
- Lead poisoning
- Pyridoxine deficiency

DISEASES OF WHITE BLOOD CELLS, LYMPH NODES, SPLEEN, AND THYMUS

219. Ans. (a) Parasitic infections *Ref: Harsh Mohan Textbook of Pathology 6th ed. p 350*

A rise in the blood monocytes above 800/μl is termed monocytosis. Some common causes of monocytosis are as follows:

- Certain bacterial infections, e.g. tuberculosis, subacute bacterial endocarditis, syphilis.
- Viral infections

- Protozoal and rickettsial infections, e.g. malaria, typhus, trypanosomiasis, kala-azar.
- Convalescence from acute infection.
- Haematopoietic disorders, e.g. monocytic leukaemia, lymphomas, myeloproliferative disorders, multiple myeloma, lipid storage disease.
- Malignancies, e.g. cancer of the ovary, stomach, breast.
- Granulomatous diseases, e.g. sarcoidosis, inflammatory bowel disease.
- Collagen-vascular diseases

220. Ans. (a) Neutrophilic leucocytes *Ref: Harsh Mohan Textbook of Pathology 6th ed. p 348*

The normal functions of neutrophils are as under:

- Chemotaxis or cell mobilisation in which the cell is attracted towards bacteria or at the site of inflammation.
- Phagocytosis in which the foreign particulate material of tiny sizes is phagocytosed by actively motile neutrophils; thus PMNs act as microphages compared to function of monocytes as macrophages.
- Killing of the microorganism is mediated by oxygen-dependent and oxygen-independent pathways

221. Ans. (c) Platelet disorder *Ref: Essential of Medicine for dental student by Tripathi p 69*

Spontaneous gingival bleeding is common when platelet cound is below 20.000/mm3 during oral prophylaxis.

222. Ans. (d) Myelofibrosis *Ref: http://en.wikipedia.org/wiki/Alkaline_phosphatase#Leukocyte_alkaline_phosphatase*

Leukocyte alkaline phosphatase (LAP) is found within white blood cells. White blood cell levels of LAP can help in the diagnosis of certain conditions.

- Higher levels are seen in polycythemia vera (PV), essential thrombocytosis (ET), primary myelofibrosis (PM), and the leukemoid reaction.
- Lower levels are found in chronic myelogenous leukemia (CML), paroxysmal nocturnal hemoglobinuria (PNH) and acute myelogenous leukaemia (AML). Myelofibrosis, also known as osteomyelofibrosis and primary myelofibrosis is a disorder of the bone marrow. It is currently classified as a myeloproliferative disease, in which the proliferation of an abnormal clone of hematopoietic progenitor cells in the bone marrow and other sites results in fibrosis, or the replacement of the marrow with collagenous connective tissue fibers.

223. Ans. (c) Lactoferrin *Ref: Harsh Mohan Textbook of Pathology 6th ed. p 142, 347*

A polymorphonuclear neutrophil (PMN), commonly called polymorph or neutrophil, is 12-15 μm in diameter. It consists of a characteristic dense nucleus, having 2-5 lobes and pale cytoplasm containing numerous fine violet-pink granules. These lysosomal granules contain several enzymes and are of 2 types: Primary or azurophilic granules are large and coarse and appear early at the promyelocyte stage. These granules contain lysozyme, hydrolases, elastase, myeloperoxidase (MPO), cathepsin-G, cationic proteins, bacterial permeability increasing protein (BPI), and microbicidal protein called defensins. Secondary or specific granules are smaller and more numerous. These appear later at myelocyte stage, are MPOnegative and contain lactoferrin, NADPH oxidase, histaminase, vitamin B12 binding protein, and receptors for chemoattractants and for laminin.

224. Ans. (c) Steroids *Ref: http://en.wikipedia.org/wiki/leukocytosis*

Leukocytosis is very common in acutely ill patients. It occurs in response to a wide variety of conditions, including viral, bacterial, fungal, or parasitic infection, cancer, hemorrhage, and exposure to certain medications or chemicals including steroids. For lung diseases, such as pneumonia and tuberculosis, WBC count is very important for the diagnosis of the disease, as leukocytosis is usually present. The mechanism that causes leukocytosis can be of several forms: an increased release of leukocytes from bone marrow storage pools, decreased margination of leukocytes onto vessel walls, decreased extravasation of leukocytes from the vessels into tissues, or an increase in number of precursor cells in the marrow.

Certain medications, including corticosteroids, lithium and beta agonists, may cause leukocytosis.

Causes of leukocytosis

Neutrophilic leukocytosis (neutrophilia)	• Acute bacterial infections, especially pyogenic infections • Sterile inflammation – Tissue necrosis - Myocardial infarction - Burns
Eosinophilic leukocytosis (eosinophilia)	• Allergic disorders – Asthma – Hay fever – Drug allergies – Allergic skin diseases - Pemphigus - Dermatitis herpetiformis • Parasitic infections • Some forms of malignancy – Hodgkin's lymphoma – Some forms of Non-Hodgkin lymphoma • Systemic autoimmune diseases (e.g. SLE) • Some forms of vasculitis • Cholesterol embolism (transiently)
Basophilic leukocytosis basophilia	(rare) • Myeloproliferative disease, e.g. chronic myelogenous leukemia
Monocytosis	• Chronic infections – Tuberculosis – Bacterial endocarditis – Rickettsiosis – Malaria • Systemic autoimmune diseases, e.g. SLE • Inflammatory bowel diseases, e.g. ulcerative colitis
Lymphocytosis	• Chronic infections – Tuberculosis – Brucellosis

225. Ans. (a) Brain *Ref: Harsh Mohan Textbook of Pathology 6th ed. p 62*

Feature	*T cells*	*B cells*
1. Origin	Bone marrow → Thymus	Bone marrow → Bursa (in fowl): Mucosa-associated lymphoid tissue (MALT)
2. Lifespan	Small T cells: Months to years T cell blasts: Several days	Small B cells: Less than 1 month B cell blasts: Several days
3. Location		
• Lymph nodes	Perifollicular (paracortical)	Germinal centres, medullary cords
• Spleen	Periarteriolar	Germinal centres, red pulp
• Peyer's patches	Perifollicular	Central follicles

Contd...

Contd...

Feature	*T cells*	*B cells*
4. Presence in circulation	75–80%	10-15%
5. Surface markers		
• Ag receptors	Present	Absent
• Surface Ig	Absent	Present
• Fc receptor	Absent	Present
• Complement receptor	Absent	Present
• Rosettes	E-rosettes (sheep erythrocytes)	EAC-rosettes (mouse erythrocytes)
• CD markers	T_H cells CD4, 3, 7, 2	CD 19, 20, 21, 23
	T_S cells CD8, 3, 7, 2	
Functions	• CMI via cytotoxic T cells positive for CD3 and CD4	• Role in humoral immunity by synthesis of specific antibodies (Igs)
	• Delayed hypersensitivity via CD4+ T cells	• Precursors of plasma cells
	• Immunoregulation of other T cells, B cells and stem cells via T helper (CD4+) or T suppressor (CD8+) cells	

226. Ans. (b) Acute promyelocytic leukemia *Ref: Robbins Pathologic Basis of Disease 7th ed. p 335, 657*

Several vascular and hematologic manifestations may appear in association with a variety of forms of cancer. Migratory thrombophlebitis (Trousseau syndrome) may be encountered in association with deep-seated cancers, most often carcinomas of the pancreas or lung. Disseminated intravascular coagulation may complicate a diversity of clinical disorders. Acute disseminated intravascular coagulation is most commonly associated with acute promyelocytic leukemia and prostatic adenocarcinoma. Bland, small, nonbacterial fibrinous vegetations sometimes form on the cardiac valve leaflets (more often on left-sided valves), particularly in patients with advanced mucin-secreting adenocarcinomas. These lesions are called nonbacterial thrombotic endocarditis. The vegetations are potential sources of emboli that can further complicate the course of cancer. Among cancers, acute promyelocytic leukemia and carcinomas of the lung, pancreas, colon, and stomach are most frequently associated with DIC. These tumors release of a variety of thromboplastic substances, including tissue factors, proteolytic enzymes, mucin, and other undefined tumor products.

227. Ans. (a) Decreased absolute neutrophil count *Ref: http://en.wikipedia.org/wiki/Agranulocytosis#Diagnosis*

Agranulocytosis, also known as agranulosis or granulopenia, is an acute condition involving a severe and dangerous leukopenia (lowered white blood cell count), most commonly of neutrophils causing a neutropenia in the circulating blood. It represents a severe lack of one major class of infection-fighting white blood cells. People with this condition are at very high risk of serious infections due to their suppressed immune system. The diagnosis is made after a complete blood count, a routine blood test. The absolute neutrophil count in this test will be below 500, and can reach 0 cells/mm^3. Other kinds of blood cells are typically present in normal numbers. To formally diagnose agranulocytosis, other pathologies with a similar presentation must be excluded, such as aplastic anemia, paroxysmal nocturnal hemoglobinuria, myelodysplasia and leukemias. This requires a bone marrow examination that shows normocellular (normal amounts and types of cells) blood marrow with underdeveloped promyelocytes. These underdeveloped promyelocytes, if fully matured, would have been the missing granulocytes.

228. Ans. (c) Polycythemia vera

Refer explanation of 222

229. Ans. (b) Leukocytosis

Refer explanation of 224

230. Ans. (b) Myeloblast *Ref: Robbins Pathologic Basis of Disease 7th ed. p 692, 694*

Auer rods are clumps of azurophilic granular material that form elongated needles seen in the cytoplasm of leukemic blasts. They can be seen in the leukemic blasts of acute myeloid leukemia with maturation and acute promyelocytic leukemia (known as acute myeloid leukemia M2 and M3, in the FAB classification, respectively) and in high grade myelodysplastic syndromes and myeloproliferative syndromes. They are composed of fused lysosomes/primary neutrophilic granules and contain peroxidase, lysosomal enzymes, and large crystalline inclusions. Morphologically, the Auer 'rods' come in all sizes and shapes. They have been described as needle-shapes with pointed ends (most common), comma-shapes, and diamond-shapes; others were long and rectangular. Occasional corkscrew forms and rare granular Auer bodies were also noted. More appropriately, they can be referred to as Auer bodies.

231. Ans. (d) Left supra-clavicular nodes *Ref: Harsh Mohan Textbook of Pathology 6th ed. p 557*

Involvement of left supraclavicular lymph node, Virchow or Troisier's sign, is sometimes the presenting feature of gastric carcinoma. Virchow's node (or signal node) is a lymph node in the left supraclavicular fossa (the area above the left clavicle). It takes its supply from lymph vessels in the abdominal cavity. Virchow's node is also sometimes coined 'the seat of the devil' given its ominous association with malignant disease. The finding of an enlarged, hard node (also referred to as Troisier's sign) has long been regarded as strongly indicative of the presence of cancer in the abdomen, specifically gastric cancer that has spread through the lymph vessels.

232. Ans. (c) Agranulocytosis

Refer explanation of 227

LUNG

233. Ans. (c) Neck flexion *Ref: Lung Function Test Made Easy p 12*

Depresion of the Jaw with flexion of the neck produce a mean decrease in the dead space

234. Ans. (a) The surfactant will be reduced *Ref: Robbins Pathologic Basis of Disease 7th ed. p 767*

Pneumothorax refers to air or gas in the pleural cavities and may be spontaneous, traumatic, or therapeutic. Spontaneous pneumothorax may complicate any form of pulmonary disease that causes rupture of an alveolus. An abscess cavity that communicates either directly with the pleural space or with the lung interstitial tissue may also lead to the escape of air. In the latter circumstance, the air may dissect through the lung substance or back through the mediastinum (interstitial emphysema), eventually entering the pleural cavity. Pneumothorax is most commonly associated with emphysema, asthma, and tuberculosis.

235. Ans. (b) Brachial artery *Ref: Pfenninger and Fowler's Procedures for primary care p 120.*

236. Ans. (b) 12 times per minute *Ref: Malamed p 138-7th/ed.*

237. Ans. (c) Middle of the lower part of the sternum *Ref: Harrisons Principles of Internal Medicine, 18th ed. p 2243*

Chest compression is based on the assumption that cardiac compression allows the heart to maintain a pump function by sequential filling and emptying of its chambers, with competent valves maintaining forward direction of flow. The palm of one hand is placed over the middle of the lower part of the sternum, with the heel of the other resting on the dorsum of the lower hand. The sternum is depressed, with the arms remaining straight, at a rate of approximately 100 per minute. Sufficient force is applied to depress the sternum 45 cm, and relaxation is abrupt.

238. Ans. (b) Red hepatisation *Ref: Robbins Pathologic Basis of Disease 7th ed. p 750*

In lobar pneumonia, four stages of the inflammatory response have classically been described: Congestion, red hepatization, gray hepatization, and resolution. Present-day effective antibiotic therapy frequently slows or halts the progression.

- In the first stage of congestion, the lung is heavy, boggy, and red. It is characterized by vascular engorgement, intra-alveolar fluid with few neutrophils, and often the presence of numerous bacteria.
- The stage of red hepatization that follows is characterized by massive confluent exudation with red cells (congestion), neutrophils, and fibrin filling the alveolar spaces. On gross examination, the lobe now appears distinctly red, firm, and airless, with a liver-like consistency, hence the term hepatization.
- The stage of gray hepatization follows with progressive disintegration of red cells and the persistence of a fibrinosuppurative exudate, giving the gross appearance of a grayish brown, dry surface.
- In the final stage of resolution, the consolidated exudates within the alveolar spaces undergoes progressive enzymatic digestion to produce a granular, semifluid, debris that is resorbed, ingested by macrophages, coughed up, or organized by fibroblasts growing into it.

HEAD AND NECK

239. Ans. (a) Aberrant sebaceous glands *Ref: Harsh Mohan Textbook of Pathology 6th ed. p 522*

- Fordyce's granules: Fordyce's granules are symmetric, small, light yellow macular spots on the lips and buccal mucosa and represent collections of sebaceous glands. They remain undeveloped until puberty but occur quite commonly in adults.

240. Ans. (c) Submandibular *Ref: Robbins Pathologic Basis of Disease 7th ed. p 790*

Nonspecific bacterial sialadenitis, most often involving the major salivary glands, particularly the submandibular glands, is a common condition, usually secondary to ductal obstruction produced by stones (sialolithiasis). The stone formation is sometimes related to obstruction of the orifices of the salivary glands by impacted food debris or by edema about the orifice after some injury. Frequently, the stones are of obscure origin.

241. Ans. (a) Pleomorphic adenoma *Ref: Robbins Pathologic Basis of Disease 7th ed. p 791*

Pleomorphic Adenoma

Because of their remarkable histologic diversity, these neoplasms have also been called mixed tumors. They represent about 60% of tumors in the parotid, are less common in the submandibular glands, and are relatively rare in the minor salivary glands. They are benign tumors that are derived from a mixture of ductal (epithelial) and myoepithelial cells, and therefore they show both epithelial and mesenchymal differentiation. They also reveal epithelial elements dispersed throughout a matrix along with varying degrees of myxoid, hyaline, chondroid (cartilaginous), and even osseous tissue. In some tumors, the epithelial elements predominate; in others, they are present only in widely dispersed foci.

242. Ans. (a) Lichen planus *Ref: Robbins Pathologic Basis of Disease 7th ed. p 1258*

Lichen planus

'Pruritic, purple, polygonal papules' are the presenting signs of this disorder of the skin and mucous membranes. Lichen planus is self-limiting and generally resolves spontaneously 1 to 2 years after onset, often leaving zones of postinflammatory hyperpigmentation. Oral lesions may persist for years. Lichen planus is characterized histologically by a dense, continuous infiltrate of lymphocytes along the dermoepidermal junction. The lymphocytes are intimately associated with basal keratinocytes, which show degeneration, necrosis, and a resemblance in size and contour to more mature cells of the stratum spinosum (squamatization). A consequence of this destructive infiltration of lymphocytes is a redefinition of the normal, smoothly undulating configuration of the dermoepidermal interface to a more angulated zigzag contour (saw-toothing).

243. Ans. (b) Cyst in floor of mouth *Ref: Robbins Pathologic Basis of Disease 7th ed. p 790*

Mucocele. This is the most common lesion of the salivary glands and it results from either blockage or rupture of a salivary gland duct, with consequent leakage of saliva into the surrounding connective tissue stroma. Mucoceles are most often found on the lower lip and are the result of trauma. Histologically, mucoceles demonstrate a cystlike space that is lined by inflammatory granulation tissue or by fibrous connective tissue. The cystic spaces are filled with mucin as well as inflammatory cells, particularly macrophages. A ranula is histologically identical to a mucocele. However, this term is reserved for mucoceles that arise when the duct of the sublingual gland has been damaged. A ranula can become extremely large and develop into a 'plunging ranula' when it dissects its way through the connective tissue stroma connecting the two bellies of the mylohyoid muscle.

244. Ans. (c) Mucicarmine stain

Stain	*Component/Tissue*	*Dyes*	*Interpretation*
• Amyloid			
– Congo red with polarising light	Amyloid	Congo red	Green-birefringence: Amyloid
– Toluidine blue	Amyloid	Toluidine blue	Orthochromatic blue: Amyloid
• Carbohydrates			
– Periodic acid-Schiff (PAS)	Carbohydrates (particularly glycogen), all mucins	Periodic acid, Schiff reagent (basic fuchsin)	Glycogen and other carbohydrates: Magenta Nuclei: Blue
– Mucicarmine/Best's carmine	Acidic mucin	Carmine	Mucin: Red Nuclei: Blue
– Alcian blue (AB)	Acidic mucin	Alcian blue (at pH 2.5)	Acid mucin: Blue Nuclei: Red
– Combined AB-PAS	Neutral mucin	Alcian blue	Acid mucin: Blue Neutral mucin: Magenta Nuclei: Pale blue
• Connective Tissues			
– Van Gieson's	Extracellular collagen	Picric acid, acid fuchsin, celestin blue-haemalum	Nuclei: Blue/black Collagen: Red Other tissues: Yellow
– Masson's trichrome	Extracellular collagen	Acid fuchsin, phosphomolybdic acid, methyl blue, celestin blue-haemalum	Nuclei: Blue/black cytoplasm, muscle, red cells: Red collagen: Blue

GASTROINTESTINAL TRACT

245. Ans. (c) Urinary copper excretion is less than 100 μg/day *Ref: Robbins Pathologic Basis of Disease 7th ed. p 910*
Harrisons Principles of Internal Medicine, 18th Ed. p 3188

This autosomal-recessive disorder is marked by the accumulation of toxic levels of copper in many tissues and organs, principally the liver, brain and eye. Wilson's disease is an autosomal recessive disorder caused by mutations in the ATP7B gene, a membrane-bound, copper-transporting ATPase. Urine copper is an important diagnostic tool, but it must be collected carefully to avoid contamination. Symptomatic patients invariably have urine copper levels > 1.6 μmol (>100 μg) per 24 h. Heterozygotes have values < 1.3 μmol (<80 μg) per 24 h. About half of presymptomatic patients who are ultimately affected have diagnostically elevated urine copper values, but the other half are in an intermediate range between 0.9 and 1.6 μmol (60 and 100 μg) per 24 h. Because heterozygotes may have values up to 1.3 μmol (80 μg) per 24 h, patients in this range may require a liver biopsy for definitive diagnosis. All other options are correct.

246. Ans. (b) Increased urinary excretion of copper

Wilson's disease, also termed by a more descriptive designation of hepatolenticular degeneration, is an autosomal recessive inherited disease of copper metabolism, characterised by toxic accumulation of copper in many tissues, chiefly the liver, brain and eye. These accumulations lead to the triad of features:

- Cirrhosis of the liver.
- Bilateral degeneration of the basal ganglia of the brain.
- Greenish-brown pigmented rings in the periphery of the cornea (Kayser-Fleischer rings).

Biochemical abnormalities in Wilson's disease include the following:

- Decreased serum ceruloplasmin (due to impaired synthesis of apoceruloplasmin in damaged liver and defective mobilisation of copper from hepatocellular lysosomes).
- Increased hepatic copper in liver biopsy (due to excessive accumulation of copper in the liver).
- Increased urinary excretion of copper.
- However, serum copper levels are of no diagnostic help and may vary from low-to-normal-to-high depending upon the stage of disease.

247. Ans. (c) Muscularis propria *Ref: Robbins Pathologic Basis of Disease 7th ed. p 870*

The histologic criterion for the diagnosis of acute appendicitis is neutrophilic infiltration of the muscularis propria. Usually, neutrophils and ulcerations are also present within the mucosa. Since drainage of an exudate into the appendix from alimentary tract infection may also induce a mucosal neutrophilic infiltrate, evidence of muscular wall inflammation is requisite for the diagnosis.

LIVER AND BILIARY TRACT

248. Ans. (c) Right iliac fossa *Ref: Differential diagnosis of acute pain p 233 by stanley*

- Pain due to gallstone is referred to the epigastrium or the right-hypochondrium. It may radiate throughout the abdomen, often extending into the chest and to the right shoulder.

249. Ans. (a) HbeAg *Ref: Robbins Pathologic Basis of Disease 7th ed. p 893*

Serologic Diagnosis: After exposure to HBV, the long asymptomatic 4- to 26-week incubation period (mean: 6 to 8 weeks) is followed by acute disease lasting many weeks to months. Most patients experience a self-limited illness:

- HBsAg appears before the onset of symptoms, peaks during overt disease, and then declines to undetectable levels in 3 to 6 months.

- HBeAg, HBV-DNA, and DNA polymerase appear in the serum soon after HBsAg, and all signify active viral replication.
- IgM anti-HBc becomes detectable in serum shortly before the onset of symptoms, concurrent with the onset of elevation of serum aminotransferases. Over months, the IgM antibody is replaced by IgG anti-HBc.
- Anti-HBe is detectable shortly after the disappearance of HBeAg, implying that the acute infection has peaked and the disease is on the wane.
- IgG anti-HBs does not rise until the acute disease is over and is usually not detectable for a few weeks to several months after the disappearance of HBsAg. Anti-HBs may persist for life, conferring protection; this is the basis for current vaccination strategies using noninfectious HBsAg. The carrier state is defined by the presence of HBsAg in serum for 6 months or longer after initial detection. The presence of HBsAg alone does not necessarily indicate replication of complete virions, and patients may be asymptomatic and without liver damage. In contrast, chronic replication of HBV virions is characterized by persistence of circulating HBsAg, HBeAg, and HBV DNA, usually with anti-HBc and occasionally with anti-HBs. Ideally answer should be IgM anti-HBc but since that option is not given, closer answer is HBeAg.

250. Ans. (d) HBsAg

Refer explanation 249

251. Ans. (c) Pancreatic carcinoma *Ref: Harsh Mohan Textbook of Pathology 6th ed. p 599*

Extrahepatic cholestasis: Extrahepatic cholestasis results from mechanical obstruction to large bile ducts outside the liver or within the porta hepatis. The common causes are gallstones, inflammatory strictures, carcinoma head of pancreas, tumours of bile duct, sclerosing cholangitis and congenital atresia of extrahepatic ducts. The obstruction may be complete and sudden with eventual progressive obstructive jaundice, or the obstruction may be partial and incomplete resulting in intermittent jaundice. The features of extrahepatic cholestasis (obstructive jaundice), like in intrahepatic cholestasis, are: predominant conjugated hyperbilirubinaemia, bilirubinuria, elevated serum bile acids causing intense pruritus, high serum alkaline phosphatase and hyperlipidaemia.

252. Ans. (a) Increased bilirubin in urine

Refer explanation 251

253. Ans. (c) Hepatocellular jaundice *Ref: Harsh Mohan Textbook of Pathology 6th ed. p 610*

The most common consequence of all hepatotropic viruses is acute inflammatory involvement of the entire liver. In general, type A, B, C, D and E run similar clinical course and show identical pathologic findings. Clinically, acute hepatitis is categorised into 4 phases: Incubation period. It varies among different hepatotropic viruses: for hepatitis A it is about 4 weeks (15-45 days); for hepatitis B the average is 10 weeks (30-180 days); for hepatitis D about 6 weeks (30-50 days); for hepatitis C the mean incubation period is about 7 weeks (20-90 days), and for hepatitis E it is 2-8 weeks (15-60 days). Pre-icteric phase: This phase is marked by prodromal constitutional symptoms that include anorexia, nausea, vomiting, fatigue, malaise, distaste for smoking, arthralgia and headache. Icteric phase: The prodromal period is heralded by the onset of clinical jaundice and the constitutional symptoms diminish. Other features include dark-coloured urine due to bilirubinuria, clay-coloured stools due to cholestasis, pruritus as a result of elevated serum bile acids, loss of weight and abdominal discomfort due to enlarged, tender liver. The diagnosis is based on deranged liver function tests. Post-icteric phase: The icteric phase lasting for about 1 to 4 weeks is usually followed by clinical and biochemical recovery in 2 to 12 weeks. The recovery phase is more prolonged in hepatitis B and hepatitis C. Up to 1% cases of acute hepatitis may develop severe form of the disease (fulminant hepatitis), and 5-10% of cases progress on to chronic hepatitis.

254. Ans. (d) Increased breakdown of red cells *Ref: Harsh Mohan Textbook of Pathology 6th ed. p 598*

Unconjugated Hyperbilirubinaemia

This form of jaundice can result from the following three sets of conditions:

(i) Increased bilirubin production (Haemolytic, acholuric or prehepatic jaundice)

- Intra- and extravascular haemolysis
- Ineffective erythropoiesis

(ii) Decreased hepatic uptake

- Drugs
- Prolonged starvation
- Sepsis

(iii) Decreased bilirubin conjugation

- Hereditary disorders (e.g. Gilbert's syndrome, Crigler-Najjar syndrome)
- Acquired defects

Haemolytic jaundice

This results from excessive red cell destruction as occurs in intra and extravascular haemolysis or due to ineffective erythropoiesis. There is increased release of haemoglobin from excessive breakdown of red cells that leads to overproduction of bilirubin. Hyperbilirubinaemia develops when the capacity of the liver to conjugate large amount of bilirubin is exceeded.

255. Ans. (c) Chronic rental failure *Ref: Harsh Mohan Textbook of Pathology 6th ed. p 594,595*

5'-Nucleotidase is another phosphatase derived from the liver. Its determination is useful to distinguish alkaline phosphatase of hepatic origin from that of bony tissue.

- Liver function tests are as follows:

Tests	*Significance*
• Tests for manufacture and excretion of bile	
– Bilirubin	
- Serum bilirubin	Increased in hepatocellular, obstructive and haemolytic disease, Gilbert's disease
- In faeces	Absent in biliary obstruction
- In urine	Conjugated bilirubinuria in patients of hepatitis
– Urobilinogen	Increased in hepatocellular and haemolytic diseases, absent in biliary obstruction
– Bile acid (Bile salts):	Increased in serum and detectable in urine in cholestasis
• Serum enzyme assays	
– Alkaline phosphatase	Increased in hepatobiliary disease (highest in biliary obstruction), bone diseases, pregnancy
– γ-Glutamyl transpeptidase (γ-GT)	Rise parallels alkaline phosphatase but is specific for hepatobiliary diseases
– Transaminases:	
- SGOT (AST)	Increased in tissue injury to liver as well as to other tissues like in myocardial infarction
- SGPT (ALT)	Increase is fairly specific for liver cell injury

Contd...

Contd...

Tests	*Significance*
– Other enzymes	
- 5′-Nucleotidase	Rise parallels alkaline phosphatase but more specific for diseases of hepatic origin
- Lactic dehydrogenase	Increased in tumours involving the liver
- Cholinesterase	Decreased in hepatocellular disease, malnutrition
• Tests for metabolic functions	
– Amino acid and protein metabolism:	
- Serum proteins (total, A/G ratio, protein electrophoresis)	Hypoalbuminaemia in hepatocellular diseases; hyperglobulinaemia in cirrhosis and chronic active hepatitis
- Immunoglobulins	Nonspecific alterations in IgA, IgG and IgM
- Clotting factors	Prothrombin time and partial thromboplastin time prolonged in patients with hepatocellular disease
- Serum ammonia	Increased in acute fulminant hepatitis, cirrhosis, hepatic encephalopathy
- Aminoaciduria	In fulminant hepatitis
– Lipid and lipoprotein metabolism:	
Blood lipids (total serum cholesterol, triglycerides and lipoprotein fractions)	Increased in cholestasis, decreased in acute and chronic diffuse liver disease and in malnutrition
– Carbohydrate mtabolism:	
Blood glucose and GTT	Decreased in hepatic necrosis
• Immunologic tests	
– Nonspecific immunologic reactions	
- Smooth muscle antibody	In hepatic necrosis
- Mitochondrial antibody	In primary biliary cirrhosis
- Antinuclear antibody and LE cell test	In chronic active hepatitis
– Antibodies to specific etiologic agents:	
- Antibodies to hepatitis B (HBsAg, HBc, HBeAg)	In hepatitis B
- Amoeba antibodies	Amoebic liver abscess
• Ancillary diagnostic tests	
– Ultrasound examination	Cholestasis of various etiologies; SOLs, US-guided-FNAC/liver biopsy
– FNAC and/or percutaneous liver biopsy	Unknown cause of hepatocellular disease, hepatomegaly and splenomegaly; long-standing hepatitis; PUO and SOLs of the liver

256. Ans. (d) Albumin *Ref: Refer explanation of Chapter 18 Q 255*

Serum proteins. Liver cells synthesise albumin, fibrinogen, prothrombin, alpha-1-antitrypsin, haptoglobin, ceruloplasmin, transferrin, alpha fetoproteins and acute phase reactant proteins. The blood levels of these plasma proteins are decreased in extensive liver damage. Hypoalbuminaemia may occur in liver diseases having significant destruction of hepatocytes. Hyperglobulinaemia may be present in chronic inflammatory disorders such as in cirrhosis and chronic hepatitis.

257. Ans. (c) Prolonged bleeding *Ref: Harsh Mohan Textbook of Pathology 6th ed. p 595*

Clotting factors: Hepatic synthetic function of several clotting factors can be assessed by a few simple coagulation tests. Prothrombin time and partial thromboplastin time, both of which reflect the activities of various clotting factors, are prolonged in patients with hepatocellular disease. Prothrombin time is dependent upon both- hepatic synthesis of clotting factors and intestinal uptake of vitamin K, a fat soluble vitamin. Hence, main complication during extraction in liver disease is prolonged bleeding.

258. Ans. (c) 6 months *Ref: Harsh Mohan Textbook of Pathology 6th ed. p 511*

Chronic hepatitis is defined as continuing or relapsing hepatic disease for more than 6 months with symptoms along with biochemical, serologic and histopathologic evidence of inflammation and necrosis. Majority of cases of chronic hepatitis are the result of infection with hepatotropic viruses hepatitis B, hepatitis C and combined hepatitis B and hepatitis D infection. However, some non-viral causes of chronic hepatitis include: Wilson's disease, α-1-antitrypsin deficiency, chronic alcoholism, drug-induced injury and autoimmune diseases. The last named gives rise to autoimmune or lupoid hepatitis which is characterised by positive serum autoantibodies (e.g. antinuclear, anti-smooth muscle and anti-mitochondrial) and a positive LE cell test but negative for serologic markers of viral hepatitis.

PANCREAS

259. Ans. (d) Fibre *Ref: Clin Excell Nurse Pract. 2000 Sep;4(5):272-6.*

Dietary fiber and type 2 diabetes.

Dietary fiber shows promise in the management of type 2 DM. The inclusion of sufficient dietary fiber in a meal flattens the postprandial glycemic and insulinemic excursions and favorably influences plasma lipid levels in patients with type 2 DM. Water-soluble fiber appears to have a greater potential to reduce postprandial blood glucose, insulin, and serum lipid levels than insoluble fiber. Viscosity of the dietary fiber is important; the greater the viscosity, the greater the effect. Possible mechanisms for metabolic improvements with dietary fiber include delay of glucose absorption, increase in hepatic extraction of insulin, increased insulin sensitivity at the cellular level, and binding of bile acids. Patients with type 2 DM should increase their dietary fiber intake to 20 to 35 g/d and be aware of the considerations when increasing fiber intake.

KIDNEY

260. Ans. (d) Impotence *Ref: Wassertheil-Smoller S, Blaufox MD, Oberman A, et al. Effect of antihypertensives on sexual function and quality of life: the TAIM study. Ann Intern Med. 1991;114:613-620.*

Adverse effects of thiazide and thiazide-like diuretics on male sexual function, including decreased libido, erectile dysfunction, and difficult ejaculation have been reported in several studies with an incidence that varies from 3%-32%.

261. Ans. (c) Nephrotic syndrome *Ref: http://en.wikipedia.org/wiki/Hyponatremia#Causes*

Hypervolemic hyponatremia: Both sodium and water content increase—Increase in sodium content leads to hypervolemia and water content to hyponatremia. Total body water and sodium are regulated independently.

- Cirrhosis of the liver
- Congestive heart failure
- Nephrotic syndrome in the kidneys
- Massive edema of any cause

262. Ans. (c) Mu heavy chain disease *Ref: Hematology. 2004 Apr;9(2):135-7.*

Mu-heavy chain disease associated with systemic amyloidosis

The diagnosis of m-heavy chain disease was based on findings of mu-heavy chain fragments in the serum. Bence Jones proteinuria and vacuolated plasma cells in the bone marrow.

263. Ans. (b) Neurofibroma

Ref: Robbins Pathologic Basis of Disease 7th ed. p 502, Harsh Mohan Textbook of Pathology 6th ed. p 800

Urine VMA is associated with neuroblastoma and pheochromocytoma. About 90% of neuroblastomas, regardless of location, produce catecholamines (similar to the catecholamines associated with pheochromocytomas), which are an important diagnostic feature (i.e. elevated blood levels of catecholamines and elevated urine levels of metabolites, vanillylmandelic acid [VMA], and homovanillic acid [HVA]).

264. Ans. (a) Metabolic acidosis *Ref: Harsh Mohan Textbook of Pathology 6th ed. p 104*

Metabolic Acidosis

A fall in the blood pH due to metabolic component is brought about by fall of bicarbonate level and excess of H+ ions in the blood. This occurs in the following situations:

- Production of large amounts of lactic acid (lactic acidosis), e.g. in vigorous exercise, shock.
- Uncontrolled diabetes mellitus (diabetic ketoacidosis). Starvation.
- Chronic renal failure.
- Therapeutic administration of ammonium chloride or acetazolamide (diamox). High blood levels of H+ ions in metabolic acidosis stimulate the respiratory centre so that the breathing is deep and rapid (air hunger or Kussmaul's respiration). There is fall in the plasma bicarbonate levels.

265. Ans. (b) Red cell casts *Ref: Robbins Pathologic Basis of Disease 7th ed. p 973; Harsh Mohan Textbook of Pathology 6th ed. p 662*

Acute glomerulonephritis: This group of glomerular diseases is characterized anatomically by inflammatory alterations in the glomeruli and clinically by the syndrome of acute nephritis. The nephritic patient usually presents with hematuria, red cell casts in the urine, azotemia oliguria, and mild to moderate hypertension. The patient also commonly has proteinuria and edema, but these are not as severe as those encountered in the nephrotic syndrome.

266. Ans. (c) Multiple myeloma *Ref: Harsh Mohan Textbook of Pathology 6th ed. p 683*

The diagnosis of multiple myeloma is made by classic triad of features:

- Marrow plasmacytosis of more than 10%
- Radiologic evidence of lytic bony lesions
- Demonstration of serum and/or urine M component.

There is rise in the total serum protein concentration due to paraproteinaemia but normal serum immunoglobulins (IgG, IgA and IgM) and albumin are depressed. Paraproteins are abnormal immunoglobulins or their parts circulating in plasma and excreted in urine. About two-third cases of myeloma excrete Bence Jones (light chain) proteins in the urine, consisting of either kappa (κ) or lambda (λ) light chains, along with presence of Bence Jones paraproteins in the serum. On serum electrophoresis, the paraprotein usually appears as a single narrow homogeneous M-band component, most commonly in the region of γ-globulin.

267. Ans. (a) Kidney *Ref: Robbins Pathologic Basis of Disease 7th ed. p 1018*

The three classic diagnostic features of renal cell carcinoma are costovertebral pain, palpable mass, and hematuria, but these are seen in only 10% of cases. The most reliable of the three is hematuria, but it is usually intermittent and may be microscopic; thus, the tumor may remain silent until it attains a large size. At this time, it gives rise to generalized constitutional symptoms, such as fever, malaise, weakness, and weight loss. This pattern of asymptomatic growth occurs in many patients, so the tumor may have reached a diameter of more than 10 cm when it is discovered.

One of the common characteristics of this tumor is its tendency to metastasize widely before giving rise to any local symptoms or signs. In 25% of new patients with renal cell carcinoma, there is radiologic evidence of metastases at the time of presentation. The most common locations of metastasis are the lungs (more than 50%) and bones (33%), followed in order by the regional lymph nodes, liver and adrenals, and brain.

268. Ans. (c) Nodular glomerulosclerosis *Ref: Robbins Pathologic Basis of Disease 7th ed. p 991*

Diabetic nephropathy (nephropatia diabetica), also known as Kimmelstiel-Wilson syndrome, or nodular diabetic glomerulosclerosis and intercapillary glomerulonephritis, is a progressive kidney disease caused by angiopathy of capillaries in the kidney glomeruli. It is characterized by nephrotic syndrome and diffuse glomerulosclerosis. It is due to longstanding diabetes mellitus, and is a prime indication for dialysis in many Western countries. It is classified as a microvascular complication of diabetes.

Section C Maharahstra/Manipal/PGI

269. Ans. (d) All of the above *Ref: Harsh Mohan Textbook of Pathology 6th ed. p 662*

Feature	*Acute nephritic syndrome*	*Nephrotic syndrome*
• Proteinuria	Mild (< 3 gm per 24 hrs)	Heavy (> 3 gm per 24 hrs)
• Hypoalbuminaemia	Uncommon	Present
• Oedema	Mild, in loose tissue	Marked, generalised peripheral
• Mechanism of oedema	Na^+ and water retention	↓ Plasma osmotic pressure, Na^+ and water retention
• Haematuria	Present, microscopic	Absent
• Hypertension	Present	Present in advanced disease
• Hyperlipidaemia	Absent	Present
• Lipiduria	Absent	Present
• Oliguria	Present	Present in advanced disease
• Hypercoagulability	Absent	Present

270. Ans. (b) Bence jones proteins *Ref: http://medical-dictionary.thefreedictionary.com/Bence+Jones+protein+test*

A routine urinalysis will not detect Bence Jones proteins. There are several methods used by laboratories to detect and measure these proteins. The classic Bence Jones reaction involves heating urine to 140°F (60°C). At this temperature, the Bence Jones proteins will clump. The clumping disappears if the urine is further heated to boiling and reappears when the urine is cooled. Other clumping procedures using salts, acids, and other chemicals are also used to detect these proteins. These types of test will reveal whether or not Bence Jones proteins are present, but not how much is present. This protein is seen in multiple myeloma.

FEMALE GENITAL TRACT

271. Ans. (d) Hormonal study *Ref: Hum Reprod 2000;15(12):2478-2482.*

Prediction of Ovulation by Urinary Hormone Measurements with the home use ClearPlan® Fertility Monitor: Comparison with Transvaginal Ultrasound Scans and Serum Hormone Measurements

The luteinizing hormone is always present in urine and increases 24-48 hours prior to ovulation. The LH surge triggers ovulation, which is the release of an egg from one of your ovaries. Ovulation is the most fertile time of the cycle. Ovulation tests are approximately 99% accurate in detecting the LH surge. The WHO funded subsequent studies in order to evaluate the measurement of urinary hormones as a simple, reliable method to predict ovulation and determine the limits of the potentially fertile period. Oestrone-3-glucuronide was selected as the urinary oestrogen metabolite that best predicted the start of the potentially fertile period and was shown quantitatively to be the most important parameter (Branch et al., 1982). Urinary LH was chosen as the best method for predicting imminent ovulation (WHO, 1983).

ENDOCRINE SYSTEM

272. Ans. (b) Hyperthyroidism *Ref: Harsh Mohan Textbook of Pathology 6th ed. p 802*

Clinical features: Patients with hyperthyroidism have a slow and insidious onset, varying in severity from case to case. The usual symptoms are emotional instability, nervousness, palpitation, fatigue, weight loss in spite of good appetite, heat intolerance, perspiration, menstrual disturbances and fine tremors of the outstretched hands. Cardiac manifestations in the form of tachycardia, palpitations and cardiomegaly are invariably present in hyperthyroidism. The skin of these patients is warm, moist and flushed. Weakness of skeletal muscles and osteoporosis are common. Typical eye changes in the form of exophthalmos are a common feature in Graves' disease. Serum levels of T3 and T4 are elevated but TSH secretion is usually inhibited. A sudden spurt in the severity of hyperthyroidism termed 'thyroid storm' or 'thyroid crisis' may occur in patients who have undergone subtotal thyroidectomy before adequate control of hyperthyroid state, or in a hyperthyroid patient under acute stress, trauma, and with severe infection. These patients develop high grade fever, tachycardia, cardiac arrhythmias and coma and may die of congestive heart failure or hyperpyrexia.

273. Ans. (b) Hypothyroidism *Ref: Harsh Mohan Textbook of Pathology 6th ed. p 803*

Growth hormone deficiency, diabetes mellitus and oestrogen deficiency are all related with obesity except hypothyroidism.

274. Ans. (b) Hyperthyroidism

Refer explanation 272

275. Ans. (a) Adrenal medulla *Ref: Robbins Pathologic Basis of Disease 7th ed. p 1219*

The most important diseases of the adrenal medulla are neoplasms, which include neoplasms of chromaffin cells (pheochromocytomas) and neuronal neoplasms (including neuroblastomas and more mature ganglion cell tumors).

Pheochromocytoma: Pheochromocytomas are uncommon neoplasms composed of chromaffin cells, which synthesize and release catecholamines and in some instances peptide hormones. These tumors are important because they (similar to aldosterone secreting adenomas) give rise to surgically correctable forms of hypertension. Although only about 0.1% to 0.3% of hypertensive patients have an underlying pheochromocytoma, the hypertension can be fatal when the pheochromocytoma goes unrecognized.

Pheochromocytomas usually subscribe to a convenient 'rule of 10s':

- 10% of pheochromocytomas arise in association with one of several familial syndromes. These include the MEN-2A and MEN-2B syndromes, type I neurofibromatosis, von Hippel-Lindau syndrome, and Sturge-Weber syndrome.
- 10% of pheochromocytomas are extra-adrenal, occurring in sites such as the organ of Zuckerkandl and the carotid body, where these chromaffin-negative tumors are usually called paragangliomas to distinguish them from pheochromocytomas.
- 10% of nonfamilial adrenal pheochromocytomas are bilateral; this figure may rise to 70% in cases that are associated with familial syndromes.
- 10% of adrenal pheochromocytomas are biologically malignant, although the associated hypertension represents a serious and potentially lethal complication of even 'benign ' tumors. Frank malignancy is somewhat more common (20% to 40%) in tumors arising in extra-adrenal sites.
- 10% of adrenal pheochromocytomas arise in childhood, usually the familial subtypes, and with a strong male preponderance. The nonfamilial pheochromocytomas most often occur in adults between 40 and 60 years of age, with a slight female preponderance.

276. Ans. (c) Hypothyroidism

Refer explanation 273

277. Ans. (a) Addison's disease *Ref: Harsh Mohan Textbook of Pathology 6th ed. p 798*

Primary chronic adrenocortical insufficiency (Addison's Disease) Progressive chronic destruction of more than 90% of adrenal cortex on both sides results in an uncommon clinical condition called Addison's disease.

Clinical features: Clinical manifestations develop slowly and insidiously. The usual features are as under:

- Asthenia, i.e. progressive weakness, weight loss and lethargy as the cardinal symptoms.
- Hyperpigmentation, initially most marked on exposed areas, but later involves unexposed parts and mucous membranes as well.
- Arterial hypotension.
- Vague upper gastrointestinal symptoms, such as mild loss of appetite, nausea, vomiting and upper abdominal pain.
- Lack of androgen causing loss of hair in women.
- Episodes of hypoglycaemia.
- Biochemical changes include reduced GFR, acidosis, hyperkalaemia and low levels of serum sodium, chloride and bicarbonate.

278. Ans. (c) RIA *Ref: Obstet Gynecol. 1985 Apr;65(4):545-9.*

Use of an immunoradiometric assay and a radioimmunoassay for the detection of free beta-human chorionic gonadotropin.

Radioimmunoassay (RIA) is a very sensitive in vitro assay technique used to measure concentrations of antigens (for example, hormone levels in the blood) by use of antibodies. An immunoradiometric assay and a radioimmunoassay (RIA) are used to quantitate human chorionic gonadotropin (hCG) in the serum of pregnant women. It is also used to detect testicular or gestational trophoblastic neoplasia.

279. Ans. (a) Large tongue *Ref: Harsh Mohan Textbook of Pathology 6th ed. p 793*

Hyperfunction of anterior pituitary: Three common syndromes of adenohypophyseal hyperfunction are: Gigantism and acromegaly, hyperprolactinaemia and Cushing's syndrome.

Gigantism and acromegaly: Both these clinical syndromes result from sustained excess of growth hormone (GH), most commonly by somatotroph (GH-secreting) adenoma.

Gigantism: When GH excess occurs prior to epiphyseal closure, gigantism is produced. Gigantism, therefore, occurs in prepubertal boys and girls and is much less frequent than acromegaly. The main clinical feature in gigantism is the excessive and proportionate growth of the child. There is enlargement as well as thickening of the bones resulting in considerable increase in height and enlarged thoracic cage.

Acromegaly: Acromegaly results when there is overproduction of GH in adults following cessation of bone growth and is more common than gigantism. The term 'acromegaly' means increased growth of extremities (acro=extremity). There is enlargement of hands and feet, coarseness of facial features with increase in soft tissues, prominent supraorbital ridges and a more prominent lower jaw which when clenched results in protrusion of the lower teeth in front of upper teeth (prognathism). Other features include enlargement of the tongue and lips, thickening of the skin and kyphosis. Sometimes, a few associated features such as TSH excess resulting in thyrotoxicosis, and gonadotropin insufficiency causing amenorrhoea in the females and impotence in the male, are found.

280. Ans. (a) Hyperthyroidism

Refer explanation 272

281. Ans. (a) Hyperparathyroidism *Ref: Harsh Mohan Textbook of Pathology 6th ed. p 835*

The brown tumor is a bone lesion that arises in settings of excess osteoclast activity, such as hyperparathyroidism. It is not a true neoplasm, as the term 'tumor' suggests; however, it may mimic a true neoplasm. Brown tumours consist of fibrous tissue, woven bone and supporting vasculature, but no matrix. The osteoclasts consume the trabecular bone that osteoblasts lay down and this front of reparative bone deposition followed by additional resorption can expand beyond the usual shape of the bone, involving the periosteum thus causing bone pain. Haemosiderin-laden macrophages and multinucleate giant cells appear at the areas of haemorrhages producing an appearance termed as 'brown tumour' or 'reparative giant cell granuloma of hyperparathyroidism' requiring differentiation from giant cell tumour or osteoclastoma. However, the so-called brown tumours, unlike osteoclastoma, are not true tumours but instead regress or disappear on surgical removal of hyperplastic or adenomatous parathyroid tissue.

282. Ans. (b) Parathyroid hormone related protein (PTHrP) *Ref: Robbins Pathologic Basis of Disease 7th ed. p 1184*

Hypercalcemia is one of a number of changes induced by elevated levels of PTH. Hypercalcemia is a relatively common complication of malignancy, occurring both with solid tumors, such as lung, breast, head and neck, and renal cancers, and with hematologic malignancies, notably multiple myeloma. In fact, malignancy is the most common cause of clinically apparent hypercalcemia, while primary hyperparathyroidism is a more common cause of asymptomatic elevated blood calcium. The prognosis of patients with malignancy-associated hypercalcemia is generally poor, in that it more frequently occurs in individuals with advanced cancers. Hypercalcemia of malignancy is due to increased bone resorption and subsequent release of calcium. There are two major mechanisms by which this can occur:

- Osteolytic metastases and local release of cytokines and
- Release of PTH-related protein (PTHrP).

283. Ans. (b) Elevation after complete therapy suggests recurrence in well differentiated thyroid malignancies

Ref: http://en.wikipedia.org/wiki/Thyroglobulin#Clinical_significance

Thyroglobulin levels in the blood are mainly used as a tumor marker for certain kinds of thyroid cancer (particularly papillary or follicular thyroid cancer). Thyroglobulin is not produced by medullary or anaplastic thyroid carcinoma. Circulating thyroglobulin has a half-life of 65 hours. Following thyroidectomy, it may take many weeks before thyroglobulin levels become undetectable. After thyroglobulin levels become undetectable following thyroidectomy, levels can be serially monitored. A subsequent elevation of the thyroglobulin level is an indication of recurrence of papillary or follicular thyroid carcinoma.

Section C Maharashtra/Manipal/PGI

284. Ans. (d) Sleep

Refer explanation of 272

285. Ans. (d) Exophthalmic goiter *Ref: http://en.wikipedia.org/wiki/Graves%27_disease#History*

- Graves' disease has also been called exophthalmic goiter.
- Less commonly, it has been known as Parry's disease, Begbies' disease, Flajani's disease, Flajani-Basedow syndrome, and Marsh's disease.

286. Ans. (a) Ketosis

287. Ans. (a) Medullary carcinoma of thyroid *Ref: Harsh Mohan Textbook of Pathology 6th ed. p 814*

Calcitonin: It may be used diagnostically as a tumor marker for medullary thyroid cancer, in which high calcitonin levels may be present and elevated levels after surgery may indicate recurrence. It may even be used on biopsy samples from suspicious lesions (e.g. lymph nodes that are swollen) to establish whether they are metastasis of the original cancer.

SKIN

288. Ans. (a) UVA *Ref: http://en.wikipedia.org/wiki/Ultraviolet_light_and_cancer#Harmful_Effects_on_Skin*

There are three different types of ultraviolet light UVA, UVB and UVC

- **UVA**: Ultraviolet A light has the longest wavelengths. The length of these waves ranges from 400-315 nanometers
- **UVB**: Ultraviolet B light has wavelengths shorter than UVA. The waves range from 315-280 nanometers
- **UVC**: Ultraviolet C light is the shortest of the three UV lights. The wavelengths range from 280-100 nanometers

Type of ultraviolet	*Types of cancer*	*Treatability*	*Absorbed by ozone?*
UVA	Melanoma	**(Often fatal)**	No
UVB	Squamous cell cancer skin cancer	Easily treatable	Yes

UVA rays are 95% of the ultraviolet light on earth. Most people are exposed to large amounts of UVA radiation in their lifetime. UVA rays penetrate the skin deeper than any other UV rays, it can cause the skin to age and wrinkle much faster. Just recently studies have been able to link it to skin cancer. In the basal skin layer of the epidermis there are skin cells called keratinocytes. When the keratinocytes are exposed to UVA radiation the rays can cause damage to the basal layer where most skin cancer can occur. UVA rays are the main tanning ray for tanning the skin, when exposed these rays cause damage over time. When the skin is exposed to UVA the skin darkens as it defense to prevent more damage to the DNA. A tan is just an injury to the skin's DNA. THis can cause mutations which lead to skin cancer.

BONES, JOINTS, AND SOFT-TISSUE TUMORS

289. Ans. (a) Bence Jones proteins *Ref: Refer explanation 11*

Refer explanation 11

290. Ans. (a) Ground-glass density *Ref: Robbins Pathologic Basis of Disease 7th ed. p 1300*

Fibrous dysplasia is a benign tumor that has been likened to a localized developmental arrest; all of the components of normal bone are present, but they do not differentiate into their mature structures. The lesions appear in three distinctive but sometimes overlapping clinical patterns:

- Involvement of a single bone (monostotic);
- Involvement of multiple, but never all, bones (polyostotic) and
- Polyostotic disease, associated with cafe au lait skin pigmentations and endocrine abnormalities, especially precocious puberty. Radiographically this lesion shows ground glass appearance.

291. Ans. (a) Type 4 *Ref: http://en.wikipedia.org/wiki/Collagen#Types_and_associated_disorders*

- Types of collagen

Type	*Notes*	*Disorders*
I	This is the most abundant collagen of the human body. It is present in scar tissue, the end product when tissue heals by repair. It is found in tendons, skin, artery walls, cornea, the endomysium of myofibrils, fibrocartilage, and the organic part of bones and teeth.	Osteogenesis imperfecta, Ehlers-Danlos syndrome, infantile cortical hyperostosis aka Caffey's disease

Contd...

Contd...

Type	*Notes*	*Disorders*
II	Hyaline cartilage, makes up 50% of all cartilage protein. Vitreous humour of the eye.	Collagenopathy, types II and XI
III	This is the collagen of granulation tissue, and is produced quickly by young fibroblasts before the tougher type I collagen is synthesized. Reticular fiber. Also found in artery walls, skin, intestines and the uterus.	Ehlers-Danlos syndrome, Dupuytren's contracture
IV	Basal lamina; eye lens. Also serves as part of the filtration system in capillaries and the glomeruli of nephron in the kidney.	Alport syndrome, Goodpasture's syndrome
V	Most interstitial tissue, assoc. with type I, associated with placenta	Ehlers-Danlos syndrome (classical)
VI	Most interstitial tissue, assoc. with type I, cartilage	Ulrich myopathy, Bethlem myopathy, Atopic dermatitis[40]
VII	Forms anchoring fibrils in dermoepidermal junctions	Epidermolysis bullosa dystrophica
VIII	Some endothelial cells	Posterior polymorphous corneal dystrophy 2
IX	FACIT collagen, cartilage, assoc. with type II and XI fibrils	EDM2 and EDM3
X	Hypertrophic and mineralizing cartilage	Schmid metaphyseal dysplasia
XI	Cartilage	Collagenopathy, types II and XI
XII	FACIT collagen, interacts with type I containing fibrils, decorin and glycosaminoglycans	—
XV	—	—
XVI	—	—
XVII	Transmembrane collagen, also known as BP180, a 180 kDa protein	Bullous pemphigoid and certain forms of junctional epidermolysis bullosa

In addition to the above-mentioned disorders, excessive deposition of collagen occurs in scleroderma.

292. Ans. (c) Increase in osteoid maturation time *Ref: Robbins Pathologic Basis of Disease 7th ed. p 455, 1287*

Rickets and osteomalacia represent a group of diseases of divergent causes that are characterized by a defect in matrix mineralization, most often related to a lack of vitamin D or some disturbance in its metabolism. The term rickets refers to the disorder in children in which deranged bone growth produces distinctive skeletal deformities. In the adult, the disorder is called osteomalacia because the bone that forms during the remodeling process is undemineralized. This results in osteopenia and predisposition to insufficiency fractures. In adults, the lack of vitamin D deranges the normal bone remodeling that occurs throughout life. The newly formed osteoid matrix laid down by osteoblasts is inadequately mineralized, thus producing the excess of persistent osteoid characteristic of osteomalacia.

293. Ans. (c) Multiple myeloma *Ref: Robbins Pathologic Basis of Disease 7th ed. p 679. http://en.wikipedia.org/wiki/Multiple_myeloma#Signs_and_symptoms*

Multiple myeloma (from Greek myelo-, marrow), also known as plasma cell myeloma or Kahler's disease, is a cancer of plasma cells, a type of white blood cell normally responsible for producing antibodies. In multiple myeloma, collections of abnormal plasma cells accumulate in the bone marrow, where they interfere with the production of normal blood cells. Most cases of myeloma also feature the production of a paraprotein an abnormal antibody which can cause kidney problems. Bone lesions and hypercalcemia (high blood calcium levels) are also often encountered. Myeloma develops in 14 per 100,000 people per year. It is more common in men. The peak age of incidence of multiple myeloma is between 50 and 60 years Because many organs can be affected by myeloma, the symptoms and signs vary greatly. Amnemonic sometimes used to remember the common symptoms of multiple myeloma is CRAB: C = Calcium (elevated), R = Renal failure, A = Anemia, B = Bone lesions. Myeloma has many other possible symptoms, including opportunistic infections (e.g. pneumonia.) CRAB symptoms and proliferation of monoclonal plasma cells in the bone marrow are part of the diagnostic criteria of multiple myeloma.

294. Ans. (a) Purine metabolism *Ref: Harsh Mohan Textbook of Pathology 6th ed. p 453*

Gout is a disorder of purine metabolism manifested by the following features, occurring singly or in combination:

- Increased serum uric acid concentration (hyperuricaemia).
- Recurrent attacks of characteristic type of acute arthritis in which crystals of monosodium urate monohydrate may be demonstrable in the leucocytes present in the synovial fluid.
- Aggregated deposits of monosodium urate monohydrate (tophi) in and around the joints of the extremities.
- Renal disease involving interstitial tissue and blood vessels.
- Uric acid nephrolithiasis.

The disease usually begins in 3rd decade of life and affects men more often than women. A family history of gout is present in a fairly large proportion of cases indicating role of inheritance in hyperuricaemia. Clinically, the natural history of gout comprises 4 stages: asymptomatic hyperuricaemia, acute gouty arthritis, asymptomatic intervals of intercritical periods, and chronic tophaceous stage. In addition, gout nephropathy and urate nephrolithiasis may occur.

295. Ans. (a) Smooth muscle *Ref: Harsh Mohan Textbook of Pathology 6th ed. p 867*

Rhabdomyoma and rhabdomyosarcoma are the benign and malignant tumours respectively of striated muscle. Rhabdomyoma is a rare benign soft-tissue tumour. It should not be confused with glycogen-containing lesion of the heart designated as cardiac rhabdomyoma which is probably a hamartomatous lesion and not a true tumour. Soft-tissue rhabdomyomas are predominantly located in the head and neck, most often in the upper neck, tongue, larynx and pharynx.

296. Ans. (b) Osteitis deformans *Ref: Robbins Pathologic Basis of Disease 7th ed. p 1285*

Paget Disease (Osteitis Deformans)

This unique skeletal disease can be characterized as a collage of matrix madness. At the outset, Paget disease is marked by regions of furious osteoclastic bone resorption, which is followed by a period of hectic bone formation, and then finally the bone cell activity becomes markedly diminished. This repetitive and overlapping sequence forms the basis for dividing Paget disease into:

(1) An initial osteolytic stage, followed by (2) a mixed osteoclastic-osteoblastic stage, which ends with a predominance of osteoblastic activity and evolves ultimately into (3) a burnt-out quiescent osteosclerotic stage. The histologic hallmark is the mosaic pattern of lamellar bone. This pattern, which is likened to a jigsaw puzzle, is produced by prominent cement lines that anneal haphazardly oriented units of lamellar bone.

297. Ans. (b) Plasmacytoma on tissue biopsy

Ref: http://en.wikipedia.org/wiki/Multiple_myeloma#Diagnostic_criteria

In 2003, the International Myeloma Working Group agreed on diagnostic criteria for symptomatic myeloma, asymptomatic myeloma and MGUS (monoclonal gammopathy of undetermined significance), which was subsequently updated in 2009:

- **Symptomatic myeloma:**
  - Clonal plasma cells >10% on bone marrow biopsy or (in any quantity) in a biopsy from other tissues (plasmacytoma)
  - A monoclonal protein (paraprotein) in either serum or urine (except in cases of true non-secretory myeloma)
  - Evidence of end-organ damage felt related to the plasma cell disorder (related organ or tissue impairment, ROTI, commonly referred to by the acronym 'CRAB'):
- Hypercalcemia (corrected calcium >2.75 mmol/L)
- Renal insufficiency attributable to myeloma
- Anemia (hemoglobin <10 g/dL)
- Bone lesions (lytic lesions or osteoporosis with compression fractures) recurrent infections alone in a patient who has none of the CRAB features is not sufficient to make the diagnosis of myeloma. Patients who lack CRAB features but have evidence of amyloidosis should be considered as amyloidosis and not myeloma. CRAB like abnormalities are common with numerous diseases, and it is imperative that these abnormalities are felt to be directly attributable to the related plasma cell disorder and every attempt made to rule out other underlying causes of anemia, renal failure, etc.
- **Asymptomatic/smouldering myeloma:**
  - Serum paraprotein >30 g/L and/or
  - Clonal plasma cells >10% on bone marrow biopsy and
  - No myeloma-related organ or tissue impairment
- **Monoclonal gammopathy of undetermined significance (MGUS):**
  - Serum paraprotein <30 g/L and
  - Clonal plasma cells <10% on bone marrow biopsy and
  - NO myeloma-related organ or tissue impairment Related conditions include solitary plasmacytoma (a single tumor of plasma cells, typically treated with irradiation), plasma cell dyscrasia (where only the antibodies produce symptoms, e.g. AL amyloidosis), and POEMS syndrome (peripheral neuropathy, organomegaly, endocrinopathy, monoclonal plasma cell disorder, skin changes).

298. Ans. (b) Growth continues after skeletal maturity *Ref: Robbins Pathologic Basis of Disease 7th ed. p 1296*

Osteochondroma, also known as an exostosis, is a benign cartilage-capped outgrowth that is attached to the underlying skeleton by a bony stalk. Clinically, osteochondromas present as slow-growing masses, which can be painful if they impinge on a nerve or if the stalk is fractured. In many cases, they are detected as an incidental finding. In multiple hereditary exostosis, the underlying bones may be bowed and shortened, reflecting an associated disturbance in epiphyseal growth. Osteochondromas usually stop growing at the time of growth plate closure. Rarely (<1% of cases), they give rise to a chondrosarcoma or some other type of sarcoma.

299. Ans. (c) Decreasing the osteoclast mediated resorption of bone

Ref: http://en.wikipedia.org/wiki/Bisphosphonate

Bisphosphonates are a class of drugs that prevent the loss of bone mass, used to treat osteoporosis and similar diseases. They are the most commonly prescribed drugs used to treat osteoporosis. They are called bisphosphona tes because they have two phosphonate (PO3) groups and are similar in structure to pyrophosphate. Evidence shows that they reduce the risk of osteoporotic fracture in those who have had previous fractures. Bone undergoes constant turnover and is kept in balance (homeostasis) by osteoblasts creating bone and osteoclasts destroying bone. Bisphosphonates inhibit the digestion of bone by encouraging osteoclasts to undergo apoptosis, or cell death, thereby slowing bone loss. The uses of bisphosphonates include the prevention and treatment of osteoporosis, osteitis deformans ('Paget's disease of bone'), bone metastasis (with or without hypercalcaemia), multiple myeloma, primary hyperparathyroidism, osteogenesis imperfecta, fibrous dysplasia, and other conditions that feature bone fragility.

300. Ans. (a) Fluorosis *Ref: Robbins Pathologic Basis of Disease 7th ed. p 1283*

- Categories of generalized osteoporosis,

Primary	
Postmenopausal Senile	Idiopathic
Secondary **Endocrine disorders** Hyperparathyroidism Hypo-hyperthyroidism Hypogonadism Pituitary tumors Diabetes, type 1 Addison disease	**Rheumatologic disease** **Drugs** Anticoagulants Chemotherapy Corticosteroids Anticonvulsants Alcohol
Neoplasia Multiple myeloma Carcinomatosis **Gastrointestinal** Malnutrition Malabsorption Hepatic insufficiency Vitamin C, D deficiencies	**Miscellaneous** Osteogenesis imperfecta Immobilization Pulmonary disease Homocystinuria Anemia

301. Ans. (d) Aneurysmal bone cyst *Ref: Harsh Mohan Textbook of Pathology 6th ed. p 839*

Aneurysmal bone cyst, true to its name, is an expanding osteolytic lesion filled with blood (aneurysm = dilatation, distension). When FNAC is performed on this lesion it is inconclusive because only blood cells are seen in cytology. Hence, definite diagnosis cannot be given from FNAC.

302. Ans. (d) Simple bone cyst *Ref: http://en.wikipedia.org/wiki/Bone_cyst*

The simple bone cyst is a common, benign, fluid-containing lesion, most commonly found in the metaphysis of long bones, typically the proximal humerus or femur. Pathologic fractures are common, often with minor trauma. These cysts typically resolve after skeletal maturity and not typically associated with bone tumors. The cause is unknown. These were first recognised as a distinct entity in 1910. Jaffe and Lichtenstein provided a detailed discussion of simple bone cysts in 1942. These cysts appear centrally and never eccentrically.

303. Ans. (c) Renal osteodystrophy *Ref: Radiology, February 200, Volume 230, Issue 2 (RSNA)*

The rugger jersey spine sign is said to be almost diagnostic of the osteosclerosis associated with secondary hyperparathyroidism of chronic renal failure. The major skeletal components of renal osteodystrophy that can be seen on radiographs include osteomalacia, osteosclerosis, and soft-tissue calcification. At radiography, sclerotic bands along the superior and inferior thoracic and lumbar vertebral body endplates give a striped appearance to the vertebral bodies, with a relative band of lucency at the center of each vertebral body. The alternating parallel sclerotic and lucent bands are analogous to the stripes on an English rugby sweater, from which arises the name 'rugger jersey spine'. The opaque sclerotic bands seen on the inferior and superior endplates of vertebral bodies represent accumulations of excess osteoid. Although they are deficiently mineralized, the areas of osteoid appear opaque at radiography because of their increased volume in comparison with that of normal bone. The spinal canal and intervertebral disk spaces are normal.

304. Ans. (d) Systemic lupus erythematosus *Ref: Robbins Pathologic Basis of Disease 7th ed. p 227*

The American College of Rheumatology (ACR) established eleven criteria in 1982, which were revised in 1997 as a classificatory instrument to operationalise the definition of SLE in clinical trials. They were not intended to be used to diagnose individuals and do not do well in that capacity. For the purpose of identifying patients for clinical studies, a person has SLE if any 4 out of 11 symptoms are present simultaneously or serially on two separate occasions. Useful mnemonic for remembering the diagnostic findings or symptoms of SLE is SOAP BRAIN MD (S=serositis, O=oral ulcers, A=arthritis, P=photosensitivity, pulmonary fibrosis, B=blood cells, R=renal, Raynauds, A=ANA, I=immunologic (anti-Sm, anti-dsDNA), N=neuropsych, M=malar rash, D=discoid rash), however, not in order of diagnostic importance.

- Malar rash (rash on cheeks); sensitivity = 57%; specificity = 96%.
- Discoid rash (red, scaly patches on skin that cause scarring); sensitivity = 18%; specificity = 99%
- Serositis: Pleurisy (inflammation of the membrane around the lungs) or pericarditis (inflammation of the membrane around the heart); sensitivity = 56%; specificity = 86% (pleural is more sensitive; cardiac is more specific).
- Oral ulcers (includes oral or nasopharyngeal ulcers); sensitivity = 27%; specificity = 96%.
- Arthritis: nonerosive arthritis of two or more peripheral joints, with tenderness, swelling, or effusion; sensitivity = 86%; specificity = 37%.
- Photosensitivity (exposure to ultraviolet light causes rash, or other symptoms of SLE flareups); sensitivity = 43%; specificity = 96%.
- Blood hematologic disorder hemolytic anemia (low red blood cell count) or leukopenia (white blood cell count<4000/µl), lymphopenia (<1500/µl) or thrombocytopenia (<100000/µl) in the absence of offending drug; sensitivity = 59%; specificity = 89%. Hypocomplementemia is also seen, due to either consumption of C3 and C4 by immune complex-induced inflammation or to congenitally complement deficiency, which may predispose to SLE.
- Renal disorder: More than 0.5 g per day protein in urine or cellular casts seen in urine under a microscope; sensitivity = 51%; specificity = 94%.
- Antinuclear antibody test positive; sensitivity = 99%; specificity = 49%.
- Immunologic disorder: Positive anti-Smith, anti-ds DNA, antiphospholipid antibody, and/or false positive serological test for syphilis; sensitivity = 85%; specificity = 93%. Presence of anti-ss DNA in 70% of cases (though also positive with rheumatic disease and healthy persons).
- Neurologic disorder: Seizures or psychosis; sensitivity = 20%; specificity = 98%.

Other than the ACR criteria, people with lupus may also have:
- Fever (over 100°F)
- Extreme fatigue
- Hair loss
- Fingers turning white and/or blue when cold (Raynaud's phenomenon)

305. Ans. (d) Hydroxyproline *Ref: Menopause by Rogerio p 290*

Hydroxyproline is the marker for bone resorption

PERIPHERAL NERVE AND SKELETAL MUSCLE

306. Ans. (a) Neuron *Ref: http://scienceline.ucsb.edu/getkey.php?key=1710*

It does seem weird that we can't replace nerve cells that get damaged. The answer is basically that having nerve cells reproduce can do more harm than good. Each nerve cell has a specific place in our nervous system. Its job is all about taking a signal from one specific place to another one. Adding new nerve cells would mess up these very specific connections in a very complex system. So, we trade off the ability to repair our nerves in order to avoid messing up connections.

CENTRAL NERVOUS SYSTEM

307. Ans. (a) A normal patient with normal verbal and eye response and obeys full commands
Ref: http://en.wikipedia.org/wiki/Glasgow_Coma_Scale

- Glassgow Coma Scale

	1	2	3	4	5	6
Eye	Does not open eyes	Opens eyes in response to painful stimuli	Opens eyes in response to voice	Opens eyes spontaneously	N/A	N/A
Verbal	Makes no sounds	Incomprehensible sounds	Utters inappropriate words	Confused, disoriented	Oriented, converses normally	N/A
Motor	Makes no movements	Extension to painful stimuli (decerebrate response)	Abnormal flexion to painful stimuli (decorticate response)	Flexion/ withdrawal to painful stimuli	Localizes painful stimuli	Obeys commands

The scale is composed of three tests: eye, verbal and motor responses. The three values separately as well as their sum are considered. The lowest possible GCS (the sum) is 3 (deep coma or death), while the highest is 15 (fully awake person). Individual elements as well as the sum of the score are important. Hence, the score is expressed in the form 'GCS 9 = E2 V4 M3 at 07:35'.

Generally, brain injury is classified as:
- Severe, with GCS < 8-9
- Moderate, GCS 8 or 912 (controversial)
- Minor, GCS ≥ 13.

Generally when a patient is in a decline of their GCS score, the nurse or medical staff should assess the cranial nerves and determine which of the twelve have been affected.

308. Ans. (c) Muscle twitching *Ref: http://en.wikipedia.org/wiki/Intracranial_pressure#Signs_and_symptoms*

In general, symptoms and signs that suggest a rise in ICP including headache, vomiting without nausea, ocular palsies, altered level of consciousness, back pain and papilledema. If papilledema is protracted, it may lead to visual disturbances, optic atrophy, and eventually blindness. The headache is classically a morning headache which may wake them from sleep. The brain is relatively poorly supplied by oxygen as a result of mild hypoventilation during the sleeping hours, and also cerebral oedema may worsen during the night due to the lying position. The headache is worse on coughing/sneezing/bending, and progressively worsens over time. There may also be personality or behavioral changes. In addition to the above, if mass effect is present with resulting displacement of brain tissue, additional signs may include pupillary dilatation, abducens palsies, and the Cushing's triad. Cushing's triad involves an increased systolic blood pressure, a widened pulse pressure, bradycardia, and an abnormal respiratory pattern. In children, a low heart rate is especially suggestive of high ICP. Irregular respirations occur when injury to parts of the brain interfere with the respiratory drive. Cheyne-Stokes respiration, in which breathing is rapid for a period and then absent for a period, occurs because of injury to the cerebral hemispheres or diencephalon. Hyperventilation can occur when the brain stem or tegmentum is damaged. As a rule, patients with normal blood pressure retain normal alertness with ICP of 2540 mm Hg (unless tissue shifts at the same time). Only when ICP exceeds 4050 mm Hg do CPP and cerebral perfusion decrease to a level that results in loss of consciousness. Any further elevations will lead to brain infarction and brain death. In infants and small children, the effects of ICP differ because their cranial sutures have not closed. In infants, the fontanels, or soft spots on the head where the skull bones have not yet fused, bulge when ICP gets too high. Papilledema, or the swelling of the optic disc, can be a reliable sign that ICP is elevated. Unlike other conditions that may result in the swelling of the optic disc, it is in the case of papilledema that vision may go largely unaffected.

309. Ans. (a) Flumazenil *Ref: Harrisons Principles of Internal Medicine, 18th ed. p 3554*

Flumazenil (Anexate) is a competitive benzodiazepine receptor antagonist that can be used as an antidote for benzodiazepine overdose. A specific antagonist for benzodiazepines, flumazenil at 0.2 mg/mincan be given to a maximum of 3 g/h, but it may precipitate seizures and increase intracranial pressure. Like naloxone, administration for a prolonged period is usually required since most benzodiazepines remain active for considerably longer than flumazenil.

310. Ans. (d) 15

Refer explanation of chapter 28 Q 307

311. Ans. (b) Petit mal epilepsy *Ref: http://en.wikipedia.org/wiki/Absence_seizure#Signs_and_symptoms*

Absence seizures are one of several kinds of seizures. These seizures are sometimes referred to as petit mal seizures (from the French for 'little illness', a term dating from the late 18th century). Absence seizures are characterized by a brief loss and return of consciousness not followed by a period of lethargy (post-ictal state). Impairment of consciousness is the essential symptom, and may be the only clinical symptom, but this can be combined with other manifestations. The hallmark of the absence seizures is abrupt and sudden-onset impairment of consciousness, interruption of ongoing activities, a blank stare, possibly a brief upward rotation of the eyes. If the patient is speaking, speech is slowed or interrupted; if walking, he or she stands transfixed; if eating, the food will stop on its way to the mouth. Usually, the patient will be unresponsive when addressed. In some cases, attacks are aborted when the patient is called. The attack lasts from a few seconds to half a minute, and evaporates as rapidly as it commenced. Absence seizures generally are not followed by a period of disorientation or lethargy (post-ictal state), this is in contrast to the majority of seizure disorders. Mixed forms of absence frequently occur. These seizures can happen a few times a day or in some cases hundreds of times a day, to the point that the person cannot concentrate in school or other situations requiring sustained, concentrated attention.

312. Ans. (a) Exposure and response prevention

Ref: http://en.wikipedia.org/wiki/Obsessive%E2%80%93compulsive_disorder#Management

This patient is suffering from obsessive compulsive disorder. Obsessive compulsive disorder (OCD) is an anxiety disorder characterized by intrusive thoughts that produce uneasiness, apprehension, fear, or worry; by repetitive behaviors aimed at reducing the associated anxiety; or by a combination of such obsessions and compulsions. Behavioral therapy (BT), cognitive behavioral therapy (CBT), and medications are first- line treatments for OCD. The specific technique used in BT/CBT is called exposure and ritual prevention (also known as 'exposure and response prevention') or ERP; this involves gradually learning to tolerate the anxiety associated with not performing the ritual behavior. Exposure ritual/response prevention (ERP) has a strong evidence base. It is considered the most effective treatment for OCD.

313. Ans. (b) Skinner *Ref: http://psychology.about.com/od/behavioralpsychology/a/introopcond.htm*

Operant conditioning was coined by behaviorist B.F. Skinner, which is why you may occasionally hear it referred to as Skinnerian conditioning. As a behaviorist, Skinner believed that internal thoughts and motivations could not be used to explain behavior. Instead, he suggested, we should look only at the external, observable causes of human behavior.

314. Ans. (c) In upper dorsal lesion of pons, ipsilateral sensory loss of face is present

Ref: Neurology Secrets by Joseph p 119

In upper dorsal lesion of pous, ipsilateral paralysis of muscle of mastication and sensory loss of face occurs.

EYE

315. Ans. (c) Cavernous haemangioma *Ref: http://www.ncbi.nlm.nih.gov/books/NBK13668/*

The most common benign orbital tumor of adults is the cavernous hemangioma (in contrast to the capillary hemangioma for children). Patients have slowly progressive painless proptosis with a mass indenting the globe, showing striae in the retina and a flattened globe on imaging studies. Treatment is surgical, and complete removal is possible. Other well-circumscribed lesions include neurofibromas, schwannomas, hemangiopericytomas, meningioma, and gliomas.

6 Microbiology

GENERAL MICROBIOLOGY

1. Which of the following is not used as a disinfectant? *(AIIMS Nov 2010, 2009)*
a. 12% cetrimide
b. 100% alcohol
c. 2% lysol
d. 5% chlorhexidine

2. Which one of the following is true? *(AIIMS May 2009)*
a. Agar has nutrient properties
b. Chocolate medium is a selective medium
c. Addition of selective substances in a solid medium is called enrichment medium
d. Nutrient broth is a basal medium

3. Phase-contrast microscopy is based on: *(AIIMS Nov 2009)*
a. Difference in refractive index
b. Difference in reflective index
c. Difference in scattering of light between objects
d. Difference in reflection of light between objects

4. For sterilization efficiency determination, the control used is: *(AIPG 2008)*
a. Spores of harmless bacteria
b. Spores of clostridium tetani
c. Viruses
d. None of the above

5. Microorganisms that grow best at a temperature of 2540°C are termed as: *(AIPG 2008)*
a. Thermophilic b. Cryophilic
c. Mesophilic d. None of the above

6. Which of the following regions is responsible for antibody activity?: *(AIPG 2008)*
a. Light-chain constant
b. Light-chain variable
c. Heavy-chain constant
d. Heavy-chain variable

7. Blood spills in the hospital are disinfected with: *(AIPG 2007)*
a. Quaternary ammonium compounds
b. Sodium hypochlorite
c. Plain soap and water
d. Cetavlon

8. Which of the following have maximum resistance to disinfection and antiseptics?
a. Spores *(AIIMS Nov 2012, AIPG 2013)*
b. Prions
c. Mycoplasma
d. Virus

9. Sterlization means: *(AIPG 2013)*
a. Kills all living organism in a specific environment
b. Kills all pathogenic organism
c. Deactivate the pathogenic organism but not spores
d. Deactive the spores and only pathogenic organism

10. The indicator used in autoclave is: *(AIPG 2013)*
a. Bacillus subtilis varniger
b. Clostridium tetani
c. Bacillus pumilus
d. Bacillus stearothermophilus

11. Sterlization by sunlight is effective because of: *(AIPG 2012)*
a. High wavelength light
b. Low wavelength light
c. Ultraviolet rays
d. Presence of ozone in atmosphere

12. Sterlization is: *(AIPG 2012)*
a. Deactivating all pathogenic and nonpathogenic organisms but not spores
b. Killing of all organisms
c. Killing of pathogenic organisms
d. Killing of all organisms and spores

13. Capsule of bacteria: *(AIPG 2012)*
a. Prevent their phagocytosis
b. Virulence
c. Provides oxygen
d. Not recalled

14. The efficacy of the moist-heat sterilization technique commonly used to sterilize laboratory ware and culture media is tested by using: *(COMED 2013, 2007, KCET 2009, 2006)*
a. Clostridium tetani spores
b. T-Even-Bacteriophages
c. Bacillus sterothermophilus spores
d. Browne's tubes

15. Cold sterilization refers to the process of sterilization by use of: *(COMED 2009)*
a. Ultraviolet rays
b. Ultrasonic vibrations
c. Infrared rays
d. Gamma rays

16. The major enzyme responsible for oxidative killing mechanism in neutrophils is: *(COMED 2009)*
a. Antioxidant
b. Lysozyme
c. Hypochlorous acid
d. Superoxide

17. Bacteria that grow best at temperatures below 20°C are called: *(COMED 2006)*
a. Mesophillic
b. Psychrophillic
c. Thermophillic
d. Microaerophillic

18. Glasswares are sterilized by: *(COMED 2006)*
a. Autoclaving b. Hot air oven
c. Incineration d. Formaldehyde

19. Negative staining is used to demonstrate: *(COMED 2006)*
a. Bacterial spores
b. Bacterial flagella
c. Bacterial capsule
d. Bacterial fimbriae

20. Bacteria acquire characteristics by all the following *except*: *(COMED 2006)*
a. Through plasmids
b. Incorporating part of host DNA
c. Through bacteriophages
d. Through conjugation

21. Sterlization by moist heat is used in: *(KCET 2007)*
a. Autoclave b. Hot air oven
c. Filters d. Incineration

22. Antiseptic technique in surgery was first introduced by: *(KCET 2007)*
a. Joseph Lister
b. Louis Pastuer
c. Robert Koch
d. Antony Van Leeuwenhoek

23. Which component of the cell was is responsible for endotoxic activity: *(KCET 2007)*
a. Region I
b. Region II
c. Region III
d. Boivin antigen

24. Lophotrichous flagella are seen in: *(KCET 2006)*
a. Spirilla
b. Vibrio
c. Pseudomonas
d. Kliebsiella

25. Microscope is invented by: *(KCET 2006)*
a. Louis Pasteur
b. Hippocrates
c. Robert Koch
d. Leeuwen Hoeck

26. Plasmid is transmitted to other bacteria in:
a. Transformation
b. Transduction
c. Conjugation
d. All of the above

©27. The temperature and pressure at which spores are killed during sterilization by autoclave are: *(KCET 2005)*
a. 102°C temp and pressure is 8 lb/sq. inch for 10 mins
b. 105°C temp and pressure is 15 lb/sq. inch for 12 mins
c. 110°C temp and pressure is 4 lb/sq. inch for 5 mins
d. 121°C temp and pressure is 151 lb/sq. inch for 12 mins

28. Monotrichous, lophotrichous, amphitrichous, peritrichous. These are all types of _______ in anatomy of the bacterial cell: *(KCET 2013)*
a. Flagella b. Ribosomes
c. Mesosomes d. None of the above

29. Which of the following fulfill all the criterias of Koch's postulates? *(KCET 2013)*
a. Treponema pallidum
b. Mycobacterium leprae
c. N. gonorrhoea
d. None of the above

30. Amongst the following which is an anaerobic media: *(MH 2011)*
a. Sabourad's medium
b. Robertson's cooked meat medium
c. Staurt's medium
d. Mcleod's medium

31. Most effective disinfectant/antiseptic against spores are: *(MH 2011)*
a. Gluteraldehyde
b. Iodophores
c. Alcohol
d. Chlorhexidine

32. Most common mode of drug resistance transfer in Gram-negative organism is by: *(MH 2012)*
a. Conjugation
b. Mutation
c. Transduction
d. Transformation

33. Solid culture medium for tuberculosis? *(MH 2012)*
a. Dubos
b. Pawlowsky
c. Lowenstein-Jensen medium
d. Loeffler

IMMUNOLOGY

34. Autoinfection is seen with: *(AIIMS May 2011)*
a. Ascaris lumbricoides
b. Strongyloides
c. Giardiasis
d. Gnathostoma

35. Which of the following investigations should be done immediately to best confirm a nonmatched blood transfusion reaction? *(AIIMS Nov 2010)*
a. Indirect Coomb's test
b. Direct Coomb's test
c. Antibody in patient's serum
d. Antibody in donor's serum

36. A rabbit is injected with horse serum. Two weeks later it is again injected with the same serum in the skin. The type of necrotizing skin reaction observed at the site of the second injection is:
a. Atopy *(AIIMS Nov 2010, 2008)*
b. Anaphylactic reaction
c. Serum sickness
d. Arthus reaction

37. Main function of T cells is: *(AIIMS Nov 2008)*
a. Lymphokine production and delayed hypersensitivity
b. Antigen-antibody reaction (complement activation)
c. Anaphylaxis (immediate hypersensitivity)
d. Antibiotic production

38. Which of the following immunoglobulin shows the maximum amount of immunoglobulin after secondary humoral immune response? *(AIIMS Nov 2006)*
a. IgG b. IgM
c. IgA d. IgD

39. The immunoglobulin used in the preparation of caries vaccine for the prevention of dental caries is: *(AIIMS Nov 2006)*
a. IgG b. IgA
c. IgM d. IgD

40. Heat-labile instruments for use in surgical procedures can be sterilized by: *(AIIMS May 2006)*
a. Absolute alcohol
b. Ultraviolet rays
c. Chlorine-releasing compounds
d. Ethylene oxide gas

41. Interleukins and growth factors are: *(AIIMS Nov 2005)*
a. Cytokines b. Lipoxins
c. Enzymes d. Hormones

42. The cell type that lacks in human leukocyte antigen (HLA) antigen is: *(AIIMS Nov 2005)*
a. Monocyte b. Thrombocytes
c. Neutrophil d. Red blood cells

43. The following methods of diagnosis utilize labelled antibodies, *except*: *(AIIMS May 2005)*
a. Enzyme-linked immunosorbent assay (ELISA)
b. Hemagglutination inhibition test
c. Radioimmunoassay
d. Immunofluorescence

44. Both CMI and humoral immunity are best elicited by: *(AIPGEE 2011)*
a. Polysaccharide antigen
b. Protein antigen
c. Lipid antigen
d. Adjuvant

45. Natural immunity against viruses is provided by: *(AIPG 2008)*
a. Natural killer cells
b. B cells
c. Helper T cells
d. Cytotoxic T cells

46. Which of the following human IgG subclass has maximum serum concentration? *(AIPG 2005)*
a. IgG1 b. IgG2
c. IgG3 d. IgG4

47. Which of the following immunoglobulins mediates type I hypersensitivity? *(AIPG 2005)*
a. IgA b. IgG
c. IgM d. IgE

48. NK cells act on interferon virus because: *(AIIMS Nov 2012)*
a. Expression of MHC I on cell surface receptor
b. Non-expression of MHC I on cell surface receptor
c. Expression of MHC II on cell surface receptor
d. Non-expression of MHC II on cell surface receptor

49. Patients with severe allergic reactions such as anaphylaxis require immediate therapy with: *(COMED 2013)*
a. Glucocorticoids b. Antihistamines
c. Epinephrine d. Moropine

50. Anaphylaxis refers to? *(COMED 2011)*
a. Severe reaction following re-injection of protein solutions in a sensitized individual
b. Severe reaction following primary injection of protein solutions
c. State of immunity developed by repeated injections of any foreign substance
d. The severe reaction resulting from sensitivity to common allergies

51. Alternative pathway of complement activation begin with: *(COMED 2010, AIPG 2013)*
a. C1
b. C2
c. C3
d. C5

52. The immunoglobulin which crosses placenta is: *(COMED 2010, 2009, KCET 2006)*
a. IgM b. IgA
c. IgG d. IgD

53. Which statement is true about Lyme disease? *(COMED 2010)*
a. Caused by Borrelia Vincenti
b. Transmitted by flea bite
c. Diagnosed by demonstration of specific IgM antibody
d. Etiological agent can be grown in modified Kelley's medium

54. Which one of the following does not present antigens? *(COMED 2010)*
a. NK cells
b. Dendritic cells
c. Langerhans cells
d. Macrophages

55. Tissue graft rejection can be prevented by suppression of: *(COMED 2009)*
a. Plasma antibodies
b. T-cell
c. Allergy producing mast cells and basophils
d. Macrophages

56. Antibiotic sensitivity and resistance of microorganisms is determined by: *(COMED 2009)*
a. Direct microscopy
b. Culture
c. ELISA
d. DNA probe

57. The term epitope refers to: *(COMED 2009)*
a. Compete antigen molecule
b. Hapten
c. Immunogen
d. Smallest antigenic determinant

58. In primary immune deficiency, the fraction of plasma protein reduced is: *(COMED 2008)*
a. Alpha 1 globulin
b. Alpha 2 globulin
c. Beta globulin
d. Gamma globulin

59. The following immunoglobulin is not known to fix complement: *(COMED 2007)*
a. IgE b. IgM
c. IgA d. IgG

60. Out of the following hypersensitivity reactions, in which type a single dose of the antigen can act as both the sensitizing and shocking dose: *(KCET 2011)*

a. Anaphylaxis
b. Arthus reaction
c. Serum sickness
d. Contact dermatitis

61. Negative phase is seen in ________immunity: *(KCET 2010)*

a. Active b. Passive
c. Herd d. Local

62. The cells which produce antibodies are: *(COMED 2006)*

a. Plasma cells b. Helper T cells
c. Macrophage d. Natural killer cells

63. Type of immunological response in transplant rejection is: *(COMED 2006)*

a. Type I b. Type II
c. Type III d. Type IV

64. Erythroblastosis foetalis can be prevented if the mother is injected, at parturition, with an antibody called: *(COMED 2005)*

a. Blocking antibody
b. Rh (D) immunoglobulin
c. Antilymphocyte globulin
d. Antilymphocyte serum

65. A test that can be used for typing of Type I histocompatibility antigens is: *(COMED 2005)*

a. Cell mediated lempholysis (CML)
b. Donor-recipient mixed lymphocyte response
c. Primed lymphocyte typing
d. Antibody and complement mediated cytotoxicity

66. The earliest identifiable cells of T-cell lineage during maturation are: *(KCET 2008)*

a. CD7 + Pro T cells
b. CD4 + Pre T cells
c. CD8 + Pro T cells
d. CD8 + Pre T cells

67. An immunoglobulin has only been found in mammals:

a. IgA
b. IgE
c. IgM
d. IgG

68. The same or closely related antigens may sometimes occur in different biological species class or kingdom is known as ___.

a. Self antigen
b. Organ specific antigen
c. Isoantigen
d. Heterophile antigen

69. Mediated immediate hypersensitivity reaction are called allergy:

a. IgG
b. IgM
c. IgE
d. IgA

70. Which of the following promote the growth of T-lymphote?

a. MHC I
b. MHC II
c. Both
d. None

71. Reaction of particulate antigen with its antibody is: *(MH 2009)*

a. Neutralization
b. Agglutination
c. Precipitation
d. Complement fixation

72. Direct Coombs test detects: *(MH 2014)*

a. Antigen in serum
b. Antibodies on RBC surface
c. Antigen on RBC surface
d. Antibodies in serum

BACTERIOLOGY

73. Gas gangrene is caused by all, *except*: *(AIIMS May 2011)*

a. Clostridium histolyticum
b. Clostridium novyi
c. Clostridium septicum
d. Clostridium sporogenes

74. Culture media of leptospirosis is: *(AIIMS May 2011)*

a. Korthof b. Perkin
c. Tinsdale d. Baker's

75. Which of the following is microaerophilic? *(AIIMS May 2011)*

a. Campylobacter b. Vibrio
c. Bacteriodes d. Pseudomonas

76. All of the following statements about *Staphylococcus aureus* are true, *except*: *(AIIMS Nov 2010)*
a. Most common source of infection is cross-infection from infected people
b. About 30% of population is healthy nasal carriers
c. Epidermolysis and TSS toxins are super antigens
d. Methicillin resistance is chromosomally mediated

77. Which of the following is not a part of Koch's postulate? *(AIIMS Nov 2010, 2008)*
a. Bacteria may or may not cause disease in experimental animals
b. Bacteria should be isolated from the diseased animals
c. Bacteria should be cultivable outside the animal
d. Bacteria should be able to cause the same disease or condition when inoculated in another animal

78. About pseudomonas, all are true, *except*: *(AIIMS Nov 2010, 2009)*
a. Strict aerobe
b. Can grow in disinfectant in hospital
c. Infection is mostly due to endogenous source
d. Most common organism in burn patient

79. About *Neisseria gonorrhoeae*, all are true, *except*: *(AIIMS Nov 2010, 2009)*
a. Most common cause of urethritis in males
b. All strains are susceptible to penicillin G
c. Some strains are found in disseminated form
d. Found exclusively in human beings

80. About bacteroids all are true, *except*: *(AIIMS Nov 2010, 2009)*
a. Susceptible to most of the antibiotics
b. Present mainly in mixed infection
c. Most common species is *B. fragilis*
d. Bile-resistant anaerobes

81. All are true about Widal test, *except*: *(AIIMS Nov 2010, 2009)*
a. Baseline differs depending on the endemicity of disease
b. O antibodies last longer and hence are not an indicator of recent infection
c. **H antigen** cannot differentiate between subtypes
d. **high** titer value in a single **widal test is not** confirmative

82. Average number of bacteria present in saliva is: *(AIIMS Nov 2010)*
a. 500 million/mL
b. 750 million/mL
c. 850 million/mL
d. 900 million/mL

83. A farmer presents with pustules, which show Gram-positive cocci on smear culture. The organisms show beta hemolysis and are catalase negative. To show that the identified organism is Group A streptococci, which of the following test should be done? *(AIIMS May 2010)*
a. Bacitracin sensitivity
b. Optochin sensitivity
c. Novobiocin sensitivity
d. Bile solubility

84. A young male patient presented with urinary tract infection (UTI). On urine examination, pus cells were detected but no organisms were found. Which method would be best for culture? *(AIIMS May 2010)*
a. McCoy culture
b. Thayer-Martin medium
c. LJ medium
d. Levinthal medium

85. Which of the following is true about endemic typhus? *(AIIMS May 2010)*
a. Man is the only reservoir of infection
b. Flea is a vector of the disease
c. A rash developing into an eschar is characteristic of the disease
d. Culture is the diagnostic modality

86. Which of the following organism produces a toxin that acts by adenylate cyclase? *(AIIMS May 2010)*
a. Vibrio cholerae
b. Shigella
c. Corynebacterium
d. E. coli

87. Brucella is transmitted by all, *except*: *(AIIMS May 2010)*
a. Through the placenta of animals
b. Aerosol transmission
c. Person to person
d. Eating uncooked food

88. Culture was done on a child with infective skin lesions of the leg, which showed Gram-positive cocci in chains and hemolytic colonies. Which of the following tests will best identify the organism? *(AIIMS May 2009)*

a. Bile solubility
b. Optochin sensitivity
c. Catalase positive
d. Bacitracin sensitivity

89. Which of the following is not true of Vibrio cholera? *(AIIMS May 2009)*

a. It is halophilic
b. It grows on simple media
c. Man is the only natural host
d. It can survive outside human intestine

90. An elderly male patient is presented with fever, chest pain and dry cough. Sputum culture showed growth of charcoal yeast extract medium. The organism is: *(AIIMS May 2009)*

a. H. influenza
b. Moraxella catarrhalis
c. Legionella
d. Burkholderia cepacia

91. Five friends had eaten outside at a restaurant at 2 p.m. by 6 p.m., all of them began feeling sick and three of them started vomiting. The food sample was procured and sent to a laboratory for investigation. The sample tested positive for Bacillus cereus that were present in the rice. Which of the following could possibly explain this? *(AIIMS May 2008)*

a. The bacteria multiplied in the intestinal tract
b. The spores of the bacteria multiplied in the intestinal tract
c. The heat-stable toxin was present in the food when stored at room temperature, which caused the symptoms
d. Bacteria were not involved

92. Lancefield classification is based on:

a. M protein *(AIIMS May 2008, AIPG 2007)*
b. Carbohydrate C antigen
c. Cell-wall peptidoglycan
d. T protein

93. The most commonly used selective medium for S. mutans is: *(AIIMS Nov 2007)*

a. MacConkey's medium
b. MSA
c. Nutrient agar
d. Tellurite medium

94. A 60-year-old man is diagnosed to be suffering from legionnaire's disease after he returns from attending a convention. He could have acquired it: *(AIIMS May 2006)*

a. From a person suffering from the infection while travelling in an aeroplane
b. From a chronic carrier in the convention center
c. From inhalation of the aerosols in an air-conditioned room at a convention center
d. By sharing an infected towel with a fellow delegate at the convention

95. The most common microorganism causing subacute bacterial endocarditis (SABE) after oral surgical procedure is: *(AIIMS May 2006, AIPG 2011, 2009)*

a. S. viridans
b. S. mutans
c. S. aureus
d. S. albus

96. Which one of the following is not a method of isolation of Chlamydia from clinical specimens? *(AIIMS Nov 2005)*

a. Yolk sac inoculation
b. Blood agar
c. Tissue culture using irradiated McCoy cells
d. Tissue culture using irradiated BHK cells

97. All of the following statements are true with reference to mycoplasma, *except*: *(AIIMS Nov 2005)*

a. That they are inhibited by penicillin
b. That they can reproduce in cell-free media
c. That they have an affinity for mammalian cell membranes
d. That they can pass through filters of 450 nm pore size

98. All are true about Bordetella pertussis, *except*: *(AIPGEE 2011)*

a. Infection with pertussis induces temporary natural immunity
b. At present no antitoxins are available
c. Cause disease in adults who have taken vaccine in childhood
d. The acellular vaccine is associated with high incidence of neurological symptoms

99. True statement regarding Donovanosis is: *(AIPGEE 2011)*
a. Caused by Calymmatobacterium
b. Painful ulcers
c. It contains Donovan bodies
d. Spreads by blood transmission

100. All of the following are STDs, *except*: *(AIPGEE 2011)*
a. Herpes b. Scabies
c. Candida d. Mycobacterium leprae

101. One of the following is true about tetanus acquired through traumatic wound: *(AIPGEE 2011)*
a. Clostridium tetani travels via the nerves to the anterior horn cells in the spinal cord
b. The tetanospasmin component of the exotoxin acts on the postsynaptic neurons and prevents impulse transmission
c. The patient should be given antitoxin intravenously
d. The presence of Clostridium tetani in the wound can be identified by a positive Nagler reaction

102. Which one of following is included in probiotics? *(AIPGEE 2010)*
a. E. coli
b. Bifidobacteria
c. Diphtheria
d. All of the above

103. Untrue about leptospirosis? *(AIPGEE 2010)*
a. Drug of choice is penicillin G
b. IgM antibody detectable in 5 days
c. Mortality is 515% in severe cases
d. Incubation period is 10 days

104. Which of the following is true about mycobacterium other than tuberculosis (MOTT)? *(AIPG 2009)*
a. It causes disseminated infection
b. It occurs in person with normal immunity
c. MOTT infection interferes with protection given by BCG results
d. Person to person transmission is seen

105. Gram-positive cocci that produce greenish colonies are bile insoluble and when given intraperitoneally in mice do not produce the symptoms: *(AIPG 2008)*
a. S. mitis
b. S. pyogens
c. S. pneumoniae
d. S. aureus

106. S. viridans can be distinguished from other streptococci by: *(AIPG 2008)*
a. Culture
b. Fermentation of mannitol and sorbitol
c. Hemolysis on blood agar
d. All of the above

107. Lactobacillus is a carcinogenic bacteria because: *(AIPG 2008)*
a. It is acidogenic and aciduric
b. It is most abundant in saliva
c. It is the only acidogenic bacteria in the oral cavity
d. None of the above

108. All of the following are true about Yersinia pestis, *except*: *(AIPG 2007)*
a. That it shows pleomorphic appearance
b. That it is a Gram-positive organism that forms endotoxins
c. That it is easily destroyed by exposure to heat, sunlight and drying
d. That it is nonmotile, nonsporing bacillus

109. A veterinary doctor had pyrexia of unknown origin (PUO) after handling cattles. His blood culture in special laboratory media was positive for Gram-negative short bacilli, which were oxidase positive. Which of the following organism is likely to be detected in the culture? *(AIPG 2006)*
a. Yersinia spp.
b. Francisella spp.
c. Bartonella spp.
d. Brucella spp.

110. Which one of the following statements is true regarding the pathogenicity of mycobacterial species? *(AIPG 2006)*
a. M. tuberculosis is more pathogenic than M. bovis to the humans
b. M. kansas can cause a disease indistinguishable from tuberculosis
c. M. africana infection is acquired from the environmental source
d. M. marinum is responsible for tubercular lymphadenopathy

111. All of the following organisms are known to survive intracellularly, *except*: *(AIPG 2005)*
a. Neisseria meningitides
b. Salmonella typhi
c. S. pyogenes
d. Legionella pneumophila

112. The condition that has been associated with the three 'Rs', i.e. rats, ricefields and rainfall, is: *(AIPG 2005)*

a. Leptospirosis b. Plague
c. Melioidosis d. Rodent-bite fever

113. Legionnaire's disease false is: *(AIIMS May 2012)*

a. Ab in urine is diagnostic
b. Waterborne disease
c. Can infect amoeba intracellularly
d. Human to human transmission is seen

114. With reference to bacteroides fragilis, the following statements are true *except*: *(AIIMS Nov 2012)*

a. B. fragilis is most frequent anaerobe from clinical sample from GI tract
b. B. fragilis is not uniformly sensitive to metronidazole
c. Lipopolysaccharide formed by B. fragilis is structurally and functionally different from conventional endotoxin
d. Shock and DIC are common in bacteroides bacteremia

115. The only organism associated with pyrexia of unknown origin: *(AIIMS Nov 2013)*

a. Salmonella type
b. Salmonella paratype
c. Brucella
d. Mycobacterium tuberculosis

116. Endotoxin of which Gram negative bacteria doesn't participate in natural defence mechanism: *(AIIMS Nov 2013)*

a. E. coli b. M. tuberculosis
c. V. cholera d. Klebsiella

117. The urine sample of a patient has been sent to the laboratory to look for leptospira. The specimen is to be screened by use of the: *(COMED 2013)*

a. Scanning microscope
b. Inverted microscope
c. Dark ground microscope
d. Electron microscope

118. The tissue and pus aspirate is to be collected for diagnosis of Gas gangrene. It should ideally be transported using: *(COMED 2013)*

a. Buffered glycerol saline
b. Todd-Hewin broth
c. Robertson's cooked meat medium
d. Hanks balanced salt solution

119. The most frequent nonsporing anaerobic bacilli isolated from clinical specimens is: *(COMED 2014, 2011)*

a. Bacteroides fragilis
b. Clastridium tetani
c. Prevotella melaninogenica
d. Fusobacterium nucleatum

120. Infection with Helicopter pylori is associated with: *(COMED 2014)*

a. Acute gastritis
b. Chronic gastritis
c. Eosinophillic gastritis
d. Recurrent esophagitis

121. Most commonly used treponemal test in diagnosis of syphilis is: *(COMED 2014)*

a. Treponema pallidum immobilization (TPI)
b. Treponema pallidum immune adherence (TPIA)
c. Treponema pallidum Haeagglutination (TPHA)
d. Fluoroscent treponemal antibody absorption test (FTA ABS)

122. Which one of the following enteric organisms is anaerogenic and nonmotile? *(COMED 2012)*

a. Shigella sonnel
b. Salmonella typhi
c. Proteus mirabilis
d. Klebsiella pneumonia

123. Which of the following agents of gas gangrene is capsulated? *(COMED 2012)*

a. Cl. septicum
b. Cl. novyi
c. Cl. perfingens
d. Cl. histolyticum

124. Pseudomonas aeruginosa? *(COMED 2011)*

a. Produces heat stable enterotoxin
b. Causes Shangai fever
c. Cannot be destroyed at 55 degrees at 1 hour
d. Does not produce any pigment

125. Pathogenesis of diptheria is attributed to? *(COMED 2011, 2009)*

a. Invasion b. Endotoxin
c. Exotoxin d. Capsule

126. Kveim Siltzbach test is useful in the diagnosis of: *(COMED 2009)*

a. Tuberculosis b. Sarcoidosis
c. Leprosy d. Cat scratch disease

127. **Streptococcus mutans produces an adhesive polymer from sucrose known as:** *(COMED 2009)*
a. Levans b. Lectins
c. Glucans d. Polyfructans

128. **Erysipelas is caused by:** *(COMED 2007)*
a. Group B staphylococci
b. Group A streptococci
c. Gonococci
d. Pneumococci

129. **In which phase of the bacterial growth curve involution forms of the bacteria can be observed?** *(KCET 2011)*
a. Lag phase b. Log phase
c. Stationary phase d. Phase of decline

130. **Ziehl Neelsen's staining is routinely performed from sputum samples for the detection of:** *(KCET 2011)*
a. Mycobacterium tuberculosis
b. Bacillus anthracis
c. Streptococcus pneumoniae
d. Mycoplasma pneumonia

131. **Which of the following organisms does not react with gram's stain?** *(KCET 2011)*
a. Actinomyces israelii
b. Candida albicans
c. Mycobacterium tuberculosis
d. Streptococcus mutans

132. **Xylitol is a low caloric sweetener which inhibits the growth of:** *(KCET 2010)*
a. S. mutans
b. S. pyogens
c. Lactobacillus
d. Actinomycosis

133. **Mycobacterium tuberculosis is best demonstrated by:** *(KCET 2009)*
a. Gram's stain
b. H and E stain
c. Zeihl and Neelsen stain
d. PAS stain

134. **The process of attenuation can be achieved by all *except*:** *(KCET 2009)*
a. Growing bacteria in adverse environment
b. Growing bacteria in unconventional host
c. Serial passage in an experimental host
d. Repeated cultures in artificial media

135. **The spirochete which is associated with fuso-spirochetosis is:** *(KCET 2009)*
a. Treponema pallidum
b. Treponema pertenue
c. Borrellia burgdorferi
d. Borrelia vincenti

136. **The cell wall deficient bacteria is:** *(KCET 2009, 2008)*
a. Rickettsiae b. Mycoplasma
c. Chlamydiae d. Ehrlichiae

137. **Actinomycosis is caused by:** *(COMED 2006)*
a. Virus b. Bacteria
c. Fungus d. Unknown factor

138. **Polypeptide capsule is seen in:** *(COMED 2006)*
a. Corynebacterium diptheriae
b. Clostridium welchii
c. Staphylococcus aureus
d. Bacillus anthracis

139. **Lowenstein-Jensen medium is selectively used to cultivate:** *(KCET 2008)*
a. Vibrio cholera
b. Mycobacterium tuberculosis
c. Salmonella typhi
d. Treponema pallidum

140. **Endotoxin is released from:** *(KCET 2008)*
a. C. albicans.
b. S. sanguis
c. GM negative bacteria
d. Actinomyces viscosus

141. **Gas gangrene is not caused by:** *(KCET 2006)*
a. Clostridium wechii
b. Clostridium septicum
c. Clostridium emotines
d. Clostridium tetani

142. **Diphtheria toxin acts by:** *(KCET 2006)*
a. Increasing levels of cramps
b. Inhibiting protein synthesis
c. Inhibiting acetyl choline release
d. Inhibiting glucose transport

143. **Rice water stools are seen in infections with:** *(KCET 2005)*
a. Proteus
b. Shigella
c. Vibrio cholera
d. Salmonella

144. Which of the following statement is true in the case of endotoxins? *(KCET 2013)*

a. Highly antigenic
b. Protein in nature
c. Heat stable
d. Action is often enzymatic

145. Impetigo is the staphylococcus infection of the: *(KCET 2013)*

a. Skin　b. Ear
c. Floor of the mouth　d. Eye

146. Actinomycosis is a: *(KCET 2012)*

a. Aerobic bacterial disease
b. Anaerobic bacterial disease
c. Aerobic fungal disease
d. Anaerobic fungal disease

147. Kolmer test is a screening test done for: *(KCET 2012)*

a. Syphilis　b. Tuberculosis
c. Conorrhea　d. Lymphoma

148. Transport medium for typhoid bacilli is: *(MH 2009)*

a. Bile broth　b. Selenite broth
c. Tetrathionate broth　d. All of the above

149. Bacteria which release both exotoxin and endotoxin are: *(MH 2010)*

a. C. diphtheria
b. U. tetani
c. Actinobacillus actinomycetem comitans
d. Streptococcus pyogenes

150. Which of the following stain is used in cat scratch disease for staining bacilli? *(MH 2012)*

a. Acid fast stain
b. PTAH
c. Gram stain
d. Warthin-Starry silver stain

151. Clostridium tetani are following type of bacteria: *(MH 2014)*

a. Spore bearing aerobes
b. Nonsporing aerobes
c. Sporebearing anaerobes
d. Nonsporing anaerobes

VIROLOGY

152. Dentist after suffering from jaundice due to hepatitis B has recovered since 3 months, but is not allowed to practice by medical board as he is a: *(AIIMS Nov 2009)*

a. Paradoxical carrier
b. Convalescent carrier
c. Healthy carrier
d. Inactive carrier

153. Infectious mononucleosis is caused by:

a. EBV *(AIIMS Nov 2008, AIPG 2010, KCET 2007)*
b. Herpes simplex virus (HSV)
c. CMV
d. Hantavirus

154. Bacteria are different from viruses in that the latter lead to the production of: *(AIIMS May 2008)*

a. Interferons (IFNs)　b. Endotoxins
c. Exotoxins　d. Colicins

155. Acute hepatitis B infection can be diagnosed by all of the following, *except*: *(AIIMS May 2008)*

a. The presence of hepatitis B surface Ab
b. The presence of hepatitis B surface Ag
c. The presence of IgM Ab to the core Ag
d. The presence of DNA polymerase

156. The tissue of the origin of the Kaposi's sarcoma is: *(AIIMS May 2005)*

a. Lymphoid　b. Vascular
c. Neural　d. Muscular

157. Dengue hemorrhagic fever is caused by: *(AIPGEE 2011)*

a. Virus
b. Mosquito Aedes aegypti
c. Bacteria
d. Ticks

158. With which of following types of viral hepatitis infection in pregnancy, the maternal mortality is the highest: *(AIPGEE 2011)*

a. Hepatitis A　b. Hepatitis B
c. Hepatitis C　d. Hepatitis E

159. Enzyme found in retrovirus is: *(AIPGEE 2010)*

a. Reverse transcriptase
b. RNA polymerase
c. DNA polymerase
d. Topoisomerase

160. The most common malignancy in AIDS is: *(AIPG 2009, COMED 2014)*

a. Kaposi's sarcoma
b. Hodgkin's
c. Squamous cell carcinoma
d. Non-Hodgkin's lymphoma

161. Herpangina is caused by: *(AIPG 2009)*
a. Coxsackievirus b. HSV
c. HBV d. All of the above

162. Which of the following is true? *(AIPG 2009)*
a. Hantavirus spreads by aerosolized infected urine of rodents
b. Lassa virus spreads through tick
c. Marburg virus does not spread from person to person
d. Kyasanur forest disease virus spreads by contaminated rodent excreta

163. Which of the following is the oral manifestation caused by viruses? *(AIPG 2008)*
a. Scarlet fever
b. Herpangina
c. Oral thrush
d. Vincent's angina

164. Which of the following is the characteristic of viruses? *(AIPG 2007)*
a. They are intracellular organisms
b. They affect the production of IFN and are sensitive to it
c. They reproduce by binary fission
d. They can be grown on inanimate media

165. Virus-mediated transfer of host DNA from one cell to another is known as: *(AIPG 2005)*
a. Transduction b. Transformation
c. Transcription d. Integration

166. HIV can be detected and confirmed by: *(AIPG 2005)*
a. Polymerase chain reaction (PCR)
b. ELISA
c. Latex agglutination
d. Dot blot assay

167. Viruses can be isolated from clinical samples by cultivation in the following, *except*: *(AIPG 2005)*
a. Tissue culture
b. Embryonated eggs
c. Animals
d. Chemically defined media

168. About prion true statement is: *(AIIMS May 2012)*
a. Readily inactivated by autoclave at 121°C
b. Evokes strong immunologic reaction
c. Have long incubation period
d. Contains DNA/RNA

169. Virus culture is done on: *(AIIMS Nov 2013)*
a. Embryonated egg
b. Nonembryonated egg
c. Sarboud's agar
d. Blood agar

170. Hepatitis-E virus causes: *(AIPG 2013)*
a. Acute liver failure
b. Cirrhosis
c. Chronic liver failure
d. Chronic renal failure

171. Hep-E is associated with: *(AIPG 2013)*
a. Acute liver failure
b. Acute renal failure
c. Chronic liver failure
d. Epidemics

172. Culture media for viruses: *(AIPG 2013)*
a. Sabourads agar
b. Nonembryonated hen's eggs
c. Embryonated hen's eggs
d. Blood agar

173. Which of these is not an oncogenic virus?
a. Human papillomavirus *(COMED 2013)*
b. Cytomegalovirus
c. Epstein-Barr virus
d. Hepatitis B virus

174. Indicator of viral replication in Hepatitis B infection is: *(COMED 2014)*
a. HbsAg b. HbeAg
c. IgM anti-HBc d. Anti-Hbe

175. Which of the following is DNA virus?
a. Hepatitis A virus *(COMED 2014, 2011)*
b. Hepatitis B virus
c. Hepatitis C virus
d. Hepatitis D virus

176. Which virus given below is not a teratogenic virus? *(COMED 2010)*
a. Rubella b. CMV
c. Herpes simplex d. Measles

177. All the following viruses are capable of causing human cancers *except*: *(COMED 2009)*
a. Papilloma virus
b. Hepatitis B virus
c. Epstein barr virus
d. Parvovirus B19

178. Which of the following viruses produces both intranuclear and intracytoplasmic inclusion bodies? *(COMED 2009)*
a. Chicken pox
b. Rabies
c. Small pox
d. Measles

179. Salivary protein which prevents transmission of human immunodeficiency virus via saliva is: *(COMED 2008)*
a. Sialoperoxidase
b. Secretor IgA
c. Salivary leukocyte proteinase inhibitor
d. Rich proteins

180. Which of the following infections are associated with Hodgkin's lymphoma? *(COMED 2008)*
a. Herpes simplex
b. Herpes zoster
c. Herpangina
d. Aphthous ulcer

181. Negri bodies are pathognomonic of: *(COMED 2007)*
a. CMV infection b. HSV infection
c. Poliomyelitis d. Rabies

182. Kaposi's sarcoma is of: *(COMED 2007)*
a. Bacterial origin b. Viral origin
c. Fungal origin d. Radiation origin

183. Western blot test is a confirmatory test used for the diagnosis of: *(KCET 2011)*
a. CMV b. Hepatitis B Virus
c. HIV d. Epstein barr virus

184. A young man presents with jaundice and itching. His viral serology showed active hepatitis E infection. Which of the following is true of hepatitis E? *(KCET 2011)*
a. Chronic hepatitis always occurs
b. Hepatitis E can be prevented by passive immunization
c. Transmission is by feco-oral route
d. Coinfection with hepatitis B is required for pathogenicity

185. Herpes simplex virus binds to epithelium using: *(KCET 2011)*
a. Chondroitin sulphate
b. Heparan sulphate
c. Hyaluronidase
d. Keratin sulphate

186. S4 Dane particle refers to: *(KCET 2009)*
a. Hepatitis A virus
b. Hepatitis B virus
c. Hepatitis C virus
d. Hepatitis E virus

187. Hepatitis C belongs to which one if the following virus groups: *(COMED 2005)*
a. Picorna virus b. Herpes virus
c. Hepadna virus d. Flavi virus

188. Which of the following statement about P24 antigen of HIV is not true? *(KCET 2008)*
a. It can be detected during the window period
b. Free P24 antigen disappears after the appearance of IgM response to it
c. Virus load parallels P24 titer
d. It remains during an asymptomatic phase

189. A health care professional is at maximum danger of a most concerned with developing chronic carrier state of: *(MH 2009)*
a. Hepatitis A b. Hepatitis B
c. Syphilis d. All of the above

190. Common cause of diarrhea in AIDS cases is due to: *(MH 2014)*
a. Plasmodium falciparum
b. Cryptosporidium
c. Ascaris lumbricoides
d. Taenia solium

MYCOLOGY

191. All are dimorphic fungi, *except*: *(AIIMS May 2011)*
a. Histoplasma capsulatum
b. Blastomyces dermatitidis
c. Penicillium marneffei
d. Phialophora verrucosa

192. Which of the following culture media is used for Candida albicans? *(AIIMS Nov 2006, AIPG 2008)*
a. Pongo levin medium
b. Methylene blue medium
c. Sabouraud's agar
d. All of the above

193. Mycotic abscesses are due to: *(AIPG 2006)*
a. Bacterial infection
b. Fungal infection
c. Viral infection
d. Mixed infection

194. Most fungi of medial importance belong to: *(COMED 2012)*

a. Zygomycetes b. Ascomycetes
c. Basidiomycetes d. Deuteromycetes

195. Otomycosis is caused by: *(COMED 2012)*

a. Aspergillus niger
b. Histoplasma capsulatum
c. Rhinosporidium seeberi
d. Crytococcusneoformans

196. Name the fungi which are ovoid or spherical in morphology, produces budding cells and pseudo-hyphae in culture media and in human tissues: *(KCET 2011)*

a. Histoplasma capsulatum
b. Candidia albicans
c. Blastomyces dermatitidis
d. Paracoccidioides brasiliensis

197. Following are the characteristic of Cryptococcus neoformans *except*: *(KCET 2010)*

a. Noncapsulated fungus infecting man
b. Causes meningitis
c. Melanin production related virulence
d. Basidiomycetes yeast

198. The yeast which shows thick gelatinous capsule and positive for mucicarmine is: *(KCET 2010)*

a. Cryptococcus neoformans
b. Histoplasmosis
c. Blastomycosis
d. Paracoccidiomycosis

199. Nonseptae hyphae with a tendency to branch at 90 degree angle is a characteristic of: *(KCET 2009)*

a. Mucor
b. Aspergillosis
c. Cryptococcus neoformans
d. Coccidioides immitis

200. Candial hyphae can be stained using: *(KCET 2007)*

a. Van Gieson's stain
b. Periodic acid schiff stain
c. Masson trichrome stain
d. Toluidine blue stain

201. Rapid evaluation of fungal hyphae/spores can be achieved with: *(KCET 2012)*

a. Grocott Gomari methenamine silver
b. Hematoxylin and eosin
c. KOH wet mount
d. Per iodic acid schiff

PARASITOLOGY

202. Which stage of Plasmodium vivax is infective to mosquito? *(AIIMS Nov 2010, 2009)*

a. Sporozoite b. Gametocyte
c. Merozoite d. Zygote

203. Sleeping sickness vector is *(AIPGEE 2010)*

a. Sandfly b. Tsetse fly
c. Anopheles d. House fly

204. Durck granules are seen in? *(COMED 2011)*

a. Berylliosis b. Sarcoidosis
c. Tuberculosis d. Malaria

205. Which of the following parasite causes auto-infection? *(COMED 2009)*

a. Giardia lamblia b. Isosproa belli
c. Balantidium coli d. Taenia solium

206. Schuffner's dots are seen in infection due to: *(COMED 2010)*

a. Plasmodium falciparum
b. Plasmodium vivax
c. Plasmodium malaria
d. Plasmodium ovale

207. Recurrent epidydimitis is a feature of following infection: *(KCET 2009)*

a. Wuchereria bancrofti b. Ascaris lumbricoides
c. Mumps d. Tuberculosis

208. Donavan bodies are seen in bone marrow and splenic aspiration smears in infection with: *(KCET 2005)*

a. Leishmania donovani
b. Lymphogranuloma venereum
c. Klebsiella pneumonia
d. Heamophilis ducreyi

209. Hydatid cysts are due to infection with: *(KCET 2005)*

a. Hymenilepis nana
b. Diphyllobothrium latum
c. Echinococcus granulosus
d. Ascaris Lumbricoides

210. The following clinical presentation qualify for the term "Severe Falciparum Malaria" *except*: *(MH 2014)*

a. Severe anemia
b. Acidosis
c. Pulmonary edema
d. High grade fever with rigors

MISCELLANEOUS

211. DTP vaccine is not contraindicated in: *(AIIMS Nov 2009)*
a. Immunocompromised patient
b. Progressive neurological disease
c. Severe reaction to first dose or subsequent doses
d. Uncontrolled convulsions

212. Man acts as reservoir of which enteropathogen? *(AIPG 2010)*
a. Entamoeba histolytica
b. Campylobacter jejuni
c. Salmonella
d. Treponema pallidum

213. Adjuvant used in DPT vaccine is: *(AIPG 2009)*
a. Zinc b. Manganese
c. Aluminum d. Copper

214. In the case of anemia due to falciparum which of the following is not seen? *(AIPG 2008)*
a. Hemolysis
b. Malabsorption
c. Splenomegal
d. Bone marrow suppression

215. Laboratory test for the diagnosis of ANUG is: *(AIPG 2008)*
a. Dark field
b. Tissue culture
c. Phase contrast
d. Slide preparation

216. Which of the following is a test for the detection of mRNA? *(AIPG 2008)*
a. Southern blot b. Western blot
c. Northern blot d. Eastern Blot

217. The most common pathogens responsible for nosocomial pneumonias in the ICU are: *(AIPG 2005)*
a. Gram-positive organisms
b. Gram-negative organisms
c. Mycoplasma
d. Virus infections

218. It is true regarding the normal microbial flora present on the skin and mucous membranes that: *(AIPG 2005)*
a. It cannot be eradicated by antimicrobial agents
b. It is absent in the stomach due to the acidic pH
c. It establishes in the body only after the neonatal period
d. The flora in the small bronchi is similar to that of the trachea

219. Following splenectomy in children, which one of the following is recommended? *(COMED 2012)*
a. Hepatitis B vaccination
b. Typhoid vaccination
c. Pneumococcal vaccination
d. Regular follow- up

220. The vaccine currently used against hepatitis B infection is: *(COMED 2012)*
a. Killed pooled serum
b. Live attenuated
c. Recombinant
d. Synthetic vaccine

221. Injection abscess due to use of contaminated vaccines occur in infections caused by? *(COMED 2012)*
a. M. kansasii
b. M. ulcerans
c. M. chelonae
d. M. smegmatis

222. Hospital wastes should ideally be disposed by: *(KCET 2010)*
a. Burial b. Composting
c. Incineration d. Trench method

223. The abundant glycoprotein in the basement membrane and which has binding domain for both ECM and cell-surface receptor is: *(KCET 2010)*
a. Laminin b. Fibronectin
c. Ecadherins d. Tenascin

224. The transmembrane adhesive molecules present in hemidesmosomes which specifically binds to basal lamina glycoprotein laminin are: *(KCET 2010)*
a. Integrin alpha-6 beta-4
b. Catenins desmoplakin
c. Cadherins desmoglein
d. Alpha and Beta catenin

225. Ability of a material to elicit as appropriate biological response in a given application in the body is called: *(KCET 2010)*
a. Biocompatibility
b. Biointegration

c. Antigen-antibody reaction
d. Sensitization

226. The yeast which shows thick gelatinous capsule and positive for mucicarmine is: *(KCET 2010)*
a. Cryptococcus neoformans
b. Histoplasmosis
c. Blastomycosis
d. Paracoccidiomycosis

227. The degradation of P53 through ubiquitous-dependent proteolysis by the binding of high-risk HPV protein is: *(KCET 2010)*
a. E6 and E7 b. E7
c. E6 d. E6, E7 and E8

228. Most common fungus in diabetics is: *(COMED 2006)*
a. Cryptococcus b. Aspergillus
c. Rhodotorula d. Nocardia

229. Collagen contains aminoacid which inhibits alpha-helix formation: *(MH 2010)*
a. Glycine
b. Proline
c. Hydroxy proline
d. Thiamine

230. Which of the following is related to Jarisch-Herxheimer reaction? *(MH 2012)*
a. Interaction of drug and bacterial endotoxins
b. Seen in sulphonamides action
c. Both of the above
d. None of the above

231. A full course of immunization against, tetanus with 3 doses of tetanus toxoid, confers immunity for how many years? *(MH 2012)*
a. 20 b. 10
c. 5 d. 15

Answers with Explanations

GENERAL MICROBIOLOGY

1. Ans. (b) 100% alcohol *Ref: Ananthnarayan, 8th ed. p 36*

Alcohols

Mode of action: Alcohols dehydrate cells, disrupt membranes and cause coagulation of protein.

Examples: Ethyl alcohol, isopropyl alcohol and methyl alcohol.

Application: A 70% aqueous solution is more effective at killing microbes than absolute alcohols. 70% ethyl alcohol (spirit) is used as antiseptic on skin. Isopropyl alcohol is preferred to ethanol. It can also be used to disinfect surfaces. It is used to disinfect clinical thermometers. Methyl alcohol kills fungal spores, hence, is useful in disinfecting inoculation hoods.

Disadvantages: Skin irritant, volatile (evaporates rapidly), inflammable.

ALDEHYDES:

Mode of action: Acts through alkylation of amino-, carboxyl- or hydroxyl group, and probably damages nucleic acids. It kills all microorganisms, including spores.

Examples: Formaldehyde, gluteraldehyde

Application: 40% formaldehyde (formalin) is used for surface disinfection and fumigation of rooms, chambers, operation theatres, biological safety cabinets, wards, sick rooms etc. Fumigation is achieved by boiling formalin, heating paraformaldehyde or treating formalin with potassium permanganate. 2% gluteraldehyde is used to sterilize thermometers, cystoscopes, bronchoscopes, centrifuges, anasethetic equipments, etc.

Disadvantages: Vapors are irritating (must be neutralized by ammonia), has poor penetration, leaves non-volatile residue, activity is reduced in the presence of protein. Gluteraldehyde requires alkaline pH and only those articles that are wettable can be sterilized.

PHENOL:

Mode of action: Act by disruption of membranes, precipitation of proteins and inactivation of enzymes.

Examples: 5% phenol, 1–3% cresol, 2% lysol (a saponified cresol), hexachlorophene, chlorhexidine, chloroxylenol (dettol).

Applications: Joseph Lister used it to prevent infection of surgical wounds. Phenols are coal-tar derivatives. They act as disinfectants at high concentration and as antiseptics at low concentrations. They are bactericidal, fungicidal, mycobactericidal but are inactive against spores and most viruses. They are not readily inactivated by organic matter.. Chlorhexidine can be used in an isopropanol solution for skin disinfection, or as an aqueous solution for wound irrigation. It is often used as an antiseptic hand wash. 20% Chlorhexidine gluconate solution is used for pre-operative hand and skin preparation and for general skin disinfection.

Triclosan is an organic phenyl ether with good activity against Gram-positive bacteria and effective to some extent against many Gram-negative bacteria including pseudomonas. It also has fair activity on fungi and viruses.

Disadvantages: It is toxic, corrosive and skin irritant. Chlorhexidine is inactivated by anionic soaps. Chloroxylenol is inactivated by hard water.

2. Ans. (d) Nutrient broth is a basal medium *Ref: Ananthnarayan, 8th ed. p 39*

Agar

- Approx 2% of agar is used to prepare solid media.
- Agar is derived from the polysaccharide agarose

- It has no nutritive value.
- The growth of bacteria is not affected by it.
- It is hydrolysed at high acid or alkaline ph and high temperature.
- A gelatinous material derived from certain marine algae (seaweeds).
- It is used as a base for bacterial culture media and as a stabilizer and thickener in many food products.
- Melts at 98°C and sets at 42°C

Nutrient broth:

- Nutrient agar is formed when 2% agar is added to nutrient broth
- Nutrient broth is a simple or basal media.
- Nutrient broth is used for the general cultivation of less fastidious microorganisms, can be enriched with blood or other biological fluids.
- Composition:
  - Ingredients Gm/Liter
  - Peptic digest of animal tissue 5.000
  - Sodium chloride 5.000
  - Beef extract 1.500
  - Yeast extract 1.500
  - Final pH (at 25°C) 7.4 ± 0.2

  **Formula adjusted, standardized to suit performance parameters

Enriched media

- When blood, serum or egg is added to the basal media, an enriched media is formed.
- E.g. chocolate agar, egg media and blood agar.

Enrichment media

- An enrichment culture is a medium with specific and known qualities that favors the growth of a particular microorganism.
- The enrichment culture's environment will support the growth of a selected microorganism, while inhibiting the growth of others.
- Tetrathionate broth: Tetrathionate inhibits coliforms and allows typhoidparatyphoid bacilli to grow.
- Selenite F broth: For dysentery bacilli.

3. Ans. (a) Difference in refractive index *Ref: Ananthnarayan, 8th ed. p 12*

- The phase contrast microscopy is based on the principle that rays of slight move at different refractive index.
- The phase contrast moicroscopy amplifies the slight difference in the refractive index in the microbial cells and converts it to a difference in contrast and makes the structure clearly visible within the cells.

4. Ans. (b) Spores of clostridium tetani *Ref: Ananthnarayan, 8th ed. p 32*

Sterilization	*Control organism*
• Autoclave	*Bacillus stearothermophilus*
• Hot air oven	*Clostridium tetani*
• Ionizing radiation	*Bacillus pumilus*
• Ethylene oxide	*Bacillus globigii*

5. Ans. (c) Mesophilic *Ref: Ananthnarayan, 8th ed. p 26*

Temperature ranges of microorganisms

Microorganisms can be grouped into broad (but not very precise) categories, according to their temperature ranges for growth.

- **Psychrophiles** (cold-loving) can grow at 0°C, and some even as low as –10°C; their upper limit is often about 25°C.
- **Mesophiles** grow in the moderate temperature range, from about 20°C (or lower) to 45°C.
- **Thermophiles** are heat-loving, with an optimum growth temperature of 50° or more, a maximum of up to 70°C or more, and a minimum of about 20°C.
- **Hyperthermophiles** have an optimum above 75°C and thus can grow at the highest temperatures tolerated by any organism. An extreme example is the genus Pyrodictium, found on geothermally heated areas of the seabed. It has a temperature minimum of 82°, optimum of 105° and growth maximum of 110°C.

Mesophiles are the the most common bacteria. Saprophytes grow best around 30 and the parasitic species around 37C. Every species grows over a wide range. Saprophytic have a wider range than parasitic species. Two species may have an optimum at 37, but one may grow from 5 to 45 and the othr may only grow from 25 to 40.

6. Ans. (b) Light-chain variable and (d) Heavy-chain variable *Ref: Ananthnarayan, 8th ed. p 97*

- An antibody (Ab), also known as an immunoglobulin (Ig), is a large Y-shape protein produced by B cells that is used by the immune system to identify and neutralize foreign objects, such as bacteria and viruses.
- The antibody recognizes a unique part of the foreign target, called an antigen.
- Each tip of the 'Y' of an antibody contains a paratope (a structure analogous to a lock) that is specific for one particular epitope (similarly analogous to a key) on an antigen, allowing these two structures to bind together with precision.
- Antigen-combining site of an antibody is at the amino terminus.
- It has both light and heavy chains.
- The amino acid sequence in aminoterminal is variable. This variable region determines immunological specifi city.

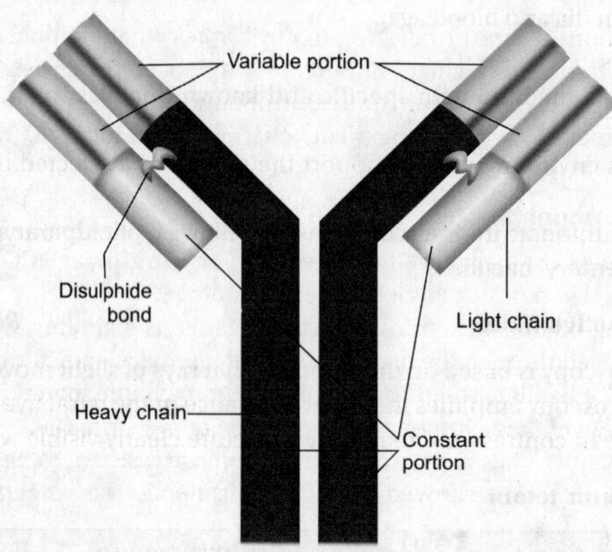

7. Ans. (b) Sodium hypochlorite *Ref: Manual of Infection Control Procedures by N. N. Daman 2nd/e, p 70 books.google.co.in/books?isbn=0521687012*

Blood spills or other human body fluids that occur inside or in the outside environment need to be decontaminated to prevent the potential transmission of communicable disease.

Sodium hypochlorite

- Sodium hypochlorite has broad spectrum antimicrobial activity; however, it is inactivated in the presence of organic matter. It is used for the treatment of water, disinfection of laundry items, dental appliances and clean environmental surfaces.

- Clinical uses in health-care facilities include:
  - Hyperchlorination of potable water to prevent Legionella colonization
  - Chlorination of water distribution systems used in hemodialysis centers
  - Cleaning of environmental surfaces
  - Disinfection of laundry
  - Local use to decontaminate blood spills
  - Disinfection of equipment
  - Decontamination of medical waste prior to disposal
  - Dental therapy

8. Ans. (a) Spores *Ref: Ananthnarayan, 8th ed. p 30, 38*

Disinfectants:

- These are substances that are applied to nonliving objects to destroy microorganisms that are living on the objects.
- Disinfection does not necessarily kill all microorganisms, especially resistant bacterial spores.
- Disinfectants work by destroying the cell wall of microbes or interfering with the metabolism.
- Disinfectants are frequently used in hospitals, dental surgeries, kitchens, and bathrooms to kill infectious organisms.

Antiseptics

- These are antimicrobial substances that are applied to living tissue/skin to reduce the possibility of infection, sepsis, or putrefaction.

9. Ans. (a) Kills all living organism in a specific environment *Ref: Ananthnarayan, 8th ed. p 30*

- Sterilization (or sterilisation) is a term referring to any process that eliminates (removes) or kills all forms of microbial life, including transmissible agents (such as fungi, bacteria, viruses, spore forms, etc.) present on a surface, contained in a fluid, in medication, or in a compound such as biological culture media.
- Sterilization can be achieved by applying heat, chemicals, irradiation, high pressure, and filtration or combinations thereof.

10. Ans. (d) Bacillus stearothermophilus *Ref: Ananthnarayan, 8th ed. p 34*

- Bacillus stearothermophilus is a thermophilic bacteria which can grow at 65°C and above. The spores are highly heat resistant and are used to monitor autoclave performance.
- Sterilization is the freeing of an article from all living organisms including viable spores. Sterilization quality control can only be achieved through the use of calibrated biological indicators (endospores).
- These indicators consist of bacillus stearothermophilus spores impregnated on chromatography paper strips, individually placed into envelopes. Number of spores present per strip: 106.
- These organisms are difficult to destroy because they are more resistant to heat than other vegetative bacteria and viruses. Therefore, if they are destroyed during sterilization, it is assumed that all other life forms are also destroyed.
- This test is considered the most sensitive check of the autoclaves efficiency.

11. Ans. (c) Ultraviolet rays *Ref: Ananthnarayan, 8th ed. p 31*

- Sunlight is the one of the physical agent of sterilization due to its content of UV light and heat rays.
- It has a very good bactericidal activity due to its ultraviolet rays.
- Bacteria suspended in water are destroyed due to exposure to sunlight.

12. Ans. (d) Killing of all organisms and spores *Ref: Ananthnarayan, 8th ed. p 30*

Sterilization (or sterilisation) is a term referring to any process that eliminates (removes) or kills all forms of microbial life, including transmissible agents (such as fungi, bacteria, viruses, spore forms, etc.) present on a surface, contained in a fluid, in medication, or in a compound, such as biological culture media. Sterilization can be achieved by applying heat, chemicals, irradiation, high pressure, and filtration.

13. Ans. (a) Prevent their phagocytosis *Ref: Ananthnarayan, 8th ed. p 19*

- The cell capsule is a very large structure of some prokaryotic cells, such as bacterial cells.
- It is a polysaccharide layer that lies outside the cell envelope of bacteria, and is thus deemed part of the outer envelope of a bacterial cell. It is a well organized layer, not easily washed off, and it can be the cause of various diseases.
- The capsule which can be found in both Gram-negative bacteria and Gram-positive bacteria should not be confused with the second lipid membrane (or bacterial outer membrane), which contains lipopolysaccharides and lipoproteins and is found only in Gram-negative bacteria.
- The capsule is considered a virulence factor because it enhances the ability of bacteria to cause disease (e.g. prevents phagocytosis). The capsule can protect cells from engulfment by eukaryotic cells, such as macrophages.
- A capsule-specific antibody may be required for phagocytosis to occur.
- Capsules also contain water which protects bacteria against desiccation.

14. Ans. (c) Bacillus sterothermophilus spores *Ref: Ananthnarayan, 8th ed. p 34*

Sterilization control

For determining the efficacy of moist heat sterilization, spores of Bacillus stearothermophilus are used as the test organism. It is a thermophilic organism with an optimum growth temperature of 55-60°C and its spores require an exposure of 12 minutes at 121°C to be killed. Paper strips impregnated with 106 spores are dried at room temperature and placed in paper envelops. These envelops are inserted in different parts of the load. After sterilization, the strips are inoculated into a suitable recovering medium and incubated for the sterility test at 55°C for five days.

15. Ans. (d) Gamma rays *Ref: Ananthanarayan and Paniker's, 8th ed. p 35*

Ionising radiation: X-rays, gamma rays and cosmic rays are highly lethal to DNA and other vital constituent. They have very high penetrative power. **Since there is no appreciable increase in temperature in this method, it is referred as cold sterilization.**

Gamma rays are formed with the self disintegration of Cobalt-60 (60Co) or cesium-137 (137Cs).

It is a high penetrating and commonly used sterilization method. It is generally used for the sterilization of gaseous, liquid, solid materials, homogeneous and heterogeneous systems and disposable medical equipment, such as syringes, needles, cannulas, density materials, cosmetics and i.v. sets.

Method of sterilization of important materials

Materials	*Methods*
• All suture materials except catgut	Autoclave
• Catgut	Ionizing radiation
• Rubber gloves, surgical instruments and most of culture media	Autoclave
• Forceps, scalpels, scissors, needles	Hot air oven
• Disposable syringes	Ethylene oxide
• Suture materials	Glutaraldehyde
• Hospital wastes	Incinerator
• Vaccines/serum/antibiotic solutions	Filtration
• Operation theaters	Fumigation with formalin
• Preparation of the skin for surgery	Iodine, spirit, savlon, chlorhexidine
• Absorbent points, broaches files and other RC instrument	Hot-salt sterilizer of Glass bead sterilizer
• Cotton pliers, cement spatulas	Immersing in 5.2% sodium hypochlorite for 1 min
• Gutta-percha cone	
• Sugar media	Tyndallization or intermittent sterilization
• Loeffler's serum slop Lowenstein Jensen's medium	Inspissator
• Dental Hand piece	Dry heat, chemiclave and autoclave **[Ethylene oxide is contraindicated]**

16. Ans. (b) Lysozyme *Ref: Robbins, Basic Pathology, 8th ed. p 39*

Killing and degradation of microbes: The culmination of the phagocytosis of microbes is killing and degradation of the ingested particles. The key steps in this reaction are the production of microbicidal substances within lysosomes and fusion of the lysosomes with phagosomes, thus selectively exposing the ingested particles to the destructive mechanisms of the leukocytes. The most important microbicidal substance are reactive oxygen species (ROS) and lysosomal enzymes.

17. Ans. (b) Psychrophillic *Ref: Ananthanarayan and Paniker's, 8th ed. p 26*

Refer: Ans no. 5

18. Ans. (b) Hot air oven *Ref: Ananthanarayan and Paniker's, 8th ed. p 31*

- Hot air ovens are electrical devices used in sterilization.
- They were originally developed by Pasteur.
- The oven uses dry heat to sterilize articles. Generally, they can be operated from 50 to 300°C (122 to 572°F) .
- There is a thermostat controlling the temperature.
- It is one of the most common method used for sterilization. Glass wares, swab sticks, all-glass syringes, powder and oily substances are sterilized in hot air oven.
- For sterilization, a temperature of 160°C is maintained (holding) for one hour. Spores are killed at this temperature. It leads to sterilization.

19. Ans. (c) Bacterial capsule *Ref: Ananthanarayan and Paniker's, 8th ed. p 14*

Indirect (negative) staining

- The acidic dye nigrosine will be used to visualize the capsule or sheath that surrounds some bacteria in a process called negative staining.
- Capsules are composed primarily of polysaccharides or glycoproteins and are gelatinous in texture
- They are readily destroyed by heating and hence direct staining methods cannot be utilized. In general, the size and shape of microorganisms is often less distorted with indirect staining procedures, especially when sampled from a broth culture.
- Therefore negative staining is useful whenever the morphology of individual bacteria is in question. **Morphology** can often be determined with confidence with only the high dry lens. Consider that this procedure does not necessarily kill the organism, so be careful.
- After preparing a clean, greaseless slide, a small drop of nigrosine is mixed with a small drop from a broth culture or with a quantity of dry material.
- The drop is spread across the slide using the edge of another slide as a spreader. This same procedure is used for blood smears.

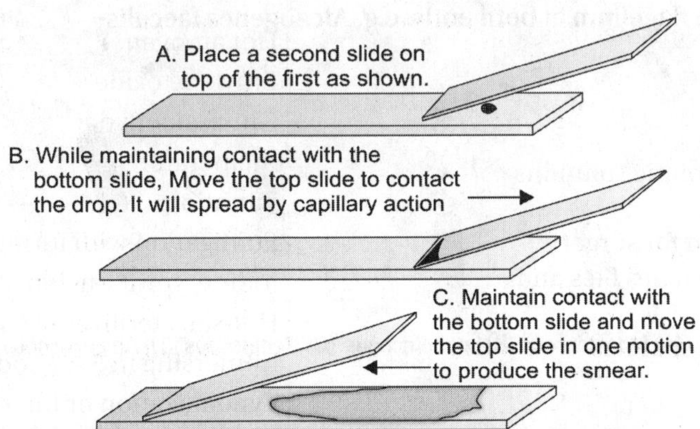

After air drying, the smear is observed using the high dry lens, or oil immersion if desired. The smear will be most dense where the nigrosine dye was deposited on the slide. Somewhere along the tapered spear the density will be ideal. The background should be blue-gray. Bacteria will be evident by the absence of any color.

20. Ans. (b) Incorporating part of host DNA *Ref: Ananthanarayan and Paniker's, 8th ed.*

In bacteria, the transmission of genetic material is through transformation, transduction, and conjugation.

21. Ans. (d) Incineration *Ref: Ananthanarayan and Paniker's, 8th ed. p 32*

- Moist heat sterilization is the process of sterilizing objects with hot air that is heavily laden with water vapor, which is essentially the definition of hot steam.
- A better method to sterilize objects which is commonly used in hospitals is autoclaving.
- The moist heat from an autoclave kills virtually all microorganisms by denaturing their proteins.

22. Ans. (a) Joseph Lister *Ref: Ananthanarayan and Paniker's, 8th ed. pg 4*

- Antiseptics are antimicrobial substances that are applied to living tissue/skin to reduce the possibility of infection, sepsis, or putrefaction.
- Joseph Lister discovered antiseptic.
- Dr. Joseph Lister revolutionized surgery in the late 19th century by introducing antiseptic methods that drastically reduced the incidence of infection and death, dramatically improving patient health while enabling surgical knowledge and approaches to advance rapidly.
- Lister's antiseptic system, explained first in the Lancet in 1867, relied on carbolic acid as an antiseptic to exclude airborne infection.

23. Ans. (b) Region II *Ref: Ananthanarayan and Paniker's, 8th ed. p 18*

The lipopolysaccharide consist of 3 regions:

- **Region I**—it is the polysaccharide portion which determine the O antigen specificity.
- **Region II**—it is the core polysaccharide
- **Region III**—it is the glycolipid portion and it is responsible for the endotoxic activity.

24. Ans. (a) Spirilla *Ref: Ananthanarayan and Paniker's, 8th ed. p 20*

Flagella

They are long, whip-like appendages that move the bacteria toward nutrients and other attractants. The long filament of flagella is composed of many subunits of a single protein, flagellin, arranged in several intertwined chains. The energy for movement, the proton motive force, is provided by ATP.

There are four types of flagellar arrangement:

1. Monotrichous: Single polar flagellum, e.g. Vibrio cholerae (Mneomonics: Mono means one)
2. Amphitrichous: Single flagellum at both ends, e.g. Alcaligenes faecalis

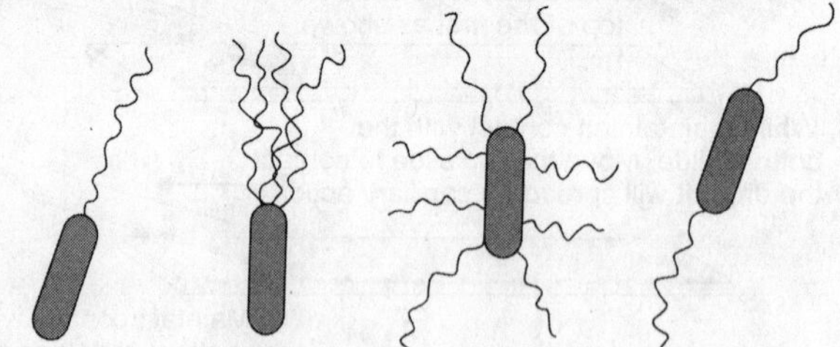

(A) Monotrichous polar (B) Lophotrichous (C) Peritrichous (D) Amphitrichous

3. Lophotrichous: Tuft of flagella at one or both ends, e.g. spirilla
4. Peritrichous: Flagella surrounding the cell, e.g. typhoid bacilli

25. Ans. (d) Leeuwen Hoeck *Ref: Ananthanarayan and Paniker's, 8th ed. p 8*

- In 1675, Leeuwen Hoeck made a simple microscope.
- He is commonly known as "the Father of Microbiology", and considered to be the first microbiologist.

26. Ans. (c) Conjugation *Ref: Ananthanarayan and Paniker's, 8th ed. p 60*

- Conjugation is the direct transfer of DNA from one bacterial cell to another bacterial cell. The transferred DNA is a plasmid, a circle of DNA that is distinct from the main bacterial chromosome.
- The transfer of the plasmid take advantage of the complementary nature of double stranded DNA.
- One strand of the plasmid is transferred and the other remains in the original cell. Both strands have the complementary stranded added so that each cell ends up with a complete plasmid.

27. Ans. (d) 121°C temp and pressure is 151 lb/sq. inch for 12 mins
Ref: Ananthanarayan and Paniker's, 8th ed. p 32, 34

Autoclaving

- This is the means of moist heat sterilization. It is a method of choice for sterilization of instruments as it reliably eliminates even resistant, spore forming micro-organisms, fungi, viruses, along with vegetative micro-organisms. It works on the principle of 'steam under pressure'. It provides moist heat in the form of saturated steam under pressure.
- The pressure increases the boiling point of water. Roughly for every 5 lbs pressure, the boiling point of water rises by 100°C by increasing the latent heat of energy for boiling of water. Hence at 15 pressure, the boiling point of water rises to 121°C.

The temperature pressure and sterilization time ratio is as follows:

Pressure	*Temperature*	*Time*
15 psi	121°C	20 mins
20 psi	134°C	3–5 mins (flash method)

Articles that can be sterilized

- Instruments, gauze, cotton, linen, needles, syringes, catheters, drains, autoclavable hand pieces, gloves, etc.

Articles that cannot be sterilized

- Powders, oils, greases, thermolabile material like electrical cords of micromotors, fibreoptic cable, etc.

Advantages: Simple, economical and reliable.

Disadvantages: Tends to corrode the instruments, makes sharp instruments dull.

28. Ans. (a) Flagella *Ref: Ananthanarayan and Paniker's, 8th ed. p 20*

Refer: Ans No. 24

29. Ans. (d) None of the above *Ref: Ananthanarayan and Paniker's, 8th ed. p 6*

Koch's postulates are four criteria designed to establish a causal relationship between a microbe and a disease. Koch applied the postulates to describe the etiology of cholera and tuberculosis

Koch's postulates are the following:

- The microorganism must be found in abundance in all organisms suffering from the disease, but should not be found in healthy organisms.
- The microorganism must be isolated from a diseased organism and grown in pure culture.
- The cultured microorganism should cause disease when introduced into a healthy organism.
- The microorganism must be reisolated from the inoculated, diseased experimental host and identified as being identical to the original specific causative agent.

Here, Treponema pallidum and Mycobacterium leprae could not be cultivated in vitro and Neisseria gonorrheae does not posses any animal model hence the answer will be none of the above.

30. Ans. (b) Robertson's cooked meat medium *Ref: Anantnarayan, 6th ed. p 37*

Also know:

- In 1916, Robertson developed a cooked meat medium for use in the cultivation of certain anaerobes isolated from wounds.
- The present formulation for cooked meat medium is a modification of Robertson's original formula.
- Cooked meat medium is used for the cultivation and maintenance of clostridia and for determining proteolytic activity of anaerobes.
- It supports the growth of most spore forming and non-spore forming obligate anaerobes and may be used for a variety of purposes including the maintenance of stock cultures.
- This medium is also useful as an enrichment broth as backup to plated media or for cultivating anaerobes that may be present in small numbers in a population and as a subculture medium for determination of proteolysis (meat digestion) and spore formation by Clostridium species.
- Enriched media
  - Blood agar, chocolate agar and egg media
- Enrichment media
  - Tetrathionnate broth for typhoid-paratyphoid
- Selenite F both for dysentery bacilli S
  - Selective media
  - Dosoxychoclate citrate medium for dysentery bacilli
- Indicator media
  - McLeods medium for diphtheria bacillus
- Differential media
  - Negler medium for Lecithinase activity
- Sugar media
- Transport media
  - Stuart's medium

31. Ans. (a) Gluteraldehyde *Ref: Anantnarayan, 8th ed. p 29*

- Gluteraldehyde is an agent for high level of disinfection
- Used at 2% dilution
- Extremely irritant
- Action similar to formaldehyde
- Acts by denaturation of cell proteins by reacting with cell components.
- Disinfection time: 10 minutes; sterlization: 10–12 hours
- Active against spores

Also note:

- Iodophores and chlorhexidine are moderately active against spores
- Alchohols don't have any action against spores. They are most active at 70–80% conc.

32. Ans. (a) Conjugation *Ref: Anantanarayan, 6th ed. p 54-55*

Conjugative transfer of bacterial plasmids is the most efficient way of horizontal gene spread, and it is therefore considered one of the major reasons for the increase in the number of bacteria exhibiting multiple-antibiotic resistance. Thus, conjugation and spread of antibiotic resistance represents a severe problem in antibiotic treatment, especially of immunosuppressed patients and in intensive care units.

While conjugation in gram-negative bacteria has been studied in great detail over the last decades, the transfer mechanisms of antibiotic resistance plasmids in Gram-positive bacteria remained obscure.

This plasmid is of great medical importance as it is responsible for the spread of multiple drug resistance among bacteria.

33. Ans. (c) Lowenstein-Jensen medium *Ref: Ananthanaryan, 8th ed. p 348*

- The solid medium most widely employed for routine culture is the Lowenstein-Jensen.
- The several liquid media described. Dubos' Middlebrook's, Proskauer and Beck's, Sula's and Sauton's are more common. Liquid media are not generally employed for routine cultivation, but are used for sensitivity testing, chemical analyses and preparation of antigens and vaccines.
- Diffuse growth is obtained in Dubos medium containing Tween-80 (sorbitan monooleate).

IMMUNOLOGY

34. Ans. (b) Strongyloides *Ref: Harrison, 17th ed. p. 1322*

- The term autoinfection refers to the ability of certain parasites, particularly helminths, to establish a life cycle within the host, eliminating the need for an intermediate stage, and secondary hosts.
- Strongyloidiasis for example involves premature transformation of noninfective larvae in infective larvae, which can then penetrate the intestinal mucosa (internal autoinfection) or the skin of the perineal area (external autoinfection). Infection can be maintained by repeated migratory cycles for the remainder of the person's life.

Organisms capable of this

- Strongyloides stercoralis
- Enterobius vermicularis
- Hymenolepis nana.
- Taenia solium

35. Ans. (b) Direct Coomb's test *Ref: Ananthnarayan, 8th ed. p 188*

A Coombs test is either of two clinical blood tests used in immunohematology and immunology. The two Coomb's tests are:

- The direct Coomb's test (DCT, also known as direct antiglobulin test or DAT)
- The indirect Coomb's test (also known as indirect antiglobulin test or IAT)

Direct Coomb's test

- During post-transfusion blood sample from patient, it should be done to detect antibodies directed against the transferred red blood cells.
- A positive direct Coomb's test suggests that the patient has an antibody directed against the transfused red blood cells.
- At blood bank, every post-transfusion sample should be tested for evidence of hemolysis, a direct Coomb's test should be performed.

Hemolytic transfusion reactions

- A positive direct antiglobulin test result may be the first indication of an immune response to a recent transfusion.
- The patient's developing antibodies will coat transfused RBCs bearing the corresponding antigen, resulting in a positive direct antiglobulin test result.
- Antibodies appear within 7–10 days after a primary exposure or within 1–2 days of a secondary response.
- Antibodies can shorten the survival of previously or subsequently transfused RBCs.

36. Ans. (d) Arthus reaction *Ref: Ananthnarayan, 8th ed. p 166*

- In immunology, the arthus reaction is a type of local type III hypersensitivity reaction.
- Type III hypersensitivity reactions are immune complex-mediated, and involve the deposition of antigen/antibody complexes
- Arthus repeatedly injected horse serum subcutaneously into rabbits, after first injection he does not find any reaction but when he inject it second time, he found that there was edema, induration and hemorrhagic necrosis.
- Further injections eventually led to gangrene

37. Ans. (a) Lymphokine production and delayed hypersensitivity *Ref: Ananthnarayan, 8th ed. p 168*

- Lymphocytes are cells present in peripheral blood, lymph, lymphoid organ and many other tissue.
- It is small and round in shape.
- There are T and B lymphocytes. Nature of immune response depends on the type of lymphocytes.
- T cell is responsible to produce lymphokines and cell mediated immunity where as B cell divide and transform into plasma cell (synthesize immunoglobulins).
- T cells are involved in cell-mediated immunity, whereas B cells are primarily responsible for humoral immunity (relating to antibodies).
- **Cell mediated immunity participates in:**
  - Delayed hypersensitivity
  - Transplantation immunity
  - Immunosurveillance
  - Immunity against cancer
  - Autoimmune diseases, e.g. thyroiditis

38. Ans. (a) IgG *Ref: Ananthnarayan, 8th ed. p 139*

- **Humoral immunity** (also called the antibody-mediated system) is the aspect of immunity that is mediated by macromolecules (as opposed to cell-mediated immunity) found in extracellular fluids, such as secreted antibodies, complement proteins and certain antimicrobial peptides.
- The antibody response to an antigen is of two types:
  - Primary immune response
  - Secondary immune response

Primary response	*Secondary response*
• Slow, sluggish, short lived	• Prompt, powerful, prolonged
• Long lag phase	• Short or negligible lag phase
• Low titer of antibodies	• Higher level of antibodies
• Not persist for long	• Long lasting
• IgM antibody predominantly seen	• IgG antibody predominantly seen

39. Ans. (b) IgA *Ref: Ananthnarayan, 8th ed. p 89*

- **IgA** is a major component of local immunity.
- **Secretory IgA** is a type of IgA, it is produced locally by plasma cellor through secretory gland.
- Secretory IgA is the principal immune component of major and minor gland salivary secretions and thus would be considered to be the primary mediator of adaptive immunity in the salivary milieu apart from other immunoglobulins like IgG and IgM. which are derived from the gingival circular fluid.
- The salivary IgA may act as specific agglutinin acting with the bacterial surface receptors and inhibiting colonization and subsequent caries formation.

40. Ans. (d) Ethylene oxide gas *Ref: Ananthnarayan, 8th ed. p 37*

Ethylene oxide

- Ethylene oxide gas is appropriate to use for sterilization of instruments/equipment made from heat labile materials or those devices that contain electronic components.
- The time required to process the instrument is dependent on the temperature, humidity and concentration level of the gas.

- The gas must penetrate the packaging and reach all surfaces of the instrument/equipment requiring sterilization.
- The time for such a process is between 12 hours to over 24 hours. Because EO is toxic, this gas is restricted in health care facilities and must be used according to strict guidelines to ensure staff safety.
- The manufacturer's instructions must be followed for the packaging, sterilization process, validation and aeration process.
- It is highly inflammable and in concentration s in air greater than 3% is highly explosive. Its explosive tendency is decreased by adding CO_2 or N, to a concentration of 10%.

41. Ans. (a) Cytokines *Ref: Ananthnarayan, 8th ed. p 146*

- The term "cytokine" is derived from a combination of two Greek words 'cyto' meaning cell and 'kinos' meaning movement. Cytokines are cell signalling molecules that aid cell to cell communication in immune responses and stimulate the movement of cells toward sites of inflammation, infection and trauma.

These include:

- Monokines, cytokines produced by mononuclear phagocytic cells
- Lymphokines, cytokines produced by activated lymphocytes, especially Th cells
- Interleukins, cytokines that act as mediators between leukocytes.

Examples include:

- Interleukins (IL1-IL13)
- CSF (colony-stimulating factor)
- TNF (tumor necrosis factor)
- IFNs (Interferons)
- Others
- TGF-B (transforming growth factor-B)
- LIF (leukemia inhibitory factor)

42. Ans. (d) Red blood cells *Ref: Ananthnarayan, 8th ed. p 134*

- The human leukocyte antigen (HLA) system is the name of the loci of genes that encode for major histocompatibility complex (MHC) in humans.
- The super-locus contains a large number of genes related to immune system function in humans.
- This group of genes resides on chromosome 6, and encodes cell-surface antigen-presenting proteins and has many other functions.

They have three separate groups of genes:

HLA class I antigens (A, B, C) are located on the surface of virtually all nucleated cells.

- It is involved in graft rejection, cytolysis and components of hormone receptors.
- A test that can be used for typing of class I histocompatibility antigens is antibody and complement—mediate cytotoxicity (microcytotoxicity).

HLA class II antigens are situated on cells of immune system, e.g. macrophages, activated T cells, B cells, etc.

- It is involved in graft versus host reaction.
- Since serotyping is not possible for HLA DR antigen, it is detected by mixed lymphocytic reactions (MLRs) and primed lymphocyte typing.

HLA class III includes complementary components associated with C3 formation, heat-shock proteins, etc.

RBCs are nonnucleated; it does not have HLA class I, as their function is not defensive.

43. Ans. (b) Hemagglutination inhibition test *Ref: Ananthnarayan, 8th ed. p 389*

Serological diagnosis of mycoplasma

- **Most sensitive**
  - Immunofluorescence
  - Hemagglutination inhibition
  - Metabolic hemagglutination
- **Less sensitive**
  - Complement fixation
  - Indirect hemagglutination
- **Nonspecific serological test**
  - Streptococcus MG
  - Cold agglutination tests

Hence, hemagglutination inhibition test is used to detect mycoplasmal or viral infection.

44. Ans. (b) Protein antigen *Ref: Ananthnarayan, 8th ed. p*

45. Ans. (a) Natural killer cells *Ref: Ananthnarayan, 8th ed. p 86*

Natural killer cells

- Natural killer cells (or NK cells) are a type of cytotoxic lymphocyte critical to the innate immune system.
- The role NK cells play is analogous to that of cytotoxic T cells in the vertebrate adaptive immune response.
- NK cells provide rapid responses to virally infected cells and respond to tumor formation, acting at around 3 days after infection.
- Typically immune cells detect MHC presented on infected cell surfaces, triggering cytokine release, causing lysis or apoptosis.
- NK cell activity is inversely proportionate to MHC class I expression on the surface of nucleated cells.
- Virus infection downregulates the MHC class I expression in the infected nucleated body cell. Hence, such virus infected cells are prone to killing by NK cell.
- NK cells are derived from bone marrow.
- Functionally active NK cells are found in spleen and cells in lymph node are immature.
- The ability for NK cells to act in both the innate and adaptive immune response.

46. Ans. (a) IgG1 *Ref: Ananthnarayan, 8th ed. p 98*

- Immunoglobulin G (IgG) is an antibody isotype.
- It is a protein complex composed of four peptide chains: two identical heavy chains and two identical light chains arranged in a Y-shape typical of antibody monomers.
- Each IgG has two antigen binding sites.
- IgG is the most abundant antibody isotype found in the circulation.
- IgG molecules are synthesized and secreted by plasma B cells.

There are four IgG subclasses (IgG1, 2, 3, and 4) in humans, named in order of their abundance in serum (IgG1 being the most abundant).

Name	*Percent*	*Crosses placenta easily*	*Complement activator*	*Binds to Fc receptor on phagocytic cells*
IgG1	66%	Yes (1.47)†	Second-highest	High affinity
IgG2	23%	No (0.8)†	Third-highest	Extremely low affinity
IgG3	7%	Yes (1.17)†	Highest	High affinity
IgG4	4%	Yes (1.15)†	No	Intermediate affinity

47. Ans. (d) IgE *Ref: Ananthnarayan, 8th ed. p 162*

- Type I hypersensitivity (or immediate hypersensitivity) is an allergic reaction provoked by re-exposure to a specific type of antigen referred to as an allergen.
- The difference between a normal infectious immune response and a type 1 hypersensitivity response is that in type 1 hypersensitivity the antibody is IgE instead of IgA, IgG, or IgM.
- Type 1 hypersensitivity can be further classified into an immediate and late-phase reaction. The immediate hypersensitivity reaction occurs minutes after exposure and includes release of vasoactive amines and lipid mediators, whereas the late-phase reaction occurs 24 hours after exposure and includes the release of cytokines.

Treatment usually involves adrenaline (epinephrine), antihistamines, and corticosteroids. If the entire body gets involved, then anaphylaxis can take place, which is an acute, systemic reaction that can prove fatal.

Overview of mediators released by mast cells in type 1 hypersensitivity, and their actions	
Vasodilation and increased permeability	• Histamine • PAF • Leukotriene C4, D4 and E4 • Prostaglandin D2 • Neutral proteases
Smooth muscle spasm	• Histamine • PAF • Leukotriene C4, D4 and E4 • Prostaglandin
Leukocyte extravasation	• Cytokines (e.g. chemokines and TNF) • Leukotriene B4 • Chemotactic factors for neutrophils and eosinophils

48. Ans. (b) Non-expression of MHC I on cell surface receptor *Ref: Ananthnarayan, 8th ed. p 86*

Refer Ans no. 12

49. Ans. (c) Epinephrine DOC in certain situation *Ref: Ananthnarayan, 8th ed. p 164*

Epinephrine is DOC in certain situation

- In human beings, fatal anaphylaxis is fortunately rare. Symptoms and signs of anaphylactic shock begin with itching of the scalp and tongue, flushing of the skin over the whole body and difficulty in breathing due to bronchial spasm. There may be nausea, vomiting, abdominal pain and diarrhea, sometimes with blood in the stool. Acute hypotension, loss of consciousness and death follow. Human anaphylaxis, once commonly associated with heterologous serum therapy, is now seen mostly following injection of antibiotics or other drugs. Insect stings can also cause anaphylaxis in human beings. Prompt treatment with adrenaline can be life-saving. Adrenaline is to be administrated, 0.5 ml of a 1 in 1000 solution, subcutaneously or intramuscularly, the dose being repeated up to a total of 2 ml over 15 minutes, if necessary.
- Cutaneous anaphylaxis: When a small shocking dose of an antigen is administrated intradermally to a sensitized host, there will be a local wheal-and-flare response (local anaphylaxis). The wheal is a pale, central area of puffiness due to edema, which is surrounded by a flare caused by hyperemia and subsequent erythema. Cutaneous anaphylaxis (skin test for type I hypersensitivity) is useful in testing for hypersensitivity and in identifying the allergen responsible in atopic diseases. In highly sensitized individuals even the skin test may lead to serious and even fatal reactions. Hence, a syringe loaded with adrenaline should always be kept ready whenever a skin test is performed to detect anaphylactic hypersensitivity.

50. Ans. (a) Severe reaction following reinjection of protein solutions in a sensitized individual

Ref: Ananthnarayan, 8th ed. p 161-166

Few important points about anaphylaxis

- Also called as Type I or IgE mediated hypersensitivity reaction
- Chronic form is called as atopy
- 1st does acts as sensitization dose
- Antigen as well as hapten induces anaphylaxis
- 2nd dose is termed as shocking dose
- Tissue affected is known as larger tissue or shock organs
- Treatment adrenaline 0.5 ml at 1:1000 ratio intramuscular repeated till 2 ml over 15 min, if necessary
- Primary mediator histamine, serotonin chemotactic factor heparin
- Secondary mediator prostaglandin, platelet activating factor

51. Ans. (c) C3

Ref: Ananthanarayan and Paniker's, 7th ed. p 111-112

- Complement is a complex of nine different fractions called C1 to C9, the c cascade can be triggered by two pathways
- Classical pathway first step is the binding of C1 to the antigen antibody complex.
- Alternate or properdin pathway first step in the alternate pathway is the binding of C3 b to an activator.
- The component system.

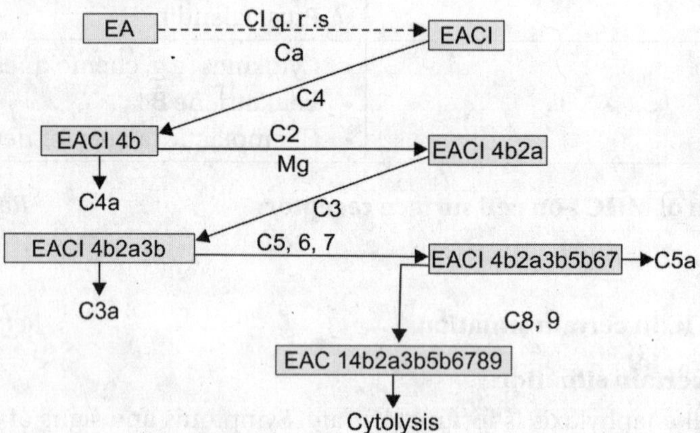

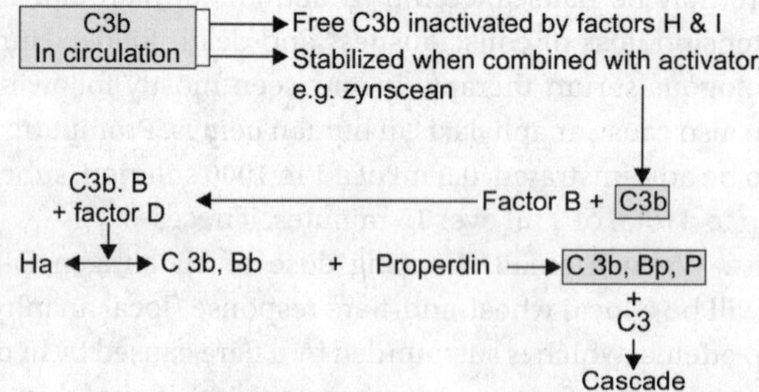

52. Ans. (c) IgG

Ref: Ananthanarayan and Pankiker's, 7th ed. p 88

IgG is a major serum immunoglobulin consisting about 80% of the total four subclasses of IgG have been recognized.

Class	Percentage of Ig	Half life	Important points
IgG	So (max)	23 days (max)	• Major serum immunoglobulin. • Normal serum concentration is 8–16 mg per ml. • Only immunoglobulin that can cross the placenta and provides natural passive immunity to newborn. • Classical complement fixation is positive. • Smallest immunoglobulin. • Also known as warm immunoglobulin. • Predominant immunoglobulin in the gingival fluid (OCF).
IgM	5–8	5 days	• Earliest immunoglobulin synthesized by fetus in response to infection. • Oldest immunoglobulin class. • Presence of IgM in the newborn indicates intrauterine infection and is useful in diagnosis of congenital infection, such as syphilis, rubella, HIV infection. • Activates classical complement pathway. • Also known as cold immunoglobulin. • Both IgG and IgM are involved in type II or cytotoxic type of hypersensitivity reaction.
IgA	10-13	6 days	• Predominant immunoglobulin in saliva. • Occurs in two forms, i.e. serum IgA and category secretory IgA. Secratory IgA is synthesized from mucosal or glandular epithelium and protects IgA from proteolysis. • Present in exocrine secretions. • Activates alternative pathway of complement fixation. • Both IgA and IgG are secreted in milk. • Caries vaccine is prepared based on action of IgA in the oral cavity.
IgE	1	2–8 days	• Has unique property of heat labiality, i.e. inactivated at 56°C in 1 hour. • Has affinity for mast cells off same species. • Mediates prausunitz-Kustner reactions, a method to detect atopic antibody. • Responsible for anaphylactic type of hypersensitivity reaction, e.g. contact dermatitis. • Chiefly produced in linings of respiratory and intestinal tracts. • IgE is believed to have special role in parasitic infection.
IgD	1 (min)	1–5 (min)	• Structurally resemble IgG • IgD and IgM serve as recognition for antibody production or suppression.

53. Ans. (c) and (d) Diagnosed by demonstration of specific IgM antibody; Etiological agent can be grown in modified Kelley's medium *Ref: Ananthanarayan and Paniker's, 7th ed. p 389*

Lyme disease: Borrelia Burgdorferi

- It is caused by Borrelia burgdorferi transmitted by the bite of Ixodid ticks.
- B. burgdorferi is a fastidious bacterium which can be grown in a modified Kelly's (BSK) medium, after incubation for two weeks or more, optimally at 33°C.
- Laboratory diagnosis can be made by isolation of the borrelia or by serology. The borrelia has been isolated from ticks as well as from skin lesions, CSF and blood of patients, but culture is too slow and difficult to be of use in

diagnosis. Serological tests, such as ELISA and IF, have been described and immunoblotting recommended for confirmation.

54. Ans. (a) NK cells *Ref: Ananthanarayan and Paniker's, 7th ed. p 126*

- NK cells posses spontaneous cytotoxicity toward various target cells, mainly malignant and virus infected cells. Their cytotoxicity is not antibody dependent or MHC restricted NK activity is natural or non-immune as it does not require sensitization by prior antigenic contact, NK cells therefore from part of the innate immune system.
- They bind to the glycoprotein receptors on the surface of autologous as well as allergenic target cells and release several cytolytic factors.
- NK cells activity is augmented by interferon. They are considered to be important in immune surveillance and neutral defense against virus infected and malignant mutans cells.

55. Ans. (b) T-cell *Ref: Ananthanarayan and Paniker's, 8th ed. p 180, 181*

- **Graft-versus-Host Reaction:** Graft rejection is due to the reaction of the host to the grafted tissue (host- versus-graft response). The contrary situation, in which the graft mounts an immune response against the antigens of the host, is known as the graft-versus-host (GVH) reaction.

  The GVH reaction occurs when the following conditions are present:

  1. The graft contains immune-competent T cells.
  2. The recipient possesses transplantation antigens that are absent in the graft.
  3. The recipient must not reject the graft.

  Hence the rejection can be prevented by the suppression of T cells.

- **Examples of situations leading to the GVH reaction are:**

  a. Allograft in a recipient in whom specific immunological tolerance has been induced.
  b. Adult lymphocytes injected into an immunologically deficient recipient. The immunological deficiency may be due to immaturity (newborn) of immune-suppression.
  c. F1 hybrid receiving a transplant from any one parental strain.

  The major clinical features of the GVH reaction in animals are retardation of growth, emaciation, diarrhea, hepatosplenomegaly, lymphoid atrophy and anemia, terminating fatally. The syndrome has been called runt disease.

56. Ans. (b) Culture *Ref: Ananthanarayan and Paniker's, 8th ed. p 44*

In the clinical laboratory, the indications for culture are mainly to:

- Isolate bacteria in pure culture
- Demonstrate their properties
- Obtain sufficient growth for preparation of antigens and for other tests
- Type isolates by methods such as bacteriophage and bacteriocin susceptibility
- Determine sensitivity to antibiotics
- Estimate viable counts
- Maintain stock cultures.

57. Ans. (d) Smallest antigenic determinant *Ref: Ananthanarayan and Paniker's, 8th ed. p 91-92*

- **Complete antigen** is able to induce antibody formation and produce a specific and observable reaction with antibody so produced.
- **Haptens** are substances which are incapable of inducing antibody formation by them but can react specifically with antibodies.
- **Epitope smallest unit of antigenicity or antigenic determinant:** It is that small area on the antigen, usually consisting of 4 to 5 amino acid or monosaccharide residues possessing a specific chemical structure, electrical charges and spatial configuration, capable of sensitising an immunocyte and of reacting with its complementary site on the specific antibody or T-cell receptor.
- **Paratope:** The combining area on the antibody molecule, corresponding to the epitope.

58. Ans. (d) Gamma globulin *Ref: Ananthanarayan and Paniker's, 7th ed. p 152,153*

In primary immunodeficiencies, such as humoral immunodeficiencies and B cell defects, hypogamma globulinemia is seen, i.e. gammaglobulin is reduced. Its management consists of the maintainence of an adequate level of immunoglobulins. This can be achieved with an initial administration of gammaglobulin.

59. Ans. (a) IgE *Ref: Ananthanarayan and Paniker's, 8th ed. p 118*

A. IgG

i. Structure

All IgGs are monomers (7S immunoglobulin). The subclasses differ in the number of disulfide bonds and length of the hinge region.

ii. Properties

IgG is the most versatile immunoglobulin because it is capable of carrying out all of the functions of immunoglobulin molecules.

- IgG is the major Ig in serum—75% of serum Ig is IgG
- IgG is the major Ig in extravascular spaces
- Placental transfer: IgG is the only class of Ig that crosses the placenta. Transfer is mediated by a receptor on placental cells for the Fc region of IgG. Not all subclasses cross equally well.
- IgG2 does not cross well.
- Fixes complement: Not all subclasses fix equally well; IgG4 does not fix complement
- Binding to cells: Macrophages, monocytes, PMNs and some lymphocytes have Fc receptors for the Fc region of IgG. Not all subclasses bind equally well; IgG2 and IgG4 do not bind to Fc receptors. A consequence of binding to the Fc receptors on PMNs, monocytes and macrophages is that the cell can now internalize the antigen better. The antibody has prepared the antigen for eating by the phagocytic cells. The term opsonin is used to describe substances that enhance phagocytosis. IgG is a good opsonin. Binding of IgG to Fc receptors on other types of cells results in the activation of other functions.

B. IgM

i. Structure

IgM normally exists as a pentamer (19S immunoglobulin) but it can also exist as a monomer. In the pentameric form all heavy chains and all light chains are identical. This chain functions in polymerization of the molecule into a pentamer.

ii. Properties

- IgM is the third most common serum Ig.
- IgM is the first Ig to be made by the fetus and the first Ig to be made by a virgin B cells when it is stimulated by antigen.
- As a consequence of its pentameric structure, IgM is a good complement fixing Ig. Thus, IgM antibodies are very efficient in leading to the lysis of microorganisms.
- As a consequence of its structure, IgM is also a good agglutinating Ig . Thus, IgM antibodies are very good in clumping microorganisms for eventual elimination from the body.
- IgM binds to some cells via Fc receptors.
- B cell surface Ig

C. IgA

i. Structure

When IgA exits as a dimer, a J chain is associated with it.When IgA is found in secretions is also has another protein associated with it called the secretory piece or T piece; sIgA is sometimes referred to as 11S immunoglobulin.

ii. Properties

- IgA is the 2nd most common serum Ig.
- IgA is the major class of Ig in secretions—tears, saliva, colostrum, mucus. Since it is found in secretions secretory IgA is important in local (mucosal) immunity.
- Normally, IgA does not fix complement, unless aggregated.
- IgA can binding to some cells—PMNs and some lymphocytes.

D. IgD

i. Structure

IgD exists only as a monomer.

ii. Properties

- IgD is found in low levels in serum; its role in serum uncertain.
- IgD is primarily found on B cell surfaces where it functions as a receptor for antigen. IgD on the surface of B cells has extra-amino acids at C-terminal end for anchoring to the membrane. It also associates with the Ig-alpha and Ig-beta chains.
- IgD does not bind complement.

E. IgE

i. Structure

IgE exists as a monomer and has an extra domain in the constant region.

ii. Properties

- IgE is the least common serum Ig since it binds very tightly to Fc receptors on basophils and mast cells even before interacting with antigen.
- Involved in allergic reactions—As a consequence of its binding to basophils an mast cells, IgE is involved in allergic reactions. Binding of the allergen to the IgE on the cells results in the release of various pharmacological mediators that result in allergic symptoms.
- IgE also plays a role in parasitic helminth diseases. Since serum IgE levels rise in parasitic diseases, measuring IgE levels is helpful in diagnosing parasitic infections. Eosinophils have Fc receptors for IgE and binding of eosinophils to IgE-coated helminths results in killing of the parasite.
- IgE does not fix complement.

60. Ans. (c) Serum sickness *Ref: Ananthanarayan, 8th ed. p 165*

- Serum sickness in humans is a reaction to proteins in antiserum derived from a nonhuman animal source, occurring 410 days after exposure. It is a type of hypersensitivity, specifically immune complex hypersensitivity (type III). The term serum sickness-like reaction (SSLR) is occasionally used to refer to similar illnesses that arise from the introduction of certain non-protein substances. It was first characterized by Clemens von Pirquet and Béla Schick in 1906.
- When an antiserum is given, the human immune system can mistake the proteins present for harmful antigens. The body produces antibodies, which combine with these proteins to form immune complexes. These complexes enter walls of blood vessels and initiate an inflammatory response. They can also cause more reactions resulting in typical symptoms of serum sickness. This results in hypocomplementemia, a low C3 level in serum.
- Serum sickness differs from other type of hypersensitivity reaction in that a single dose of the antigen can severe as both the sensitizing and shocking dose.
- Seen more commonly following penicillin or other antibiotics injections.

61. Ans. (a) Active *Ref: Ananthanarayan and Paniker's, 8th ed. p 87*

Comparison of active and passive immunity

Active immunity	*Passive immunity*
Produced actively by host's immune system	Received passively. No active host participation
Induced by infection or by immunogens	Readymade antibody transferred
Durable effective protection	Transient, less effective
Immunity effective only after lag period	Immediate immunity
Immunological memory present	No memory
Booster effect on subsequent dose	Subsequent dose less effective
'Negative phase' may occur	No negative phase
Not applicable in the immunodeficient	Applicable in the immunodeficient

62. Ans. (a) Plasma cells *Ref: Ananthanarayan and Paniker's, 8th ed. p 96*

- Antibodies (immunoglobulins) are made by plasma cells.
- Antibodies are proteins that attach to, and help to destroy, germs such as bacteria and viruses.
- Normally, plasma cells make many different antibodies, each able to attack different bacteria and viruses.

63. Ans. (d) Type IV *Ref: The Immune Response: Basic and Clinical Principles, 1st ed. p957*
http://books.google.co.in/books?id=2AaJqNl1QIYCandp=PA957&dq=immunological+response+in+trans pla nt+rejection+is+by+type+IV&hl=en&sa=X&ei=aV0VU6ziMYKwiAeT2YA4&ved.=0CCoQ6AEwAA#v=o nepage&q=immunological%20response%20in%20transplant%20rejection%20is%20by%20type%20IV&f=false

- Transplantation is the process of taking cells, tissue or organs called a graft from one individual and placing them into another individual.
- A major barrier to transplantation is the process of rejection, in which the recipients immune system recognizes the graft as foreign and attack it.
- Sometime delayed hypersensitivity (type IV) also be the cause of some disease. It includes:
  - Allergic contact dermatitis
  - Hypersensitivity pneumonitis
  - Transplant rejection
  - Autoimmune disorder

64. Ans. (b) Rh (D) immunoglobulin *Ref: Ananthanarayan and Paniker's, 8th ed. p 190, 191*

- Rh incompatibility is a condition that develops when a pregnant woman has Rh-negative blood and the baby in her womb has Rh-positive blood.
- During pregnancy, red blood cells from the unborn baby can cross into the mother's bloodstream through the placenta.
- The use of special immunoglobulins called RhoGHAM,in order to prevent Erythroblastosis foetalis.

65. Ans. (d) Antibody and complement mediated cytotoxicity *Ref: Ananthanarayan and Paniker's, 8th ed. p 133,134*

- All nucleated cells in the body express HLA Class I molecules (A, B, and Cw), whereas HLA Class II (DR, DP and DQ) molecule expression is limited to B cells, antigen-presenting cells, and activated microvascular endothelial cells.
- HLA-1 are the principal antigen involved in graft rejection and cell mediated cytolysis.
- It may function as components of hormone recepters.

66. Ans. (a) CD7 + Pro T cells *Ref: Ananthanarayan, 7th ed. p 123*

T cell precursors from the yolk sac, fetal liver and bone marrow migrate to the thymus during the embryonic and postnatal stages. The earliest identifiable cells of T lineage are the CD7+ pro-T cells, which acquire CD2 on entering the thymus. They synthesis CD3 in the cytoplasm and become pre-T cells.

67. Ans. (c) IgM *Ref: Ananthanarayan and Paniker's, 8th ed. p 100*

Immunoglobulin E (IgE)

- It is a class of antibody (or immunoglobulin (Ig) that has been found only in mammals.
- IgE exists as monomers consisting of two heavy chains and two light chains.
- IgE's main function is immunity to parasites, such as parasitic worms like Schistosoma mansoni, Trichinella spiralis, and Fasciola hepatica.
- IgE may also be important during immune defense against certain protozoan parasites, such as Plasmodium falciparum.
- IgE also plays an essential role in type I hypersensitivity, which manifests various allergic diseases, such as allergic asthma, most types of sinusitis, allergic rhinitis, food allergy, and some types of chronic urticaria and atopic dermatitis.
- IgE also plays a pivotal role in allergic conditions, such as anaphylactic reactions to certain drugs, bee stings, and antigen preparations used in specific desensitization immunotherapy.

68. Ans. (d) Heterophile antigens *Ref: Ananthnarayan, 8th ed. p 93*

- Same or closely related antigens present in different biological species, classes, and kingdom are known as heterophile antigens
- Also known as heterogenetic antigen.
- The Weil-felix reaction in typhous fever, paul bunnel test in mononucleosis, and the cold agglutinin test in primary atypical pneumonia are the example of it.

69. Ans. (c) IgE antibodies *Ref: Ananthanarayan, 7th ed. p 159*

- Immediate hypersensitivity is an IgE antibody and mast cellmediated reaction to certain antigens that causes rapid vascular leakage and mucosal secretions, often followed by inflammation. IgE-mediated immediate hypersensitivity reactions are also called allergy, atopy.
- The sequence of events in the development of immediate hypersensitivity reactions begins with the activation of TH2 cells and the production of IgE antibodies in response to an antigen, binding of the IgE to Fc receptors of mast cells, then on subsequent exposure to the antigen, cross-linking of the bound IgE by the antigen and release of mast cell mediators

70. Ans. (b) MHC II *Ref: Ananthnarayan, 8th ed. p 130*

- Helper cells or inducer cells are CD4 cells.
- They have MHC class II restriction where as CD8 cells have MHC Class I restriction.
- It stimulate or promote the growth of T lymphocyte and macrophage.

71. Ans. (b) Agglutination *Ref: Ananthnarayan, 7th ed. p 98*

- **Agglutination reaction**: When a particular antigen is mixed with its antibody in the presence of electrolytes at a suitable temperature and pH, the particles are clumped.
  - Agglutination occurs optimally when antigen and antibody react in equivalent proportions
  - For example, Slide agglutination: Blood grouping
- Coomb's test (antiglobulin): Detection of anti Rh antibodies
- Tube agglutination: For serological diagnosis of typhoid, brucellosis and typhus fever.
- Various antigen-antibody reaction:
  - Precipitation reaction: e.g. VDRL test
  - Complement fixation test: e.g. Wassermann test for diagnosis of syphilis
  - Neutralization test

Note: Agglutination is more sensitive than precipitation for detection of antibodies.

72. Ans. (b) Antibodies on RBC surface *Ref: Ananthnarayan, 8th ed. p 188*

Refer Ans. 2

BACTERIOLOGY

73. Ans. (d) Clostridium sporogenes *Ref: Ananthnarayan, 8th ed. p 255*

- Gas gangrene (also known as 'Clostridial myonecrosis' and 'Myonecrosis') is a bacterial infection that produces gas in tissues in gangrene. It is a deadly form of gangrene.
- Causes of gas gangrene: Cl perfringens is encountered 60%, Cl novyi and Cl septicum is 20–40% and Cl histolyticum is less often.
- Treatment is usually debridement and excision, with amputation necessary in many cases. Antibiotics alone are not effective because they do not penetrate ischemic muscles sufficiently to be effective. However, penicillin is given as an adjuvant treatment to surgery. In addition to surgery and antibiotics, hyperbaric oxygen therapy (HBOT) is used and acts to inhibit the growth of and kill the anaerobic C. perfringens.

74. Ans. (a) Korthof *Ref: Ananthnarayan, 8th ed. p 382*

- Leptospirosis also known as Weil's syndrome, canicola fever, canefield fever, nanukayami fever, 7-day fever, Rat Catcher's Yellows, Fort Bragg fever, black jaundice, and Pretibial fever
- It is caused by infection with bacteria of the genus Leptospira and affects humans as well as other animals.
- On infection the microorganism can be found in blood and Cerebrospinal fluid (CSF) for the first 7 to 10 days (invoking serologically identifiable reactions) and then moving to the kidneys.
- After 7 to 10 days the microorganism can be found in fresh urine. Hence, early diagnostic efforts include testing a serum or blood sample serologically with a panel of different strains.
  - Media used for leptospirosis organism
  - Fletcher medium
  - Korthof medium
  - Stuart's medium
  - Ellinghausen Mecullough Johnson Harris medium (EMJH) a semisynthetic fever

75. Ans. (a) Campylobacter *Ref: Ananthnarayan, 8th ed. p 398*

- A microaerophile is a microorganism that requires oxygen to survive, but requires environments containing lower levels of oxygen than are present in the atmosphere (i.e. <21% O_2; typically 2-10% O_2).
- Many microaerophiles are also capnophiles, as they require an elevated concentration of carbon dioxide.

List of microaerophile bacteria are:

Borrelia burgdorferi

- Borrelia burgdorferi is a spiral-shaped bacterium responsible for Lyme disease in cattle and humans.
- The microorganism is mostly transmitted by ticks, but also by fleas, mosquitoes and mites.

Helicobacter pylori

- Helicobacter pylori is a gram negative spiral rod, motile bacteria.
- Helicobacter pylori causes digestive problems such as gastritis, peptic ulcers (sores in the stomach or first part of the small intestine), and even cancer.

Campylobacter

- Campylobacter are gram negative rods, typically coma shaped bacteria.
- Campylobacter causes food poisoning.
- Symptoms include diarrhea, vomiting, stomach pains and cramps and fever.
- Most infected people recover without treatment within two to five days, but some cases require the use of antibiotics.

76. Ans. (a) Most common source of infection is cross-infection from infected people *Ref: Harrison's 17th ed. p 873*

- S. aureus is a facultative anaerobic Gram-positive coccal bacterium, also known as "golden staph" and Oro staphira

- Most commonly, the individuals who suffered from staphylococcal infection are affected due to their own colonizing strains. Where as it is also listed under nosocomial infection hence it may also be acquired from the environment as well as other person.
- Toxic shock syndrome toxin (TSST-1) and staphylococcal enterotoxins are consider as a super antigen.
- Epidermolytic toxin is not considered as super antigen but it is responsible for staphylococcal scalded skin syndrome.
- Anterior nares is the susceptible site for their colonization(about 30% of population)
- Methicillin resistance is chromosomal mec (SCCmec) mediated -penicillin binding protein PBP-2a synthesized by mecA gene.

77. Ans. (a) Bacteria may or may not cause disease in experimental animals *Ref: Ananthnarayan, 8th ed. p 5*

- Koch's postulates are four criteria designed to establish a causal relationship between a microbe and a disease.
- The postulates were formulated byRobert Koch and Friedrich Loeffler in 1884 and refined and published by Koch in 1890.
- Koch applied the postulates to establish the etiology of cholera and tuberculosis, but they have been generalized to other diseases.
- **Koch's postulates are the following:**
  - The microorganism must be found in abundance in all organisms suffering from the disease, but should not be found in healthy organisms.
  - The microorganism must be isolated from a diseased organism and grown in pure culture.
  - The cultured microorganism should cause disease when introduced into a healthy organism.
  - The microorganism must be reisolated from the inoculated, diseased experimental host and identified as being identical to the original specific causative agent.

78. Ans. (c) Infection is mostly due to endogenous source *Ref: Ananthnarayan, 8th ed. p 315*

Pseudomonas aeruginosa

- It is a slender, nonsporulating, actively motile, aerobic Gram-negative bacteria.
- It is a obligate aerobe, but have the ability to grow anaerobically in the presence of nitrates.
- Pyocyanin and fluorescein (pyoverdin) are two best known pigment produces by it. Apart from it ,it also produces pyorubin and pyomelanin.
- It can grow in antiseptic solutions such as dettol, cetrimide, etc.
- In hospital, it may cause generalised as well as localised infection, due to its resistance to common antiseptics and antibiotics.
- It is the most common as well as serious cause of infection in burns patient.
- It give positive catalase and oxidase test
- Being Gram-negative bacteria, most Pseudomonas spp. are naturally resistant to penicillin.

Endogenous infection caused by an infectious agent that is already present in the body, but has previously been inapparent or dormant, e.g. Tuberculosis.

79. Ans. (b) All strains are susceptible to penicillin G *Ref: Ananthnarayan, 8th ed. p 230*

- Neisseria gonorrhoeae, also known as gonococcus is a species of Gram-negative coffee bean-shaped diplococci bacteria responsible for the sexually transmitted infection gonorrhea.
- It was first described by Neisser in 1879 in gonorrheal pus.
- Neisseria are fastidious Gram-negative cocci that require nutrient supplementation to grow in laboratory cultures.
- To be specific, they grow on chocolate agar with carbon dioxide and Muller-Hinton agar.
- These cocci are facultatively intracellular and typically appear in pairs (diplococci), in the shape of coffee beans.
- It is a delicate bacteria, which can be killed by heat, drying, and antiseptics.

- Adhesion of gonococci by pili to the mucous membrane.
- In males, urethritis is usually seen with painful micturition.
- In females, primary infection is in endocervix and extends to urethra and vaginawith mucopurulent discharge.
- Earlier all strains are sensitive to penicillin but by the time susceptibility decreased due to the penicillinase producing N gonorrhoeae.
- Incubation period is 2-8 days
- It is a strict parasite and can't live outside the body (become dead within 2 hrs).

80. Ans. (a) Susceptible to most of the antibiotics *Ref: Ananthnarayan, 8th ed. p 269*

- Bacteroids are anaerobic, gram-negative bacilli belongs to Bacteroidaceae family.
- It is non motile, nonsporing, strict anaerobe, possessing pleomorphism, (i.e. appears in branching forms, slender rods, or coccobacilli)
- It may appears single, pair or in short chains
- Normally they inhabitants of intestinal, respiratory or female genital tracts.
- Most frequent species is B. fragilis
- The species of anaerobes most frequently isolated from clinical infections are Bacteroides.
- B.fragilis is most commonly isolated from blood, pleural, and peritoneal fluid, CSF, brain abcess, wounds, and urogenital infection.
- In general, bacteroides are resistant to a wide variety of antibiotics β-lactams, aminoglycosides, and recently many species have acquired resistance to erythromycin and tetracycline.
- Bacteroids are susceptible to metronidazole, chloramphenicol and clindamycin.

81. Ans. (b) O antibodies last longer and hence are not an indicator of recent infection
Ref: Ananthnarayan, 8th ed. p 296

- Widal test is the most commonly used agglutination test for the detection of salmonella antibodies in patients sera
- It measures H and O aglutinins for typhoid and paratyphoid bacilli
- **Two types of tubes are used in it as:**
  - Dreyer's tube—H agglutination (connical bottom)
  - Flix tube—O agglutination (round bottom)
- **Appearance:**
  - H agglutination appears as a loose, woolly clump of cotton.
  - Agglutination appears as a granular, irregular disc.
- It is usually done after the first week of the disease.
- H agglutinins persist tonger than O agglutinins

Significant titer: A titer of 1 in 100 or more for O and 1 in 200 or more for H is usually taken as a diagnostic titer.

82. Ans. (b) 750 million/mL *Ref: Advances in Applied Microbiology, Vol 8 , p 226*

- Saliva is a watery substance located in the mouths of organisms, secreted by the salivary glands.
- Human saliva is 99.5% water, while the other 0.5% consists of electrolytes, mucus, glycoproteins, enzymes, and antibacterial compounds, such as secretory IgA and lysozyme.
- The enzymes found in saliva are essential in beginning the process of digestion of dietary starches and fats.
- Saliva has both a mechanical cleansing action and a specific (immunoglobulins, e.g. IgA) and non-specific immunologic action (e.g. lysozyme, lactoferrin and myeloperoxidase).
- These factors control the micro-organisms that survive in the mouth. It also has a protective function, helping to prevent dental plaque build-up on the teeth and washing away adhered food particles.
- Salivary glands secrete about 1,500 ml of saliva on a daily basis.
- Microscopic counts in saliva show an average of 750 million mircro-organisms per milliliter. With the temperature in the oral cavity around 98.6° Fahrenheit, the mouth is the perfect environment for mircro-organisms to live.
- Salivary enzymes are urease (derived from microbes) and ptyalin (causes degradation of starch).

83. Ans. (a) Bacitracin sensitivity *Ref: Ananthnarayan, 8th ed. p 673*

- Streptococci are Gram-positive, nonmotile, nonsporeforming, catalase-negative cocci that occur in pairs or chains.
- Group A streptococci have a hyaluronic acid capsule.
- It is highly sensitive to bacitracin hence it is used to differentiate between various beta-hemolytic streptococci.
- Other important facts about Group A beta-hemolytic streptococci:
  - Catalase and coagulase negative
  - PYR test positive
  - On blood agar colonies are pinpoint sized (head-sized colonies Staphylococcus aureus)
  - M-protein is the single most important virulent factor.

84. Ans. (a) McCoy culture *Ref: Ananthnarayan, 8th ed. p 418*

- Chlamydia infection is a common sexually transmitted infection in humans caused by the bacterium Chlamydia trachomatis.
- The term Chlamydia infection can also refer to infection caused by any species belonging to the bacterial family Chlamydiaceae. C. trachomatis is found only in humans.
- Chlamydia is a major infectious cause of human genital and eye disease.
- Chlamydia infection is one of the most common sexually transmitted infections worldwide
- In men, infection of the urethra (urethritis) is usually symptomatic, causing a white discharge from the penis with or without pain on urinating (dysuria)
- Cell cultures commonly used for isolation of chlamydia are as follows:
  - McCoy
  - HeLa cells

85. Ans. (b) Flea is a vector of the disease *Ref: Ananthnarayan, 8th ed. p 407*

- Endemic typhus fever is a disease caused by bacteria called Rickettsia typhi or bacteria called Rickettsia felis.
- Endemic typhus fever occurs worldwide, most commonly among people in contact with rats or areas where rats live. Disease also occurs among people to live near or have contact with other small mammals (such as opossums)
- Endemic typhus fever is not directly spread from person-to-person.
- Disease is spread by rat fleas infected with the bacteria that cause endemic typhus fever. Rat fleas become infected when they feed on the blood of a rat with endemic typhus fever.
- Common symptoms of endemic typhus fever include low-grade fever, mild headache, tiredness, joint pain and muscle aches.
- Culture is not a preferred method for diagnosis of endemic typhus.
- Heterophile Weil-Felix reaction: Endemic typhus agglutinate OX19 and sometimes OX2 also.

86. Ans. (a) Vibrio cholerae *Ref: Ananthnarayan, 8th ed. p 307*

- Vibrio cholerae is a "comma" shaped Gram-negative bacteria with a single, polar flagellum for movement.
- There are numerous strains of V. cholerae, some of which are pathogenic and some of which are not.
- Cholera toxin is similar to the heat labile toxin of E coli.
- Biochemical reactions: Oxidase +ve, sucrose fermenter (yellow colonies on TCBS), string test +ve, cholera red reaction.
- Cholerae vibrios are susceptible to heat, drying and acids but resist high alkalinity.
- Vibrio cholerae produce- cholera toxin,a peptid that irreversibly activates Gs by Covalently adding an ADP-ribose moiety to specific arginine residue. This leads to continuous activation of adenylate cyclase and dramatic increase in CAMP levels intestinal epthelial cells.

87. Ans. (c) Person to person *Ref: Ananthnarayan, 8th ed. p 342-345*

- Brucella is a genus of Gram-negative bacteria named after David Bruce (1855–1931).
- They are small (0.5 to 0.7 by 0.6 to 1.5 µm), non-motile, non-encapsulated coccobacilli, which function as facultative intracellular parasites.
- Brucella melitensis is the most pathogenic form, B. abortus and B. suis are of intermediate pathogenicity.
- Brucella is the cause of brucellosis, which is a zoonosis.
- Human brucellosis is usually not transmitted from human to human.
- people become infected by contact with fluids from infected animals (sheep, cattle or pigs) or derived food products like unpasteurized milk and cheese.
- Brucellosis is also considered an occupational disease because of a higher incidence in people working with animals (slaughterhouse cases).
- People may also be infected by inhalation of contaminated dust or aerosols, and as such the CDC has labeled brucella as highly weaponizable.

88. Ans. (d) Bacitracin sensitivity *Ref: Ananthnarayan, 8th ed. p 207*

The description of microorganismsn given in the question indicates that the infective skin leison is due to the GpA β-hemolytic streptococci as it is a Gram-positive cocci arranged in chains and hemolytic (attack red blood cells) in nature. It is a catalase negative.

Refer Ans no. 11

89. Ans. (a) It is halophilic *Ref: Ananthnarayan, 8th ed. p 312*

Genus Vibrio:

- Curved Gram negative rods (coma-shaped), motile by polar flagellum, they are either:
- Halophilic, require 8.5% and the isolated human pathogens included are:
  - V. parahaemolyticum: Self limited enteritis from contaminated seafood.
  - V. vulnificus: Wound infection
- Non-halophilic, the most important pathogens are:
  - V. cholera: Cholera
  - Noncholera Vibrio (Nonagglutinable vibrio): Sever enteritis

General characteristics of V. cholera

- Actively motile Gram negative, curved rod.
- Ferment glucose, sucrose and mannose but require few days to ferment mannitol.
- All are oxidase positive
- Optimum pH required (8.5)
- Cholera is transmitted by fecal contamination of water and food from human sources.
- Biochemical reactions: oxidase positive, sucrose fermenter (yellow colonies on TCBS), string test positive and cholera red reaction.
- Cholera vibrios are susceptible to heat, drying and acids but resist high alkalinity.

90. Ans. (c) Legionella *Ref: Ananthnarayan, 8th ed. p 400*

- The genus Legionella is a pathogenic group of gram negative bacteria, that includes the species L. pneumophila, causing Legionellosis (all illnesses caused by Legionella) including a pneumonia type illness called Legionnaires Disease and a mild flu like illness called Pontiac fever.
- Legionella acquired its name after a July 1976 outbreak of a then-unknown "mystery disease" sickened 221 persons, causing 34 deaths. The outbreak was first noticed among people attending a convention of the American Legionan association of US military veterans in Philadelphia.
- It was characterised by fever, cough, and chest pain.

- Incubation period is 2-10 days.
- Legionella is traditionally detected by culture on buffered charcoal yeast extract (BCYE) agar. Legionella requires the presence of cysteine and iron to grow and therefore does not grow on common blood agar media
- New techniques for the rapid detection of Legionella in water samples are emerging including the use of polymerase chain reaction (PCR) and rapid immunological assays. These technologies can typically provide much faster results.
- Legionella live within amoebae and other protozoan in the natural environment.
- Person-to-person transmission of Legionella has not been demonstrate

91. Ans. (c) The heat-stable toxin was present in the food when stored at room temperature, which caused the symptoms *Ref: Ananthnarayan, 8th ed. p 247*

- **Bacillus cereus** is an endemic, soil-dwelling, Gram-positive, rod-shaped, beta hemolytic bacterium.
- Some strains are harmful to humans and cause foodborne illness, while other strains can be beneficial as probiotics for animals.
- It is the cause of "Fried Rice Syndrome," as the bacteria is classically contracted from fried rice dishes that have been sitting at room temperature for hours (such as at a buffet)
- Ingestion of bacillus cereus leads to two types of illness, diarrheal and emetic (vomiting) syndrome.
  - **The diarrheal type** is associated with a wide range of foods, has an 8- to 16.5-hour incubation time, and is associated with diarrhea and gastrointestinal pain. Also known as the 'long-incubation' form of B. cereus food poisoning, it might be difficult to differentiate from poisoning caused by Clostridium perfringens.
  - **The 'emetic' form** is commonly caused by rice that is not cooked for a time and temperature sufficient to kill any spores present, then improperly refrigerated. It can produce a toxin, cereulide, which is not inactivated by later reheating. This form leads to nausea and vomiting 15 hours after consumption. It can be difficult to distinguish from other short-term bacterial foodborne pathogens such as Staphylococcus aureus.

92. Ans. (b) Carbohydrate C antigen *Ref: Ananthnarayan, 8th ed. p 205*

- The system was created by Rebecca Lancefield and remains her biggest contribution to medical science
- Lancefield grouping is a method of grouping beta-hemolytic bacteria based on the carbohydrate (c) composition of bacterial antigens found on their cell walls.
- Group A streptococci are further classified by serological typing of (M) proteins into Griffith types (1, 2, 3, etc.).

93. Ans. (b) MSA *Ref: Shafer's, 7th ed. p 468*

- Mitis Salivarius Agar is a selective streptococcal medium having 20% sucrose and 0.2 U bacitracin/ml.
- The growth of most non-S. mutans colonies is suppressed by Bacitracin present in the medium.

94. Ans. (c) From inhalation of the aerosols in an air-conditioned room at a convention center *Ref: Ananthnarayan, 8th ed. p 400*

Legionnaires's disease

- Caused by Legionella pneumophilla.
- It may be epidemic or sporadic.
- Incubation period is 2-10 days.
- Legionella lives in natural as well as artificial water sources, such as mud, stagnant water, hot spring, cooling towers, air conditioner, shower heads, etc.
- Human infection is due to inhalation of aerosol produced by artificial water containing items act as disseminators which are discussed in above point.
- No animal reservoir exists.
- Infection is limited to human being.
- No carrier state is present.
- Man to man transmission is not occur.

- **Laboratory diagnosis:**
  - Culture of transtracheal aspirate in BYCE is most sensitive and specific
  - Direct fluorescence stain is the most sensitive option for visualization in tissues and
  - Urinary Legionella antigen testing is rapid inexpensive and the second-most sensitive and a specific test.
  - Clinical syndrome: Pontiac fever, mild self-limiting infl uenza like illness.

95. Ans. (c) S. aureus *Ref: Shafer's, 6th ed. p 512*

- Subacute bacterial endocarditis is an infection of the inner lining of the heart and the heart valves.
- It is very serious because it can cause destruction of the heart tissue.
- It is usually caused by a form of streptococci viridans bacteria that normally live in the mouth and throat. Other strains of streptococci (bovis and equines) can also cause subacute endocarditis, usually in patients who have a form of gastrointestinal cancer. Additional causes are Enterococci (urinary tract infections) and coagulase negative staphylococci such as Staphylococcus epidermidis (skin).
- **Signs of SABE:**
  - Unexplained fever
  - Night sweats
  - Poor appetite
  - Muscle and joint aches
  - No energy
  - Weight loss
  - Back or chest pain
  - Unusual rashes
- The standard treatment is with a minimum of four weeks of high-dose intravenous penicillin with an aminoglycoside, such as gentamicin.

96. Ans. (b) Blood agar *Ref: Ananthnarayan, 8th ed. p 417, 418*

Isolation of Chlamydia

- By inoculation in yolk sac, as Chlamydia grows in yolk sac of 6–8 day old chick embryo.
- In a tissue culture isolation, procedure involved irradiated Mc Coy, HeLa cells and BHK-21 cells.
- Inoculation into experimental animal.
- Cell culture used for isolation are penetrated by irradiation or chemicals, such as 5-iodo, 2-deoxyuridine or cycloheximide to enhance its replication.

97. Ans. (a) That they are inhibited by penicillin *Ref: Ananthnarayan, 8th ed. p 388*

Mycoplasma

- Mycoplasma refers to a genus of bacteria that lack a cell wall.
- Without a cell wall, they are unaffected by many common antibiotics, such as penicillin or other beta-lactam antibiotics that target cell wall synthesis.
- They can be parasitic or saprotrophic.
- Several species are pathogenic in humans, including M. pneumoniae, which is an important cause of atypical pneumonia and other respiratory disorders, and M. genitalium, which is believed to be involved in pelvic inflammatory diseases.
- It is a pleomorphic organisms.
- The granules may be coccoid, ballon, disc, ring, or star forms.
- The filaments are slender, varying in lengths and show true branching.
- Multiplied by binary fission.
- They are Gram negative but are better stained by Giemsa.
- It can be treated by tetracycline and erythromycin.

98. Ans. (d) The acellular vaccine is associated with high incidence of neurological symptoms

Ref: Ananthnarayan, 8th ed. p 335-339

- Bordetella pertussis is a Gram-negative, aerobic coccobacillus capsulate, non motile of the genus Bordetella, and the causative agent of pertussis or whooping cough.
- B. pertussis is pleomorphic, nonmotile, nonsporing, capsulated, fimbriated coccobacilli, which show Bipolar metachromatic granules on staining with toluidine blue.
- Bordetella pertussis is a highly communicable agent and is transmitted person-to-person via airborne droplets or direct contact with discharges from the respiratory mucous membranes of an infected person.
- It colonizes the respiratory tract including the mouth, nose, throat and beginning of the lungs of young children worldwide. The bacteria bind to ciliated cells in the respiratory mucosa by producing adhesions.
- The bacterium is spread by airborne droplets; its incubation period is seven to 14 days.
- B. pertussis has the ability to inhibit the function of the host's immune system. The toxin, known as pertussis toxin (or PTx), inhibits G protein coupling that regulates an adenylate cyclase-mediated conversion of ATP to cyclic AMP. The end result is phagocytes convert too much ATP to cyclic AMP, which can cause disturbances in cellular signaling mechanisms, and prevent phagocytes from correctly responding to an infection.
- The infection occurs mostly in children under the age of one when they are unimmunized, or children with faded immunity, normally around the ages 11 through 18.
- The signs and symptoms are similar to a common cold: runny nose, sneezing, mild cough, and low-grade fever. The patient becomes most contagious during the catarrhal stage of infection, normally two weeks after the coughing begins. It may become airborne when the person cough.
- A nasopharyngeal or an oropharynx swab is sent to the bacteriology laboratory for Gram stain (Gram negative, coccobacilli, diplococci arrangement), growth on Bordet-Gengou agar or BCYE plate with added cephalosporin to select for the organism, which shows mercury-drop-like colonies
- The organism is oxidase positive, but urease, nitrate reductase, and citrate negative. It is also nonmotile
- Cellular vaccine causes high incidence of neurological symptoms and not the acellular vaccine.

99. Ans. (a) Caused by Calymmatobacterium *Ref: Ananthnarayan, 8th ed. p 396*

- Granuloma inguinale is a sexually transmitted infection (STI) caused by the bacteria Calymmatobacterium or Klebsiella granulomatis.
- It is characterised by lesions on the genitals or perianal area that start as raised nodules (granulomas) and then erode to form beefy-red velvety heaped-up ulcers that gradually increase in size.
- Granuloma inguinale is also called Donovanosis. Donovan bodies are cellular components that are seen when scrapings from the edge of the lesions are viewed under a microscope.
- After contracting the infection it may take from 1 week to 3 months for any signs and symptoms to appear. There are several types of lesions that may occur and symptoms are mild.
  - The nodular type consists of soft lumps that are typically beefy red in colour and tend to bleed easily. These are usually painless despite ulceration.
  - The hypertrophic or verrucous type consists of large dry warty masses that resemble genital warts .
  - The necrotic type presents as dry ulcers that evolve into scarred areas
- In the early stages it may be difficult to differentiate granuloma inguinale from chancroid. In the later stages, the condition may look likelymphogranuloma venereum. It may also be confused with other conditions, such as penile or vulvar cancer or syphilis.

100. Ans. (d) Mycobacterium leprae *Ref: Ananthnarayan, 8th ed. p 365*

Transmission

The risks and transmission probabilities of sexually transmitted diseases are summarized as:

Bacterial

- Chancroid (Haemophilus ducreyi)
- Chlamydia (Chlamydia trachomatis)

- Gonorrhea (Neisseria gonorrhoeae), colloquially known as "the clap"
- Granuloma inguinale or (Klebsiella granulomatis)
- Syphilis (Treponema pallidum)

Fungal

- Candidiasis (yeast infection)

Viral

- Viral hepatitis (Hepatitis B virus)saliva, venereal fluids. (Note: Hepatitis A and Hepatitis E are transmitted via the fecal-oral route; Hepatitis Cis rarely sexually transmittable,[19] and the route of transmission of Hepatitis D (only if infected with B) is uncertain, but may include sexual transmission.[20][21][22])
- Herpes simplex (Herpes simplex virus 1, 2) skin and mucosal, transmissible with or without visible blisters
- HIV (human immunodeficiency virus) venereal fluids, semen, breast milk, blood
- HPV (human papillomavirus) skin and mucosal contact. 'High risk' types of HPV cause almost all cervical cancers, as well as some anal, penile, and vulvar cancer. Some other types of HPV cause genital warts.
- Molluscum contagiosum (molluscum contagiosum virus MCV) close contact.

Parasites

- Crab louse, colloquially known as "crabs" or "pubic lice" (Pthirus pubis)
- Scabies (Sarcoptes scabiei).

Protozoal

- Trichomoniasis (Trichomonas vaginalis), colloquially known as "trich"
- **Leprosy or Hansen's disease (HD) is a chronic disease caused by the bacteria Mycobacterium leprae and Mycobacterium lepromatosis.**

101. Ans. (c) The patient should be given antitoxin intravenously *Ref: Ananthnarayan, 8th ed. p 260*

- Tetanus is caused by Cl tetani.
- It is distributed in the intestines of human being, and animals as well as soil.
- It is a gram positive, slender bacillus, occurs singly or sometime arranged in chains, obligate anaerobe.
- It grows well in Robertson's cooked meat broth.
- It produces at least two distinct toxins alpha hemolysin (tetanolysin) and a powerful neurotoxin (tetanospasmin).
- Toxin produced locally is absorbed by the motor nerve and it goes to CNS.
- The incubation period is 2 days to several weeks (6-12 days).
- Commonly it occurs in rural area and developing country.
- Anti tetanus serum should be given IV, when tetanus acquired through traumatic wound.

102. Ans. (c) Diphtheria *Ref: Microbiological Safety and Quality of Food, Vol 1, P 253*
http://books.google.co.in/books?id=lks9dALNzZAC&pg=PA257&dq=bifidobacteria+ PROBIOTIC&hl=en&sa=X&ei =0DEIU6nTDISXigeH0YGQDw&ved=0CDUQ6AEw Ag#v=onepage&q=bifidobacteria%20PROBIOTIC&f=false

Probiotic

- Probiotic bacteria favourably alter the intestinal microflora balance, inhibit the growth of harmful bacteria, promote good digestion, boost immune function, and increase resistance to infection.
- People with flourishing intestinal colonies of beneficial bacteria are better equipped to fight the growth of disease-causing bacteria.
- Lactobacilli and bifidobacteria maintain a healthy balance of intestinal flora by producing organic compoundssuch as lactic acid, hydrogen peroxide, and acetic acidthat increase the acidity of the intestine and inhibit the reproduction of many harmful bacteria.
- Probiotic bacteria also produce substances called bacteriocins, which act as natural antibiotics to kill undesirable microorganisms.

103. Ans. (b) IgM antibody detectable in 5 days *Ref: Ananthnarayan, 8th ed. p 381-385*

Leptospirosis

- Leptospirosis is caused by various species of Leptospira, a spirochete in the family Leptospiraceae, order Spirochaetales.
- Leptospirosis can be transmitted either directly between hosts or indirectly in the environment.
- Leptospira spp. can be ingested in contaminated food or water, spread in aerosolized urine or water, or transmitted by direct contact with the skin. The organisms usually enter the body through mucous membranes or abraded skin.
- Leptospira spp. do not multiply outside the host. In the environment, they require high humidity for survival and are killed by dehydration or temperatures greater than 50°C.
- Leptospira species can be inactivated by 1% sodium hypochlorite, 70% ethanol, glutaraldehyde, formaldehyde, detergents and acid. This organism is sensitive to moist heat (121°C for a minimum of 15 min) and is also killed by pasteurization.
- The incubation period in humans is usually 10 days, with a range of 2 to 29 days.
- Leptospirosis can be diagnosed by culture, detection of antigens or nucleic acids, or serology. Serum chemistry values and analysis of the CSF may support the diagnosis.
- The most commonly used serologic tests are the microscopic agglutination test (MAT, previously known as the agglutination-lysis test) or ELISAs.
- ELISA is used and deter IgM which is produced and become detectors as early as 3 days of illness.
- Antibiotics used in humans include doxycycline, ampicillin, amoxicillin, penicillin and erythromycin.
- Mortality is 515% in severe cases.

104. Ans. (c) MOTT infection interferes with protection given by BCG results *Ref: Ananthnarayan, 8th ed. p 362*

- Human disease is believed to be acquired from environmental exposures, and unlike tuberculosis and leprosy, there has been no evidence of animal-to-human or human-to-human transmission of NTM,
- The most common clinical manifestation of NTM disease is lung disease, but lymphatic, skin/soft tissue, and disseminated disease are also important.
- They cause opportunistic infections in persons with low immunity.
- They interfere with protection given by BCG vaccine.

105. Ans. (a) S. mitis *Ref: Ananthnarayan, 8th ed. p 205*

Streptococci and staphylococci can be differentiate simply by a catalase test, Streptococci are catalase negative, whereas staphylococci are catalase positive.

106. Ans. (c) Hemolysis on blood agar *Ref: Ananthnarayan, 8th ed. P 216*

- The viridans streptococci are a large group of commensal streptococcal bacteria species that are either α-hemolytic, producing a green coloration on blood agar plates (hence the name "viridans", from Latin "vĭridis", green), or nonhemolytic.
- Viridans streptococci can be differentiated from Streptococcus pneumoniae using an optochin test, as viridans streptococci are optochin resistant;
- Viridans streptococci have the unique ability to synthesize dextrans from glucose, which allows them to adhere to fibrin-platelet aggregates at damaged heart valves.

107. Ans. (a) It is acidogenic and aciduric *Ref: Shafer's Textbook of Oral Pathology, 7th ed. p 468*

- Streptococcus mutans and Lactobacillus are acidogenic and aciduric meaning that they can produce acids which can dissolve the tooth substance (calcium phosphate in the form of hydroxyapatite crystals) and that they can survive and even produce acids in a low pH environment.

- Compared to other oral flora, Streptococcus mutans and Lactobacillus are cariogenic and have enzymes with greater resistance to acid.
- They also have greater capacities of the cells to extrude protons from the cytoplasm.
- The most important enzyme for extrusion of protons is ATPase.
- This enzyme is found in higher amounts and is working at lower pH with S. mutans and Lactobacillus.

108. Ans. (a) That it shows pleomorphic appearance *Ref: Ananthnarayan, 8th ed. p 321*

- Yersinia pestis (formerly Pasteurella pestis) is a Gram-negative rod-shaped coccobacillus, non-motile a facultative anaerobic bacterium that can infect humans and other animals.
- Human Y. pestis infection takes three main forms: pneumonic, septicemic, and bubonic plagues.
- Y. pestis with bipolar staining giving it a safety pin appearance.
- Similar to other Yersinia members, it tests negative for urease, lactose fermentation, and indole.
- The closest relative is the gastrointestinal pathogen Yersinia pseudotuberculosis, and more distantly Yersinia enterocolitica.
- The transmission of Y. pestis by fleas is well characterized.
- Flea bites allow for the bacteria to pass the skin barrier
- The traditional first line treatment for Y. pestis has been streptomycin, chloramphenicol, tetracycline, and fluoroquinolones.
- Y. pestis has been used as a biological weapon in World War II, when on October 4, 1940, a Japanese airplane flying over Chushien, Chekiang Province, China released rice and wheat plus rat fleas carrying Y. pestis. A second plane load was released 3 weeks later. These actions led to a local plague that killed 121 people. Leon A. Fox from the U.S. Army Medical Corps had suggested a similar approach in 1933 proposing to drop infested rats from planes.

109. Ans. (d) Brucella spp. *Ref: Ananthnarayan, 8th ed. p 341-346*

- Brucella is a genus of Gram-negative bacteria named after David Bruce (1855–1931).
- They are small (0.5 to 0.7 by 0.6 to 1.5 μm), non-motile, non-encapsulated coccobacilli, which function as facultative intracellular parasites.
- Brucella is the cause of brucellosis, which is a zoonosis.
- It is transmitted by ingesting contaminated food (such as unpasteurized milk products), direct contact with an infected animal, or inhalation of aerosols.
- Transmission from human to human, for example through sexual intercourse or from mother to child, is exceedingly rare, but possible.
- Brucella is isolated from a blood culture on Castaneda medium. Prolonged incubation (up to 6 weeks) may be required as they are slow-growing, but on modern automated machines the cultures often show positive results within seven days.
- On Gram stain they appear as dense clumps of Gram-negative coccobacilli.
- Oxidase and catalase tests are positive for most members of the genus Brucella.
- Human brucellosis is usually not transmitted from human to human; people become infected by contact with fluids from infected animals (sheep, cattle or pigs) or derived food products like unpasteurized milk and cheese.
- Brucellosis is also considered an occupational disease because of a higher incidence in people working with animals.
- **Yersinia spp.** grows on ordinary media and is oxidase negative.
- **Francisella spp.** is mainly transmitted via rabbits and rodents and not cattle.
- **Bartonella spp.** is oxidase negative.

110. Ans. (b) M. kansas can cause a disease indistinguishable from tuberculosis *Ref: Ananthnarayan, 8th ed. p 359*

M. Kansasii

- M. kansasii causes lung disease that is clinically indistinguishable from tuberculosis.
- Symptoms may be less severe and more chronic than Mycobacterium tuberculosis infection.

- Asymptomatic M. kansasii infection occurs in a small proportion (16%) of affected patients
- The most common symptoms of pulmonary M. kansasii infection include cough (91%), sputum production (85%), weight loss (53%), breathlessness (51%), chest pain (34%), hemoptysis (32%), and fever or sweats (17%).
- Cutaneous M. kansasii infection resembles sporotrichosis secondary to local lymphatic spread. Cutaneous lesions may include nodules, pustules, verrucous lesions, erythematous plaques, abscesses, and ulcers.
- M. kansasii infection manifests late in the course of HIV disease. The lung is the organ most commonly involved. Commonly reported symptoms include fever, chills, night sweats, productive or nonproductive cough, weight loss, fatigue, dyspnea, and chest pain.

111. Ans. (c) S. pyogenes *Ref: Ananthnarayan, 8th ed. p 225*

- Streptococcus pyogenes is an aerobic, gram-positive extracellular bacterium.
- It is made up of non-motile, non-sporing cocci that are less then 2 μm in length and that form chains and large colonies greater then 0.5 mm in size.
- It has a β-hemolytic growth pattern on blood agar and there are over 60 different strains of the bacterium.
- This bacterium is responsible for a wide array of infections. It can cause streptococcal sore throat which is characterized by fever, enlarged tonsils, tonsillar exudate, sensitive cervical lymph nodes and malaise.
- Transmission via respiratory droplets, hand contact with nasal discharge and skin contact with impetigo lesions are the most important modes of transmission.
- The incubation period is usually 1–3 days.
- The bacterium can be spread to cattle and then back to humans through raw milk as well as through contaminated food sources (salads, milk, eggs).

112. Ans. (a) Leptospirosis *Ref: Ananthnarayan, 8th ed. p 381-385*

- Leptospirosis is a zoonosis with a worldwide distribution.
- Water is an important vehicle in their transmission.
- Epidemics of leptospirosis may result from exposure to flood waters contaminated by urine from infected animals.
- Leptrospira are excreted in urine of infected animals for a long time. Rats, mice and voles particularly R. novergicus and Mus musculus are Reservoirs.
- Human infection is usually caused by occupational exposure to the urine of infected animals, eg agricultural and live stock farmers, worker in rice fields.
- Leisure time activities such as swimming and fishing also carry risks.
- Leptospira shed in urine and can survive for weeks in soil and water heavy rainfall can leads to high level of contamination of soil of that area. Potential contamination of water occurs.

113. Ans. (d) Human to human transmission is seen *Ref: Ananthnarayan, 8th ed. p 400*

Refer Ans no. 22

114. Ans. (d) Shock and DIC are common in bacteroides bacteremia *Ref: Ananthnarayan, 8th ed. p 267*

Bacteroides:

- Gram negative anaerobic bacilli
- Most common anaerobic pathogen isolated from clinical specimens
- They are nonsporing, nonmotile, strict anaerobe, show pleomorphism.
- It grows well in brain heart infusion agar have 10% CO_2 in anaerobic atmosphere.
- Virulence factors include capsular polysaccharides and lipopolysaccharide endotoxin
- Lipopolysaccharide endotoxin is much less toxic compared to other gram negative bacteria
- Hence infections do not directly produce signs of sepsis, which is common in other gram negative bacteria
- Some are resistant to metronidazole

Remember-

B. fragilis—only Gram ve without typical endotoxin
Listeria—only Gram +ve with endotoxin.

115. Ans. (d) Mycobacterium tuberculosis *Ref: Ananthnarayan, 8th ed. , p 355*

Pyrexia of unknown origin (PUO) refers to a condition in which the patient has an elevated temperature but despite investigations by a physician no explanation has been found.

- In 1961 Petersdorf and Beeson suggested the following criteria for PUO:
  - Fever higher than 38.3°C (101°F) on several occasions
  - Persisting without diagnosis for at least 3 weeks
  - At least 1 week's investigation in hospital

Common causes of pyrexia of unknown origin

Most cases are unusual presentations of common diseases as: tuberculosis, endocarditis, gallbladder disease and HIV infection.

116. Ans. (c) V. cholera *Ref: Ananthnarayan, 8th ed. p- 307*

Vibrio cholerae

- Vibrio cholerae is a Gram-negative, comma-shaped, facultative anaerobic organism and has a flagellum at one cell pole.
- Natural infection with cholera occurs in humans only.
- The endotoxin produced by Cholerae does not play any role in the natural pathogenesis.

Endotoxins are part of the outer membrane of the cell wall of Gram-negative bacteria. Endotoxin is invariably associated with Gram-negative bacteria whether the organisms are pathogenic or not. Gram-negative pathogens such as Escherichia coli, Salmonella, Shigella, Pseudomonas, Neisseria, Haemophilus influenzae, Bordetella pertussis and Vibrio cholerae.

117. Ans. (c) Dark ground microscope *Ref: Anathanarayan, 8th ed. p 381-385*

- Leptospires are actively motile, delicate spirochetes, possessing a large number of closely wound spirals and characteristic hooked ends. They are too thin to be seen under the light microscope (leptos, meaning fine or thin). Several leptospires are saprophytic, while many are parasitic in rodents and other animals.

Examination of urine: During the second week of the disease Leptospires appear in the urine and there for 4-6 weeks. The urine should be examined immediately after voiding as leptospires readily undergo lysis in acid urine. Centrifuged deposit of the urine may be examined under dark ground illumination. Direct culture of urine is seldom successful because of contamination.

Therapy: Leptospires are sensitive to penicillin and tetracyclines, Penicillin is given as IV, 1-2 million units 6 hourly for 7 days in serious cases. A mild Jarisch-Herxheimar reaction may occur in some. Doxycycline 200 mg orally given once a week is effective in prophylaxis.

118. Ans. (c) Robertson's cooked meat medium *Ref: Aananthnarayan, 8th ed. p 251*

Cultural characteristics of clostridia are:

As the gas Gangrene is caused by Clostria perfringes

It is an anaerobe microorganism. Oxygen is not actively toxic to the bacillus and cultures do not die on exposure to air. It grows pH range of 5.5-8.0 and temperature range of 20-50°C. If can be utilized for obtaining pure cultures of CI perfringens. Robertson's cooked meat broth inoculated with mixtures of Cl perfringens and other bacteria and incubated at 45°C for 4–6 hours serves as enrichment. Subcultures from this transferred to blood agar plates yield pure or predominant growth of Cl perfringens.

Clostridia as human pathogens

	Viridans streptococci	*Streptococcus pneumoniae*
Solubility in bile	Insoluble	Soluble
Fermentation of inulin	Not a fermenter	Fermenter with acid production
Sensitivity to optochin	Not sensitive	Sensitive
Pathogenicity to mice	Nonpathogenic	Pathogenic
Quellung test	Negative	Positive

119. Ans. (a) Bacteroides fragilis *Ref: Ananthnarayan, 8th ed. p 269*

- B. fragilis is gram negative anaerobic bacilius and is most frequent non-sporing anaerobe isolated from clinical specimens like blood pleural space, peritoneal cavity, brain abscess and CSF wounds.
- Bacteroides fragilis is a Gram-negative bacillus bacterium species, and an obligate anaerobe of the gut
- B. fragilis group is the most commonly isolated Bacteroidaceae in anaerobic infections, especially those that originate from the gastrointestinal flora.
- B. fragilis is the most prevalent organism in the B. fragilis group, accounting for 41% to 78% of the isolates of the group.
- The B. fragilis group is the species of Bacteroidaceae isolated with greatest frequency in clinical specimens.
- These organisms are resistant to penicillin by virtue of production of beta-lactamase, and by other unknown factors.

120. Ans. (a) Acute gastritis *Ref: Medical KDT, 6th ed. p 637*

- Helicobacter pylori (H. pylori) is a bacterium that causes chronic inflammation of the inner lining of the stomach (gastritis) in humans. This bacterium also is considered as a common cause of ulcers worldwide.
- H. pylori infection is most likely acquired by ingesting contaminated food and water, and through person to person contact.
- The infection is more common in crowded living conditions with poor sanitation.
- Helicobacter pylori, previously named Campylobacter pylori, is a Gram-negative, microaerophilic bacterium found in the stomach.
- The standard first-line therapy is a one week "triple therapy" consisting of proton pump inhibitors such as omeprazole and the antibiotics clarithromycin and amoxicillin.

121. Ans. (d) Fluoroscent treponemal antibody absorption test (FTA ABS) *Ref: Ananthnarayan, 8th ed. p 376*

Syphilis tests detect antibodies to the bacterium that causes syphilis (Treponema pallidum) in blood, body fluid, or tissue. The tests are used to screen or to confirm a syphilis infection.

Syphilis is a sexually transmitted infection (STI) that is usually spread during sexual contact, including kissing or oral sex.

Tests used to screen for syphilis include:

- Venereal disease research laboratory (VDRL) test. The VDRL test checks for an antibody that can be produced in people who have syphilis. This antibody is not produced as a reaction to the syphilis bacteria specifically, so this test is sometimes not accurate. The VDRL test may be done on a sample of blood or spinal fluid. The VDRL test is not very useful for detecting syphilis in very early or advanced stages.
- Rapid plasma reagin (RPR) test. The RPR test also detects syphilis antibodies.
- Enzyme immunoassay (EIA) test. This is a newer blood test that checks for antibodies to the bacteria that cause syphilis. A positive EIA test should be confirmed with either the VDRL or RPR tests.

Tests used to diagnose syphilis include:

- Fluorescent treponemal antibody absorption (FTA-ABS) test. The FTA-ABS test checks for antibodies to the bacteria that cause syphilis and can be used to detect syphilis except during the first 3 to 4 weeks after exposure to syphilis bacteria. The test can be done on a sample of blood or spinal fluid. It is one of the most commonly used treponemal test to diagnose syphilis.
- Treponema pallidum particle agglutination assay (TPPA): The TPPA test is used to confirm a syphilis infection after another method tests positive for the syphilis bacteria. This test detects antibodies to the bacteria that cause syphilis. This test is not done on spinal fluid.
- Darkfield microscopy: This test uses a special microscope to examine a sample of fluid or tissue from an open sore (chancre) for the syphilis bacteria. This test is used mainly to diagnose syphilis in an early stage.
- Microhemagglutination assay (MHA-TP): The MHA-TP is used to confirm a syphilis infection after another method tests positive for the syphilis bacteria.

122. Ans. (a) Shigelia sonnei *Ref: Ananthnarayan, 8th ed. p 283*

123. Ans. (c) C1 perfingens *Ref: Ananthnarayan, 8th ed. p 251*

- Cl. Perfringens is a capsulated, nonmotile, Gram positive bacillus with straight, parallel sides and rounded ends.
- It is the most important clostridia causing gas gangrene.
- It is an amaerobic organisms but can also grow in microaerophillie condition.
- Robertson's cooled meat medium show its good growth.

124. Ans. (b) Causes Shanghai fever *Ref: Ananthanaryan-, 8th ed. p 315*

- It is a Gram-negative, aerobic, cocco-bacillus bacterium with unipolar motility.
- An opportunistic human pathogen, P. aeruginosa is also an opportunistic pathogen of plants.
- P. aeruginosa is the type species of the genus Pseudomonas (Migula). P. aeruginosa secretes a variety of pigments, including pyocyanin (blue-green), pyoverdine (yellow-green and fluorescent), and pyorubin (red-brown). King, Ward, and Raney developed Pseudomonas Agar P (King A medium) for enhancing pyocyanin and pyorubin production, and Pseudomonas Agar F (King B medium) for enhancing fluorescein production.
- Pseudomonas aeruginosa causes Shaghai fever.
- Shanghai fever is a sporadic community-acquired disease of previously healthy infants that manifests as sepsis associated with P. aeruginosa enteric disease. Both host and microbial factors play a role in pathogenesis.

125. Ans. (c) Exotoxin *Ref: Anantanarayan, 8th ed. p 240*

- Diphtheria toxin is an exotoxin secreted by Corynebacterium diphtheriae, the pathogen bacterium that causes diphtheria. Unusually, the toxin geneis encoded by a bacteriophage (a virus that infects bacteria).
- The toxin causes the disease diphtheria in humans by gaining entry into the cell cytoplasm and inhibiting protein synthesis.
- Virulent strains of diphtheria releases a powerful exotoxin.
- The pathogenic effects of diphtheria are attributed to this toxic only.
- **It consists of two fragments**

A. The gas gangrene group: 1. Established pathogens 2. Less pathogenic 3. Doubtful pathogens	Cl perfringens Cl septicum, Cl novyi Cl histolyticum, Cl fallax Cl bifermentans, Cl sporogenes
B. Tetanus:	Cl tetani
C. Food poisoning: 1. Gastroenteritis 2. Necrotizing enteritis 3. Botulism	Cl perfringens (Type A) Cl perfringens (Type C) Cl botulinum
D. Acute colitis:	Cl difficile

- The diphtheria toxin is labile. Prolonged storage, incubation at 37°C for 4-6 weeks, treatment with 0.2–0.4 percent formalin or acid pH converts it to toxoid.
- The toxigenicity of the diphtheria bacillus depends on the presence in it of corynephages (tox+), which act as the genetic determinant controlling toxin production. Nontoxigenic strains may be rendered toxigenic by infecting them with beta phage or some other toxlarger phage. This is known as lysogenic or phage conversion.
- Toxin production is also influenced by the concentration of iron in the medium. The optimum level of iron for toxin production is 0.1 mg per litre, while a concentration of 0.5 mg per litre inhibits the formation of toxin.
- The diphtheria toxin acts by inhibiting protein dinucleotide by inactivating the elongation factor, FF-2
- It has a special affinity for certain tissues such as the myocardium, adrenals and nerve endings.

126. Ans. (b) Sarcoidosis *Ref: Harsh Mohan, 3rd ed. p 134 and Shafer's, 5th ed. p 923*

KVIEM'S test is a useful intradermal diagnostic test. The antigen prepared for involved lymph node or spleen is injected intradermally. In a positive test, nodular lesion appears in 3–6 weeks at the inoculation site which on microscopic examination shows presence of non-caseating granulomas.

Sarcoidosis is described as a multisystem granulomatous disease of unknown origin, characterized by the formation of uniform, discrete, compact, non-caseating epitheloid granuloma. It is more common in black than in whites.

An intracutaneous test for diagnosis of sarcoidosis the Kvein-Siltzbach test has been devised utilizing a suppression of human known sarcoidal tissue as the test agent.

Identification tests for different conditions

Shigella sonnei	Nonmotile and anaerogenic
Salmonella typhi	Motile, aerobic and facultative anaerobes
Proteus mirabilis	Motile
Klebsiella pneumoniae	Nonmotile of aerogenic

127. Ans. (c) Glucans *Ref: Ananthanarayan and Paniker's, 7th ed. p 215*

- S. mutans (so called because it assumes a bacillary form in acid environments) is important in the causation of dental caries. It breaks down dietary sucrose, producing acid and a tough adhesive dextran.
- The acid damages dentine and the dextrans bind together food debris, epithelial cells, mucus and bacteria to form dental plaques, which lead to caries.
- Dextran is a type of glucan.

128. Ans. (b) Group A streptococci *Ref: Ananthanarayan and Paniker's, 8th ed. p 209*

- Erysipelas is an acute infection of the upper dermis and superficial lymphatics, usually caused by streptococcus bacteria.
- Erysipelas is more superficial than cellulitis, and is typically more raised and demarcated.
- Patients typically develop symptoms including high fevers, shaking, chills, fatigue, headaches, vomiting, and general illness within 48 hours of the initial infection.
- The erythematous skin lesion enlarges rapidly and has a sharply demarcated raised edge.
- It appears as a red, swollen, warm, hardened and painful rash, similar in consistency to an orange peel.
- More severe infections can result in vesicles, bullae, and petechiae, with possible skin necrosis.
- Lymph nodes may be swollen, and lymphedema may occur.
- Occasionally, a red streak extending to the lymph node can be seen.
- Most cases of erysipelas are due to Streptococcus pyogenes (also known as beta- hemolytic group A streptococci), although non-group A streptococci can also be the causative agent.
- Erysipelas infections can enter the skin through minor trauma, insect bites, dog bites, eczema, surgical incisions and ulcers, and often originate from strep bacteria in the subject's own nasal passages.
- Erysipelas does not affect subcutaneous tissue. It does not release pus, only serum or serous fluid.

129. Ans. (d) Phase of decline *Ref: Ananthanarayan, 7th ed. p 21*

Bacterial growth can be modeled with four different phases:

i. Lag phase:
- No appreciable increase in number
- There may be increase in size of the cell
- Bacteria has maximum cell size towards the end of this phase

ii. Exponential or Log (logarithmic phase):
- Characterized by cell doubling
- The number of new bacteria appearing per unit time is proportional to the present population
- Plotting the natural logarithm of cell number against time produces a straight line.
- Cells are smaller and stains uniformly

iii. Stationary phase:
- The growth rate slows as a result of nutrient depletion and accumulation of toxic products.
- Value of constant as the rate of bacterial growth is equal to the rate of bacterial death.
- Cells show irregular gram staining due to presence of intracellular storage granules.
- Sporulation occurs in this stage.

iv. Death phase or phase of decline:
- Bacteria run out of nutrients and die.
- Involution occurs in this phase.

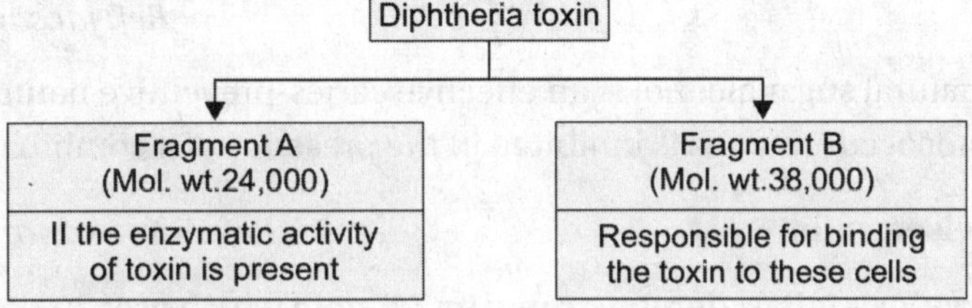

130. Ans. (a) Mycobacterium tuberculosis *Ref: Ananthanarayan, 8th ed. p 351*

- The Ziehl-Neelsen stain, also known as the acid-fast stain, was first described by two German doctors: the bacteriologist Franz Ziehl (18591926) and the pathologist Friedrich Neelsen (18541898).
- It is a special bacteriological stain used to identify acid-fast organisms, mainly Mycobacteria.
- Mycobacterium tuberculosis is the most important of this group because it is responsible for tuberculosis (TB).
- Other important Mycobacterium species involved in human disease are Mycobacterium leprae, Mycobacterium kansasii, Mycobacterium marinum, and members of the Mycobacterium avium complex.
- Acid fast organisms like Mycobacterium contain large amounts of lipid substances within their cell walls called mycolic acids. These acids resist staining by ordinary methods such as a Gram stains.
- It can also be used to stain a few other bacteria, such as Nocardia.
- The reagents used are Ziehl-Neelsen carbol fuchsin, acid alcohol, and methylene blue.
- Acid-fast bacilli will be bright red after staining.

131. Ans. (c) Mycobacterium tuberculosis *Ref: Ananthanarayan, 8th ed. p 351*

Mycobacterium tuberculosis is a acid fast bacilli so obviously will not take up gram stain hence answer of exclusion.

Also know about Gram stain:
- Gram staining (or Gram's method) is a method of differentiating bacterial species into two large groups (Gram-positive and Gram-negative). The name comes from its inventor, Hans Christian Gram.

- Gram staining differentiates bacteria by the chemical and physical properties of their cell walls by detecting peptidoglycan, which is present in a thick layer in Gram-positive bacteria.
- A Gram-positive results in a purple-blue color while a Gram-negative results in a pink-red color.
- The Gram stain is almost always the first step in the identification of a bacterial organism.
- Gram-positive bacteria generally have a single membrane (monoderm) surrounded by a thick peptidoglycan. This rule is followed by two phylaFirmicutes (except for the classes Mollicutes and Negativicutes) and the Actinobacteria. In contrast, members of the Chloroflexi (green non-sulfur bacteria) are monoderms but possess a thin or absent (class Dehalococcoidetes) peptidoglycan and can stain negative, positive or indeterminate. Members of the Deinococcus-Thermus group, stain positive but are diderms with a thick peptidoglycan.
- Historically, the Gram-positive forms made up the phylum Firmicutes, a name now used for the largest group. It includes many well-known genera, such as Bacillus, Listeria, Staphylococcus, Streptococcus, Enterococcus, and Clostridium. It has also been expanded to include the Mollicutes, bacteria like Mycoplasma that lack cell walls and so cannot be stained by Gram, but are derived from such forms.
- Normally, if Gram's stain is done on acid-fast bacteria they show up as if they are Gram-positive, mostly because of their thick cell wall.
- Gram-negative bacteria generally possess a thin layer of peptidoglycan between two membranes (diderms). Most bacterial phyla are Gram-negative, including the cyanobacteria, spirochaetes and green sulfur bacteria, and most Proteobacteria and Escherichia coli (Exceptions being some members of the Rickettsiales and the insect-endosymbionts of the Enterobacteriales.

132. Ans. (a) S. mutans *Ref: jdr.sagepub.com/content/81/6/380.full*

- Xylitol, a 5 carbon natural sugar alcohol is an effective caries-preventive natural carbohydrate sweetener.
- The growth of streptococcus mutans is inhibited in the presence of a combination of dietary sugars and xylitol.

133. Ans. (c) Zeihl and Neelsen stain *Ref: Ananthanarayan and Paniker's, 8th ed. p 348*

Mycobacterium tuberculosis is best demonstrated by ZN stain which uses 20% acid. PAS stain is for fungus. Gram's stain is for bacteria. ZN with 5% acid is used to stain mycobacterium leprae known as Wade fite stain.

134. Ans. (c) Serial passage in an experimental host *Ref: Ananthanarayan and Paniker's, 8th ed. p 78*

Attenuation is reduction in virulence of microorganisms. It can be achieved by:

- Passage through unfavorable host.
- Repeated cultures in artificial media.
- Growth at high temperature.
- Growth in presence of weak antiseptic.
- Prolonged storage in culture.

Enhancement of virulence is called exaltation.

135. Ans. (d) Borrelia vincenti *Ref: Ananthanarayan and Paniker's, 8th ed. p 380-381*

Fusospirochetosis - It is the symbiotic infection by Borrelia vincenti and fusifrom bacilli (Fusobacterium fusiforme), e.g. fusopirochetal infection of small intestine, Vincent's angina and ulcerative gingivostomatitis.

About other options

- **Treponema pallidum** causes **syphilis.**
- **Treponema pertenue** causes **yaws.**
- **Borellia burgdorferi** causes **Lyme disease.**

136. Ans. (b) Mycoplasma *Ref: Ananthanarayan and Paniker's, 8th ed. p 387*

Mycoplasmas are a group of bacteria that are devoid of cell walls and so are highly pleomorphic, with no fixed shape or size. They lack even cell wall precursors like muramic acid or diaminopimelic acid. The cell are bounded by a soft trilaminar unit membrane containing sterols. Because of their plasticity, they can pass through bacterial filters and have often been mistaken for viruses. The first member of the group was the organism causing bovine pleuropneumonia, isolated by Nacard and Roux (1898).

137. Ans. (b) Bacteria *Ref: Ananthanarayan and Paniker's, 8th ed. p 319*

- Actinomycosis is an infectious bacterial disease caused by Actinomyces species such as Actinomyces israelii or A. gerencseriae.
- The disease is characterised by the formation of painful abscesses in the mouth, lungs, or gastrointestinal tract.
- Actinomycosis abscesses grow larger as the disease progresses, often over months.
- In severe cases, they may penetrate the surrounding bone and muscle to the skin, where they break open and leak large amounts of pus, which often contains characteristic granules (sulphur granules).
- The purulent leakage via the sinus cavities contains "sulphur granules," not actually sulphur-containing but resembling such particles.
- Actinomyces bacteria are generally sensitive to penicillin, which is frequently used to treat actinomycosis.
- In cases of penicillin allergy, doxycyclin is used. Sulfonamides such as sulfamethoxazole may be used as an alternative regimen at a total daily dosage of 2–4 gm.

138. Ans. (d) Bacillus anthracis *Ref: Ananthanarayan and Paniker's, 8th ed. p 244*

- Bacillus anthracis is an encapsulated, endospore-forming, gram-positive rod and is the causative agent of anthrax
- Bacillus anthracis is surrounded by a polypeptide capsule composed of poly- gamma-D-glutamic acid (γDPGA).
- Pathogenicity of B. anthracis depends upon elaboration of both toxins and capsule.
- The B. anthracis capsule consists of a repeating epitope structure, is of high molecular weight, and is likely resistant to degradation.

139. Ans. (b) Mycobacterium tuberculosis *Ref: Ananthanarayan, 7th ed. p 352*

Lowenstein-Jansen (LJ) medium is the selective media for mycobacterium tuberculosis.

Composition of the Lowenstein-Jensen medium

1. Coagulated hen's egg
2. Mineral salt solution
3. Asparagine
4. Malachite green-selective agent which inhibits other bacteria

140. Ans. (c) GM negative bacteria *Ref: Ananthanarayan, 7th ed. p 67-68*

Differences between exotoxin and endotoxin

	Exotoxin	*Endotoxin*
1.	Proteins	Lipopolys accharide
2.	Produced mainly by Gram-positive bacteria and by some gram-negative bacteria like shiga, vibrio, E. coli	Produced by Gram-negative bacteria
3.	Heat labile	Heat stable
4.	Highly antigenic	Weakly antigenic
5.	Specific action	Nonspecific action
6.	Active in minute doses	Active in large doses

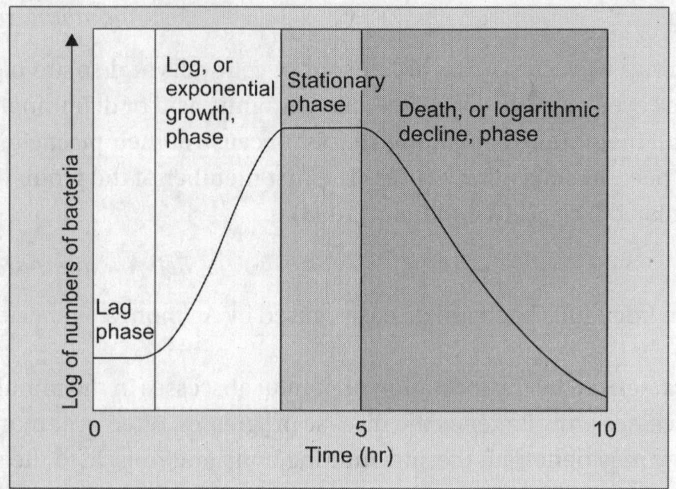

141. Ans. (d) Clostridium tetani

Gas Gangrene is not caused by clostridium tetani.

142. Ans. (b) Inhibiting protein synthesis *Ref: Anantanarayan, 8th ed. p 240*

Diphtheria toxin acts by inhibition protein synthesis

143. Ans. (c) Vibrio cholera *Ref: Anantanarayan, 8th ed. p 306*

- Cholera is an infection of the small intestine caused by the bacterium Vibrio cholerae.
- The main symptoms are watery diarrhea and vomiting.
- Transmission occurs primarily by drinking water or eating food that has been contaminated by the feces (waste product) of an infected person, including one with no apparent symptoms.
- The primary symptoms of cholera are profuse diarrhea and vomiting of clear fluid. These symptoms usually start suddenly, half a day to five days after ingestion of the bacteria.
- The diarrhea is frequently described as "rice water" in nature and may have a fishy odor.

144. Ans. (c) Heat stable *Ref: Anantanarayan, 8th ed. p 67, 68*

Endotoxin are heat stable while exotoxins are heat labile

145. Ans. (a) Skin *Ref: Anantanarayan, 8th ed. p 199*

- Impetigo, one of the most common skin infections among kids, usually produces blisters or sores on the face, neck, hands, and diaper area.
- This contagious superficial skin infection is generally caused by one of two bacteria: Staphylococcus aureus or Streptococcus pyogenes (also called group A streptococcus, which also causes strep throat). Methicillin-resistant Staphylococcus aureus (MRSA) is also becoming an important cause of impetigo.

Test	*Bacteria*
1. Naggler's reaction	Clostridia
2. Satellitism	H. influenza
3. Dick test or Scheultz—Charlton reaction	Streptococci
4. Elek's test, Schick test	Diphtheria
5. Milk ring test	Brucellosis
6. Kveim-Siltzback test	Sarcoidosis
7. String test	Vibrio cholera

Contd...

Contd...

Test	*Bacteria*
8. Montoux test	Tuberculosis
9. Koch's phenomenon	Tuberculosis
10. Cosoni's test	Hydatid cyst (parasite)

- The two types of impetigo are bullous impetigo (large blisters) and non-bullous impetigo (crusted) impetigo. The non-bullous or crusted form is most common. It's usually caused by S. aureus but can also be caused by infection with group A streptococcus. Non-bullous begins as tiny blisters, which eventually burst and leave small wet patches of red skin that may weep fluid. Gradually, a tan or yellowish-brown crust covers the affected area, making it look like it has been coated with honey or brown sugar.

146. Ans. (b) Anaerobic bacterial disease *Ref: Shafer's, 5th ed. p 445*

- A chronic suppurative and granulomatous disease of the cervico-facial, thoracic or abdominal areas
- Caused by gram positive, non motile, non sporing, non capsulated, anaerobic actinomyces.
- Actinomyces bacteria are generally sensitive to penicillin, which is frequently used to treat actinomycosis. In cases of penicillin allergy, doxycyclin is used.

147. Ans (a) Syphillis *Ref: Ghom, 1st ed. p 97*

- Kolmer test is a screening test done for syphilis.
- American physician. Kolmer investigated the fields of bacteriology, immunology, chemotherapy, and syphilology. He developed the Kolmer test in 1922 as a modification of the Wassermann test.
- It is a complement fixation test for the diagnosis of syphilis.

148. Ans. (a) Bile broth *Ref: Anathnarayan, 7th ed. p 37-290*

For diagnosis of typhoid bacilli, blood is collected and is inoculated and is inoculated into a bile broth culture bottle.

- Selenite F broth and tetrathionate broth are enrichment media
- Wilson and Blair Bismuth sulphite medium are selective media

149. Ans. (c) Actinobacillus actinomycetem comitans *Ref: Essential Microbiology for Dentistry Samaranayake, 2nd ed. p 113*

- A number of virulence factors including lipopolysaccharide (endotoxin), a leucotoxin, collagenase and protease cleaving IgG have been isolated from Aa
- The leucotoxin in particular thought to play a significant role in subverting the host immune response in the gingival crevice
- Together with other co-agents, Aa is involved in LAP and destructive periodontal disease in adults

150. Ans. (d) Warthin Starry silver stain *Ref: Ananthnarayan, 8th ed. p 412*

- A febrile illness with lymphadenopathy following a cat scratch had been known for long under the name cat scratch disease.
- B henselae has been isolated from the blood of patients, in blood media after prolonged incubation and is now considered as its causative agent. It can be demonstrated in lymph node biopsy smears and section by Warthin-Starry staining.

151. Ans (c) Spore bearing anaerobes *Ref: Ananthnarayan, 8th ed. p 256, 257*

- Clostridium tetani is an anaerobic bacterium of the genus species Clostridium. Like other Clostridium genus species, it is Gram-positive, and its appearance on a gram stain resembles tennis rackets or drumsticks.

- C. tetani is found as spores in soil or in the gastrointestinal tract of animals.
- C. tetani produces a potent biological toxin, tetanospasmin, and is the causative agent of tetanus, a disease characterized by painful muscular spasms that can lead to respiratory failure and, in up to 40% of cases, death.
- C. tetani is a rod-shaped, obligate anaerobe which stains Gram positive in fresh cultures; established cultures may stain Gram negative.
- During vegetative growth, the organism cannot survive in the presence of oxygen, is heat-sensitive and exhibits flagellar motility.
- As the bacterium matures, it develops a terminal spore, which gives the organism its characteristic appearance. C. tetanispores are extremely hardy as they are resistant to heat and most antiseptics.
- The spores are distributed widely in manure-treated soils.

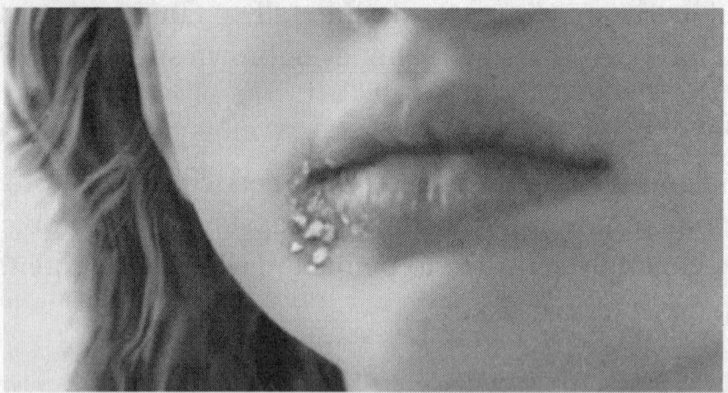

VIROLOGY

152. Ans. (d) Inactive carrier *Ref: Ananthnarayan, 8th ed. p 542-544*

- Hepatitis B is an infectious illness of the liver caused by the hepatitis B virus (HBV) that affects hominoidea, including humans.
- The virus is transmitted by exposure to infectious blood or body fluids such as semen and vaginal fluids, while viral DNA has been detected in the saliva, tears, and urine of chronic carriers.
- Acute infection with hepatitis B virus is associated with acute viral hepatitis an illness that begins with general ill-health, loss of appetite, nausea, vomiting, body aches, mild fever, and dark urine, and then progresses to development of jaundice
- Chronic infection with hepatitis B virus either may be asymptomatic or may be associated with a chronic inflammation of the liver (chronic hepatitis), leading to cirrhosis over a period of several years. This type of infection dramatically increases the incidence of hepatocellular carcinoma (liver cancer).
- Hepatitis B virus DNA persists in the body after infection, and in some people the disease recurs.
- Inactive carriers forms the largest group in chronic HBV infected patients. HBV reactivation is usually asymptomatic but on occasion can mimic acute viral hepatitis.
- Although reactivation can occur spontaneously.
- Dentist have been responsible for small outbreak and is not allowed to practice by medical board if he is an inactive carrier because there will be chances of reactivation and transmission of disease.

153. Ans. (a) EBV *Ref: Ananthnarayan, 8th ed. p 476*

- Infectious mononucleosis also known as mono, glandular fever (and sometimes colloquially as the kissing disease from its oral transmission) is an infectious, widespread viral disease caused by the EpsteinBarr virus.
- Especially in adolescents and young adults, the disease is characterized by fever, sore throat and fatigue, lymphadenopathy along with several other possible signs and symptoms.
- Incubation period is 4–8 weeks.
- Sometime it may also caused by cytomegalovirus and toxoplasmosis.

Epstein Barr virus (EBV)

- It is best known as the cause of infectious mononucleosis (glandular fever).
- It is also associated with particular forms of cancer, such as Hodgkin's lymphoma, Burkitt's lymphoma, nasopharyngeal carcinoma, and conditions associated with human immunodeficiency virus (HIV) such as hairy leukoplakia and central nervous system lymphomas.
- There is evidence that infection with the virus is associated with a higher risk of certain autoimmune diseases, especially dermatomyositis, systemic lupus erythematosus, rheumatoid arthritis, Sjögren's syndrome,and multiple sclerosis
- Infection with EBV occurs by the oral transfer of saliva and genital secretions

154. Ans. (a) Interferons (IFNs) *Ref: Ananthnarayan, 8th ed. p 447*

Interferon

- Interferons play an important role in the first line of defense against viral infections. They are part of the non-specific immune system and are induced at an early stage in viral infection before the specific immune system has had time to respond.

Therapeutic uses of interferon:

- Interferons-alpha and -beta have been used to treat various viral infections. One currently approved use for various types of interferon-a is in the treatment of certain cases of acute and chronic hepatitis C and chronic hepatitis B.
- Interferon-gamma has been used to treat a variety of disease in which macrophage activation might play an important role in recovery, e.g. lepromatous leprosy, leishmaniasis, toxoplasmosis.
- Since interferons have antiproliferative effects, they have also been used to treat certain tumors, such as melanoma and Kaposi's sarcoma.

155. Ans. (a) The presence of hepatitis B surface Ab *Ref: Ananthnarayan, 8th ed. p 543*

Laboratory diagnosis for type B Hepatitis

- The first marker visible in blood after infection is HBsAg.
- Anti-HBs protective antibody and its presence demonstrates immunity in the patient as it remain for very long period in blood.
- Anti-HBc appears 12 weeks before anti-HBc. It is an useful indication as it remains lifelong. IgM antibody is seen in acute cases (recent infection). After 6 months, IgG is seen in chronic cases (remote infection).
- Viral replication and infectivity is indicated by HbeAg and HBV DNA.
- HBV DNA levels in serum helps to access the progress of patients with chronic hepatitis under antiviral chemotherapy.

156. Ans. (b) Vascular *Ref: Shafer's, 6th ed. p 163, 164*

- Kaposi's sarcoma is a vascular tumor that manifests as nodular lesions on the skin and, to a lesser extent, visceral organs.
- Kaposi's sarcoma is the most common neoplasm encountered in HIV-infected patients, and disproportionately involves men who have sex with men.
- Kaposi's sarcoma is a tumor caused by human herpesvirus 8 (HHV8, also known as Kaposi's sarcoma-associated herpesvirus, KSHV). It was originally described by Moritz Kaposi.
- It is characterized by soft purplish plaques and papules in skin.
- These typically start on the feet and ankles and then slowly spread across the skin of the legs, hands and arms.

157. Ans. (a) Virus *Ref: Ananthnarayan, 8th ed. p 131*

Dengue hemorrhagic fever

- Dengue hemorrhagic fever is a severe, potentially deadly infection spread by mosquitos, mainly the species Aedes aegypti.

- Four different dengue viruses are known to cause dengue hemorrhagic fever. Dengue hemorrhagic fever occurs when a person is bitten by a mosquito that is infected with the virus.
- They include the following genera:
  - **Genus Flavivirus**—yellow fever virus, west nile virus, dengue fever, Japanese encephalitis, tick-borne encephalitis
  - **Genus Hepacivirus**—type species Hepatitis C virus, the single member
  - **Genus Hepatitis G virus**—GB agent and hepatitis G virus (HGV)
  - **Genus Pestivirus**—type species Bovine virus diarrhoea, others include classical swine fever or hog cholera contains viruses infecting nonhuman mammals.
- Early symptoms of dengue hemorrhagic fever are similar to those of dengue fever. But after several days the patient becomes irritable, restless, and sweaty. These symptoms are followed by a shock-like state.
- Bleeding appears as tiny spots of blood on the skin (petechiae) and larger patches of blood under the skin (ecchymoses). Minor injuries can cause bleeding.
- Shock can lead to death. If the patient survives, recovery begins after a one-day crisis period.
- **Early symptoms include:**
  - Decreased appetite
  - Fever
  - Headache
  - Joint or muscle aches
  - Malaise
  - Vomiting
- **Acute phase symptoms include:**
  - Restlessness followed by:
  - Ecchymosis
  - Generalized rash
  - Petechiae
  - Worsening of earlier symptoms
  - Shock-like state
  - Cold, clammy extremities
  - Sweating

Treatment

- Because dengue hemorrhagic fever is caused by a virus for which there is no known cure or vaccine, the only treatment is to treat the symptoms.
  - A transfusion of fresh blood or platelets can correct bleeding problems
  - Intravenous (IV) fluids and electrolytes are also used to correct electrolyte imbalances
  - Oxygen therapy may be needed to treat abnormally low blood oxygen
  - Rehydration with intravenous (IV) fluids is often necessary to treat dehydration
  - Supportive care in an intensive care unit/environment

158. Ans. (d) Hepatitis E *Ref: Ananthnarayan, 8th ed. p 546*

- **Hepatitis** E is a viral hepatitis (liver inflammation) caused by infection with a virus called hepatitis E virus (HEV).
- HEV is a positive-sense single-stranded RNA icosahedral virus.
- HEV has a fecal-oral transmission route.
- The incidence of hepatitis E is highest in juveniles and adults between the ages of 15 and 40.
- Hepatitis E occasionally develops into an acute, severe liver disease, and is fatal in about 2% of all cases.
- Clinically, it is comparable to hepatitis A, but in pregnant women the disease is more often severe and is associated with a clinical syndrome called fulminant hepatic failure. Pregnant women, especially those in the third trimester, suffer an elevated mortality rate from the disease of around 20%.

- The incubation period of hepatitis E varies from 3 to 8 weeks.
- After a short prodromal phase symptoms lasting from days to weeks follow. They may include jaundice, fatigue and nausea.
- The symptomatic phase coincides with elevated hepatic aminotransferase levels.

159. Ans. (a) Reverse transcriptase *Ref: Ananthnarayan, 8th ed. p 565*

Reverse transcriptase

- Reverse transcriptase is a common name for an enzyme that functions as a RNA- dependent DNA polymerase.
- They are encoded by retroviruses, where they copy the viral RNA genome into DNA prior to its integration into host cells.

Reverse transcriptases have two activities:

- DNA polymerase activity: In the retroviral life cycle, reverse transcriptase copies only RNA, but, as used in the laboratory, it will transcribe both single-stranded RNA and single-stranded DNA templates with essentially equivalent efficiency. In both cases, an RNA or DNA primer is required to initiate synthesis.
- RNase H activity: RNase H is a ribonuclease that degrades the RNA from RNA- DNA hybrids, such as are formed during reverse transcription of an RNA template. This enzyme functions as both an endonuclease and exonuclease in hydrolyzing its target.

All retroviruses have a reverse transcriptase, but the enzymes that are available commercially are derived from one of two retroviruses, either by purification from the virus or expression in E. coli.

160. Ans. (a) Kaposi's sarcoma *Ref: Ananthnarayan, 8th ed. p 575; Shafer's, 6th ed. p 354*

Kaposi's sarcoma (KS)

- There are five form out of which HIV-associated KS is called an epidemic KS.
- In pathogenesis of kaposi's sarcoma Human herpes virus type 8 is involved.
- It is particularly common in HIV-positive gay population.
- Non-Hodgkin's lymphoma is the second commonest after kaposis sarcoma

Opportunistic infections and malignancies typically associated with HIV infection are as follows:

Viral

- CMV
- Herpes simplex
- Malignancies

Parasitic

- Pneumocystis carinii pneumonia
- Toxoplasmosis
- Cryptosporidiosis

Mycotic

- Candidiasis
- Cryptococcosis
- Aspergillosis
- Histoplasmosis

Bacterial

- Mycobacterial infections, TB and nontuberculous infections
- Salmonellosis
- Campylobacter infections
- Nocardia and actinomycetes infections

161. Ans. (a) Coxsackievirus *Ref: Shafer's, 6th ed. p 339*

- Herpangina, also called mouth blisters, is the name of a painful mouth infection caused by cox sackieviruses. Usually, herpangina is produced by one particular strain of coxsackie virus A.
- Most cases of herpangina occur in the summer, affecting mostly children. However, it occasionally occurs in adolescents and adults. It was first characterized in 1920.

Clinical feature

- Most commonly affects infants and young children
- Typically occurs during the summer
- Typically spreads via the fecal-oral route or via the respiratory droplets.
- Fatigue will last about three to four days after treatment.
- Associated with small vesicular or ulcerative lesions on the posterior oropharyngeal structures (enanthem).
- Symptoms include sudden fever with sore throat, headache, loss of appetite, and often neck pain.

Treatment

- Treatment is usually supportive only, as the disease is self-limiting and usually runs its course in less than a week.
- Drinking cold beverages, especially milk and eating ice cream are recommended. Hot and high acidity beverages are to be avoided.
- No Antiviral medications exist for Coxsackie A or other Enteroviruses.

162. Ans. (a) Hantavirus spreads by aerosolized infected urine of rodents *Ref: Ananthnarayan, 8th ed. p 522*

- Hantaviruses are single-stranded, enveloped, negative sense RNA viruses in the Bunyaviridae family.
- Humans may become infected with hantaviruses through contact with rodent urine, saliva, or feces.
- Some strains of hantaviruses cause potentially fatal diseases in humans, such as Hantavirus hemorrhagic fever with renal syndrome (HFRS) and hantavirus pulmonary syndrome (HPS), while others have not been associated with known human disease.
- In HFRS the main effect is in the blood vessels while in HPS most symptoms are associated with the lungs.
- In HFRS, there are increased vascular permeability and decreased blood pressure due to endothelial dysfunction and the most dramatic damage is seen in the kidneys, whereas in HPS, the lungs, spleen, and gallbladder are most affected.
- The Korean Army is one of the largest consumers of the hantavirus vaccine, second only to public health centers.
- No hantavirus vaccine has been approved for use in the US, and no WHO-approved vaccine has gained widespread acceptance.
- Option B Lassa virus is zoonotic (transmitted from animals), in that it spreads to man from rodents, specifically multi-mammate rats
- Option C Marburg hemorrhagic fever is a rare viral disease that occurs primarily in countries in East and Central Africa. The virus has the potential to spread from person to person, especially among health-care staff and family members who care for patients with Marburg VHF.
- Option D Monkeys become infected with KFDV through the bite of infected ticks; the virus is then transmitted to other ticks feeding on infected monkeys.

163. Ans. (b) Herpangina *Ref: Ananthnarayan, 8th ed. p 489*

- Herpangina, also called mouth blisters, is the name of a painful mouth infection caused by coxsackie viruses.
- Usually, herpangina is produced by one particular strain of coxsackie virus A (and the term "herpangina virus" refers to coxsackievirus A) but it can also be caused by coxsackievirus B or echoviruses.
- Most cases of herpangina occur in the summer, affecting mostly children. However, it occasionally occurs in adolescents and adults.
- It was first characterized in 1920

- A small number of lesions (usually 2-6) form in the back area of the mouth, particularly the soft palate or tonsillar pillars.
- The lesions progress initially from red macules to vesicles and lastly to ulcerations which can be 2–4 mm in size.
- The lesions heal in 7–10 days.

164. Ans. (b) They affect the production of IFN and are sensitive to it *Ref: Ananthnarayan, 8th ed. p 447*

General Characteristics of Viruses:

- Viruses are a cellular, non-cytoplasmic infectious agents.
- They are smaller than bacteria, and this can pass through bacteriological filter.
- Viruses are transmissible from disease to healthy organisms.
- All viruses are obligate intracellular parasites and can multiply only within the living host cells.
- Viruses contain only a single type of nucleic acid either DNA or RNA.
- Viruses are host specific that they infect only a single species and definite cells of the host organisms.
- Viruses are effective in very small doses. They are highly resistant to germicides and extremes of physical conditions.
- Many viruses have evolved mechanisms to resist interferon activity. They circumvent the IFN response by blocking downstream signaling events that occur after the cytokine binds to its receptor, by preventing further IFN production, and by inhibiting the functions of proteins that are induced by IFN.
- They do not show growth, development, nutrition, reproduction, etc. on inanimate object.

165. Ans. (a) Transduction *Ref: Ananthnarayan, 8th ed. p 63*

Transduction

- It is the process by which DNA is transferred from one bacterium to another by a virus.
- It also refers to the process whereby foreign DNA is introduced into another cell via a viral vector.
- Transduction is a common tool used by molecular biologists to stably introduce a foreign gene into a host cell's genome.

Transformation

- It is the transfer of genetic information through agency of free DNA. It was the first type to be discovered.
- Transformation occurs naturally in some species of bacteria, but it can also be effected by artificial means in other cells.
- Transformation was first demonstrated in 1928 by British bacteriologist Frederick Griffith.

Transcription

- It is the synthesis of RNA from a DNA template by the enzyme RNA polymerase.

Conjugation

- Bacterial conjugation is the transfer of genetic material (plasmid) between bacterial cells by direct cell-to-cell contact or by a bridge-like connection between two cells.
- During conjugation the donor cell provides a conjugative or mobilizable genetic element that is most often a plasmid or transposon.
- The genetic information transferred is often beneficial to the recipient. Benefits may include antibiotic resistance, xenobiotic tolerance or the ability to use new metabolites.

166. Ans. (a) Polymerase chain reaction (PCR) *Ref: Ananthnarayan, 8th ed. p 577*

Polymerase chain reaction

- It is the gold standard for diagnosis in all stages of HIV.
- Reverse transcriptase PCR (RT-PCR) is sensitive for viral nucleic acid (RNA).
- It can detect a single copy of RNA or proviral DNA from infected cells.

- It is both a sensitive and a specific test.
- Rest of the options are used for the detection of HIV and not confirmation.

HIV testing in neonate

- Due to passively transferred IgG from mother IgM, ELISA is advisable.

HIV testing during window period (seronegative infective stage)

- p24 ELISA
- Viral isolation
- PCR (DNA PCR or RT PCR)

Laboratory diagnosis of HIV

Nonspecific tests	*Specific tests*
• Reversal of CD4:CD8 ratio (from 2:1 to 1:2) • Increased B2 microglobulin • Increased serum neoptrin	Antibody detection • E/R/S: ELISA/rapid/sample • Western blot Antigen detection • P24 detection by ELISA during window period (p24 by sandwich ELISA is the test of choice in the window period). Culture

For research purposes.

RNA detection • RT-PCR • NASBA

167. Ans. (d) Chemically defined media *Ref: Ananthnarayan, 8th ed. p 450*

Methods for Cultivation of Virus:

Since the viruses are obligate intracellular parasites, they cannot be grown on any inanimate culture medium. Viruses can be cultivated within suitable hosts, such as a living cell. Generally three methods are employed for the virus cultivation.

- Inoculation of virus into animals
- Inoculation of virus into embryonated eggs
- Tissue culture

168. Ans. (c) Have long incubation period *Ref: Ananthnarayan, 8th ed. p 553*

Prion diseases

- Prion disease represents a group of conditions that affect the nervous system in humans and animals.
- In people, these conditions impair brain function as:
  - Changes in memory, personality, and behavior
  - A decline in intellectual function (dementia)
  - And abnormal movements, particularly difficulty with coordinating movements (ataxia).
- The signs and symptoms of prion disease typically begin in adulthood and worsen with time, leading to death within a few months to several years.
- Prion diseases in both humans and animals are characterised by a long latent phase or incubation period (i.e. 5–10 years) which is determined by many factors including our genes.

Humans are susceptible to several prion diseases such as:

- CJD: Creutzfeld-Jacob Disease
- GSS: Gerstmann-Straussler-Scheinker syndrome
- FFI: Fatal familial insomnia

- Kuru
- Alpers syndrome

169. Ans. (a) Embryonated egg *Ref: Ananthnarayan, 8th ed. p 450*

Most of the virus can be cultivated in

- Experimental animal
- Embryonated egg
- Tissue culture

170. Ans. (a) Acute liver failure *Ref: Ananthnarayan, 8th ed. p 546*

Acute liver failure can occurs due to Hepatitis E.

171. Ans. (a) Acute liver failure *Ref: Ananthnarayan, 8th ed. p 546*

Refer Ans no. 170.

172. Ans. (c) Embryonated hen's eggs *Ref: Ananthnarayan, 8th ed. p 546*

Refer Ans no. 169.

173. Ans. (b) Cytomegalovirus *Ref: Anathanarayan, 8th ed. p 563*

RNA viruses	
A. Retroviruses	1. Avian leukosis viruses
	2. Murine leukosis viruses
	3. Murine mammary tumor virus
	4. Leukosis-sarcoma virus of various animals
	5. Human T cell leukemia viruses
DNA viruses	
A. Papovavirus	1. Papillomaviruses of human beings, rabbits and other animals
	2. Polyomavirus
	3. Simian virus 40
	4. BK and JV viruses
B. Poxvirus	1. Molluscum contagiosum
	2. Yaba virus
	3. Shope
C. Adenovirus	Many human and nonhuman types
D. Herpes virus	1. Marek's disease virus
	2. Lucke's frog tumor virus
	3. Herpes virus pan, papio, ateles and saimiri
	4. Epstein-Barr virus
	5. Herpes simplex virus types 1 and 2
	6. Cytomegalovirus
E. Hepatitis B and C viruses	

174. Ans. (b) HbeAg *Ref: Ananthnarayan, 8th ed. p 543*

Indicator for viral replication in hepatitis B infection is HbeAg.

175. Ans. (b) Hepatitis B virus *Ref: Ananthnarayan, 8th ed. p 539*

- Hepatitis B is an infectious illness of the liver caused by the hepatitis B virus (HBV)
- The virus is transmitted by exposure to infectious blood or body fluids such as semen and vaginal fluids, while viral DNA has been detected in the saliva, tears, and urine of chronic carriers.
- Hepatitis B virus is a hepadna virus: hepa from hepatotropic (attracted to the liver) and dna because it is a DNA virus and it has a circular genome of partially double-stranded DNA.
- Components: It consists of HBsAg; HBcAg (HBeAg is a splice variant); Hepatitis B virus DNA polymerase; HBx. The function of this protein is not yet well known, but evidence suggests it plays a part in the activation of the viral transcription process

176. Ans. (d) Measles *Ref: Harrison's, 24th ed. p 48*

Following virus is Teratogenic:

- Cytomegalovirus most common congenital infection.
- Rubella.
- Herpes virus.
- Parvo virus.
- HIV infection.

177. Ans. (d) Parvovirus B 19 *Ref: Ananthanarayan and Paniker's, 8th ed. p 564*

Viruses associated with human cancer

Virus family	*Human papilloma virus*	*Types of cancer*
Papovaviridae	Human papilloma virus	Cervical, vulvar, penile cancers Squamous cell carcinoma
Herpesviridae	EB virus	Nasopharyngeal carcinoma African Burkitt's lymphoma B cell lymphoma, cervical carcinoma
Hepadnaviridae	Hepatitis B virus	Hepatocellular carcinoma
Flaviviridae	Hepatitis C virus	
Retroviridae	HTL virus	Adult T cell leukemia

178. Ans. (d) Measles *Ref: Ananthanarayan and Paniker's, 8th ed. p 444*

The most characteristic histological feature in virus infected cells is the appearance of inclusion bodies. Inclusion bodies are structures with distinct size, shape, location and staining properties that can be demonstrated in virus infected cells under the light microscope. They may be situated in:

- Cytoplasm (as with poxviruses)
- Nucleus (herpes viruses)
- Both (measles virus)

179. Ans. (c) Salivary leukocyte proteinase inhibitor *Ref: Ananthanarayan and Paniker's, 7th ed. p 402*

Salivary leukocyte proteinase inhibitor is a protein present in saliva and has anti-HIV activity and therefore prevents transmission of HIV via saliva.

Common modes of transmission of HIV are as follows:

1. Sexual intercourse
2. Through blood and blood products
3. Through tissue and organ donation
4. Through injections, injuries and shared needles by drug addicts
5. From infected mother to baby which may be trans-placental during birth, after birth or through breast milk

180. Ans. (b) Herpes zoster *Ref: Ananthanarayan and Paniker's, 8th ed. p 473 and Robbins, 8th ed. p 456*

Herpes zoster is a common infection in immune-compromised patients and those patients with certain malignancies, e.g. Hodgkin's disease and malignant lymphoma.

Herpes Zoster (Shingles, Zona)

- The name is derived from Herpein, meaning to creep; zoster, meaning girdle.
- The rash is typically unilateral and confined to the area supplied by a single sensory ganglion. The most common sites are the areas innervated by spinal cord segments D3 to L2 and the trigeminal nerve, particularly, its ophthalmic branch. The lesions are identical in nature to varicella lesions, except for their limited distribution. The rash heals in about two weeks. Pain and paresthesia at the affected area may persist for weeks or months. Other complications are lower motor neuron paralysis which sometimes ensues, meningoencephalitis and generalized zoster where the lesions are scattered widely, perhaps due to hematogenous dissemination of the virus. Herpes zoster ophthalmicus is a common and troublesome presentation. The Ramsay Hunt syndrome is a rare form of zoster affecting the facial nerve, with eruption on the tympanic membrane and the external auditory canal, and often a facial palsy. Chronic or recurrent zoster is often seen in the HIV infected.

181. Ans. (d) Rabies *Ref: Ananthnarayan, 8th ed. p 526*

- Negri bodies are eosinophilic, sharply outlined, pathognomonic inclusion bodies (210 μm in diameter) found in the cytoplasm of certain nerve cells containing the virus of rabies, especially in Ammon's horn of the hippocampus.
- They are also often found in the cerebellar cortex of postmortem brain samples of rabies victims. They consist of ribonuclear proteins produced by the virus.

182. Ans. (b) Viral origin *Ref: Ananthnarayan, 8th ed. p 477*

- Kaposi's sarcoma is a tumor caused by human herpesvirus 8 (HHV8, also known as Kaposi's sarcoma-associated herpesvirus, KSHV).
- It became more widely known as one of the AIDS-defining illnesses in the 1980s.
- Kaposi's sarcoma (KS) is a systemic disease that can present with cutaneous lesions with or without internal involvement
- In AIDS patients, Kaposi sarcoma is considered an opportunistic infection, a disease that is able to gain a foothold in the body because the immune system has been weakened.

183. Ans. (c) HIV *Ref: Ananthanarayan, 8th ed. p 592*

- The western blot (sometimes called the protein immunoblot) is a widely accepted analytical technique used to detect specific proteins in the given sample of tissue homogenate or extract.
- It uses gel electrophoresis to separate native proteins by 3D structure or denatured proteins by the length of the polypeptide. The proteins are then transferred to a membrane (typically nitrocellulose or PVDF), where they are stained with antibodies specific to the target protein.
- There are now many reagent companies that specialize in providing antibodies (both monoclonal and polyclonal antibodies) against tens of thousands of different proteins.

- Commercial antibodies can be expensive, although the unbound antibody can be reused between experiments. This method is used in the fields of molecular biology, biochemistry, immunogenetics and other molecular biology disciplines.

Other related techniques include using antibodies to detect proteins in tissues and cells by immunostaining and enzyme-linked immunosorbent assay (ELISA).

184. Ans. (c) Transmission is by feco-oral route *Ref: Ananthanarayan, 8th ed. p 545*

	A	*B*	*C*	*D*	*E*
Type	27 nm RNA Picorvirus	47 nm DNA Hepadnavirus	30–60 nm RNA–Flavivirus	35–37 nm RNA	32–34 nm RNA
Mode of infection	Fecal-oral	Percutaneous sexual, vertical	Percutaneous	Percutaneous	Fecal-oral
Age	Children	Any age	Adults	Adults	Young adult
Incubation period	15–45 days	30–180 days	15–160 days	30–180 days	15–60 days
Carrier state	Nil	Common	Present	Nil (only with HBV)	Nil
Oncogenecity	—	Present after neonatal infection	Present after neonatal infection	—	
Prevalence	Common	Common	Probably common	Endemic	Only in developing countries
Prophylaxis	Ig and vaccine	Ig and vaccine	Nil	HBV vaccine	Nil
Severity of illness	Acute mild	Insidious and occasionally serious	Insidious and moderate	Insidious and occasionally serious	Mild but severe pregnancy

185. Ans. (b) Heparan sulphate *Ref: Ananthnarayan, 8th ed. p 468*

- Entry of HSV into the host cell involves interactions of several glycoproteins on the surface of the enveloped virus, with receptors on the surface of the host cell. The envelope covering the virus particle, when bound to specific receptors on the cell surface, will fuse with the host cell membrane and create an opening, or pore, through which the virus enters the host cell.
- The sequential stages of HSV entry are analogous to those of other viruses. At first, complementary receptors on the virus and the cell surface bring the viral and cell membranes into proximity. In an intermediate state, the two membranes begin to merge, forming a hemifusion state.
- Finally, a stable entry pore is formed through which the viral envelope contents are introduced to the host cell. In the case of a herpes virus, initial interactions occur when a viral envelope glycoprotein called glycoprotein C (gC) binds to a cell surface particle called heparan sulfate.
- A second glycoprotein, glycoprotein D (gD), binds specifically to at least one of three known entry receptors. These include herpes virus entry mediator (HVEM), nectin-1 and 3-O sulfated heparan sulfate.
- The receptor provides a strong, fixed attachment to the host cell. These interactions bring the membrane surfaces into mutual proximity and allow for other glycoproteins embedded in the viral envelope to interact with other cell surface molecules.

- Once bound to the HVEM, gD changes its conformation and interacts with viral glycoproteins H (gH) and L (gL), which form a complex. The interaction of these membrane proteins results in the hemifusion state. Afterward, gB interaction with the gH/gL complex creates an entry pore for the viral capsid.
- Glycoprotein B interacts with glycosaminoglycans on the surface of the host cell.

186. Ans. (b) Hepatitis B Virus *Ref: Ananthnarayan and Paniker's, 8th ed. p 539*

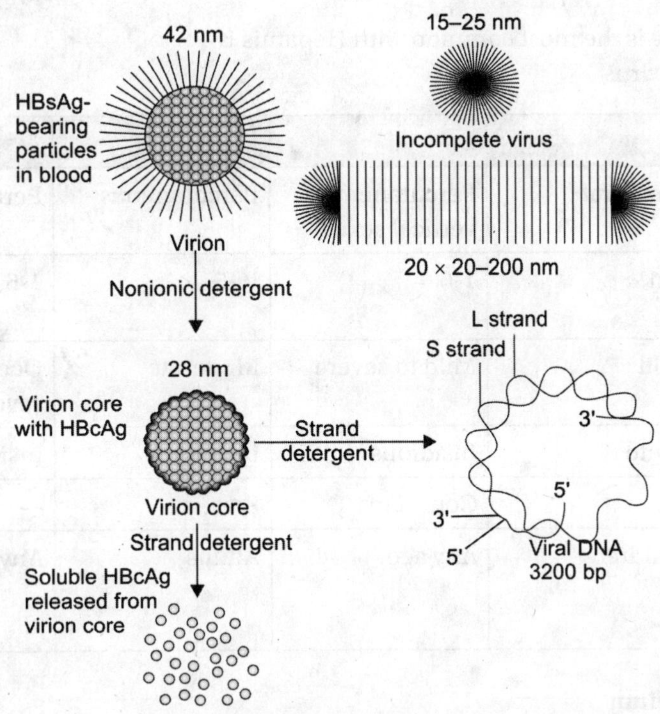

Hepatitis B virus

Under the electron microscope, sera from type B hepatitis patients show three types of particles. The most abundant form is a spherical particle, 22 nm in diameter. The second type of particle is filamentous or tubular with a diameter of 22 nm and of varying length. These two particles are antigenically identical and are surface components of HBV (HBsAg) which are produced in great excess. The third type of particle, for fewer in number, is a double- walled spherical structure, 42 nm in diameter. This particle is the complete hepatitis B virus. It was first described by Dane in 1970 and so is known as the Dane particle.

187. Ans. (d) Flavi virus *Ref: Ananthnarayan and Paniker's, 8th ed. p 545*

- Hepatitis C is an infectious disease affecting primarily the liver, caused by the hepatitis C virus (HCV).
- The hepatitis C virus (HCV) is a small, enveloped, single-stranded, positive-sense RNA virus. It is a member of the Hepacivirus genus in the family Flaviviridae. The half life of the virus particles in the serum is around 3 hours and may be as short as 45 minutes.
- The infection is often asymptomatic, but chronic infection can lead to scarring of the liver and ultimately to cirrhosis, which is generally apparent after many years. In some cases, those with cirrhosis will go on to develop liver failure, liver cancer or life-threatening esophageal and gastric varices.
- HCV is spread primarily by blood-to-blood contact associated with intravenous drug use, poorly sterilized medical equipment and transfusions. An estimated 150200 million people worldwide are infected with hepatitis C.
- Those who develop cirrhosis or liver cancer may require a liver transplant. Hepatitis C is the leading reason for liver transplantation, though the virus usually recurs after transplantation.
- No vaccine against hepatitis C is available.

188. Ans. (d) It remains during an asymptomatic phase *Ref: Ananthanarayan, 7th ed. p 584*

The major core antigen is p24 which can be detected in serum during the early stages of HIV infection before antibodies appear. Late in the course of infection, the decline of free anti-p24 antibody and reappearance of p24 antigen in circulation point to exacerbation of the illness.

189. Ans. (b) Hepatitis B *Ref: Anathnarayan,, 7th ed. p 550-560*

- Chronic carrier state is the most common with Hepatitis B
- HBV is bloodborne virus

	A	B	C	D	E
Mode of infection	Feco-oral	Percutaneous vertical sexual	Percutaneous	Percutaneous	Feco-oral
Incubation period (mouths)	½-1½	1-6	½-5	1-6	½-2
Illness	Mild	Mild to severe	Moderate	Occasionally severe	Mild
Onset	Acute	Insidious	Insidious	Insidious	Acute
Carrier state	—	Common	Present	—	—
Age affected	Children	Any age	Adults	Any age	Young adult and especially pregnant ladies

190. Ans. (b) Cryptosporidium *Ref: Anathnarayan, 8th ed. p 575*

- Cryptosporidium was the most common pathogen causing diarrhoea in AIDS cases.
- Cryptosporidium spp. cause diarrhoea in a number of different ways, including malabsorption.
- In normal subjects the infection is confined to the small intestine but in the immunocompromised (for example, AIDS and congenital immunodeficiency), it may spread to the biliary tree.
- Cryptosporidium is the organism most commonly isolated in HIV-positive patients presenting with diarrhea. Treatment is symptomatic, with fluid rehydration, electrolyte correction and management of any pain.

The parasite is transmitted by environmentally hardy microbial cysts (oocysts) that, once ingested, exist in the small intestine and result in an infection of intestinal epithelial tissue.

MYCOLOGY

191. Ans. (d) Phialophora verrucosa *Ref: Medical Microbiolog by William L, 1st ed. p 184*

Dimorphic fungi

- These fungi have two growth forms i.e they can grow either as yeast or mold depending on environmental conditions and temperatures.
- At room temperature, it grows as a mold.
- At body temperature, it grows as a yeast.

Examples of dimorphic fungi are:

1. Candida albicans (not other candidas)
2. Coccidiodes immitis

3. Paracoccidiomyces brasiliensis
4. Blastomyces dermatidis
5. Sporothrix schenki
6. Pencillium marfenii
7. Histoplasma capsulatum

192. Ans. (c) Sabouraud's agar *Ref: Ananthnarayan, 8th ed. p 601*

Most common culture media in mycology are:

- Sabouraud's glucose agar
- Czapek-Dox medium
- Corn meal agar

Stains used for demonstration of fungus in tissue section:

- Period acid schiff
- Methanamine silver

Candida albicans

- Candida albicans is a diploid fungus that grows both as yeast and filamentous cells and a causal agent of opportunistic oral and genital infections in humans.
- C. albicans is commensal and a constituent of the normal gut flora comprising microorganisms that live in the human mouth and gastrointestinal tract.
- C. albicans lives in 80% of the human population without causing harmful effects, although overgrowth of the fungus results in candidiasis (candidosis).

193. Ans. (b) Fungal infection *Ref: Infections of the Central Nervous System, 3rd ed. p 713 (books.google.co.in/books?isbn=0781743273)*

Mycoses is the term used for fungal infections, ie. superficial mycoses and systemic mycoses.

Mycotic abscess:

- It is an abscess caused by fungus.
- Soft cystic mass with slight inflammation caused by hyaline and dematiaceous fungi and nocardia species.

194. Ans. (d) Deuteromycetes *Ref: Ananthnarayana, 8th ed. p 601*

Based on the fungus spore formation, it is classified as:

- Phycomycetes lower fungi.
- Ascomycetes higher fungi
- Basidomycetes higher fungi
- Fungi imperfecti (Deuteromycetes or hypomycetes)
  - Its sexual phase have not been identified
  - Most fungi of medical importance belong to this group.

195. Ans. (a) Aspergillus niger *Ref: Aanthanarayan, 8th ed. p 614*

- Species of aspergilla generally A. Niger and A. fumigates is the causative agent of a fungal infection of the external ear is Otomycosis.
- Symptoms are itching and pain, may lead to deafness.

196. Ans. (b) Candidia albicans *Ref: Ananthanarayan, 8th ed. p 616*

- Although often referred to as 'dimorphic', C. albicans is in fact polyphenic. When cultured in standard yeast laboratory medium, C. albicans grows as ovoid 'yeast' cells.

- However, mild environmental changes in temperature and pH can result in a morphological shift to pseudohyphal growth.
- Pseudohyphae share many similarities with yeast cells, but their role during candidiasis remains unknown.
- When C. albicans cells are grown in a medium that mimics the physiological environment of a human host, they grow as "true" hyphae.
- Its ability to form hyphae has been proposed as a virulence factor, as these structures are often observed invading tissue, and strains that are unable to form hyphae are defective in causing infection.

197. Ans. (a) Noncapsulated fungus infecting man *Ref: Ananthanarayan and Paniker's, 8th ed. p 610*

- Cryptococcosis (torulosis) is a subacute or chronic infection caused by the yeast Cryptococcus neoformans. It is a round or ovoid budding cell, 4-20 μm in diameter, with a prominent polysaccharide capsule. It is a soil saprophyte and is particularly abundant in the feces of pigeons and other birds.
- Cryptococcal meningitis is the most serious type of infection and can resemble tuberculous or other chronic types of meningitis. Its onset is insidious and the course slow and progressive. It is often seen in AIDS.
- Two perfect stages of the fungus have been discovered. They belong to the class Basidiomycetes and have been termed Filobasidiella neoformans and F basilispora.
- Four serological types of cryptococcal capsular polysaccharide-A, B, C and D have been identified.

198. Ans. (a) Cryptococcus neoformans *Ref: D.R. Arora and Hina Arora, 2nd ed. p 370*

C. neoformans is true yeast. Both in the tissues and culture at room temperature as well as at 37°C, only budding yeasts are seen. Diagnosis is established by demonstration of budding yeast cells in CSF, sputum, pus or brain tissue by direct microscopy, culture and serological tests for capsular antigen. The direct microscopy of CSF, mixed with a drop of India ink or nigrosin shows round budding yeast cells, 4-10 μm in diameter. The organisms are surrounded by a wide refractile gelatinous capsule that may be twice the size of the yeast cell. In India ink preparation, it appears as a clear halo around the yeast cells. Sputum, pus and brain tissue should be examined after digestion in KOH. The histopathological examination of biopsy material can be done by staining with Mayer's mucicarmine. PAS, GMS and H and E staining.

199. Ans. (a) Mucor *Ref: Ananthanarayan and Paniker's, 8th ed. p 610-614*

- Mucormycosis shows broad nonseptate hyphae with right angle branching. It has a propensity for vascular invasion.
- Aspergillosis shows thin, septate hyphae with acute angle branching.
- Both these hyphae are positive for periodic acid Schiff (PAS) and silver methinamine.
- Cryptococcosis shows capsulated oval yeast forms. It has a thick gelatinous capsule showing red positivity with mucicarmine. It commonly affects CNS in which gelatinous masses of fungus expand perivascular Virchow-Robbin spaces within grey matter.
- Candida shows psuedohyphae and yeast forms and commonly affects immunocompromised patients.
- Coccidioidomycosis is an infection caused by the dimorphic fungus Coccidioides immitis.
- The fungus is dimorphic, occurring in the tissue as a yeast and in culture (both at 37°C at room temperature) as the mycelial form. The tissue form is a spherule, 15-75 μm in diameter, with a thick doubly refractile wall and filled with endospores. The mycelial phase consists of hyphae which fragment into arthrospores that are highly infectious. Cultures should be handled with particular care as they may cause laboratory infection.

200. Ans. (b) Periodic acid schiff stain *Ref: Ananthanarayan and Paniker's, 8th ed. p 601*

- Special investigations to detect the presence of candida species include oral swabs, oral rinse or oral smears.
- Smears are collected by gentle scraping of the lesion with a spatula or tongue blade and the resulting debris directly applied to a glass slide.
- Oral swabs are taken if culture is required. Some recommend that swabs be taken from 3 different oral sites.
- Smears and biopsies are usually stained with Periodic acid-Schiff, which stains cabohydrate in fungal cell walls magenta.
- Gram staining is also used as Candida stains strongly strongly Gram +ve

201. Ans. (c) KOH wet mount *Ref: Parija, 1st ed. p 629*

- Potassium hydroxide (KOH) is widely used in the wet mount preparation of various clinical specimens for demonstration of fungi and fungal elements.
- Fungus in the vagina is often detected through a vaginal wet mount like KOH.

PARASITOLOGY

202. Ans. (b) Gametocyte *Ref: Sherman. Malaria, 1998 ed. p 578.*

- Malaria is caused by obligate intracellular protozoan parasites of genus plasmodium.
- Plasmodium vivax gametocytes is injective to mosquitoes, while sporozoites is injective to humans.

203. Ans. (b) Tsetse fly *Ref: Vector Control: Methods for use by Individuals and Communities, 1st ed. p 148*

- Sleeping sickness is a parasitic, vector-borne disease, carried by the tsetse fly and prevalent in sub-Saharan Africa.
- Leishmaniasis is caused by a wide range of parasites that are transmitted by an even wider range of sand fly vectors.
- The Anopheles mosquito is known universally as the Malaria Mosquito species because it is considered the primary vector of the disease.
- Housefly Typhoid, cholera, dysentery, parasitic infections.

204. Ans. (d) Malaria *Ref: Ananthanaryana, 8th ed. p 694*

This question seems to be a printing mistake; instead of Durck granule it should be Durcks granuloma which is seen in malignant cerebral malaria.

- There are numerous petechial hemorrhages in white matter. Infarction, necrosis and large hemorrhages are however, rare.
- In many patients focal ring hemorrhages are seen centered on small sub-cortical vessels (Oo et al., 1987; Boonpucknavig et al., 1990; Riganti et al., 1990).
- The reparative process following the ring hemorrhage leads to a small nodule or Dürck's granuloma, composed of micro-glial cells aggregated around the area of demyelination associated with the vessel.
- An inflammatory cell response was generally lacking in cases examined by Macpherson et al. (1985) and Pongponratn et al. (2003).
- Although fibrin thrombi have been described in the vessels, they are not common and some detailed studies have failed to detect them. Students also note the malarial parasite life cycle, it is important, questions are often asked on life-cycle of malaria especially.

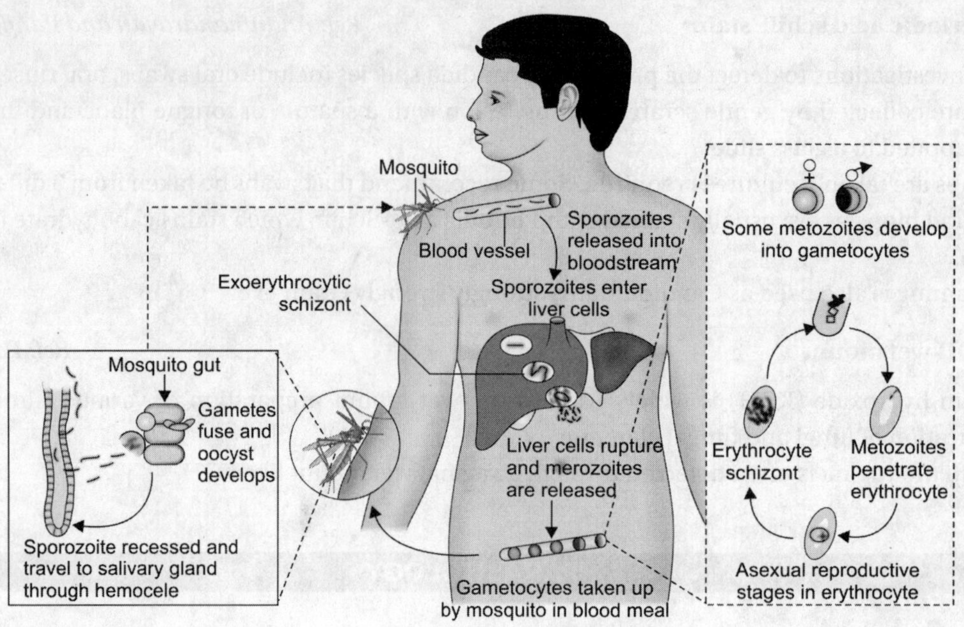

205. Ans. (d) Taenia solium *Ref: Paniker's, 5th ed. p 173*

Parasite causing autoinfection:

Always remember CHEST

C: Cryptosporidium

H: Hymenolepsis nana

E: Enterobius vermicularis

S: Strongyloids stercoralis

T: Taenia solium (cysticercosis)

206. Ans. (b and d) Plasmodium vivax and Plasmodium ovale *Ref: DR Arora and Hina Arora, 2nd ed. p 391*

Different characters of plasmodia of man

	P. viax	*P. falciparum*	*P. malariae*	*P. ovale*
1. Forms in peripheral blood	Trophozoites, schizonts and gametocytes.	Rings and crescents (gametocytes)	Trophozoites, schizonts and gametocytes	Trophozoites, schizonts and gametocytes
2. Early trophozoite or ring stage	Large 2.5 µm in diameter, usually one prominent chromatin dot, sometime two, cytoplasm opposite the chromatin dot thicker, usually one and often two rings in one red blood cell	Small, delicate 1.25-1.5 µm in diameter often with two chromatin dots, two rings in one red blood cell common. Some parasites lie along the red cell membrane. These are known as accole forms	Similar to that of P. vivax.	

Contd...

Contd...

	P. viax	*P. falciparum*	*P. malariae*	*P. ovale*
3. Late trophozoite	Large, markedly amoeboid, prominent vacuole	Medium-sized, compact rarely amoeboid, vacuole inconspicuous	Small, compact band-shaped, not amocboid, vacuole inconspicuous	Small, compact, not amoeboid, vacuole inconspicuous
4. Schizont	Large, 9-10 µm in diameter, almost fills an enlarged red blood cell	Small, 4.5-5.0 µm in diameter, fills two-thirds of normal sized red blood cell	Small, 6.5-7.0 µm in diameter, almost fills a normal sized red blood cell	Small 6.2 µm in diameter, fills about three-quarters of slightly enlarged red blood cell
5. Number of merozoites	14-24	14-32	6-12	6-12
6. Micro gametocytes	Spherical, compact, no vacuole, diffuse chromatin, diffuse coarse pigment, cytoplasm stains light blue	Crescent-shaped chromatin diffuse, pigment scattered in large grains	Similar to that of P. vivax but smaller	Similar to that of P. vivax but smaller
7. Macrogametocytes	Spherical, compact, larger than micro-grametocyte, compact chromatin, pigment same, cytoplasm stains dark blue	Crescent-shaped, longer and more slender, chromatin compact, pigment more compact, cytoplasm stains dark blue	Similar to that of P. vivax but smaller	Similar to that of P. vivax but smaller
8. Malaria pigment	Yellowish brown	Dark-brown	Dark-brown	Dark-brown
9. Age of red blood cells invaded	Young	All age (young and old)	Old	Young
10. Alterations in infected red cell	Enlarge; pale and the portion of the cytoplasm not occupied by the parasite shows a dotted or stippled appearance, called Schuffner's dots. With Leishman stain the appear as fine pink granules.	Normal size and possesses 6-12 Maurer's dots Which stains brick-red with Leishman stain.	Normal size and may occasionally show fine stippling (Ziemann's dots) on prolonged staining.	Enlarged, pale Schuffner's dots appear early and infected cell may be oval
11. Duration of erythrocytic schizogony	48 hours	36-48 hours	72 hours	48 hours

207. Ans. (a) Wuchereria bancrofti *Ref: Internet*

- The pathogenesis of W. bancrofti infection is dependent on the immune system and inflammatory responses of the host. After infection, the worms will mature within 68 months; male and female worms will mate and then release the microfilariae. These microfilariae worms can be released for up to ten years.

- Asymptomatic Phase: Usually consists of high microfilaremia infection and individuals show no symptoms of being infected. This occurs due to the cytokine IL-4 suppressing the activity of TH1 cells in our immune system. This can occur for years until the inflammatory reaction rises again.
- Inflammatory (Acute) Phase: The antigens from the female adult worms elicit inflammatory responses. The worms in the lymph channels disrupt the flow of the lymph causing lymphedema: The individual will exhibit fever, chills, skin infections, painful lymph nodes, and tender skin of the lymphedematous extremity.

These symptoms often lessen after 57 days. Other symptoms that may occur include: orchitis-inflammation of the testes, which is accompanied by painful immediate enlargement and epididymitis-which is the inflammation of the spermatic cord.

- Obstructive (chronic) phase: Marked by lymph varices, lymph scrotum, hydrocele, chyluria (lymph in urine), and elephantiasis. Microfilariae are not normally present in this phase. A key feature of this phase is scar formation from affected tissue areas. Other features include thickening of the skin and elephantiasis, which develops gradually with the attack of the lymphatic system. Elephantiasis affects men mainly in the legs, arms, and scrotum. In women, the legs and arms are affected.

208. Ans. (a) Leishmania donovani *Ref: en.wikiped.ia.org/wiki/Leishmaniasis*

- Leishmaniasis is a disease caused by protozoan parasites of the genus Leishmania and spread by the bite of certain types of sandflies.
- The disease can present in three main ways as: cutaneous leishmaniasis, mucocutaneous leishmaniasis and visceral leishmaniasis.
  - **Cutaneous leishmaniasis**—The cutaneous form presents with skin ulcers
  - **Mucocutaneous leishmaniasis**—mucocutaneous form presents with ulcers of the skin, mouth and nose and
  - **Visceral leishmaniasis**—the viceral form starts with skin ulcers and than latter presents with fever, low red blood cells, and a large spleen and liver.
- Leishmaniasis is diagnosed in the hematology laboratory by direct visualization of the amastigotes (Leishman-Donovan bodies).

209. Ans. (c) Echinococcus granulosus *Ref: Ananthanaryana, 8th ed. p 694*

Hydatid disease in man is caused mainly by infection by the larval stage of the dog tapeworm Echinococcus granulosus.

Pathophysiology

There are four types of echinococcosis, of which the first two are the most common and therefore the most important, the third rare and the fourth extremely rare

- **Cystic echinococcosis** due to E. granulosus—this is also known as hydatid disease or hydatidosis and is the most common type by far
- **Alveolar echinococcosis** due to E. multilocularis: this type is uncommon but the most virulent.
- **Polycystic echinococcosis** due to E. vogeli.
- **Unicystic echinococcosis** caused by infection with E. oligarthrus

210. Ans. (d) High grade fever with rigors *Ref: http://www.malariasite.com/malaria/Complications2.htm*

The common clinical features of severe falciparum malaria were cerebral malaria, metabolic acidosis, acute renal failure, respiratory distress, severe anemia, thrombocytopenia, coagulopathy, hypotension, hyperbilirubinemia, hepatic encephalopathy, hypoglycaemia and convulsions

MISCELLANEOUS

211. Ans. (a) Immunocompromised patient *Ref: Ananthnarayan, 8th ed. p 622*

- DPT refers to a class of combination vaccines against three infectious diseases in humans: diphtheria, pertussis (whooping cough), and tetanus.
- The vaccine components include diphtheria and tetanus toxoids and killed whole cells of the organism that causes pertussis (wP).
- DTP vaccination can be given to a immunocompromised patient, if the patient is on immunosuppressive drugs. If the immunosuppressive therapy is going to be discontinued, then DTP vaccination can be postponed for at least 1 month.
- Contraindications include:
  - An immediate anaphylactic reaction.
  - Encephalopathy: An acute, severe CNS disorder occurring < 7 days following vaccination.
  - Progressive neurological

Recommended immunization schedule followed in India

Sl no.	*Age*	*Disease*	*Vaccination*	*Remarks*
1	At birth	Hepatitis B	HEP B vaccine 1	
2	At birth	Polio	Oral PV 0 dose	
3	Birth to 6 week	Tuberculosis	BCG	
4	4-6 weeks	Hepatitis B	HEP B Vaccine II	
5	6 weeks	Diphtheria pertusis tetanus polio	DPT-I OPV-I	
6	10 weeks	Diphtheria pertusis tetanus polio hepatitis B	DPT-II OPV-II HEP B vaccine III*	Delhi Govt recommendation
7	14 weeks	Diphtheria pertusis tetanus polio	DPT-III OPV-III HEP B vaccine IV*	Delhi Govt recommendation
8	24 weeks	Hepatitis B	HEP B vaccine III*	IAP recommendation
9	9-12 months	Polio measles	OPV-IV measles	
10	15-18 months	Mumps measles rubella	MMR*	
11	18 months	Diphtheria pertusis tetanus polio	DPT-Booster I OPV-V	Recommended by Delhi Govt and IAP only
12	24 months	Typhoid	Typhoid*	IAP recommendation
13	4-5 years	Diphtheria pertusis tetanus polio	DPT booster-II OPV-VI	

212. Ans. (a) Entamoeba histolytica *Ref: Wastewater Aerosols and Disease: Proceedings of a Symposium ..., Vol. 1, p 24 http://books.google.co.in/books?id=HAdSAAAAMAAJ&pg=P A24&dq=Man+acts+as +reservoir+of+Entamoeba+histolytica+enteropathogen&hl=en&sa=X&ei=EjcIU4OX MMGAiQeAkYDIBw&ve d=0CCoQ6AEwAA#v=onepage&q=Man%20acts%20as%2 0reservoir%20of%20Entamoeba%20histolytica%20 enteropathogen&f=false*

Organisms	*Disease*	*Reservoir*
Salmonella	Typhoid and salmonellosis	Man, domestic and wild animals
E. coli	Gastroenteritis	Man, domestic animals
Entamoeba histolytica	Amebiasis	Man
Giardia lambia	Giardiasis	Man

213. Ans. (c) Aluminum *Ref: Ananthnarayan, 8th ed. p 238*

- A vaccine adjuvant is a substance that is added to the vaccine to increase the body's immune response to the vaccine.
- Aluminum salts, such as aluminum hydroxide, aluminum phosphate, and aluminum potassium sulfate have been used in vaccines for more than 70 years.
- In DPT vaccine, aluminium phosphate and aluminium hydroxide are used as adjuvants.
- The adjuvant aluminum is present in US childhood vaccines that prevent hepatitis A, hepatitis B, diphtheria-tetanus-pertussis (DTaP, Tdap) Haemophilus influenzae type b (Hib), human papillomavirus (HPV) and pneumococcus infection.
- Live attenuated (weakened) viral vaccines that prevent measles, mumps, rubella, chickenpox, and rotavirus do not contain adjuvants. An inactivated (non-live) vaccine that prevents polio (inactivated polio vaccine, or IPV) does not contain adjuvant. Seasonal influenza vaccines used in the United States do not contain adjuvants.

214. Ans. (c) Splenomegal *Ref: Ananthnarayan, 8th ed. p 238*

215. Ans. (b) Tissue culture

Ref: Oral Medicine and Pathology by Saman Warnakulasuriya, WM Tilakaratna, 1st ed. p 375

- Acute necrotizing ulcerative gingivitis (ANUG; colloquially known as trench mouth) is a common, non-contagious infection of the gums with sudden onset.
- The main features are painful, bleeding gums, and ulceration of interdental papillae (the sections of gum between adjacent teeth).
- The causative organisms are mostly anaerobic bacteria, particularly Fusobacteria and Spirocaete species.
- Predisposing factors include poor oral hygiene, smoking, malnutrition, psychological stress and immuno-suppression (sub-optimal functioning of the immune system).
- Laboratory test for the diagnosis of ANUG includes:
  - The viral isolation by the tissue culture
  - Cytological examination
  - Direct fluorescent antibody test
  - Serological assay
  - DNA detection by PCR based methodology.

216. Ans. (c) Northern blot *Ref: Harper's, 28th ed. p 393*

Northern blot

- The northern blot is a mlecular technique used in molecular biology research to study gene expression by detection of RNA (or isolated mRNA) in a sample
- The term 'northern blot' actually refers specifically to the capillary transfer of RNA from the electrophoresis gel to the blotting membrane
- Northern blotting allows one to observe a particular gene's expression pattern between tissues, organs, developmental stages, environmental stress levels, pathogen infection, and over the course of treatment.
- The technique has been used to show overexpression of oncogenes and downregulation of tumor-suppressor genes in cancerous cells when compared to 'normal' tissue as well as the gene expression in the rejection of transplanted organs.

Southern blot

- A southern blot is a method routinely used in molecular biology for detection of a specific DNA sequence in DNA samples.
- Southern blotting combines transfer of electrophoresis-separated DNA fragments to a filter membrane and subsequent fragment detection by probe hybridization.

Western blot

- The western blot (sometimes called the protein immunoblot) is a widely accepted analytical technique used to detect specific proteins in a sample of tissue homogenate or extract.
- It uses gel electrophoresis to separate native proteins by 3D structure or denatured proteins by the length of the polypeptide.

Medical diagnostic applications

- The confirmatory HIV test employs a western blot to detect anti-HIV antibody in a human serum sample. Proteins from known HIV-infected cells are separated and blotted on a membrane as above. Then, the serum to be tested is applied in the primary antibody incubation step; free antibody is washed away, and a secondary anti-human antibody linked to an enzyme signal is added. The stained bands then indicate the proteins to which the patient's serum contains antibody.
- A western blot is also used as the definitive test for Bovine spongiform encephalopathy (BSE, commonly referred to as 'mad cow disease').
- Some forms of Lyme disease testing employ western blotting.
- Western blot can also be used as a confirmatory test for Hepatitis B infection.
- In veterinary medicine, western blot is sometimes used to confirm FIV+ status in cats.

217. Ans. (b) Gram-negative organisms *Ref: Ananthnarayan, 8th ed. p 629*

Nosocomial infection

- It is an infection whose development is favored by a hospital environment, such as one acquired by a patient during a hospital visit or one developing among hospital staff. Such infections include fungal and bacterial infections and are aggravated by the reduced resistance of individual patients.
- The Gram-negative bacilli vary in the frequencies that they cause the 4 most frequent types of hospital-acquired infection: pneumonia, surgical site infection (SSI), urinary tract infection (UTI), and bloodstream infection (BSI)

Common nosocomial infections in ICU

- Pneumonia (including ventilator and aspiration pneumonia)
- Bacteremia (including indwelling catheter-related infections)
- Urinary tract infections.
- Clostridium difficile diarrhea
- Infected decubitus ulcers

Nosocomial pneumonia

- Hospital-acquired pneumonia (HAP) or nosocomial pneumonia refers to any pneumonia contracted by a patient in a hospital at least 4872 hours after being admitted.
- It is thus distinguished from community-acquired pneumonia. It is usually caused by a bacterial infection, rather than a virus.
- HAP is the second most common nosocomial infection (after urinary tract infections) and accounts for 1520% of the total.
- It is the most common cause of death among nosocomial infections and is the primary cause of death in intensive care units.
- Gram-negative aerobes (65.9%) remained the most frequently reported bacterial pathogens associated with pneumonia.

218. Ans. (a) It cannot be eradicated by antimicrobial agents *Ref: Ananthnarayan, 8th ed. p 587*

Facts regarding normal flora of skin and mucous membranes

- They cannot be eradicated by antimicrobial agents. It can only decrease the number of organisms
- They are present even in the acidic pH of stomach
- They are present even at birth as within 12 hours of birth, α-hemolytic streptococci are found in the upper respiratory tract.
- The flora of the small bronchi are different from those present in the trachea because the small bronchi and alveoli are sterile.

219. Ans. (c) Pneumococcal vaccination *Ref: Ananthanarayana, 8th ed. p 223*

Pneumococcal vaccination is only recommended to the patient, who is at high risk of pneumococoal infection such as patient with:

- Absent or dysfunction of spleen
- Sickle cell anemia
- Coliac disease
- Cronic renal, liver, lung and heart diseases
- Diabetes mellilus
- HIV injection

Note: It is not recommended in children under 2 years of age.

220. Ans. (c) Recombinant *Ref: Harrisons, 17th ed. p 1947*

- Recombinant vaccine derived from recornbinant yeast.
- Currently it is divides into 2 as pre exposure and post exposure.
- Pre exposure prophylaxis against hepatits B is meant for person who are frequently exposed as heath worker hemodialysis patient and staff.
- Post exposure prophylaxis is meant for persons suffer from hepatitis B injection.
- True avoidable recombinant hepatitis B vaccination are: (1) Recombivax HB, (2) Engeri XB.

221. Ans. (c) M chelonae *Ref: Anantanarayan, 8th ed. p 367*

M. Chelonae:

- Mycobacterium chelonae is a species of the phylum actinobacteria (Gram-positive bacteria with high guanine and cytosine content, one of the dominant phyla of all bacteria), belonging to the genus mycobacterium. Mycobacterium chelonae is a rapidly growing mycobacterium, that is found all throughout the environment including sewage and tap water. It can occasionally cause opportunistic infections of humans.
- It is grouped in Runyon group IV
- They are the organisms which form outbreaks of abscess when vaccines are injected which are contaminated with M Chelonae or M fortuitum.

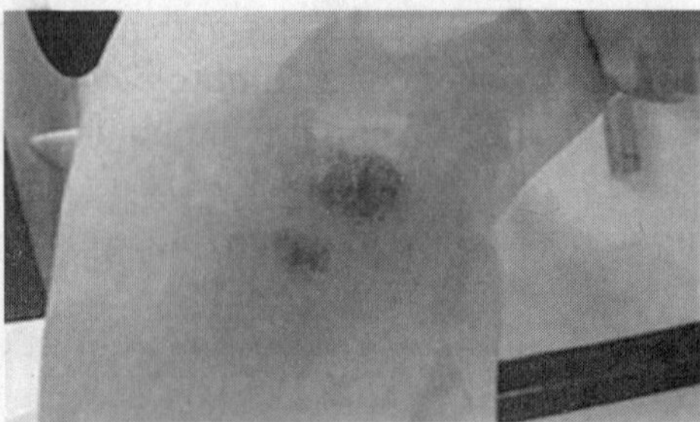

Mycobacterium chelonae abscesses associated with biomesotherapy, an alternative therapy practice (The abscesses are at the biomesotherapy injection site).

222. Ans. (c) Incineration *Ref: Ananthanarayan and Paniker's, 8th ed. p 627-628*

Waste Treatment

- Several methods of waste treatment are available and the choice of methods is based on the item of waste and the facilities available. The place of final disposal may be in the premises or away from crowded areas if possible. Some of the methods are indicated below.
- Chemical disinfection is a very useful method for many items, particularly in small places like clinics. It is also an important preliminary process before final treatment with some materials. For example, contaminated materials like sputum or pus are to be disinfected before being buried or autoclaved.
- Deep burial where large areas of uninhabited land are available this is convenient. Materials after chemical disinfection are put in deep trenches, covered with lime and filled with soil. This is a safe method for disposal of sharps also.
- Incineration is a safe method of treating large solid infectious waste, particularly anatomy waste and amputated limbs, animal carcasses and the like. The incinerator subjects them to very high heat, converting them to ash, which would be only about a tenth of the original volume. However, it is expensive and is generally used only by very large establishments.
- Autoclaving is widely used in laboratories and clinics for treating infectious waste before disposal.
- This is another useful method of sterilization of small volume waste at the point of generation. This cannot be used for animal or human body parts, metal items or toxic or radioactive material

Liquid waste pathological, chemical and toxic liquid waste should be appropriately treated with disinfectants or reagents and neutralized before flushing into the sewer.

223. Ans. (a) Laminin *Ref: Satyanarayana, 3rd ed. p 489-490 and Orban's 12th ed. p 341*

- The basal lamina of glomerular membrane (of renal cells) contains laminin. In fact, laminin is one of the first extracellular proteins synthesized during embryogenesis. It is actively involved in neuronal growth and nerve regeneration. In the patients of Alzheimer's disease, high concentrations of laminin are found.
- Laminin-5 in its assembled form ($\alpha3\beta3\gamma2$) is speculated to support cell adhesion, unlike its unassembled form. The latter form is a soluble ($\gamma2$) monomeric form. The laminin $\gamma2$ chain is now regarded as one of the typical invasion marker. This form does not contain any integrin binding site. A recent study has shown the release of domain III in the short arm of the $\gamma2$ chain by MT1-MMP, which shows ability to bind with EGFR.

224. Ans. (a) Integrin α-6 and β-4 *Ref: Tencate's, 7th ed. p 61-62*

The transmembrane adhesive molecules present in hemi desmosomes which specifically binds to basal lamina glycoprotein laminin are Integrin alpha-6 and beta-4.

225. Ans. (a) Biocompatibility *Ref: Phillip's, 11th ed. p 171*

- Allergy abnormal antigen, antibody reaction to a substance that is harmless to most individual (see Hypersensitivity)
- Biocompatibility Ability at a material to elicit an appropriate biological response in a given application in the body.
- Biointegration Process in which bone or other living tissue becomes integrated with an implanted material with no intervening space.
- Sensitization Process that produces an allergy antibody, which reacts specifically to the causative foreign substance.

226. Ans. (a) Cryptococcus neoformans *Ref: D.R. Arora and Hina Arora, 2nd ed. p 370*

C. neoformans is true yeast. Both in the tissues and culture at room temperature as well as at 37°C, only budding yeasts are seen. Diagnosis is established by demonstration of budding yeast cells in CSF, sputum, pus or brain tissue by direct microscopy, culture and serological tests for capsular antigen. The direct microscopy of CSF, mixed with a drop of India ink or nigrosin shows round budding yeast cells, 4-10 μm in diameter. The organisms are surrounded by a wide refractile gelatinous capsule that may be twice the size of the yeast cell. In India ink preparation, it appears as a clear halo around the yeast cells. Sputum, pus and brain tissue should be examined after digestion in KOH. The histopathological examination of biopsy material can be done by staining with Mayer's mucicarmine. PAS, GMS and H & E staining.

227. Ans. (c) E6 *Ref: Robbins, Basic Pathology, 8th ed. p 212*

Human Papilloma virus

The oncogenic potential of HPV can be related to products of two early viral genes.

E6 and E7, Together, they interact with a variety of growth regulating proteins encoded by protooncogenes and tumor suppressor genes. The E7 protein binds to the retinoblastoma protein and displaces the E2F transcription factors that are normally sequestered by RB, promoting progression through the cell cycle. Interestingly, E7 protein from high-risk HPV types has a higher affinity for RB than does E7 from low-risk HPV types. E7 also inactivates the CDK is CDKN1A/p21 and CDNK1B/p27. E7 protein from high-risk HPV types (types 16,18 and 21) also bind and presumably activate cyclins E and A. The E6 protein has complementary effects. It binds to and mediates the degradation of p53 and BAX, a pro-apoptotic member of the BCL2 family and it activates telomerase. In analogy with E7, E6 from high-risk HPV types has a higher affinity for p53 than E6 from low-risk HPV types. Interestingly, in benign warts the HPV genome is maintained in a nonintegrated episomal form, while in cancers the HPV genome is randomly integrated into the host genome. Integration interrupts the viral DNA, resulting in over-expression of the oncoproteins E6 and E7. Furthermore, cells in which the viral genome has integrated show significantly more genomic instability.

228. Ans. (b) Aspergillus *Ref: http://www.tsim.org.tw/journal/jour22-1/08.pdf*

Invasive pulmonary aspergillosis

- Invasive pulmonary aspergillosis (IPA) usually only affects people with lowered immunity, such as those who have received a bone marrow transplant or cancer treatment, diabetes or those with HIV or AIDS.
- It's the most serious type of aspergillosis.
- Aspergillus have a tendency to invade blood vessels.
- In people with a severely weakened immune system, the fungus can spread through the bloodstream from the lungs to the brain, eyes, heart or kidneys.

229. Ans. (a) Glycine *Ref: http://en.wikiped.ia.org/wiki/Alpha_helix*

- Different amino-acid sequences have different propensities for forming α-helical structure
- Methionine, alanine, leucine, uncharged glutamate and Lysin (MALEK) have especially high helix forming propensity
- Proline and glycine poor helix forming propensity
- Glycine tends to disrupt helices because its high conformational flexibility makes it entropically expensive to adopt the relatively constrained α-helical structure
- Proline either breaks or kinks a helix or both because it cannot donate an amide hydrogen bond

230. Ans. (a) Interaction of drug and bacterial endotoxins *Ref: KDT, 6th ed. p 698, 756*

- The Jarisch-Herxheimer reaction is a reaction to endotoxins released by the death of harmful organisms within the body.
- Jarisch-Harxheimer reaction resembles bacterial sepsis and can occur after initiation antibacterials such as penicillin or tetracycline, or treatment of tick borne relapsing fever.

- Typically, the death of these bacteria and the associated release of endotoxins occurs faster than the body can remove the toxins. It manifests as fever, chilis, rigor, hypotension, headache, tachycardia, hyperventilation, vasodilation with flushing, myalgla (muscle pain) and exacerbation of skin lesions.
- The intensity of the reaction indicates the severity of inflammation. Reactions commonly occur within two hours of drug administration, but are usually self limiting.
- Jarisch-Harxheimer reaction has been reported by people with bronchitis, hypothyroidism, pneumonia, crohn's disease, borrelia infection.

231. Ans. (b) 10 *Ref: Ananthanarayan, 8th ed. p 260*

- Tetanus Toxoid, for intramuscular or subcutaneous use, is a sterile solution of toxoid in isotonic sodium chloride solution. The vaccine is clear or slightly turbid in appearance.
- A course of immunization consist of three doses of tetanus toxoid, with an interval of 4–6 weeks between the first two injections and the third dose 6 months later (or as per recommendations of the National Immunization Programme).
- A full course of immunization confers immunity for a period of at least ten years. A 'booster dose' of toxoid is recommended after ten years.

7 Dental Anatomy, Physiology and Occlusion

INTRODUCTION TO DENTAL ANATOMY

No questions were asked from this chapter.

DEVELOPMENT AND ERUPTION OF TOOTH

1. Which of the following is true about calcification of dentin? *(AIIMS Nov 2010)*
a. Calcification of primary teeth is almost complete at the time of birth
b. Calcification of all primary teeth and few permanent teeth complete at birth
c. Calcification of permanent teeth starts at birth
d. Calcification of primary teeth starts around birth

2. Tooth eruption occurs when root formation is completed: *(AIIMS Nov 2006)*
a. 25% b. 50%
c. 75% d. 100%

3. Tooth eruption starts at which Nolla's stage? *(AIIMS Nov 2006)*
a. 6 b. 7
c. 8 d. 5

4. When is the first evidence of calcification of primary teeth? *(AIPG 2005)*
a. 4 months in utero
b. 4 and ½ months in utero
c. 5 months in utero
d. 6 months in utero

5. Relative to primary mandibular incisors, permanent mandibular incisors erupt: *(AIPG2005)*
a. Lingually b. Facially
c. Distally d. Mesially

6. The last primary tooth to be replaced by a permanent tooth is usually: *(AIPG 2005)*
a. Maxillary canine
b. Mandibular canine
c. Maxillary first molar
d. Mandibular second molar

7. Successor of permanent teeth develops from: *(COMED 2011)*
a. Buccal extension of dental lamina
b. Lingual extension of dental lamina
c. Distal extension of dental lamina
d. Main or parent dental lamina

8. Tooth eruption generally occurs when root development is complete by: *(COMED 2011)*
a. 30% b. 10%
c. 75% d. 100%

9. The first evidence of calcification of anterior teeth begins approximately between: *(COMED 2007)*
a. 14 to 17 weeks in utero
b. 09 to 12 weeks in utero
c. 06 to 009 weeks in utero
d. 17 to 20 weeks in utero

10. The human permanent anterior teeth show how many developmental lobes? *(COMED 2007)*
a. One lobe b. Two lobes
c. Three lobes d. Four lobes

11. The teeth that are retained for the longest period of time are: *(COMED 2006)*
a. Maxillary incisors
b. Maxillary canines
c. Mandibular incisors
d. Mandibular canines

12. The optimal time for a molar tooth to be erupt is when: *(KCET 2013)*
a. Two third of a root is complete
b. Half of root is complete
c. One third of the root is complete
d. Full root length is complete

13. During the development of tooth, sound coalescence of the lobes result in: *(KCET 2013)*
a. Grooves b. Fissures
c. Cusps d. All of the above

14. Any one of the rounded protuberances on incisal ridges of newly erupted incisor is called: *(KCET 2009)*
a. Tubercle b. Cusp
c. Mamelon d. Fossa

15. Number of line angles to anterior teeth: *(KCET 2008)*
a. 4 line angles
b. 8 line angles
c. 6 line angles
d. 10 line angles

16. Tooth transition period starts approximately at the age of
a. 6 months b. 6 years
c. 2 years d. 12 years

17. According to Cushion: Hammock theory, which of the following is responsible for the eruption of tooth.
a. Ligament at the base of the socket
b. Ligament at the middle of the socket
c. Periodontal ligaments
d. Pulpal pressure and pulpal growth

THE PRIMARY TEETH

18. The primary tooth is whiter than the permanent tooth because: *(AIIMS Nov 2010, 2008)*
a. Of thin dentin in primary teeth
b. The difference in crystalline structure of enamel makes the refractive index different
c. Of contrast with the surrounding tissue
d. Of the lighter color of the enamel

19. Resorption of deciduous central incisor starts at: *(AIIMS Nov 2010, AIPG 2013)*
a. 3 years b. 4 years
c. 5 years d. 6 years

20. The sharpest and highest cusp on primary first molar tooth is: *(AIIMS May 2010, 2007)*
a. Mesiobuccal b. Mesiolingual
c. Distobuccal d. Distolingual

21. The pulp of the first primary molar contains: *(AIIMS May 2006)*
a. Four pulp horns and three root canals
b. Three pulp horns and three root canals
c. Two pulp horns and two root canals
d. Two pulp horns and three root canals

22. The truth about primary teeth is: *(AIPG 2009)*
a. Furcation is close to the cervical line
b. Pulp chambers are large
c. Roots are narrowed and thin
d. All of the above

23. The pulp of mandibular deciduous first molar has: *(AIPG 2008)*
a. Four pulp horns and three root canals
b. Two pulp horns and two root canals
c. Three pulp horns and three root canals
d. Two pulp horns and three root canals

24. Which of the following factors are primarily contributory to the shedding of deciduous teeth:
a. Hydrostatic pressure *(COMED 2007)*
b. Vascular pressure
c. Oncotic pressure
d. Masticatory pressure

FORENSICS, COMPARATIVE ANATOMY, GEOMETRICES AND FORMS AND FUNCTIONS

25. A primitive basic tooth form having a single conical crown and a single root is known as: *(AIIMS May 2010, 2007, AIPG 2007)*
a. Haplodont
b. Heterodont
c. Acrodont
d. Thecodont

26. The curve of occlusion that touches the buccal and the lingual surfaces of the mandibular buccal teeth is called as: *(AIIMS Nov 2006)*
a. Curve of Wilson
b. Curve of Monsoon
c. Curve of Spee
d. Catenary curve

27. Linear curve running from anterior to posterior: *(AIIMS Nov 2012)*
a. Curve of Wilson
b. Curve of Spee
c. Curve of Monson
d. Bonwill curve

28. According to scientists, the experiments prove that: *(AIIMS Nov 2013)*
a. Head and tail both are resistant to dissolution
b. Head and tail both are not resistant to dissolution
c. Head is more resistant to disolution
d. Tail is more resistant to disolution

29. The Human Teeth are: *(KCET 2005)*
a. Haplodont b. Triconodont
c. Bunodont d. All of the above

OROFACIAL COMPLEX: FORMS AND FUNCTIONS

30. The embrasure in the following areas is continuous with the interproximal spaces between the teeth: *(COMED 2013)*
a. Labial and lingual
b. Lingual and occlusal
c. Incisal and occlusal
d. Labial and occlusal

THE PERMANENT MAXILLARY INCISORS

31. Maximum variation in the tooth mass is seen in: *(AIIMS May 2010)*
a. Maxillary lateral incisor and 3rd molar
b. Maxillary lateral incisor and canine
c. Maxillary canine and 3rd molar
d. Maxillary 1st molar and canine

32. The permanent anterior tooth that most often shows variation in size is the: *(AIPG 2005)*
a. Mandibular canine
b. Mandibular central incisor
c. Maxillary canine
d. Maxillary lateral incisor

33. The first evidence of calcification of a permanent maxillary central incisor takes place at the age of: *(COMED 2010)*
a. 2-3 months b. 3-4 months
c. 6-7 months d. 8-9 months

34. The number of point angles in a permanent maxillary central incisor is: *(COMED 2009)*
a. Two b. Four
c. Six d. Eight

35. Following eruption, the root of the maxillary central incisor completes development at what approximate age? *(COMED 2008)*
a. 7 years b. 8 years
c. 9 years d. 10 years

36. Maxillary lateral incisor is smaller than the maxillary central incisor on all aspects except which one of the following: *(COMED 2007)*
a. Crown length
b. Mesiodistal crown width
c. Faciolingual crown width
d. Root length

37. Which of the following teeth have a mesiodistal dimension greater than the cervicoincisal dimensions? *(KCET 2011)*
a. Permanent maxillary central incisor
b. Primary lower central incisor
c. Primary lower lateral incisor
d. Primary maxillary central incisor

THE PERMANENT MANDIBULAR INCISORS

No questions were asked from this chapter.

THE PERMANENT MAXILLARY AND MANDIBULAR CANINE

38. Dentin islands are frequently found in the root canals of which of the following permanent teeth? *(AIIMS May 2010, AIPG 2010)*
a. Maxillary first molar and maxillary second premolar
b. Maxillary second premolar and mandibular canine
c. Maxillary lateral incisor and canine
d. Maxillary first molar and mandibular canine

39. The most steep cusp inclines are seen in: *(AIIMS Nov 2006)*
a. Maxillary first premolar
b. Mandibular second premolar
c. Maxillary first molar
d. Mandibular first molar

40. Cervical cross-section of maxillary first premolar is: *(AIIMS May 2005)*
a. Rectangular
b. Kidney shape
c. Oval
d. Square

41. The maxillary first premolar will typically demonstrate which of the following pulpal configuration? *(COMED 2010)*
a. Single root with one root canal
b. A double root with one root canal
c. A double root with two root canals
d. One root with three root canals

42. Mesial developmental depression is the characteristics feature of: *(COMED 2006, KCET 2006)*
a. Maxillary first premolar
b. Maxillary 2nd premolar
c. Mandibular 1st premolar
d. Mandibular 2nd premolar

43. Occlusal aspect of the maxillary first premolar is roughly: *(KCET 2008)*
a. Octagonal b. Trapezoidal
c. Hexagonal d. Rhomboidal

44. Mesial marginal developmental groove is present in: *(MH 2009)*
a. Deciduous maxillary 1st molar
b. Maxillary 1st premolar
c. Mandibular 1st premolar
d. Maxillary lateral incisor

THE PERMANENT MAXILLARY MOLAR

45. Which of the following cusp is associated with cusp of carabelli in permanent maxillary first molar? *(COMED 2010, KCET 2011)*
a. Mesiobuccal b. Mesiopalatal
c. Distobuccal d. Distopalatal

46. According to Schour and Massler, the crown completion of both the permanent maxillary and mandibular 1st molars is by the age of: *(COMED 2007)*
a. $1^{1/2}$-2 years
b. $2^{1/2}$-3 years
c. 3 to 4 years
d. 4 to 5 years

47. Oblique ridge of permanent maxillary first molar connects: *(KCET 2008)*
a. Mesiobuccal cusp and distobuccal cusp
b. Distobuccal cusp and mesiolingual cusp
c. Mesiolingual cusp and distolingual cusp
d. Mesiobuccal cusp and distolingual cusp

48. Which of the listed teeth has got four major cusps? *(KCET 2010)*
a. Mandibular molar
b. Maxillary 1st molar
c. Maxillary 2nd molar
d. Mandibular 2nd premolar

49. Longest root in the permanent maxillary molar is: *(KCET 2007)*
a. Buccal b. Lingual
c. Mesiobuccal d. Distobuccal

50. The Oblique ridge runs from the distobuccal cusp to:
a. Mesiobuccal
b. Mesiolingual
c. Distolingual cusp
d. None of the above

51. The fourth canal in maxillary first molar is commonly located in: *(COMED 2014)*
a. Distobuccal b. Palatal
c. Mesiobuccal d. Distolingual

52. Single antagonist is seen only with: *(MH 2010)*
a. Maxillary 1st molar
b. Mandibular 1st molar
c. Mandibular 3rd molar
d. Maxillary 3rd molar

THE PERMANENT MANDIBULAR PREMOLAR

53. The premolar with the occlusal groove pattern that may simulate the letter 'Y' is: *(AIIMS May 2010, 2007)*
a. Mandibular first premolar
b. Mandibular second premolar
c. Maxillary first premolar
d. Maxillary second premolar

54. The Y-shaped occlusal pattern appears in: *(AIPG 2007)*
a. Mandibular first premolar
b. Maxillary second premolar
c. Maxillary first premolar
d. Mandibular second premolar

55. Which of the following teeth is most likely to be congenitally missing? *(AIPG 2005)*
a. Maxillary central incisor
b. Mandibular canine
c. Mandibular second premolar
d. Maxillary first premolar

56. Most common teeth in mandibular arch that displaced out due to arch discrepancy is: *(AIPG 2013)*
a. 2nd Premolar b. Canine
c. 1st Molar d. 1st Premolar

57. Mesiolingual developmental groove is seen in:
a. Mandibular first premolar
b. Mandibular second premolar
c. Maxillary first premolar
d. Maxillary second premolar

58. "Y" shaped arrangement of central groove is seen on the occlusal surface of: *(KCET 2012, 2011)*
a. Permanent maxillary first premolar
b. Permanent maxillary second premolar
c. Permanent mandibular first premolar
d. Permanent mandibular second premolar

59. Bifurcation and trifurcation are most commonly observed in :

a. Permanent maxillary first premolar
b. Permanent maxillary second premolar
c. Permanent mandibular first premolar
d. Permanent mandibular second premolar

THE PERMANENT MANDIBULAR MOLAR

60. What is the geometrical outline of crowns of mandibular molar when viewed from proximal aspect? *(COMED 2011, COMED 2009)*

a. Trapezoid
b. Triangle
c. Rhomboid
d. Rectangle

61. The number of point angles in a permanent mandibular first molar is: *(COMED 2008)*

a. 4 b. 6
c. 8 d. 10

62. Roots of the permanent mandibular 1st molar are: *(KCET 2007)*

a. Mesiobuccal, Distobuccal and Lingual
b. Mesiolingual, Distolingual and Buccal
c. Mesial and Distal
d. Buccal and Lingual

PULP CHAMBERS AND CANALS

No questions were asked from this chapter

DENTO-OSSEOUS STRUCTURE, BLOOD VESSELS, AND NERVES

63. Mobility of teeth in carcinoma of Maxillary sinus is due to involvement by tumor of: *(COMED 2011)*

a. Anterior wall of Sinus
b. Posterior wall of Sinus
c. Roof of the Sinus
d. Floor of Sinus

THE TEMPOROMANDIBULAR JOINTS, MUSCLES, TEETH, AND THEIR FUNCTIONS

64. To protrude the mandible the following muscles will contract in conjunction with controlled stabilizing of the opening muscles: *(KCET 2006)*

a. Outer and inner of temporalis
b. Contraction of posterior fibers of temporalis and geniohyoid
c. Lateral and medial pterygoid muscles
d. Mylohyoid and temporalis

OCCLUSION

No questions were asked from this chapter

Answers with Explanations

DEVELOPMENT AND ERUPTION OF TOOTH

1. Ans. (c) Calcification of permanent teeth starts at birth *Ref: Wheeler's Dental Anatomy, 8th ed. p 51*

- At the age of 6 to 8 months in utero, the calcification of primary teeth starts.
- Initial calcification of permanent teeth starts at birth for 1st molar and the last permanent tooth, which shows initial classification in 3rd molar at the age of 8 years.
- At stage 8 of Nolla's stage, most of the tooth pierces the alveolar mucosa.

2. Ans. (c) 75% *Ref: Shobha Tandon*

- At the time of clinical eruption root formation is approximately three quarter (i.e. ¾ or 75%) is complete.

3. Ans. (c) 8 *Ref: Shobha Tandon, 2nd ed. p 91*

- When crown formation is completed the tooth starts to erupt in the oral cavity.

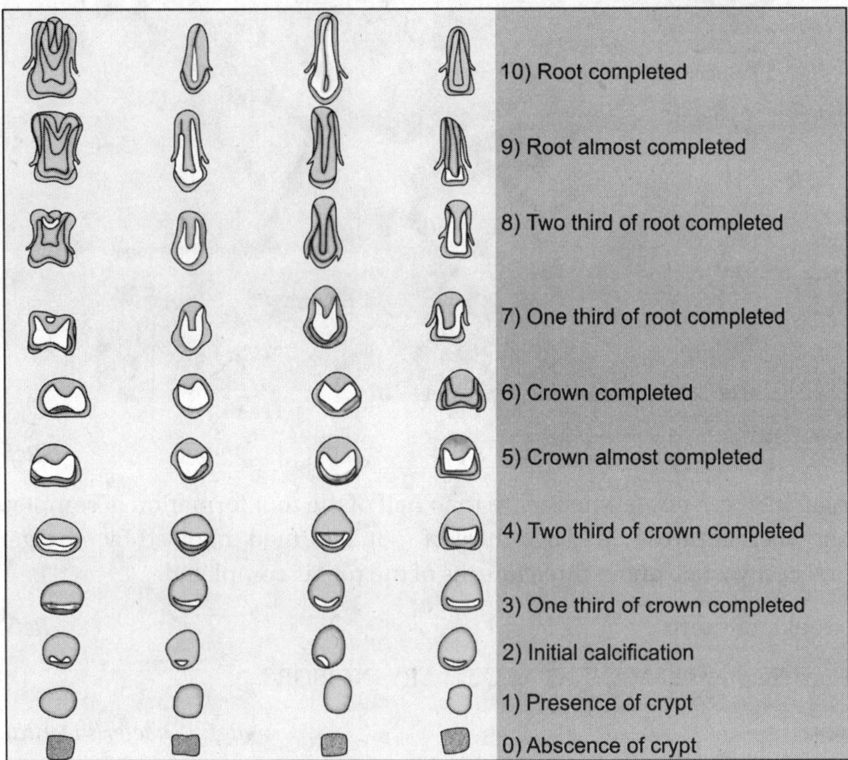

4. Ans. (a) 4 months in utero *Ref: Wheeler's Dental Anatomy, 8th ed. p 53*

Refer Ans no. 33 from chapter PERMANENT MAXILLARY INCISORS:

5. Ans. (a) Lingually *Ref: Wheeler's Dental Anatomy, 8th ed. p 44*

- The follicles of the incisors and canines are located lingual to deciduous roots.
- Generally permanent incisors erupt lingually to deciduous incisors in case the latter are not shed.

6. Ans. (a) Maxillary canine *Ref: Wheeler's Dental Anatomy, 8th ed. p 45*

Order of permanent tooth eruption

- First molars
- Mandibular central and lateral incisors
- Maxillary central incisor
- Maxillary lateral incisor
- Mandibular canines
- First premolars
- Second premolars
- Maxillary canines
- Second molars
- Third molars

Maxillary canine are last succedaneous teeth to erupt

7. Ans. (b) Lingual extension of dental lamina *Ref: Orban's, 12th ed. p 31*

- Lingual extension of the dental lamina is termed as successional lamina which is formed at 5th months in utero to 10th month of age and gives rise to permanent teeth.

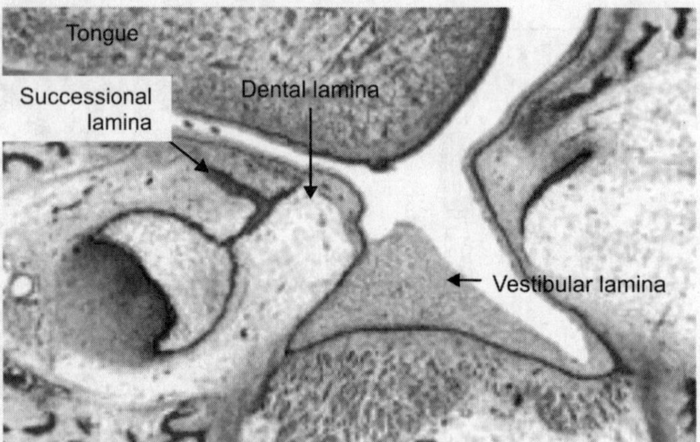

8. Ans. (c) 75% *Ref Wheeler's, 6th ed. p 38*

The eruption permanent teeth occur when more than half of the root formation is complete. Passage through the alveolar crest occur when approximately two third of root is formed followed by emergencies through alveolar gingival into the oral cavity when about three fourths of the root is completed.

9. Ans. (a) 14 to 17 weeks in utero *Ref: Wheeler's, 8th ed. p 53*

Refer Ans no. 33 from chapter PERMANENT MAXILLARY INCISORS:

10. Ans. (d) Four lobes *Ref: Wheeler's Dental Anatomy, 8th ed. p 42*

- All anterior teeth are formed from four centers of development, referred to as lobes.
- Three are located on the facial side of the tooth, and one on the lingual side.
- The cingulum forms from this lingual lobe of development.
- Mamelons are usually found as three small bumps on the incisal edges of anterior teeth. They are the remnants of three lobes of formation of these teeth.

11. Ans. (b) Maxillary canines *Ref: Wheeler's Dental Anatomy, 8th ed. p 45*

Refer Ans No. 6

12. Ans. (a) Two third of a root is complete *Ref: Wheeler's, 6th ed. p 38*

Refer Ans No. 8

13. Ans. (a) Grooves *Ref: Wheeler's, 8th ed. p 44*

A developmental groove: Is a shallow groove or line between the primary parts of the crown or root.

A supplemental groove: Less distinct. It is also a shallow linear depression on the surface of a tooth but is supplemental to developmental groove.

14. Ans. (c) Mamelon *Ref: Wheeler's, 8th ed. p 13*

- The incisor terminates incisally in rounded emineneces known as mamelons. These mamelons are prominent on newly erupted incisors, soon after eruption they are worn off gradually by use unless escaped through malocclusion.
- Mamelons important esthetic characteristics along with translucency give tooth life like appearance.

15. Ans. (c) 6 line angles *Ref: Wheeler's, 8th ed. p 14-15*

The line angles of the anterior teeth are as follows:

Mesiolabial	distolingual
Distolabial	labioincisal
Mesiolingual	linguoincisal

The line angles of the posterior teeth are as follows:

Mesiobuccal	mesio-occlusal
Distobuccal	disto-occlusal
mesiolingual	bucco-occlusal
distolingual	linguo occlusal

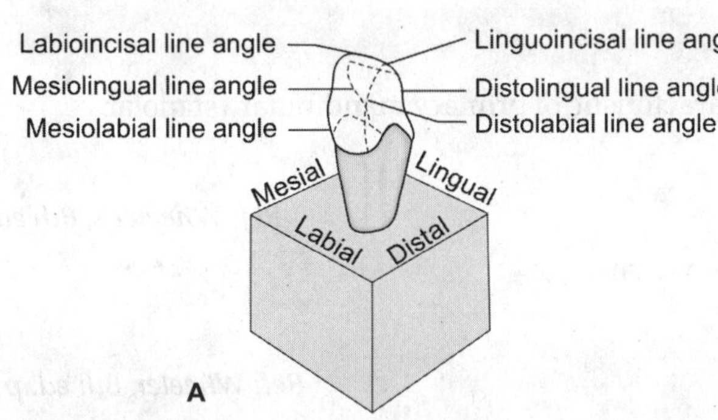

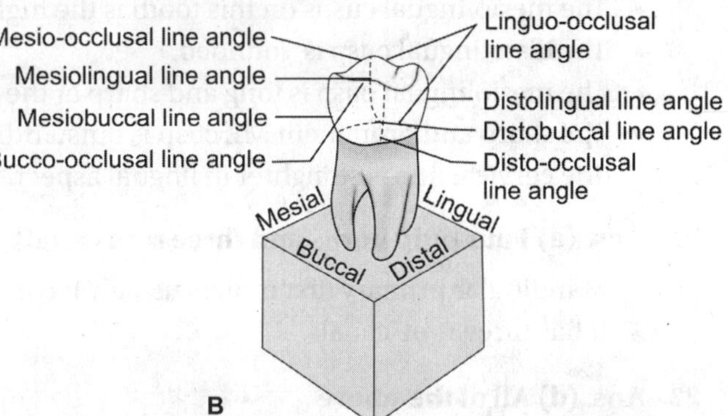

16. Ans. (c) 2 years *Ref: Wheeler's, 8th ed. p 1*

- It is the period when permanent as well as deciduous tooth are present in mouth.
- When children enter the tooth transition period, their deciduous teeth will loosen due to the resorption of the roots and will sequentially fall off.
- The permanent teeth will gradually erupt into the space left by the deciduous teeth.
- Tooth transition period starts approximately at the age of 6, and ends around the age of 12 or 13.

17. Ans. (a) Ligament at the base of the socket *Ref: Textbook of Craniofacial Growth by Sridhar, 1st ed. p 119*

Cushion Hammock theory:

- Proposed by Harry Sicher and was widely taught between 1930's to 1950's.
- According to it, a ligament below the tooth was responsible for eruption.

- This Hammock ligament does not extend across the socket, but only separates the pulp from the follicle.
- Ligament straddling the base of the socket like a sling from one bony wall to other.

THE PRIMARY TEETH

18. Ans. (b) The difference in crystalline structure of enamel makes the refractive index different

Ref: Wheeler's, 8th ed. p 70

- Primary and permanent teeth have a similar enamel prism structure except at the tooth surface.
- Primary teeth are more likely to have prismless surface zone than are permanent teeth.
- Enamel is twice as thick in permanent teeth as in primary teeth.
- Enamel formed postnatally is more highly pigmented than enamel formed prenatally.
- Despite this pigmentation, the enamel of primary teeth is whiter than that of permanent teeth. This is also believed to be because the difference in crystalline structure of enamel makes the refractive index different.

19. Ans. (b) 4 years *Ref: Oral Development and Histology by James K Avery, 3rd ed. p 132*

Deciduous Tooth	*Root Completion*	*Root Resorption Begins*	*Root Resorption Completed*
Central incisor	1.5 - 2 years	4 years	7 years
Lateral incisor	1.5 - 2 years	5 years	8 years
Canine	2.5 - 3 years	8 years	11 years
First molar	2 - 2.5 years	7 years	10 years
Second molar	3 years	7 years	11 years

20. Ans. (b) Mesiolingual *Ref: Wheeler's, 8th ed. p 93*

- The mesiolingual cusps on this tooth is the highest and largest of the cusps.
- The distolingual cusp is rounded.
- The mesiolingual cusp is long and sharp at the tip.
- The sharp and prominent ML cusp is outstanding characteristic of primary mandibular 1st molar.
- The cervical line is straighter in lingual aspect.

21. Ans. (a) Four pulp horns and three root canals *Ref: Wheeler's, 8th ed. p 72*

- Mandibular primary first molars usually have four pulp horns.
- It has three root canals.

22. Ans. (d) All of the above *Ref: Wheeler, 8th ed. p 67-71*

- Deciduous teeth are fewer in number and smaller in size but the deciduous molars are wider mesiodistally than the premolars. The deciduous anteriors are narrower mesiodistally than their permanent successors.
- Their enamel is thinner and whiter in appearance.
- The crowns are rounded. The deciduous teeth are constricted at the neck (cervix).
- The roots of deciduous anterior teeth are longer and narrower than the roots of their permanent successors.
- The roots of deciduous molars are longer and more slender than the roots of the permanent molars. Also, they flare greatly.
- The cervical ridges of enamel seen on deciduous teeth are more prominent than on the permanent teeth. This 'bulge' is very pronounced at the mesiobuccal of deciduous first molars.
- Deciduous cervical enamel rods incline incisally/occlusally.
- The pulp horns are high, and the pulp chambers are large.
- Primary roots are narrow and long when compared with crown width and length.

23. Ans. (a) Four pulp horns and three root canals *Ref: Wheeler', 8th ed. p 72*

Refer Ans no. 21

24. Ans. (d) Masticatory pressure *Ref: Tencate's 7th/ed, p 279*

- Pressure from the permanent tooth plays a very important role in the shedding of deciduous.
- Increasing the masticatory forces will accelerate the exfoliation.
- Masticatory forces also determine the pattern and rate of deciduous tooth shedding.

FORENSICS, COMPARATIVE ANATOMY, GEOMETRICES AND FORMS AND FUNCTIONS

25. Ans. (a) Haplodont *Ref: Wheeler's, 8th ed. p 101*

- Homodont: All teeth have same shape
- Heterodont:Different types of teeth
- Acrodont: Teeth attached to crest of bone
- Pleurodont: Teeth attached to inner margins of bone
- Thecodont: Teeth are inserted in a bony socket
- Haplodont: Teeth with single conical cusp and single root
- Monophyodont: One set of dentition for entire life
- Diphyodont: Two sets of dentition in life
- Polyphyodont: Many sets of teeth or more than two sets of teeth in life
- Bunodont: Primitive teeth with simple conical cusps

26. Ans. (a) Curve of Wilson *Ref: Glossary of Prosthodontic Terms, Vol. 1, 94, p 28*

Curve of Wilson

- It is a curve that contacts the buccal and lingual cusp tips of the mandibular buccal teeth.
- It is medio-lateral on each side of the arch and it is due to lingual inclination of mandibular posteriors.
- It is concave for mandibular and convex for maxillary teeth.
- It is a cross arch, cross tooth curve and indicates the difference between supporting and non supporting cusp in occlusion.

27. Ans. (b) Curve of Spee *Ref: Wheeler's, 8th ed. p 454*

Curve of Spee

- The Curve of Spee is an anatomic curvature of the occlusal alignment of the teeth, beginning at the tip of the lower canine, following the buccal cusps of the natural premolars and molars and continuing to the anterior border of the ramus.
- It is named for the German embryologist Ferdinand Graf von Spee (1855–1937), who was first to describe the anatomic relations of human teeth in the sagittal plane.

28. Ans. (d) Tail is more resistant to disolution *Ref: Sturdevant's, 6th ed. p 3*

The periphery of head region and the whole tail region is more resistant to dissolution due to acid attack.

29. Ans. (c) Bunodont *Ref: Wheeler's, 8th ed. p 108*

- In bunodont molars the cusps are low and rounded hills rather than sharp peaks.
- They are most common among omnivores such as pigs, bears and humans.
- Bunodont molars are effective crushing devices and often basically quadrate in shape.

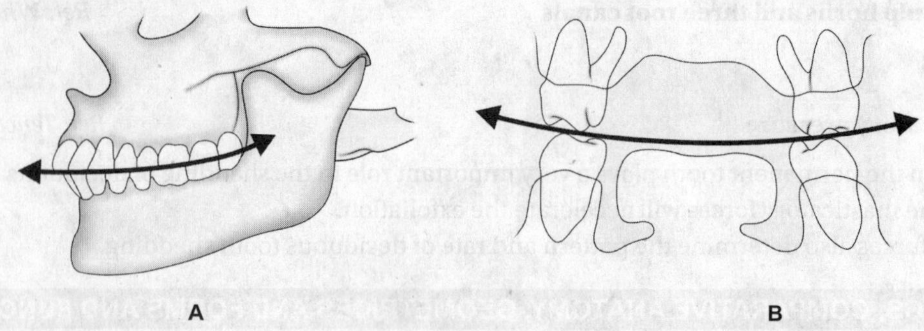

(A) Curve of Spee (B) Curve of Wilson

OROFACIAL COMPLEX: FORMS AND FUNCTIONS

30. Ans. (a) Labial and lingual *Ref: Wheeler's, 8th ed. p 130*

- When two teeth in the same arch are in contact, their curvatures adjacent to the contact areas form spillway space called embrasures. The spaces that widen out from the area of contact labially or buccally and lingually are called labial or buccal and lingual interproximal embrasures. These embrasures are continuous with the interproximal spaces between the teeth.
- Function of embrasures is to prevent food from being forced through the contact area. When teeth wear down to the contact area so that no embrasure remains, especially in the incisors, food is pushed into the contact area even when teeth are not mobile.

THE PERMANENT MAXILLARY INCISORS

31. Ans. (a) Maxillary lateral incisor and 3rd molar *Ref: Wheeler's, 8th ed. p 161*

- Maxillary lateral incisor and 3rd molar shows maximum variation in the tooth mass. Maxillary Lateral Incisor
- Most common missing tooth next to third molars
- Tooth in maxillary arch, which can be extracted by pure rotation
- Usually have abnormal relation with adjacent teeth
- Infection is usually palatal apical third of root curves distally and palatally
- Dens in dente most common in this tooth

32. Ans. (d) Maxillary lateral incisor *Ref: Wheeler's, 8th ed. p 161*

- Maxillary lateral incisor is the permanent anterior tooth that most often shows variation in size whereas third molar is the permanent posterior tooth that most often shows variation in size and shape.

33. Ans. (b) 3-4 months *Ref: Wheeler's, 8th ed. p 53*

Chronology of human dentition

Dentition	*Tooth*	*First evidence of calcification*	*Crown completed*	*Eruption*	*Root completed*
		Weeks in utero	*Months*	*Months*[a,b]	*Years*
Primary (Upper)	I1	14 (13-16)	1½	10 (8-12)	1½
	I2	16 (14⅔-16½)[b]	2½	11 (9-13)	2
	C	17 (15-18)[b]	9	19 (16-22)	3¼
	m1	15½ (14½-17)	6	16 (13-19)♂ (14-18) ♀	2½
	m2	19 (16-23½)	11	29 (25-33)	3

Contd...

Contd...

Dentition	*Tooth*	*First evidence of calcification*	*Crown completed*	*Eruption*	*Root completed*
		Weeks in utero	*Months*	*Months*[a,b]	*Years*
Primary (Lower)	I1	14 (13-16)	2½	8 (6-10)	1½
	12	16(14⅔-)[b]	3	13 (10-16)	1½
	C	17 (16–)[b]	9	20 (17-23)	3¼
	m1	15½ (14½-17)	5½	16 (14-18)	2¼
	m2	18 (17-19½)	10	27 (23-31) ♂ (24-30) ♀	3
Permanent (Upper)	I1	3-4 mo	4-5 yr	7-8 yr	10
	12	10-12 mo	4-5 yr	8-9 yr	11
	C	4-5 mo	6-7 yr	11-12 yr	13-15
	P1	1½-1¾ yr	5-6 yr	10-11 yr	12-13
	P2	2-2¼ yr	6-7 yr	10-12 yr	12-14
	M1	At birth	2½-3 yr	6-7 yr	9-10
	M2	2½-3 yr	7-8 yr	12-13 yr	14-16
	M3	7-9 yr	12-16 yr	17-21 yr	18-25
Permanent (Lower)	I1	3-4 mo	4-5 yr	6-7 yr	9
	I2	3-4 mo	4-5 yr	7-8 yr	10
	C	4-5 mo	6-7 yr	9-10 yr	12-14
	P1	1¾ -2 yr	5-6 yr	10-12 yr	12-13
	P2	2¼-2½ yr	6-7 yr	11-12 yr	13-14
	M1	At birth	2½–3 yr	6-7 yr	9-10
	M2	2½-3 yr	7-8 yr	11-13 yr	14-15
	M3	8-10 yr	12-16 yr	17-21 yr	18-25

34. Ans. (b) Four *Ref: Wheeler's, 8th ed. p 15*

A line angle is formed by the junction of two surfaces

Line angle of maxillary central incisor (6)	
• Mesiolabial	• Distolingual
• Mesiolingual	• Distoincisal
• Mesioincisal	• Distolabial
Line angle of Posterior teeth (8)	
• Mesiobuccal	• Mesio-occlusal
• Distobuccal	• Disto-occlusal
• Mesiolingual	• Bucco-occlusal
• Distolingual	• Linguo-occlusal

A point angle is formed by junction of three surfaces

In anterior teeth (4)	
• Mesiolabioincisal	• Mesiolinguoincisal
• Distolabioincisal	• Distolinguoincisal
In posterior teeth (4)	
Mesiobucco-occlusal	• Mesiolinguo-occlusal
Distobucco-occlusal	• Distolinguo-occlusal

35. Ans. (d) 10 years *Ref: Wheeler's, 8th ed. p 45*

Chronology of Permanent Teeth

	Tooth	*First evidence of calcification*	*Crown completed (years)*	*Emergence (eruption) (years)*	*Root completed (years)*
CI	8, 9	3-4 mo	4-5	7-8	10
LI	7,10	10-12 mo	4-5	8-9	11
C	6, 11	4-5 mo	6-7	11-12	13-15
P1	5, 12	1½ -1¾ yr	5-6	10-11	12-13
P2	4, 13	2-2¼ yr	6-7	10-12	12-14
M1	3, 14	At birth	2½-3	6-7	9-10
M2	2, 15	2½-3 yr	7-8	12-13	14-16
M3	1,16	7-9 yr	12-16	17-21	18-25
	Maxillary teeth 1 2 3 4 5 6 7 8 9 10 11 12 13 14 15 16 32 31 30 29 28 27 26 25 24 23 22 21 20 19 18 17				
Right	Mandibular Teeth				Left
CI	24, 25	3-4 mo	4-5	6-7	9
LI	23, 26	3-4 mo	4-5	7-8	10
C	22, 27	4-5 mo	6-7	9-10	12-14
P1	21, 28	1¼-2 yr	5-6	10-12	12-13
P2	20, 29	2¼-2½ yr	6-7	11-12	13-14
M1	19, 30	At birth	2½ - 3	6-7	9-10
M2	18, 31	2½ -3 yr	7-8	11-13	14-15
M3	17, 32	8-10 yr	12-16	17-21	18-25

36. Ans. (d) Root length *Ref: Wheeler's, 8th ed. p 161*

Maxillary lateral incisor is smaller in all dimensions in comparison to maxillary central incisor except root length, i.e. 13 mm (same as maxillary central incisors).

37. Ans. (d) Primary maxillary central incisor *Ref: Wheeler's, 8th ed. p 79*

- The overall length of the deciduous maxillary central incisor is 16 mm on average, with the crown being 6 mm and the root being 10 mm. In comparison to the permanent maxillary central incisor, the ratio of the root length to the crown length is greater in the deciduous tooth.
- The diameter of the crown mesiodistally is greater than the length cervicoincisally, which makes the tooth appear wider rather than taller from a labial viewpoint.
- The marginal ridges and the cingulum of the tooth are well-developed. The cingulum reaches incisally a great length and is large enough to create small fossa on either side of it.
- and crown of a tooth. On the mesial and distal surfaces, the cervical line curves incisally, which is also seen in the permanent maxillary central incisor.
- The root of this tooth is cone-shaped with a rounded apex. Most of the surfaces are smooth, but the mesial surface of the root may have a developmental groove or a concavity

THE PERMANENT MAXILLARY AND MANDIBULAR CANINE

38. Ans. (b) Maxillary second premolar and mandibular canine

Ref: www2.sci.u-szeged.hu/ABS/2002/Acta%20HPa/4671.pdf

- A dentinal island may be found in any tooth that demonstrates an extremely wide labiolingual dimension and a narrow mesiodistal dimension.
- Some teeth possess dentinal islands in the apical third of the root; this situation essentially forces the clinician to these as two-canaled teeth.
- Dentin islands are frequently found in the root canals of Maxillary second premolar and mandibular canine

39. Ans. (a) Maxillary first premolar *Ref: Wheeler's, 8th ed. p 215*

- The mandibular and maxillary second premolar possess less sharp cusps in compare to others.
- Their cusps articulate with opposing teeth when the jaws brought together, that's why, it is more efficient as grinding teeth and hence in this way, it functions like molar.

40. Ans. (b) Kidney shape *Ref: Wheeler's, 8th ed. p 345*

Cervical cross section	*Outline form*
Maxillary 1st premolar	Kidney shape
Maxillary 2nd premolar	Oval
Maxillary 1st molar	Rhomboidal
Maxillary 2nd molar	Angulation of the outline form
Mandibular 1st premolar	Oval, rectangular or triangular
Mandibular 2nd premolar	Oval, rectangular or triangular
Mandibular 1st molar	Quadrilateral
Mandibular 2nd molar	Triangular

41. Ans. (c) A double root with two root canals *Ref: Wheeler's, 8th ed. p 217*

Most maxillary first premolars have two roots and two pulp canals. When only one root is present, two pulp canals are usually found anyway.

42. Ans. (a) Maxillary first premolar *Ref: Wheeler's, 8th ed. p 226*

Maxillary First Premolar

Chronology:

Eruption of deciduous: (Replaces max 1st molar

Eruption of permanent: 10-11 years

Calcification initiation: 1.5-2.5 years

Mesial:

- Outline is trapezoidal.
- Cusp tip is located within confines of root surfaces
  - mesial cusp ridge is longer than its distal cusp ridge - only tooth where mesioincisal is longer than the distoincisal
- Both cusps are visible, and the buccal cusp is 1 mm taller, straighter, and less pointed than lingual cusp (more convex)

- mesial concavity is below contact point (middle 1/3) allows easy distinguish from distal
- mesial developmental depression/concavity present, note maxillary second premolars do not have this
- mesial marginal ridge developmental groove is present. (This distinguish from max. second premolar)

43. Ans. (c) Hexagonal *Ref: Wheeler's, 8th ed. p 227-228*

The occlusal aspect of the maxillary first premolar resembles roughly a six-sided or hexagonal figure. The six sides are made up of the mesiobuccal, which is mesial to the buccal ridge; mesial; mesiolingual, which is mesial to the lingual ridge; distolingual; distal; and distobuccal. This hexagonal figure, however, is not equilateral. The two buccal sides are nearly equal. The mesial side is shorter than the distal side and the mesiolingual side is shorter than the distolingual side.

44. Ans. (b) Maxillary 1st premolar *Ref: Wheeler's, 8th ed. p 227-229*

The mesial marginal developmental groove present in the maxillary first premolar crosses the mesial marginal ridge and ends on the mesial surface of crown.

THE PERMANENT MAXILLARY MOLAR

45. Ans. (b) Mesiopalatal *Ref: Wheeler's, 8th ed. p 276*

- In maximum 1st molars the four major cusps are well developed, with the small minor, or fifth cusp appearing on the lingual surface of the mesiolingual cusp near the mesiolingual line angle of the crown. The fifth cusp may be indistinct, or all the cusp form may be absent. The mesiolingual cusp is the largest cusp; it is followed in point of size by the mesiobuccal, distolingual, distobuccal and fifth cusps.
- Developmental, only three major cusps can be considered as primary, the mesiolingual cusp and the two buccal cusps. The distolingual cusp is common to all of the maxillary molars; any other additional one such as the cusp of Carabelli on first molars must be regarded as secondary.
- 60% of population may have a 5th cusp called cusp of carabelli on mesial half of mesiopalatal cusp. Cusp of carabelli is also seen in maxillary deciduous second molar. The cusp ridge of 5th cusp or cusp of carabelli is approximately 2 mm cervical to the cusp ridge of mesiopalatal cusp.

46. Ans. (b) $2^{1/2}$-3 years *Ref: Wheeler's, 8th ed. p 53*

Refer Ans no. 33 from chapter PERMANENT MAXILLARY INCISORS:

47. Ans. (b) Distobuccal cusp and mesiolingual cusp *Ref: Wheeler's, 8th ed. p 277*

The oblique ridge is a ridge that crosses the occlusal surface obliquely. The union of the triangular ridge of the distobuccal cusp and the distal ridge of the mesiolingual cusp forms it. This ridge is reduced in height in the center of the occlusal surface, being about on a level with the marginal ridges of the occlusal surface.

48. Ans. (b) Maxillary 1st molar *Ref: Wheeler's, 8th ed. p 263*

- The maxillary molars have large crowns with four well-formed cusps.
- They have three roots, two buccal and one lingual.
- The lingual root is the largest.
- The crowns have two buccal cusps and two lingual cusps.

49. Ans. (b) Lingual *Ref: Wheeler's, 8th ed. p 263*

Also refer ans no. 48

The maxillary first molar normally has three roots.

- The Mesiobuccal Root is broad buccolingually and has prominent depressions or flutings on its mesial and distal surfaces. The internal canal morphology is highly variable, but the majority of the mesiobuccal roots contain two canals.

- The Distobuccal Root is generally rounded or ovoid in cross section and usually contains a single canal.
- The Palatal Root (lingual root) is more broad mesiodistally than buccolingually and ovoidal in shape but normally contains only a single canal. Although the palatal root generally appears straight on radiographs, there is usually a buccal curvature in the apical third. Depressions on the buccal and palatal surfaces of the palatal root can be present but are generally shallow.

50. Ans. (b) Mesiolingual *Ref: Wheeler's, 8th ed. p 277*

Also Refer Ans no. 47

A crest on the occlusal surface of upper molars comprising the distal cusp ridge of the mesiolingual cusp and the triangular ridge of the distobuccal cusp.

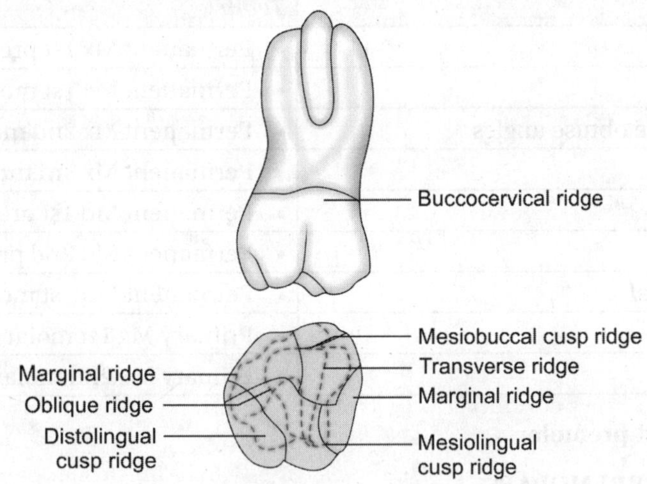

51. Ans. (c) Mesiobuccal *Ref: Grossman, 12th ed. p 192*

The maxillary first molar normally has three roots:

- The Mesiobuccal Root is broad buccolingually and has prominent depressions or flutings on its mesial and distal surfaces. The internal canal morphology is highly variable, but the majority of the mesiobuccal roots contain two canals.
- The Distobuccal Root is generally rounded or ovoid in cross section and usually contains a single canal.
- The Palatal Root is more broad mesiodistally than buccolingually and ovoidal in shape but normally contains only a single canal. Although the palatal root generally appears straight on radiographs, there is usually a buccal curvature in the apical third. Depressions on the buccal and palatal surfaces of the palatal root can be present but are generally shallow.There are prominent depressions found on the distal aspect of the mesiobuccal roots. Depressions can also be found on the furcal side of the distobuccal and palatal roots. The overall average length of the maxillary first molar is 20.5 mm with an average crown length of 7.5 mm and an average root length of 13 mm.

52. Ans. (d) Maxillary 3rd molar *Ref: Color Atlas of Human Anatomy, Vol. 2, 5th ed.*

- The 2 mandibular central incisors and 2 mandibular lateral incisors appear quite similar although the lateral incisor is larger
- The opposite situation exists in the maxilla, where the central is larger than the lateral incisor
- As the smallest tooth in the dentition, the mandibular central incisor has only one antagonist
- This tooth and the maxillary 3rd molar are the only teeth that have one antagonist, all the others have two.

THE PERMANENT MANDIBULAR PREMOLAR

53. Ans. (b) Mandibular second premolar *Ref: Wheeler's, 8th ed. p 260*

MANDIBULAR SECOND PREMOLAR

- The mandibular second premolar most commonly has three cusps but can have two as well.
- The three cusp variety has one large cusp on the buccal with two smaller lingual cusps.
- The mesiolingual cusp is twice the size of the disolingual cusp.
- The occlusal table (the area bounded by the cusps, cusp ridges, and marginal ridges) is rectangular. The groove pattern is shaped like a "Y" with the tail pointed to the lingual and placed between the distolingual and mesiolingual cusps one third of the distance form the distal to the mesial.

Shape of occlusal surface	*Tooth*
• Hexagonal	• Permanent Mx 1st premolar
• Rhomboidal	• Permanent Mx 1st molar
• Rhomboidal with more obtuse angles	• Permanent Mx 2nd molar
• Heart shape	• Permanent Mx 3rd molar
• Diamond	• Permanent Md 1st premolar
• Square	• Permanent Md 2nd premolar
• Hexagonal/Trapezoidal	• Permanent Md 1st molar
• Rectangular	• Primary Mx 1st molar
• Rhomboidal	• Primary Mx 2nd molar

54. Ans. (b) Maxillary second premolar *Ref: Wheeler's, 8th ed. p 260*

MANDIBULAR SECOND PREMOLAR

Facial: From this aspect, the tooth somewhat resembles the first, but the buccal cusp is less pronounced. The tooth is larger than the first.

Lingual: The most common is the three-cusp form which has two lingual cusps. The mesial of those is the larger of the two.

Proximal: The buccal cusp is shorter than the first. The lingual cusp (or cusps) are much better developed than the first and give the lingual a full well-developed profile.

Occlusal: The two or three cusp versions become clearly evident. In the three- cusp version, the developmental grooves present a distinctive 'Y' shape and have a central pit. In the two cusp version, a single developmental groove crosses the transverse ridge from mesial to distal.

Root: The mandibular second premolar has a single root that is usually larger than that of the first premolar.

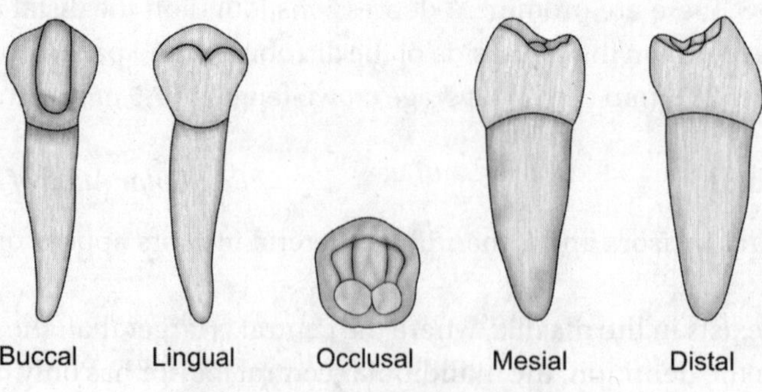

Mandibular right second premolar

55. Ans. (c) Mandibular second premolar *Ref: Shafer's, 6th ed. p 46*

Mandibular second premolars are the second most common missing teeth next to third molars, and are absent in 2.5% to 5% of the population.

TREATMENT IN SUCH CASES:

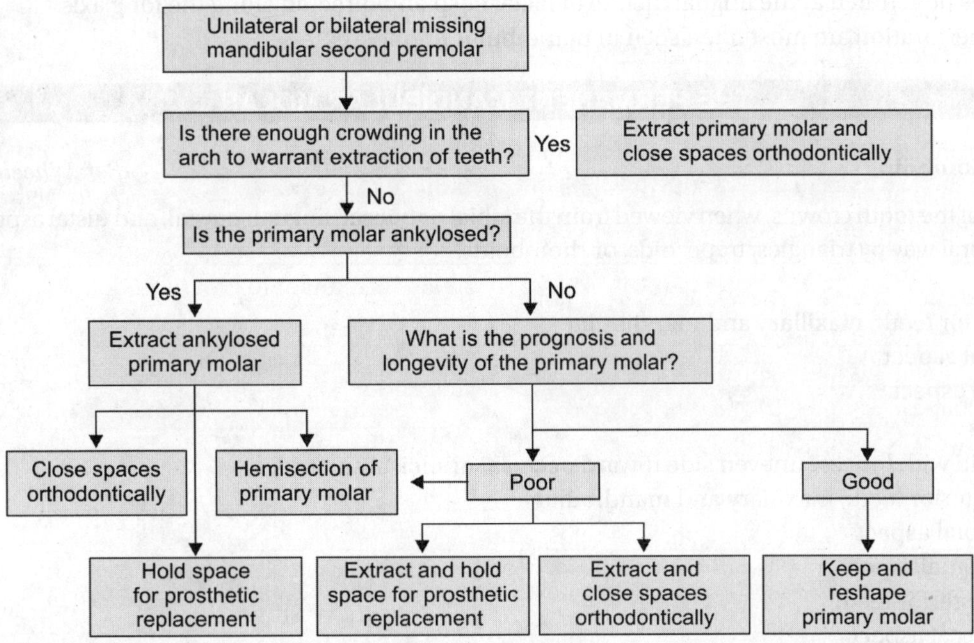

56. Ans. (a) 2nd Premolar *Ref: Balaji, 3rd ed. p 392*

The most frequently absent teeth in children are mandibular second premolars, maxillary lateral incisors and maxillary second premolars.

57. Ans. (a) Mandibular first premolar *Ref: Wheeler's, 8th ed. p 247, 260, 226-227, 236*

- Characteristic features of the mandibular first premolar is the mesiolingual developmental groove. This groove acts as a line of demarcation between the mesiobuccal lobe and the lingual lobe and extends into the mesial fossa of the occlusal surface.
- A distinguishing feature of maxillary 1st premolar is found on the mesial surface of the crown. Immediately cervical to the mesial contact area, centered on the mesial surface and bordered buccally and lingually by the mesiobuccally and mesiolingual line angles, is a marked depression called the mesial developmental depression. This mesial concavity continues apically beyond the cervical line, join a deep developmental depression between the roots, and ends at the root bifurcation.
- No developmental depression is evident on the mesial surface of the crown as on the first premolar; the crown surface is convex instead. A shallow developmental groove appears on the single tapered root.

58. Ans. (d) Permanent mandibular second premolar *Ref: Wheeler's, 6th ed. p 213*

- The mandibular second premolar most commonly has three cusps. The three cusp variety has one large cusp on the buccal with two smaller lingual cusps.
- The occlusal table (the area bounded by the cusps, cusp ridges, and marginal ridges) is rectangular. The groove pattern is shaped like a "Y" with the tail pointed to the lingual and placed between the distolingual and mesio-lingual cusps one third of the distance form the distal to the mesial.

59. Ans. (c) Permanent mandibular first premolar *Ref: Ingle's 5th ed. p 751*

Mandibular 1st Premolar

- Smallest of all the premolars
- The crown of mandibular 1st premolar lingual till of 30° to the long axis of root. To compensate for the tilt, the enamel is penetrated at the lingual incline of facial cusp and directed along the long axis.
- Lateral perforation are most often seen in mandibular premolars.

THE PERMANENT MANDIBULAR MOLAR

60. Ans. (c) Rhomboid *Ref: Wheeler's, 8th ed. p 112*

- Outline of the tooth crowns, when viewed from the labial or buccal, lingual, mesial, and distal aspects are described in a general way by triangles, trapezoids, or rhomboids.

Triangles

- Six anterior teeth, maxillary and mandibular
  - Mesial aspect
  - Distal aspect

Trapezoids

- Trapezoid with longest uneven side toward occlusal or incisal surface.
  - All anterior teeth, maxillary and mandibular
    - Labial aspect
    - Lingual aspect
  - All posterior teeth
    - Buccal aspect
    - Lingual aspect
- Trapezoid with shortest uneven side toward occlusal surface.
  - All maxillary posterior teeth
    - Mesial aspect
    - Distal aspect

61. Ans. (a) 4 *Ref: Wheeler's, 8th ed. p 15,16*

The point angles of the posterior teeth are as follows:

Mesiobucco-occlusal	mesiolinguo-occlusal
Distobucco-occlusal	distolinguo-occlusal

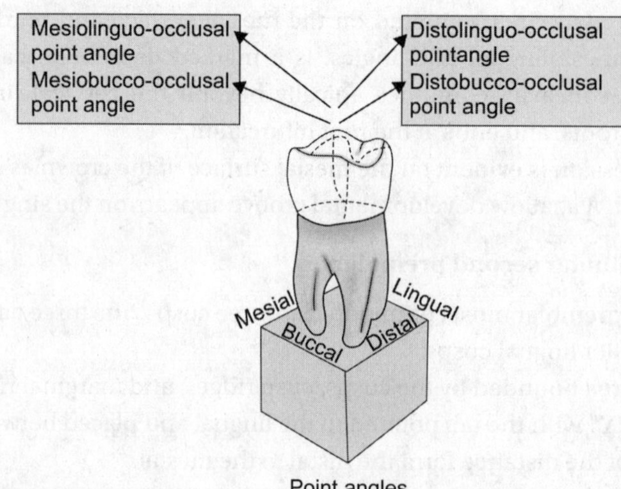

Point angles

62. Ans. (c) Mesial and Distal *Ref: Wheeler's, 8th ed. p 297*

- The mandibular first molar has five cusps: the mesiobuccal (MB, toward midline and cheek), mesiolingual (ML, toward midline and tongue), distolingual (DL, away from midline and towards tongue), distobuccal (DB, away from midline and toward cheek), and distal (D, away from midline), listed in order of decreasing size.
- Listed in order of decreasing height they are: ML, DL, DF, MF, and D.
- It possess two roots i.e., mesial and distal.
- Both roots have flutings but they are more prominent on the mesial root.
- The mesial root is broader buccolingually and its apex is more blunted.
- The mandibular first molars are the most common carious teeth and the most common teeth to undergo endodontic treatment or extraction. Up to 45% of all extracted teeth are mandibular first molars.

DENTO-OSSEOUS STRUCTURE, BLOOD VESSELS, AND NERVES

63. Ans. (d) Floor of Sinus *Ref: Orban's, 12th ed. p 433 & Wheeler's, 8th ed. p 386-387*

- Now students this common sense based question which nobody should miss out or get incorrect. The floor of maxillary sinus is closer to the maxillary posterior tooth.
- Hence when the carcinoma involves the floor, the mobility can be found in the maxillary posterior teeth.

THE TEMPOROMANDIBULAR JOINTS, MUSCLES, TEETH, AND THEIR FUNCTIONS

64. Ans. (c) Lateral and medial pterygoid muscles *Ref: Wheeler's, 8th ed. p 430*

- **To protrude the mandible without occlusal contact is achieved by contraction of lateral pterygoid.**
  - Medial pterygoid.
  - Masseter.
- **To protrude the mandible against resistance is achieved by contraction of:**
  - Lateral pterygoid.
  - Medial pterygoid.
  - Suprahyoid muscle.
- **To protrude the mandible with the teeth in occlusion is done by contraction of:**
  - Pterygoid muscle.
  - Masseter.
- **To protrude as well as to open the mouth, the muscle helps is:**
  - Medial pterygoid muscle.
  - Lateral pterygoid muscle.
  - Masseter muscle.
  - Temporalis muscle.

8 Oral Histology and Embryology

DEVELOPMENT AND GROWTH OF TEETH

1. Which deficiency affects tooth development? *(AIPG 2009)*
a. Vitamin A
b. Carbohydrates
c. Vitamin E
d. Vitamin B

2. The cells of the enamel organ which differentiate into future ameloblasts are: *(COMED 2013)*
a. Cells of inner enamel epithelium
b. Cells of outer enamel epithelium
c. Cells of stellate reticulum
d. Cells of stratum intermedium

3. In the open position of the mandible, the intercisal distance in males is approximately: *(COMED 2012)*
a. 28 mm b. 38 mm
c. 48 mm d. 58 mm

4. Which structure dictates the furcation formation in a tooth? *(COMED 2008)*
a. Enamel knot
b. Enamel niche
c. Hertwig's epithelial root sheath
d. Enamel cord

5. Morphological stages of tooth development are explained based on: *(COMED 2005)*
a. Shape of enamel organ
b. Shape of tooth germ
c. Functions of enamel organ
d. Shape of dental papilla

6. The first sign of tooth development in human being is seen around: *(KCET 2012, 2011)*
a. 12th week of intrauterine life
b. 6th week of intrauterine life
c. 6th week of life
d. At birth

7. The formation of hard tissue initiates in the: *(KCET 2005)*
a. Bud Stage
b. Cap Stage
c. Advanced Bell Stage
d. Early Bell Stage

ENAMEL

8. Maximum amount of phosphate is seen in: *(AIIMS Nov 2009)*
a. Enamel
b. Dentin
c. Cementum
d. Bone

9. Highest phosphate concentration in calcified and noncalcified tissues of oral cavity is found in: *(AIIMS Nov 2009)*
a. Bone
b. Dentin
c. Gingiva
d. Enamel

10. Deciduous teeth are differentiated from the permanent teeth by: *(AIIMS Nov 2006)*
a. Enamel prismatic arrangement
b. Dentinal tubule arrangement
c. Primary and secondary dentin
d. Mineral content

11. The final secretion of ameloblasts is: *(AIIMS Nov 2005)*
a. Enamel matrix
b. Enamel cuticle
c. Tomes layer
d. Enamel pellicle

12. The width of enamel over incisors is: *(AIIMS Nov 2005)*
a. 2 mm b. 2.5 mm
c. 2.3 mm d. 3 mm

13. **Enamel lamellae. True is:** *(AIIMS Nov 2013)*
   a. Enamel molecules uniformly arranged
   b. Enamel rod from enamel to dentin
   c. Dentinal tubules from dentin to enamel
   d. Outer elevation on enamel surface

14. **Water content in enamel:** *(AIIMS Nov 2013)*
   a. 2 to 3% b. 6 to 7%
   c. 10 to 12% d. 20 to 25%

15. **Phosphate ion concentration is maximum in:**
   a. Enamel b. Dentin *(AIPG 2010)*
   c. Cementum d. Bone

16. **What lines become prominent after carious process?** *(AIPG 2009)*
   a. Hunter Schreger bands
   b. Incremental lines of Retzius
   c. Incremental lines of Pickerill
   d. Incremental lines of Owen

17. **Least calcified structure is:** *(AIPG 2008)*
   a. Enamel lamella and gnarled enamel
   b. Enamel lamella and enamel prisms
   c. Enamel lamella and incremental lines
   d. Enamel lamella and perikymata

18. **What is the thickness of the layer of prismless enamel found in primary teeth?** *(AIPG 2005)*
   a. 25 mm b. 50 mm
   c. 75 mm d. 100 mm

19. **Striae of Retzius:** *(COMED 2011)*
   a. Are not found in permanent teeth
   b. Represent the daily growth rate of enamel
   c. Result from temporary constriction of Tomes process
   d. Has more number of crystals

20. **The maximum rate of eruption, as the tooth cusps reach the surface epithelium is around (Micrometers/day):** *(COMED 2011)*
   a. 100 b. 75
   c. 50 d. 25

21. **Which of this DOES NOT contain Collagen?** *(COMED 2009)*
   a. Enamel b. Dentin
   c. Bone d. Cementum

22. **The average width of enamel rods is:** *(COMED 2009)*
   a. 10 μm b. 5 μm
   c. 2 μm d. 0.5 μm

23. **The 'key hole' pattern appearance in the cross section is feature of:** *(COMED 2008)*
   a. Aprismatic enamel
   b. Prismatic enamel
   c. Intertubular dentin
   d. Intratubular dentin

24. **The shallow furrows on the enamel surface, where striae of Retzius end are known as:***(COMED 2008)*
   a. Cracks
   b. Pellicle
   c. Perikymata
   d. Enamel lamellae

25. **Tome's process is part of:** *(COMED 2008)*
   a. Radicular dentin b. Odontoblasts
   c. Ameloblasts d. Osteoblasts

26. **The class of low molecular weight calcium binding proteins seen predominantly in developing enamel are:** *(COMED 2007)*
   a. Enamelin b. Amelogenin
   c. Tuftelin d. Ameloplakin

27. **Gnarled enamel is seen in:** *(COMED 2006)*
   a. Proximal surface of tooth
   b. Cervical region of tooth
   c. Cusp tip of tooth
   d. All of the above

28. **Perikymata are believed to be the external manifestations of:** *(COMED 2005)*
   a. Diazones b. Striae of Retzius
   c. Parazones d. Prismless Enamel

29. **The cells of the enamel organ that are characterized by an exceptionally high activity of enzyme alkaline phosphatase:** *(KCET 2012)*
   a. Outer enamel epithelium
   b. Inner enamel epithelium
   c. Stratum intermedium
   d. Stellate reticulum

30. **Dark bands that are present in enamel rods at interval of 4 mm are:** *(KCET 2011)*
   a. Neonatal bands b. Cross striations
   c. Striae of retzius d. Hunter-Schreger bands

31. **This structure is created by the plane of section cutting through a curved lateral lamina so that the mesenchyme appears to be surrounded by the dental epithelium:** *(MH 2011)*
   a. Enamel niche b. Enamel cord
   c. Enamel knot d. Enamel sac

32. Nonamelogenin protein which is associated with enamel formation: *(MH 2011)*

a. Enamelin
b. Tuftelin
c. Steatherin
d. Sulfated glycoprotein

DENTIN

33. Greatest portion of the tooth is formed by: *(AIIMS Nov 2009)*

a. Dentin
b. Enamel
c. Cementum
d. Pulp

34. The type of dentine formed in slowly advancing enamel caries with rapid involvement of dentin is: *(AIIMS Nov 2009)*

a. Secondary
b. Sclerotic
c. Reparative
d. Tertiary

35. Which of the following is not true about the calcio-traumatic line? *(AIIMS Nov 2006)*

a. It represents the death of the primary odontoblastic cells
b. It remains even after the caries removal and reparative dentin formation
c. It is formed by active pluripotent stem cells that are transferred from the inner active layers
d. It is the developmental oblique line that is represented by alternate primary and secondary dentin formation

36. All of the following are true about the dentinal tubules *except*: *(AIIMS Nov 2006)*

a. Inner pulpal layer contains more dentinal tubules than the outer dentinal layer
b. The diameter of dentinal tubule ranges from 5 to 7 μm
c. The diameter of dentinal tubule is more at the pulpal layer than the outer layer
d. The bonding is more on the inner layer of dentin compared to the outer surface

37. The disturbances occurred during 'calcification' stage of tooth development are seen as: *(AIIMS May 2006)*

a. Peg lateral
b. Microdontia
c. Supernumerary tooth
d. Interglobular dentin

38. von Korff's fibers are present in: *(AIIMS Nov 2005)*

a. Circumpulpal dentin
b. Mantle dentin
c. Peritubular dentin
d. Interglobular dentin

39. True about Tome's fibers: *(AIIMS Nov 2013)*

a. Cytoplasmic extensions of dentinal tubules
b. Periodontal fibers extendng into root dentine
c. Collagen fibers in dentine
d. Periodontal fibers ending into root cementum

40. Lost odontoblast is replaced from mesenchymal cell within: *(AIPG 2010)*

a. 15 days
b. 1 month
c. 1 week
d. 46 week

41. In recent caries, one can mistake a radiolucent line below the DEJ for: *(AIPG 2008)*

a. Hunter-Schreger bands
b. Lines of Retzius
c. Tomes granular layer
d. Mach bands

42. The most widely accepted theory for dentinal hypersensitivity is: *(AIPG 2008)*

a. Hydrodynamic
b. Neural
c. Viscoelastic
d. Odontoblastic conduction

43. The average diameter of coronal dentinal tubules near the pulp is: *(AIPG 2005)*

a. 0.2–0.5 μm
b. 2–3 μm
c. 0.2–0.3 μm
d. 4–7 μm

44. One of the following statements is unique about circumpulpal dentin: *(COMED 2011)*

a. Collagen fibers are oriented perpendicular to DEJ
b. von Korff fibers are present
c. Contain phosphophoryn
d. Requires matrix vesicle for mineralization

45. Matrix vesicles: *(COMED 2009)*

a. Are found in mantle dentin
b. Contain collagen
c. Produce alkaline phosphatase
d. Inhibit mineralization

46. In adult tooth, the type of dentin present underlying dentin enamel junction is: *(COMED 2008)*

a. Predentin
b. Mantle dentin
c. Interglobular dentin
d. Tertiary dentin

47. What line is formed when primary curvatures of dentinal tubules meet? *(COMED 2005)*
a. Schreger line
b. Contour line of Owen
c. von Ebner's line
d. Imbrication lines of Pickerel

48. The inner organic lining of the calcified dentinal tubule is called: *(KCET 2012)*
a. Lamina lucida b. Lamina limitans
c. Lamina densa d. Lamina dura

49. In reflected light, dead tracts are seen as: *(KCET 2011)*
a. White zones
b. Black zones
c. Purple zones
d. A combination of white & black zones

50. The term 'dead tract' in dentin was coined by: *(KCET 2009)*
a. Robinson b. Silverman
c. Sir Wilfred fish d. Silverstone

51. Which of the following types of dentin is continuously produced throughout the life? *(MH 2012)*
a. Interglobular dentin
b. Intertubular dentin
c. Intratubular dentin
d. Mantle dentin

PULP

52. Histologically, the dental pulp most closely resembles what type of tissue? *(AIIMS Nov 2010, 2008)*
a. Nerve tissue
b. Vascular tissue
c. Granulation tissue
d. Loose connective tissue

53. Nerve supply in pulp is: *(AIIMS May 2013)*
a. Sympathetic and afferent postganglionic
b. Parasympathetic postganglionic
c. Motor sympathetic and autonomic
d. Motor only

54. Which of the following statements regarding pulp stones are true? *(COMED 2012)*
a. Pulp stones are due to metastatic calcification
b. Pulp stones are due to dystrophic calcification
c. Pulp stones are usually of true denticles type
d. Pulp stones are usually embedded in dentine

55. Characteristic thistle tube shaped appearance of pulp chambers of single rooted teeth are seen in: *(COMED 2012)*
a. Type I dentinogenesis imperfecta
b. Type II dentinogenesis imperfecta
c. Type II dentine dysplasia
d. Type I dentine dysplasia

56. The subodontoblastic plexus of Rashkow occupies: *(COMED 2010)*
a. Cell free zone of weil
b. Odontoblastic zone
c. Cell rich zone
d. Core of the pulp

57. Pulp responds to all stimuli by pain because it has only: *(COMED 2009)*
a. Free nerve endings
b. Krause end bulbs
c. Pacinian corpuscle
d. Ruffians corpuscle

58. Cells occurring in greater number in pulp are: *(COMED 2008, 2014)*
a. Cementoblasts b. Fibroblasts
c. Osteoblasts d. Ameloblasts

59. The diameter of the largest arterial vessels in the pulp range from: *(COMED 2007)*
a. 50 to 100 micrometer
b. 101 to 150 micrometer
c. 151 to 200 micrometer
d. 201 to 250 micrometer

60. The 'Plexus of Rachkow' is present in which of the following zones in pulp? *(COMED 2005)*
a. Cell free zone
b. Cell rich zone
c. Odontoblastic zone
d. Pulp core

61. Sharp momentary pain elicited by pulp is caused by: *(KCET 2005)*
a. A delta fibers b. C Fibers
c. A alpha fibers d. None of the above

62. Cell rich zone of the pulp is named after: *(MH 2011)*
a. Weil
b. Hohl
c. Miller
d. Fitzgerald

CEMENTUM

63. Less calcified among the type of cementum is: *(AIIMS May 2010, AIPG 2010)*
a. Cellular cementum
b. Acellular cementum
c. Cementoid
d. Incremental line

64. Inorganic content of cementum is: *(COMED 2012, 2008)*
a. 45% to 50%
b. 50% to 55%
c. 55% to 60%
d. 60% to 65%

65. Which is the most common type of cementoenamel junction seen in the teeth? *(COMED 2010)*
a. Edge to edge or butt joint type
b. Gap type
c. Cementum overlapping enamel
d. Enamel overlapping cementum

66. Cellular cementum is: *(COMED 2010)*
a. First formed cementum
b. Less calcified than acellular type
c. More calcified than acellular type
d. Less irregular

67. Collagen fibrils have a transverse striation with a characteristic periodicity of: *(COMED 2009)*
a. 64 cm
b. 64 nm (640 Å)
c. 640 μm (64000 Å)
d. 640 nm (6400 Å)

68. Fusion of cementum and alveolar bone with the obliteration of periodontal ligament is called: *(KCET 2012)*
a. Avulsion
b. Extrusion
c. Ankylosis
d. Luxation

69. Intermediate cementum is: *(KCET 2010)*
a. Highly defined cellular zone near cementodentinal junction
b. Highly defined fibrillar zone near cementodentinal junction
c. Poorly defined zone near cementodentinal junction
d. Both a and b

70. Cementum and enamel meet edge to edge in percentage of cases: *(KCET 2010)*
a. 5–10 percent
b. 30 percent
c. 60–65 percent
d. 100 percent

PERIODONTAL LIGAMENT

71. The type of collagen found in principle fibres is: *(AIIMS Nov 2007)*
a. Type I
b. Type II
c. Type III
d. Type IV

72. The fibres attached to adjacent teeth are: *(AIPG 2011)*
a. Transseptal
b. Apical
c. Oblique
d. Horizontal

73. Apical PDL fibres arise from: *(AIPG 2008)*
a. The crest of alveolar bone
b. The apical end of root
c. The middle third of root
d. Junctional epithelium

74. Epithelial cell rests of Malassez are seen in: *(COMED 2009)*
a. Enamel
b. Cementum
c. Alveolar bone
d. Periodontal ligament

75. Cementicles are calcified masses sometimes seen in the: *(COMED 2008)*
a. Pulp
b. Bone
c. Periodontal ligament
d. Cementum

76. With age, the elastic fiber content of periodontal ligament: *(COMED 2007)*
a. Remains the same
b. Increases
c. Decreases
d. Either increases or decreases

77. Elaunin fibers are found in: *(COMED 2007)*
a. Gingiva
b. Cementum
c. Alveolar bone
d. PDL

78. Cell rests of Malassez are found in: *(COMED 2006)*
a. Enamel
b. Dentin
c. Pulp
d. PDL

BONE

79. Which is the predominant factor in the formation of the alveolar process? *(AIPG 2005)*
a. Eruption of teeth
b. Normal process of growth
c. Lengthening of the condyle
d. Overall growth of the bodies of the maxilla and the mandible

80. The cortical plates are thickest in the: *(COMED 2012)*
a. Premolar and molar region of the maxilla on the buccal side
b. Premolar and molar region of the maxilla on the lingual side
c. Premolar and molar region of the mandible on the lingual side
d. Premolar and molar region of the mandible on the buccal side

81. Interdependency of osteoblasts and osteoclasts in bone remodeling is called as: *(COMED 2009)*
a. Lacunae
b. Coupling
c. Reversal lines
d. Canaliculi

82. Canals of Zuckerkandl and Hirschfeld are seen in: *(COMED 2009)*
a. Spongy bone
b. Cribriform plate of alveolar bone
c. Interdental and interradicular septa of alveolar bone
d. Cortical plates of alveolar bone

83. Bundle bone is a part of: *(COMED 2009)*
a. Periodontal ligament
b. Alveolar bone
c. Cementum
d. Long bones

84. When osteoblasts lay new bone from outside to inside in an osteon, the active formation area is called: *(COMED 2007)*
a. Haversian cone
b. Filling cone
c. Cutting cone
d. Howship's cone

85. Basic metabolic unit of bone is: *(COMED 2006)*
a. Osteon b. Osteoblast
c. Osteocyte d. Osteoclast

86. Which of the following influence the ability of osteoclast to resorb bone matrix? *(KCET 2010)*
a. Cathepsin K and carbonic anhydrase
b. Alkaline phosphatase
c. Both a and b
d. Matrix metalloproteinase

87. Fatty/Yellow bone marrow is seen in: *(MH 2009)*
a. Alveolar bone
b. Maxillary tuberosity
c. Condyle
d. Angle of mandible

ORAL MUCOUS MEMBRANE

88. Which of the following does not contain taste buds? *(AIIMS Nov 2011)*
a. Circumvallate papillae
b. Filiform papillae
c. Fungiform papillae
d. Foliate papillae

89. Least sensitive to pain: *(AIIMS Nov 2011, AIPG 2012)*
a. Buccal mucosa b. Gingiva
c. Lip d. Labial mucosa

90. In which part of oral cavity mucous membrane is the thinnest? *(AIPG 2005)*
a. Soft palate
b. Labial mucosa
c. Floor of mouth
d. Buccal mucosa

91. The cell type of periodontium that plays a role in pathogenesis as well as healing is: *(COMED 2011)*
a. Epithelial
b. Langerhans
c. Fibroblast
d. Mast cell

92. Membrane coating granules may: *(COMED 2010)*
a. Appear as circular with an amorphous core in keratinized epithelium
b. Originate from Golgi system
c. Packed with tonofilaments
d. Helps in adhesion of fully keratinized epithelial cells

93. Keratohyalin granules are seen in: *(COMED 2009)*
a. Stratum basale
b. Stratum spinosum
c. Stratum corneum
d. Stratum granulosum

94. Buccal Mucosa is: *(COMED 2009)*
a. Keratinized
b. Nonkeratinized
c. Parakeratinised
d. Orthokeratinised

95. Granules seen in the stratum granulosum of keratinized oral mucosa are known as: *(COMED 2007)*
a. Keratohyalin granules
b. Zymogen granules
c. Membrane coating granules
d. Birbeck granules

96. In which of the following the mucosa is keratinized? *(COMED 2005)*
a. Hard palate
b. Buccal mucosa
c. Labial mucosa
d. Soft palate

97. Which of the following are non keratinocytes? *(COMED 2005)*
a. Langhans cells
b. Red blood cells
c. Langerhans cells
d. Grey cells

98. Glands of Blandin and Nuhn are the: *(COMED 2005)*
a. Palatine glands in the posterolateral region of hard palate
b. Anterior lingual glands located near the apex of the tongue
c. Labial and buccal glands
d. Glossopalatine glands

99. Merkel cells are found in which of the following tissue? *(KCET 2011)*
a. Epidermis
b. Papillary layer of dermis
c. Reticular layer of dermis
d. Hypodermis

100. The functions of myoepithelial cells may be: *(KCET 2010)*
a. Initiating contraction
b. Support for the end piece during active secretion of saliva
c. Provide signals to the acinar secretory cells for structural organization
d. All of the above

101. Progenitor cells of oral epithelium lies in: *(MH 2012)*
a. Basal layer
b. Spinous layer
c. Granular layer
d. Cornified layer

102. All of the following are nonkeratinocytes *except*: *(MH 2012)*
a. Merkel's cells
b. Langerhans cell
c. Melanocytes
d. Macrophage

103. Myoepithelial cells are present in: *(MH 2010)*
a. Secretory ducts
b. Intercalated ducts
c. Intermediate ducts
d. Secretory and intercalated ducts

104. Most active in protein synthesis: *(MH 2009)*
a. Basal cells
b. Prickle cells
c. Granular cells
d. Melanocytes

SALIVARY GLANDS

105. Tuft cells are receptors seen on: *(AIIMS Nov 2011)*
a. TMJ
b. Lining of max sinus
c. Cell rich zone
d. Excretory duct of salivary gland

106. The glands of Von Ebner empty into a deep groove running around: *(COMED 2009)*
a. Foliate papilla
b. Circumvallate papilla
c. Filiform papilla
d. Fungiform papilla

107. Which papillae are completely keratinized? *(COMED 2009)*
a. Fungiform
b. Filiform
c. Circumvallate
d. Foliate

108. Where do we see 'Actin' and 'Myosin'? *(COMED 2005)*

a. Serous cells
b. Mucous cells
c. Myoepithelial cells
d. Demilunes

109. "Von Ebner" salivary glands are serous glands present in association with: *(KCET 2012, 2011)*

a. Filiform papilla
b. Circumvallate papilla
c. Foliate papilla
d. Fungiform papilla

110. Stratification specific keratins present in gingival epithelium are: *(KCET 2010)*

a. K1, K2 b. K10, K12
c. K16, K6 d. K5, K14

111. The higher level clear cell present in the oral epithelium: *(KCET 2009)*

a. Melanocyte
b. Lymphocyte
c. Merkel cells
d. Langerhans cells

112. Salivary glands are absent in which part of the palate? *(MH 2011)*

a. Anterior part of the hard palate
b. Posterior part of the hard palate
c. Soft palate
d. Uvula

GINGIVA

113. Width of attached gingiva is least in:

a. Maxillary central incisor *(AIIMS May 2006)*
b. Maxillary 1st premolar
c. Mandibular 1st premolar
d. Mandibular central incisor

114. Dendritic cells located in basal and supraspinous layer are: *(AIPG 2010)*

a. Basket cells b. Melanocytes
c. Keratinocytes d. Merkel cells

115. The gingiva covering the hard palate is: *(KCET 2013)*

a. Masticatory mucosa
c. Lining mucosa
b. Specialized mucosa
d. All of the above

116. Junctional epithelium is: *(KCET 2008)*

a. Keratinized
b. Nonkeratinized
c. Hyperkeratinized
d. Parakeratinized

SHEDDING OF THE DECIDUOUS TEETH

117. In a dried skull, holes on the lingual aspects of the deciduous teeth are called: *(COMED 2011, 2009)*

a. Volkmann canals
b. Canals of Hirschfel and Zuckerkandl
c. Haversian canals
d. Gubernacular canals

TEMPOROMANDIBULAR JOINT

118. Nerve endings of temporomandibular joint, confined to ligaments associated with the joint: *(COMED 2011)*

a. Ruffini corpuscles
b. Pacini corpuscles
c. Golgi tendon organs
d. Free nerve endings

119. The initial B cells of synovial membrane of temporomandibular joint are: *(COMED 2011)*

a. Fibroblast like
b. Macrophage like
c. Lymphocyte like
d. Plasma like

HISTOCHEMISTRY OF ORAL TISSUE

120. Osteoclasts show an intensive activity of which of the following enzymes? *(COMED 2007)*

a. Alkaline phosphatase
b. Acid phosphatase
c. Esterase
d. Carbonic anhydrase

MISCELLANEOUS

121. The type of collagen present in hyaline cartilage is: *(AIPG 2008)*

a. Type I
b. Type II
c. Type III
d. Type IV

122. In which part of oral cavity mucous membrane is the thinnest? *(AIPG 2005)*
a. Soft palate
b. Labial mucosa
c. Floor of mouth
d. Buccal mucosa

123. Pigmentation of the permanent teeth may develop if tetracyclines are given between the ages of: *(COMED 2013)*
a. 5 and 7 years
b. 0.2 and 5 years
c. 6 and 10 years
d. 10 and 12 years

124. Fiber group which prevent the extrusion of the tooth is: *(COMED 2012)*
a. Alveolar crest group
b. Transseptal group
c. Oblique group
d. Horizontal group

125. Lymph from the teeth drains into all of the following nodes *except*: *(COMED 2012)*
a. Sub mandibular nodes
b. Retropharyngeal nodes
c. Deep cervical nodes
d. Sub mental nodes

126. Human beings are: *(COMED 2008)*
a. Monophyodonts
b. Polyphyodonts
c. Homodonts
d. Diphyodonts

127. Which type of collagen fibers demonstrate 'chicken wire' configuration? *(COMED 2007)*
a. Type I
b. Type II
c. Type III
d. Type IV

128. Which of the following is expected when the tooth is lost? *(KCET 2013)*
a. Decrease in trabecular pattern
b. Loss of bone width
c. Loss of bone height
d. All of the above

129. Which of the portions of the intra articular disc is the thinnest? *(KCET 2013)*
a. Anterior
b. Intermediate
c. Posterior
d. Retrodiscal

130. Mandibular foramen is situated at the: *(KCET 2013)*
a. Lower level than the occlusal plane of the primary teeth
b. Higher level than the occlusal plane of the primary teeth
c. At the level of the occlusal plane
d. At the level of the buccal vestibule

131. Facial occlusal line in the maxillary arch is formed by: *(KCET 2012)*
a. Stamp cusps
b. Centric holding cusps
c. Supporting cusps
d. Non-supporting cusps

132. Dental DNA is only: *(MH 2009)*
a. Obtained from the odontoblasts
b. Obtained from cells of pulp
c. Identification of individuals is not only use
d. All of the above

Answers with Explanations

DEVELOPMENT AND GROWTH OF TEETH

1. Ans. (a) Vitamin A *Ref: Orban's, 12th ed. p 50*

- During vitamin A deficiency, the ameloblast fail to differentiate properly.
- If the vitamin A deficiency is severe, ameloblast cells will become completely atrophied, resulting in an absence of enamel formation.

2. Ans. (a) Cells of inner enamel epithelium *Ref: Orban's, 12th ed. p 28-29*

Inner enamel epithelium

- The inner enamel epithelium consists of a single layer of cells that differentiate prior to amelogenesis into tall columnar cells called ameloblasts.
- The cells of the inner enamel epithelium exert an organizing influence on the underlying mesenchymal cells in the dental papilla, which later differentiate into odontoblasts.
- **Stratum intermedium** a few layers of squamous cells from the stratum intermedium, between the inner enamel epithelium and the stellate reticulum.
- This layer seems to be essential to enamel formation.
- It is absent in the part of the tooth germ that outlines the root portions of the tooth which does not form enamel.

Stellate reticulum

- The stellate reticulum expands due to increase in the amount of intercellular fluid. The cells are star shaped, with long processes.

Outer enamel epithelium

- The cells of the outer enamel epithelium flatten to a low cuboidal form.

3. Ans. (c) 48 mm *Ref: Orban's, 12th ed. p 34*

- Normally in the open position of the mandible, the interincisal distance in males and females is approximately 48 mm and 45.5 mm respectively.
- When the mouth is opened unusually wide during yawning, the head of the mandible may slip forward into the infratemporal fossa causing articular dislocation of the joint.

4. Ans. (c) Hertwig's epithelial root sheath *Ref: Orban's, 12th ed. p 138-140*

- There is pronounced difference in development of Hertwig's epithelial root sheath in teeth with one root and in those with more roots.
- Prior to beginning of root formation Hertwig's epithelial root sheath forms a diaphragm by proliferation of inner and outer enamel cells dictated by sheath forms furcation; therefore, accordingly number of roots are formed.

5. Ans. (a) Shape of enamel organ *Ref: Orban's, 12th ed. p 24*

- Tooth development or odontogenesis is the complex process by which teeth form from embryonic cells, grow and erupt into the mouth.
- The tooth germ is an aggregation of cells that eventually forms a tooth.
- These cells are derived from the ectoderm of the first branchial arch and the ectomesenchyme of the neural crest.
- Development of tooth is a continuous process and the Morphological stages of tooth development are explained based on Shape of enamel organ (epithelial part of tooth germ)

- Morphological stages of tooth development are:
  - Bud stage
  - Cap stage
  - Bell stage

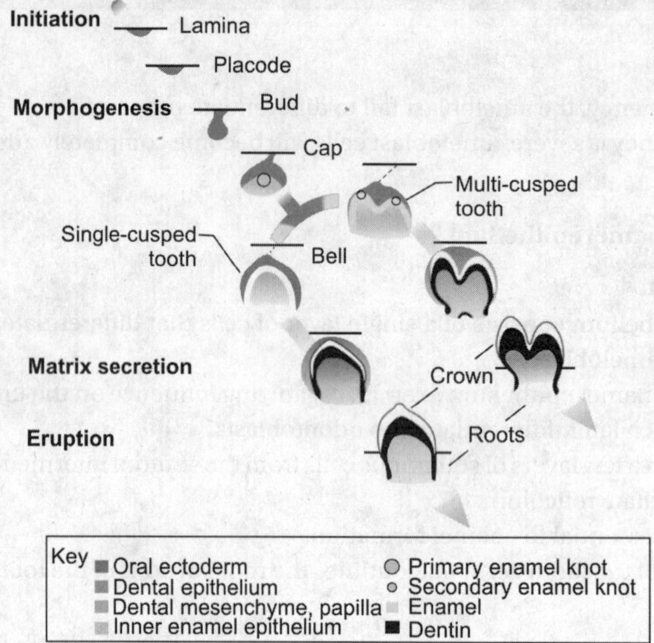

6. Ans. (b) 6th week of intrauterine life *Ref: Orban's, 12th ed. p 46*

- Tooth development begins in the 6th week I.U as a U-shaped thickening of the oral epithelium. These structures, called dental laminae, are placed along the length of the upper and lower jaw. Dental laminae soon give rise to the ten proliferation centers called tooth buds which penetrate into underlying mesenchyme. Tooth buds soon develop a cup-shaped enamel organ due to the invagination of the mesenchyme condensation called the dental papilla.
- Evidence of development of the human tooth can be observed as early as the sixth week of embryonic life.
- The first macroscopic indication of morphologic development occurs at approximately 11 weeks in utero.

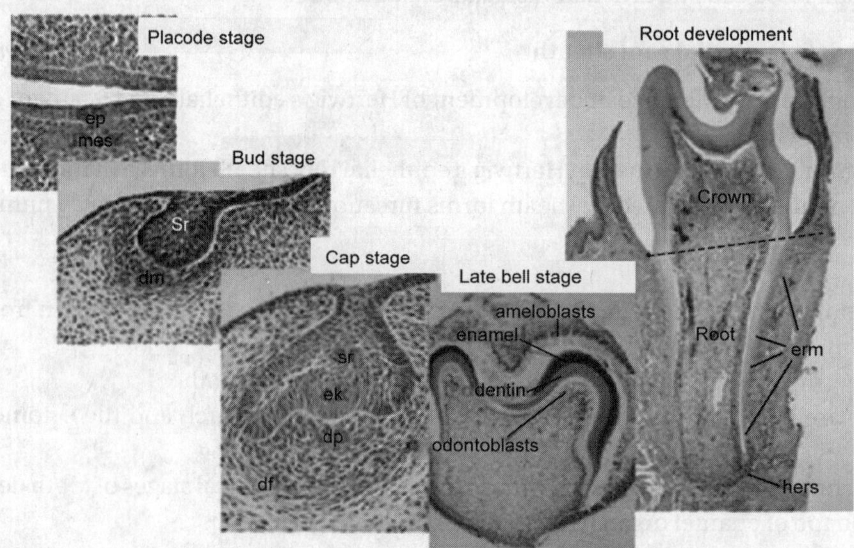

7. Ans. (d) Early Bell Stage *Ref: Orban's 12th ed. p 28*

Advanced bell stage

- Hard tissues, including enamel and dentin, develop during the next stage of tooth development. This stage is called the crown, or maturation stage by some researchers. Important cellular changes occur at this time. In prior stages, all of the IEE cells were dividing to increase the overall size of the tooth bud, but rapid dividing, called mitosis, stops during the crown stage at the location where the cusps of the teeth form. The first mineralized hard tissues form at this location. At the same time, the IEE cells change in shape from cuboidal to columnar and become preameloblasts. The nuclei of these cells move closer to the stratum intermedium and away from the dental papilla as they become polarized
- After dentin formation begins, the cells of the IEE secrete an organic matrix against the dentin. This matrix immediately mineralizes and becomes the initial layer of the tooth's enamel. Outside the dentin are the newly formed ameloblasts in response to the formation of dentin, which are cells that continue the process of enamel formation; therefore, enamel formation moves outwards, adding new material to the outer surface of the developing tooth.

You must remember the following:

- Hard tissue formation starts at the late stages of the bell stage
- Differentiation of cells into odontoblasts and ameloblasts
- Dentin is formed before enamel
- Dentin initiates the formation of enamel

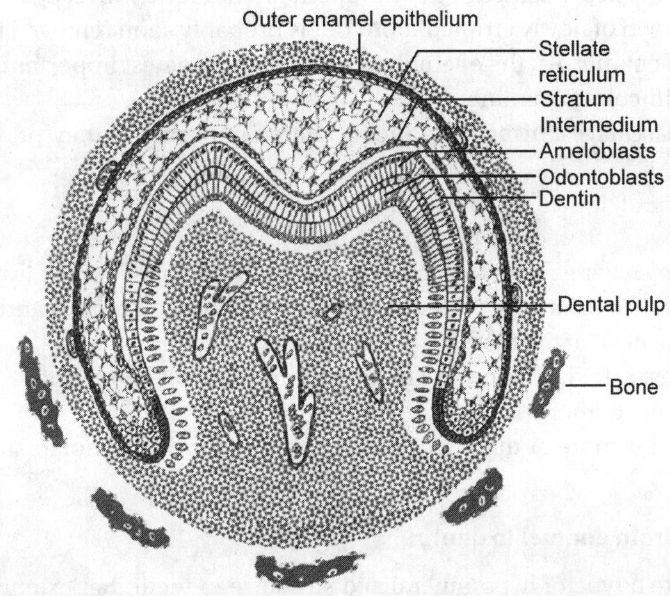

ENAMEL

8. Ans. (a) Enamel *Ref: Orban's, 12th ed. p 50, 107, 180*

- Tooth enamel is one of the four major tissues that make up the tooth in humans.
- It is the hardest substance in the human body and contains the highest percentage of minerals, 96% with water and organic material composing the rest.
- The primary mineral is hydroxyapatite, which is a crystalline calcium phosphate.
- Enamel does not contain collagen, as found in other hard tissues such as dentin and bone, but it does contain two unique classes of proteins—amelogenins and enamelins.
- Enamel is avascular and has no nerve supply within it.

Remember:
- Highest phosphate concentration: Enamel
- Highest carbonate concentration: Bone
- Highest magnesium concentration: Dentin
- Highest fluorine concentration: Cementum

9. Ans. (d) Enamel

Refer Ans. 8

10. Ans. (a) Enamel prismatic arrangement *Ref: Orban's, 12th ed. p 50*

- The deciduous teeth are differentiated from permanent teeth by enamel prismatic arrangement.
- Due to this, enamel rods causes a change in the refractive index of the enamel, thereby altering the overall brightness of the tooth.
- Aprismatic layer in permanent enamel is approximately four times thinner than that deciduous enamel.
- This layer, present on the outermost surface, shows increased mineralization (increased inorganic content) owing to thicker outer layer in deciduous teeth.
- This layer brings more opaqueness or whiteness to the deciduous teeth as compared to the permanent teeth.

11. Ans. (b) Enamel cuticle *Ref: Orban's, 12th ed. p 54*

- Delicate membrane called Nasmyth's membrane named after its investigator or the primary enamel cuticle covers the entire crown of newly erupted tooth but is probably soon removed by mastication.
- The surface layer of enamel, i.e. the enamel cuticle is of the greatest importance in the initial caries attack.
- Enamel cuticle is difficult to examine.
- When the ameloblast have finished producing the enamel prism, they produce a thin continuous layer of enamel cuticle.

12. Ans. (a) 2 mm *Ref: Orban's, 12th ed. p 46*

- A protective covering having variable thickness covers the crown of a tooth is termed as enamel.
- Thickness of enamel 2 to 2.5 mm is present on the cusps of human molars and premolars.
- It is knife edge at the neck of the tooth.
- Enamel is the hardest calcified tissue due to its high mineral salt in our body.
- The specific gravity of enamel is 2.8.
- Thickness of enamel is more at the lingual surface of the maxillary molars and buccal surface of mandibular molars.

13. Ans. (b) Enamel rod from enamel to dentin *Ref: Orban's, 12th ed. p 54*

- Enamel lamellae are a type of hypomineralized structure in teeth that extend either from the dentinoenamel junction (DEJ) to the surface of the enamel, or vice versa.
- It is a thin leaf like structure.
- Enamel lamella sometimes may extend to or penetrate into the dentin.
- In essence, they are prominent linear enamel defects but are of no clinical consequence.
- These structures contain proteins, proteoglycans, and lipids.

14. Ans. (a) 2 to 3% *Ref: Orban's, 12th ed. p 46*

Composition of Enamel:
- Enamel consists of approximately 96% of inorganic material and 4% of organic material by weight.
- It consists of approximately 12% of inorganic material and 88% of organic material and water by volume.
- Organic material forms the matrix while inorganic comprises of various minerals.

Tissue	*Inorganic*	*Organic*
Enamel	96%	4%
Dentin	70%	30%
Cementum	45 to 50%	50 to 55%

15. Ans. (a) Enamel *Ref: Orban's, 12th ed. p 50, 107, 180*

- It is the hardest substance in the human body and contains the highest percentage of minerals, 96%, with water and organic material composing the rest.
- The primary mineral is hydroxyapatite, which is a crystalline calcium phosphate.
- Enamel is formed on the tooth while the tooth is developing within the gum, before it erupts into the mouth.
- Once fully formed, it does not contain blood vessels or nerves.
- Remineralization of teeth can repair damage to the tooth to a certain degree but damage beyond that cannot be repaired by the body.
- The maintenance and repair of human tooth enamel is one of the primary concerns of dentistry.

16. Ans. (b) Incremental lines of Retzius *Ref: Orban's, 12th ed. p 51*

- Striae of Retzius are incremental lines that appear brown in a stained section of mature enamel.
- These lines are composed of bands or cross striations on the enamel rods that, when combined in longitudinal sections, seem to transverse the enamel rods.
- Formed from changes in diameter of Tomes' processes, these incremental lines demonstrate the growth of enamel, similar to the annual rings on a tree on transverse sections of enamel.
- Incremental lines of Retzius become more prominent during abnormal condition such as carious process.
- Mean daily rate of enamel formation is about 3.5 microns. It increases inner to outer enamel and decreases from incisal/cuspal region to cervical enamel.

17. Ans. (c) Enamel lamella and incremental lines *Ref: Orban's, 12th ed. p 51 56*

Mineralized structures of enamel:

- Enamel rods (enamel prisms)
- Structureless enamel
- Perikymata lines
- Gnarled enamel

Hypomineralized structures of enamel:

- Enamel spindle
- Hunter-Schreger bands
- Incremental lines of retzius
- Enamel tufts
- Enamel lamellae
- Neonatal lines

18. Ans. (a) 25 mm *Ref: Orban's, 12th ed. p 51*

- The prismless enamel is the structureless enamel present as a surface layer of enamel.
- It is 30 µm thick in permanent as well as deciduous tooth.
- The thickness of prismless enamel in different areas of the same tooth is variable.
- There are significant differences in the micromorphological appearance of prismless enamel between the primary and permanent teeth.
- A laminated band is found in primary prismless enamel whereas a scale like shape is observed in permanent teeth.

19. Ans. (b) Represent the daily growth rate of enamel *Ref: Tencate's, 7th ed. p 192 and Orban's, 12th ed. p 60-61*

- Striae of Retzius is found in permanent teeth, so option a is ruled out.
- It is either hypomineralized or hypermineralized.
- It is definitely not due to temporary constriction of tomes process.
- Now Tencate says it due to the weekly rhythm of enamel deposition and Orbans says is the rhythmic apposition of enamel during its formation.
- Although the word 'daily' is not mentioned in either of the two texts still option 2 seems to be nearly correct. Hence the answer.

20. Ans. (b) 75 *Ref: Orban's, 12th ed. p 98*

- Intraosseous eruption occurs at 1-10 µm/day.
- Later it can increase to a maximum of 75 µm/day.

21. Ans. (a) Enamel *Ref: Orban's, 12th ed. p 46*

- The enamel consists mainly of inorganic material (96%) and only a small amount of organic substance and water.
- Chemical analyses of matrix of mature enamel indicate that the amino acid composition is not closely related to keratin and different from collagen, they generally contain high percentage of serine, glutamic acid and glycine.

22. Ans. (b) 5 µm *Ref: Orban's, 12th ed. p 46*

Enamel rods measurements are:

Length - 9 µm [Remember LBD-954]
Breadth - 5 µm
Diameter - 4 µm

23. Ans. (b) Prismatic enamel *Ref: Orban's, 12th ed. p 47*

- Many areas of human enamel seem to contain rods surrounded by rod sheaths and separated by interrod substance a more common pattern is a keyhole- or paddle-shaped prism in human enamel.

24. Ans. (c) Perikymata *Ref: Orban's, 12th ed. p 52*

Perikymata are transverse, wavelike grooves, believed to be the external manifestations of the striae of Retzius. They are continuous around a tooth and usually lie parallel to each other and to the cementoenamel junction.

25. Ans. (c) Ameloblasts *Ref: Orban's, 12th ed. p 69*

The surfaces of the ameloblasts facing the developing enamel are not smooth. There is an interdigitation of the cells and the enamel rods that they produce. This interdigitation is partly a result of the fact that the long axes of the ameloblasts are not parallel to the long axes of the rods. The projections of the ameloblasts into the enamel matrix have been named Tomes' processes.

26. Ans. (b) Amelogenin *Ref: Orban's, 12th ed. p 334*

- There are two types of protein found in enamel, i.e. amelogenins and non-amelogenins.

Amelogenins	*Non-amelogenins*
Low molecular weight protein	High molecular weight protein
Comprise 90% enamel protein	Only 10%
They are rich in proline, histidine, glutamine and leucine	They are rich in glycine, serine, and aspartic acid

Amelogenins:

- It is the major component of enamel matrix protein.
- Amelogenins and enamelins are the two major classes and calcium binding proteins.
- Accumulate during the secretary stage of amelogenesis.

27. Ans. (c) Cusp tip of tooth *Ref: Orban's, 12th ed. p 50*

- Bundles of enamel rods appear to intertwine in a highly irregular manner in the cusp region of teeth to form gnarled enamel.
- Gnarled enamel are thought to give extra strength to enamel.
- This is especially needed for functional cusp tips.
- It is less likely that enamel would fracture at the cusp tips due to their gnarled enamel.
- These are the clinical significance of gnarled enamel.

28. Ans. (b) Striae of Retzius *Ref: Orban's, 12th ed. p 52*

- Perikymata, enamel surface manifestations of internal structures are known as Striae of Retzius.
- These structures, external and internal, are thought to be deposited in a time ordered sequence and to provide an indication of the time frame of development of lateral or cervical enamel.
- These are transverse, wave like grooves, parallel to one another as well as CEJ.
- Number of perikymata near the CEJ is 30 per mm which is reduced to 10 per mm at the region of incisal or occlusal edge.

29. Ans. (c) Stratum intermedium *Ref: Orban's, 12th ed. p 394*

- The stratum intermedium in a developing tooth is a layer of two or three cells between the inner enamel epithelium and the newly forming cells of the stellate reticulum. It first appears during the early bell stage of tooth development, at around the 14th week of intrauterine life. The stratum intermedium has a notably high alkaline phosphatase activity. This layer, along with the inner enamel epithelium, is responsible for the tooth enamel formation. ANS-39. Actinomycosis
- A chronic suppurative and granulomatous disease of the cervico-facial, thoracic or abdominal areas
- Caused by gram positive, non-motile, non-sporing, non-capsulated, anaerobic actinomyces.
- Actinomyces bacteria are generally sensitive to penicillin, which is frequently used to treat actinomycosis. In cases of penicillin allergy, doxycycline is used.

30. Ans. (b) Cross striations *Ref: Orban's, 12th ed. p 57*

- Each enamel rod is made up of segments separated by dark lines that give it a striated appearance.
- Becomes more visible on application of mild acids
- More pronounced in insufficiently calcified enamel
- Rods are segmented because matrix is formed in a rhythmic manner. The rods exhibits cross-striations with periodicity of 4 μm, representing the amount of enamel deposited daily during odontogenesis.

31. Ans. (a) Enamel niche *Ref: Tencate's, 7th ed. p 90, 91*

- The enamel niche is a structure that appears in a histologic slide of a developing tooth from sectioning the slide in a single plane.
- The enamel organ looks to be connected to the oral epithelium by two or more strands of dental lamina.
- The enamel niche is the name of the mesenchymal cells which look to be surrounded by the strands of the dental lamina.
- In actuality, there is no mesenchyme completely surrounded by dental lamina. These cases are a result from the dental lamina being a curved structure while the slide contains tissue taken in one plane.

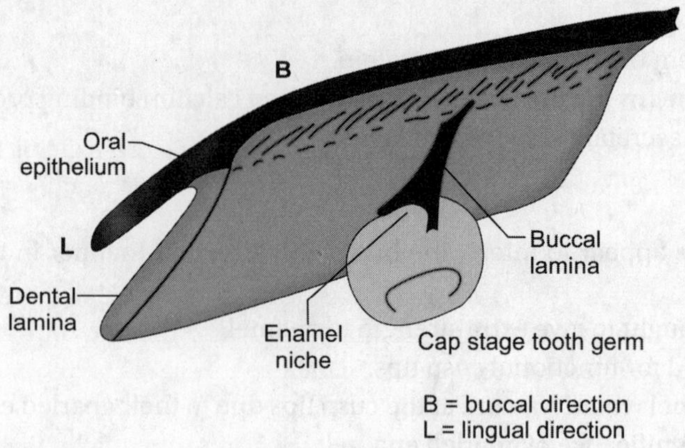

32. Ans. (a) Enamelin *Ref: Tencate's, 7th ed. p 175*

- Enamelin is a protein in humans that is encoded by the ENAM gene. Dental enamel is a highly mineralized tissue with 85% of its volume occupied by unusually large, highly organized, hydroxyapatite crystals.
- This highly organized and unusual structure is thought to be rigorously controlled in ameloblasts through the interaction of a number of organic matrix molecules that include enamelin, amelogenin (AMELX; MIM 300391), ameloblastin (AMBN; MIM 601259), tuftelin (TUFT1; MIM 600087), dentin sialophosphoprotein (DSPP; MIM 125485), and a variety of enzymes.
- Enamelin is the largest protein in the enamel matrix of developing teeth and comprises approximately 5% of total enamel matrix protein.
- Mutations in the ENAM gene can give rise to autosomal dominant Amelogenesis imperfecta, indicating a role in Amelogenesis.

Also know about Proteins of Enamel:

- Mature proteins
- Immature protein
- **Enamelins (Nonamelogenin/Anionic)**
- Ameloblastin
- Tuftelin
- Proteinases
- Sulfated
- Derived
- **Amelogenin**
- Multiple alternatively spliced proteins.

DENTIN

33. Ans. (a) Dentin *Ref: Orban's, 12th ed. p 84*

- Dentin is the main portion or body of the tooth.
- It provides the bulk as well as general form of the tooth.
- Dentin is wrapped in an envelope of enamel which cover the crown and an envelop of cementum, which covers the root.
- Dentin is a hard, dense, calcified tissue.
- Its chemical composition is:
  - Inorganic—70%.
  - Organic and water—30%.

34. Ans. (b) Sclerotic *Ref: Orban's, 12th ed. p 99*

Tertiary dentin or Sclerotic dentin

- Tertiary dentin is dentin formed as a reaction to external stimulation such as cavities.
- It is of two types, either reactionary, where dentin is formed from a pre-existing odontoblast, or reparative, where newly differentiated odontoblast-like cells are formed due to the death of the original odontoblasts, from a pulpal progenitor cell.
- Tertiary dentin is only formed by an odontoblast directly affected by a stimulus; therefore, the architecture and structure depend on the intensity and duration of the stimulus, e.g., if the stimulus is a carious lesion, there is extensive destruction of dentin and damage to the pulp, due to the differentiation of bacterial metabolites and toxins. Thus, tertiary dentin is deposited rapidly, with a sparse and irregular tubular pattern and some cellular inclusions; in this case it is referred to as 'osteodentin'
- The hardness of sclerotic dentin formed due to aging is harder than that of found below carious lesions.

35. Ans. (d) It is the developmental oblique line that is represented by alternate primary and secondary dentin formation *Ref: Shafer's, 6th ed. p 519*

Calcitraumatic Line

- It forms in response to recent, injury in odontoblast or delayed mineralization due to deep caries penetration.
- It also divides dentin into original primary dentin or subsequent irritation dentin.
- Bacterial are concentrated in calciotraumatic line.

36. Ans. (b) The diameter of dentinal tubule ranges from 5 to 7 μm *Ref: Orban's, 12th ed. p 85*

- The course follows a gentle curve in the crown, less so in the root, where it resembles S in shape.
- Starting at right angles from the pulpal surface, the first convexity of this doubly curved course is directed toward the apex of the tooth.
- These tubules end perpendicular to the dentinoenamel and dentinocementum junctions.
- Near the root tip and along the incisal edges and cusps the tubules are almost straight.
- The ratio between the outer and inner surfaces of dentin is about 5:1.
- The ratio between the numbers of tubules per unit area on the pulpal and outer surfaces of dentin is about 4:1.
- There are more tubules per unit area in the crown than in the root.
- The dentinal tubules have lateral branches throughout dentin, which are termed canaliculi or microtubules.
- A few dentinal tubules extend through the dentinoenamel junction into the enamel. These are termed enamel spindles.
- They are larger in diameter near the pulp cavity (3–4 μm) and smaller at the outer ends (1 μm).
- At the pulpal and surface of the dentin, the number of tubules is between 50,000 and 90,000 mm^2.

37. Ans. (d) Interglobular dentin *Ref: Orban's, 12th ed. p 95, 96*

- In areas where both primary and secondary mineralization have occurred with complete crystalline fusion, these appear as lighter rounded areas on a stained section of dentin and are considered globular dentin.
- In contrast, the darker arc like areas in a stained section of dentin are considered interglobular dentin.
- In these areas, only primary mineralization has occurred within the predentin, and the globules of dentin do not fuse completely.
- Thus, interglobular dentin is slightly less mineralized than globular dentin.
- The dentinal tubules pass through the interglobular dentin and helps to detect the defect of mineralization.

38. Ans. (b) Mantle dentin *Ref: Orban's, 12th ed. p 89, 90, 102*

Mental Dentin

- It is a type of primary dentin.
- It lies under DEJ as it is a first formed dentin and provides the cushioning effect to the tooth.

- It is 20 micrometer thick.
- The fibrils are perpendicular to DEJ and made by larger collagen type III.
- The larger diameter collagen fibers are argyrophilic (silver stained and termed as von korff's fibers).

39. Ans. (a) Cytoplasmic extensions of dentinal tubules *Ref: Tencate's, 7th ed. p 201*

- A very long and often branched process emerges from the apical pole of each odontoblasts is termed as Tomes fibers.
- Tomes fibers and dentinal tubules are responsible for transport of nutrients to the dentin.
- Some tomes fibers may penetrate for short distances into the enamel.

40. Ans. (a) 15 days *Ref: Sturdevant's, 5th ed. p 26*

- Reparative or tertiary dentin is formed by replacement or secondary odontoblast in response to intense irritation caused by attrition, abrasion, erosion trauma, caries.
- Some operative procedures and other irritants when tomes processes are cutted within 1.5 mm from the pulp.
- The cutted fibers die along with the corresponding odontoblasts, leaving dead tracts.
- New odontoblasts are differentiated from mesenchymal cells of the pulp in about 15 days, and these replacement odontoblasts lay down the reparative dentin. It is confined to the localized irritated area of the pulp cavity wall, becomes apparent microscopically about month from inception of stimulus, structurally it vary from well-organized tubular dentin to very irregular atubular dentin (more often) depending on the severity of stimulus.
- Reparative dentin is a defense reaction to an area of injury when the odontoblastic processes are cut not more than 1.5 mm peripheral of the pulp using high speed with air-water coolant, if more depth; the processes and corresponding odontoblasts die, and no reparative dentin results.

41. Ans. (d) Mach bands *Ref: Essentials of Dental Radiography, 1st ed. p 419*

Mach band: Where there is a sharply defined difference in density such as the dentoenamel junction, the dentin may appear more radiolucent as the DEJ is approached. This can contribute to a false positive reading and unnecessary restoration of sound tooth structure.

Conditions resembling caries:

- Non-Metallic restorations
- Cervical burnout
- Mach band
- Attrition and Abrasion
- Indirect pulp capping

42. Ans. (a) Hydrodynamic *Ref: Orban's, 12th ed. p 96*

Dentinal hypersensitivity:

- Dentinal hypersensitivity (DH) is a common clinical condition usually associated with exposed dentinal surfaces.
- It can affect patients of any age group and most commonly affects the canines and premolars of both the arches.
- It is clinically described as an exaggerated response to application of a stimulus to exposed dentine, regardless of its location.
- 'Dentine hypersensitivity is characterized by short, sharp pain arising from exposed dentine in response to stimuli, typically thermal, evaporative, tactile, osmotic or chemical and which cannot be ascribed to any other dental defect or pathology'.

Theories of pain transmission through dentin:

- Direct nerve stimulation,
- Dentinal receptor (transducer/modulation),

- Hydrodynamic, and
- Direct ionic diffusion hypothesis.

Fluid hydrodynamic theory:

- It states that the flow of fluid in dentinal tubules trigger receptors within the tooth.
- Various stimuli such as heat, cold, air blast, desiccation or mechanical or osmotic pressure affect fluid movement in dentinal tubules.
- This fluid movement, inward or outward, stimulates pain mechanism
- It is the most widely accepted theory explaining tooth sensitivity.

43. Ans. (b) 2–3 μm *Ref: Orban, 12th ed. p 85*

Facts about dentin:

- Thickness of dentin is 3–10 μm or more.
- Average diameter of tubules at dentino enamel junction is 0.5–0.9 μm, but this increases to 23 μm at the pulp.
- Number of dentinal tubules near the pulp is 50,000–90,000 while near DEJ it is 15,000–20,000.

44. Ans. (c) Contain phosphophoryn *Ref: Orban's, 12th ed. p 90*

Circumpulpal dentin forms the remaining primary dentin or bulk of the tooth. It is the circumpulpal dentin that represents all of the dentin formed before root completion. The collagen fibrils in circumpulpal dentin are much smaller in diameter (0.05 μm) and are more closely packed together compared to the mantle dentin. The circumpulpal dentin may contain slightly more mineral than mantle dentin.

45. Ans. (a) Are found in mantle dentin *Ref: Orban's, 12th ed. p 89-90*

Mantle dentin

- It is the name of the first formed dentin in the crown underlying the DEJ
- It is the outer or most peripheral part of the primary dentin and is about 20 μm thick. It is bounded by the DEJ and the zone of interglobular dentin
- The fibrils formed in this zone are perpendicular to the DEJ and the organic matrix is composing of larger collagen fibrils than are present in the rest of primary dentin.
- Mantle dentin comprises of various vesicles of first site of calcification of dentin matrix. These matrix vesicles are surrounded by forming enamel matrix on one side and odontoblast process on the pulpal side.

46. Ans. (b) Mantle dentin *Ref: Orban's, 12th ed. p 89*

Mantle dentin is the name of the first-formed dentin in the crown underlying the dentinoenamel junction. This zone below the DE junction is soft and this provides cushioning effect to the tooth. It is thus the outer or most peripheral part of the primary dentin and is about 20 μm thick.

47. Ans. (a) Schreger line *Ref: http://oralhistology-viva.blogspot.in/2013/10/dentin.html*

- Lines associated with primary curvature of dentin is Schreger line. It differentiates primary and secondary dentin
- Lines associated with secondary curvature of dentin is Contour line of Owen; neonatal line
- Short period deposition of incremental lines in dentin are commonly called as Von Ebner's line.
- The coarser long period lines in dentin are called as Andresen lines.
- Between two Andresen lines in dentin, there are 6 to 10 pairs number of Von Ebner lines.

48. Ans. (c) Lamina densa *Ref: Orban's, 12th ed. p 65*

- The lamina limitans is the innermost surface of the dentinal tubule (that exist in dentin) that lies in intimate contact with the long process of the odontoblast. It is hypocalcified and appears electron-dense in electron microscopy. It is composed of a fibrous outer layer and a membranous inner layer. It was previously known as the sheath of Neumann.

49. Ans. (b) Black zones *Ref: Orban's, 12th ed. p 125*

- The normal odontoblastic processes disintegrate due to caries, attrition, and erosion or during formation of ground section which is filled with air.
- These degenerated odontoblastic processes give rise to dead tracks which appear black in transmitted light and white in reflected light.
- More commonly seen in pulpal horn areas due to crowding of odontoblasts in these areas whereas sclerotic dentin appears light in transmitted light and black in reflected light.

50. Ans. (b) Silverman *Ref: Ten Cate's Oral Histology, 7th ed. p 236-237*

- Dead tract in dentin was coined by Sir Wilfred fish.
- In ground section of normal dentin the odontoblast process disintegrate and the empty tubules are filled with air. They appear black in transmitted and white in reflected light.
- These areas demonstrate decreased sensitivity and appear to a greater extent in older teeth. Dead tracts are probably the initial step in formation of sclerotic dentin.

The evidence that exposed dentine always dies is as follows:

- Such dentine is insensitive right through to the secondary dentine.
- The injured dentine is found experimentally to be shut off from the pulp in such a way that fluids cannot enter it. It thus lacks the necessary body fluids to support life.
- Under an injury the primary dentine is seen to stop abruptly at the original pulp margin, and to be sealed off with a homogeneous barrier of lime salts before the tubules of the secondary dentine start. The tubules of the secondary dentine take origin below this homogeneous layer in fine branches and obviously have no connexion with the injured primary tubules.

The injured tubules although walled off from the pulp remain permeable from the mouth and have therefore not died by slow calcification.

51. Ans. (c) Intratubular dentin *Ref: Internet*

Intratubular dentin is produced continuously throughout the life sealing the lumen of tubule.

PULP

52. Ans. (d) Loose connective tissue *Ref: Grossman, 12th ed. p 16, 17*

- Dental pulp is an unmineralized oral tissue composed of soft connective tissue, vascular, lymphatic and nervous elements that occupies the central pulp cavity of each tooth.
- Pulp has a soft, gelatinous consistency.
- The majority of pulp (75–80%) is water.
- The pulp cavity extends down through the root of the tooth as the root canal which opens into the periodontium via the apical foramen. The blood vessels, nerves etc. of dental pulp enter and leave the tooth through this foramen.
- Developmentally and functionally, pulp and dentin are closely related. Both are products of the neural crest-derived connective tissue that formed the dental papilla.

Histology of Dental Pulp

Dental pulp is a loose connective tissue with an appearance similar to mucoid CT. It contains the components common to all connective tissues:

- **Cells:** Fibroblasts and undifferentiated mesenchymal cells as well as other cell types (macrophages, lymphocytes, etc.) required for the maintenance and defense of the tissue.

- **Fibrous matrix:** Collagen fibers, type I and II, are present in an unbundled and randomly dispersed fashion, higher in density around blood vessels and nerves. Type I collagen is thought to be produced by the odontoblasts as dentin, secreted by these cells, is composed of type I collagen. Type II is probably produced by the pulp fibroblasts as this type increases in frequency with the age of the tooth. Older pulp contains more collagen of both the bundled and diffuse types.
- **Ground substance**: the environment that surrounds both cells and fibers of the pulp is rich in proteoglycans, glycoproteins and large amounts of water.
- The large number of undifferentiated mesenchymal cells (present as perivascular cells) within the pulp facilitates the recruitment of newly differentiating cells to replace others when they are lost—specifically odontoblasts.

Functions of the Pulp:

- Formative: Elaboration of dentin to form the tooth.
- Protective: Protection against and repairing of the effects of noxious stimuli.
- Nutritive: Preserving the vitality of all the cellular elements.
- Sensory: Perception of stimuli.

53. Ans. (a) Sympathetic and afferent postganglionic *Ref: Ingle's Endodontics, 6th ed. p 137*

- Comparatively less is known about parasympathetic innervation in dental pulp.
- Postganglionic sympathetic nerve travel with the internal carotid nerve, join the trigeminal nerve at the ganglion and supply teeth and supporting structure via the maxillary and mandibular division of t5th CN.

54. Ans. (b) Pulp stones are due to dystrophic calcification *Ref: Orban's Oral Histology and Embryology, 12th ed. p 129*

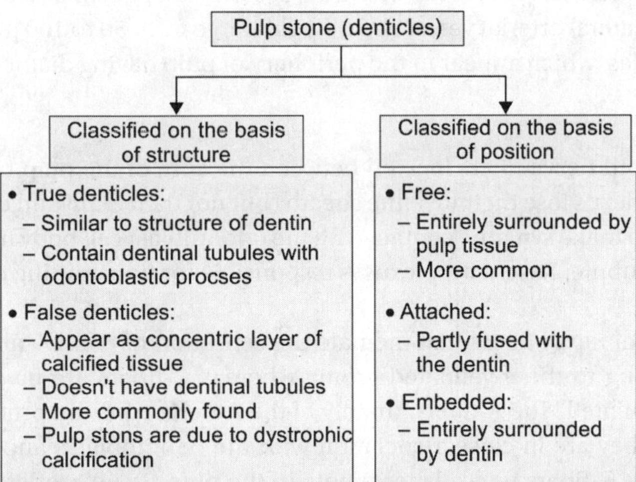

55. Ans. (c) Type II dentine dysplasia *Ref: Shafer, 6th ed. p 56, 57*

Dentin dysplasia is characterized by normal enamel but atypical dentin formation and pulp morphology. It is divided into two as:

1. Radicular dentin dysplasia (Type I)
2. Coronal dentin dysplasia (Type II)
   - Radiologically in Type I, the pulp is completely obliterated in primary tooth while in permanent crescent shaped pulpal remnants may be seen.
   - In Type II, the pulp chamber shows thistle tube appearance.

56. Ans. (a) Cell free zone of weil *Ref: Orban's, 12th ed. p 124*

- The peripheral axons form a network of nerves located adjacent to the cell-rich zone. This is termed the parietal layer of nerves, also known as the plexus of Raschkow.

- Nerve enter the pulp through the apical foramen and each nerve fiber is estimated to produce at least 8 terminal branches, which ultimately contribute to an extensive plexus of nerves in the cell free zone just below the cell bodies of the odontoblasts. This plexus of nerves are called sub odontoblastic plexus of Raschkow and it occupies the cell free zone of weil.

57. Ans. (a) Free nerve endings *Ref: Orban's, 12th ed. p 123,124*

- The majority of the nerves that enter the pulp are non-myelinated. They are found in close association with the blood.
- They are found in close association with the blood vessels of the pulp and are sympathetic in nature.
- Pulp lacks the receptors of heat, touch, pressure or chemicals and proprioception. Any stimulus will elicit only pain in the form of response due to presence of free nerve endings.

58. Ans. (b) Fibroblasts *Ref: Orban's, 12th ed. p 112*

The pulp organ consists of specialized connective tissue because it lacks elastic fibers. Fibroblasts are the most numerous cell types in the pulp. As their name implies, they function in collagen fiber formation throughout the pulp during the life of the tooth.

59. Ans. (a) 50 to 100 micrometer *Ref: Orban's, 12th ed. p 120*

- The pulp organ is highly vascularized.
- The rate of blood flow in pulp is more rapid in compare to other areas of the body. It is around 0.3 to 1 mm per second in arterioles while in venules it is 0.15 mm/second and in capillaries about 0.08 mm.
- The diameter of the lateral arterial vessels in the pulp range from 50 to 100 μm.
- The terminal arterioles, which appear in the periphery of pulp having diameter 10 to 15 μm.

60. Ans. (a) Cell free zone *Ref: Orban's, 12th ed. p 124*

- A plexus of myelinated nerve fibers located between the core of the pulp of the tooth and the cell-rich zone; axons of Raschkow plexus lose their myeline sheath (but not their Schwann cells) as they penetrate the cell-rich and cell-free zones to make synaptic contact with the odontoblast cell body in the pulp or odontoblastic process within the dentinal tubule; Raschkow plexus is responsible for transmitting pain sensation from the pulp of the tooth.
- There are two types of nerve fibers that mediate the sensation of pain: A-fibers conduct rapid and sharp pain sensations and belong to the myelinated group, whereas C-fibers are involved in dull aching pain and are thinner and unmyelinated. The A-fibers, mainly of the A-delta type, are preferentially located in the periphery of the pulp, where they are in close association with the odontoblasts and extend fibers to many but not all dentinal tubules. The C-fibers typically terminate in the pulp tissue proper, either as free nerve endings or as branches around blood vessels.

61. Ans. (a) A delta fibers *Ref: Orban's, 12th ed. p 134*

- Dental pulp is a highly innervated tissue that contains sensory trigeminal afferent axons
- The 2 types of sensory nerve fibers in the pulp are: myelinated A fibers (A-delta and A-beta fibers) and unmyelinated C fibers.
- Ninety percent of the A fibers are A-delta fibers, which are mainly located at the pulpdentin border in the coronal portion of the pulp and concentrated in the pulp horns.
- The C fibers are located in the core of the pulp, or the pulp proper, and extend into the cell-free zone underneath the odontoblastic layer.
- Sympathetic efferent fibers regulate the blood flow.
- Aδ-fibers are more affected by the reduction of blood flow than C-fibers, because they are more sensitive to hypoxia.

- The A fibers are mainly stimulated by an application of cold, producing sharp pain, whereas stimulation of the C fibers produces a dull aching pain.
- The location of the C fibers within the nerve bundles in the core or central region of the pulp may explain the diffuse pain, called referred pain.

62. Ans. (b) Hohl *Ref: Seltzer, 1st ed. p 56*

- Hohl's cell rich zone contains undifferentiated mesenchymal cells which are progenitor cells for formation or odontoblastic cells
- Miller gave the term 'liquefaction foci' is caries zones
- Fitzgerald and Keyes had provided the first evidence that dental caries was an infectious, transmissible disease induced by the Strep Mutants, Cardiogenic Diet and Susceptible tooth.

CEMENTUM

63. Ans. (a) Cellular cementum *Ref: Orban's, 12th ed. p 137 143*

- Cellular cementum is formed after the tooth reaches occlusal plane.
- It is more irregular.
- Cellular cementum is located at the apical half of the root.
- Cellular cementum is less calcified than acellular cementum.
- Cellular cementum grows at a faster rate.

64. Ans. (a) 45% to 50% *Ref: Orban's Oral Histology and Embryology, 12th ed. p 137*

On a dry weight basis, cementum from fully formed permanent teeth contains about 45–50% inorganic substances and 50–55% organic material and water. The inorganic portion consist mainly of calcium and phosphate in the form of hydroxyapatite.

65. Ans. (c) Cementum overlapping enamel *Ref: Orban's, 12th ed. p 192-193*

Cement enamel junction:

- In about 60–65% of cases cementum overlaps the enamel.
- In about 30% there is an edge to edge butt joint.
- In 5–10% the cementum and enamel fail to meet.

66. Ans. (b) Less calcified than acellular type *Ref: Orban's, 11th ed. p 184-187*

Cementum is thinnest at CEJ and thickest toward the apex.

Acellular cementum	*Cellular cementum*
• First formed cementum • It is cementum, i.e. formed before the both reaches the occlusal plane. It covers the cervical third or half of root • Sharpey's fibers make up most of the structure of acellular cementum which has a principle role in supporting tooth • More calcified than cellular cementum • Do not contain cementocytes	• Formed after the tooth reaches the occlusal plane • It is more irregular and contains cementocytes in lacunae • Cellular cementum is more frequent on the apical half • It is always thickest around the apex and by its growth, contributes to the length of root

67. Ans. (c) 640 µm 64000 Å *Ref: Orban's, 12th ed. p 147*

The crystals associated with collagen fibrils are arranged in an orderly fashion with their long axes paralleling the fibril long axes and in rows conforming to the 64 nm (640 Å) striation pattern.

- Normally all collagen fibrils have a transverse striation of 64 nm periodicity but afibrillar cementum is an exception. It does not possess collagen fibrils with a 64 nm periodicity.

68. Ans. (c) Ankylosis *Ref: Shafer's, 6th ed. p 527*

- Fusion of cementum and alveolar bone with obliteration of the periodontal ligament is termed as Ankylosis.
- It occurs in teeth with cemental resorption which suggest, it may represent a form of abnormal repair.

69. Ans. (c) Poorly defined zone near cementodentinal junction *Ref: Carranza, 10th ed. p 76*

Intermediate cementum is a poorly defined zone near the cementodentinal junction of certain teeth that appears to contain cellular remnants of Hertwig's sheath embedded in calcified ground substance.

70. Ans. (b) 30 percent *Ref: Orban's, 12th ed. p 147*

- The relation between cementum and enamel at the cervical region of teeth is variable. In approximately 30% of all teeth, cementum meets the cervical end of enamel in a relatively sharp line. In about 10% of the teeth, enamel and cementum do not meet.
- In approximately 60% of the teeth, cementum overlaps the cervical end of enamel for a short distance.

PERIODONTAL LIGAMENT

71. Ans. (a) Type I *Ref: Orban's, 12th ed. p 171*

- The most important elements of the periodontal ligament are the principal fibers, which are collagenous, are arranged in bundles, and follow a wavy course when viewed in longitudinal sections.
- Terminal portions of the principal fibers that insert into cementum and bone are termed Sharpey's fibers.
- The principal fiber bundles consist of individual fibers that form a continuous anastomosing network between tooth and bone.

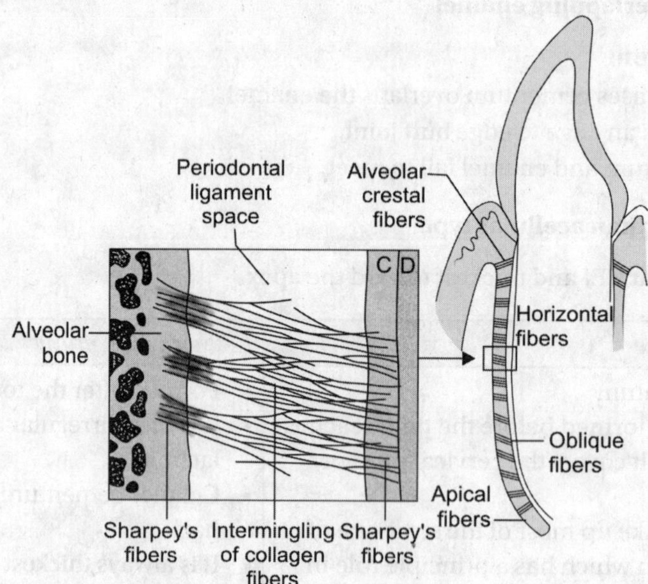

- Collagen is a protein composed of different amino acids, the most important of which are glycine, proline, hydroxylysine, and hydroxyproline.

- The amount of collagen in a tissue can be determined by its hydroxyproline content
- The principal fibers are composed mainly of collagen type I, whereas reticular fibers are composed of collagen type III. Collagen type IV is found in the basal lamina.
- More than 70% of PDL collagen is type I
- The principal fibers of the periodontal ligament are arranged in six groups that develop sequentially in the developing root:
  1. The transseptal
  2. Alveolar crest
  3. Horizontal
  4. Oblique
  5. Apical, and
  6. Interradicular fibers.

72. Ans. (a) Transseptal *Ref: Orban's, 12th ed. p 172*

Refer Ans no. 73

73. Ans. (b) The apical end of root *Ref: Orban's, 12th ed. p 172*

Fibers of PDL:

- Alveolar crest fibers: Alveolar crest fibers (I)run from the cervical part of the root to the alveolar bone crest
- Horizontal fibers: Horizontal fibers attach to the cementum apical to the alveolar crest fibers and run perpendicularly from the root of the tooth to the alveolar bone.
- Oblique fibers: Oblique fibers are the most numerous fibers in the periodontal ligament, running from cementum in an oblique direction to insert into bone coronally.
- Apical fibers: Apical fibers are found radiating from cementum around the apex of the root to the bone, forming base of the socket or alveolus.
- Interradicular fibers: Interradicular fibers are only found between the roots of multirooted teeth, such as premolars and molars. They also attach from the cementum and insert to the nearby alveolar bone.
- Transseptal fibers: Transseptal fibers extend interproximally over the alveolar bone crest and are embedded in the cementum of adjacent teeth; they form an interdental ligament. These fibers keep all the teeth aligned. These fibers may be considered as belonging to the gingival tissue because they do not have an osseous attachment.

74. Ans. (d) Periodontal ligament *Ref: Orban's, 12th ed. p 167 and Carranza, 10th ed. p 70-71*

- Epithelial rests of Malassez: The periodontal ligament contains epithelial cells that are found close to the cementum. These cells were first described by Malassez in 1884 and are the remnants of the epithelium of Hertwig's epithelial root sheath.
- Although the periodontal ligament does not contain mature elastin, two immature forms are found: oxytalan and elaunin. The so-called oxytalan fibers run parallel to the root surface in a vertical direction and bend to attach to the cementum in the cervical third of the root. They are thought to regulate vascular flow. An elastic meshwork has been described in the periodontal ligament as being composed of many elastin lamellae with peripheral oxytalan fibers and elaunin fibers. Oxytalan fibers have been shown to develop de novo in the regenerated periodontal ligament.
- The principal fibers are remodeled by the periodontal ligament cells to adapt to physiologic needs and in response to different stimuli.
- In addition to these fiber types, small collagen fibers associated with the larger principal collagen fibers have been described. These fibers run in all directions, forming a plexus called the indifferent fiber plexus.

75. Ans. (c) Periodontal ligament *Ref: Orban's, 12th ed. p 177*

- Calcified bodies called cementicles are sometimes found in the periodontal ligament. These bodies are seen in older individuals, and they may remain free in the connective tissue, they may fuse into large calcified masses, or they may be joined with the cementum.

76. Ans. (b) Increases *Ref: Carranza, 10th ed. p 95*

PDL (Age related changes in PDL)

- Decreased number of fibroblasts.
- Decreased organic matrix production and epithelial cell rest.
- Increased amount of elastic fibers.

77. Ans. (d) PDL *Ref: Orban's, 12th ed. p 173*

- Elaunin is a component of elastic fibers formed from the deposition of elastin between oxytalan fibers.
- It is found in the periodontal ligament and in the connective tissue of the dermis, particularly in association with sweat glands.
- Actually elastic fibers of periodontal ligament are composed of elastic, elaunin, and oxytalan fibers.
- Elaunin fibers are believed to be an immature form of elastic fibers and are made up of bundles of microfibrils intermingled with small amounts of elastin.

78. Ans. (d) PDL *Ref: Orban's, 12th ed. p 167 and Carranza, 10th ed. p 70-71*

Refer Ans No. 74

- In dentistry, the epithelial cell rests of Malassez or epithelial rests of Malassez are part of the periodontal ligament cells around a tooth.
- They are discrete clusters of residual cells from Hertwig's epithelial root sheath (HERS) that didn't completely disappear.
- It is considered that these cell rests proliferate to form epithelial lining of various odontogenic cysts such as radicular cyst under the influence of various stimuli.

BONE

79. Ans. (a) Eruption of teeth *Ref: Orban's, 12th ed. p 200*

- Whenever the movement of teeth is attempted through orthodontics, an area of bone undercompressive force from a tooth moving towards it has a high osteoclast level, creates bone resorption. Similarly area under tension from periodontal ligaments creates new bone.
- During the eruption of teeth, an alveolar process is developed and when the tooth exfoliates the alveolar process degeneration will start.

80. Ans. (d) Premolar and molar region of the mandible on the buccal side *Ref: Orban's Oral Histology and Embryology, 12th ed. p 201*

- They are thickest in the premolar and molar region of the lower jaw, especially on the buccal side.
- The cortical plates, continuous with the compact layers of the maxillary and mandibular body, are generally much thinner in the maxilla, than in the mandible
- In the maxilla, the outer cortical plate is perforated by many small openings through which blood and lymph vessels pass.
- In the region of the anterior teeth of both jaws, the supporting bone usually is very thin.

81. Ans. (b) Coupling *Ref: Carranza, 10th ed. p 81*

Bone Remodeling:

- It is the major pathway of bony changes in shape, resistance to forces, repair or wounds and calcium and phosphate homeostasis in the body. Indeed, the coupling of bone resorption with bone formation constitutes one of the fundamental principles by which bone is necessarily remodeled throughout its life.
- Bone remodeling involves the co-ordination of activities of cells from two distinct lineages, the osteoblasts and the osteoclasts, which form and resorb the mineralized connective tissues of bone
- Regulation of bone remodeling is a complex process involving hormones and local factors acting in an autocrine and a paracrine manner on the generation and activity of differentiated bone cells.
- Osteoclasts have resorbed organic matrix release various osteogenic substrates, which are covalently bound to collagen and this in turn stimulates the differentiation of osteoblasts, which ultimately deposit bone. This interdependency of osteoblast and osteoclasts in remodeling is called coupling.
- Ten cate's described the sequence of events in the resorptive process as follows:
  - Attachment of osteoclasts to the mineralized surface of bone
  - Creation of a sealed acidic environment through action of the proton pumps which demineralizes bone and organic matrix.
  - Degradation of the exposed organic matrix to its constituent amino acids by the action of released enzymes such as acid phosphatase and cathepsin
  - Sequestering of mineral ions and amino acids within the osteoclast.

82. Ans. (c) Interdental and interradicular septa of alveolar bone *Ref: Orban's, 12th ed. p 201*

The alveolar bone proper, which forms the inner wall of the socket, is perforated by many openings that carry branches of the interalveolar nerves and blood vessels into the periodontal ligament, and it is therefore called the cribriform plate. Bone between the teeth is called interdental septum and is composed entirely of cribriform plate. The interdental and interradicular septa contain the perforating canals of Zuckerkandl and Hirschfeld (nutrient canals) which house the interdental and interradicular arteries, veins, lymph vessels and nerves.

83. Ans. (b) Alveolar bone *Ref: Orban's, 12th ed. p 200,201*

- The Alveolar bone proper consists partly of lamellated and partly of bundle bone.
- Bundle bone is that bone in which the principal fibers of the periodontal ligament are anchored. The term bundle bone was chosen because the bundles of the principal fibers continue into the bone as sharpey's fibers.
- It contains fewer fibrils than does lamellated bone, therefore it appears dark in routine hematoxylin and eosin stained section.

84. Ans. (b) Filling cone *Ref: Ten Cate's, 7th ed. p 139*

Cutting Cone:

- When an osteoclast creates a resorption channel while moving through compact bone. The leading edge of resorption is known as cutting cone.
- Characterized by Howship's lacunae.

Filling Bone:

- It is the area where osteoclast lay down new bone from outside to inside in an osteon.
- When the formation of new bone proceeds, many osteoblast will turn into osteoclast.

85. Ans. (a) Osteon *Ref: Orban's, 12th ed. p 189*

- The basic functional unit of mature compact bone is an osteon.
- This allows the effective metabolism of bone cells surrounded by rings of mineral salts.
- This functional unit is also known as Haversian canal.

- Each osteon consists of concentric layers, or lamellae of compact bone tissue that surround a central canal, the haversian canal.
- The haversian canal contains the bone's nerve and blood supplies. The boundary of an osteon is the cement line.
- Osteons are connected to each other and the periosteum by oblique channels called volkmann's canals or

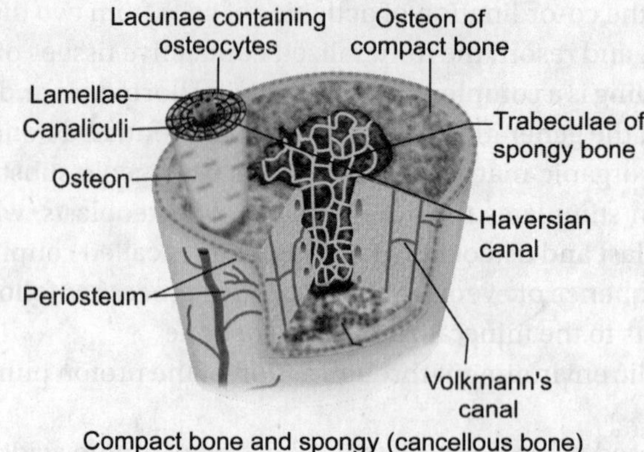

Compact bone and spongy (cancellous bone)

86. Ans. (a) Cathepsin K and carbonic anhydrase *Ref: Drug News Perspectives 2004;17(1):19*

Cathepsin K and Carbonic anhydrase plays a critical role in the degradation of bone and appears to be a limiting step in osteoclastic bone resorption.

87. Ans. (a) Alveolar bone *Ref: Orban's, 11th ed. p 247 and Carranza, 10th ed. p 82 and 8th ed. p 44*

- The marrow spaces in the alveolar process may contain hematopoietic marrow, but usually they contain fatty marrow. In the condylar process, in the angle of the mandible, in the maxillary tuberosity, and in other isolated foci, hematopoietic cellular marrow is found.
- Bone marrow: In the embryo and newborn the cavities of all bones are occupied by red hematoipoietic marrow. The red marrow gradually undergoes a physiologic change to the fatty or yellow inactive type of marrow. In adult the marrow of jaw is normally of the latter type, and red marrow is found only in the ribs, sternum, vertebrate, skull, and humerus. However, foci of red bone marrow are occasionally seen in the jaws, often accompanied by resorption of bony trabeculae. Common locations are the maxillary tuberosity, the maxillary and mandibular molar and premolar areas, and the mandibular symphysis and ramus angle, which may be visible radiographically as zones of radiolucency.

ORAL MUCOUS MEMBRANE

88. Ans. (b) Filiform papillae *Ref: Orban's, 12th ed. p 237*

- Taste buds contain the receptors for taste.
- They are located around the small structures on the upper surface of the tongue, soft palate, upper esophagus and epiglottis, which are called papillae.

The majority of taste buds on the tongue sit on raised protrusions of the tongue surface called papillae. There are four types of papillae present in the human tongue:

- Fungiform papillae—as the name suggests, these are slightly mushroom-shaped if looked at in longitudinal section. These are present mostly at the dorsal surface of the tongue, as well as at the sides. Innervated by facial nerve.
- Filiform papillae—these are thin, long papillae 'V'-shaped cones that do not contain taste buds but are the most numerous. These papillae are mechanical and not involved in gustation. They are characterized by increased keratinization. It lacks taste buds.

- Foliate papillae—these are ridges and grooves towards the posterior part of the tongue found at the lateral borders. Innervated by facial nerve (anterior papillae) and glossopharyngeal nerve (posterior papillae).
- Circumvallate papillae—there are only about 10 to 14 of these papillae on most people, and they are present at the back of the oral part of the tongue. They are arranged in a circular-shaped row just in front of the sulcus terminalis of the tongue. They are associated with ducts of Von Ebner's glands, and are innervated by the glossopharyngeal nerve.

Taste buds are only present in circumvallate, fungiform papillae and soft palate.

89. Ans. (a) Buccal mucosa *Ref: Oral Development and Histology by James Avery, 3rd ed. Table 16.2*

Sensation	*Least*	*Moderate*	*Greatest*
Pain	Buccal mucosa	Anterior tongue, gingiva	Lips, pharynx, base of tongue teeth
Heat	Ventral tongue palate	Anterior teeth	Lips
Cold	Buccal mucosa, Dorsum tongue	Base and ventral tongue	Lips and posterior palate
Touch	Base of tongue, buccal mucosa	Gingiva	Lips, tips of tongue, anterior palate

90. Ans. (c) Floor of mouth *Ref: Orban's, 12th ed. p 236*

Part of oral cavity	*Epithelium present*	*Lamina propria*	*Submucosa*
Soft palate	Thin (150 μm), nonkeratinized stratified squamous epithelium	Thick, having numerous short papillae highly vascular	Diffuse tissue having minor salivary glands.
Floor of the mouth	Very thin (100 μm), nonkeratinized stratified squamous epithelium	Short papillae, some elastic fibers highly vascular	Loose fibrous connective tissue having fat and minor salivary glands.
Labial and buccal mucosa	Very thick (500 μm), non keratinized stratified squamous epithelium	Long slender papillae, dense fibrous connective tissue having collagen and elastic as well. Rich vascular supply.	Mucosa is firmly attached to underlying muscle by collagen and elastin, minor salivary glands and some sebaceous glands.

91. Ans. (c) Fibroblast *Ref: Orban's, 12th ed. p 213*

- Fibroblasts: As we all know, fibroblasts performs the function of secretion of collagen fibers. Also they possess lysosomes which contain collagen of periodontal ligaments under digestion process. Hence they are capable of both synthesis and resorption of soft connective tissue.
- Langerhans cells are antigen presenting cells which identify a foreign antigen and represent it to CD4 helper cells.

92. Ans. (b) Originate from Golgi system *Ref: Orban's, 12th ed. p 218*

In the stratum granulosum the cell surfaces become more regular and more closely applied to adjacent cell surfaces. At the same time the lamellar granule, a small organelle (also known as keratinosome, odland body, or membrane-coating granule) forms in the upper spinous and granular cell layers. The membrane coating granules are glycolipids. It has an internal lamellate structure. Lamellar granules discharge their contents into the intercellular space forming an intercellular lamellar material, which contributes to the permeability barrier.

93. Ans. (d) Stratum granulosum *Ref: Orban's, 12th ed. p 218, 219*

Stratum granulosum contains flatter and wider cells. These cells are larger than spinous cells. Sometimes dense networks of tonofilaments and keratohyalin granules are seen. They contain at least two types of proteins one that is rich in the amino acid histidine. It functions in the stratum corneum as a keratin filament matrix protein.

1. The nuclei show signs of degeneration and pyknosis. This layer still synthesizes protein.
2. In the stratum granulosum the cell surfaces become more regular and more closely applied to adjacent cell surface.
3. Lamellae granule (Keratinosome, odland body, or membrane coating granule) present in upper spinous and granular cell layer. It has internal lamellated structure. It discharge their contents into the intercellular space, forming an intercellular lamellar material, which contributes to the permeability barrier. This barrier forms at the junction of granular and cornified cell layers.

94. Ans. (b) Non-keratinized *Ref: Orban's, 12th ed. p 210, 211 and Orban's, 11th ed. p 283*

Classification of Oral Mucosa

Basing classification on these functional criteria, the oral mucosa may be divided into three major types:

1. Masticatory mucosa (gingiva and hard palate)
2. Lining or reflecting mucosa (lip, cheek, vestibular fornix, alveolar mucosa, floor of mouth and soft palate)
3. Specialized mucosa (dorsum of the tongue and taste buds)

Keratinzed area	Masticatory mucosa, i.e. Hard palate and gingiva Vermilion border of lip
Nonkeratinized area	Lining mucosa, i.e. lip, cheek, buccal mucosa, alveolar mucosa and floor of mouth. Soft palate, vestibular mucosa
Specialized mucosa	Dorsal lingual mucosa

95. Ans. (a) Keratohyalin granules *Ref: Orban's, 12th ed. p 218, 219*

Refer Ans no. 93 of same chapter

- Keratohyalin is a protein structure found in granules in the stratum granulosum of the epidermis, which may be involved in keratinization, and in Hassall's corpuscles in the thymus.
- In H and E stained sections, they are large deeply stained granules found in the cytoplasm of epithelial cells in keratinized oral mucosa.

96. Ans. (a) Hard palate *Ref: Orban's, 12th ed. p 227*

Oral mucous membrane may be divided into the following way:

- **Keratinized area**
  - Masticatory mucosa—gingival, hard palate.
  - Vermillion border of lip
- **Nonkeratinized area**
  - Lining mucosa lip, cheek, vestibular fornix, alveolar mucosa, inferior surface of tongue, floor of oral cavity, soft palate.

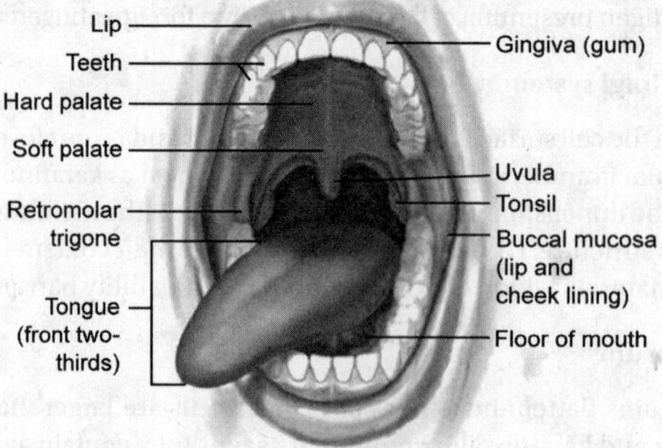

Anatomy of the oral cavity

- Specialized mucosa- Dorsal lingual mucosa taste buds.

- **Hard Palate**
  - The hard palate is a thin horizontal bony plate of the skull, located in the roof of the mouth. It spans the arch formed by the upper teeth.
  - It is formed by the palatine process of the maxilla and horizontal plate of palatine bone.
  - It forms a partition between the nasal passages and the mouth.
  - It is covered by stratified squamous well keratinized mucosa which is tightly fixed to the periosteum.

97. Ans. (c) Langerhans cells *Ref: Orban's, 12th ed. p 221*

- Langerhans cells are dendritic cells (antigen-presenting immune cells) of the skin and mucosa, and contain large granules called Birbeck granules.
- They are present in all layers of the epidermis, but are most prominent in the stratum spinosum.
- It is hematopoieic in origin.
- It is involved in immune response

98. Ans. (b) Anterior lingual glands located near the apex of the tongue *Ref: Orban's, 12th ed. p 271*

- Von Ebner's glands are exocrine glands found in the mouth. More specifically, they are serous salivary glands which reside adjacent to the moats surrounding the circumvallate papillae in the posterior one-third of the tongue, anterior to the terminal sulcus.
- Anterior lingual glands located near the apex of the tongue is the Glands of Blandin and Nuhn

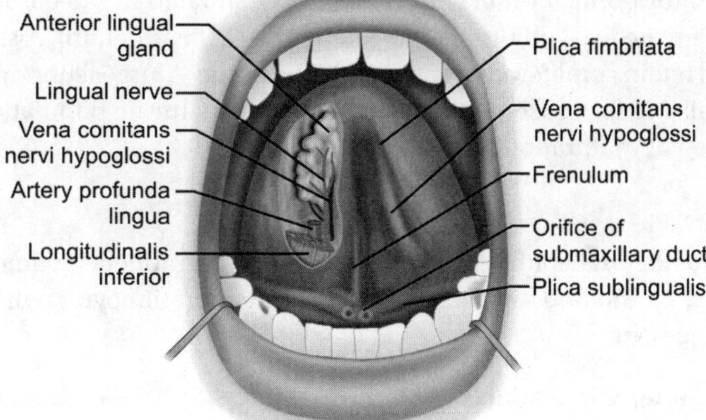

99. Ans. (a) Epidermis *Ref: Orban's, 12th ed. p 297*

- Oral epithelium contains three types of cells apart from normal keratinocytes. These are:
  - Melanocytes (derived from neural crest)
  - Langerhans cells (originated in bone marrow) and
  - Merkel cells
    - Merkel cells or Merkel-Ranvier cells are oval receptor cells found in the skin of vertebrates that have synaptic contacts with somatosensory afferents.
    - They are associated with the sense of light touch discrimination of shapes and textures. They can turn malignant and form the skin tumor known as Merkel cell carcinoma.
    - It has been reported that they are derived from neural crest cells; however, more recent experiments in mammals have indicated that they are in fact epithelial in origin.
    - Merkel cells are found in the skin and some parts of the mucosa of all vertebrates.
    - In mammalian skin, they are clear cells found in the stratum basale (at the bottom of sweat duct ridges) of the epidermis approximately 10 μm in diameter.

- They also occur in epidermal invaginations of the plantar foot surface called rete ridges.
- Most often, they are associated with sensory nerve endings, when they are known as Merkel nerve endings (also called a Merkel cell-neurite complex). They are associated with slowly adapting (SA1) somatosensory nerve fibers.

100. Ans. (d) All of the above *Ref: Orban's, 12th ed. p 263,264*

- Myoepithelial (ME) cells are closely related to the secretory and intercalated duct cells.
- Their appearance is reminiscent of a basket cradling the secretory unit, hence the terms 'basket cell'.
- ME cells contain cytokeratin intermediate filament and contractile actin filaments. These can be used to help identify then using immunocytochemistry. The presence of cytokeratin confirms the epithelial origin of myoepithelial cells.
- The functions related to ME cells indicate clearly that ME cells actively can:
  - Accelerate the initial outflow of saliva from the acini.
  - Reduce luminal volume in the intercalated ducts. May shorten and widen the ducts helping to maintain their patency.
  - Contribute to secretory pressure in the acini or duct.
  - Support the underlying parenchyma and reduce the back permeation of fluid. Help salivary flow to overcome increase in peripheral resistance of the ducts.

101. Ans. (a) Basal layer *Ref: Carranza, 10th ed. p 966*

In epithelium, a progenitor population of cells (stem cells), situated in the basal layer, provides new cells. These cells of the basal layer are the least differentiated cells of the oral epithelium. A small subpopulation of these cells produce basal cells and retains proliferative potential of the tissue. A larger subpopulation of these cells (amplifying cells) produce cells available for subsequent maturation. This maturing population of cells continually undergo a process of differentiation or maturation

102. Ans. (d) Macrophage *Ref: Carranza, 10th ed. p 49*

The principal cell type of the oral epithelium as well as of other stratified squamous epithelia, is the keratinocyte. Other cells found in the epithelium are the clear cells or nonkeratinocytes, which include the langerhans cells, merkel's cells, and melanocyte.

103. Ans. (d) Secretory and intercalated ducts *Ref: Ten Cate's Oral Histology, 6th ed. p 314*

- Myoepithelial cells are contractile cells associated with salivary glands
- Located between the basal lamina and the secretory or duct cells and are joined to the cells by desmosomes.
- They are derived from epithelium

104. Ans. (b) Prickle cells *Ref: Orban's, 11th ed. p 269-281*

- The spinous (prickle) cells resemble a cocklebur or sticker that has each spine ending at a desmosome. Of the four layers, the spinous cells are the most active in protein synthesis.'
- Keratinizing oral epithelium has four layers: basal, spinous, granular, and comified. These are also referred to in Latin as stratum basale, stratum spinosum, stratum granulosum, and stratum corneum.

Stratum Basale:

- The Basal layer is made up of cells that synthesize DNA and undergo mitosis, thus providing new cells. New cells are generated in the basal layer.
- However, some mitotic figure may be seen in spinous cells just beyond the basal layer. These cells have become determined as they leave the basal layer. The basal cells and the parabasal spinous cells are referred to as the 'stratum germinativum', but only the basal cells can divide.

- The serrated basal cells are a single layer of cuboid or high cuboid cells that have protoplasmic processes (pedicles) projecting from their basal surfaces towards the connective tissue.
- Specialized structures called 'Hemidesmosomes,' which abut on the basal lamina, are found on the basal surface. They consist of a single attachment plaque, the adjacent plasma membrane, and an associated extracellular structure that appears to attach the epithelium to the connective tissue.
- The 'Basal lamina' is made up of a clear zone (lamina lucida) just below the epithelial cells and a dark zone (lamina densa) beyond the lamina lucida thus far has been shown to contain laminin and bullous pemphigoid antigen. Laminin is a large, triple-chain molecule (Mr = 106). It and type IV collagen promote epithelial cell growth and guide epithelial cell movement through chemotaxis.
- 'Basement membrane' promotes differentiation. It also promotes peripheral nerve regeneration and growth, and tends to prevent metastases. The lamina densa contains type IV collagen and an antigen bound by the antibody KF-1. Below the lamina densa is a fibrillar zone (sub-lamina densa fibrils) that is not of epithelial origin.

SALIVARY GLANDS

105. Ans. (d) Excretory duct of salivary gland *Ref: Tencate's Oral Histology, 7th ed. p 309*

- These are the small type of cells which are present in Excretory duct and to some extent in striated duct.
- They are also known as Caveolated or Brush cell.
- They have long stiff microvilli and represent some type of unknown receptor.
- The nerve ending may end adjacent to these cells.

106. Ans. (b) Circumvallate papilla *Ref: Orban's, 12th ed. p 271, 272*

Lingual glands	
Anterior glands	*Posterior glands*
• The anterior lingual glands (**glands of Blandin and Nuhn**) are located near the apex of the tongue • They are chiefly mucous in nature and open on the **ventral surface of the tongue near lingual frenum**	1. The posterior lingual mucous glands are located lateral and posterior to the vallate papillae and in association with lingual tonsil. They are purely mucous and their duct open into dorsal surface of the tongue 2. Posterior lingual serous glands (**Von Ebner's glands**). They are purely serous and are present in between muscle fibers of tongue below vallate papillae. Their duct open into trough of the **circumvallate papillae**

107. Ans. (b) Filiform *Ref: B.D. Chaurasia for Dental Students, p 271*

Foliate papillae	Present on lateral border of the posterior of tongue and contains taste buds
Filiform papillae	Keratinizes thread like and do not contain taste buds
Fungiform papillae	Mushroom shaped, round, reddish with few taste buds
Circumvallate papillae	Present in front of V-shaped sulcus terminalis, 8-10 in number, longest and contain many taste buds.

108. Ans. (c) Myoepithelial cells *Ref: Orban's, 12th ed. p 263*

- Myoepithelial cells are contractile cells associated with the secretary and pieces and intercalated duct of the salivary glands.
- It is very much similar to smooth muscle cell but are derived from epithelium.

- Myoepithelial cells processes are filled filaments of actin, myosin and related proteins.
- These are stellate and spider like cells having flattened nucleus.

109. Ans. (b) Circumvallate papilla *Ref: Orban's, 12th ed. p 306*

- Ebner's glands, also Von Ebner's glands are exocrine glands found in the mouth. More specifically, they are serous salivary glands which reside adjacent to the moats surrounding the circumvallate papillae in the posterior one-third of the tongue, anterior to the terminal sulcus.
- Von Ebner's glands (also called gustatory glands) are named after Anton Gilbert Victor von Ebner, Ritter von Rosenstein, who was an Austrian histologist.
- As mentioned above, these glands are located around circumvallate and foliate papillae in the tongue. They secrete lingual lipase, beginning the process of lipid hydrolysis in the mouth.
- These glands empty their serous secretion into the base of the moats located around the foliate and circumvallate papillae. This secretion presumably flushes material from the moat to enable the taste buds to respond rapidly to changing stimuli.
- The Von Ebner glands are innervated by Cranial Nerve IX, the glossopharyngeal nerve. Also know—Glands of tongue are divided into various groups.
- Anterior regions are mucous in nature while posterior are mixed.
- Anterior lingual glands (glands of Blandin and Nuhn) are located near apex of tongue.
- Posterior lingual mucous glands are located near apex of tongue.
- Posterior lingual mucous glands are located lateral and posterior to vallate papillae and opens onto dorsal surface of tongue. The posterior lingual serous glands (von Ebner's) are located below vallate papillae and their ducts opens into the trough of vallate papillae and at the rudimentary foliate papillae on the sides of tongue.

110. Ans. (d) K5, K14 *Ref: Carranza's, 10th ed. p 52*

Type of keratin	*Specification*
K1- K2, K10 to K12	Epidermal-type differentiation
K6 and K16	Highly proliferative epithelia
K5 and K 14	Stratification—specific cytokeratins
K19	Parakeratinized areas

111. Ans. (d) Langerhans cells *Ref: Orban's, 12th ed. p 221*

Langerhans cell is another clear cell or dendritic cell found in upper layers of the skin and mucosal epithelium restricted to zones of orthokeratinization. There is correlation in occurrence of stratum granulosum and langerhans cells. The cell has convoluted nucleus and characteristic, rodlike granules.

112. Ans. (a) Anterior part of the hard palate *Ref: Orban's, 12th ed. p 284, 285, 302*

- The mucosa covering the hard palate exhibits a distinct keratinized layer—the stratum corneum (A). In addition, capillaries (B) loop up into the connective tissue papillae (C).
- A characteristic feature of keratinized regions in the oral cavity is the presence of relatively high connective tissue papillae projecting into the overlying epithelium. High connective tissue papillae are associated with keratinized epithelium. This form of keratinization in the oral cavity is referred to as orthokeratinized stratified squamous epithelium
- The anterolateral part of hard palate is also known as fatty zone and posterolateral is also known as glandular zone.

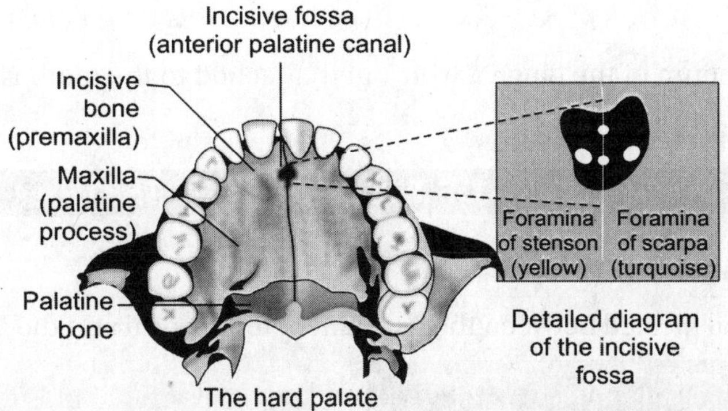

GINGIVA

113. Ans. (c) Mandibular 1st premolar *Ref: Carranza, 10th ed. p 47*

- Continuation of marginal gingival give rise to attached gingival.
- Attached gingival is tightly bounded to the underlying periosteum of alveolar bone. It is firm and resilient in nature.
- The distance between the mucogingival junction and the bottom of the gingival sulcus is termed as width of attached gingival.
- Width of attached gingival is:
- Greatest—In the incisor, i.e. (3.5 to 4.5 mm in maxilla, 3.3 to 3.9 in mandible.
- Narrower—In the posterior, i.e. (1.9 mm in maxilla, 1.8 mm in mandibular premolar)
- Width of attached gingival increases with age and also in supraerupted teeth.

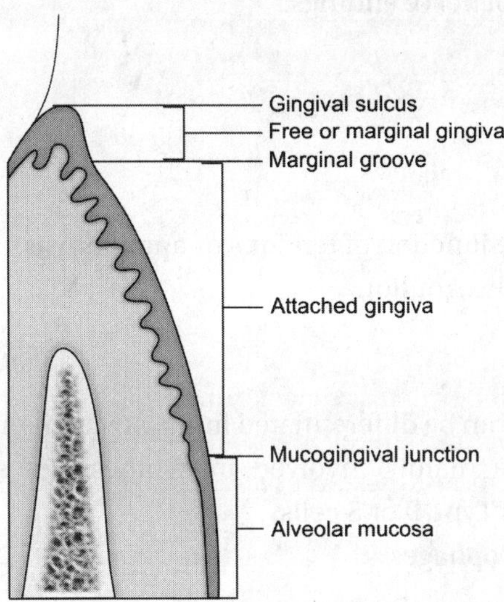

114. Ans. (b) Melanocytes *Ref: Carranza, 10th ed. p 51*

- Melanocyte is a type of nonkeratinocyte cell present in the basal and spinous layers of the gingival epithelium.
- It is a type of dendritic cell.
- They synthesize melanin in melanosomes.

115. Ans. (a) Masticatory mucosa *Ref: Orban's, 12th ed. p 227*

Refer Ans No. 96 of Chapter Oral Mucous Membrane

116. Ans. (b) Nonkeratinized *Ref: Orban's, 12th ed. p 241*

The nonkeratinized epithelium of the gingiva which gets attached to the tooth is called junctional or attachment epithelium.

SHEDDING OF THE DECIDUOUS TEETH

117. Ans. (d) Gubernacular canals *Ref: Tencates, 7th ed. p 270*

- Definition: A small canal located between the permanent tooth germ and the apex of the deciduous tooth.

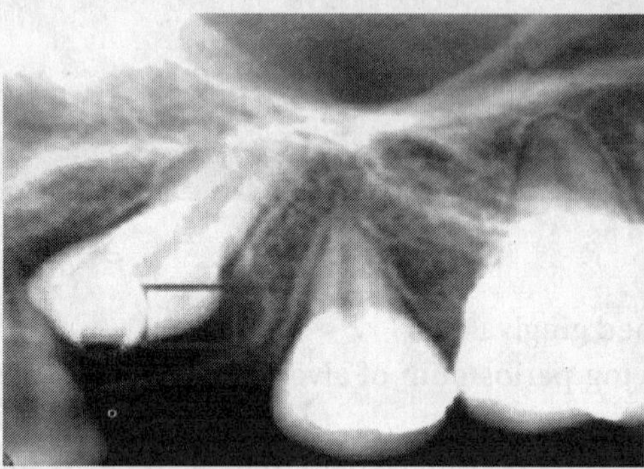

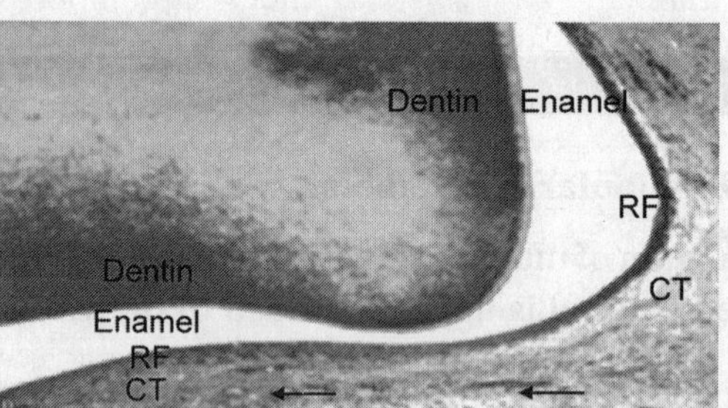

TEMPOROMANDIBULAR JOINT

118. Ans. (c) Golgi tendon organs *Ref: Tencate's, 5th ed. p 390-385*

Innervations of TMJ has four type of nerve endings:

Type I: Ruffini's corpuscles

Type II: Pacini's corpuscles

Type III: Golgi tendon organs

Type IV: Free nerve endings

- Golgi tendons are situated at the junction of tendons or aponeurosis.
- Free nerve endings have wider distribution.

119. Ans. (a) Fibroblast like *Ref: Raymond J Fonseca 1st ed. p 13, Internet*

- Histologically two types of cells can be differentiated in a synovial membrane of TMJ based on the RNA content.
- Cells like fibroblast which are mainly involved in synthesis of sub-intimal collagen proteoglycan and glycoproteins and are termed as Type B or S cells.
- The other types of cells are macrophages.

Also note about TMJ: TMJ pain is generally due to one of four reasons–

- The most common cause of TMJ pain is myofascial pain dysfunction syndrome, primarily involving the muscles of mastication.
- Internal derangements is defined as an abnormal relationship of the disc to any of the other components of the TMJ. Disc displacement is an example of internal derangement.
- Degenerative joint disease, otherwise known as osteoarthritis is the organic degeneration of the articular surfaces within the TMJ.
- TMJ pain remains one of the most reliable diagnostic criteria for temporal arteritis.

HISTOCHEMISTRY OF ORAL TISSUE

120. Ans. (b) Acid phosphatase *Ref: Orban's, 12th ed. p 337*

- An intense acid phosphatase activity is seen in the osteoclast cell, which is present in bone.
- Acid phosphatase shows the same characteristic in odontoclast in resorbing dentin.
- Acid phosphatase activity in human gingival seems related to the degree of keratinization. The pulp organ is highly vascularized.
- The rate of blood flow in pulp is more rapid in compare to other areas of the body. It is around 0.3 to 1 mm per second in arterioles while in venules it is 0.15 mm/ second and in capillaries about 0.08 mm.
- The diameter of the lateral arterial vessels in the pulp range from 50 to 100 μm.
- The terminal arterioles, which appear in the periphery of pulp having diameter 10 to 15 μm.
- PDL (Age related changes in PDL)
- Decreased number of fibroblasts.
- Decreased organic matrix production and epithelial cell rest.
- Increased amount of elastic fibers.
- Pulp

MISCELLANEOUS

121. Ans. (b) Type II *Ref: Dynamics of Bone and Cartilage Metabolism: Principles and Clinical Applications, p 10*

Hyaline Cartilage:

- The matrix of hyaline cartilage appears glassy in the living state: hence, the name hyaline (Gr. hyalos, glassy).
- Throughout the cartilage matrix are spaces called lacunae.
- Located within these lacunae are the chondrocytes.
- Hyaline cartilage is not a simple, inert, homogeneous substance but a complex living tissue.
- It provides a low-friction surface, participates in lubricating synovial joints, and distributes applied forces to the underlying bone.
- Although its capacity for repair is limited, under normal circumstances it shows no evidence of abrasive wear over a lifetime.
- An exception is articular cartilage, which, in many individuals, breaks down with age.
- The macromolecules of hyaline cartilage matrix consist of collagen (predominantly type II fibrils and other cartilage-specific collagen molecules), proteoglycan aggregates containing GAGs, and multiadhesive glycoproteins (noncollagenous proteins).

122. Ans. (c) Floor of mouth *Ref: Orban's, 12th ed. p 236*

Part of oral cavity	*Epithelium present*	*Lamina propria*	*Submucosa*
Soft palate	Thin (150 μm), Nonkeratinized stratified squamous epithelium	Thick, having numerous short papillae highly vascular	Diffuse tissue having minor salivary glands
Floor of the mouth	Very thin (100 μm), nonkeratinized stratified squamous epithelium	Short papillae, some elastic fibers, highly vascular	Loose fibrous connective tissue, having fat and minor salivary glands
Labial and buccal mucosa	Very thick (500 μm), non keratinized stratified squamous epithelium	Long slender papillae, dense fibrous connective tissue having collagen and elastic as well. Rich vascular supply	Mucosa is firmly attached to underlying muscle by collagen and elastin, minor salivary glands and some sebaceous glands

123. Ans. (b) 0.2 and 5 years *Ref: Sturdevant, 5th ed. p 639 and Wheelers, 8th ed. p 45*

- Antibiotics drug tetracycline can cause the generalized type of intrinsic discoloration. The severity of the staining depends on the dose, duration of exposure to the drug, and type of tetracycline analogue used. Different types of tetracyclines induce different types of discoloration varying from yellow orange to dark blue gray. Due to staining from tetracycline type drugs most frequently occurs at an early age and is caused by ingestion of the drug during development of the permanent teeth.

Chronology of permanent teeth					
	Tooth	*First evidence of calcification*	*Crown completed (Years)*	*Emergence (eruption) (Years)*	*Root completed (Years)*
CI	8, 9	3-4 mo	4-5	7-8	10
LI	7,10	10-12 mo	4-5	8-9	11
C	6, 11	4-5 mo	6-7	11-12	13-15
P1	5, 12	1½ -1¾ yr	5-6	10-11	12-13
P2	4, 13	2-2¼ yr	6-7	10-12	12-14
M1	3, 14	At birth	2½ - 3	6-7	9-10
M2	2, 15	2½ - 3 yr	7-8	12-13	14-16
M3	1,16	7-9 yr	12-16	17-21	18-25
Right		*Maxillary teeth* 1 2 3 4 5 6 7 8 9 10 11 12 13 14 15 16 32 31 30 29 28 27 26 25 24 23 22 21 20 19 18 17 *Mandibular teeth*			*Left*
CI	24, 25	3-4 mo	4-5	6-7	9
LI	23, 26	3-4 mo	4-5	7-8	10
C	22, 27	4-5 mo	6-7	9-10	12-14
P1	21, 28	1¼-2 yr	5-6	10-12	12-13
P2	20, 29	2¼-2½ yr	6-7	11-12	13-14
M1	19, 30	At birth	2½-3	6-7	9-10
M2	18, 31	2½-3 yr	7-8	11-13	14-15
M3	17, 32	8-10 yr	12-16	17-21	18-25

124. Ans. (a) Alveolar crest group *Ref: Carranza's, 10th ed. p 70*

- Alveologingival group extend from the alveolar crest to the lamina propria of the gingiva.
- Dentogingivial group and alveologingival group are also called attached gingival group and free gingival

125. Ans. (c) Deep cervical nodes *Ref: B.D.C, 5th ed. p 191*

- The group of lymph nodes which drain lymph from the teeth are submandibular nodes. Submental lymph nodes drain lymph from tongue and floor of the mouth which could also be considered as appropriate option.
- The entire lymph from head and neck drains ultimately into the deep cervical nodes. So deep cervical nodes is also correct option.
- Retropharyngeal nodes, drain the pharynx, auditory tube, nose and palate. So these nodes does not drain teeth.

126. Ans. (d) Diphyodonts *Ref: Shobha Tandon, 2nd ed. p 88*

Diphyodont	Two sets of teeth	Human beings
Monophyodont	One set of teeth	Sheep, Goat
Polyphyodont	Teeth replaced throughout life	Shark
Homodont	A single type of teeth present	—
Heterodont	Various types of teeth	Human beings
Acrodont	Teeth attached to the jaw by a connective tissue	—
Pleurodont	Teeth are set inside the jaw	—
Thecodont	Teeth are inserted in a bony socket	—

127. Ans. (d) Type IV *Ref: Tencate's, 5th ed. p 69*

Based on their domain organization and other structural features collagens may be categorized as:-

- Fibril-forming collagens represented by types I, II, III, V, XI, XXIV, and XXVII
- Collagens capable of forming hexagonal network (e.g., VIII, X)
- Basement membrane collagens represented by IV collagen.
- Collagens that assemble into beaded filaments (e.g., type VI)
- Anchoring fiber-forming collagens (e.g., VII).
- Plasma membrane-spanning types XIII, XVII, XXIII, and XXV collagens.
- Collagens with unique domain organization, represented by types XV and XVIII.

Type IV collagen:

- It neither form fibrils nor fibers
- It contains frequent non helical sequences.
- It aggregates in a sheet like, chicken wire configuration.

128. Ans. (d) All of the above *Ref: McCracken's Removable partial Prosthodontic, 11th ed. p 208 or Oral Medicine by Ghom, 1st ed. p 462*

When the tooth is lost, there will be:

- Trabecular pattern become less dense in compare to normal.
- There will be loss of height as well as width of alveolar bone.

129. Ans. (b) Intermediate *Ref: Oral Anatomy, Histology and Embryology by Berkovitz, p 254*

The inter articular disk or meniscus is a fibrous tissue and is divided into 3 parts:

- Thicker anterior section called anterior band
- Middle thinnest intermediate zone
- Thickest posterior section called posterior band

130. Ans. (a) Lower level than the occlusal plane of the primary teeth *Ref: BD Chaurasia, 3rd ed. p 32*

The mandibular foramen lies a little above the center of ramus at the level of occlusal surface of the teeth. It leads into the mandibular canal which descends into the body of mandible and opens at mental foramen.

131. Ans. (d) Nonsupporting cusps *Ref: Sturdevant's, 4th ed. p 38*

- Facial occlusal line in the maxillary arch is formed by nonsupporting cusps.

132. Ans. (d) All of the above *Ref: www.ncbi.nlm.nih.gov ›... › J Forensic Dent Sci 2(2); Jul-Dec 2010*

- Dental DNA:
  As DNA can be extracted from any tissue in human
  - Can be extracted from pulp tissue
  - Odontoblast (part of the pulpal tissue)
  - PDL
  - Alveolar bone
- **Dental DNA can be used for:**
  - Individual identification
  - Age identification
  - Sex identification

9 Oral Pathology

DEVELOPMENT AND DISTURBANCES

1. Enamel demineralization starts at pH? *(MHCET 2012)*

a. 3.5–4.5
b. 4.3–4.5
c. 4.9–5.1
d. 5.2–5.5

2. The most initial sign of fluorosis? *(MHCET 2012)*

a. Brown discoloration
b. Enamel opacity
c. Pitting
d. All of the above

3. Hypoplasia due to local trauma: *(MHCET 2012)*

a. Turner's tooth
b. Klinefelter syndrome
c. Turner's syndrome
d. Congenital syndrome

4. Yellow green pigmentation of teeth is seen in? *(MHCET 2012)*

a. Tetracycline
b. Erthroblastosis fetalis
c. Porphyria
d. Internal resorption

5. This condition is due to a defect in the normal keratinization of the oral mucosa: *(COMEDK 2013)*

a. Erythema multiforme
b. White sponge nevus
c. Incontinentia pigment
d. Systemic sclerosis

6. Enlargement of crown at the expense of root is called: *(COMEDK 2013)*

a. Microdontia
b. Dens evaginatus
c. Taurodontism
d. Dens invaginatus

7. In hypodontia, the most commonly affected tooth is: *(COMEDK 2014)*

a. Permanent third molar
b. Permanent second premolar
c. Permanent lateral incisor
d. Permanent Canine

8. The abnormalities of tooth morphology in cleft lip and palate patients are mostly observed in Primary and permanent: *(COMEDK 2014)*

a. Mandibular molars
b. Maxillary incisors
c. Maxillary molars
d. Mandibular incisors

9. Chromosome number related to dentinogenesis imperfecta: *(AIIMS May 2015)*

a. Chromosome no 4
b. Chromosome no 6
c. Chromosome no 10
d. Chromosome no 11

10. Till what age tetracycline should not be given to prevent discoloration? *(AIIMS May 2013)*

a. 3 years
b. 8 years
c. 12 years
d. 18 years

11. Minimum dosage of tetracycline which will show tooth discoloration is: *(AIIMS May 2013)*

a. 5 mg/kg body weight
b. 20 mg/kg body weight
c. 50 mg/kg body weight
d. 80 mg/kg body weight

12. Most characteristic feature of mandibulofacial dysostosis is: *(AIIMS May 2013)*

a. Normal hearing
b. Normal vision with coloboma
c. Mandibular prognathism
d. Vertical maxillary excess

13. Which of the following is true microdontia of lateral incisor? *(AIIMS May 2014)*
a. Peg lateral
b. Natal teeth
c. Mulberry teeth
d. Hutchinson's teeth

14. Patient having extra X chromosomes exhibit: *(AIIMS May 2014)*
a. Dilaceration
b. Taurodontism
c. Cheesy molars
d. Mulburry molars

15. Tooth bud spilts into 2 giving rise to 2 crowns with a single root: *(AIIMS Nov 2012)*
a. Fusion
b. Gemination
c. Concrescene
d. Twinning

16. Non ulcerated, pigmented fast growing lesion on maxillary alveolar ridge of infant is: *(AIIMS Nov 2013)*
a. Oral melanotic macule
b. Rhabdomyoma
c. Melanotic neuroectodermal tumor
d. Congential epulis

17. Which of the following is correct about cleft-lip and cleft palate? *(AIIMS Nov 2014)*
a. Polygenic trait
b. Monogenic trait
c. Multifactorial trait
d. Sex linked trait

18. A 1-year-old male patient normal at the time of birth is having copious discharge, coarse facial features, thick lips, large tongue, large bulging head and flattened nose. On examination it was found that he has enlarged liver and spleen. What will be the diagnosis? *(AIIMS Nov 2014)*
a. Proteus syndrome
b. Hurler's syndrome
c. Hypothyroidism
d. Beckwith - Wiedemann syndrome

19. White discoloration seen on recently erupted permanent central incisor of a child who had suffered injury in deciduous teeth 3 years back. Likely diagnosis is: *(AIPGEE 2013)*
a. Turner hypoplasia
b. Hypophosphatasia
c. Tetracycline stains
d. Pulpal trauma

20. Developmental cysts arise due to: *(AIPGEE 2013)*
a. Inclusion of epithelial cells between embryonic fusion lines
b. Inclusion of bony structures
c. Inclusion of squamous cell between fusion lines
d. Arise from connective tissue

21. A union of the roots of adjacent teeth through the cementum is referred to as: *(AIPGEE 2013)*
a. Fusion
b. Sclerosis
c. Gemination
d. Concrescence

22. Primary enamel hypoplasia is a disturbance of: *(AIPGEE 2013)*
a. Ectoderm
b. Mesoderm
c. Endodoerm
d. Ectoderm and mesoderm

23. Hypodontia seen in all *except*: *(AIPGEE 2013)*
a. Ectodermal dysplasia
b. Osteopetrosis
c. Craniofacial dysostosis
d. Papillon Lefevre syndrome

24. In Down's syndrome, child who is mentally retarded have most probably: *(AIPGEE 2013)*
a. Robertsonian translocation
b. Trisomy 21
c. Mosaicism
d. Deleted 21

25. Taurodontism Bull's teeth are formed by: *(AIPGEE 2014)*
a. Failure of invagination at proper horizontal location of HERS
b. Invagination of stellate reticulum into enamel organ
c. Fusion of the HERS
d. High fluoride content in blood

26. High attachment of tongue's ventral surface to floor of mouth: *(AIPGEE 2014)*
a. Ankyloglossia
b. Microglossia

c. Macroglossia
d. None of the above

27. Supernumerary tooth, tooth within a tooth is most commonly seen in: *(AIPGEE 2014)*
a. Maxillary lateral incisor
b. Mandibular lateral and central incisor
c. Mandibular 2nd premolar
d. Mandibular incisors

28. Hutchinsons triad includes all of the following *except*: *(AIPGEE 2015)*
a. Peg lateral
b. Hypoplasia of molar teeth
c. Eight nerve deafness
d. Interstitial keratitis

29. Endoderm, mesoderm and ectoderm all germ layers are present in which of the following? *(AIPGEE 2015)*
a. Teratoma
b. Dermoid cyst
c. Radicular cyst
d. Ameloblastoma

30. A patient has normal maxillary and mandibular primary teeth but permanent teeth in maxillary and mandibular anterior region are smaller than normal. Which of the following is true about it? *(AIPGEE 2015)*
a. Hypomaturation
b. Hypocalcification
c. Generalized developmental
d. Focal developmental

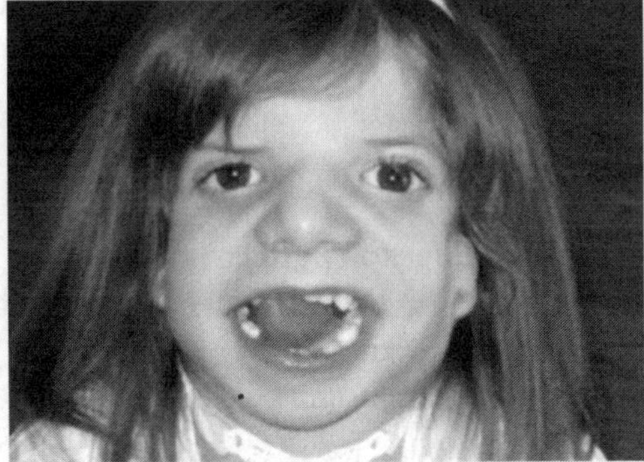

31. What is the most likely condition depicted above? *(Andhra Pradesh 2015)*
a. Downs syndrome
b. Williams syndrome
c. Treacher Collins syndrome
d. Pierre Robin syndrome

32. Parry Romberg syndrome is associated with: *(Andhra Pradesh 2015)*
a. Hemifacial atrophy b. Micrognathia
c. Cleft palate d. Small tongue

33. The syndrome associated with predisposition for squamous cell carcinoma of pharyngeal region is: *(Andhra Pradesh 2015)*
a. Osler-Weber-Rendu syndrome
b. Plummer-Vinson syndrome
c. Sturge-Weber syndrome
d. Turners syndrome

34. Delayed eruption of teeth is seen in all the following conditions *except*: *(Andhra Pradesh 2015)*
a. De lange syndrome
b. Gardner's syndrome
c. Hyperthyroidism
d. Chondroectodermal dysplasia

35. Melkersson-Rosenthal syndrome does not have: *(J&K 2015)*
a. Facial paralysis b. Hemifacial hypotrophy
c. Scrotal tongue d. Cheilitis granulomatosa

36. 'Mottled enamel' in dental fluorosis is due to: *(J&K 2015)*
a. Excess fluoride affecting the ameloblasts during the tooth formations stage
b. Excess fluoride affecting the odontoblasts during the tooth formation stage
c. Decreased ingestion of fluoride affecting both ameloblasts and odontoblasts during the tooth formation stage
d. None of the above

37. Following are true about thyroglossal cyst *except*:
a. Often occur in children; they may also present in adults
b. Rarely may contain only functioning thyroid tissue
c. Treated surgically by Sistrunks operation
d. Moves downwards on tongue protrusion

38. The characteristic histological appearance of 'Lava flowing around boulders' is seen in:
a. Dentinogenesis imperfecta
b. Amelogenesis imperfecta
c. Regional odontodysplasia
d. Dentin dysplasia

39. Eagle's syndrome is characterized by: *(AB Shetty 2015)*
a. Elongation of mastoid process
b. Elongation of styloid process
c. Absence of cingulum on incisors
d. Osteomalacia

40. Neonatal teeth are those teeth which: *(AB Shetty 2015)*
a. Are present during birth
b. Indicate abnormal erupting pattern
c. Erupt during first 30 days after birth
d. None of these

41. In amelogenesis imperfecta, the defects are primarily seen in: *(AB Shetty 2015)*
a. Dentine b. Enamel
c. Cementum d. Entire root

42. Dens evaginatus is characterized by: *(AB Shetty 2015)*
a. Dentin dysplasia
b. Enamel cracks
c. Dentinal hypersensitivity
d. Accessory cusp

43. The gene most commonly associated with carcino facial dysostosis is: *(AB Shetty 2015)*
a. Hox gene
b. Fibroblasts growth factor receptor 2 and 3
c. Epithelial growth factor
d. ROR 2 gene

44. One of the features of Pierre Robin syndrome is: *(AB Shetty 2015)*
a. Mandibular micrognathia
b. Maxillary vertical excess
c. Mandibular prognathia
d. Mandibular asymmetry

45. Turner's tooth is most common feature of which permanent teeth? *(Tamil Nadu 2015)*
a. Maxillary central incisor
b. Maxillary canine
c. Maxillary premolar
d. Mandibular molar

46. Ghost teeth are seen in: *(Tamil Nadu 2015)*
a. Regional odontodysplasia
b. Amelogenesis imperfecta
c. Dentinogenesis imperfecta
d. Dentin dysplasia

47. Natal teeth is the teeth which: *(Tamil Nadu 2015)*
a. Erupts within 30 days after birth
b. Erupts at birth
c. Erupts within a year after birth
d. Erupts within 90 days after birth

48. Bohn's nodules are typically seen in: *(AB Shetty 2015)*
a. New born babies
b. Old people with edentulous arch
c. Young children in the age of 3 to 7 years
d. Women during pregnancy

BENIGN AND MALIGNANT TUMORS

49. Benign lymphoepithelial lesion is seen in: *(MHCET 2012)*
a. Mikulicz disease
b. Kimura's disease
c. Kuttner tumor
d. Hodgkin's disease

50. Fibroma combined with glandular tissue is: *(COMEDK 2013)*
a. Neurofibroma
b. Fibroademona
c. Fibrolipoma
d. Fibromyoma

51. A 13-year-old boy presents with a large mixed lytic and blastic mass in the metaphyseal region of the lower end of femur. The most likely diagnosis is: *(COMEDK 2013)*
a. Ewing's sarcoma
b. Osteosarcoma
c. Chondrosarcoma
d. Giant cell tumor

52. Sun burst radiograph pattern is seen in? *(COMEDK 2014)*
a. Osteogenic sarcoma
b. Osteogenic carcinoma
c. Ameloblastoma
d. Fibrous dysplasia

53. The most common variety of soft tissues sarcoma is: *(COMEDK 2014)*
a. Rhabdomyosarcoma
b. Liposarcoma

c. Malignant fibrous histiocytoma
d. Synovial sarcoma

54. Kiolocytes are seen in all *except*: *(MHCET 2014)*
a. Verruca vulgaris
b. Condyloma accuminatum
c. Actinic keratosis
d. Squamous papilloma

55. Which is low grade malignancy of salivary gland? *(AIIMS May 2015)*
a. Ductal adenocarcinoma
b. Acinic cell carcinoma
c. Pleomorphic adenoma
d. Mucoepidermoid carcinoma

56. A 35-year-old patient is diagnosed with class III development with mandibular deviation, developing crossbite, spicule growth on right condyle with increased radiopacity and pointing toward lateral pterygoid muscle. Most likely the diagnosis is: *(AIIMS Nov 2012)*
a. Osteoma
b. Osteoid osteoma
c. Osteochondroma
d. Condylar hyperplasia

57. A patient comes with less than 2 cm bony swelling which is associated with severe pain and the pain responds to salicylates. The most probable diagnosis of the swelling is: *(AIIMS Nov 2012)*
a. Osteoma
b. Osteoid osteoma
c. Osteochondroma
d. Osteoblastoma

58. Commonly used staging system for tumor, TNM system. The TNM stands for: *(AIIMS Nov 2014)*
a. Tumor necrosis metastasis
b. Tumor node metastasis
c. Tumor node malformation
d. Treatment node metastasis

59. Tobacco chewer and smoker develop oral cancer. Biopsy of oral ulcer histologically similar to: *(AIPGEE 2013)*
a. Adenocarcinoma
b. Squamous cell carcinoma
c. Oat cell carcinoma
d. Verrucous carcinoma

60. A child is having pedunclated, exophytic, irregular, finger-like projection and hyperkeratotic lesion seen on lower lip, same type of lesion is observed on dorsal side of left thumb and on right side of thumb. The most likely diagnosis is: *(AIPGEE 2014)*
a. Papilloma
b. Carcinoma in situ
c. Keratoacanthoma
d. Verrucous carcinoma

61. A patient with osteomas of bone, desmoids tumors, multiple polyposis of large intestine, supernumerary tooth: *(AIPGEE 2014)*
a. Cowden syndrome
b. Pierre Jegher's syndrome
c. Perie-Robbin syndrome
d. Gardner's syndrome

62. The picture depicts which one of the following conditions: *(Andhra Pradesh 2015)*

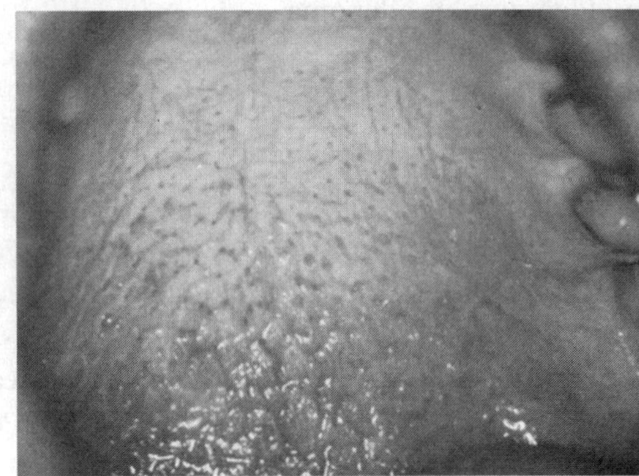

a. Denture stomatitis
b. Nicotinic stomatitis
c. Amyloidosis
d. Leukoplakia

63. 'Swiss cheese' pattern is seen in: *(J&K 2015)*
a. Adenoid cystic carcinoma
b. Pleomorphic adenoma
c. Warthin tumor
d. Mikulicz's disease

64. Bull's eye appearance could be seen in which of the following lesion radiographically: *(J&K 2015)*
a. Osteoblastoma
b. Cementoblastoma
c. Osteoid osteoma
d. Osteopetrosis

65. Which among the following tumors will have coarse, curved septa which originates from the normal bone that has been trapped within the bone? The septa can remodel into curved shapes providing a radiographic honeycomb or soap bubble pattern: *(J&K 2015)*
a. Odontogenic myxoma
b. Radicular cyst
c. Adenomatoid odontogenic tumor
d. Ameloblastoma

66. Tumor which spreads through perineural space is: *(J&K 2015)*
a. Pleomorphic adenoma
b. Basal cell carcinoma
c. Adenoid cystic carcinoma
d. Canalicular adenoma

67. Epithelial myoepithelium most commonly resembles ____ histologically: *(J&K 2015)*
a. Mucoepidermoid carcinoma
b. Pleomorphic adenoma
c. Adenocarcinoma
d. Mucus retention cyst

68. Verocaxy bodies are seen in:
a. Traumatic neuroma
b. Ameloblastoma
c. Schwannoma
d. Metastatic carcinoma

69. Longitudinal ridging of nails is usually seen in cases of: *(AB Shetty 2015)*
a. Lichen planus
b. Iron deficiency
c. Neurofibromatosis
d. Psoriasis

70. Reed Sternberg cells are characteristic of: *(AB Shetty 2015)*
a. Megaloblastc anemia
b. Non-Hodgkin's lymphoma
c. Hodgkin's disease
d. Pernicious anemia

71. Which of the following is true about smoking associated melanosis? *(AB Shetty 2015)*
a. It affects men more than women
b. More commonly seen in floor of the mouth
c. It affects females more commonly than males
d. None of these

72. 'Spindle cell carcinoma' is a type of: *(AB Shetty 2015)*
a. Basal cell carcinoma
b. Squamous cell carcinoma
c. Melanoma
d. Osteosarcoma

73. Which of the following otherwise called as *Phakomatosis* Or *Phakomatosis* is seen with association of? *(Tamil Nadu 2015)*
a. Sturge-Weber syndrome
b. Angiosarcoma
c. Nasopharyngeal sarcoma
d. Hemangioma

74. Absence of C1-esterase inhibitor leads to: *(Tamil Nadu 2015)*
a. Angioneuroticedema
b. Leukoedema
c. Angiofibroticedema
d. Papillary cystadenoma

75. Which of these locations has high potential for malignancy in leukoplakia? *(Tamil Nadu 2015)*
a. Floor of mouth b. Buccal mucosa
c. Lip d. Gingivobuccal complex

76. Rodent ulcer is other name for: *(Tamil Nadu 2015)*
a. Basal cell carcinoma
b. Squamous cell carcinoma
c. Adenocarcinoma
d. Verrucous carcinoma

77. Grading of tumor is based on: *(Tamil Nadu 2015)*
a. Metastasis
b. Histological differentiation
c. Tumor size of primary tumor
d. All of the above

78. Lip cancer most common in: *(Tamil Nadu 2015)*
a. Upper lip b. Lower lip
c. Commisures d. Labial mucosa

SALIVARY GLAND

79. A salivary gland tumor which histologically shows a double layer of epithelial cells based on a reactive lymphoid stroma is: *(COMEDK 2013)*
a. Pleomorphic adenoma
b. Mucoepidermoid carcinoma

c. Acinic cell tumor
d. Warthin tumor

80. Intra oral pleomorphic adenoma usually occurs in: *(COMEDK 2013)*
a. Buccal mucosa
b. Upper lip
c. Floor of the mouth
d. Palate

81. Commonest tumor of parotid salivary gland is: *(COMEDK 2013)*
a. Pleomorphic adenoma
b. Warthin tumor
c. Acinic cell carcinoma
d. Mucoepidermoid carcinoma

82. Most common malignant tumor of parotid gland: *(AIIMS Nov 2012)*
a. Mucoepidermoid CA
b. Pleomorphic adenoma
c. Odontogenic myxoma
d. Adenoid cystic carcinoma

83. The salivary gland tumor which is associated with smoking: *(Andhra Pradesh 2015)*
a. Ductal papilloma
b. Cannicular adenoma
c. Warthin tumor
d. Pleomorphic adenoma

84. The soft, fluctuating, transluscent bluish lesion depicted in the following picture could be due to: *(Andhra Pradesh 2015)*
a. Ranula b. Mucocoele
c. Gingival cyst d. Hemangioma

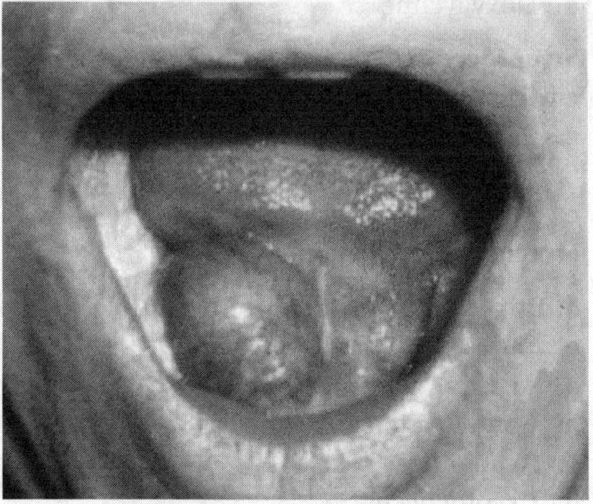

85. Sialolith found in salivary glands are primarily composed of: *(Andhra Pradesh 2015)*
a. Zinc apatite
b. Fluoroapatite
c. Hydroxyapatite
d. Potassium apatite

86. Which is a benign, self-limiting, reactive, inflammatory disorder of the salivary glands? *(Andhra Pradesh 2015)*
a. Extravasation mucocoele
b. Allergic sialadenitis
c. Chronic sclerosing sialadenitis
d. Necrotizing sialometaplasia

87. The most common salivary gland tumor is: *(AB Shetty 2015)*
a. Mucoepidermoid carcinoma
b. Warthin tumor
c. Adenoid cystic carcinoma
d. Pleomorphic adenoma

88. Papillary cystadenoma Lymphatosum seen in which salivary gland: *(TAMIL NADU 2015)*
a. Parotid
b. Submandibular
c. Sublingual
d. Minor salivary glands

BACTERIAL, VIRAL AND MYCOTIC INFECTIONS

89. Critical pH of saliva below this pH, the inorganic material of the tooth may dissolve in caries. The critical pH value is: *(COMEDK 2013)*
a. 6.5 b. 5.5
c. 7.5 d. 6.0

90. The sugar implicated in the etiology of dental caries is: *(COMEDK 2013)*
a. Glucose b. Fructose
c. Maltose d. Sucrose

91. Ludwig's angina is caused due to pus collection in? *(COMEDK 2014)*
a. Submandibular region
b. Parotid region
c. Cardiac muscle
d. Nasal cavity

92. Gingival enlargement is associated with? *(COMEDK 2014)*

a. Anemia
b. Hyperpigmentation
c. Leukemia
d. Hyperthyroidism

93. Antibiotic stomatitis is the other name for: *(COMEDK 2014)*

a. Acute atrophic candidiasis
b. Chronic atrophic candidiasis
c. Chronic hyperplastic candidiasis
d. Acute pseudomembranous candidiasis

94. The explosive and widespread form of secondary syphilis in immune-compromised individual is known as: *(COMEDK 2014)*

a. Condylomatalata
b. Mucous patches
c. Lues maligna
d. Lupus vulgaris

95. Pastia lines in scarlet fever are: *(MHCET 2014)*

a. White lines on the dorsum of tongue
b. Seen bilaterally on the buccal mucosa
c. Present on the skin fold secondary to capillary fragility
d. Seen when white and red strawberry tongue is seen simultaneously

96. Patient with oral bullae on H/E examination ballooning degeneration is present, lipschutz bodies and nucleons 5–8 microns is seen what is the diagnosis? *(AIIMS May 2015)*

a. Oral herpes
b. Herpangina
c. Kala azar
d. Herpes zoster

97. Condition which is unusual to have gingival involvement? *(AIIMS May 2014)*

a. Pyogenic granuloma
b. Primary herpes
c. Pemphigoid
d. Recurrent aphthae

98. Specific auto-inoculation is seen in which of the following? *(AIIMS May 2014)*

a. Human papilloma virus
b. Ameloblastoma
c. Bullous pemphigoid
d. Lichen planus

99. Median rhomboid glossitis is due to? *(AIIMS May 2014)*

a. Atrophy of filliform papillae
b. Absence of fungiform papillae
c. Ectodermal covering with absence of mucosa
d. Non-fusion of mesodermal thickening and retraction of tuberculum impar

100. Primary herpes can be best diagnosed by: *(AIIMS Nov 2012)*

a. Smear stained by Giemsa staining
b. Fluorescent staining
c. Smear by routine cytology staining
d. Smear stained by Wright's stain

101. Which of the following is an unusual finding in gingiva? *(AIIMS Nov 2012)*

a. Primary herpes
b. Recurrent aphthae
c. Pyogenic granuloma
d. Erythema multiforme

102. White patch seen on buccal mucosa consisting of pseudomycelia and chlamydospores with desquamated epithelium seen under microscope is suggestive of: *(AIIMS Nov 2012)*

a. Candidiasis
b. Histoplasmosis
c. Sporothrix infection
d. Cryptococcosis

103. Patient diagnosed with trench mouth. Antibiotic of choice: *(AIIMS Nov 2012)*

a. Penicillin + H_2O_2 mouthwash
b. Chloramphenicol
c. Tetracycline
d. Doxycycline

104. Streptoccocus differ by other bacteria in causing caries, in: *(AIPGEE 2013)*

a. Production of extracellular polysaccharides
b. Acid production
c. Mannitol fermentation
d. Sucrose fermentation

105. Multiple sinus at angle of mandible with yellow granules in them, diagnosis is: *(AIPGEE 2013)*

a. Actinomycosis
b. Candida albicans
c. Aspergillus
d. Cryptococcus

106. Fever blisters are due to: *(AIPGEE 2014)*
a. Primary infection of herpes simplex
b. Varicella zoster
c. CMV
d. Reactivation of HSV 1

107. Primary herpes zoster is caused by: *(AIPGEE 2014)*
a. Varicella zoster b. CMV
c. EBV d. Herpes virus

108. In which of the following angular cheilitis may be seen: *(AIPGEE 2014)*
a. Human papilloma virus
b. Candida albicans
c. Tuberculosis
d. CMV

109. Herpetic paronychia is the involvement of the: *(AIPGEE 2015)*
a. Nail b. Skin
c. Hair d. Tongue

110. HIV affects by altering: *(AIPGEE 2015)*
a. Ratio of helper T cell to NK cell
b. Ratio of T cell to B cell
c. Degree of T cells
d. Ratio of CD4 cells to CD8 cells

111. Which of the following have the association between hepatitis C? *(AIPGEE 2015)*
a. Lichen planus b. Leukoplakia
c. Gingivitis d. Erythroplakia

112. Which of the following is the viral disease of parotid gland but it usually affect only once in a lifetime? *(AIPGEE 2015)*
a. Mumps b. Herpes simplex
c. Secondary herpes d. Sjögren's syndrome

113. Molluscum contagiosum is a: *(Andhra Pradesh 2015)*
a. Ricketsial disease b. Bacterial disease
c. Fungal disease d. Viral disease

114. The feature that distinguishes lesions of herpes zoster from other vesiculo bullous lesions is: *(Andhra Pradesh 2015)*
a. Prominent crusting of vesicles
b. Subepidermal bulla formation
c. Severe burning pain
d. They are unilateral

115. One of the following cells are HPV virus altered cells: *(Andhra Pradesh 2015)*
a. Giant cells
b. Target cells
c. Keratinocytes
d. Koilocytes

116. Noma is: *(Andhra Pradesh 2015)*
a. Fibrous dysplasia
b. Pyogenic granuloma
c. Vincents angina
d. Cancrum oris

117. Mycosis fungoides is a: *(Andhra Pradesh 2015)*
a. Fungal infection
b. T cell lymphoma
c. Papillitis
d. Paracytic infection

118. Which of the following is not a type of candidiasis? *(J&K 2015)*
a. Chronic plaque type non-scrapable
b. Median rhomboid glossitis
c. Plaque type
d. Angular chelitis

119. Higoumenaki's sign is seen in: *(Kerala 2015)*
a. AIDS
b. Infective endocarditis
c. Fracture mandible
d. Congenital syphilis

120. 'Mickey mouse ears' is a histological feature of: *(Kerala 2015)*
a. Candidiasis
b. Paracoccidioidomycosis
c. Leptospirosis
d. Tuberculosis

121. The causative organism of oral hairy leukoplakia is: *(Kerala 2015)*
a. Herpes simples virus
b. Epstein barr virus
c. Human immunodeficiency virus
d. Mucor species

122. Which of the following viruses have been implicated in the pathogenesis of some head and neck cancer? *(AB Shetty 2015)*
a. Human papilloma b. Epstein Barr
c. Both a and b d. None of these

123. Cancrum oris is otherwise called as: *(AB Shetty 2015)*
a. Oral cancer
b. Chronic ulcerative gingivitis
c. Noma
d. Chronic periodontitis

124. Herpes simplex infection of oral cavity is predominantly caused by virus: *(AB Shetty 2015)*
a. HSV-1
b. HSV-2
c. HSV-3
d. HSV-4

125. 'Osteoradionecrosis' is: *(AB Shetty 2015)*
a. A form of osteomyelitis
b. A form of necrosis caused following heavy dose of radiation
c. Characterized by painful infection
d. All of these

126. Unerupted teeth are not affected by caries because: *(AB Shetty 2015)*
a. Host defense mechanism
b. Presence of Nasmyth's membrane
c. They are free from bacterial infection
d. None of these

127. 'Mulberry molars' is a characteristic feature of: *(AB Shetty 2015)*
a. Acquired syphilis
b. Ectodermal dysplasia
c. Congenital syphilis
d. Amelogenesis imperfecta

128. Mild mucositis is defined as: *(AB Shetty 2015)*
a. Severe erythema, no ulceration, mild pain
b. No erythema, mild ulceration, no pain
c. Mild erythema, no ulceration, mild pain
d. None of these

129. The first evidence of caries activity in enamel is: *(M.P. 2015)*
a. Black discoloration
b. Catch on probing
c. White spot lesion
d. Radiolucency in radiograph

130. A condition which has been found in approximately 90% of AIDS patients is: *(M.P. 2015)*
a. Oral candidiasis
b. Oral hairy leukoplakia
c. Kaposi's sarcoma
d. Atypical ulcers

131. Hand foot and mouth disease is caused by: *(TAMIL NADU 2015)*
a. CAV 16
b. CAV 9
c. CAV 10
d. CAV 4

132. Koplik spots seen in:
a. Measles
b. Mumps
c. Herpangina
d. Rubella

PULP AND PERIAPICAL TISSUE

133. A 25-year-old male comes with a complaint of throbbing pain in the upper part of the cheek or entire side of face, heavy feeling in the face, which exacerbates on bending down and with associated pyrexia. The most probable diagnosis is: *(COMEDK 2013)*
a. Acute dento alveolar abscess in relation to upper 2nd molar
b. Irreversible pulpitis in relation to upper 2nd molar
c. Acute maxillary sinusitis
d. Acute periodontal abscess in relation to upper molar

134. In a pericoronal abscess related to distoangular impacted third molar, the infection may spread to: *(COMEDK 2013)*
a. Submasseteric space
b. Buccal space
c. Sublingual space
d. Submental space

135. Serum alkaline phosphatase in increased in all *except*: *(AIIMS Nov 2012)*
a. Paget's disease
b. Fibrous dysplasia
c. Osteomyelitis
d. Hyperparathyroidism

136. A 15-year patient with mild pain in 46 region, radiograph shows mild expansion of cortical bone, cortex is intact and onion skin appearance is: *(AIPGEE 2014)*
a. Ewing's sarcoma
b. Osteosarcoma
c. Periostitis ossificans
d. Not recalled

137. True about involcrum in osteomyelitis? *(AIPGEE 2014)*
a. Extracted dead bone
b. Newly formed bone surrounding dead bone

c. New bone fill the cavity space
d. Dead bone covered by new bone

PHYSICAL AND CHEMICAL INJURY

DISEASE OF BONE AND JOINT

138. Serum alkaline phosphatase level is elevated in: *(COMEDK 2013)*
a. Paget's disease
b. Infantile cortical hyperostosis
c. Cleidocranial dysplasia
d. Pierre Robin syndrome

139. Blue sclera may be seen in all type of osteogenesis imperfect *except*: *(MHCET 2014)*
a. type I
b. type II
c. type III
d. type IV

140. True about papillon leferve syndrome is: *(MHCET 2014)*
a. Autosomal dominant disorder
b. Characterized by palmer planter hyperkeratosis
c. Mutation in cathepsin C gene
d. All of the above

141. Bilateral mandibular involvement seen in: *(AIIMS May 2014)*
a. Cherubism
b. Osteoma
c. Central giant cell granuloma
d. Lichen planus

142. In case of brittle bone syndrome, defect lies in: *(AIIMS Nov 2012)*
a. Procollagen synthesis/production of collagen
b. Decreased bone formation
c. Increased osteoclastic activity
d. Polymerization of collagen

143. Osteosarcoma can arise from? *(AIPGEE 2014)*
a. Paget and cherubism
b. Cherubism and osteopetrosis
c. Paget and polyostotic fibrous dysplasia
d. Polyostotic fibrous dyplasia and cherubism

144. How can you distinguish between fibrous dysplasia and hemifacial hypertrophy? *(AIPGEE 2014)*
a. Changes in face size
b. Size of tooth and rate of eruption
c. Difference in the distance between anatomical soft tissue landmarks relative to midline
d. Change in palatal structures

145. A 30-year-old patient having chronic pain of long duration with radiographic appearance of endosteal bone formation and sclerosed bone is likely to be: *(AIPGEE 2014)*
a. Ewing's sarcoma
b. Garry's osteomyelitis
c. Chronic focal sclerosing osteomyelitis
d. Acute osteomyelitis

146. Ectodermal dysplasia is characterized by: *(Bihar 2015)*
a. Xerostomia
b. Microdontia
c. Anodontia
d. Moist skin

147. Most common complication of rheumatoid arthritis involving TMJ is: *(J&K 2015)*
a. Ankylosis
b. Subluxation
c. Osteoma of condyle
d. Recurrent dislocation

BLOOD DISEASE

148. Oral and dermal manifestations are seen in which type of leukemia? *(AIPGEE 2014)*
a. Aleukemic leukemia
b. Monocytic leukemia
c. Lymphocytic leukemia
d. Myelocytic leukemia

149. Christmas disease is due to deficiency of: *(AIPGEE 2014)*
a. Hageman factor
b. Platelets
c. Plasma thromboplastin antecedent
d. Plasma thromboplastin component

150. Cooley's Anemia is also known as: *(AIPGEE 2014)*
a. Beta thalassemia major
b. Beta thalassemia minor
c. Pernicious anemia
d. Aplastic anemia

151. _____ is also referred as the 'disease of kings': *(AB Shetty 2015)*
a. Hemophilia
b. Hodgkin's lymphoma
c. Leukoplakia
d. Thrombocytopenia

SKIN DISEASE

152. Lesion seen in erythema multiforme minor? *(MHCET 2012)*
a. No skin involvement
b. Less than 10% skin involvement
c. More than 10% skin involvement
d. Depends on the severity of the disease

153. A lady comes to the clinic with a 11-year-old child complaining of recurent ulcers in the mouth since previous some days and also complains of desquamation on hand and feet. Patient should be checked for which of the following dermatological disease? *(AIPGEE 2015)*
a. Psoriasis b. DLE
c. SLE d. Phemphigoid

154. Among which of the following disorders, high values of anti-smith antibodies and ANA could be appreciated together? *(J&K 2015)*
a. Rheumatoid arthritis
b. Systemic sclerosis
c. Mixed connective tissue disorder
d. SLE

155. A positive pathergy test, erythema nodosum genital ulceration are components of which of the following syndrome? *(J&K 2015)*
a. MAGIC syndrome b. PFAPA syndrome
c. Sweet's syndrome d. Bechet's syndrome

156. Gorlin sign is appreciated in which of the following syndrome? *(J&K 2015)*
a. Ehlers-Danlos syndrome
b. Osler-Weber-Rendu syndrome
c. Darier's disease
d. Cole-Engman syndrome

157. 'Suprabasilar split' is a characteristic feature of:
a. Bullous pemphigoid
b. Systemic sclerosis
c. Oral submucous fibrosis
d. Pemphigus vulgaris

158. Pemphigus is characterized by: *(AB Shetty 2015)*
a. Acanthosis
b. Hyperorthokeratosis
c. Acantholysis
d. Hyperparakeratosis

159. Erythema multiforme is: *(AB Shetty 2015)*
a. A bacterial infection
b. Acute inflammatory disease
c. Viral disease
d. Neoplastic disorder

160. 'TARGET' or 'IRIS' lesions are pathognomonic of which of the following disease? *(M.P. 2015)*
a. Lichen planus b. Erythema multiforme
c. RAS d. ANUG

DISEASE OF NERVE AND MUSCLE

161. Transcutaneous electrical nerve stimulation is a treatment modality for: *(Andhra Pradesh 2015)*
a. Myofascial pain
b. Subcondylar fractures
c. Internal derangement of TM joint
d. Scleroderma

162. Features of trigeminal neuralgia do not include: *(Andhra Pradesh 2015)*
a. Paresthesia
b. Refractory period
c. Presence of trigger zone
d. Paroxysmal pain

ODONTOGENIC CYST AND TUMOR

163. Not an odontogenic tumor? *(MHCET 2012)*
a. Osteoid osteoma
b. Lipoma
c. Giant cell tumor
d. All of the above

164. Corrugated collagenous rings surrounding lymphocytes and plasma cells in the wall of inflammatory cyst are: *(MHCET 2014)*
a. Hyaline bodies
b. Rushton bodies
c. Howell-Jolly bodies
d. Papenhiemer bodies

165. The cyst that remains behind after the removal of the tooth is: *(MHCET 2014)*
a. Lateral periodontal cyst
b. Residual cyst
c. Radicular cyst
d. None of the above

166. Most common cyst associated with adjoining vital teeth? *(AIIMS May 2014)*

a. Periapical cyst b. Globulomaxillary cyst
c. Lateral cyst d. Dentigerous cyst

167. A 40 years old lady presents with ameloblastoma in mandibular molar region. Histopathological features reveal: *(AIIMS Nov 2012)*

a. Central loose tissue with mitotic figures
b. Peripheral palisading cells with central loose stellate reticulum
c. Peripheral palisading cells with artifact stroma
d. Central palisading cells which fails to differentiate

168. Histologic feature of ameloblastoma: *(AIIMS Nov 2012)*

a. Peripheral palisading epithelium with central loose stratum intermedium
b. Central loose tissue with mitotic figures
c. Stellate reticulum in center with mitotic bodies with dysplastic features
d. Palisading peripheral epithelium with artefacts

169. A middle age male patient came with the swelling in lower right posterior region of the jaw. On histopathologic examination it was diagnosed as ameloblastoma. Which of the following histological picture is likely to be present? *(AIIMS Nov 2014)*

a. Central loose stellate reticulum shows marked nuclear atypia and numerous mitotic figure
b. Peripheral palisading with central loose stellate reticulum
c. Peripheral palisading with central stroma retraction artifact
d. Central palisading cells which fails to differentiate

170. Most aggressive type of cyst causing the hollowing of the mandible: *(AIPGEE 2012)*

a. Dentigerous cyst
b. Periapical cyst
c. Incisive canal cyst
d. Globulomaxillary cyst

171. Which one is also called as premaxillary maxillary cyst? *(AIPGEE 2012)*

a. Globulomaxillary cyst
b. Nasoplatine duct cyst
c. Median palatal cyst
d. Traumatic bone cyst

172. Most potential aggressive and destructive cyst: *(AIPGEE 2013)*

a. Dentigerous cyst
b. Globulomaxillary cyst
c. Periapical cyst
d. Incisive canal cyst

173. Cyst present along the median raphe of hard palate and appeared to arise from entrapped epithelial remnants? *(AIPGEE 2014)*

a. Epstein pearls
b. Dental lamina
c. Bohn's nodules
d. Gingival cyst of adult

174. Cyst arising due to degeneration of stellate reticulum in place of tooth? *(AIPGEE 2014)*

a. Primordial cyst
b. Dentigerous cyst
c. Lateral periodontal cyst
d. Globulomaxillary cyst

175. Which of the following is not true about dentigerous cyst? *(AIPGEE 2015)*

a. Associated with erupted third molar
b. OPG is diagnostic for it
c. Usually unilocular swelling
d. Multiple dentigerous cysts associated with impacted tooth

176. Radicular cyst is often associated with: *(Andhra Pradesh 2015)*

a. Pericoronal infection
b. Non-vital tooth
c. Vital tooth
d. Teeth with deep caries

177. Eruption cyst or hematoma is a type of: *(J&K 2015)*

a. Odontogenic keratocyst
b. Primordial cyst
c. Fibroma
d. Dentigerous cyst

178. The odontogenic cyst which is associated with the nevoid basal cell carcinoma syndrome is:

a. Radicular cyst
b. Dentigerous cyst
c. Odontogenic keratocyst
d. Nasopalatine cyst

179. The most common odontogenic cyst is: *(AB Shetty 2015)*
a. The periapical (radicular cyst)
b. Dentigerous cyst
c. Calcifying odontogenic cyst
d. Eruption cyst

180. 'Pindborg' tumor is otherwise known as: *(AB Shetty 2015)*
a. Periapical ameoblastoma
b. Adenoameloblastoma
c. Calcifying epithelial odontogenic tumor
d. Ameloblastic fibroma

181. 'Rushton bodies' are usually seen in: *(AB Shetty 2015)*
a. Ameloblastoma
b. Squamous cell carcinoma of tongue
c. Dentigerous cyst
d. Paget's disease

REGRESSIVE ALTERATION OF TEETH

182. The term Localized acute Alveolar Osteomyelitis is also used to describe: *(COMEDK 2014)*
a. Dry socket
b. Garre's osteomyelitis
c. Sclerotic cemental masses
d. Florid osseous dysplasia

183. In a patient there are some cavities on cervical aspect of the tooth with some fracture line over the tooth surface. Which of the following is the most probable diagnosis? *(AIPGEE 2015)*
a. Non-carious cervical lesion
b. Abfraction
c. Abrasion
d. Erosion

184. 'Pink spot' is associated with: *(J&K 2015)*
a. External resorption b. Internal resorption
c. Pulpal necrosis d. Root resorption

185. Pink disease is caused due to toxicity of which metal?
a. Mercury b. Silver
c. Lead d. Bismuth

MISCELLANEOUS

186. In biopsy true about formalin as fixative is all *except*: *(AIIMS May 2013)*
a. To prevent autolysis
b. To make tissue rigid
c. To kill micro organisms
d. 2% formalin is used

187. The tooth with epithelial structure at level of the alveolar gingiva in two-month-old child without any radiographic evidence of roots. Treatment is: *(AIIMS May 2014)*
a. Surgically remove it under LA
b. Let it remain as it is future tooth and root formation occurs at around 6 months
c. Preserve it and reassure the parents
d. Extract if mobile under GA

188. The fixative used in histopathalogy: *(AIIMS Nov 2014)*
a. 10% buffered neutral formalin
b. Bouins fixative
c. Glutarldehyde
d. Ethyl alcohol

189. Painful sensation from non-noxious stimuli is: *(AIPGEE 2013)*
a. Allodynia b. Hyperesthesia
c. Dysthesisa d. Paresthesia

190. Riga-Fede disease is associated with? *(AIPGEE 2014)*
a. Natal teeth b. Multiple impacted teeth
c. Permanent incisor d. Primary incisor

191. A patient complains of pain and redness in all over the mouth after using the new tooth paste few days back which of the following is the treatment of choice for this patient? *(AIPGEE 2015)*
a. Topical beclamethasone
b. Topical antifungal agents
c. Topical triclosan
d. Antibiotic administration

192. Which of the following is true regarding brush cytology? *(AIPGEE 2015)*
a. Tissue obtained by using the brush at the border and rotating 1 or 2 turns
b. Tissue obtained by using the brush at the border and rotating 7 or 8 turns
c. In the center of lesion till bleeding occurs
d. Tissue obtained by rubbing the brush on wound

193. Which of the following type of epithelium is present over tongue? *(J&K 2015)*
a. Keratinized specialized
b. Non-keratinized specialized
c. Keratinized stratified
d. Non-keratinized stratified specialized

194. The clinical condition shown by the arrow in the below picture depicts: *(Andhra Pradesh 2015)*
a. Amalgam tattoo b. Late ecchymotic lesion
c. Necrosis of gingiva d. Pigmentation

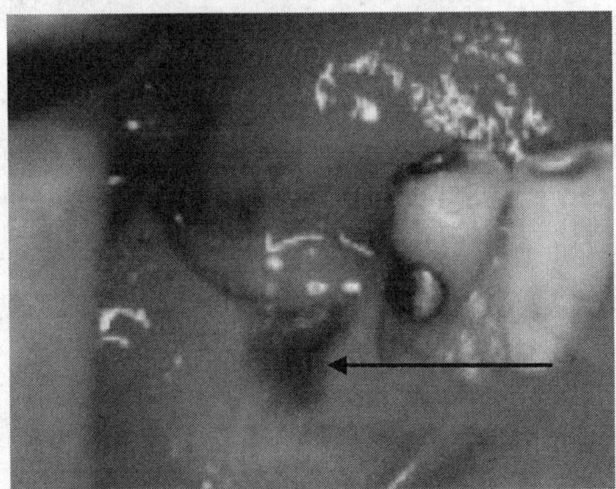

195. The study of tooth prints is also called as:
a. Dermatoglyphics
b. Ameloglyphics
c. Dentinoglyphics
d. Cementopglyphics

196. Dental profiling is also called as:
a. Comparative identification
b. Reconstructive identification
c. Positive identification
d. Oral autopsy

197. Which one of the following is a metric dental feature?
a. Shovelling
b. Caravelli's trait
c. Mandibular moral groove pattern
d. Root length of maxillary canine

198. 'Pyostomatitisvegetans' could be a oral manifestation of:
a. Coronary artery disease
b. Ulcerative colitis
c. Chronic kidney disease
d. Transient bacteremia

ORAL ASPECT OF METABOLIC DISEASE

199. Osteitis fibroma cystica: *(MHCET 2012)*
a. Associated with hypoparathyrodism
b. Associated with hyperparathyrodism
c. Associated with Paget's disease
d. Seen in cherubism

200. Giant cells lesions and loss of lamina dura is seen in: *(MHCET 2012)*
a. Hyperparathyroidism
b. Hypothyroidism
c. Hyperthyroidism
d. Hypoparathyroidism

201. The protein found in the amyloid deposits in senile systemic amyloidosis is: *(COMEDK 2013)*
a. AL protein b. α2 microglobulin
c. α amyloid protein d. Transthyretin

202. Brown tumor: *(AIPGEE 2013)*
a. Hyperparathyroidism
b. Pigmented vilionodular synovitis
c. Osteomalacia
d. Neurofibromatosis

203. Hyperbilirubinemia associated tooth discoloration is called: *(AIPGEE 2014)*
a. Chlordontia b. Onchronosis
c. Leongs tooth d. Pink tooth of mummery

204. Which of the following is most likely to be associated with deficiency of vitamin D?
a. Decreased rate of eruption *(AIPGEE 2015)*
b. Bowed leg
c. Hyperurea
d. Osteoporosis

205. Scorbutic gingivitis has marked clinical manifestations as: *(J&K 2015)*
a. Spontaneous hemorrhage
b. Severe pain
c. Involvement of marginal gingival tissue and papillae
d. All of the above

206. Iron deficiency anemia is characterized by presence of: *(AB Shetty 2015)*
a. Glossodynia b. Hairy tongue
c. Ulcerative gingivitis d. Erythematous tongue

207. One of the oral manifestation of mercury poisoning is: *(AB Shetty 2015)*
a. Increased salivation
b. Decreased salivation
c. Increased pigmentation
d. Halitosis

208. 'Hunter's glossitis' is a feature of: *(AB Shetty 2015)*
a. Leukemia b. Sickle cell anemia
c. Pernicious anemia d. HIV infection

Answers with Explanations

DEVELOPMENT AND DISTURBANCES

1. Ans. (d) 5.2-5.5 *Ref: Shafer's 6th ed. Pg. 426*

The pH at which any particular saliva ceases to be saturated with calcium phosphate is referred to as the 'Critical pH' below this value, the inorganic material of the tooth may dissolve. Critical pH varies according to the calcium and phosphate concentration, but it is usually about 5.5.

2. Ans. (b) Enamel opacity *Ref: Shafer's 6 ed. Pg. 52*

The amount of fluoride level in the drinking water determines the grades of hypoplasia

Optimum level of fluoride: 1 ppm

Fluorosis occurs >2 ppm

Normal

Questionable: white flecking

Very Mild: white opaque areas involving 25% of tooth surface

Mild white opaque areas involving 50% of tooth surface

Moderate: all surface

Severe: corroded with brown stains

3. Ans. (a) Turner's tooth *Ref: Shafer's 6th ed. Pg. 52*

- Enamel hypoplasia due to local infection or trauma. A type of hypoplasia occasionally seen is unusual in that only a single tooth is involved, most commonly one of the permanent maxillary incisors or a maxillary or mandibular premolar.
- The single teeth are frequently referred to as 'Turner's tooth' and the condition is called 'Turner's hypoplasia'.

4. Ans. (b) Erythroblastosis fetalis *Ref: Naville's 2nd ed. Pg. 814-815*

Mesentice lines	Brown stain at cervical 3rd in children who are immune to caries
Yellow	Brown black which fluorescence under uv light tetracyclines
Pink	Internal resorption
Orange stain	By pigment producing microorganism
Green stain	Due to enamel cuticle of nasmyth membrane
Yellow green	Erythroblastosis fetalis
Red brown	Porphyria

5. Ans. (b) White sponge nevus *Ref: Cowson Odell 8th ed. Pg. 256*

White sponge naevus

White sponge naevus is a developmental anomaly inherited as an autosomal dominant trait, it is caused by mutation in keratin genes.

Clinical features

The affected mucosa is white, soft and irregularly thickened. The abnormality is usually bilateral but only affects the lining. There are no defined borders and the edge fade imperceptibly into normal tissue. The anus and vagina can also be affected.

Pathology

The epithelium is hyperplastic, with uniform acanthosis and the rete ridges have a smooth lower border. Shaggy hyperparakeratosis and intracellular edema with abnormally prominent epithelial cell membranes produce a so called basket weave appearance. There is no dysplasia and inflammatory cells.

Management

The main requirement is to reassure the patient of the benign nature of the condition.

6. Ans. (c) Taurodontism *Ref: Shafer's 6th ed. Pg. 43-44*

Taurodontism

The term 'Taurodontism' was coined by Sir Arthur Keith in 1913 to describe a dental anomaly in which the body of the tooth is enlarged at the expense of the roots. The term means 'bull-like' teeth. Shaw classified taurodont teeth into hypotaurodont, mesotaurodont, and hypertaurodont forms, with hypertaurodontism being the extreme form in which the bifurcation or trifurcation occurs near the apices of the roots and hypotaurodontism being the mildest form.

In addition, it has been reported that many patients with the Klinefelter syndrome.

- Taurodontism may affect either the deciduous or permanent dentition, but permanent tooth involvement is more common.
- The condition may be unilateral.

The pulp chamber is extremely large with a much greater apico-occlusal height than normal radiographic picture is quite striking and characteristic.

No special treatment is necessary for this anomaly.

7. Ans. (a) Permanent third molar *Ref: Shafer's 6th ed. Pg. 46*

Hypodontia is more common in the permanent dentition but when the primary dentition is affected, the permanent dentition is affected in 75–80% of cases. Most patients lack 1 or 2 permanent teeth. It most often affects the permanent third molars with up to 10–30% of the population missing these teeth. Lateral incisor-premolar hypodontia is the second most common form of the disease, affecting mainly mandibular second premolars (32% of cases) and then maxillary lateral incisors (27% of cases).

8. Ans. (b) Maxillary incisors *Ref: Shafer's 6th ed. Pg. 16*

Cleft lip and palate (CLP) has become a major public health problem affecting one in every 500–1,000 births worldwide. It is the fourth most common birth defect and the most common congenital defect of the face. These patients are likely to have significant dental problems that require attention of various specialties in dentistry. Embryologically, the formation of tooth germs and the occurrence of cleft lip (CL) and/or cleft palate (CP) defects have a close relationship both in terms of timing and anatomical position. The odontogenic epithelium over the premaxillary and mandibular processes can be identified as early as the fifth embryonic week, while CL and/or CP anomalies are believed to occur during the fourth and seventh week period. By the 38th day, fusion of the frontonasal, maxillary and mandibular process is complete and specific odontogenic growth centers for primary central incisors and their permanent successors become evident. Various phenomena, including delayed tooth development, morphological anomalies in both sets of dentition, delayed eruption of permanent maxillary incisors, reduced tooth dimension and variations in tooth number, have been reported in cleft populations. Jordan et al. (1966) have described supernumerary teeth, congenitally missing teeth, T-cingulum and peg-shaped teeth and thick curved hypoplastic incisors in CLP children.

9. Ans. (a) Chromosome no 4 *Ref: AIIMS SRship July 2014*
Shafer's Textbook of Oral Pathology 6th ed. Pg. 54

Dentinogenesis imperfecta is an autosomal dominant condition affecting both deciduous and permanent teeth. The gene maps to chromosome number 4. It encodes a protein called **dentin sialophosphoprotein (DSPP; 4q21.3)**. Dentinogenesis imperfecta 2 may be an allelic variant of dentinogenesis imperfecta 1 (a different mutation in the same gene), both genes map to the same region on chromosome number 4.

10. Ans. (b) 8 year *Ref: Neville's Oral and Maxillofacial Pathology 3rd ed. Pg. 73; Shafer's Textbook of Oral Pathology 7th ed. Pg. 560*

'The drug and its homologues can cross the placental barrier, therefore administration should, if possible be avoided during pregnancy and in children upto 8 years of age.' - Neville

Tetracycline Discoloration:

Due to formation of a complex with calcium ions in the surface of the microcrystals of hydroxyapatite in bone and tooth substance.

Tetracycline and its homologues have a selective affinity for deposition in bone and tooth substance, possibly through the formation of a complex with calcium ions in the surface of the microcrystals of hydroxyapatite.

The severity of the staining by tetracycline is determined by the stage of tooth development at the time of drug administration. Dosage, the length of time over which administration occurred, and the form of the tetracycline. The critical period for tetracycline-induced discoloration (A/c to Moffitt).

Dentition	*Teeth*	*Critical period*
Deciduous	Incisors (maxillary and mandibular)	4 months in utero to 3 months postpartum
	Canines (maxillary and mandibular)	5 months in utero to 9 months postpartum
Permanent	Incisors (maxillary and mandibular)	3–7 months postpartum to 7 years of age
	Canines (maxillary and mandibular)	

Binding of minocycline to certain types of collagenous tissues like dentin, dental pulp, bone, and dermis, results in oxidation and produces the discoloration. The stained pulp is seen through the overlying translucent dentin and enamel.

Clinical Features:

Tetracycline itself fluoresces under ultraviolet lightand, accordingly, the teeth involved by its discoloration also fluoresce a bright yellow under ultraviolet light.

It has been shown that the dentin is more heavily stained than the enamel.

Drugs	*Appearance*
Tetracycline	Yellowish or brownish-gray discoloration, most pronounced at the time of eruption of the teeth
Oxytetracycline	Yellowish color
Chlortetracycline	Brownish-gray color

Minocycline hydrochloride causes discoloration of the skin, nails, conjunctiva, bone, and teeth. Palate or anterior alveolar mucosa has a distinctive blue-gray appearance due to the black bone showing through the thin, translucent mucosa. The incisal edge of the fully erupted teeth reveal a blue-gray discoloration, with the middle one-third being maximally involved and the exposed roots of the erupted teeth reveal dark green discoloration. The roots of developing teeth show a dark black color.

11. Ans. (b) 20 mg/kg body weight *Ref: Ghom 2nd ed. Pg. 149*

- Discoloration of either deciduous or permanent teeth may occur as a result of prophylactic or therapeutic regimen instituted for pregnant females or infants.
- The minimum amount required to produce discoloration is 21 mg/kg body weight. It is deposited during mineralization.
- Physicians should prescribe other antibiotics where possible for children under 8 years of age or for women in the last trimester of pregnancy.

12. Ans. (b) Normal vision with coloboma *Ref: Neville's Oral and Maxillofacial Pathology 3rd ed. Pg. 45; Shafer's Textbook of Oral Pathology 7th ed. Pg. 720*

Mandibulofacial Dysostosis (Treacher Collins-Franceschetti Syndrome)

- The syndrome is thought to result from *a retardation or failure of differentiation of maxillary mesoderm at and after the 50 mm stage of the embryo.*
- The gene for Treacher-Collins syndrome was mapped to *chromosome 5q32–q33.1.*

Clinical Features:

- **Antimongoloid palpebral fissures with a coloboma** of the outer portion of the lower lids, and deficiency of the eyelashes (and sometimes the upper lids).
- **Hypoplasia** of the facial bones, especially of the malar bones and mandible.
- Malformation of the external ear, and occasionally of the middle and internal ears.
- **Macrostomia, high palate** (sometimes cleft) and abnormal position and malocclusion of the teeth.
- Blind fistulas between the angles of the ears and the angles of the mouth.
- Atypical hair growth in the form of a tongue-shaped process of the hairline extending toward the cheeks.
- Other anomalies such as facial clefts and skeletal deformities.
- The characteristic faces of the patients have often been described as being ***bird like or fish like in nature.***

13. Ans. (a) Peg laterals *Ref: Neville's Oral and Maxillofacial Pathology 3rd ed. Pg. 83; Shafer's Textbook of Oral Pathology 7th ed. Pg. 39-40*

Microdontia

Microdontia is the condition in which one or more teeth are smaller than normal in size. When all teeth are involved, it is called generalized microdontia and when only a few teeth are involved it is called localized or focal microdontia.

Types of Microdontia:

True Generalized Microdontia

- When all the teeth in both arches are uniformly and measurably smaller than normal the condition is known as true generalized microdontia.
- This is an extremely uncommon condition and can be seen in pituitary dwarfism.
- True generalized microdontia can also be associated with other congenital defects like Down syndrome and congenital heart disease, etc.

Relative Generalized Microdontia

- Relative generalized microdontia is the condition in which teeth of normal size may look smaller, if they are placed in an abnormally large maxilla or mandible.
- In such cases larger size of the jaws give an illusion of microdontia although the teeth are not really small.

Focal/isolated Microdontia

- When one or two teeth in the jaw are measurably smaller in size while rest of the teeth are normal, the condition is called focal microdontia.
- *Maxillary lateral incisors and maxillary third molars are the most frequently involved teeth in focal microdontia.*
- When *maxillary lateral incisors are involved, the teeth often appear 'cone' or 'peg' shaped and are often designated as peg laterals.*
- These peg laterals carry an autosomal dominant type.

14. Ans. (b) Taurodontism *Ref: Neville's Oral and Maxillofacial Pathology 3rd ed. Pg. 94; Shafer's Textbook of Oral Pathology 7th ed. Pg. 48*

'Patients with the Klinefelter syndrome (males whose sex chromosome constitution includes one or more extra X chromosomes) exhibit taurodontism, but it is not a constant feature of this syndrome'.

Taurodontism ('bull-like' teeth)

- The termoriginated by Sir Arthur Keith (1913) for a tooth in which the body of the tooth is enlarged at the expense of the roots.
- Taurodontism is an enlargement of the body and pulp chamber of a multirooted tooth with apical displacement of the pulpal floor and bifurcation of the roots.
- This pattern of molar formation has been found in ancient Neanderthals and the overall shape of the taurodont resembles that of the molar teeth of cud-chewing animals (Tauro = bull and dont = tooth).
- Classification according to the degree of apical displacement of the pulpal floor (by Shaw): 3 forms—1. Hypotaurodont (mildest form), 2. mesotaurodont, and 3. hypertaurodont forms (extreme form in which the bifurcation or trifurcation occurs near the apices of the roots).
- A variety of possible causes of taurodontism have been enumerated by Mangion as follows: (1) a specialized or retrograde character, (2) a primitive pattern, (3) a Mendelian recessive trait, (4) an atavistic feature, and (5) a mutation resulting from odontoblastic deficiency during dentinogenesis of the roots.
- Hammer and his associates believe that the taurodont is caused by failure of Hertwig's epithelial sheath to invaginate at the proper horizontal level.
- Clinical features:
  - The affected tooth in taurodontism exhibits large crown with elongated pulp chamber and short rudimentary root.
  - The affected tooth is usually rectangular in shape with minimum constriction at the cervical area; moreover the furcation area of the tooth is more apically placed than normal.
  - The tooth often has a greater apico-occlusal height and the level of furcation of the roots is situated much below the cervical area.
  - In taurodontism the affected tooth generally exhibit certain morphologic changes.
  - This defect can involve both sexes equally.
  - Taurodontism commonly affects the multirooted permanent molars and sometimes the premolars. It is rarely seen in the primary dentition.
- This dental anomaly may sometimes be associated with some craniofacial deformities, e.g. Down syndrome, Klinefelter syndrome, amelogenesis imperfecta and Poly-X syndrome, etc.
- Patients with hypodontia may have taurodontism in about 30% cases.

Syndromes Associated with Taurodontism

1. Ameloge nesis imperfecta, hypoplastic, type IE
2. Ameloge nesis imperfecta-taurodontism, type IV
3. Cranioectodermal
4. Ectodermal dysplasia
5. Hyperphosphata siaoligophrenia taurodontism
6. Hypophosphatasia
7. Klinefelter
8. Microdontia-taurodontia-dens invaginatus
9. Microcephalic dwarfism-taurodontism
10. Oculodentodigital dysplasia/
11. Oral-facial-digital, type II
12. Rapp-Hodgkin
13. Scanty hair-oligodontia-taurodontia
14. Sex chromosomal aberrations (e.g., XXX, XYY)
15. Down
16. Tricho-dento-osseous, types I, II, and III

Points to Remember

Radiographic changes in various tooth abnormalities	
Germination (incomplete)	Two crowns with one root.
Dilacerations	Sharp bend in the tooth (mostly root).
Dens-in-dente	Tooth within a tooth.
Taurodontism	Large crown with small root, too much apically placed bifurcation.
Concrescence	Joining of roots of many teeth with obliteration of periodontal ligament space.
Amelogenesis imperfecta	Little or no enamel on tooth.
Dentinogenesis imperfecta	Obliteration of pulp chamber.
Dentinogenesis imperfecta type III	Abnormally large pulp with thin shell of enamel and dentin surrounding the pulp.
Ghost tooth	Decreased radiodensity of tooth; abnormally large pulp chamber.
Hypercementosis	Bulbous root.
Dentin dysplasia	Abnormally short, blunt root, molar roots appear 'w' shaped.
Supernumerary tooth	Mostly small and conical shaped.
Pit and fissure caries	Triangular-shaped radiolucency with it's base toward DE junction.
Smooth surface caries	Triangular-shaped radiolucency with it's base toward surface of the tooth.
External resorption of tooth	Moth-eaten irregular destruction of root surface.
Internal resorption	Well-defined spherical radioluceny of dentine in continuation with the pulp.
Compound odontome	Multiple miniature teeth projecting from a single focus.

15. Ans. (b) Gemination

Ref: Neville's Oral and Maxillofacial Pathology 3rd ed. Pg. 8 4; Shafer's Textbook of Oral Pathology 7th ed. Pg. 40

Germination

- Developmental disturbance in shape of teeth.
- Arises from an attempt at division of single tooth germ by an invagination.
- Incomplete formation of two teeth, two completely or incompletely separated crown (bifid crown) and have single root and root canal.
- Seen in both deciduous and permanent teeth.

Tweening

- Term given by Levitas
- The term designate for the structure produced by division of tooth germ resulting into one normal and one supernumerary tooth.

Fusion

- Term given by Levitas
- Teeth arise through the union of two normally separated tooth germ.
- Fusion may be either complete or incomplete depending upon the stage of development. The dentin however is always confluent in true fusion.
- The tooth may have separate or fused root canal, seen in both deciduous and permanent teeth.

Concrescence

- Term given by Levitas
- Developmental disturbance in shape of the teeth in which fusion of teeth occurs after root formation completed, teeth are united by cementum only.

Note: Double teeth (germination and fusion) occurs in both the primary and permanent dentition with higher frequency in anterior and maxillary region. In both dentition, incisors and canines are the most commonly affected teeth. Germination is more common in maxilla, while fusion is more frequent in mandible.

16. Ans. (c) Melanotic neuroectodermal tumor *Ref: Neville's Oral and Maxillofacial Pathology 3rd ed. Pg. 533; Shafer's Textbook of Oral Pathology 7th ed. Pg. 204*

Melanotic Neuroectodermal Tumor of Infancy

- Rareosteolytic-pigmented neoplasm of neural crest origin.
- Usually occurs within the first year of life (1-6 month), with equal sex predilection.
- It is generally accepted that this lesion is of neural crest origin.
- Anterior maxillary ridge is the most common site, where it classically appears as a rapidly growing non-ulcerated darkly pigmented lesion.
- The tumor often destroys the underlying bone and may be associated with displacement of the teeth. May be associated with osteogenic reactions, which gives '*Sun Ray*' radiographic pattern.
- Laboratory Values:
  - All the hematological and blood chemistry values are within the normal range
  - High urinary levels of vanillylmandelic acid (VMA) often are found in patients with melanotic neuroectoderm al tumor of infancy.
  - These levels may return to normal once the tumor has been resected. This find ing supports the hypothesis of neural crest origin because other tumors from this tissue (e.g. neuroblastoma, retinoblastoma, pheochromocytoma, ganglioneuroblastoma) often secrete norepinephrine—like hormones that are metabolized to VMA and excreted in the urine.

17. Ans. (c) Multifactorial trait *Ref: Robbins & Cotron's Pathologic Basis of Disease 7th ed. Pg. 474; Burkit's Oral Medicine 11th ed. Pg. 558; Neville's Oral and Maxillofacial Pathology 3rd ed. Pg. 2; Shafer's Textbook of Oral Pathology 7th ed. Pg. 18*

According to Robbins 7th ed./474

Multifactorial Causes

'The genetic and environmental factors just discussed account for no more than half of human congenital anomalies. They causes the vast majority of birth defect, including some common disorders such as cleft lip and cleft palate, remain unknown, in these anomalies, it would appears that inheritance of a certain numbers of mutant genes and their interaction with the environment is required before the disorder is expressed.' - Robbins/474

According to Burkit's Oral Medicine 11th ed./558

Multifactorial Diseases and Disorders

'The etiology, pathogenesis, manifestations, management, and treatment outcomes of complex human diseases or multifactorial genetic disorders represent a dynamic interplay between regulatory and structural genes and environmental and behavioral factors. **The results from international, multicenter studies of cleft lip and/or palate suggest that many genes (e.g. MSX1, interferon regulatory factor 6 [IRE6]) and their expression are coupled with several environmental factors**.'- Burkit/558

According to Neville's Oral and Maxillofacial Pathology 3rd ed. Pg. 2

- Genetic and environmental causes of Nonsyndromic orofacial Clefts:
- Genetic factors
  - Gene- SKI/MTHFR, TGFB2/TGFA/MSX1/PVRL1/TGFB3/GABRB3/RARA/BCL3
- Environmental factors
  - Maternal alcohol consumption, maternal cigarette smoking, folic acid deficiency, corticosteroid use, anticonvulcent therapy

According to Shafer's Textbook of Oral Pathology 7th ed. Pg. 18

- Craniofacial anomalies (CFA) are a diverse group of deformities in the growth of the head and facial bones.
- There is no single factor that causes these abnormalities. Instead, there are many factors that may contribute to their.

Cleft Lip and Cleft Palate

- The term cleft lip and palate is commonly used to represent two types of malformation, i.e., cleft lip with or without cleft palate (CL/P) and cleft palate (CP).
- **Etiology**
- It has been clearly established that two separate and distinct entities exist: Cleft lip with or without associated cleft palate, and Isolated cleft palate.
- Heredity is undoubtedly one of the most important factors to be considered in the etiology of these malformations. However, there is increasing evidence that environmental factors are important as well.
- This has been discussed by Bhatia, who pointed out that the possible main modes of transmission are either by a single mutant gene, producing a large effect, or by a number of genes (polygenic inheritance), each producing a small effect which together create this condition. The most common is hereditary, its nature being most probably polygenic (determined by several different genes acting together).
- Despite the numerous clinical and experimental investigations, the etiology of cleft palate in the human being is still largely unknown. It must be concluded; however, that heredity is probably the most important single factor.

Guys!!

Hence, from the above description the most appropriate response for the etiology of cleft-lip and cleft palate is — Multifactorial.

18. Ans. (b) Hurler's syndrome *Ref: Neville's Oral and Maxillofacial Pathology 3rd ed. Pg. 817; Shafer's Textbook of oral pathology 7th ed. Page no. 630-631*

Hurler's Syndrome: (Mucopolysaccharidosis I, MPS IH, gargoylism)

- A chromosomal abnormality occurs in chromosome arm 4p16.3.
- Hurler's syndrome is a disturbance of mucopolysaccharide metabolism.
- Inherited as an autosomal recessive trait.

Clinical Features

- The disease usually becomes apparent within the first two years of life.
- The head appears large and the facial characteristics are quite typical, consisting of:
  - a prominent forehead, broad saddle nose and wide nostrils, hypertelorism, puffy eyelids with coarse bushy eyebrows, thick lips, large tongue, open mouth, and nasal congestion with noisy breathing.[Q]
- Progressive corneal clouding.
- Hepatosplenomegaly.
- A short neck and spinal abnormalities.
- 'Claw hand' due to flexion contractures.
- These dwarfed individuals are mentally retarded.

Oral Manifestations

- Shortening and broadening of the mandible with prominent gonions, a wide intergonial distance.
- Localized areas of bone destruction in the jaws may be found.
- The teeth are small, widely spaced, and mishappen.
- Delay eruption of teeth.
- Gingival hyperplasia may be present.
- The tongue is also characteristically enlarged.

Histologic Features

- There is excessive accumulation of intracellular mucopolysaccharide in many tissues and organs throughout the body including the liver, spleen, reticuloendothelial system, nervous system, cartilage, bone, and heart.
- Abnormal deposits are also found in many sites, with involved fibroblasts assuming the appearance of Hurler cells' or clear or gargoyle cells.
- The Hurler cells are relatively large, with metachromatically staining cytoplasm which is either agranular or finely granular, often with crescent-shaped nuclei.[Q]

Laboratory Findings

- There is an elevated level of mucopolysaccharides in the urine.
- Metachromatic granules or **Reilly bodies**[Q] can often be demonstrated in the cytoplasm of circulating lymphocytes.

Treatment

- There is no treatment for the disease.

19. Ans. (a) Turner hypoplasia *Ref: Neville's Oral and Maxillofacial Pathology 3rd ed. Pg. 56; Shafer's Textbook of Oral Pathology 7th ed. Pg. 52-54*

Enamel Hypoplasia due to Local Infection or Trauma:

- A type of hypoplasia occasionally seen is unusual in that **only a single tooth** is involved, most commonly one of the permanent maxillary incisors or a maxillary or mandibular premolar.
- There may be any degree of hypoplasia, ranging from a mild, brownish discoloration of the enamel to a severe pitting and irregularity of the tooth crown.
- These single teeth are frequently referred to as **'Turner's teeth,'** and the condition is called **'Turner's hypoplasia.'**
- **A similar type of hypoplasia may follow trauma to a deciduous tooth, particularly when the deciduous tooth has been driven into the alveolus and has disturbed the permanent tooth bud.** If this permanent tooth crown is still being formed, the resulting injury may be manifested as a yellowish or brownish stain or pigmentation of the enamel, usually on the labial surface, or as a true hypoplastic pitting defect or deformity. This form of dental injury has been discussed by Via, who has pointed out that a disturbance either in matrix formation or in calcification can occur, depending chiefly upon the stage of tooth formation at the time of injury.

20. Ans. (a) Inclusion of epithelial cells between embryonic fusion lines *Ref: Neville's Oral and Maxillofacial Pathology 3rd ed. Pg. 25; Shafer's Textbook of Oral Pathology 7th ed. Pg. 63*

Kramer (1974) has defined a cyst as 'a pathological cavity having fluid, semifluid or gaseous contents and which is not created by the accumulation of pus.' Most cysts, but not all, are lined by epithelium.

Fissural (Inclusion, Developmental) Cysts of Oral Region

- Number of different types of fissural (or inclusion) cysts of bone occur in the jaws and have generally been considered arising, as the name would indicate, along the lines of fusion of various bones or embryonic processes.
- These are true cysts (i.e. pathologic cavities lined by epithelium, usually containing fluid or semisolid material).
- The epithelium being derived from epithelial cells which are entrapped between embryonic processes of bones at union lines.
- These fissural cysts may be classified: (1) median anterior maxillary cyst, (2) median palatal cyst, (3) globulomaxillary cyst, and (4) median mandibular cyst.
- There are several additional developmental cysts derived from embryologic structures or faults which involve the oral or adjacent soft tissue structures.
- These may be listed as: (1) nasoalveolar cyst, (2) palatal cysts of the neonate, (3) thyroglossal tract cyst, (4) benign cervical lymphoepithelial cyst, (5) epidermoid and dermoid cyst, and (6) heterotopic oral gastrointestinal cyst.

21. Ans. (d) Concrescence *Ref: Neville's Oral and Maxillofacial Pathology 3rd ed. Pg. 84-86; Shafer's Textbook of Oral pathology 7th ed. Pg. 40-41]*

Germination:

- Developmental disturbance in shape of teeth.
- Arises from an attempt at division of single tooth germ by an invagination.
- Incomplete formation of two teeth, two completely or incompletely separated crown (bifid crown) and have single root and root canal.
- Seen in both deciduous and permanent teeth.

Tweening:

- Term given by Levitas
- The term designate for the structure produced by division of tooth germ resulting into one normal and one supernumerary tooth.

Fusion:

- Term given by Levitas
- Teeth arise through the union of two normally separated tooth germ.
- Fusion may be either complete or incomplete depending upon the stage of development. The dentin however is always confluent in true fusion.
- The tooth may have separate or fused root canal, seen in both deciduous and permanent teeth.

Concrescence:

- Term given by Levitas
- Developmental disturbance in shape of the teeth in which fusion of teeth occurs after root formation completed, teeth are united by cementum only.

Note: Double teeth (germination and fusion) occurs in both the primary and permanent dentition with higher frequency in anterior and maxillary region. In both dentition, incisors and canines are the most commonly affected teeth. Germination is more common in maxilla, while fusion is more frequent in mandible.

22. Ans. (a) Ectoderm *Ref: Albert schuurs's Pathology of the Hard Dental Tissues, Pg. 52; Neville's Oral and Maxillofacial Pathology 3rd ed. Pg. 99-101; Shafer's Textbook of Oral pathology 7th ed. Pg. 49*

- Hypoplasia is a quantitative development defect caused by failure of matrix production or insufficient deposition of proteins on the outside of the developing enamel surface.
- Hypocalcification is a qualitative developmental deficiency that arise due to interruption in the resorption of the organic enamel matrix or a deficiency in the active calcium transport through the ameloblasts, and/or failure of maturation.
- The principal expressions of pathologic amelogenesis are hypoplasia, which is manifested by pitting, furrowing, or even total absence of the enamel, and hypocalcification, in the form of opaque or chalky areas on normally contoured enamel surfaces.
- The causes of such defective enamel formation can be systemic, local, or genetic.
- The most common systemic influences are nutritional deficiencies, endocrinopathies, febrile diseases, and certain chemical intoxications.
- Since it has been realized that enamel development occurs in two phases, that is, matrix formation and maturation
- If matrix formation is affected, enamel hypoplasia will ensue and defect of the enamel is found.
- If maturation is lacking or incomplete, hypocalcification of the enamel results and deficiency in the mineral content of the enamel is found.

23. Ans. (b) Osteopetrosis *Ref: Neville's Oral and Maxillofacial Pathology 3rd ed. Pg. 78*

Syndrome Associated with Hypodontia

- Ankyloglossia superior
- Book
- Cockayne
- Coffin-Lowry
- Cranio-oculo-dental
- Crouzon
- Down
- Ectodermal dysplasia
- Ectodermal dysplasia, cleft lip, cleft palate
- Ehlers-Danlos
- Ellis-van Creveld
- Focal dermal hypoplasia
- Freire-Mala
- Frontometaphyseal dysplasia
- Goldenhar
- Gorlin
- Gorlin-Chaudhry-Moss
- Hallermann-Streiff
- Hanhart
- Hurler
- Hypoglossia-hypodactylia
- Incontinentia pigmenti
- Johanson-Blizzard
- Lipoid proteinosis
- Marshall-White
- Melanoleukoderma
- Monilethrix-anodontia
- Oral-facial-digital type I
- Otodental dysplasia
- Palmoplantar keratosis, hypotrichosis, cysts of eyelid
- Progeria
- Rieger
- Robinson
- Rothmund-Thomson
- Sturge-Weber
- Tooth-and-nail
- Turner

Syndrome Associated with Hyperdontia

- Apert
- Angio-osteohypertrophy
- Cleidocranial dysplasia
- Craniometaphyseal dysplasia
- Crouzon
- Curtius
- Down

- Ehlers-Danlos
- Ellis-van Creveld
- Fabry-Anderson
- Fucosidosis
- Gardner
- Hallermann-Streiff
- Incontinentia pigmenti
- Klippel-Trenaunay-Weber
- Laband
- Leopard
- Nance-Horan
- Oral-Facial-digital types I and III
- Sturge-Weber
- Tricho-rhino-phalangeal

24. Ans. (b) Trisomy 21 *Ref: Shafer's Textbook of Oral pathology 7th ed. Pg. 728*

Down Syndrome (Down syndrome, trisomy 21 syndrome, mongolism, congenital acromicria syndrome):

- Down syndrome is a frequent form of mental retardation associated with characteristic morphologic features (mongolism) and many somatic abnormalities due to a number of chromosomal aberrations.
- Three cytogenetic variants cause Down syndrome:

Types/cytogenetic variants	*Cytogenetic pathology*	*Incidences/cases (%)*
Trisomy 21	• Typical trisomy 21 with 47 chromosomes	95%
Chromosomal translocation type (Children with the translocation type of Down syndrome are more commonly born to mothers over 30 years of age)	• Appear to be only 46 chromosomes, although the extra chromosome material of number 21 is translocated to another chromosome of G or D group, either 21/22 translocation or 21/21 translocation	3%
Chromosomal mosaicism	• Result of chromosomal mosaicism	2%

Clinical Features:

- Down syndrome is the most common autosomal abnormality.
- The major features of Down syndrome are mental retardation (IQ of 25–50).
- Characteristic head appearance includes:
  - Small head (brachycephaly)
  - Flat facies with increased interocular distance (hypertelorism)
  - Depressed nasal bridge
  - Flat occiput and
  - Broad short neck.
- Ocular anomalies includes:
  - Narrow, upward and outward slanting of the palpebral fissures
  - Medial epicanthal folds
  - Strabismus
  - Cataract and
  - Retinal detachment.
- Skeletal anomalies include:

- Short stature
- Broad and short hands, feet, and digits
- Short curved fifth finger (dysplasia of the midphalanx)
- Clinodactyly of the fifth finger
- Dysplasia of the pelvis
- Joint laxity
- A wide gap between the first and second toes
- Atlanto-occipital instability

- Muscle hypotonia in newborns with decreased response to normal stimuli has been reported.
- Oral Manifestations—Small mouth with protrusion of the tongue (macroglossia), scrotal tongue, hypoplasia of the maxilla, delayed tooth eruption, partial anodontia, enamel hypoplasia, juvenile periodontitis, and cleft lip or palate (rare) are noticed commonly.

25. Ans. (a) Failure of invagination at proper horizontal location of HERS *Ref: Neville's Oral and Maxillofacial Pathology 3rd ed. Pg. 94;Shafer's Textbook of Oral Pathology 7th ed. Pg. 48*

Taurodontism ('bull-like' teeth)

- The termoriginated by Sir Arthur Keith (1913) for a tooth in which thebody of the tooth is enlarged at the expense of the roots.
- Taurodontism is an enlargement of the body and pulp chamber of a multirooted tooth with apical displacement of the pulpal floor and bi furcation of the roots.
- This pattern of molar formation has been found in ancient Neanderthals and the overall shape of the taurodont resembles that of the molar teeth of cud-chewtng animals (Tauro = bull and dont = tooth).
- Classification according to the degree of apical displacement of the pulpal floor(by Shaw): 3 forms- 1. Hypotaurodont (mildest form) 2. mesotaurodont, and 3. hypertaurodont forms (extreme form in which thebifurcation or trifurcation occurs near the apices of the roots).
- A variety of possible causes of taurodontism have beenenumerated by Mangion as follows: (1) a specialized orretrograde character, (2) a primitive pattern, (3) a Mendelian recessive trait, (4) an atavistic feature, and (5) a mutationresulting from odontoblastic deficiency during dentinogenesisof the roots.
- Hammer and his associates believe that thetaurodont is caused by failure of Hertwig's epithelial sheathto invaginate at the proper horizontal level.
- Clinical features:
  - The affected tooth in taurodontism exhibits large crown with elongated pulp chamber and short rudimentary root.
  - The affected tooth is usually rectangular in shape with minimum constriction at the cervical area; moreover the furcation area of the tooth is more apically placed than normal.
  - The tooth often has a greater apico-occlusal height and the level of furcation of the roots is situated much below the cervical area.
  - In taurodontism the affected tooth generally exhibit certain morphologic changes.
  - This defect can involve both sexes equally.
  - Taurodontism commonly affects the multirooted permanent molars and sometimes the premolars. It is rarely seen in the primary dentition.
    - This dental anomaly may sometimes be associated with some craniofacial deformities, e.g. Down syndrome, Klinefelter syndrome, amelogenesis imperfecta and Poly-X syndrome, etc.
    - Patients with hypodontia may have taurodontism in about 30% cases.

Syndromes Associated with Taurodontism

- Ameloge nesis imperfecta, hypoplastic, type IE
- Ameloge nesis imperfecta-taurodontism, type IV
- Cranioectodermal
- Ectodermal dysplasia
- Hyperphosphata siaoligophrenia• taurodontism
- Hypophosphatasia
- Klinefelter
- Microdontia-taurodontia-dens invaginatus
- Microcephalic dwarfism-taurodontism
- Oculodentodigital dysplasia
- Oral-facial-digital, type II
- Rapp-Hodgkin
- **Scanty hair-oligodontia-tau rod ont ia**
- Sex chromoso mal aberrations (e.g., XXX, XYY)
- Down
- 'Tricho-dento-osseous, types I, II, and III

Points to Remember:

Radiographic changes in various tooth abnormalities	
Germination (incomplete)	Two crowns with one root.
Dilacerations	Sharp bend in the tooth (mostly root).
Dens-in-dente	Tooth within a tooth.
Taurodontism	Large crown with small root, too much apically placed bifurcation.
Concrescence	Joining of roots of many teeth with obliteration of periodontal ligament space.
Amelogenesis imperfecta	Little or no enamel on tooth.
Dentinogenesis imperfecta	Obliteration of pulp chamber.
Dentinogenesis imperfecta	Abnormally large pulp with thin shell of enamel and dentin surrounding **type III** the pulp.
Ghost tooth	Decreased radiodensity of tooth; abnormally large pulp chamber.
Hypercementosis	Bulbous root.
Dentin dysplasia	Abnormally short, blunt root, molar roots appear 'w' shaped.
Supernumerary tooth	Mostly small and conical shaped.
Pit and fissure caries	Triangular-shaped radiolucency with it's base toward DE junction.
Smooth surface caries	Triangular-shaped radiolucency with it's base toward surface of the tooth.
External resorption of tooth	Moth-eaten irregular destruction of root surface.
Internal resorption	Well-defined spherical radioluceny of dentine in continuation with the pulp.
Compound odontome	Multiple miniature teeth projecting from a single focus.

26. Ans. (a) Ankyloglossia *Ref: Neville's Oral and Maxillofacial Pathology 3rd ed. Pg. 11; Shafer's Textbook of oral pathology 7th ed. Pg, 28]*

ANKYLOGLOSSIA

Definition

- Ankyloglossia can be defined as a congenital developmental condition characterized by **fixation of the tongue to the floor of the mouth**; causing restricted tongue mobility.
- During functional movements, the tip of the normal tongue should touch the anterior palate but in case of ankyloglossia, it fails to reach up to that limit.

- Complete ankyloglossia is an extremely rare condition, however partial ankyloglossia, which is otherwise known as '**tongue-tie**' is a relatively common developmental anomaly of the tongue.
- The tongue tie occurs either due to a short and thick lingual frenulum (a membrane connecting the undersurface of the tongue to the floor of the mouth) or due to a frenulum, which attaches too near to the tip of the tongue.

Clinical Features

- Ankyloglossia affects the males more frequently than females (2.6:1)
- Although most affected individuals can perform tongue functions almost normally, the restricted tongue mobility in ankyloglossia may sometimes cause the following problems:
  - Speech disorders—patient cannot properly pronounciate certain consonants and diphthongs such as L, R, T, D, N, TH, SH, Z, etc.
  - Patient pronounciates the word 'lemonade' as wemonade.
  - Infants feel difficulty in sucking breast milk.
  - Deformities in dental occlusion especially development of open bite and mandibular prognathism, etc.
  - Difficulty in swallowing food and maintaining oral hygiene.
  - Tension in the anterior lingual gingiva in tongue-tie may initiate some localized gingival or periodontal diseases near the site of frenal attachment (e.g. gingival recession and persistent gap between lower incisors).
  - Difficulty in kissing, licking one's lips, eating icecream cones and performing tongue tricks.

Ankyloglossia may occur sometimes in association with the following syndromes:

- Ankyloglossum spurious syndrome
- Van der Woude syndrome
- Fraser's syndrome
- Rainbow's syndrome
- Orofacial digital syndrome, etc.

Treatment

Partial ankyloglossia in most of the cases does not require any treatment, however in severe cases of ankyloglossia, surgical correction (frenulctomy) of the lingual frenulum is done to free the tongue. Sometimes, the offending frenulum may tear spontaneously resulting in freeing of tongue.

27. Ans (a) Maxillary lateral incisor *Ref: Neville's Oral and Maxillofacial Pathology 3rd ed. Pg. 90; Shafer's Textbook of Oral Pathology 7th ed.Pg. 43*

Dens in Dente (Dens invaginatus, dilated composite odontome)

The 'dens in dente' is a developmental variation which is thought to arise as a result of an invagination in the surface of tooth crown before calcification has occurred.

Several proposedcauses include -an increased localized external pressure, focal growth retardation, and focal growth stimulation in certain areas of the tooth bud.

The permanent maxillary lateral incisors are the teeth mostfrequently involved, and in the majority of cases the 'dens in dente' appears to represent simply an accentuation in the development of the lingual pit.

Dens in dente is often broadly divided into two types—coronal type and radicular type.

Coronal type; Coronal type of dens in dente occurs when the invagination or folding occurs on the crown portion of the tooth. The coronal type is further divided into three subtypes, which are as follows:

Type I—The invagination within the crown of the tooth.

Type II—The invagination extends below the cemento enamel junction (CEJ) of tooth but it may 01 may not communicate with the pulp.

Type III—The invagination extends through the rootand perforates in the apical or lateral radicular arear Radicular type: In case of dens in dente if the invagination occurs in the root portion of the tooth Radicuar Type: In case of dens in dente if the invagination occurs in the root portion of the tooth it is called radicular type and the condition It is called the radicular type and the condition presumably occurs due to folding of the Hertwig's sheath during the development of root.

The term 'dens in dente, ' originally applied to a severe invagination that gave the appearance of a tooth within a tooth, is actually a misnomer, but it has continued in usage. In the mild form, there is a deep invagination.

Dens-in-dente refers to a folding or invagination of the surface of the tooth toward pulp; which begins before the calcification of the tooth and eventually after calcification the defect produces a typical appearance of a "tooth within a tooth". Shafer's

28. Ans. (a) Peg lateral *Ref: Neville's Oral and Maxillofacial Pathology 3rd ed. Pg. 190-192; Shafer's Textbook of Oral Pathology 7th ed. Pg. 52, 303*

Enamel Hypoplasia due to Congenital Syphilis:

- The hypoplasia due to congenital syphilis is presents a characteristic, almost pathognomonic, appearance.
- This hypoplasia involves the maxillary and mandibular permanent incisors and the first molars.
- The anterior teeth affected are sometimes called 'Hutchinson's teeth, ' while the molars have been referred to as 'mulberry molars' (Moon's molars, Fournier's molars).
- Characteristically, the upper central incisor is 'screw-driver' shaped, the mesial and distal surfaces of the crown tapering and converging toward the incisal edge of the tooth rather than toward the cervical margin. In addition, the incisal edge is usually notched.
- The mandibular central and lateral incisors may be similarly involved, although the maxillary lateral incisor may be normal.
- The cause of the tapering and notching of the maxillary incisor due to the absence of the central tubercle or calcification center.
- The crowns of the first molars in congenital syphilis are irregular and the enamel of the occlusal surface and occlusal third of the tooth appears to be arranged in an agglomerate mass of globules rather than in well-formed cusps.
- The crown is narrower on the occlusal surface than at the cervical margin.

Review Topic: SYPHILIS

- It is also called as '*Lues*'.
- It occurs most exclusively by venereal contact, in overcrowded living and primitive housing conditions.
- **Classification**
  - Acquired syphilis
    - Primary
    - Secondary
    - Tertiary
    - Quaternary syphilis/Latent phase
      - Early syphilis—primary syphilis, secondary syphilis and the early latent phase of the disease.
      - Late syphilis—late latent and tertiary are grouped as late syphilis.
  - Congenital syphilis-
- Clinical features
  - **PRIMARY SYPHILIS**
    - Lesion develops at the site of inoculation (genitalia) approximately 3 weeks after contact with infection.
    - Extragenital sites of involvement include fingers, perianal region, and lips, tonsils and intraoral structures such as tongue and palate
    - Painless indurated ulcer with rolled out margin (Choncre), which heals in weeks spontaneously.

- Regional lymphadenopathy (non-suppurative)
- Acartilagenous consistency
- Indurated lesion (Chanchre)
- Single lesion
- Exudate with discharging serous fluid

– **SECONDARY SYPHILIS**
- Develops 3 to 6 weeks after primary lesion.
- Condylomata lata—elevated broad base verrucal white plaque.
- Assoc. lesions—Fever and generalized lymphadenopathy, which is painless, discrete and non-adherent to the surrounding tissues.
- Mucous patch—Fine macular or papular rash, sometimes accompanied by alopecia, circinate lesions on face.
- Pruritic papules—The lesions either resolve completely or leave residual areas of hypo or hyper-pigmentation.
- Spirochetemia (highly infective stage), Headache, anorexia, pain in joints and muscles.

– **TERTIARY SYPHILIS**
- Gumma—There are two types of gumma, i.e. central and cortical.
- It is a chronic granulomatous and usually localized lesion, which later ulcerates which may be nodular.
- Punched out ulcer with vertical walls and dull red granulomatous base.
- Cutaneous lesions heal slowly and leave behind tissue paper like scars.
- Single cerebral gumma may produce symptoms suggestive of brain tumor.
- **Tabes dorsalis**
  - ◆ Loss of positional sense of lower extremities and walks with a slapping step.
  - ◆ Burning and pricking sensation of the extremities, paresthesia, or at times, actual anesthesia of the part may accompany the characteristic gait.
- **Positive Romberg's sign**
  - ◆ Person is unable to stand erect unaided with his eyes closed.
  - ◆ Short, shooting, knife-like pains may be experienced in the abdominal region called 'tabetic crises', which results from involvement of the dorsal root ganglion.
- **Charcoat** ***joint***—trophic changes consist of deep perforating ulcers and painless destruction of larger joints.
- **Argyll Robertson Pupil**—*Pupils that react to accommodation but not to light.* (**A**ccommodation **R**eflex – **P**resent & **P**upillary **R**eflex - **A**bsent)
- **Cardiovascular Syphilis**—Involvement of CVS in tertiary syphilis affects aorta and aortic valve and 80% of deaths occur due to it. Medial necrosis and destruction of elastic tissue occurs in the wall of large blood vessels.

CONGENITAL SYPHILIS

- It is infection of fetus established by the passage of spirochetes from mother, through the placenta.
- *T. pellidum* usually do not infects the fetus in syphilitic mother before 5th month of pregnancy. Becoz; the layer of cylindrical langerhans cells of early placenta, which are intact until after 4th month, langerhans cells layer than begins to atrophy.
  – Manifested within the first 2 years of life as:
  - Generalized spirochetamia.
  - Rhinitis and chronic nasal discharge with maculo-papular eruptions.
  - The lesions can be seen in spleen, kidney, bones and cns.
  - Bullae, vesicles and superficial desquamation with cracking and scaling of reddened soles and palms, petechiae, mucus patches and condyloma latum.
  – Manifested after the first 2 years of life as:

- **Hutchinson's triad:**
  - **Interstitial keratitis (inflammatory reaction in the cornea),**
  - **VIIIth nerve deafness,**
  - **Dental abnormalities- mulburry molar, screwdriver shaped incisor**
- Arthropathy (*Clutton's joint*)
- Gummatous destruction of palate and nasal septum develop.
- Anterior tibial bowing (*Saber shins*)
- Higoumenaki's sign—Irregular thickening of sternoclavicular portion of clavicle.
- Unexplained nerve deafness, retinal and corneal damage can also occur.
- Postrhagadic scarring and syphilitic rhagades:
  - Are linear lesions found around oral opening (*perioral creases*).
  - Result from diffuse leutic involvement of the skin in these areas from 3rd to 7th week after birth.
  - Appear as red or copper-colored linear areas covered with a soft crust.
- Saddle nose- due to destruction of vomer.

29. Ans. (a) Teratoma *Ref: Robbins & Cotron's Pathologic Basis of Disease 7th ed. Pg. 271; Neville's Oral and Maxillofacial Pathology 3rd ed. Pg. 34; Marx & Stern's Oral and Maxillofacial Pathology 1st ed. Pg.*

Hyperplasias

- Hyperplasias may produce tissue masses referred to as tumors.
- They represent a limited cellular proliferation.
- Like hamartomas, they cease growth at some point.
- Unlike true neoplasms, they lack the capacity for autonomous growth.
- They may resemble neoplasms clinically and histologically by virtue of their increased cellularity.
- The evolution of these lesions is usually initiated and controlled by an identifiable stimulus; however, the process stops when the stimulus is removed.

Choristomas

- Choristomas are similar to hamartomas except that they are dysmorphic proliferations of tissue that are not native to the site.
- Each tissue has a limited proliferation.
- The more commonly seen ectopic sebaceous glands known as Fordyce granules and salivary gland tissue within lymph nodes may also be considered choristomas.

Teratomas

- Teratomas, which are often thought of as hamartomas or choristomas, are actually true neoplasms with the capacity for continual growth.
- They are neoplasias that arise from multiple germ layers and thus produce tissues that are foreign to the part in which they develop.
- They arises from totipotent cells such as those normally present in the ovary and testis and sometimes abnormally present in sequestered midline embryonic rests.
- They are distinct from other neoplasias that may also show tissue diversity, such as pleomorphic adenomas of salivary glands, which are derived from native tissue.
- The majority of teratomas occur within the ovary, where they are usually benign, or in the testes, where they are predominantly malignant.
- Teratomas also are seen in the neck, the jaws, and the floor of the mouth on rare occasions.
- One tumor of particular interest is the benign cystic teratoma of the ovary. Because of its origin from three germ layers, it will form various components of skin (including hair and sebaceous glands), teeth, and bone.

30. Ans. (c) Generalized developmental *Ref: Neville's Oral and Maxillofacial Pathology 3rd ed. Pg. 83; Shafer's Textbook of oral Pathology 7th ed. Pg. 39-40*

Microdontia

Microdontia is the condition in which one or more teeth are smaller than normal in size. When all teeth are involved, it is called generalized microdontia and when only a few teeth are involved it is called localized or focal microdontia.

Types of Microdontia:

True Generalized Microdontia

- When all the teeth in both arches are uniformly and measurably smaller than normal the condition is known as true generalized microdontia.
- This is an extremely uncommon condition and can be seen in pituitary dwarfism.
- True generalized microdontia can also be associated with other congenital defects like down syndrome and congenital heart disease, etc.

Relative Generalized Microdontia

- Relative generalized microdontia is the condition in which teeth of normal size may look smaller, if they are placed in an abnormally large maxilla or mandible.
- In such cases larger size of the jaws give an illusion of microdontia although the teeth are not really small.

Focal/isolated Microdontia

- When one or two teeth in the jaw are measurably smaller in size while rests of the teeth are normal, the condition is called focal microdontia.
- Maxillary lateral incisors and maxillary third molars are the most frequently involved teeth in focal microdontia.

31. Ans. (c) Treacher Collins syndrome *Ref: Oral and Maxillofacial Pathology by Neville 3rd ed. Pg. 40*

(Synonym: mandibulo facial dysostosis, Franceschetti-Zwahlen-Klein syndrome)

Defects of structures derived from first and second arch.

Features:

- Coloboma of outer canthus of eye
- Downward slanting of palpebral fissures
- Depressed middle third of face (including zygoma, maxillary sinuses)
- Hypoplasia of condylar and coronoid process and mandibular bone
- Retrognathic chin
- Hypoplasia of nasopharynx, hypopharynx and parotid gland may be seen .
- Improper tongue positioning

32. Ans. (a) Hemifacial atrophy *Ref: Oral and Maxillofacial Pathology by Neville 3rd ed. Pg. 40*

Progressive hemifacial atrophy is an uncommon and poorly understood degenerative condition characterized by atrophic changes affecting one side of the face.

33. Ans. (b) Plummer Vinson syndrome *Ref: Oral and Maxillofacial Pathology by Neville 3rd ed. Pg. 828*

Plummer-Vinson Syndrome (Paterson-Kelly syndrome or sideropenic dysphasia) is a rare condition characterized by iron-deficiency anemia, seen in conjunction with glossitis and dysphasia.

There are usually abnormal bands of tissue in the esophagus called esophageal webs which have higher chances to turn into dysplasia or malignancy.

Koilonychia: brittle or spoon shaped nails seen.

34. Ans. (c) Hyperthyroidism *Ref: Shafer's Textbook of Oral Pathology 6th ed. Pg. 650*

Delayed eruption is seen in the conditions like:

- Rickets
- Down syndrome
- Hypothyroidism
- Cleidocranial dysplasia
- Achondroplasia
- Cherubism

In hyperthyroidism, premature shedding of deciduous teeth and accelerated eruptionof permanent teeth is seen.

35. Ans. (b) Hemifacial hypotrophy *Ref: Shafer's Textbook of Oral Pathology 5th ed. Pg. 28*

Melkerson-Rosenthal syndrome

Has a triad of features—Facial paralysis, Chelitis granulomatosa and fissured tongue also known as scrotal tongue. If only Chelitis granulomatosa is present the condition is called Meischer'schelitis.

36. Ans. (a) Excess fluoride affecting the ameloblasts during the tooth formations stage

Mottled enamel-enamel hypoplasia due to fluoride.

Due to disturbance of the ameloblasts during the formative stage of tooth development.

Interference with the calcification process of the matrix.

Mottled teeth.

37. Ans. (d) Moves downwards on tongue protrusion *Ref: Shafers 6th ed. Pg. 67, Bailey and Love 26th ed. Pg. 702*

Thyroglossal tract cyst—The thyroid gland descends early in fetal life from the base of the tongue toward its position in the lower neck with the isthmus lying over the 2nd and 3rd tracheal rings. Thyroglossal duct cyst found anywhere in or adjacent to the midline from the tongue base to the thyroid isthmus. Rarely, a thyroglossal cyst may contain the only functioning thyroid tissue in the body.

Physical examination shows that the cyst elevates on swallowing or on protruding the tongue, this occurs because the cyst or tract is tethered to the hyoid bone. Thyroglossal cyst treated surgically by Sistrunk operation.

38. Ans. (d) Dentia dysplasia *Ref: Shafer's 6th ed. Pg. 57*

Type I radicular dentin dyaplasia

Normal dentinal tubules formation appears to be blocked, so that new dentin forms around obstacles and takes the characteristic appearance described as 'lava flowing around boulders' and this pattern of 'cascades of dentin' results from repetitive attempts to form root structure.

39. Ans. (b) Elongation of styloid process

According to key given by A.B. Shetty answer is (3)

Eagle's syndrome is characterized by craniofacial or cervical pain due to an elongated styloid process or calcified stylohyoid ligament. Patients with Eagle's syndrome may present with a sore throat, ear pain, or even with foreign body symptoms in the pharynx secondary to pharyngeal and cervical nerve interactions. Eagle first described clinical findings of this syndrome in 1937.

40. Ans. (c) Erupt during first 30 days after birth

According to key given by A.B. Shetty answer is (2)

Teeth which are present in the oral cavity at the time of birth are called natal teeth and neonatal teeth are those that erupt during the first 30 days of life. The teeth which erupt after 30 days and much before their normal time of eruption (usually one to three and half months after birth) are termed as early infancy teeth.

1. Natal teeth are said to be three times more common than neonatal teeth.
2. Natal and neonatal teeth are rarely seen in very premature babies.

41. Ans. (b) Enamel

The term "amelogenesis imperfecta" (AI) is the developmental enamel defects inherited primarily as defects of the enamel only.

42. Ans. (d) Accessory cusp

Dens evaginatus is a disturbance in tooth formation that appears clinically as an accessory occlusal tuberculated cusp composed of enamel and dentin, usually enclosing pulp tissue. The tubercle often fractures or is worn away, with subsequent pulp exposure leading to pulpal inflammation, necrosis, and periapical inflammation.

It is also referred to as tuberculated cusp, accessory tubercle, occlusal tuberculated premolar, Leong's premolar, evaginatusodontoma, and occlusal pearl.

43. Ans. (b) Fibroblasts growth factor receptor 2 and 3

According to key given by A.B. Shetty answer is (3)

Crouzon syndrome is an autosomal dominant genetic disorder known as a branchial arch syndrome. Specifically, this syndrome affects the first branchial (or pharyngeal) arch, which is the precursor of the maxilla and mandible. Since the branchial arches are important developmental features in a growing embryo, disturbances in their development create lasting and widespread effects. First called 'craniofacial dysostosis,' the disorder was characterized by a number of clinical features. This syndrome is caused by a mutation in the fibroblast growth factorreceptor II and III, located on chromosome 10. Breaking down the name, 'craniofacial' refers to the skull and face, and 'dysostosis' refers to malformation of bone.

Now known as Crouzon syndrome, the disease can be described by the rudimentary meanings of its former name. What occurs in the disease is that an infant's skull and facial bones, while in development, fuse early or are unable to expand. Thus, normal bone growth cannot occur. Fusion of different sutures leads to different patterns of growth of the skull. Examples include: trigonocephaly (fusion of the metopic suture), brachycephaly (fusion of the coronal suture), dolichocephaly (fusion of the sagittal suture), plagiocephaly (unilateral premature closure of lambdoid and coronal sutures), oxycephaly (fusion of coronal and lambdoidal sutures), Kleeblattschaedel (premature closure of all sutures).

44. Ans. (a) Mandibular micrognathia

Pierre Robin syndrome, is a congenital condition of facial abnormalities in humans. PRS is a sequence, i.e. a chain of certain developmental malformations, one entailing the next. Pierre Robin sequence may be caused by genetic anomalies at chromosomes 2, 11, or 17.

PRS is characterized by an unusually small mandible (micrognathia), posterior displacement or retraction of the tongue (glossoptosis), and upper airway obstruction. Incomplete closure of the roof of the mouth (cleft palate) is present in the majority of patients, and is commonly U-shaped.

45. Ans. (a) Maxillary central incisor *Ref: Shafers Textbook of Oral Pathology 6th ed. Pg. 72*

Turner's hypoplasia:

- A type of hypoplasia that involves only a single tooth, most commonly one of the permanent maxillary incisors or a maxillary or mandibular premolar.
- There may be any degree of hypoplasia, ranging from a mild brownish discoloration of the enamel to a severe pitting and irregularity of the tooth crown.
- These single teeth are frequently referred to as 'Turner teeth,' and the condition is called 'Turner's hypoplasia.'

46. Ans. (a) Regional odontodysplasia *Ref: Shafers Textbook of Oral Pathology 6th ed. Pg. 57*

Regional Odontodysplasia

(Also known as Odontodysplasia, odontogenic dysplasia, odontogenesisimperfecta, ghost teeth)

This is an unusual dental anomaly in which one or several teeth in a localized area are affected in an unusual manner.

Apparently, the maxillary teeth are involved more frequently than the mandibular, the most frequently affected teeth being the maxillary permanent central incisor, lateral incisor and cuspid.

The etiology of this disease is unknown inasmuch as there is no history of trauma or systemic illness.

The radiographically unique characteristics are, showing a marked reduction in a radiodensity so that the teeth assume a 'ghost' appearance. Both the enamel and dentin appear very thin and the pulp chamber is exceedingly large. The enamel layer often is not evident.

47. Ans. (a) Erupts within 30 days after birth *Ref: Textbook Of Pedodontics by Shobha Tandon 1st ed. Pg. 107*

Natal teeth: Infants occasionally are born with structures which appear to be erupted teeth, usually in the mandibular incisor area. These structures must be distinguished from true deciduous teeth, or the so called natal **teeth described by Massler,** which may have erupted by the time of birth.

Neonatal teeth: Teeth Erupted **within 30 days** after birth are called as neonatal teeth, and they are usually premature deciduous dentition (usually mandibular incisors) rather than supernumerary teeth (10% of cases).

48. Ans. (a) New born babies

Bohn's nodules are smooth whitish bumps or cysts which are sometimes found in the mouths of newborns. They are found at the junction of the hard and soft palate, and along lingual and buccal parts of the dental ridges, away from the midline. These nodules are 1–3 mm in size, and filled with keratin.

The nodes are a result of cystic degeneration of epithelial rests of the dental lamina (rests of Serres). They are benign, and usually disappear within the first three months of life. Bohn's nodules are similar in appearance to Epstein's pearls, which develop on the roof of the mouth in midline.

BENIGN AND MALIGNANT TUMORS

49. Ans. (a) Mikulicz disease *Ref: Shafer's 6th ed. Pg. 245*

Mikulicz disease is a beningn lymphoepithelial lesion

Mikulicz disease is a chronic condition characterized by the abnormal enlargement of the salivary and lacrimal glands. The tonsils and other glands in the soft tissue of the face and neck may also be involved.with reduced lacrimation and salivation.

Mukulicz syndrome is Mikulicz disease along with known disease.

50. Ans. (b) Fibroadenoma *Ref: Robin 6th ed. Pg. 742, Shafer's 6th ed. Pg. 138, 198*

Fibroadenomas of the breast are lumps composed of fibrous and glandular tissue. Because breast cancer can also appear as a lump, doctors may recommend a tissue sample (biopsy) to rule out cancer in older patients. Unlike typical lumps from breast cancer, fibroadenomas are easy to move, with clearly defined edges.

Fibroadenomas are sometimes called **breast mice** or a **breast mouse** owing to their high mobility in the breast.

A fibroadenoma is usually diagnosed through clinical examination, ultrasound or mammography, and often a needle biopsy sample of the lump.

51. Ans. (b) Osteosarcoma *Ref: Shafer's 6th ed. Pg. 169*

- Osteosarcoma is the third most common cancer in adolescent use. It is arise from a primitive mesenchymal bone forming cells and is characterized by production of osteoid.

- Clinical features: osteosarcoma is a bone tumor that can occur in any bone. It most commonly occurs in the long bone of the extremities near metaphyseal growth plate. The most common sites are femur and humerus. Other significant locations are the skull or jaw (8%) and pelvis (8%).
- Osteosarcoma occurs chiefly in young person's the majority between 10 and 25 years.

52. Ans. (a) Osteogenic sarcoma

- Sunburst (sunray) pattern—The radiographic pattern produced when thin bony trabeculae extend away from the cortical plate in a perpendicular fashion. The sunburst (sunray) pattern is commonly associated with osteogenic sarcoma.

Shafer's Textbook of Oral Pathology 6th ed. Pg. 172

53. Ans. (c) Malignant fibrous histiocytoma *Ref: Shafer's 6th ed. Pg. 159*

The most common soft tissue sarcoma in adults is malignant fibrous histiocytoma, which occurs most often in order adults (50 to 70 years). It is a malignant tumor involving soft tissue and rarely bone that is likely derived from undifferentiated mesenchymal cells.

54. Ans (c) Actinic keratosis *Ref: Shafer's 6th ed. Pg. 80*

HPV altered epithelial cells with perinuclear space and nuclear piknosis is known as koilocytes

Lesions caused by HPV is: squamous papilloma

Verruca vulgaris

Condyloma accuminatum

Oral squamous cell carcinoma

Carcinoma of cervix

55. Ans. (b) Acinic cell carcinoma *Ref: Neville 3rd ed. Pg. 419*

Because many of these tumors act in a nonaggressive fashion and are associated with a good prognosis, this neoplasm formerly was called **acinic cell tumor**, a nonspecific designation that did not indocate whether the lesion was benign or malignant. However, because some of these tumors do metastasize or recur and cause death, it is generally agreed today that acinic cell adenocarcinoma should be considered a **low-grade malignancy**.

Also, it is the **third** most common malignant salivary gland epithelial neoplasm after mucoepidermoid carcinoma and adenocarcinoma. (Shafer's Textbook of Oral Pathology; 6th ed.; Page 231)

56. Ans. (c) Osteochondroma *Ref: White and Pharoh 6th ed. Pg. 500-501*

- The most common benign intrinsic tumors affecting the TMJ are osteomas, osteochondromas, Langerhans histiocytosis, and osteoblastomas. **The most common benign tumor is the osteochondroma.**
- The clinical examination may reveal facial asymmetry, malocclusion, and deviation of the mandible to the unaffected side; these may be accompanied by symptoms of TMJ dysfunction.
- Condylar tumors cause condylar enlargement that often is irregular in outline. The trabecular pattern may be altered, resulting new abnormal bone formation, which may increase the radiopacity of the condyle with abnormal trabeculae. An osteoma or osteochondroma appears as an abnormal, pedunculated mass attached to the condyle.
- Osteochondromas often extend from the anterior or superior surface of the condyle.
- Condylar neoplasms may simulate unilateral condylar hyperplasia because of condylar enlargement, although osteomas and osteochondromas give an irregular appearance, such as bulbous or globular expansion of the condyle or, more commonly, a pedunculated growth. Also, the characteristic condylar shape and proportions are better preserved in condylar hyperplasia.

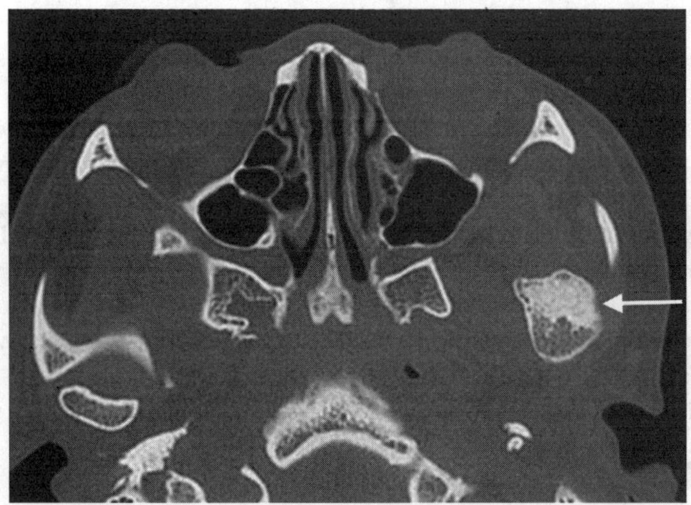

Axial bone algorithm CT image of an osteochondroma extending from the anterior surface of the left condylar head (arrow)

57. Ans. (b) Osteoid osteoma *Ref: Neville's Oral and Maxillofacial Pathology 3rd ed. Pg. 653; Shafer's Textbook of Oral Pathology 7th ed. Pg. 155-157*

'Osteoblastoma and osteoid osteoma are closely related benign bone tumors that arises from osteoblast. Histopathologically osteoid osteoma contains a concentration of peripheral nerve, not seen in other fibro-osseous neoplasm. Produces prostaglandins that results in significant pain and relived by prostaglandin inhibitors (NSAIDs).'

Osteoid osteoma	*Osteoblastoma*
Age: Younger (before 10 years)	Age: middle age (before 30 years)
Male:female = 2:1	Slight female predominance
Histopathologically, associated with nidus of peripheral nerve	No such association
Size: < 2 cm	Size: > 2 cm
Classic feature—Pain (sharp, nocturnal), due to prostaglandins, and relieved by NSAID	More generalized pain; less likely to relieved by NSAID

58. Ans. (b) Tumor node metastasis *Ref: Robbins & Cotron's Pathologic Basis of Disease 7th ed. Pg. 335; Neville's Oral and Maxillofacial Pathology 3rd ed. Pg. 419; Shafer's Textbook of Oral Pathology 7th ed. Pg. 113*

GRADING AND STAGING OF TUMORS

- Systems have been developed to express, at least in semiquantitative terms, the level of differentiation, or grade, and extent of spread of a cancer within the patient, or stage, as parameters of the clinical gravity of the disease.

Grading:

- Grading of a cancer is based on the degree of differentiation of the tumor cells and, in some cancers, the number of mitoses or architectural features.
- Grading schemes have evolved for each type of malignancy, and generally range from two categories (low grade and high grade) to four categories.
- Criteria for the individual grades vary with each form of neoplasia.
- To judge the extent to which the tumor cells resemble or fail to resemble their normal counterparts.

Staging:

- The staging of cancers is based on the size of the primary lesion, its extent of spread to regional lymph nodes, and the presence or absence of blood-borne metastases.
- The major staging system currently in use is the American Joint Committee on Cancer Staging.
- This system uses a classification called the **TNM system**, '**T** for primary tumor, **N** for regional lymph node involvement, and **M** for metastases'.
- The TNM staging varies for each specific form of cancer, but there are general principles. With increasing size the primary lesion is characterized as T1 to T4.
- T0 is used to indicate an in situ lesion.
- N0 would mean no nodal involvement, whereas N1 to N3 would denote involvement of an increasing number and range of nodes.
- M0 signifies no distant metastases, whereas M1 or sometimes M2 indicates the presence of metastases and some judgment as to their number.
- The staging has proved to be of greater clinical value than grading.

TNM clinical staging categories for oral squamous cell carcinoma

		Five-year relative survival rate	
Stage	*TNM classification*	*Oral cavity*	*Lip*
Stage I	$T_1 N_0 M_0$	68%	83%
Stage II	$T_2 N_0 M_0$	53%	73%
Stage III	$T_1 N_1 M_0$	41%	62%
	$T_2 N_1 M_0$		
	$T_3 N_0 M_0$, $T_3 N_1 M_0$		
Stage IV		27%	47%
IVA	$T_{4a} N_0$ or $N_1 M_0$ T_1, T_2, T_3 or $T_{4a} N_2 M_0$		
IVB	Any T $N_3 M_0$ or T_{4b} any N M_0		
IVC	Any T any N M_1		

59. Ans. (b) Squamous cell carcinoma *Ref: Neville's Oral and Maxillofacial Pathology 3rd ed. Pg. ??; Shafer's Textbook of Oral pathology 7th ed. Pg. 103-106*

Epidermoid Carcinoma (Squamous cell carcinoma):

'A malignant epithelial neoplasm exhibiting squamous differentiation as characterized by the formation of keratin and/or the presence of intercellular bridges' (Pindborg JJ et al., 1997)

Most common malignant neoplasm of the oral cavity.

Incidences: In India, oral cancer,

- Ranks first among all cancer cases in males and is the third most common among females.
- Male-female ratio (≈ 2:1) for oral carcinoma, except for carcinoma of the vermilion border of the lower lip (strong male predominance).
- Majority of oral cancers are unequivocally associated with tobacco-chewing habits.
- Of the areas of the oral cavity, the mortality rate is lowest for lip cancer and highest for the tongue.

Also know: National Cancer Registry Programme (NCRP)

- Was initiated in 1982, with three population-based (Mumbai, Bangalore and Chennai), and three hospital-based registries (at Chandigarh, Dibrugarh and Thiruvananthapuram).
- At present the network has
  - **Six population-based** cancer registry at—Mumbai, Bangalore and Chennai with new extension of urban population-based cancer registries at Bhopal and Delhi; rural population-based cancer registry at Barshi.
  - **Five hospital-based** cancer registries at—Dibrugarh, Thiruvananthapuram, Mumbai, Bangalore and Chennai.
  - The Chandigarh registry functioned till 1992.
  - Data from cancer registries helped in highlighting the magnitude and common sites of cancer in India, and was useful in planning the National Cancer Control Programme.

60. Ans. (a) Papilloma *Ref: Neville's Oral and Maxillofacial Pathology 3rd ed. Pg. 364; Shafer's Textbook of Oral Pathology 7th ed. Pg. 81*

PAPILLOMA

Papilloma is a common benign neoplasm of the oral cavity, arising from the epithelial tissue. It is characterized by an exophytic papillary growth with a typical **'cauliflower like'** appearance. This lesion constitutes about 2% of all oral neoplasms and it is believed by many investigators that they are caused by Human papilloma virus (HPV). HPV virus subtypes 6 and 11 have been detected from neoplastic tissues of papilloma.

CLINICAL FEATURES

Age: Any age but mostly third, fourth and fifth decade.

Sex: Both sexes are equally affected.

Site: Tongue, lips, buccal mucosa, gingiva, hard and soft plate, etc.

CLINICAL PRESENTATION

- Clinically, papilloma appears as a slow growing, exophytic, soft, usually pedunculated, painless, nodular growth often with a typical **'cauliflower-like' appearance.**
- Papillomas often characteristically have numerous finger-like projections on their surface, which can be either blunt or pointed.
- Because of these projections, the Papilloma often appears as an ovoid swelling with a rough, corrugated surface.
- The size of the lesion is usually small and that varies from few millimeters to about one centimeter in diameter.
- The base of the lesion can be either **pedunculated or sessile (broad based)** but Papilloma is mostly a well-circumscribed growth.
- The lesion is mostly white in color and is firm in consistency as the surface is highly keratinized.
- Sometimes superficial ulceration and secondary infection may occur especially in those lesions in the oral cavity, which are often subjected to trauma.
- A papilloma with non-keratinized surface may also occur and in such cases it will appear pinkish or greyish in color and moreover, this type of lesion is usually softer in consistency.
- Multiple papillomas may sometimes coalesce together and form a large lesion in the oral cavity and the condition is commonly known as 'papillomatosis'.
- *Papillomatosis of oral mucosa may sometimes occur in association with skin disorders, e.g. Focal dermal hypoplasia syndrome, Nevus unius lateris, Cowden syndrome and Acanthosis nigricans, etc.*
- 'Nevus unius lateris' is a dermal condition in which papillomatous growths can be seen in the trunk and limbs, with a unilateral distribution.

HISTOPATHOLOGICAL FEATURES

- **Proliferating keratinized stratified squamous epithelium in the form of multiple fingers-like projections.**
- **Every single finger-like projection has a fibrovascular connective tissue core in the center, which contains few inflammatory cells.**
- **The covering squamous epithelium shows hyperkeratosis and acanthosis. Thickening of the keratin is seen in lesions which are clinically whiter.**
- **Although most of the papillary projections are long and finger-like, there can be some projections, which are short, round and blunt.**
- **In the spinus cell layer 'koilocytes' are sometimes seen, these are virus-altered epithelial clear cells with small dark (pyknotic) nuclei.**
- **In some lesions, slightly increased mitotic activity can be seen in the basal layer of the epithelium, which results in mild epithelial hyperplasia.**

61. Ans. (d) Gardner's syndrome *Ref: Neville's Oral and Maxillofacial Pathology 3rd ed. Pg. 651; Shafer's Textbook of Oral Pathology 7th ed. Pg. 48*

Gardner's syndrome:

- Gardner's syndrome is an interesting disease complex, reviewed by Fader and his associates and by Duncan and his associates.
- It is also characterized by the occurrence of multiple impacted supernumerary teeth.
- This syndrome consists of *[Mnemonic: pM MODI]*: (1) Multiple polyposis of the large intestine, (2) Multiple epidermoid or sebaceous cysts of the skin, particularly on the scalp and back, (3) Osteomas of the bones, including long bones, skull, and jaws, (4) occasional occurrence of Desmoid tumors, and (5) Impacted supernumerary and permanent teeth.
- It is due to a single pleiotropic gene and has an autosomal dominant pattern of inheritance, with complete penetrance and variable expression.
- The responsible gene has been mapped to the long arm of chromosome 5 and has been identified as the adenomatous polyposis coli (APC) tumor suppressor gene.

62. Ans. (b) Nicotinic stomatitis *Ref: Shafer's Textbook of Oral Pathology 7th ed. Pg. 96*

Stomatitis nicotina or **pipe smoker's palate** is first manifested by **redness and inflammation of the palate**. Palate develops multinodular appearance with a small red spot in the center of each tiny nodule, representing the dilated and sometimes partially blocked orifice of an accessory palatal salivary gland duct around which inflammatory cell infiltration is prominent.

The epithelium around the ducts shows excessive thickening and keratinization.

63. Ans. (a) Adenoid cystic carcinoma

Also known as cylindroma.

Has the tendancy to spread through perineural spaces and usually invades well beyond the clinically apparent borders.

The cribriform growth pattern shows epithelial cell nests that form multiple cylindrical cystlike patterns resembling a swiss cheese or honey comb pattern, which is the most classic pattern.

High tendency for recurrence.

64. Ans. (c) Osteoid osteoma

Benign tumor of the bone

Etiology unknown

Chief symptom—severe, unrelenting and sharp pain.

Radiographically, it presents a pathognomonic picture characterized by a small ovoid or round radiolucent area surrounded by a rim of sclerotic bone, known as bull's eye appearance.
Osteoblastoma—no distinct radiographic feature

Osteopetrosis—rugger jersey sign (vertebrae becomes extremely dense with alternating bands)

65. Ans. (d) Ameloblastoma

Ameloblastoma-true neoplasm of the enamel organ type tissue.

Usually Unicentric, nonfunctional, intermittent in growth, anatomically benign and clinically persistant.

Second most common odontogenic neoplasm
Most common-odontoma.

Radiographic features-classic mulitlocular cystlike lesion, exhibits a compartmented appearance with septa of bone extending into the radiolucent tumor mass.

Honeycomb or soap bubble patten.

66. Ans. (c) Adenoid cystic carcinoma

Also known as cylindroma.

Has the tendancy to spread through perineural spaces and usually invades well beyond the clinically apparent borders.

The cribriform growth pattern shows epithelial cell nests that form multiple cylindrical cystlike patterns resembling a swiss cheese or honey comb pattern, which is the most classic pattern.

High tendency for recurrence.

67. Ans. (b) Pleomorphic adenoma

Pleomorphic adenoma is a benign neoplasm consisting of cells exhibiting the ability to differentiate to epithelial (ductal and non ductal) cells and mesenchymal (chondroid, myxoid and osseous) cells.
Most common salivary gland tumor.

Its postulated that the myoepithelial cells are responsible for the morphologic diversity of the lesion including the production of the fibrous, mucinous, chondroid and osseous areas.

68. Ans. (c) Schwannoma *Ref: Shafer's-6th ed. Pg. 200*

Schwannomas are benign peripheral nerve sheath neoplasms composed almost entirely of Schwann cells and are diagnosed histopathologically by the presence of singular architectural patterns called Antoni A and Antoni B areas. These were described first in 1920 by the Swedish neurologist Nils Antoni. The Antoni A tissue is highly cellular and made up of palisades of Schwann cell nuclei, a pattern first described in 1910 by the Uruguayan neuro-pathologist Jose Verocay and are known as Verocay bodies.

69. Ans. (a) Lichen planus

Longitudinal ridging (onychorrhexis) is the most common sign of lichen planus in the nail.

Nail lichen planus (NLP) is characterized by thinning, longitudinal ridging and distal splitting of the nail plate. Although mild NLP is usually asymptomatic, deformation of the fingernails is cosmetically distressing. Failure to treat NLP results in nail loss or permanent nail dystrophy in some cases. Therefore the condition should be treated effectively in its early stage. NLP is usually resistant to topical corticosteroid therapy, but successful treatment has been reported with intralesional or systemic administration of corticosteroids.

70. Ans. (c) Hodgkin's disease

According to key given by A.B. Shetty answer is (2)

Reed–Sternberg cells (also known as lacunar histiocytes for certain types) are different giant cells found with light microscopy in biopsies from individuals with Hodgkin's lymphoma (aka Hodgkin's disease; a type of lymphoma). They are usually derived from B lymphocytes, classically considered crippled germinal center B cells, meaning they have not undergone hypermutation to express their antibody.

Reed–Sternberg cells are large and are either multinucleated or have a bilobed nucleus with prominent eosinophilic inclusion-like nucleoli (thus resembling an 'owl's eye' appearance). Reed–Sternberg cells are CD30 and CD15 positive, usually negative for CD20 and CD45. The presence of these cells is necessary in the diagnosis of Hodgkin's lymphoma—the absence of Reed–Sternberg cells has very highnegative predictive value. They can also be found in reactive lymphadenopathy (such as infectious mononucleosis, carbamazepine associated lymphadenopathy) and very rarely in other types of non-Hodgkin lymphomas.

71. Ans. (c) It affects females more commonly than males

Smoker's melanosis (see Right) is increased tissue pigmentation, or darkening, due to irritation from tobacco smoke. Typically this pigmentation occurs on the gingiva (gums) of the upper and lower front teeth. The amount of pigmentation increases with greater tobacco use, and is more common in females; it occurs in 5.0–22% of cigarette and pipe smokers. There is no treatment for smoker's melanosis; however, tissues typically return to normal color in 6 to 36 months after quitting smoking.

72. Ans. (b) Squamous cell carcinoma

According to key given by A.B. Shetty answer is (3)

Spindle cell carcinoma (squamous cell carcinoma)

A carcinoma within which there are some elements resembling a squamous cell carcinoma that are associated with a spindle cell component. In a true Spindle cell carcinoma, the malignant spindle shaped cell should be demonstrably of epithelial origin and derived from the squamous cell component of the carcinoma.

73. Ans. (a) Sturge-Weber syndrome *Ref: Shafers 6th ed. Pg. 144 and Oral Manifestations of Neurological Disorders. Dental Hypothesis, 2014 Vol. 5; 2 Pg. 78-79]*

Sturge-Weber syndrome is associated with congenital hamartomatous malformations that affect the eye, skin and CNS. It is characterized by venous angiomas of the leptomeninges with ipsilateral angiomatous lesions of the face, skull, jaw and soft tissues. The port wine nevi are usually the first component observed at birth, exclusive to the skin area supplied by trigeminal nerve. The oral features include angiomatous lesions of the gingiva and the buccal mucosa. According to Can J Neurol Sci 2008 Jul;35(3):301-7; Sturge Weber syndrome: the facial nevus flammeus was unilateral in 63.5% and blilateral in 31% and absent in 5.5% of the patients with leptomeningeal angiomas.

Phakomatoses (or neuro-oculo-cutaneous syndromes, neurocutaneous disorders) are multisystem disorders that have characteristic central nervous system, ocular and cutaneous lesions of variable severity. The common neurocutaneous (phakomatosis) diseases include Sturge-Weber syndrome, tuberous sclerosis, and neurofibromatosis of von Recklinghausen and incontinentia pigmenti. These diseases are frequently remains unnoticeable but have significant direct relationship to oral cavity and orofacial structures.

74. Ans. (a) Angioneuroticedema *Ref: Shafers Textbook of Oral Pathology 6th ed. Pg. 928*

Angioedema is a diffuse edematous swelling of the soft tissues commonly involving the subcutaneous and submucosal connective tissues.

Quincks describing this disorder as early as in 1882, related the changes observed to an alteration in vascular permeability, so called **Quinck's edema.**

Mast cell degranulation, which leads to histamine release and the typical manifestations, is seen commonly in IgE-mediated hypersensitivity reactions caused by drugs, foods, Plants, dust, and inhalants.

- Hereditary form; Two rare autosomal dominant hereditary forms are seen.

Type I, comprising 85% of the cases, is caused by a quantitative reduction in the inhibitor that prevents the transformation of C1 to C1 esterase. Without adequate levels of this inhibitor (C1-INH), C1 esterase cleaves C4 and C2 and results in angioedema.

Type 2 exhibits normal levels of C1-INH, but the inhibitor is non-functional.

- Acquired form: Seen in association with certain type of lymphoproliferative diseases in patients who develop specific antibodies.

Angioedema manifests as a soft, nontender, diffuse edematous swelling of relatively rapid onset, which may be solitary or multiple, most commonly involving the face around the lips, chin, eyes, lips, tongue, pharynx, and larynx.

75. Ans. (a) Floor of mouth *Ref: Burket's oral medicine 11 th ed pg no 102]*

Oral leukoplakia lesions of the tongue and the floor of the mouth account for more than 90% of cases that show dysplasia or carcinoma.

Modified classification for oral leukoplakia	
L1	Size of Leukoplakia < 2 cm
L2	Size of Leukoplakia 2-4 cm
L3	Size of Leukoplakia >4 cm
Lx	Size of Leukoplakia not specified
P0	No epithelial dysplasia
P1	Distinct epithelial dysplasia
Px	Epithelial dysplasia not specified in pathology report

OLEP (oral leukoplakia) staging system	
Stage 1	L1PO
Stage 2	L2PO
Stage 3	L3PO (OR) L1L2P1
Stage 4	L3P1

76. Ans. (a) Basal cell carcinoma *Ref: Shafers Textbook of Oral Pathology 6th ed. Pg. 141, 142*

Basal Cell Carcinoma (also called **rodent ulcer**)

The most common malignancy in humans, BCC develops most frequently on the exposed surface of the skin, the face and the scalp in middle-aged or elderly persons.

It is slow growing and rarely metastasizes, but is can cause significant local destruction and disfigurement if neglected or treated inadequately.

BCC is most frequently seen in the **middle third of the face**, but may occur anywhere on the **sun-exposed part of skin**. It does not arise from oral mucosa and is never seen in the oral cavity unless it arrives there by invasion and infiltration from a skin surface.

77. Ans. (d) All of the above *Ref: Shafers Textbook of Oral Pathology 6th ed. Pg. 108*

Clinical Staging of Carcinomas of Head and Neck (TNM System)

In a patient with carcinoma, clinical staging is used to designate the extent of the disease and to determine the most appropriate treatment necessary for that patient during that particular stage of the disease.

Finally the method helps in making an overall evaluation regarding the prognosis of the disease.

The designation used in the TNM system are as follows:

T for primary tumor

N for regional lymph node

M for distant metastatis

All these criterias incorporated in the system are major factors, which definitely influence the prognosis of the disease.

Another clinical staging system has been introduced in recent times, which is called the STNMP system. In this system, two new variables have been included besides the original TNM factors and these are—'S' (site of the tumor) and 'P' (Pathology of the tumor).

According to many investigators, the STNMP staging system has promised considerable improvement regarding the prognostic evaluation and differentiation of a tumor over the TNM system.

TNM System: Definition and staging groups

T- Primary Tumor

TX – Primary tumor can be assessed

T0 – No evidence of primary tumor

TIS – Carcinoma – in situ

T1 – Tumor size -2 cm or less in greasted dimension

T3 – Tumor size more than 4 cm in greatest dimension

T4 – Tumor invades adjacent structures

N – Regional Lymph Node

NX – Regional lymph nodes cannot be assessed

N0 – No regional lymph node metastasis

N1 – Metastasis in single ipsilateral lymph node, 3 cm or less in greatest dimension

N2 – Metastasis in single ipsilateral lymph node, more than 3 cm but less than 6 cm in greatest dimension, or in multiple ipsilateral nodes or in bilateral or contralateral nodes (none more than 6 cm in greatest dimension).

N2a - Metastasis in single ipsilateral lymph node, more than 3 cm but less than 6 cm in greatest dimension.

N2b - Metastasis in single ipsilateral lymph node, none more than 6 cm in greatest dimension.

N2c - Metastasis in bilateral or contralateral lymph node, none more than 6 cm in greatest dimension.

N3 - Metastasis in lymph node, more than 6 cm in greatest dimension.

M – Distant Metastasis

MX – Presence of distant metastatis cannot be assessed

M0 – No distant metastasis

M1 – Clinical or radiographic evidence of metastasis

TNM clinical staging of oral carcinoma

	T	*N*	*M*
Stage 0	Tis	N0	M0
Stage I	T1	N0	M0
Stage II	T2	N0	M0
Stage III	T1	N1	M0
	T2	N1	M0
	T3	N0 N1	M0
Stage IV	T4	N0 N1	M0
	Any T	N2 N3	M0

78. Ans. (a) Upper lip *Ref: Shafers Textbook of Oral Pathology 6th ed. Pg. 541*

It is significantly observed that the **mucoceles are restricted almost entirely to the lower lip**, seldom found on the upper lip, while **accessory salivary gland and other neoplasms of the lips are almost universally found on the upper lip** and only rarely on the lower lip.

SALIVARY GLAND

79. Ans. (d) Warthin tumor *Ref: Shafer's 6th ed. Pg. 226*

Warthin's Tumor (Papillary cystadenoma lymphomatosum, adenolymphoma)

Histologic Featues

Microscopic features

The tumor consist of two histologic components: epithelial and lymphoid tissue.

- The cysts are lined by papillary proliferations.
- The inner layer cells are tall columnar with fine granule and eosinophilic cytoplasm hyperchromatic nuclei.
- The outer layer cells are oncocytic triangular and occasionally fusiform basaloid cells.
- Focal areas of squamous metaplasia and mucous cell prosoplasia may be seen. There is frequently.
- An eosinophilic coagulum present within the cystic spaces, which appears as chocolate-colored fluid in the gross specimen.

80. Ans. (d) Palate *Ref: Shafer's 6th ed. Pg. 219-221*

- Plemorphic adenoma is a benign neoplasm consisting of cells hasthe ability to differentiate to epithelial (ductal and nonductal) cells and mesenchymal (chondroid, myxoid and ossesou) cells.
- Pleomorphic adenoma is the most common tumor of salivary glands. The parotid gland is the most common site of the pleomorphic adenoma.
- Approximately 8% of pleomorphic adenomas involve the minor salivary glands, the palate is the most common site of minor salivary gland involvement.
- The palatal glands are frequently the site of origin of this type of tumors.
- The palatal pleomorphic adenoma may appear fixed to the underlying bone, but is not invasive.

81. Ans. (a) Pleomorphic adenoma *Ref: Shafer's 6th ed. Pg. 220, 226, 231, 232*

- Pleomorphic adenoma is the most common salivary gland tumor.
- Warthin tumor is the second most common tumor in the salivary glands. This tumor was first recognized by Albrecht in 1910 later described by Warthin in 1929.
- Acinic cell carcinoma is the thin most common malignant salivary gland epithelial neoplasm mucoepidermoid.

82. Ans. (a) Mucoepidermoid CA *Ref: Neville's Oral and Maxillofacial Pathology 3rd ed. Pg. 487*
Shafer's Textbook of Oral Pathology 7th ed. Pg. 235

Mucoepidermoid Carcinoma

- Mucoepidermoid carcinoma is a malignant epithelial tumor composed of both mucus-secreting cells and epidermoid-type.
- Site—The parotid gland is the most common site of occurrence.
- Palate (Intraorally m/c site)
- It is the most common malignant neoplasm observed in the major and minor salivary glands.
- It is the most common malignant salivary gland tumor of children.
- Histologically the mucoepidermoid carcinoma is composed of mucous secreting cells, epidermoid type (squamous) cells and intermediate cells (basaloid cells or maternal cell).

- Grading:
  - Low-grade tumors—is not completely encapsulated and show well formed glandular structures and prominent mucin filled cystic spaces, minimal cellular atypia and a high proportion of mucous cells, cyst formation prominent.
  - Intermediate-grade tumors—have solid areas of epidermoid cells or squamous cells with intermediate basaloid cells. All cell types are present, but intermediate cells predominate.

High-grade tumors are not encapsulated and consist of cells present as solid nests and cords of intermediate basaloid cells and epidermoid cells. Prominent nuclear pleomorphism and mitotic activity is noted. Facial nerve paralysis is frequent in parotid tumors.

83. Ans. (c) Warthin tumor *Ref: Oral and Maxillofacial Pathology by Neville 3rd ed. Pg. 482*

Synonym: papillary cystadenoma lymphomatosum

Warthin tumor is a benign neoplasm that occurs almost exclusively in the parotid gland.

It represents the second most common benign tumor of parotid gland.

A number of studies have demonstrated a strong association between the development of this tumor and smoking. Smokers have eightfold greater risk for Warthin tumor than nonsmoker.

84. Ans. (a) Ranula *Ref: Shafer's Textbook of Oral Pathology 6th ed. Pg. 543*

Ranula is a form of large mucocele frequently associated with sublingual gland. Thus it causes the swelling in the floor of the mouth below the tomgue.

The name is so as it resembles frog's belly.

The mucocele mostly originates due to rupture of salivary duct following trauma that results in pooling of saliva and consequent swelling.

It is of two types:

a. Extravasation mucocele: more common type
b. Retention mucocele: true retention cyst

85. Ans. (c) Hydroxyapatite *Ref: Burket's Oral Medicine 11th ed. Pg. 201*

The sialolith are usually crystalline in nature and are composed primarily of hydroxyapatite. The chemical composition is calcium phosphate and carbon, with trace amounts of magnesium potassium chloride and ammonium.

50% of parotid gland and 20% of sublingual gland sialolith are poorly calcified, which are radiographically not detectable.

86. Ans. (d) Necrotizing sialometaplasia *Ref: Shafer's Textbook of Oral Pathology 6th ed. Pg. 256*

Necrotizing sialometaplasia is a benign, inflammatory reaction of salivary gland that mimics a salivary gland malignancy.

Etiology is mostly due to **local ischemia**.

Most common intraoral site is palate followed by buccal mucosa and the type of necrosis is coagulative necrosis. **Similar type of lesions in skin are called as syringometaplasia.**

87. Ans. (d) Pleomorphic adenoma

Pleomorphic adenoma is a common benign salivary gland neoplasm characterized by neoplastic proliferation of parenchymatous glandular cells along with myoepithelial components, having a malignant potentiality. It is the most common type of salivary gland tumor and the most common tumor of the parotid gland. It derives its name from the architectural pleomorphism (variable appearance) seen by light microscopy. It is also known as 'Mixed tumor, salivary gland type', which describes its pleomorphic appearance as opposed to its dual origin from epithelial and myoepithelial elements.

88. Ans. (a) Parotid *Ref: Shafers Textbook of Oral Pathology 6th ed Pg. 319*

Warthin Tumor (synonyms: Papillary cystadenoma lymphomatosum, adenolymphoma)
Warthin tumor is the second most common tumor in the salivary glands. This unusual type of salivary gland tumor occurs almost exclusively in the parotid gland, although occasional cases have been reported in the submaxillary gland. The intraoral accessory salivary glands are rarely affected.

BACTERIAL, VIRAL AND MYCOTIC INFECTIONS

89. Ans. (b) 5.5 *Ref: Shafer's 6th ed. Pg. 426*

The pH at which any particular saliva creases to be saturated with calcium and phosphate is referred to as the 'critical pH'; below this value, the inorganic material of the tooth may dissolve. It is considered as 5.5 because at this pH the calcium and phosphate concentration varies.

90. Ans. (d) Sucrose *Ref: Shafer's 6th ed. Pg. 430-431*

- The carbohydrates available in human diets principally are starches, sucrose and some lactose; with less glucose, fructose or maltose.
- Sucrose is primarily responsible in the pathogenesis of dental caries.
- The key role of sucrose as a dietary substrate in the caries process on smooth surfaces S. mutans directly utilized sucrose via PTS.
- The intercellular product sucrose 6-phosphate is then cleaved by a sucrose 6-phosphate hydrolase, which give rise to glucose 6-phosphate and fructose. The sucrose 6-phosphate has dual specificity for sucrose 6- phosphate and sucrose.

91. Ans. (a) Submandibular region

Ludwig's Angina

- The distinct clinical entity of Ludwigs angina is characterized by a deep, lender swelling of both the submandibular and sublingual spaces, swelling of the flour of the mouth, and elevation of the tongue.
- This condition is usually a nonsuppurative cellulitis that originates in the submandibular space and spreads rapidly toward the floor of the mouth. It is caused almost exclusively from mandibular molar teeth because their root apices may reach below the mylohyoid ridge. An apical infection may spread directly to the submandibular space, and from there it may extend to adjacent regions by continuity. The subperiosteal implant does not extend below this structure beyond the first molar, so the risk of infection below the muscle is reduced. The main danger from this infection is asphyxiation as a result of rapidly increasing respiratory embarrassment caused by swelling and displacement of the tongue backward and edema of the glottis. Early in the disease there is no pus. and thus no fluctuation. If pus does form, it will be found between the mylohyoid and geniohyoid or between the geniohyoid and genioglossus. This will make swallowing and speech more difficult.
- Bilateral incisions of the submandibular spaces with a blunt dissection into the submental region are needed. An incision into the submental space through the mylohyoid muscle should also be made. A clamp is inserted toward the base of the tongue to explore the sublingual space. The through and through drainage through submandibular space should be done.

'Contemporary Implant Dentistry by Carl E. Misch Spread of Dental Infection in Head and Neck, Page 507'

92. Ans. (c) Leukemia

- Perioral and intraoral Characteristics: Oral findings in all types of leukemia include increased gingival or periodontal infections, increased gingival bleeding, unexplained petechiae or purpura in the oral soft tissues. and gingival enlargement due to leukemic infiltrate Gingival enlargement is seen most often in CML. Many patients seek dental care prior to medical tare because of the rapid decline in oral health and appearance of the tissues.

'Shafer's Textbook of Oral Pathology (6th Edition) - Page 394, by R. Rajendran'

93. Ans. (a) Acute atrophic Candidiasis *Ref: Textbook of Oral Pathology by Anil Ghom 1st ed. Pg. 507*

- Acute pseudomembranous candidiasis (thrush) is a common infection in the young, elderly, or debilitated. The white plaques arc easily removable and contain candidal hyphae, spores, epithelial cells, and polymorphs.
- Acutc atrophic candidiasis also is known as antibiotic sore mouth because it frequently occurs during antibiotic therapy. This condition is a response to the suppression of the normal bacterial flora and is characterized by widespread erythematous stomatitis with accompanying depapillation of the tongue.

94. Ans. (c) Lues maligna *Ref: Purkait 3rd ed. Pg. 325, Nevelle 3rd ed. Pg. 190*

Condylomata lata: Papillary lesions in seconday syphilis that resemble viral papillomas.

Lues maligna: Explosive and widespread form of secondary syphilis in immunocompromised patients. It most commonly affect patient with low CD 4 cell counts.

95. Ans. (c) Present on skin fold secondary to capillary fragility *Ref: Shafer's 6th ed. Pg. 311*

Scarlet fever is cause by b-hemolytic streptococci, streptococci pyogens.

It is characterized by bright skin rashes after 2–3 days of infection, which are particularly prominent on skin fold as a result of toxic injury to the vascular epithelium leading to dilatation of blood vessels and hyperemia, prominent rashes in the area of skin fold is known as pastia lines.

Small papules of normal color erupt through this rashes giving a characteristic sand paper feel appearance.

Oral lesion: first white strawberry tongue and then raspberry tongue.

96. Ans. (a) Oral herpes *Ref: Shafer's Textbook of Oral Pathology 6th ed. Pg. 336*

Clinical Features: The disease occurring in children is frequently the primary attack and is characterized by the development of fever, irritability, headache, pain upon swallowing and regional lymphadenopathy. Within a few days, the mouth becomes painful and the gingival which is intensely inflamed appears erythematous and edematous. The lips, tongue, buccal mucosa, palate, pharynx and tonsils may also be involved. Shortly, yellowish, fluid-filled vesicles develop. These rupture and form shallow, ragged, extremely painful ulcers covered by a gray membrane and surrounded by an erythematous halo. The ulcers vary considerably in size, ranging from very tiny lesions to lesions measuring several millimeters or even a centimeter in diameter. They healspontaneously within 7–14 days and leave no scar.

Histologic Features: The infected cells are swollen and have pale eosinophilic cytoplasm and large vesicular nuclei, described as 'ballooning degeneration,' while others characteristically contain intranuclear inclusions known as Lipschutz bodies. These are eosinophilic, ovoid, homogeneous structures within the nucleus, which tend to displace the nucleolus and nuclear chromatin peripherally. The displacement of chromatin often produces a peri-inclusion halo.

97. Ans. (d) Recurrent Aphthae *Ref: Neville's Oral and Maxillofacial Pathology 3rd ed. Pg. 242, 333, 518, 777 Shafer's Textbook of Oral Pathology 7th ed. Pg. 334, 342, 667, 815*

Pyogenic Granuloma (Granuloma pyogenicum)

- *It is a distinctive clinical entity originating as a response of the tissues to a nonspecific infection.*
- *Pyogenic granuloma arises as a result of some minor trauma to the tissues, which provides a pathway for the invasion of nonspecific types of microorganisms (either staphylococci or streptococci)*
- *The pyogenic granuloma of the oral cavity arises most frequently on the gingiva accounting around 75% of all cases. It may also occur on the lips, tongue and buccal mucosa, and occasionally on other areas.*
- *The lesions are more common in the facial aspect than the lingual or palatal aspects of gingiva and can occur involving both sides including interdental papilla.*

Acute herpaticgingivostomatitis (primary herpes):

- *Transmitted bydroplet spread or contact with the lesions.*
- *It affects childrenand young adults.*
- *It rarely occurs before the age of six months, apparently because of the presence of circulating antibodies inthe infant derived from the mother.*
- *Within a few days of infection, the mouth becomes painful and the gingiva which isintensely inflamed appears erythematous and edematous. The lips, tongue, buccal mucosa, palate, pharynx, and tonsils may also be involved.*
- *Lesions heal spontaneously within 7–14 days andleave no scar.*

Recurrent aphthous:

Characterized by the development of painful, recurring solitary or multiple ulcerations of the oral mucosa.

The typical 'Anitschkow cell' ina cytologic smear from the margin of an aphthous ulcer.

Classified into four chief varieties:

- *Recurrent aphthousminor (canker' sore)-most common form of the disease, occurs somewhat more frequently in women than in men.*
- *The most common sites of occurrence are the buccal and labial mucosa, buccal and lingual sulci, tongue, soft palate, pharynx, gingiva, and all locations of labile mucosa not bound to periosteum (D/D: recurrent intraoral herpes simplex infection).*
- *Recurrent aphthous major—occurrence of large painful ulcers, on the lips, cheeks, tongue, soft palate, and fauces and cause severe pain and dysphagia.*
- *Recurrent herpetiform ulcerations and*
- *Behcet's syndrome.*

All the options mentioned do show gingival involvement, but according to Neville's Oral and maxillofacial Pathology 3rd ed. Page no. 333.

In minor aphthous ulceration:

- *The buccal and labial mucosae are the most commonly involved sites, followed by the ventral surface of the tongue, mucobuccal fold, floor of the mouth and soft palate.*
- *Involvement of keratinized mucosa (e.g. hard palate, gingiva, dorsal surface of the tongue and vermilion border) is rare and usually represents extension from adjacent non-keratinized epithelium.*

98. Ans. (a) Human papilloma virus *Ref: Neville's Oral and Maxillofacial Pathology 3rd ed. Pg. 363; Shafer's Textbook of Oral Pathology 7th ed. Pg. 81-82]*

Papilloma

Papilloma is a common benign neoplasm of the oral cavity, arising from the epithelial tissue. It is characterized by an exophytic papillary growth with a typical 'cauliflower-like' appearance. It is caused by Human papilloma virus (HPV). HPV virus subtypes 6 and 11 have been detected from neoplastic tissues of papilloma.

C/F:

- A slow growing, exophytic, soft, usually pedunculated, painless, nodular growth often with a typical 'cauliflower-like' appearance.
- Have numerous finger-like projections on their surface which gives ovoid swelling with a rough, corrugated surface appearance.
- Papilloma is mostly a well-circumscribed growth.
- Multiple papillomas may sometimes coalesce together and form a large lesion in the oral cavity and the condition is commonly known as 'papillomatosis'.
- Papillomatosis of oral mucosa may sometimes occur in association with skin disorders, e.g. Focal dermal hypoplasia syndrome, Nevus uniuslateris, Cowden syndrome and Acanthosisnigricans, etc.
- 'Nevus uniuslateris' is a dermal condition in which papillomatous growths can be seen in the trunk and limbs, with a unilateral distribution.

Histopathologically, in the spinus cell layer 'koilocytes' are sometimes seen, these are virus-altered epithelial clear cells with small dark (pyknotic) nuclei.

99. Ans. (d) Non-fusion of mesodermal thickening and retraction of tuberculum impar *Ref: Neville's Oral and Maxillofacial Pathology 3rd ed. Pg. 216; Shafer's Textbook of Oral Pathology 7th ed. Pg. 31-32*

'Other forms of erythematous candidiasis are usually asymptomatic and chronic. Included in this category is the condition known as central papillary atrophy of the tongue or median rhomboid glossitis. In the past, this was thought to be a developmental defect of the tongue, occurring in 0.01% to 1.00% of adult. *The lesion was supposed to have resulted from failure of the embryonic tuberculum impar to covered by the lateral processes of the tongue.*'- Neville's 3rd ed./216

'The posterior dorsal point of fusion is occasionally defective, leaving a rhomboid-shaped, smooth erythematous mucosa lacking in papillae or taste buds. This median rhomboid glossitis (central papillary atrophy, posterior lingual papillary atrophy) is a focal area of susceptibility to recurring or chronic atrophic candidiasis, prompting a recent shift towards the use of posterior midline atrophic candidiasis as a more appropriate diagnostic term.'- Shafer's 7th ed./31-32

Also know:

- *Some patients even develop a similar lesion on the midline of the palate just opposite to the tongue lesion and it occurs due to repeated contact with the infected tongue surface to the palate (kissing lesion).*
- Microscopically, median rhomboid glossitis presents the following features:
  - Loss of both filliform and fungiform papilla.
  - There may be presence of acanthosis with elongation of rete-ridges.
  - Pseudoepitheliomatous hyperplasia may be quite pronounced.
  - No treatment is basically required for this lesion. Antifungal agents and antiseptic gurgles are used to relieve the erythema and irritation in the area.

100. Ans. (b) Fluorescent staining *Ref: Burket's Oral Medicine 11th ed. Pg. 45*

- HSV can be identified from scrapings from the base of lesions (especially vesicles) smeared onto glass slides. These can be stained with **Wright, Giemsa (Tzanck preparation), or Papanicolaou stain** to demonstrate the characteristic multinucleated giant cells or intranuclear inclusions. This does not distinguish between HSV or VZV.
- A similar smear preparation can be used for the direct fluorescent antigen detection test using a monoclonal antibody against HSV conjugated to a fluorescent compound such as fluorescein. **Direct fluorescent antigen testing is more accurate than routine cytology.**

101. Ans. (b) Recurrent aphthae *Ref: Neville's Oral and maxillofacial Pathology 3rd ed. Pg. 242, 333, 518, 777; Shafer's Textbook of Oral Pathology 7th ed. Pg. 334, 342, 667, 815*

Pyogenic Granuloma (Granuloma pyogenicum)

- It is a distinctive clinical entity originating as a response of the tissues to a nonspecific infection.
- Pyogenic granuloma arises as a result of some minor trauma to the tissues, which provides a pathway for the invasion of nonspecific types of microorganisms (either staphylococci or streptococci)
- The pyogenic granuloma of the oral cavity arises most frequently on the gingiva accounting around 75% of all cases. It may also occur on the lips, tongue and buccal mucosa, and occasionally on other areas.
- The lesions are more common in the facial aspect than the lingual or palatal aspects of gingiva and can occur involving both sides including interdental papilla.

Acute herpatic gingivostomatitis (primary herpes)

- Transmitted by droplet spread or contact with the lesions.
- It affects children and young adults.
- It rarely occurs before the age of six months, apparently because of the presence of circulating antibodies in the infant derived from the mother.
- Within a few days of infection, the mouth becomes painful and the gingiva which is intensely inflamed appears erythematous and edematous. The lips, tongue, buccal mucosa, palate, pharynx, and tonsils may also be involved.
- Lesions heal spontaneously within 7–14 days and leave no scar.

Recurrent aphthous

- Characterized by the development of painful, recurring solitary or multiple ulcerations of the oral mucosa.
- The typical Anitschkow cell in a cytologic smear from the margin of an aphthous ulcer.

Classified into four chief varieties:

- Recurrent aphthous minor (canker' sore)—most common form of the disease, occurs somewhat more frequently in women than in men.
- The most common sites of occurrence are the buccal and labial mucosa, buccal and lingual sulci, tongue, soft palate, pharynx, gingiva, and all locations of labile mucosa not bound to periosteum (D/D: recurrent intraoral herpes simplex infection).
- Recurrent aphthous major—occurrence of large painful ulcers, on the lips, cheeks, tongue, soft palate, and fauces and cause severe pain and dysphagia.
- Recurrent herpetiform ulcerations and
- Behcet's syndrome.

All the options mentioned do show gingival involvement, but according to Neville's Oral and maxillofacial Pathology 3rd ed. Page no. 333.

In minor aphthous ulceration:

- The buccal and labial mucosae are the most commonly involved sites, followed by the ventral surface of the tongue, mucobuccal fold, floor of the mouth and soft palate.
- Involvement of keratinized mucosa (e.g. hard palate, gingiva, dorsal surface of the tongue and vermilion border) is rare and usually represents extension from adjacent non-keratinized epithelium.

102. Ans. (a) Candidiasis *Ref: Neville's Oral and Maxillofacial Pathology 3rd ed. Pg. 220; Shafer's Textbook of Oral Pathology 7th ed. Pg. 371*

Candidiasis: (Candidosis, moniliasis, thrush)

- Candidiasis is caused by a yeast-like fungus, Candida (Monilia) albicans.
- Candida exists in three forms namely, pseudohyphae, yeast, and chlamydospore forms.
- It reproduces by asexual budding and forms pseudohyphae.
- These species grow rapidly at 25–37°C.
- In general, candida species differ from one another but can be identified by the formation of pseudohyphae or by biochemical test.
- This disease is said to be the most opportunistic infection in the world.

Pseudomembranous Candidiasis

- It is also known as thrush and is one of the most common forms of the candidiasis.
- It may occur at any age, but is especially prone to occur in the debilitated or the chronically ill patients (immune suppression especially HIV infection, or systemic corticosteroid therapy) or in infants.
- The oral lesions are characterized by:
  - The appearance of soft, white, slightly elevated plaques most frequently occurring on the buccal mucosa and tongue.
  - The plaques, resembling as milk curds, consist chiefly of tangled masses of fungal hyphae with intermingled desquamated epithelium, keratin, fibrin, necrotic debris, leukocytes, and bacteria.
  - The white plaque can usually be wiped away with a gauze, leaving either a relatively normal appearing mucosa or an erythematous area.

Erythematous Candidiasis

- Also known as antibiotic sore mouth, includes central papillary atrophy of the tongue and cheilocandidiasis.
- It usually occurs as a sequela to a course of broad spectrum antibiotics, corticosteroids.
- Appear red or erythematous (due to increased vascularity) rather than white, thus resembling the pseudomembranous type in which the white membrane has been wiped off.
- It is only variety of oral candidiasis, which is consistently painful.

Chronic Hyperplastic Candidiasis: (Candidal leukoplakia)

- This is often spoken of as the 'leukoplakia' type of candidiasis.
- The oral lesions consist of firm, white persistent plaques, usually on the lips, tongue, and cheeks and appear similar to leukoplakia.

Denture Stomatitis: (Chronic atrophic candidiasis)

- Better known as denture sore mouth, a diffuse erythema and edema of the denture-bearing area, often occurring with angular cheilitis.
- May be the most common form of the oral disease.

103. Ans. (a) Penicillin + H_2O_2 mouthwash *Ref: Neville's Oral and Maxillofacial Pathology 3rd ed. Pg. 159; Shafer's Textbook of Oral Pathology 7th ed. Pg. 395; Burket's oral Medicine Diagnosis & Treatment 11th ed. Pg. 53*

Necrotizing Ulcerative Gingivitis: (Vincent's infection, trench mouth)

- Manifests both acute and recurrent (subacute) phases; a chronic stage also has been described.
- Inflammatory condition involves primarily the free gingival margin, the crest of the gingiva, and the interdental papillae.
- The lesions spread to the soft palate and tonsillar areas, and in such instances the term vincent's angina has been applied.
- The diagnostic triad consists of—pain, interdental ulceration, and gingival bleeding.
- Frequently occurs in an epidemic pattern, sweeping through groups of persons in close contact, especially those living under similar conditions.
- It is an endogenous, polymicrobial infection causing destructive inflammation due to the coexistence of several predisposing factors.
- Caused by a fusiform bacillus and Borrelia vincentii—a spirochete.
- The disease is characterized by:
  - The development of painful, hyperemic gingiva and sharply punched-out crater like erosions of the interdental papillae of sudden onset.
  - The ulcerated remnants of the papillae and the free gingiva bleed when touched and generally become covered by a grayish green, necrotic pseudomembrane.
- Treatment:
  - The affected area is treated best with debridement by scaling, curettage or ultrasonic instrument (except when contraindicated as in HIV +ve Pts.).

– Frequent rinse with chlorhexidine, warm salt water or diluted hydrogen peroxide are beneficial.
– Antibiotics (Metronidazole and Penicillin, are DOC) are useful adjunct.

104. Ans. (a) Production of extracellular polysaccharides *Ref: Shafer's Textbook of Oral Pathology 7th ed. Pg. 424*

Streptococcus mutans

- First isolated in 1924 by Clarke and coined the term Streptococcus mutans.
- Are catalase negative, gram-positive cocci forming short to medium chains.
- On mitis salivarius agar, they grow as highly convex colonies.
- Unlike other oral streptococci, most strains of S. mutans can be selectively cultured in mitis salivarius agar containing 20% sucrose and 0.2% units/mL of bacitracin.
- **Characteristically, S. mutans synthesizes insoluble polysaccharides from sucrose.**
- It is homofermentative and is more aciduric than other oral streptococci.

105. Ans. (a) Actinomycosis *Ref: Neville's Oral and Maxillofacial Pathology 3rd ed. Pg. 203-204; Shafer's Textbook of Oral pathology 7th ed. Pg. 324-325]*

Actinomycosis

- Actinomycosis is a chronic granulomatous suppurative and fibrosing disease caused by Actinomyces- an anaerobic or microaerophilic, gram-positive, non-acid fast and branched filamentous bacteria.
- They are a normal saprophytic component of oral flora, colon, and vagina and none are known to be recoverable from the environment.
- Common sp. Isolated from actinomycotic lesion are—A. israelii. A. viscous, A. odonolyticus, A. naeslundii or A. myeri.
- The characteristic pattern of disease is formation of abscesses that tends to drain by the formation of sinus tracts. If the pus from abscess examined under glass slide, it shows the typical 'sulfur granules' or colonies of organism which appear in the suppurative materials as tiny yellow grain.
- Actinomycosis is classified anatomically according to the location of the lesions:
  – Cervicofacial forms
  – Abdominal forms
  – Pulmonary forms

Notes:

- Localized abscess without the associated chronic fibrosing reaction have been reported in soft tissue that has received minor trauma. The tongue is the most common site.
- Another infection that produced sulfur granules is Botryomycosis.

106. Ans. (d) Reactivation of HSV 1 *Ref: Regezi's Oral Pathology: Clinical Pathologic Correlation; Burkit, Oral Medicine 11th ed. Pg. 234*

Herpes Simplex Infections

Herpes simplex virus (HSV) infections are common vesicular eruptions of the skin and mucosa. They occur in two forms—systemic or primary—and may be localized or secondary in nature. Both forms are self-limited, but recurrences of the secondary form are common because the virus can be sequestered within ganglionic tissue in a latent state. Control rather than cure is the usual goal of treatment.

Pathogenesis

Physical contact with an infected individual is the typical route of HSV inoculation for a seronegative individual who has not been previously exposed to the virus or possibly for someone with a low titer ofprotective antibody to HSV.

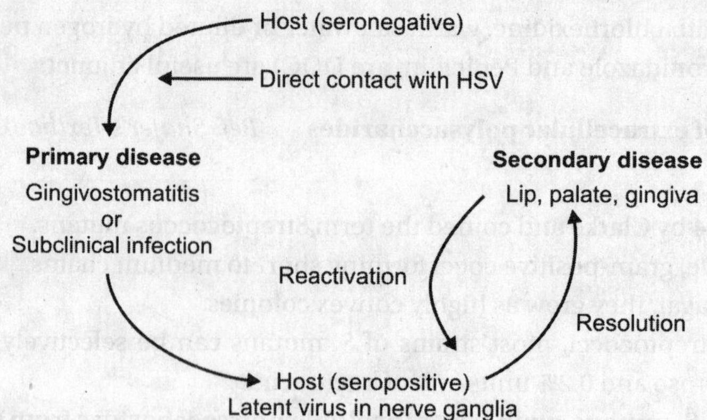

The incubation period after exposure ranges from several days to 2 weeks. In overt primary disease a vesiculo ulcerative eruption (primary gingivostomatitis) typically occurs in the oral and perioral tissues. The focus of eruption is expected at the original site of contact. After resolution of primary herpetic gingivostomatitis, the virus is believed to migrate, through some unknown mechanism, along the periaxon sheath of the trigeminal nerve to the trigeminal ganglion, where it is capable of remaining in a latent or sequestered state. During latency no infectious virus is produced; there is expression of early, but not late, genes; and there is no free virus. No major histocompatibility (MHC) antigens are expressed, so there is no T-cell response during latency.

Reactivation of virus may follow exposure to sunlight ('fever blisters'), exposure to cold ('cold sores'), trauma, stress, or immunosuppression causing a secondary or recurrent infection.

107. Ans. (a) Varicella zoster *Ref: Regezi's Oral Pathology: Clinical Pathologic correlation; Neville's Oral and Maxillofacial Pathology 3rd ed. Pg. 250; Shafer's Textbook of Oral Pathology 7th ed. Pg. 350*

Herpes Zoster: (Shingles, zona)

Herpes zoster is caused by reactivation of the latent V-Z virus which had been acquired during a previous attack of chickenpox. In essence, a primary infection by the V-Z virus results clinically in chickenpox, while a recurrent infection results clinically in herpes zoster.

The fact that herpes zoster is sporadic in occurrence whereas varicella is seasonal further supports the belief that herpes zoster is not a result of a primary exogenous infection.

Herpes zoster is an acute infectious viral disease of an extremely painful and incapacitating nature which is characterized by inflammation of dorsal root ganglia, or extra-medullary cranial nerve ganglia, associated with vesicular eruptions of the skin or mucous membranes in areas supplied by the affected sensory nerves.

Clinical Features:

The disease is most common in adult life and affects males and females with equal frequency.

Occasionally, herpes zoster may resemble the lesions of herpes simplex, but the two diseases can be separated since the zoster virus cannot be transmitted to animals, e.g. the rabbit cornea, as can the simplex virus. It is a common infection in immunocompromised patients and those with certain malignancies, including Hodgkin's disease and the malignant lymphomas, and can be life-threatening if the viscera become involved.

Herpes zoster may involve the face by infection of the trigeminal nerve. This usually consists of unilateral involvement of skin areas supplied by either the ophthalmic, maxillary or mandibular nerves. Lesions of the oral mucosa are fairly common, and extremely painful vesicles may be found on the buccal mucosa, tongue, uvula, pharynx, and larynx.

Hunt's syndrome (James Ramsay Hunt's syndrome): zoster infection of the geniculate ganglion, with the involvement of the external ear and oral mucosa.

108. Ans. (b) Candida albicans *Ref: Neville's Oral and Maxillofacial Pathology 3rd ed. Pg. 216; Shafer's Textbook of Oral Pathology 7th ed. Pg. 925*

Angular cheilitis is a multifactorial disease affecting the commissure of the lips and is commonly seen in denture wearers.

This common condition of the lip has been associated with several predisposing factors such as:

- Infection: majority of infections are Candida-associated, with nearly 20% of the cases arising due to *Candida albicans* alone, 60% due to a combined infection with *Candida albicans* and *Staphylococcus aureus*, and 20% due to *Staphylococcus aureus* alone.
- Nutritional deficiencies: such as iron deficiency anemia, vitamin B, or folic acid efficiency have been strongly implicated in angular cheilitis, referred to as perléche.
- Reduced vertical dimension of the mouth as seen in old age and in long-term denture wearers.
- Other uncommon predisposing factors include diabetes, neutropenia, and AIDS.

109. Ans. (a) Nail *Ref: Neville's Oral and Maxillofacial Pathology 3rd ed. Pg. 244; Shafer's Textbook of Oral Pathology 7th ed. Pg. 342-343; Regezi's Oral Pathology: Clinical Pathologic Correlation; Burkit, Oral Medicine 11th ed. Pg. 234*

- 'Less common presentation of HSV-1 do occurs. Infection of the **thumbs or fingers** is known as—**herpetic whitlow (herpetic paronychia)**, which may occurs as a result of self-inoculation in children with orofacial herpes.'- *Neville 3rd ed. Page no. 244*
- '**Herpetic whitlow** occurs in **fingers** due to autoinoculation. Also, as pointed out by Rowe and his coworkers, recurrent lesions of **the fingers or hands (herpetic whitlow)** and eyes may be encountered in these professional groups more frequently than in the general population.' *Shafer's 7th ed. Page no. 342-343*
- 'In ***Secondary herpes simplex infection*** multiple small ulcers preceded by vesicles; prodromal symptoms of tingling, burning, or pain; most common on lip, intraorally on palate and attached gingiva; adults and young adults usually affected; very common; ***called herpetic whitlow when occurs around fingernail***.' - *Regezi's 5th ed. Page no. 0-3*

Topic Review: Herpes Simplex Infections

- Herpes simplex virus (HSV) infections are common vesicular eruptions of the skin and mucosa.
- They occur in two forms—systemic or primary—and may be localized or secondary in nature.
- Both forms are self-limited, but recurrences of the secondary form are common because the virus can be sequestered within ganglionic tissue in a latent state.
- Control rather than cure is the usual goal of treatment.
- **Pathogenesis:**
  - Physical contact with an infected individual is the typical route of HSV inoculation for a sero negative individual who has not been previously exposed to the virus or possibly for someone with a low titer of protective antibody to HSV.

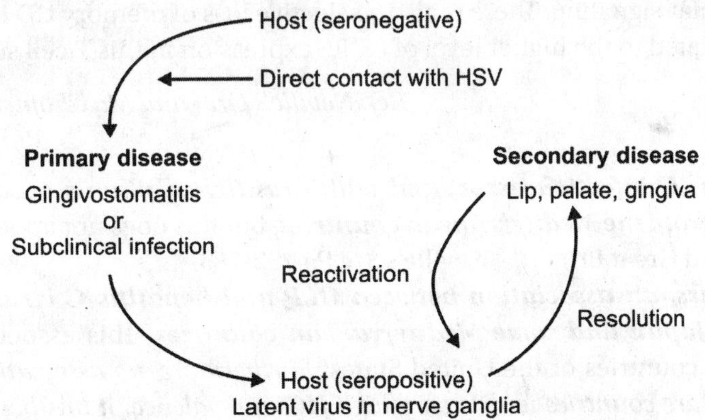

- The incubation period after exposure ranges from several days to 2 weeks.
- In overt primary disease a vesiculo-ulcerative eruption (primary gingivostomatitis) typically occurs in the oral and perioral tissues.
- The focus of eruption is expected at the original site of contact. After resolution of primary herpetic gingivostomatitis, the virus is believed to migrate, through some unknown mechanism, along the periaxon sheath of the trigeminal nerve to the trigeminal ganglion, where it is capable of remaining in a latent or sequestered state.
- During latency no infectious virus is produced; there is expression of early, but not late, genes; and there is no free virus.
- No major histocompatibility (MHC) antigens are expressed, so there is no T-cell response during latency.
- Reactivation of virus may follow exposure to sunlight ('fever blisters'), exposure to cold ('cold sores'), trauma, stress, or immunosuppression causing a secondary or recurrent infection.
- Herpes genitalis, caused by HSV-2, is a relatively common disease of the uterine cervix, vagina, vulva, and penis.
- Herpetic meningoencephalitis is a serious form of this infection, characterized by sudden fever and symptoms of increased intracranial pressure. Paralysis of various muscle groups occurs, while convulsions and even death may ensue.
- Herpetic conjunctivitis, or keratoconjunctivitis, is a rather common disease and is characterized by swelling and congestion of the palpebral conjunctiva, although keratitis and corneal ulceration also may occur. Herpetic vesicles of the eyelids are typical, but these eye lesions usually heal rapidly.
- Herpetic eczema (Kaposi's varicelliform eruption) is an epidermal form of the herpetic infection superimposed upon a pre-existing eczema (possibly an example of anachoresis) and is characterized by diffuse vesicular lesions of the skin, usually of an extremely serious nature.
- Disseminated herpes simplex of the newborn is a relatively uncommon disease in which the newborn baby acquires the infection during passage through the birth canal of a mother who is suffering from herpetic vulvovaginitis.
- Herpetic whitlow occurs in fingers due to autoinoculation.
- Herpes gladiatorum or scrumpox; a cutaneous herpetic lesion occurs in wrestlers and rugby players.
- Herpes barbae; a herpeticlesion occuring on beard region.

110. Ans. (d) Ratio of CD4 cells to CD8 cells *Ref: Robbins Pathology 8th ed. Pg. 160*

- The loss of CD4+ cells leads to an inversion of the CD4: CD8. Ratio is close to 2, patient with AIDS have a ratio of 0.5. Such inversion is a common finding in AIDS, but it may also occur in other viral infections and is therefore not diagnostic.
- Although marked reduction in CD4+ T cells is a hallmark of AIDS and can account for much of the immune deficiency late in the course of HIV infection, there is also compelling evidence for qualitative defects in T cell function that can be detected even in asymptomatic HIV infected person.
- Such defects include reduced antigen induced T cell proliferation, impaired T_h1 cytokine production, and abnormal intracellular signaling. There is also a selective loss of memory CD4+ T cells early in the course of the disease, possible related to the higher level of CCR5 expression in this T cell subset.

111. Ans. (a) Lichen planus *Ref: Neville's Oral and Maxillofacial Pathology 3rd ed. Pg. 782-783; Burkit, Oral Medicine 11th ed. Pg. 90*

- ***'Report of hepatitis C infection associated with oral lichen planus occasionally have appeared in the literature, usually from the Mediterranean countries,*** but this does not appear to be significant association in the United States and Great Britain.' - Neville's 3/e Pg 782-783
- ***'During recent years, an association between OLP and hepatitis C virus (HCV) has been described in populations from Japan and some Mediterranean countries.*** This association has not been observed in northern European countries or the United States. *Furthermore, no association has been reported from Egypt and Nigeria, which are countries with a very high HCV prevalence. It has been postulated that the association*

may be related to a genetic variability between countries. This is in part supported by the observation that specific alleles of the major histocompatibilty complex, such as HLA-DR6, are more prevalent in Italian patients with HCV-related OLP. However, ***no comprehensive explanation has been provided regarding the association between OLP and HCV.***' – Burkit's 11/e Pg 90

112. Ans. (a) Mumps *Ref: Neville's Oral and Maxillofacial Pathology 3rd ed. Pg. 263; Shafer's Textbook of Oral Pathology 7th ed. Pg. 351-352*

- 'Although most authorities assume that ***natural infections is associated with lifelong immunity, rare cases of recurrent mumps have been well documented*** in patients with a confirmed history of prior natural infection.' *– Neville's 3rd ed. Page no. 263*
- 'As the disease is contagious before the onset of parotitis, isolation of patient is not possible to prevent the infection. ***Once infected, patients develop a lifelong immunity against the disease but recurrence is also reported.***' - Shafer's 7th ed. Page no. 351-352

Review Topic: Mumps (Epidemic parotitis)

- Mumps is an acute contagious viral infection (family: Paramyxovirus, genus: Rubulavirus) characterized chiefly by unilateral or bilateral swelling exocrine gland, usually the parotid salivary glands.
- The submaxillary and sublingual glands are occasionally involved, but seldom without parotid involvement also.
- Other than salivary glands, it may also involve nerves meninges, pancreas and gonads.
- Although it is usually a disease of childhood, mumps may also affect adults, and in such cases there is a greater tendency for complications to develop (epididymoorchitis in postpubertal males; oophoritis and mastitis in postpubertal females; meningioencephalitis, pancreatitis).
- Mumps has an incubation period of two to three weeks.
- Epidemiology.
  - The incubation period varies from 14 to 18 days with the extreme of one to four weeks.
  - Mumps is transmitted through the respiratory route.
  - It can *be isolated from the saliva of the infected patients either* ***seven days before the onset of parotitis or nine days after its onset.***
  - Most cases were unrecognized because of the absence of parotid swelling.
  - ***Once infected, patients develop a lifelong immunity against the disease but recurrence is also reported.***
- Pathogenesis:
  - Once transmitted through droplet nuclei or saliva or fomites, it starts replicating in the respiratory epithelium.
  - It spreads to local lymph nodes and subsequently develops viremia.
  - The affected area shows perivascular and interstitial mononuclear cell infiltrates with edema.
  - Necrosis of acinar and epithelial duct cells is seen in salivary glands and in the germinal epithelium of seminiferous tubules.
- Clinical Features:
  - The disease is usually preceded by the onset of headache, chills, moderate fever, vomiting, and pain below the ear.
  - These symptoms are followed by a firm, somewhat rubbery or elastic swelling of the salivary glands, frequently elevating the ear, which usually lasts about one week.
  - The salivary gland involvement produces pain upon mastication.
  - Bilateral parotid involvement occurs in about 70% of the cases.
  - Pain and tenderness may be severe during the rapid phase of parotid enlargement and swelling reaches its maximum in about three days.
  - The submandibular gland may also involve separately or in conjunction with the parotid gland.
  - The involvement of the sublingual gland is

113. Ans. (d) Viral disease *Ref: Oral and Maxillofacial Pathology by Neville 3rd ed. Pg. 371*

Molluscum contagiosum is a virus induced epithelial hyperplasia produced by molluscum contagiosum virus, a member of the DNA poxvirus group.

It affects mainly young adults and children.

Histopathological findings: Molluscum contagiosum appears as a localized lobular proliferation of surface stratified squamous epithelium. The central portion of each lobule is filled with bloated keratinocytes that contain large, intranuclear, **basophilic viral inclusions** called **molluscun bodies** (or **Henderson–paterson bodies**).

114. Ans. (d) They are unilateral *Ref: Shafer's Textbook of Oral Pathology, 6th ed. Pg. 345*

Primary infection with Varicella Zoster Virus, an α-herpesvirus, leads to varicella (chicken pox).

The virus remains latent in dorsal root ganglia or ganglia of cranial nerves. Reactivation produces herpes zoster. In herpes zoster the most sites involved are the areas innervated by spinal cord segments D3 to L2 and the trigeminal nerve, particularly its ophthalmic branch.

Postherpetic neuralgia is a morbid sequela of herpes zoster infection.

Herpes zoster lesion:

- Crops of vesicles in a dermatomal or zosteriform pattern
- Unilateral, linear and clustered distribution of ulcers and vesicles and scabsin a dermatome
- Lesions followed by prodromal symptoms like fever or lynphadenopathy.

115. Ans. (d) Koilocytes *Ref: Oral and Maxillofacial Pathology by Neville. 3rd ed. Pg. 366-367*

Microscopic feature of HPV infection:

Prickle cells often demonstrate pyknotic, crinkled (or raisinlike) nuclei surrounded by clear zones called koilocytes.

Koilocytes may be less prominent in oral lesions but prominent in genital lesions.

Ultrastructural examination reveals virions within the cytoplasm or nuclie of koilocytes, and the virus can also be demonstrated by immunohistochemical analysis, in situ hybridization, and PCR technique.

116. Ans. (c) Vincents angina *Ref: Shafer's Textbook of Oral Pathology, 6th ed. Pg. 326*

Noma is rapidly spreading gangrene of oro facial region, and is caused by Vincent's organisms.

117. Ans. (a) Fungal infection *Ref: Oral and Maxillofacial Pathology by Neville 3rd ed. Pg. 598*

It is also called as **cutaneous T cell lymphoma.**

It is a **fungal** infection.

it has **three stages**: eczematous (erythematous), plaque and tumor stage

Sezary syndrome is an aggressive expression of mycosis fungoids that represents a dermatopathic T-cell leukemia.

118. Ans. (c) Plaque type

Classification of candidiasis by Samaranayake (1991)

Primary	Secondary
1. Acute forms	Oral manifestations of systemic mucocutaneous
a. Pseudomembranous	Candidiasis
b. Erythematous	
2. Chronic forms	
a. Hyperplastic	

b. Candida associated lesions
   Denture stomatitits
   Angular chelitis
   Median rhomboid glossitis

119. Ans. (d) Congenital syphilis *Ref: Shafer's 6th ed. Pg. 324*

Higouménakis' sign is a unilateral enlargement of the sternoclavicular portion of the clavicle, seen in congenital syphilis. It is an end result of neonatal periostitis. The sign was first described by George Higoumenakis in 1927.

120. Ans. (b) Paracoccidioidomycosis *Ref: Greenfield's Neuropathy Vol. 2 8th ed. Pg. 1499*

Paracoccidioidomycosis brasiliensis is endemic in Latin America from mexico to argentina. It is primary a lung infection, with dissemination to other organs, including uncommonly the CNS. The organisms enters the body through the periodontal tissue and subsequently reach the regional lymph nodes, producing a severe lymphadenopathy. The organisms is histologically characteristic, with multiple small yeast budding from a central medium sized yeast resembling Mickey mouse ears.

121. Ans. (b) Epstein barr virus *Ref: Shafer's 6th ed. Pg. 354*

- Oral hairy leukoplakia presents with the corrugated surface of the epithelium on the lateral margin of the tongue.
- It is exclusively seen in young homosexual males.
- Epstein barr virus can trigger OHL. It is hypothesized that EBV present at the basal epithelial of the lateral margin of the tongue.
- It represents as a painless, faint white vertical streaks or thickened and furrowed areas with a shaggy keratotic surface with vertical striation imparting a corrugated appearance.
- EBV can be demonstrated by in situ hybridization, PCR or immunohistochemistry.
- Antiviral agents like acyclovir, desciclovir and ganciclovir, results in clinical improvement.

122. Ans. (c) Both a and b

Three viruses have been associated with head and neck cancer are human papilloma virus (HPV), herpes simplex virus (HSV) and epstein barrvirus (EBV).

HPV may be associated with tumor of the oral cavity, oropharynx and larynx. There is a clear association between EBV and nasopharyngeal cancer.

123. Ans. (c) Noma

According to key given by A.B. Shetty answer is (b)

Cancrumoris, also called noma, is a gangrenous stomatitis. It is a rapidly spreading gangrene of oral amd facial tissue occurring usually in debilitated or nutritionally deficient person. Noma means spreading sore. It is chiefly seen in children.

124. Ans. (a) HSV-1

Herpes viruses

- HSV 1 predominantly affects the face, lips the oral cavity and upper body skin.
- HSV 2 affects predominantly genitals and skin of the lower half f the body.

125. Ans. (d) All of these

Osteoradionecrosis is an acute form of osteomyelitis with formation of sequestrum due to refractory infection and necrosis of the bone. The condition occurs secondary to radiation—induced damage of the intraosseous blood vessels. Osteoradionecrosis generally occurs if the radiation dose in the body exceeds 60 Gy.

Osteoradionecrosis is characterized by ulceration, severe pain, swelling and formation of drainage sinuses or fistulas on the alveolar ridge. Exudation of pus from the area and presence of severe foul smell.

126. Ans. (c) They are free from bacterial infection

According to key given by A.B. Shetty answer is (b)

The evidence for the role of bacteria in the genesis of caries in animal and human models has been studied, leading to the following conclusions:

1. Teeth free from bacterial infection, either in germ-free animals or unerupted teeth in humans, do not develop caries.
2. Antibiotics are effective in reducing caries in animals and humans.
3. Oral bacteria can demineralize enamel in vitro and produce lesions similar to naturally occurring caries.
4. Specific bacteria can be isolated and identified from plaque over various carious lesions.

127. Ans. (c) Congenital syphilis

According to key given by A.B. Shetty answer is (b)

A malformed first molar characterized by dwarfing of the cusps and hypertrophy of the enamel surrounding the cusp with agglomeration ofmasses of globules, giving it the appearance of a mulberry. It is seen in congenital syphilis. Also called mulberry tooth.

Symptoms of congenital syphilis include:

- Blunted upper incisor teeth known as Hutchinson's teeth
- Inflammation of the cornea known as interstitial keratitis
- Deafness from auditory nerve disease
- Frontal bossing (prominence of the brow ridge)
- Saddle nose (collapse of the bony part of nose)
- Hard palate defect
- Swollen knees
- Saber shins
- Short maxillae
- Protruding mandible

128. Ans. (d) None of these

Oral mucositis is defined as the inflammation and ulceration of the oral mucosa. In patients with cancer, it can be induced by chemotherapy and/or radiation therapy.1-4 Although the incidence of mucositis varies depending on the location of the tumor and the course of treatment, occurrence of the condition is highest among patients with cancers of the head and neck, with approximately 80% of these patients developing mucositis.

Mild mucositis is defined as mild erythema, no mucosal ulcerations, and no pain; the patient is able to swallow.

129. Ans. (c) White spot lesion *Ref: Shafer's Textbook of Oral Pathology 6th ed. Pg. 442*

On smooth enamel surface, the earliest microscopic appearance of incipient caries is the appearance of an area of decalcification beneath the dental plaque which resembles a smooth chalky white area. This is referred to as a 'White Spot'. Enamel surface overlying the white spot is hard and shiny and cannot be distinguished from the surface of adjacent sound enamel using the sharp explorer point.

Some information and clinical relevance:

- Caries prone patients usually have extensive deposits of plaque on the teeth, which must be removed before clinical examination. On clean, dry teeth, the earliest evidence of caries on the smooth enamel surface of a crown is a white spot. These lesions usually are observed on the facial and lingual surfaces of the teeth. White spots are chalky white, opaque areas that are revealed only when tooth surface is desiccated and are termed incipient caries. These areas of enamel lose their translucency because of the extensive subsurface porosity caused by demineralization. Care must be excised to distinguish white spots of incipient caries from developmental white spot hypocalcifications of enamel. **Incipient caries partially and totally disappears visually when the enamel is hydrated (wet), whereas hypocalcified enamel is affected less by drying and wetting.**

- Hypocalcifiedenamel does not represent a clinical problem except when its appearance is objectionable esthetically. The surface texture of an incipient lesion is unaltered and is undetectable by tactile examination with an explorer. A more advanced lesion develops a rough surface that is softer than the affected normal enamel. Softened chalky enamel that can be chipped away with an explorer is a sign of active caries. Injudicious use of an explorer tip can cause actual cavitation for a previously non cavitated incipient area, requiring, in most cases, restorative interventions.
- Incipient lesions sometimes can be seen on radiographs as a faint radiolucency, limited to the superficial enamel.

Ref: Sturdevant's Art Rand Science of Operative Dentistry by Theodore Roberson, Harald O. Heymann

130. Ans. (a) Oral candidiasis *Ref:Shafer's Textbook of Oral Pathology, 6th ed. Pg. 491*

Oral candidiasis is the most common opportunistic infection in HIV, of which pseudomembranous type is more prevalently seen.

131. Ans. (a) CAV 16 *Ref: Shafer's Textbook of Oral Pathology 6th ed Pg. 474*

Hand, foot and mouth disease is an epidemic infection, first reported by Robinson and coworkers in 1958. It is caused by the enterovirus Coxsackie A16 and has been reported to be caused less frequently by types A5 and A6 and occasionally even by B2, B5 or enterovirus 71.

The disease is primarily one affecting young children. Between the ages of six months and five years.

It is characterized by tlopapuhe appearance of maculopapular, exanthematous, and vesicular lesions of the skin, particularly involving the hands, feet, legs, arms, and occasionally the buttocks.

A sore mouth and refusal to eat is one of the most common findings in the disease. This is due to the small, multiple vesicular and ulcerative oral lessons that are more numerous than seen in herpangina.

132. Ans. (a) Measles *Ref: Shafer's Textbook of Oral Pathology 6th ed. Pg. 341*

In measles (Rubeola) the oral lesions are prodromal occurs 2–3 days before the cutaneous rash. These lesions are pathognomonic of the disease and are known as 'Koplik's spots'. These spots occur in 97% of cases, but seldom noticed unless the parents or dentists watches carefully and disappears after the onset of rash.

PULP AND PERIAPICAL TISSUE

133. Ans. (c) Acute maxillary sinusitis *Ref: Shafer's 6th ed. Pg. 509*

As all of the signs and symptoms indicate that the patient suffers from maxillary sinusitis.

Acute Maxillary Sinusitis

It occurs due to acute periapical abscess of a chronic inflammatory periapical lesion, a latent chronic sinusitis may be occur by extraction of a maxillary bicuspid or molar and perforation of the sinus. S. pneumonia, H. influenza, are occurs in acute sinusitis.

Clinical Features

- Patients with acute maxillary sinusitis suffer from moderate to severe pain with swelling.
- Pain may be referred to various areas, including the cheek, posterior teeth, and ear.
- Sometimes patient may feel numbness in maxillary molars and premolars. Sinus pain increases when the patient bends over or is supine.

- The patient may complain of a discharge of pus into the nose and often a fetid breath.
- Fever and malaise are usually present.

134. Ans. (a) Submasseteric space *Ref: Shafer's 6th ed. Pg. 506-507*

Boundaries: If is present between the master muscle and the lateral surface of the mandibular ramus. The submasseteric space is a narrow space that parallels the middle attachment by extending upward and backward between the middle and deep attachments. The posterior boundary of this space is the parotid gland and anterorly it adjoins the retromolar fossa.

Clinical features: infection of this space. The patient may suffer from severe trismus and pain and there may be facial swelling. The patient is often seriously ill.

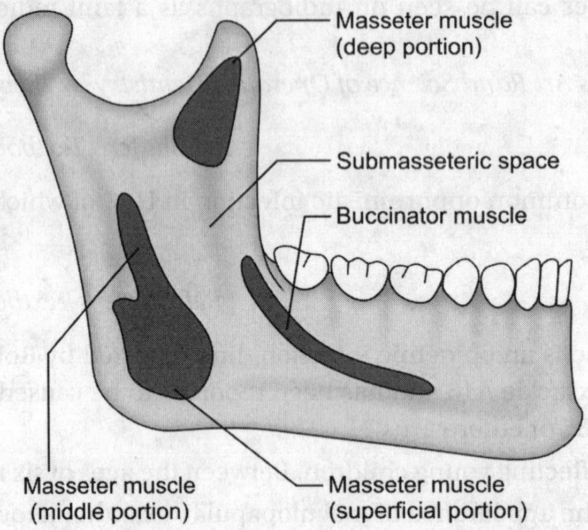

Lateral surface of the mandible showing the location of the submasseteric space.
Redrawn for GM Bransby – Zachary: the submasseteric space Br Dent J. 84; 10, 1948.

Buccal Space: The buccal space is reported to be the most commonly involved fascial space by dental abscesses,

Sublingual space: The infection may arise directly by perforating the lingual cortical palate above the mylohyoid attachment or by extension from other spaces, primarily the submandibular space.

Submental space: The spread of the infection is similar to that in the submandibular and sublingual spaces.

135. Ans. (c) Osteomyelitis *Ref: Neville's Oral and Maxillofacial Pathology 3rd ed. Pg. 625, Shafer's Textbook of Oral Pathology 7th ed. Pg. 708, 711, 733, Harrison, 17th ed. Pg. ....*

Increased alkaline phosphatase level is seen in:

- Paget's disease
- Hyperparathyroidism
- Caffey disease
- Fibrous dysplasia
- The normal serum alkaline phosphatase consists of many distinct isoenzymes found in the liver, bone, placenta and less commonly small intestine. Patients over age 60 can have a mildly elevated alkaline phosphatase. It is also nonpathologically elevated in children and adolescents undergoing rapid bone growth, because of bone alkaline phosphatase and late in normal pregnancies due to the influx of placental alkaline phosphatase.
- Alkaline phosphatase elevations greater than four times normal occur primarily in patients with cholestatic liver disorders, infiltrative liver diseases such as cancer and amyloidosis and bone conditions characterized by rapid bone turnover (e.g Paget's disease). In bone diseases elevation is due to increased amounts of the bone isoenzymes.

- Other conditions that cause isolated elevations of the alkaline phosphatase include Hodgkin's disease, diabetes, hyperthyroidism, congestive heart failure, amyloidosis and inflammatory bowel disease.

136. Ans. (c) Periostitis ossificans *Ref: Neville's Oral and Maxillofacial Pathology 3rd ed. Pg. 148-150; Shafer's Textbook of Oral Pathology 7th ed. Pg. 498*

'MRI imaging has been employed using T2 weighted images to display abnormal bone marrow edema which again lifts the periosteum from the bone surface and stimulates the periosteum to form a second layer of bone. This is detected radiographically as a second radiopaque line almost parallel to the first and separated from it by a radiolucent band. This process may continue and may result in several lines (an onion-skin appearance), and eventually a massive amount of new bone may be formed.' *-White and Pharoah*

Chronic Osteomyelitis with Proliferative Periostitis: (Garrè's chronic nonsuppurative sclerosing osteitis, periostitis ossificans)

- Periostitis ossificans was first described by German Physician Carl Garrè in 1893 as an irritation induced focal thickening of the periosteum and cortical bone of tibia. In 1955, Pell reported the first case involving the jaws.
- Proliferative periostitis represents a periosteal raction to the presence of inflammation.
- The affected periosteal forms several rows of reactive vital bone that parallel each other and expand the surface of the altered bone.
- For this lesion to develop a peculiar combination of circumstances must coexist:
  - The periosteum must possess a high potential for osteoblastic activity (this requirement is satisfied in young patients).
  - A chronic infection must be present.
  - A fine balance must be maintained between the resistance of the host and the number and virulence of organisms present, so the infection can continue at a low chronic stage invasive enough to stimulate new periosteal bone formation but not severe enough to induce bone resorption.
- Clinical features: It is seen almost exclusively in children and rarely in patients over 30 years of age. In the jaws occurs almost exclusively in the mandible in children and young adults, and most cases occur in the bicuspid and molar region. An infected mandibular first permanent molar is the most common etiologic factor.

Note: **Periosteal new bone formation** or neoperiostosis may occur in other conditions, such as, ***infantile cortical hyperostosis (Caffey's disease), hypervitaminosis A, syphilis, leukemia, Ewing's sarcoma, metastatic neuroblastoma, and even a fracture callus.***

137. Ans. (b) Newly formed bone surrounding dead bone *Ref: Neville's Oral and Maxillofacial Pathology 3rd ed. Pg. 142; Shafer's Textbook of Oral Pathology 7th ed. Pg. 537*

'A fragment of necrotic bone that has separated from the adjacent vital bone is termed as sequestrum. Sequestra often exhibit spontaneous exfoliation. On occasion, fragments of necrotic bone may become surrounded by new vital bone, known as an involucrum.' - Neville's

- After the acute inflammatory process occurs and local blood supply is compromised, necrosis of the en dosteal bone takes place.
- The bone fragments die and become sequestra. Osteoclastic activity is then responsible for separating the dead bone from vital bone. Devital bone tissue clinically appears dirty, whitish-gray with an opaque appcarance.
- The elevated periosteum involved in the inflammatory process still contains vital cells. These cells, once the acute phase has passed, form a new bony shell (involucrum) covering the sequestra.
- The involucrum may be penetrated by sinuses called cloacae, through which pus discharges, elevating the periosteum or forming fistula.
- A devitalized bone fragment which is dissolved from the adjacent cortical plate is called a 'sequester.'
- ***A periosteal bone reaction may cover the sequestem and turn it into an 'involucrum'. The origin of new bone deposition is the cambium layer of the periosteum.***

PHYSICAL AND CHEMICAL INJURY

DISEASE OF BONE AND JOINT

138. Ans. (a) Paget's disease *Ref: Shafer's 6th ed. Pg. 729*

- The serum calcium and serum phosphorus levels are usually within normal limits, where as the serum alkaline phosphates level may be elevated, however, to extreme limits.
- In fact, there is no other disease of bone in which the serum alkaline phosphatase level may be as high as in Paget's disease. However in the above given option disease is also associated with elevated serum alkaline phosphatase level but less than Paget's disease.

139. Ans (d) Type IV *Ref: Shafer's 6th ed Pg. 695*

Type	Description	Mode of inheritance
I	Mild	Autosomal dominant, 60% de novo
II	Severe and usually lethal in the perinatal period	Autosomal dominant, ~100% de novo
III	Considered progressive and deforming	Autosomal dominant, ~100% de novo
IV	**Deforming, but with normal sclerae**	Autosomal dominant, 60% de novo
V	Shares the same clinical features of IV, but has unique Histologic findings ('mesh-like')	Autosomal dominant
VI	Shares the same clinical features of IV, but has unique histologic findings ('fish scale')	Autosomal recessive
VII	Associated with cartilage associated protein	Autosomal recessive
VIII	Severe to lethal, associated with the protein leprecan	Autosomal recessive

140. Ans. (b) Characterized by palmer planter hyperkeratosis *Ref: Shafer's 6th ed. Pg. 702*

Papillon-Lefèvre syndrome (PLS), also known as palmoplantar keratoderma with periodontitis, is an autosomal recessive genetic disorder caused by a deficiency in cathepsin C.

PLS is characterized by periodontitis and palmoplantar keratoderma. The severe destruction of periodontium results in loss of most primary teeth by the age of 4 and most permanent teeth by age 14. Hyperkeratosis of palms and soles of feet appear in first few years of life. Destructions of periodontium follows almost immediately after the eruption of last molar tooth. The teeth are involved in roughly the same order in which they erupt.

So, Papillon-Lefèvre syndrome is characterized by palmer planter hyperkeratosis.

141. Ans. (a) Cherubism *Ref: Neville's Oral and Maxillofacial Pathology 3rd ed. Pg. 629; Shafer's Textbook of Oral Pathology 7th ed. Pg. 711*

Note: Option cherubism misspelt in original question paper

Cherubism

(Familial fibrous dysplasia of jaws, disseminated juvenile fibrous dysplasia, familial multilocular cystic disease of jaws, familial fibrous swelling of jaws)

A non-neoplastic autosomal dominant fibro-osseous lesion of the jaws involving more than one quadrant that stabilizes after the growth period. It affects the jaws of children bilaterally and symmetrically, usually producing the so-called cherubic look. According to WHO it affecting only the jaws.

The jaw lesions are usually painless and symmetric and have florid maxillary involvement. The lesions, which are firm to palpation and nontender, most commonly involve the molar to coronoid regions, the condyles always being spared, and are often associated with cervical lymphadenopathy. Enlargement of the cervical lymph nodes contributes to the patient's full-faced appearance and is said to be caused by lymphoid hyperplasia with fibrosis.

The gene related to cherubism was located on chromosome 4p16.3 (Mutations in the SH3BP2).

The reduction in osteoclast formation caused by sex steroids and the increase in plasma concentrations of estradiol and testosterone at puberty both suggest that the genetic defect responsible for the localized increase in osteoclasts in cherubism is overridden and normalized by the increased synthesis of sex steroids.

A rim of sclera may be visible beneath the iris, giving the classic 'eye to heaven' appearance.

Syndromes associated with cherubism are: Ramon syndrome, Jaffe-Campanacci syndrome, and Noonan syndrome.

Arnott's grading system used for the lesions of cherubism.

Radiologically, cherubism is characterized by bilateral multilocular cystic expansion of the jaws.

The presence of numerous unerupted teeth and the destruction of the alveolar bone may displace the teeth, producing a radiographic appearance referred to as floating tooth syndrome. There is a classic (but nonspecific) ground glass appearance because of the small, tightly compressed trabecular pattern.

Radiation therapy is contraindicated because of risk of development of postirradiation sarcoma.

142. Ans. (a) Procollagen synthesis/production of collagen *Ref: Neville's Oral and Maxillofacial Pathology 3rd ed. Pg. 613; Shafer's Textbook of Oral Pathology 7th ed. Pg. 699*

Osteogenesis imperfecta

('Brittle bones', fragilitas ossium, osteopsathyrosis, Lobstein's disease)

- The condition resulting from abnormality in the type I collagen, which most commonly manifests as fragility of bones.
- Generally recognized as representing a hereditary autosomal dominant characteristic, autosomal recessive and nonhereditary types also occur.
- Disorders arises from heterozygosity for mutations in genes that guide the formation of type I collagen: the COL1A1 gene on band 17q21 and COL1A2 gene on band 7q22.1.
- Qualitative defects (abnormal collagen I molecule) and quantitative defects (decrease in production of normal collagen I molecules) both exist in its causation.
- **Abnormal collagenous maturation results in bone with a thin cortex, fine trabeculation and diffuse osteoporosis.**

Clinical features:

- The extreme fragility and porosity of the bones, with an attendant proneness to fracture.
- The fractures heal readily, but the new bone is of a similar imperfect quality.
- The age of onset of symptoms: type I and IV occurring during infancy and type II in utero. In type III, half the cases present fracture in utero, and other half in the neonatal period.
- The sclerae are abnormally thin, and for this reason the pigmented choroid shows through and produces the bluish color. [The occurrence of pale blue sclerae may also be seen in Osteopetrosis, Fetal Rickets, Turner Syndrome, Paget's Disease, Marfan Syndrome, and Ehlers-Danlos Syndrome, as well as in Normal Infants.]

Sillence classification:

Type I: Osteogenesis imperfect

- The most common and mildest form.
- In subtype A, dentinogenesis imperfecta is absent, while in subtype B, dentinogenesis imperfecta is present.

Type II: Osteogenesis imperfect

- Exhibits extreme bone fragility and frequent fractures.
- Dentinogenesis imperfecta may be present along with small nose, micrognathia and short trunk.

Type III: Osteogenesis imperfecta

- Associated with dentinogenesis imperfecta, sclera of variable hue, limb shortening and progressive deformities, triangular facies with frontal bossing and pulmonary hypertension.

Type IV: Osteogenesis imperfecta

- In subtype A, dentinogenesis imperfecta is absent, while in subtype B, dentinogenesis imperfecta is present.
- Symptoms of both subtypes include normal sclera, normal hearing.

The basic defect appears to lie in the **organic matrix with failure of fetal collagen to be transformed into mature collagen**. Qualitative defects (abnormal collagen I molecule) and quantitative defects (decrease in production of normal collagen I molecules) both exist. There is some evidence that the progressive intermolecular cross-linkage of adjacent collagen molecules, which is an essential characteristic of normal collagen maturation, is defective in this disease.

143. Ans. (c) Paget and polyostotic fibrous dysplasia *Ref: Neville's Oral and Maxillofacial Pathology 3rd ed. Pg. 630, 660; Shafer's Textbook of Oral Pathology 7th ed. Pg. 174*

Osteosarcoma (Osteogenic sarcoma)

Osteosarcoma is the third most common cancer in adolescence, occurring less frequently than only lymphomas and brain tumors. It is thought to arise from a primitive mesenchymal bone-forming cell and is characterized by production of osteoid.

The exact cause of osteosarcoma is unknown. Exposure to radiation is the only known environmental risk factor. A genetic predisposition may exist, for example:

- Inactivating the retinoblastoma gene (deletion of chromosome 13q14)
- Bone dysplasias, including **Paget's disease, fibrous dysplasia,** enchondromatosis, and hereditary multiple exostoses.
- Li-Fraumeni syndrome (germline TP53 mutation)
- Rothmund-Thomson syndrome

Clinical and radiographic features:

- It most commonly occurs in the long bones of the extremities near metaphyseal growth plates. The most common sites are femur (42%, with 75% of tumors in the distal femur), tibia (19%, with 80% of tumors in the proximal tibia), and humerus (10%, with 90% of tumors in the proximal humerus). Other significant locations are the skull or jaw (8%) and pelvis (8%).
- Incidence is slightly higher in males than in females (1.25: 1).
- Extragnathic osteosarcoma demonstrates a bimodal age distribution (10–20 years age and >50 years age). Osteosarcoma occurs chiefly in young persons, with decreasing incidence as the age advances.
- The maxilla and mandible are involved with about equal frequency. Horizontal ramus and posterior body are more frequently involved while inferior maxillary portion involved then superior aspect.
- Swelling and pain are most common symptums.
- Spiking resorption as a result of the tapered narrowing of root.
- The classic sun burst or sun ray appearance.
- Codman's tringle—a triangular elevation of the peridontium.
- Symmetric widening of periodontal ligament (due to tumor infiltration along the periodontal ligament space).

Development of a malignant bone tumor, usually an osteosarcoma, is a recognized complication of Paget's disease. Malignant change usually development of an osteosarcoma, has been rarely associated with fibrous dysplasia. *-'Neville'*

144. Ans. (b) Size of tooth and rate of eruption *Ref: Neville's Oral and Maxillofacial Pathology 3rd ed. Pg. 636; Shafer's Textbook of Oral Pathology 7th ed. Pg. 14, 712*

Facial hemihypertrophy (Hyperplasia): A rare developmental anomaly asymmetric overgrowth of one or more body parts. Facial hemihypertrophy exhibit an enlargement which is confined to one side of the body, unilateral macroglossia and premature development, and eruption as well as an increased size of dentition. permanent teeth on the affected side are often enlarged, although not exceeding a 50% increase in size. This enlargement may involve any tooth, but seems to occur most frequently in the cuspid, premolars, and first molar. permanent teeth on the affected side develop more rapidly and erupt before their counterparts on the uninvolved side. Coincident to this phenomenon is premature shedding of the deciduous teeth. The bone of the maxilla and mandible is also enlarged, being wider and thicker, sometimes with an altered trabecular pattern.

Fibrous dysplasia

Nonhereditary disorder usually caused by a mutation in the GNAS1 gene (20q13.2

There may be expansion and deformity of the jaws, and the eruption pattern of the teeth is disturbed because of the loss of normal support of the developing teeth. The endocrine disturbance also may alter the time of eruption of the teeth.

Malformation syndromes associated with hemihyperplasia

- Beckwith-Wiedemann syndrome
- Neurofibromatosis
- Klippel-Trenaunay-Weber syndrome
- Proteus syndrome
- McCune-Albright syndrome
- Epidermal nevus syndrome
- Triploid/diploid mixoploidy
- Langer-Giedion syndrome
- Multiple exostoses syndrome
- Maffucci's syndrome
- Ollier syndrome
- Segmental odontomaxillary dysplasia
  - Because most of the striking signs of congenital hemihypertrophy are usually manifested in the orofacial region, Gorlin and Meskin (1962) suggested them help in differentiation of this condition from other entities that may simulate hypertrophy.
  - Among the conditions that closely mimic CHH as suggested by various authors are fibrous dysplasia, dyschondroplasia, congenital lymphedema, arteriovenous aneurysm, hemangioma, lymphangioma, Klippel-Trenaunay syndrome, von Recklinghausen's neurofibromatosis, malignant conditions such as osteosarocma and chondrosarcoma
  - All these conditions, however, exhibit sufficient clinical differences with CHH and should be distinguished on the basis of specific radiographs, clinical and laboratory findings.
  - ***To the unfamiliar clinician, hemihypertrophy that is localized to orofacial region can constitute a diagnostic problem.***
  - ***Deformities of the teeth and their related hard tissues in the jaw are key findings for correct diagnosis, particularly in hemihypertrophy limited to the face.***

Ref: Contemp Clin Dent 2011 Jul-Sep;2(3):261-264.

145. Ans. (c) Chronic focal sclerosing osteomyelitis *Ref: Neville's Oral and Maxillofacial Pathology 3rd ed. Pg. 147; Shafer's Textbook of Oral Pathology 7th ed. Pg. 495*

***Chronic focal sclerosing osteomyelitis or condensing osteitis is a rare non-suppurative inflammatory condition of bone characterized by sclerotic bone formation around the root apex of a nonvital tooth.** -Shafer's*

CHRONIC FOCAL SCLEROSING OSTEOMYELITIS (CONDENSING OSTEITIS)

Definition

Chronic focal sclerosing osteomyelitis or condensing osteitis is a rare non-suppurative inflammatory condition of bone characterized by sclerotic bone formation around the root apex of a nonvital tooth.

Pathogenesis

- The condition develops as a result of chronic persistent inflammation in the bone, where resistance of the tissue against infection is very high or where the virulence of the infective organisms is low.
- A low-grade inflammation in the jaw bone causes stimulation of the osteoblast cells, which results in the formation of dense trabecular bone in the area and this process is known as osteosclerosis.
- Osteosclerosis with additional bone formation may sometimes results in decreased marrow spaces.

Etiology

The disease often occurs in young individuals, having low grade sustained inflammation in the bone.

The common conditions, which can precipitate chronic focal sclerosing osteomyelitis, include the following:

- Chronic pulpitis.
- Traumatic malocclusion.

Clinical features

- The disease frequently develops in children or young adults before the age of 20 years.
- **Mandibular first molars are mostly involved** with this condition.
- The condition is mostly asymptomatic and there is no bony expansion seen.
- Majority of the lesions are discovered incidentally during routine radiographic examination of the jawbone.
- ***The associated tooth is non-vital and usually presents a large carious lesion, it is mostly asymptomatic or is associated with occasional mild pain.***

Radiological features

The lesion radiographically presents the following features:

- **Well-circumscribed radiopaque mass with uniform radiodensity; seen around the root apex of a nonvital tooth.**
- **There is no radiolucent border around the lesion** as may be seen in cemento-osseous dysplasia.
- The affected tooth exhibits an apical inflammatory process with **widening of periodontal ligament space**.
- A residual area of condensing osteitis that is seen after resolution of the inflammatory focus is known as **'bone scar'**.

Histological features

- There is usually presence of a dense mass of sclerotic bone in the lesion with little or no interstitial marrow tissue.
- Wherever the bone marrow is present it is usually fibrotic and is often infiltrated by chronic inflammatory cells.

Treatment

- The affected tooth should be treated endodontically or it should be removed.
- No treatment required for the bony lesion.
- Biopsy may be necessary to rule out metastatic malignancy

146. Ans. (c) Anodontia *Ref: Shafer's Textbook of Oral Pathology 3rd ed. Pg. 1099*

ECTODERMAL DYSPLASIA

(Hereditary ectodermal dysplasia, ectodermal dysplasia syndrome)

Ectodermal dysplasia syndrome (EDS) is a large heterogeneous group of inherited disorders, the manifestations of which could be seen in more than one ectodermal derivatives. These tissues primarily are the skin, hair, nails, eccrine glands and teeth.

Oral Manifestations

Patients with this abnormality invariably manifest anodontia or oligodontia, complete or partial absence of teeth, with frequent malformation of any teeth present, both deciduous and permanent dentitions where some teeth are present they are commonly truncated or cone shaped.

As there are fewer teeth the alveolar ridge is also deficient. The palatal arch is frequently high and a cleft may be present.

Also the salivary glands, are sometimes hypoplastic in this disease. This result in xerostomia and the protuberant lips may be dry and cracked with pseudorhagades formation. As a related phenomenon there may be hypoplasia of the nasal and pharyngeal mucous glands which leads to chronic rhinitis and/or pharyngitis, sometimes with associated dysphasia and hoarseness.

147. Ans. (a) Ankylosis

Most common cause of ankylosis of TMJ are traumatic injuries and infections in and about the joint.

RA is characterized by ingrowth of the granulation tissue to cover the articular surfaces, the invasion of cartilage and its replacement by granulation tissue, and the ultimate destruction of the articular cartilage, eventually fibrous adhesions occur; the meniscus may become eroded, and fibrous ankylosis results.

BLOOD DISEASE

148. Ans. (b) Monocytic leukemia *Ref: Shafer's Textbook of Oral Pathology 7th ed. Pg. 784; Burkit, Oral Medicine 11th ed. Greenberg Pg. 453*

Oral lesions occur in both acute and chronic forms of all types of leukemia: myeloid, lymphoid and monocytic. These manifestations are far more common; however, in the acute stage of the disease, and according to Burket, are most common in monocytic leukemia.

149. Ans. (d) Plasma thromboplastin component *Ref: A. Victor Hoffbrand et al. Postgraduate haematology; 5th ed. Pg. 825; Neville's Oral and Maxillofacial Pathology 3rd ed. Pg. 573; Shafer's Textbook of Oral Pathology 7th ed. Pg. 792*

Inherited bleeding disorders				
Disorder (synonym)	*Pathophysiology*	*Mode of inheritance*	*Molecular genetics*	*Approximate incidence per 106 population*
Hemophilia A (classical hemophilia)	Factor VIII (Plasma thromboplastinogen, AHG) deficient or Deletions	XL (in bands q28)	Inversions, defective missense, nonsense, insertions, splicing	100
Hemophilia B (Christmas disease)	Factor IX (Plasma thromboplastin component) deficient	XL (in bands q27)	Deletions, missense or defective nonsense, splicing	20
Hemophilia C (PTA deficiency)	Factor XI (Plasma thromboplastin actecedent) deficient	AD or R (chromosome 4)	Missense, nonsense	5% in Ashkenazi splicing Jews, others rare
von Willebrand's disease	von Willebrand factor	AD or AR	Deletions, missense deficient or defective nonsense	AD: 100 or more AR: 1
Note: XL, X-linked recessive; AD, autosomal dominant; AR, autosomal recessive.				

Hemophilia

Hemophilia is a group of sex-linked inherited blood disorders, characterized by prolonged clotting time. However, the bleeding time is normal. Usually, it affects the males, with the females being the carriers. Because of prolonged clotting time, even a mild trauma causes excess bleeding which can lead to death. Damage of skin while falling or extraction of a tooth may cause excess bleeding for few weeks. Easy bruising and hemorrhage in muscles and joints are also common in this disease.

Causes of hemophilia

Hemophilia occurs due to lack of formation of prothrombin activator. That is why the coagulation time is prolonged. The formation of prothrombin activator is affected due tothe deficiency of factor VIII, IX or XI.

Types of hemophilia

Depending upon the deficiency of the factor involved, hemophilia is classified into three types:

i. Hemophilia A or **classic hemophilia**: Due to the deficiency of factor VIII. 85% of people with hemophilia are affected by hemophilia A.
ii. Hemophilia B or **Christmas disease**: Due to the deficiency of factor IX. 15% of people with hemophilia are affected by hemophilia B.
iii. Hemophilia C or factor XI deficiency: Due to the deficiency of factor XI. It is a very rare bleeding disorder.

Symptoms of hemophilia

i. Spontaneous bleeding.
ii. Prolonged bleeding due to cuts, tooth extraction and surgery.
iii. Hemorrhage in gastrointestinal and urinary tracts.
iv. Bleeding in joints followed by swelling and pain.
v. Appearance of blood in urine.

Treatment for hemophilia

Effective therapy for classical hemophilia involves replacement of missing clotting factor.

Factors involved in blood clotting

Coagulation of blood occurs through a series of reactions due to the activation of a group of substances. Substances necessary for clotting are called clotting factors.

Thirteen clotting factors are identified:

Factor I Fibrinogen
Factor II Prothrombin
Factor III Thromboplastin (Tissue factor)
Factor IV Calcium
Factor V Labile factor (Proaccelerin or accelerator globulin)
Factor VI Presence has not been proved
Factor VII Stable factor
Factor VIII Antihemophilic factor (Antihemophilic globulin)
Factor IX Christmas factor
Factor X Stuart-Prower factor
Factor XI Plasma thromboplastin antecedent
Factor XII Hageman factor (Contact factor)
Factor XIII Fibrin-stabilizing factor (Fibrinase).

Clotting factors were named after the scientists who discovered them or as per the activity, except factor IX. Factor IX or Christmas factor was named after the patient in whom it was discovered.

150. Ans. (b) Beta Thalassemia minor *Ref: A. Victor Hoffbrand et al. Postgraduate Haematology; 5th ed. Pg. 88*

The thalassaemias are the commonest single-gene disorders. The condition was first recognized in 1925 by a Detroit physician, Thomas B. Cooley, who described a series of infants who became profoundly anemic and developed splenomegaly over the first-year of life. Mediterranean region, and hence invented the word 'thalassemia' from the Greek θαλασσα, meaning 'the sea.' The thalassaemias are a heterogeneous group of genetic disorders of hemoglobin synthesis, all of which result from a reduced rate of production of one or more of the globin chains of hemoglobin. They are divided into the α-, β-, δβ- or γδβ-thalassemias, according to which globin chain is produced in reduced amounts.

The β-thalassemias are the most important types of thalassemia because they are so common and usually produce severe anemiain their homozygous and compound heterozygous states.

Classification of thalassaemia	
Clinical phenotype	*Thalassemia (thal) syndrome*
Hydrops fetalis	Homozygous α-thal major→complete lack of α globin
Thalassemia major	Homozygous β or doubly heterozygous thal major → complete or almost complete lack of β globin
Thalassemia intermedia	See pg. 49
Thalassemia trait	Heterozygous β-thalassemia (β-thal minor, lack of one functional β-globin gene*) Heterozygous α-thalassemia (α-thal minor, lack of one or two α-globin genes†)
*Normal individual has two (one from each parent/on each allele); †Normal individual has four (two from each parent on each allele).	

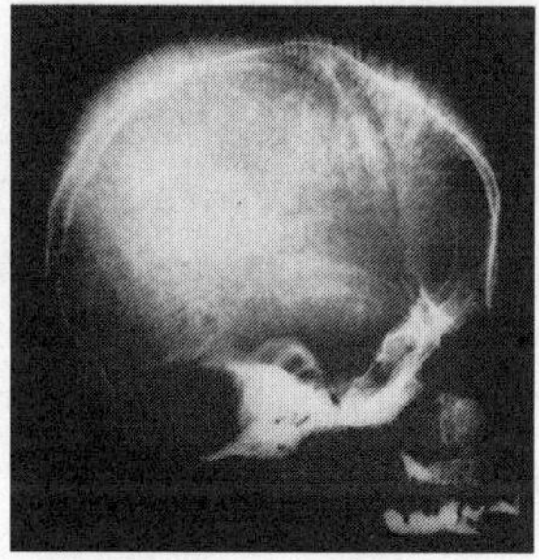

β-thalassemia major: skull X-ray showing expansion of the medullary cavity giving rise to a 'hair on end' appearance.

THALASSEMIA

- Thalassemia represents a group of disorders of hemoglobin synthesis that are characterized by reduced synthesis of either the ***alpha-globin or beta-globin chains*** of the hemoglobin molecule.
- The hemoglobin molecule is a tetramer that is composed of two alpha and two beta chains; if one of the chains is not being made in adequate quantities, the normal amount of hemoglobin cannot be made.
- Furthermore, the excess globin chains accumulate with in the erythrocyte, further compromising the structure and function of the cell.
- These abnormal erythrocytes are recognized by the spleen and selected for destruction (hemolysis).
- The net result is that the patient has ***hypochromic. microcytic anemia.***
- Because **two genes code for the beta chain and four genes code for the alpha chain,** the degree of clinical severity in these conditions can vary considerably.
- The severity depends on which specific genetic alteration is present and whether it is heterozygous or homozygous.
- **In the heterozygous state**. An adequate amount of normal hemoglobin can be made and the affected patient experiences few signs or symptoms.
- **In the homozygous state**. However. the problems arc often severe or even fatal.

Clinical and radiographic features

- ***Beta-thalassemia***
  - **If only one defective gene** for the beta-globin molecule is inherited **(thalassemia minor)**, no significant clinical manifestation are usually present.
  - **When two defective genes** for the beta-globin molecule are inherited, the patient is affected with **thalassemia major**. also **called Cooley'S anemia or Mediterranean fever**.
    - The disease is usually detected during the first year of life because a severe microcytic, hypochromic anemia develops when fetal hemoglobin synthesis ceases after 3 to 4 months of age.
    - In an attempt to maintain adequate oxygenation. The rate of hematopoiesis is greatly increased (up to 30 times normal) resulting in massive bone marrow hyperplasia, as well as hepatosplenomegaly and lymphadenopathy because of extramedullary hematopoiesis.
    - The bone marrow hyperplasia may affect the jaws especially. Producing marked but pain less enlargement of the mandible and maxilla. This results in a characteristic ***'chipmunk' facies.*** Front al bossing is also present. and a skull radiograph shows a ***prominent 'hair-an-end' appearance of the calvaria***.
- ***Alpha-thalassemia***. Alpha-thalassemia has a broader spectrum of involvement than does beta-thalassemia because there are four alpha-globin genes that may be affected.
  - With the altaration of **only one gene**, no disease can be detected.
  - With the inheritance of **two altered genes**. The condition is known as ***alpha-thalassemia trait***; these patient s have a mild degree of anemia and microcytosis that is usually not clinically significant.
  - **With three altered genes**. the term Hb (hemoglobin) II disease is applied. Patients have problems with hemolytic anemia and splenomegaiy. For patients with severe hemolysis splenectomy may be indicated.
  - **The homozygous state**, in which all **four genes are abnormal** is called ***hydrops fetalis***. This condition is typically fatal within a few hours of birth.

Treatment and prognosis

- Thalassemia major is treated today primarily by means of **blood transfusions.**
- These should be administered every 2 to 3 weeks to simulate the normal hematologic state.
- Unfortunately, with repeated blood transfusions, iron overload develops because of the constant infusion of exogenous red blood cells. This is a serious problem and often death is due to **hemochromatosis**, an abnormal deposition of iron throughout the tissues of the body.
- The heart, liver and endocrine glands are particularly affected by the toxic accumulation of iron.
- To combat this problem, an iron-chelating agent, **deferoxamine**, must be given

Note: The classical Hair on end appearance was not common in sickle cell anemia and most likely to be seen in thalassemia.

Imporatant features of thalassemia

- Rib within a rib radiological feature
- Rodent facies with mongloid features
- Presence of fessas inclusion bodies in erythrocytes.

Causes of **Hair on END** appearance

- Thalassemia
- Sickle cell anemia
- Hemangioma
- Meningioma
- Elliptocytosis
- G6PD defieciency
- Pyruvate Kinase deficiency

151. Ans. (a) Hemophilia

In hemophilia the blood does not clot normally, and even the slightest injury can cause severe bleeding. The clotting disorder is the result of a deficiency in specific blood clotting factor. Most hemophilics are male.

SKIN DISEASE

152. Ans. (b) Less than 10% skin involvement *Ref: Shafer's 6th ed. Pg. 806 and Burkets 11th ed. Pg. 55*

Erythema multiforme (EM) minor represents a localize eruption of the skin of less than 10% of skin involment with mild or no mucosal involvement. EM major and Stevens-Johnson Syndrome (SJS) are more severe mucosal and skin diseases and are potentially life-threatening disorders.

EM:

Typical target lesion

Associated with herpes infection

Lesion occurs on extremety

SJS: Atypical target lesion

Associated with medication

Lesion occurs on chest

153. Ans. (a) Psoriasis

- **Psoriasis** is uncommon in children, and seldom does a primary attack occur after the age of 45 years; it most frequently arises in the second and third decades of life. The median age at onset is 28 years. Psoriasis is slightly more common in women.**(Shafer's 7th Edition Page no. 3177)**
- The median age of onset of Psoriasis is 28 years, **but it can present from infancy to old age,** when the appearance may be atypical. The following factors in the history may help in making a diagnosis. Family history of psoriasis: 16% of the children will have psoriasis if a single parent is affected and 50% if both parents are affected. **(ABC of Dermatology 5th edition Page no. 12)**
- **Cicatricial pemphigoid** occurs nearly twice as frequently in females as it does in males with the peak **age of involvement being between 40 and 50 years. Bullous pemphigoid** is basically a disease of **elderly persons,** approximately 80% of patients being over **60 years of age**. **(Shafer's 7th ed. Page no. 3243, 3248)**
- **Systemic lupus erythematosus** is very difficult disease to diagnose in its early stages because it often appears in a nonspecific, vague fashion, frequently with periods of remission or disease inactivity. Women are affected nearly 8 to 10 times more frequently than men. **The average age at diagnosis is 31 years. (Neville 2nd Edition Page no. 689)**
- **Discoid lupus erythematosus** is a relatively common disease which, like the systemic form, occurs predominantly in the **third and fourth decades**. It is more common in women than in men. The most common sites of involvement are the face, oral mucous membranes, chest, back and extremities. **(Shafer's 7th Edition Page no. 3276)**

154. Ans. (d) SLE

SLE is an autoimmune disease characterized by autoantibodies, immune complex disorder, immune dysregulation resulting in damage to organs, including the kidney, skin, blood cells, and the CNS.

There is anemia, leukopenia, thrombocytopenia, elevated ESR, positive coombs test.

Antinuclear antibodies as well as anti-smith antibodies can also be demonstrated.

155. Ans. (d) Bechet's syndrome

Bechet's syndrome—autoimmune disorder.

Characterized chiefly by oral and genital ulcerations, ocular lesions and skin lesions.

Oral lesions—painful and resemble recurrent apthous ulcers.

Skin lesions—pustules, erythema nodosum, erythema multiforme.

156. Ans. (a) Ehler-Danlos syndrome

Ehlers-Danlos syndrome—inherited disorder with defect in collagen and connective tissue junction.

Affects skin, joints and blood vessels.

Hyperelasticity of the skin, hyperextensibility of the jointsand fragility of the skin and blood vessels resulting in excessive bruising and defective healing of skin wounds.

Rubber Man syndrome

Tongue hyperelastic, tip of the tongue touches the base of the nose-gorlin sign.

157. Ans. (d) Pemphigus vulgaris *Ref: Shafer's 6th ed. Pg. 818*

- **Pemphigus vulgaris** is a chronic blistering skin disease with skin lesions that are rarely pruritic, but which are often painful. It is classified as a type II hypersensitivity reaction, with the formation of anti-desmosome antibodies.
- It is an autoimmune disease caused by antibodies directed against both desmoglein 1 and desmoglein 3 present in desmosomes resulting in the loss of desmosomes and therefore the loss of cohesion between keratinocytes in the epidermis, classified as a type II hypersensitivity reaction (in which antibodies bind to antigens on the body's own tissues). It is characterized by extensive flaccid blisters and mucocutaneous erosions. The severity of the disease, as well as the mucosal lesions, is believed to be directly proportional to the levels of desmoglein 3.
- Transudative fluid accumulates in between the keratinocytes and basement membrane (suprabasal split), forming a blister and resulting in what is known as a positive Nikolsky's sign.
- Corticosteroids and other immunosuppressive drugs are the mainstay of treatment.

158. Ans. (c) Acantholysis

According to key given by A.B. Shetty answer is (b)

Pemphigus is a rare group of blistering autoimmune diseases that affect the skin and mucous membranes.

In pemphigus, autoantibodies form against desmoglein. Desmoglein forms the 'glue' that attaches adjacent epidermal cells via attachment points called **desmosomes**. When autoantibodies attack desmogleins, the cells become separated from each other and the epidermis becomes 'unglued', a phenomenon called acantholysis. This causes blisters that slough off and turn into sores. In some cases, these blisters can cover a significant area of the skin.

159. Ans. (c) Viral disease

Erythema multiforme (EM) is an acute, self-limited, and sometimes recurring skin condition that is considered to be a type IV hypersensitivity reaction associated with certain infections, medications, and other various triggers.

Erythema multiforme may be present within a wide spectrum of severity. Erythema multiforme minor represents a localized eruption of the skin with minimal or no mucosal involvement. The papules evolve into pathognomonic target lesions or iris lesions that appear within a 72-hour period and begin on the extremities. Lesions remain in a fixed location for at least 7 days and then begin to heal. Lesions may also appear as arcuate lesions. Precipitating factors include herpes simplex virus (HSV), Epstein-Barr virus (EBV), and histoplasmosis.

160. Ans. (b) Erythema multiforme *Ref: Shafer's Textbook of Oral Pathology, 6th ed. Pg. 806-808*

Erythema multiforme is an acute, self-limited, inflammatory mucocutaneous disease that manifests on the skin and often oral mucosa, although other mucosal surfaces, such as the genitalia may also be involved.

EM minor: Less than 10% of skin involvement and there is minimal to no mucous membrane involvement.

EM major: Extensive and characteristic skin involvement, with the oral or any other mucosa involved.

Fulminant forms of EM:

Stevens-Johnson syndrome (SJS) and toxic epidermal necrolysis [TEN (Lyell disease)]

A concentric ring like appearance of the lesions resulting from various shades of erythema, occurs in many cases of erythema multiforme and has given rise to the terms 'TARGET' or 'IRIS' or 'Bulls eye' in describing them. They are most common on the hands, wrists and ankles. Mucous membrane involvement including oral cavity is also common in EM.

Points to remember about Erythema multiforme:

Both Erythema multiformeand Stevens-Johnson syndrome are due to deposition of immune complexes in the superficial microvasculature of skin and mucosa. These immune complex diseases are mediated through **type III hypersensitivity reaction.**

DISEASE OF NERVE AND MUSCLE

161. Ans. (a) Myofascial pain *Ref: Textbook of Oral and Maxillofacial Surgery by Neelima Malik. 3rd ed. Pg. 285*

Transcutaneous electric nerve stimulation (TENS) interferes with the sensation of pain in the brain and increases blood flow to the site.

162. Ans. (a) Paresthesia *Ref: Shafer's Textbook of Oral Pathology, 6th ed. Pg. 844*

- Trigeminal neuralgia or 'Fothergill's disease' is characterized by searing, stabbing or lancinating type of pain that is initiated when the patient touches the 'trigger zone'.
- The term 'tic doulourex' is applied only when the patient suffers from spasmodic contractions of facial muscles.
- Right side of the face is commonly involved.
- Differential diagnosis of trigeminal neuralgia includes trotters syndrome and post-herpetic neuralgia.

ODONTOGENIC CYST AND TUMOR

163. Ans. (d) All of the above *Ref: Shafer's 6th, Pg. 271*

Benign tumors of odntogenic orign are:

Odontogenic epithelium with out odontogenic ectomesenchyme: ameloblastoma, CEOT, AOT.

Odontogenic epithelium with odontogenic ectomesenchyme: odontomes, ameloblastic fibroma.

Odontogenic ectomesenchyme without odontogenic epithelium: CEMENTOBLASTOMA, ODONTOGENIC MYXOMA.

164. Ans. (a) Hyaline bodies and (b) Rushton bodies *Ref: Shafer's 6 ed. Pg. 267*

Hyaline bodies/rushton bodies are found in great numbers in the wall of inflammatory cyst.

They are peculiar linear-arc shaped bodies, that are amorphous in structure, brittle in nature and eosinophilic in reaction.

165. Ans. (b) Residual cyst *Ref: Shafer's 6 ed. Pg. 269*

It is the inflammatory periapical cyst which remain behind after removal of an infected tooth.

Treatment: Curettage of the socket

166. Ans. (d) Dentigerous cyst *Ref: Neville's Oral and Maxillofacial Pathology 3rd ed. Pg. 679, 692; Shafer's Textbook of Oral Pathology 7th ed. Pg. 64, 259, 269 White and Pharoh 6th ed. Pg. 346, 361*

Option b, c and d are true as they are associated with vital teeth. But most appropriate is d because:

The term globulomaxillary cyst was used formerly. Globulomaxillary cysts are now recognized to be radicular or lateral periodontal cyst or KCOTs which means tooth can be non-vital in case of Globul maxillary cyst if it is due to radicular cyst.

Again lateral cyst can be due to lateral periodontal cyst or lateral radicular cyst. If it is due to lateral radicular cyst then tooth will be non-vital.

Repeat from Q. 87 AIPG 2014

167. Ans. (b) Peripheral palisading cells with central stellate reticulum *Ref: Neville's Oral and Maxillofacial Pathology 3rd ed. Pg. 705; Shafer's Textbook of Oral Pathology 7th ed. Pg. 280-281*

Ameloblastoma:

The ameloblastoma is a true neoplasm of enamel organ type tissue which does not undergo differentiation to the point of enamel formation.

'Usually Unicentric, Nonfunctional, Intermittent in growth, Anatomically benign and Clinically persistent' lesion (UNIAC) -Robinson

The tumor may be derived from:

- Cell rests of the enamel organ, either remnants of the dental lamina or remnants of Hertwig's sheath, the epithelial rests of Malassez.
- Epithelium of odontogenic cysts, particularly the dentigerous cyst, and odontomas.
- Disturbances of the developing enamel organ
- Basal cells of the surface epithelium of the jaws
- Heterotopic epithelium (pituitary gland)

Histologic Features: Six histopathologic subtypes:

Follicular—epithelial nest consist of core of loosely arranged angular cells resembling the stellate reticulumn of an enamel organ.

Plexiform ameloblastoma—the ameloblast like tumor cells are arranged in irregular masses, or more frequently, as a network of interconnecting strands of cells. Each of these masses or strands is bounded by a layer of columnar cells, and between these layers may be found stellate reticulum like cells.

Acanthomatous ameloblastoma—the cells occupying the position of the stellate reticulum undergo squamous metaplasia, sometimes with keratin formation in the central portion of the tumor islands.

Granular cell ameloblastoma—there is marked transformation of the cytoplasm, usually of the stellate reticulum like cells, so that it takes on a very coarse, granular, eosinophilic appearance.

Basal cell—epithelial tumor cells are more primitive and less columnar, are generally arranged in sheets, more so than in the other tumor types.

Desmoplastic ameloblastoma—characteristically, is found in a dense collagen stroma that may appear hyalinized and hypocellular. Central cells are often scant in the epithelial proliferation, and the cells making up the periphery of the strands and cords often are flattened or cuboidal rather than tall columnar in appearance.

168. Ans. (a) Peripheral palisading epithelium with central loose stratum intermedium *Ref: Neville's Oral and Maxillofacial Pathology 3rd ed. Pg. 705, 708; Shafer's Textbook of Oral Pathology 7th ed. Pg. 280-282*

Ameloblastoma:

The ameloblastoma is a true neoplasm of enamel organ type tissue which does not undergo differentiation to the point of enamel formation.

'Usually Unicentric, Nonfunctional, Intermittent in growth, Anatomically benign and Clinically persistent' lesion (UNIAC) -Robinson

The tumor may be derived from:

- Cell rests of the enamel organ, either remnants of the dental lamina or remnants of Hertwig's sheath, the epithelial rests of Malassez.
- Epithelium of odontogenic cysts, particularly the dentigerous cyst, and odontomas.
- Disturbances of the developing enamel organ
- Basal cells of the surface epithelium of the jaws
- Heterotopic epithelium (pituitary gland)

Histologic Features: Six histopathologic subtypes:

Follicular—epithelial nest consist of core of loosely arranged angular cells resembling the stellate reticulumn of an enamel organ surrounded by peripheral palisading epithelium.

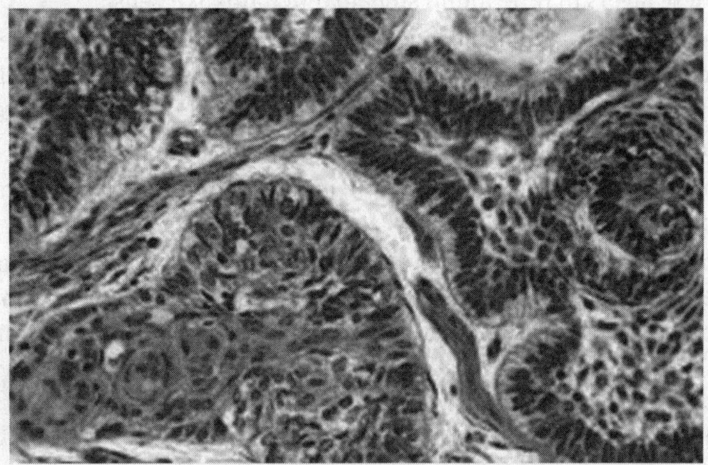

Plexiform ameloblastoma—the ameloblast like tumor cells are arranged in irregular masses, or more frequently, as a network of interconnecting strands of cells. Each of these masses or strands is bounded by a layer of columnar cells, and between these layers may be found stellate reticulum like cells.

Acanthomatous ameloblastoma—the cells occupying the position of the stellate reticulum undergo squamous metaplasia, sometimes with keratin formation in the central portion of the tumor islands.

Granular cell ameloblastoma—there is marked transformation of the cytoplasm, usually of the stellate reticulum like cells, so that it takes on a very coarse, granular, eosinophilic appearance.

Basal cell—epithelial tumor cells are more primitive and less columnar, are generally arranged in sheets, more so than in the other tumor types.

Desmoplastic ameloblastoma—characteristically, is found in a dense collagen stroma that may appear hyalinized and hypocellular. Central cells are often scant in the epithelial proliferation, and the cells making up the periphery of the strands and cords often are flattened or cuboidal rather than tall columnar in appearance.

169. Ans. (b) Peripheral palisading with central loose stellate reticulum *Ref: Neville's Oral and Maxillofacial Pathology 3rd ed. Pg. 705; Shafer's Textbook of Oral Pathology 7th ed. Pg. 280-281*

Ameloblastoma

The ameloblastoma is a true neoplasm of enamel organ type tissue which does not undergo differentiation to the point of enamel formation.

'Usually Unicentric, Nonfunctional, Intermittent in growth, Anatomically benign and Clinically persistent' lesion (UNIAC) -Robinson

The tumor may be derived from:

- Cell rests of the enamel organ, either remnants of the dental lamina or remnants of Hertwig's sheath, the epithelial rests of Malassez.
- Epithelium of odontogenic cysts, particularly the dentigerous cyst, and odontomas.
- Disturbances of the developing enamel organ
- Basal cells of the surface epithelium of the jaws
- Heterotopic epithelium (pituitary gland)

Histologic Features: Six histopathologic subtypes:

Follicular—epithelial nest consist of core of loosely arranged angular cells resembling the stellate reticulumn of an enamel organ.

Plexiform ameloblastoma—the ameloblast like tumor cells are arranged in irregular masses, or more frequently, as a network of interconnecting strands of cells. Each of these masses or strands is bounded by a layer of columnar cells, and between these layers may be found stellate reticulum like cells.

Acanthomatous ameloblastoma—the cells occupying the position of the stellate reticulum undergo squamous metaplasia, sometimes with keratin formation in the central portion of the tumor islands.

Granular cell ameloblastoma—there is marked transformation of the cytoplasm, usually of the stellate reticulum like cells, so that it takes on a very coarse, granular, eosinophilic appearance.

Basal cell—epithelial tumor cells are more primitive and less columnar, are generally arranged in sheets, more so than in the other tumor types.

Desmoplastic ameloblastoma—characteristically, is found in a dense collagen stroma that may appear hyalinized and hypocellular. Central cells are often scant in the epithelial proliferation, and the cells making up the periphery of the strands and cords often are flattened or cuboidal rather than tall columnar in appearance.

170. Ans. (a) Dentigerous cyst *Ref: Shafer 7th ed.*

Incisive canal and globulomaxillary cyst are present in maxilla.

Dentigerous cyst is more aggressive than radicular cyst.

It can cause severe expansion and hollowing of angle and ramus region of mandible.

Apart from it ameloblastoma can also arise from the lining of the cyst which is locally aggressive benign neoplasm.

171. Ans. (a) Globulomaxillary cyst *Ref Shafer's 7th ed.*

- Also known as premaxilla-maxillary cyst.
- Fissural cyst within the bone between maxillary lateral and canine.
- Radiographically appears as inverted pear shaped radiolucent area between roots of maxillary lateral and canine.

172. Ans. (a) Dentigerous cyst *Ref: Neville's Oral and Maxillofacial Pathology 3rd ed. Pg. 679-682; Shafer's Textbook of Oral pathology 7th ed. Pg. 260*

'The dentigerous cyst is **potentially capable of becoming an aggressive lesion**. Expansion of bone with subsequent facial asymmetry, extreme displacement of teeth, severe root resorption of adjacent teeth and pain are all possible sequelae brought about by continued enlargement of the cyst.'- Shafer's

Dentigerous cyst (Follicular cyst):

- An odontogenic cyst that surrounds the crown of an impacted tooth.
- Caused by fluid accumulation between the reduced enamel epithelium and the enamel surface, resulting in a cyst in which the crown is located within the lumen.
- One of the most common types of developmental odontogenic cyst, estimated to be about 20% of all jaw cysts.
- Always associated initially with the crown of an impacted, embedded or unerupted tooth.

- The most common sites of this cyst are the mandibular and maxillary third molar and maxillary cuspid areas, since these are the most commonly impacted.
- **Bilateral and multiple cysts** are usually found in association with a number of syndromes including **Cleidocranial Dysplasia** and **Maroteaux-Lamy syndrome.**
- **Potentially capable of becoming an aggressive lesion**, expansion of bone with subsequent facial asymmetry, extreme displacement of teeth, severe root resorption of adjacent teeth and pain are all possible sequelae brought about by continued enlargement of the cyst.
- Cystic involvement of an unerupted mandibular third molar may result in a 'hollowing-out' of the entire ramus extending up to the coronoid process and condyle as well as in expansion of the cortical plate due to the pressure exerted by the lesion.
- **Radiographically**, it can be suspected when the follicular space is more than 5 mm.
- The epithelial lining of dentigerous cyst might undergo neoplastic transformation to:
  - Ameloblastoma
  - Squamous cell carcinoma
  - Intraosseous mucoepidermoid carcinoma.

173. Ans. (a) Epstein pearls *Ref: Neville's Oral and maxillofacial Pathology 3rd ed. Pg. 691; Shafer's Textbook of Oral Pathology 7th ed. Pg. 67, 267*

Gingival cyst of the newborn has the microscopic appearance of an epidermoid cyst, it arises from epithelial remnants of the deeply budding dental lamina during tooth development, after the fourth month in utero.

A similar palatal cyst of the newborn is commonly found in the posterior midline of the hard palate, where it arises from epithelial remnants remaining in the stroma after fusion of the palatal processes which meet medially to form the palate. As originally described, the cysts along the median raphe of the palate were called Epstein's pearls and the term Bohn's nodules was used for cysts which originated from palatal gland structures and were scattered more widely over the hard and soft palates. Today these two terms are used interchangeably for both palatal and gingival cysts of newborns.

Histologically both gingival and palatal cysts of the newborn show a thin, stratified squamous epithelium cyst lining with a routine fibrovascular connective tissue stroma, usually without an inflammatory cell infiltrate. The cystic lumen is filled with degenerated keratin, usually formed into concentric layers or onion rings and the epithelium lacks rete processes. Occasional cysts will demonstrate a communication with the surface.

174. Ans. (a) Primordial cyst *Ref: Neville's Oral and Maxillofacial Pathology 3rd ed. Pg. 691; Shafer's Textbook of Oral Pathology 7th ed. Pg. 67, 267*

The concept of meaning of the term primordial cyst often have been controversial and confusing. In the older classification of cyst widely used in the United States, the primordial cyst was considered to originate from cystic degeneration of the enamel organ epithelium before the development of dental hard tissue. Therefore, the primordial cyst occurs in place of a tooth.-*Neville's*

- The term 'primordial cyst' was first used by Robinson (1945) to describe a cyst of the jaw that he suggested was derived from the enamel organ in its early stages of devel¬opment by degeneration of the stellate reticulum before any calcified structures had been laid down.
- He stated that primordial cysts may occur in single or multiple form arising either from an enamel organ of a single tooth of the regular series or from numerous aberrant dental anlage which become cystic.
- Primordial cyst is relatively quite uncommon.
- ***It originates due to cystic degeneration and liquefaction of stellate reticulum in an enamel organ before calcification.***
- *Thus, primordial cyst occurs in the place of a tooth and is not associated with any tooth.*
- *Sometimes it can also occur in the place of a supernumerary tooth. This results in normal complement of teeth.*

- It must be emphasised that if a cystic lesion is present in the region of an edentulous area, it is more appropriate to call it as residual cyst rather than primordial cyst. Most of the residual cysts are periapical cysts or dentigerous cysts.

175. Ans. (a) Associated with erupted third molar *Ref: Shafer 6th ed. Pg. 255*

- Clinical features—This cyst is always associated initially with the crown of an impacted, embedded or unerupted tooth.
- A dentigerous cyst may also be found enclosing a complex compound odontoma or involving a supernumerary tooth. The most common sites of this cyst are the mandibular and maxillary third molar and maxillary cuspid areas, since these are the most commonly impacted teeth.
- Most lesions present in second and third decades, with slight male predilection. Most dentigerous cysts are solitary.
- Bilateral and multiple cysts are usually found in association with a number of syndromes including cleidocranial dysplasia and Maroteaux-Lamy syndrome. In the absence of these syndromes, bilateral dentigerous cysts are rare. The dentigerous cyst is potentially capable of becoming an aggressive lesion.
- Expansion of bone with subsequent facial symmetry, extreme displacement of teeth, severe root resorption of adjacent teeth and pain are all possible sequels brought about by continued enlargement of the cyst. Cystic involvement of an unerupted mandibular third molar may result in a 'hollowing out' of the entire ramus extending up to the coronoid process and condyle as well as in expansion of the cortical plate due to the pressure exerted by the lesion.

176. Ans. (b) Non-vital tooth *Ref: Shafer's Textbook of Oral Pathology 6th ed. Pg. 268*

Radicular cyst or the periapical cyst is the most common inflammatory cyst, associated with tooth necrosis and toxins released from them, hence the involved teeth are non-vital. It is the most common odontogenic cyst.

177. Ans. (d) Dentigerous cyst

Eruption cyst is defined as an odontogenic cyst with the histologic features of a dentigerous cyst that surrounds a tooth crown that has erupted through bone but not soft tissue and is clinically visible as a soft fluctuant mass on the alveolar ridges.

When the cystic cavity contains blood, it gives a blue or purple hue, hence the term eruption hematoma.

178. Ans. (c) Odontogenic keratocyst *Ref: Shafer's 6th ed. Pg. 259*

- OKC develops from dental lamina or its remnants.
- It is 3 times more likely to be found in mandible (3rd molar area).
- Male predilection during 2nd-3rd decade of life
- The OKC is the 3rd most commonly occurring odontogenic cyst and can be associated with nevoid basal cell carcinoma.
- Most of the OKC's radiographically seems as a unilocular, with well-defined peripheral margin

Histologically OKC's seems as:

- Parakeratinized corrugated or wrinkled surface.
- 6 to 10 cells thick uniform epithelium.
- 'Picket fence' or 'tomb stone' appearance is seen with a prominent palisaded, polarized basal layer of cells.
- Marsupialization or surgical enucleation is indicated.

179. Ans. (a) The periapical (radicular cyst)

The **periapical cyst** (also termed **radicular cyst**, and to a lesser extent **dental cyst**) is the most common odontogeniccyst. It is caused by pulpal necrosis secondary to dental caries or trauma. The cyst lining is derived from the cell rests of Malassez. Usually, the periapical cyst is asymptomatic, but a secondary infection can cause pain. On radiographs, it appears a radiolucency (dark area) around the apex of a tooth's root.

Radicular cyst is the most common odontogenic cystic lesion of inflammatory origin. It is also known as periapical cyst, apical periodontal cyst, root end cyst or dental cyst. It arises from epithelial residues in periodontal ligament as a result of inflammation. The inflammation usually follows death of dental pulp. Radicular cysts are found at root apices of involved teeth. These cysts may persists even after extraction of offending tooth; such cysts are called residual cysts.

180. Ans. (c) Calcifying epithelial odontogenic tumor

According to key given by A.B. Shetty answer is (b)

The **calcifying epithelial odontogenic tumor**, also known as a **Pindborg tumor** or **CEOT**, is an odontogenic tumor, first recognized by the Danish pathologist Jens Jørgen Pindborg in 1955.

It is a typically benign and slow growing, but invasive neoplasm. Intraosseous tumors (tumors within the bone) are more likely (94%) versus extraosseus tumors (6%). It is more common in the posterior mandible of adults, typically in the 4th to 5th decades. There may be a painless swelling, and it is often concurrent with an impacted tooth. On radiographs, it appears as a radiolucency (dark area) and is known for sometimes having small radiopacities (white areas) within it. Microscopically, there are deposits of amyloid-like material. The underlying nature of the amyloid-material is still unresolved. Clinically it has two types, the central and the peripheral.

181. Ans. (c) Dentigerous cyst

A dentigerous cyst is an odontogenic cyst, thought to be of developmental origin. It is associated with the crown of an unerupted (or partially erupted) tooth. The cyst cavity is lined by epithelial cells derived from the reduced enamel epithelium of the tooth forming organ. Most dentigerous cysts are solitary. Multiple/bilateral cysts are usually found in association with a number of syndromes including cleidocranial dysplasia, Maroteaux-Lamy syndrome and Gorlin-Goltz syndrome (multiple OKCs). In the absence of these syndromes, the occurrence of multiple dentigerous cysts is rare. Microscopically the cyst walls composed of fibrous tissue and lined by stratified squamous, non-keratinized epithelium with Rushton bodies.

Rushton's bodies are peculiar, linear, often curved, hyaline bodies with variable staining of uncertain origin and unknown significance, but probably of hematogenous origin, found within the lining epithelium—especially in area of inflammation.

REGRESSIVE ALTERATION OF TEETH

182. Ans. (a) Dry socket *Ref: Shafer's 6th ed. Pg. 601*

- **Dry socket** is a post-extraction complication.
- Also known as Alveolagia, Alveolitis sicca dolorosa, Localized alveolitis, Localized acute alveolar osteomyelitis.
- It is initiated by excessive trauma during extraction, presence of infection in the surgical area prior to procedure, etc.
- It occurs on the 3rd–5th day after extraction, characterized by disintegration of the clot due to the action of fibrinolytic enzymes. The patient develops severe pain.
- The treatment is only by irrigation, placement of obtundants in the socket and prescription of analgesics.

183. Ans. (b) Abfraction *Ref: Neville's Oral and Maxillofacial Pathology 3rd ed. Pg. 64; Shafer's Textbook of Oral Pathology 7th ed. Pg. 577*

- Abfraction
  - The term was coined by Grippo (1991).
  - The pathologic loss of both enamel and dentin caused by biomechanical loading forces.

- The forces could be static, such as those produced by swallowing and clenching; or cyclic, as in those generated during chewing action.
- Till recently this type of tooth loss which is mainly confined to the gingival third of the clinical crown.
- It is proposed that with each bite, occlusal forces cause the teeth to flex though little.
- Constant flexing causes enamel to break from the crown, usually on the buccal surface.

- Attrition
  - The physiologic wearing away of a tooth as a result of tooth-to-tooth contact, as in mastication.
  - This occurs only on the occlusal, incisal, and proximal surfaces of teeth.
  - This phenomenon is physiologic rather than pathologic, and it is associated with the aging process.
  - It may be seen in the deciduous dentition as well as in the permanent.
  - The first clinical manifestation may be the appearance of a small polished facet on a cusp tip or ridge or a slight flattening of an incisal edge.
- Abrasion
  - Abrasion is the pathologic wearing away of tooth substance through some abnormal mechanical process.
  - Abrasion usually occurs on the exposed root surfaces of teeth, but under certain circumstances it may be seen elsewhere, such as on incisal or proximal surfaces.
  - The most common cause of abrasion of root surfaces is the use of an abrasive dentifrice.
  - Modern dentifrices can cause remarkable wear of cementum and dentin if the toothbrush carrying the dentifrice is injudiciously used, particularly in a horizontal rather than vertical direction.
  - In such cases abrasion caused by a dentifrice manifests itself usually as a V-shaped or wedge-shaped ditch on the root side of the cementoenamel junction in teeth with some gingival recession.
  - The angle formed in the depth of the lesion, as well as that at the enamel edge, is a rather sharp one, and the exposed dentin appears highly polished.
  - Other less common forms may be related to habit or to the occupation of the patient like habitual opening of bobby pins, carpenters, shoemakers, or tailors who hold nails, tacks, or pins between their teeth.
  - The improper use of dental floss and toothpicks may produce lesions on the proximal exposed root surface.

184. Ans. (b) Internal resorption

Begins centrally within the tooth.

First described by bell in 1830.

First evidence—appearance of a pink-hued area on the crown of the tooth, which represents the hyperplastic, vascular pulp tissue filling the resorbed area and showing through the remaining overlying tooth structure.

185. Ans. (a) Mercury *Ref: Shafer's 6th ed. Pg. 557*

Pink disease

- Also termed as acrodynia or swift's disease.
- It is caused due to the toxicity of mercury either an actual mercury poisoning or an idiosyncrasy to the metal.
- Mostly seen in young infants (- < 2 years)
- The skin of hands, nose, ears, feet and cheeks becomes red or pink with a cold clammy feelings.
- It cause maculopapular rash which is extremely pruritic.
- The gingiva becomes extremely sensitive or painful and may exhibit ulceration. Mastication is difficult because of pain.
- Chelation therapy is the standard care, like dimercaprol, D-penicillamine or DMSA.

MISCELLANEOUS

186. Ans. (d) 2% formalin is used *Ref: Shafer's 7th ed. Pg. 595; Histotechnology: A Self-Instructional Text 3th edi American Society for Clinical Pathology*

***'By far the most commonly used fixative in histology is** formaldehyde. **It is usually used as a 10% Neutral Buffered Formalin (NBF), that is approx. 3.7%–4.0% formaldehyde in** phosphate buffered saline.'--American Society for Clinical Pathology*

- **Fixation is a chemical process by which** biological tissues **are preserved from decay, thereby preventing** autolysis **or** putrefaction. *(Option B is true)*
- **Fixatives are toxic to most common microorganisms** (bacteria **in particular) that might exist in a tissue sample or which might otherwise colonize the fixed tissue.** (*Options A and C are true*)
- Finally, fixatives often alter the cells or tissues on a molecular level to increase their mechanical strength or stability. This increased strength and rigidity can help preserve the morphology (shape and structure) of the sample as it is processed for further analysis.
- ***By far the most commonly used fixative in histology is** formaldehyde. **It is usually used as a 10% Neutral Buffered Formalin (NBF), that is approx. 3.7%–4.0% formaldehyde in** phosphate buffered saline.* Because formaldehyde is a gas at room temperature, formalin-formaldehyde gas dissolved in water (~37% w/v)—is used when making the former fixative.

Target	*Fixative of choice*	*Fixative to avoid*
Proteins		
	Neutral Buffered Formalin, Paraformaldehyde	Osmium Tetroxide
Enzymes	Frozen Sections	Chemical Fixatives
Lipids	Frozen Sections, Glutaraldehyde/ Osmium Tetroxide	Alcoholic fixatives, Neutral Buffered Formalin
Nucleic Acids	Alcoholic fixatives, HOPE	Aldehyde fixatives
Mucopolysaccharides	Frozen Sections	Chemical fixatives
Biogenic Amines	Bouin Solution~, Neutral Buffered Formalin	
Glycogen	Alcoholic-based fixatives	Osmium Tetroxide

187. Ans. (c) Preserve it and reassure the parents *Ref: Shafer's Textbook of Oral Pathology 7th ed. Pg. 49*

Natal teeth must be approached individually with sound clinical judgment guiding appropriate therapy. As stated, the erupted teeth in most cases represent the deciduous dentition and removal should not be performed hastily. If the teeth are mobile and at risk for aspiration, removal is indicated. If mobility is not a problem and the teeth are stable, they should be retained.—NEVILLE

Such retained remnants may subsequently develop atypical toothlike structures that require additional treatment, as reported by Nedley, Stanley, and Cohen. The preferable approach, however, is to leave the tooth in place and to explain to the parents the desirability of maintaining this tooth in the mouth because of its importance in the growth and uncomplicated eruption of the adjacent teeth.—'Mc Donald Page 183'

- **The predeciduous teeth have been described as hornified epithelial structures without roots, occurring on the gingiva over the crest of the ridge, which may be easily removed. Prematurely erupted true deciduous teeth, of course, are not to be extracted.**

- **These predeciduous** teeth have been thought to arise either from an accessory bud of the dental lamina ahead of the deciduous bud or from the bud of an accessory dental lamina.
- The concept of predeciduous teeth has been questioned by Spouge and Feasby; however. They are probably correct in believing that considering predeciduous teeth as an entity is a misinterpretation and that such structures, present at birth, undoubtedly represent only the dental lamina cyst of the newborn (q.v.). This cyst does commonly project above the crest of the ridge, is white in color and is packed within keratin, so that it appears 'hornified' and can be easily removed.
- Spouge and Feasby have pointed out that prematurely erupted teeth are often well formed and normal in all respects except that they may be somewhat mobile. These teeth should be retained even though nursing difficulties may be experienced.

188. Ans. (a) 10% buffered neutral formalin *Ref: Histotechnology: A Self-Instructional Text 3th ed. American Society for Clinical Pathology*

'By far the most commonly used fixative in histology is formaldehyde. It is usually used as a 10% Neutral Buffered Formalin (NBF), that is approx. 3.7%–4.0% formaldehyde in phosphate buffered saline.'- American Society for Clinical Pathology

- **Fixation is a chemical process by which biological tissues are preserved from decay, thereby preventing autolysis or putrefaction.** (Option B is true)
- **Fixatives are toxic to most common microorganisms (bacteria in particular) that might exist in a tissue sample or which might otherwise colonize the fixed tissue.** (Options A and C are true)
- Finally, fixatives often alter the cells or tissues on a molecular level to increase their mechanical strength or stability. This increased strength and rigidity can help preserve the morphology (shape and structure) of the sample as it is processed for further analysis.
- **By far the most commonly used fixative in histology is formaldehyde. It is usually used as a 10% Neutral Buffered Formalin (NBF), that is approx. 3.7%–4.0% formaldehyde in phosphate buffered saline.** Because formaldehyde is a gas at room temperature, formalin-formaldehyde gas dissolved in water (~37% w/v)—is used when making the former fixative.

Target	*Fixative of choice*	*Fixative to avoid*
Proteins	Neutral Buffered Formalin, Paraformaldehyde	Osmium Tetroxide
Enzymes	Frozen Sections	Chemical Fixatives
Lipids	Frozen Sections*, Glutaraldehyde/ Osmium Tetroxide	Alcoholic fixatives, Neutral Buffered Formalin
Nucleic Acids	Alcoholic fixatives, HOPE	Aldehyde fixatives
Mucopolysaccharides	Frozen Sections	Chemical fixatives
Biogenic Amines	Bouin Solution~, Neutral Buffered Formalin	
Glycogen	Alcoholic based fixatives	Osmium Tetroxide

189. Ans. (a) Allodynia *Ref: Burket's Oral Medicine, Diagnosis and Treatment 10th ed.; Dorland's Pocket Medical Dictionary 27th ed. Pg. 29*

Hyperalgesia: Is increased response to stimulus that is usually painful.

Allodynia: Is pain due to a stimulus that does not normally produce pain. Or Pain produced by non-noxious stimuli.

Hyperesthesia: Is an increased sensitivity to stimulation and does not imply a painful sensation, but rather an augmented response to a specific sensory mode (e.g. Touch, vibration, temperature).

Hyperpathia: Is a painful syndrome with increased reaction to a stimulus and an increased threshold, faulty identification and localization of stimulus, delayed and radiating sensation and after sensation may be present.

Causalgia: Is a syndrome of burning pain, allodynia and hyperpathia after a traumatic nerve lesion and is often combined with vasomotor and sudomotor (sweat sensation) dysfunction and later trophic changes.

Hypoesthesia: Decreased sensitivity to stimulation.

Hypoalgesia: Special case of hypoaesthesia in which pain response to a normally painful stimulus is diminished.

Dysesthesia: is an abnormal unpleasant sensation.

Neuralgia: Pain in the distribution of nerve.

Neuropathy: Disturbance of function or pathologic change in a nerve.

Anesthetic dolorosa: Paradoxic pain in a region of sensory loss following an injury to a cranial nerve or a nerve root (seen often after surgical treatment of trigeminal ganglion/root for neuralgia).

Glossodynia: Refers to a painful or burning feeling of the tongue.

Glossoptosis: A medical condition and abnormality which refers to the downward displacement or retraction of the tongue.

Glossopyrosis: Burning sensation in the tongue.

Stomatopyrosis: Condition characterized by a burning sensation or as pain in the mouth cavity with clinically normal oral mucosa.

190. Ans. (a) Natal teeth *Ref: Neville's Oral and Maxillofacial Pathology 3rd ed. Pg. 287; Shafer's Textbook of Oral Pathology 7th ed. Pg. 537*

Riga-Fede disease:

- *Occurs in infants between one week and one year of life.*
- *Lesions (ulceration) are usually observed on the anteroventral surface of the tongue, caused by contact with the erupting mandibular incisors.*
- *These associated teeth are usually natal or neonatal teeth.*
- *A presentation similar to Riga-Fede disease can be the initial finding in a variety of neuro logic conditions related to self-mutilation, such as familial dysautonomia (Riley-Day syndrome), congenital indifference to pain, Lesch-Nyhan syndrome, Gaucher disease, cerebral palsy, or Tourette syndrome.*

191. Ans. (a) Topical beclamethasone *Ref: Shafer's 7th ed. Pg. 2673-2377*

- There is a well-recognized group of materials which frequently cause the oral lesion of contact stomatitis or stomatitis venenata, and which for this reason are of special interest to the dentist.

  These may be classified as follows:
  - Dental or cosmetic preparations: **Dentifrices**, Mouthwashes, Denture powders, Lipstick, candy, cough drops, chewing gum.
  - Dental materials: Rubber dam, Vulcanite, Acrylic, Metal alloy base.
  - Dental therapeutic agents: Alcohols, **Antibiotics**, Iodides, Phenols, Procaine, Volatile oils.
- After contact with some material to which the patient is sensitive, the mucosa becomes remarkably inflamed and edematous, the reaction imparting a smooth, shiny appearance to the surface. When the gingiva is involved, the tissue is uniformly bright red in all quadrants, in contrast to the plaque-induced gingivitis which is more localized and usually spares attached gingiva.
- Buccal mucosa is usually puffy and dark red, revealing engorged and ejected superficial capillaries on closer examination. Small vesicles may form, but these are transient and soon rupture to form small areas of erosion and ulceration, which may become extensive in some cases. Such swollen and edematous features subject to erosion and ulceration are more common in the lips.
- **Topical antifungal agents** may cause stomatitis medicamentosa which has features similar or even worse than stomatitis venenata.
- **Triclosan** is a component of toothpaste and is one of the causes of stomatitis venenata.
- Out of the options provided only **beclamethasone** reduces inflammation and hence is the answer.

192. Ans. (c) In the center of lesion till bleeding occurs *Ref: Oral Precancer: Diagnosis and Management of Potentially Malignant Disorders Pg. 88, 89*

- A system of obtaining exfoliated cells by cell collection devices known as cytobrushes, such as the OralCDx®brush (Oral CDx Laboratories Inc., Suffern, NY, USA), has been devised to increase basal cell yield. It is best considered as a diagnostic 'step' rather than a definitive diagnostic test as an incisional biopsy must follow an abnormal result.
- More recently the Orcellex® brush (Rovers Medical Devices B.V., the Netherlands) [14], a novel cytobrush using 'thin hair technology', has been developed. The specially designed brush head, which comprises five segments of high-density fibers designed for optimal cell collection.

http://www.cdxdiagnostics.com/OralCDx.html

OralCDx Brush Biopsy Technique

- **The oral biopsy brush is firmly pressed against lesion and rotated until pinpoint bleeding is observed**.
- The brush is then rotated onto the enclosed glass slide, transferring the cellular material.
- The sample is then preserved by immediately emptying the contents of a complete fixative packet onto slide. The sample is allowed to dry for 15 minutes slide is then placed into
- The dry slide in then placed into the supplied slide holder, placed back into the box, and shipped to the lab for analysis.

http://www.roversmedicaldevices.com/index.php?pagina_id=53

Instructions for use Rovers® Orcellex®

- The Rovers® Orcellex® Brush should be rotated ten times at each individual sample site in order to obtain an adequate number of cells.
- A fresh brush must be used for each site sampled and a separate vial must be used for that sample.
- The number of turns needed is ten when collecting an individual sample from the buccal, gingival or lateral border of tongue mucosa.
- Although fewer rotations may be satisfactory in the floor of mouth mucosa in some subjects, it is advised to use ten turns because the procedure produces a consistent high cell yield.

193. Ans. (a) Keratinized specialized *Ref: Orbans' Oral Histology and Embryology 13th ed. Pg. 267; Tencat's Oral Histology Embryology and Physiology 8th ed. Pg. 302*

- *Specialized mucosa* (Dorsal lingual mucosa): The covering epithelium is *keratinized* and forms tufts at the apex of the dermal papilla. - *Orban's*

Review topic: structure of the mucosa in different regions of the oral cavity			
Region	*Covering Epithelium*	*Lamina Propria*	*Submucosa*
Lining Mucosa			
Soft palate	Thin, nonkeratinized stratified squamous epithelium; taste buds present	Thick with numerous short papillae; elastic fibers forming on elastic lamina; highly vascular with well-defined capillary network	Diffuse tissue containing numerous minor salivary glands
Ventral surface of tongue	Thin, nonkeratinized, stratified squamous epithelium	Thin with numerous short papillae and some elastic fibers; a few minor salivary glands; capillary network in subpapillary layer; reticular layer relatively avascular	Thin and irregular; may contain fat and small vessels; where absent, mucosa is bound to connective tissue surrounding tongue musculature

Contd...

Contd...

Review topic: structure of the mucosa in different regions of the oral cavity			
Region	*Covering Epithelium*	*Lamina Propria*	*Submucosa*
Floor of mouth	Very thin, nonkeratinized, stratified squamous epithelium	Short papillae; some elastic fibers; extensive vascular supply with short anastomosing capillary loops	Loose fibrous connective tissue containing fat and minor salivary glands
Alveolar mucosa	Thin, nonkeratinized, stratified squamous epithelium	Short papillae, connective tissue containing many elastic fibers; capillary loops close to the surface supplied by vessels running superficially to the periosteum	Loose connective tissue, containing thick elastic fibers attaching it to periosteum of alveolar process; minor salivary glands
Labial and buccal mucosa	Very thick, nonkeratinized, stratified squamous epithelium	Long, slender papillae; dense fibrous connective tissue containing collagen and some elastic fibers; rich vascular supply giving off anastomosing capillary loops into papillae	Mucosa firmly attached to underlying muscle by collagen and elastin; dense collagenous connective tissue with fat, minor salivary glands, sometimes sebaceous glands
Lips: vermilion Zone	Thin, orthokeratinized, stratified squamous epithelium	Numerous narrow papillae; capillary loops close to surface in papillary layer	Mucosa firmly attached to underlying muscle; some sebaceous glands in vermilion border, minor salivary gland and fat in intermediate zone
Lips: intermediate zone	Thin, parakeratinized, stratified squamous epithelium	Long, irregular papillae; elastic and collagen fibers in connective tissue	—
Masticatory Mucosa			
Gingiva	Thick, orthokeratinized or parakeratinized, stratified squamous epithelium often showing stippled surface	Long, narrow papillae; dense collagenous connective tissue; not highly vascular but has long capillary loops with numerous anastomoses	No distinct layer; mucosa firmly attached by collagen fibers to cementum and periosteum of alveolar process (mucoperiosteum)

Contd...

Contd...

Review topic: structure of the mucosa in different regions of the oral cavity			
Region	*Covering Epithelium*	*Lamina Propria*	*Submucosa*
Hard palate	Thick, orthokeratinized (often parakeratinized in parts), stratified squamous epithelium thrown into transverse palatine ridges (rugae)	Long papillae; thick, dense collagenous tissue, especially under rugae; moderate vascular supply with short capillary loops	Dense collagenous connective tissue attaching mucosa to periosteum (mucoperiosteum); fat and minor salivaryglands are packed into connective tissue in regions where mucosa overlies lateral palatine neurovascular bundles
Specialized Mucosa			
Dorsal surface of tongue	***Thick, keratinized and nonkeratinized, stratified squamous epithelium*** forming three types of lingual papillae, some bearing taste buds	Long papillae; minor salivary glands in posterior portion; rich innervation especially near taste buds; capillary plexus in papillary layer; large vessels lying deeper	No distinct layer; mucosa is bound to connective tissue surrounding musculature of tongue

194. Ans. (a) Amalgam tattoo *Ref: Oral and Maxillofacial Pathology by Neville. 3rd ed. Pg. 308*

Amalgam tattoo is also known as ***localized argyrosis***.

Amalgam can be incorporated into the oral mucosa in following ways:

- Areas of mucosal abrasion contaminated with amalgam containing fluid
- Broken pieces of amalgam may fall into extraction socket
- Dental floss contaminated with amalgam gives linear discoloration
- Amalgam from endodontic retrograde filling.

Lesions: Small asymptomatic, macular and bluish gray or even black appearance.

It is seen on gingiva, alveolar mucosa, buccal mucosa or floor of the mouth.

195. Ans. (b) Ameloglyphics *Ref: Shafer's 7th ed. figure-1.5*

Recently there is growing interest in the study of enamel rod end patterns. These enamel rod end patterns are termed as tooth prints and the study of these prints is known as **Ameloglyphics** (amelo: Enamel, glyphics: Carvings). The tooth prints are unique, exhibiting dissimilarity both between teeth of different individuals and of the same individual. This uniqueness of the tooth print could be used as a valuable tool in forensic science for personal identification.

196. Ans. (b) Reconstructive identification *Ref: Shafer's 6th ed. Pg. 872*

Dental identification procedure consist of 2 forms, i.e. comparative identification and reconstructive identification or dental profiling.

197. Ans. (d) Root length of maxillary canine *Ref: Shafer's 6th ed. Pg. 880*

Dental feature used to describe population differences are broadly categorized as:

- Metric (size)
- Non-metric (shape and feature)

Non-metric dental features include:

- Shoveling
- Carabellis trait
- Three cusped maxillary second molar
- Mandibular molar groove pattern
- Four cusped mandibular molar etc.

198. Ans. (b) Ulcerative colitis *Ref: Shafer's 6th ed. Pg. 330*

In 1949, McCarthy described the pyostomatitis vegetans as an uncommon inflammatory disease of the oral cavity. Ulcerative colitis is an idiopathic chronic inflammatory bowel disorder part or entire colon. Oral lesions of UC, pyostomatitis vegetans shows epithelium with area of ulceration of necrosis. The oral mucosa of UC looks generally erythematous with scattered pustules, hemorrhagic ulceration and abscesses. Hence, pyostomatitis vegetans may be seen as an oral manifestation of UC.

ORAL ASPECT OF METABOLIC DISEASE

199. Ans. (b) Associated with hyperparathyroidism *Ref: Shafer's 5th ed. Pg. 900-901*

- The jaw lesions of hyperparathyroidism are known as Osteitis Fibrosa Cystica (Brown tumor).
- It is characterized by excessive secretion of parathyroid hormones.
- It is mainly due to parathyroid adenoma and rarely due to carcinoma.
- Clinical features: F>M.
- Pathologic fracture may be the first symptom of the disease.
- Radio: decrease in the radiodensity of bone.
- Loss of Lamina dura.
- The jaw resembles ground glass appearance which is also seen fibrous dysplasia.

200. Ans. (a) Hyperparathyroidism *Ref: Shafer's 5th ed. Pg. 890, 891, 899*

- The jaw lesions of hyperparathyroidism are known as Osteitis Fibrosa Cystica (Brown tumor).
- It is characterized by excessive secretion of parathyroid hormones.
- It is mainly due to parathyroid adenoma and rarely due to carcinoma.
- Clinical features: F > M.
- Pathologic fracture may be the first symptom of the disease.
- Radio: decrease in the radiodensity of bone.
- Loss of Lamina dura.
- The jaw resembles ground glass appearance which is also seen fibrous dysplasia.
- Loss of lamina dura also occurs in Paget's diseases.

201. Ans. (d) Transthyretin *Ref: Robbin Pg. 167-169*

- Transthyretin (TTR) is a normal serum protein that binds and transports thyroxine and retinol.
- Transthyretin is also deposited in the heart of aged individuals (senile systemic amyloidosis) in such cases the protein is structurally normal but it accumulates at high concentrations.
- Some cases of familial amyloidosis are associated with deposits of mutant lysozyme.
- Amyloid of aging: Several well-documented forms of amyloid deposition occur with aging.

- Senile systemic amyloidosis refers to the systemic deposition of amyloid in elderly patients (usually in their 70s and 80s).
- The dominant involvement and related dysfunction of the heart form is also called senile cardiac amyloidosis.
- The amyloid in this form is composed of the normal TTR molecule.

202. Ans. (a) Hyperparathyroidism *Ref: Neville's Oral and Maxillofacial Pathology 3rd ed. Pg. 838-839; Shafer's Textbook of Oral pathology 7th ed. Pg. 654*

Hyperparathyroidism:

- Excess production of PTH.
- Two types:
  - Primary hyperparathyroidism: uncontrolled production of PTH, usually as a result of parathyroid adenoma (80%–90%) or parathyroid hyperplasia (10%–15%).
  - Secondary hyperparathyroidism—due to continuous low level of serum calcium (e.g. in chronic renal disease).
- Sign and symptoms:
  - More common in >60 years old and female patients.
  - The classic triad of signs and symptoms are described as:
    - Stones: renal calculi, metastatic calcification.
    - Bones: subperiosteal resorption of phalanges of index and middle figures.
      - **Persistent disease causes hemorrhage and hemosiderin deposition within tumors, called brown tumor**.
    - Abdominal groans: tendency for development of duodenal ulcer.

203. Ans. (a) Chlordontia *Ref: Neville's Oral and Maxillofacial Pathology 3rd ed. Pg. 72*

The extent of the dental changes correlate with the period of hyperbilirubinemia, and most patients exhibits involvement limited to the primary dentition. Occasionally cups of permanent first molar may be affected. In addition to enamel hypoplasia the affected teeth frequently demonstrate a green discoloration (chlorodontia). The color is the result of deposition of biliverdin (the breakdown product of bilirubin) and varies from yellow to deep shades of green.

Also know:

1. *Alkaptonuria* is associated with a blue black discoloration termed *ochronosis* that occurs in connective tissue, tendons and cartilages.
2. *Parkinson's diseases* patients may have *bluish discoloration of dentition.*
3. *Hyperbilirubinemia* is most commonly associated with *erythroblastosis fetalis and biliary atresia.*
4. *Leong's premolar: also called dens evaginatus, occlusal enamel pearl, evaginated odontome or occlusal tuberculated premolar*. It is an accessory cusp or a globule of enamel on the occlusalsurface between buccal and lingual cusp of premolar. It was **Extrinsic causes for tooth discoloration**
   - ***When bilirubin levels are elevated for several months, bilirubin pigments deposit throughout the body, including the teeth. In the soft tissues, the pigment is removed over time.***
   - ***However, in the hard dental tissues, the pigment becomes trapped because of the lack of metabolic activity and thus results in permanent discoloration. Histological evaluation of green-stained deciduous teeth (CHLORODONIIA) from patients with hyperbilirubinemia has shown bilirubin deposits. The other reason for green teeth is tetracycline staining.***

Note: **Ochronosis** is the syndrome caused by the accumulation of homogentisic acid in connective tissues.

A **pink tooth of Mummery**, named after British biologist James Howard Mummery, is a tooth exhibiting a pinkish hue as a result of hematologic staining of the dentin.

204. Ans. (b) Bowed Leg *Ref: Neville's Oral and maxillofacial Pathology 3rd ed. Pg. 827; Shafer's Textbook of Oral Pathology 7th ed. Pg. 636-637; Lipincott's Illustrated Review of Biochemistry 5th ed. Pg. 388.*

- ***'Since undermineralized bone is not as capable of supporting weight as normal bone, children with rickets show bowing of the legs.'*** - Shafer's 7th ed. Pg. 636
- *'Clinical manifestations of rickets include—irritability, growth retardation and prominence of costochondral junctions (rachitic rosary).* ***As the child ages and begins to put weight on the long bones of legs, significant bowing results because of the poor mineralization of the skeleton.'*** - Neville's 3rd ed. Pg. 827
- ***'Bowed legs of middle-aged man with osteomalacia, a nutritional vitamin D deficiency that results in malformation of the skeleton.'*** - Lipincott's Biochemistry 5th ed. Pg. 388.

Review Topic: *VITAMIN D*

- The D vitamins are a group of sterols that have a hormone-like function.
- The active molecule, 1,25-dihydroxycholecalciferol (1,25-diOH-D3), binds to intracellular receptor proteins. The 1,25-diOH-D3-receptor complex interacts with DNA in the nucleus of target cells in a manner similar to that of vitamin.

A. Distribution of vitamin D

- Diet: Ergocalciferol (vitamin D2), found in plants, and cholecalciferol (vitamin D3), found in animal tissues, are sources of preformed vitamin D activity. Ergocalciferol and cholecalciferol differ chemically only in the presence of an additional double bond and methyl group in the plant sterol.
- Endogenous vitamin precursor: 7-Dehydrocholesterol, an intermediate in cholesterol synthesis, is converted to cholecalciferol in the dermis and epidermis of humans exposed to sunlight. Preformed vitamin D is a dietary requirement only in individuals with limited exposure to sunlight.

B. Metabolism of vitamin D

- Formation of 1,25-diOH-D3: Vitamins D2 and D3 are not biologically active, but are converted in vivo to the active form of the D vitamin by two sequential hydroxylation reactions.

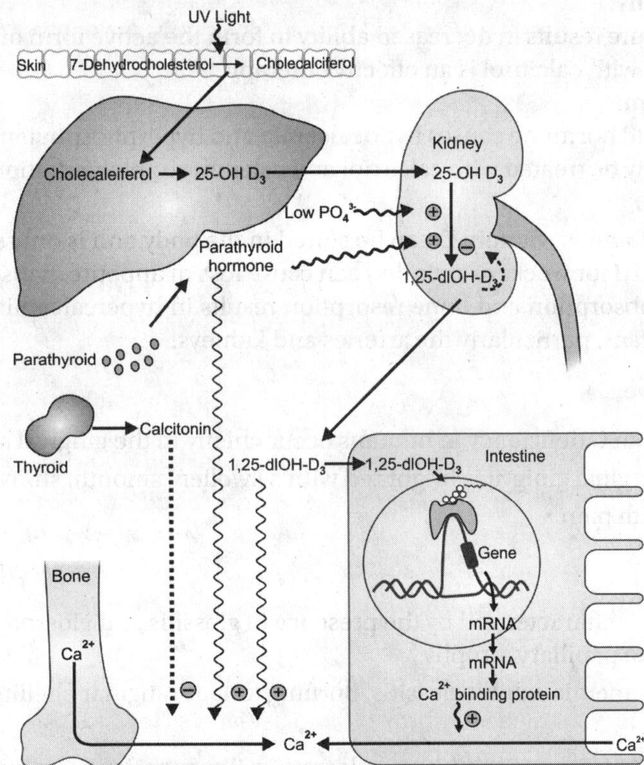

C. Function of vitamin D

- The overall function of 1,25-diOH-D_3 is to maintain adequate plasma levels of calcium.
- It performs this function by:
  - Increasing uptake of calcium by the intestine.
  - Minimizing loss of calcium by the kidney.
  - Stimulating resorption of bone when necessary.
- Effect of vitamin D on the intestine:
  - 1,25-diOH-D_3 *stimulates intestinal absorption of calcium and phosphate.*
  - 1,25-diOH-D_3 enters the intestinal cell and binds to a cytosolic receptor.
  - As a result, *calcium uptake is enhanced by an increased synthesis of a specific calcium—binding protein.*
  - Thus, the *mechanism of action of 1, 25-diOH-D_3 is typical of steroid hormones.*
- Effect of vitamin D on bone:
  - 1,25-diOH-D_3 *stimulates the mobilization of calcium and phosphate from bone* by a process that requires protein synthesis and the presence of PTH.
  - The result is an increase in plasma calcium and phosphate.
  - Thus, bone is an important reservoir of calcium that can be mobilized to maintain plasma levels.

E. *Clinical indications*

- **Nutritional rickets:**
  - Vitamin D deficiency causes a net de-mineralization of bone, resulting in ***rickets in children*** and ***osteomalacia in adults.***
  - Rickets is characterized by the continued formation of the collagen matrix of bone, but incomplete mineralization, resulting in soft, pliable bones.
  - In osteomalacia, demineralization of pre-existing bones increases their susceptibility to fracture.
  - Insufficient exposure to daylight and/or deficiencies in vitamin D consumption occur predominantly in infants and the elderly.
  - Vitamin D deficiency is more common in the northern latitudes.
- **Renal osteodystrophy**:
  - Chronic renal failure results in decreased ability to form the active form of vitamin D.
  - Supplementation with calcitriol is an effective therapy.
- **Hypoparathyroidism**:
  - Lack of parathyroid hormone causes hypocalcemia and hyperphosphatemia.
  - These patients may be treated with calcitriol and calcium supplementation.

F. Toxicity of vitamin D

- Like all fat-soluble vitamins, vitamin D can be stored in the body and is only slowly metabolized.
- High doses (100,000 IU for weeks or months) can cause loss of appetite, nausea, thirst, and stupor.
- Enhanced calcium absorption and bone resorption results in hypercalcemia, which can lead to deposition of calcium in many organs, particularly the arteries and kidneys.

205. Ans. (d) All of the above

The oral effects of vitamin C deficiency in humans occur chiefly in the gingival and periodontal tissues.

The interdental and marginal ginigva is bright red with a swollen, smooth, shiny surface.

Is usually associated with pain.

206. Ans. (a) Glossodynia

Iron deficiency anemia is characterized by the presence of glossitis and glossodynia angular cheilitis and atrophic area of the tongue due to papillary atrophy.

Patient with pernicious anemia exhibit glossitis, burning tongue, angular cheilitis, papillary atrophy and recurrent oral ulceration.

Sickle cell anemia and thalassemia exhibit oral ulceration. These patients are more likely to develop osteomyelitis.

207. Ans. (a) Increased salivation

Mercury poisoning or mercurialism is caused by ingestion or inhalation of mercury or mercury compounds due to occupational exposure or use of drugs containing mercury.

Mercury poisoning is associated with increased salivation, metallic taste, ulceration of the mouth and loosening of teeth. The pigmentation is usually found along the free marginal gingiva due to deposition of the dark sulfide compound.

Causes Pink's disease/Acrodynia/Swift disease.

208. Ans. (c) Pernicious anemia

Pernicious anemia is an autoimmune atrophic gastritis that causes a deficiency in vitamin B12 due to its malabsorption. Glossitis (Hunter's glossitis)—characterized by a slick or bald tongue, papillary atrophy, and burning sensation on contact with certain foods—is usually associated with pernicious anemia.

10 Pharmacology

GENERAL PHARMACOLOGICAL PRINCIPLES

1. Which is a prodrug? *(AIIMS May 2010, AIPG 2010)*
 a. Enalapril
 b. Clonidine
 c. Salmeterol
 d. Acetazolamide

2. Loading dose of injection depends upon: *(AIIMS Nov 2008, AIPG 2010)*
 a. The volume of distribution
 b. The plasma half-life
 c. The plasma clearance
 d. The route of administration

3. All the following statements regarding bioavailability of a drug are true, *except*: *(AIIMS Nov 2007)*
 a. It is the proportion (fraction) of unchanged drug that reaches the systemic circulation
 b. Bioavailability of an orally administered drug can be calculated by comparing the area under the curve after oral and IV administration
 c. Low oral bioavailability always and necessarily means poor absorption
 d. Bioavailability can be determined from plasma concentration or urinary excretion data

4. Which of the following properties of drug will enable it to be used in low concentrations? *(AIIMS Nov 2005)*
 a. High affinity   b. High specificity
 c. Low specificity   d. High stability

5. The time taken for the drug to decrease by 50% of its concentration when the infusion is stopped is called as: *(AIPG 2011)*
 a. Context half life
 b. Elimination half life
 c. Elimination constant
 d. Redistribution half time

6. Most important factor for calculating dose for NSAIDs in children: *(AIPG 2011)*
 a. Age of child
 b. Body weight of child
 c. Flavor of salt
 d. Extent of pain

7. Which of the following is as False statement? *(AIPG 2013)*
 a. 1 gm drug A give better effect then 3 gm drug B. Drug A is more potent than drug B
 b. Drug efficacy doesn't depend on drug dosage
 c. Drug A produces better effect that can't be produced by drug B even with max tolerated dose this implies drug A is more efficacious than drug B
 d. 1 gm of drug A produces more effect that can't be produced by 1 gm drug B so drug A is more efficacious than drug B

8. Coadministration of amoxicillin with clavulanic acid is an example of: *(AIPG 2012)*
 a. Synergism
 b. Antagonism
 c. Cumulative action
 d. Displacement

9. Phocomelia in children is caused by which drug taken by the mother during pregnancy? *(AIPG 2012)*
 a. Thalidomide
 b. Tetracycline
 c. Warfarin
 d. Chloroquine

10. In medical prescription, HS stands for: *(AIPG 2010)*
 a. At bed time
 b. At any time
 c. One teaspoon
 d. Given to the patient after retiring

11. Drug efficacy refers to: *(COMED 2006)*
a. Range of disease in which the drug is beneficial
b. Maximal intensity of response that can be reduced by the drug
c. The therapeutic dose of range of the drug
d. The therapeutic index of the drug

12. Drug metabolism can be induced by following factors, *except*: *(COMED 2006)*
a. Cigarette smoking
b. Acute alcohol ingestion
c. Exposure to insecticides
d. Consume charcoal boiled meat

13. The dose of a drug required to produce a specified effect in 50% of the population is: *(COMED 2012)*
a. Ld50
b. Td50
c. Md50
d. Ed50

14. When a drug creates an effect that is unpredictable and unique it is termed as: *(COMED 2012)*
a. Side effect
b. Toxicity effect
c. Idiosyncratic effect
d. Drug on drug effect

15. A biological experiment in which one compares the effects of two preparations by means of common biological response is known as: *(COMED 2012)*
a. Biodegradable
b. Bio experiment
c. Bio assay
d. Bio statement

16. Combination of sulfamethoxazole and trimethoprim is synergistic due to: *(COMED 2012)*
a. Enhanced entry into bacteria
b. Sequential blockade in folate metabolism
c. Inhibition of drug inactivating enzymes
d. Inhibition of drug reflex

17. The following statements are true about intravenous route of drug administration *except* that: *(KCET 2012)*
a. It is useful in emergencies
b. Aseptic precautions are required
c. Bioavailability is 100%
d. Suspensions can be administered

18. The safer way of calculating drug dosage in children is based on: *(KCET 2012)*
a. Weight
b. Body surface area
c. Basal metabolic rate
d. Chronologic age

19. Sublingual route of administration: *(KCET 2008)*
a. Has a slow onset of action
b. Does not produce systemic effect
c. Decreases drug excretion
d. Bypasses first-pass metabolism

20. Immune mediated qualitative drug intolerance is called: *(KCET 2007)*
a. Supersensitivity b. Idiosyncrasy
c. Hypersensitivity d. Hyperacidity

21. Therapeutic Index is a measure of: *(KCET 2005)*
a. Safety of a drug b. Toxicity of a drug
c. Efficacy of drug d. All of the above

22. Obtundents are: *(KCET 2005)*
a. Abrasives b. Mummifying agents
c. Sweetening agents d. Dentine desensitizers

23. True about agonists is: *(MH 2011)*
a. Affinity with intrinsic activity
b. Affinity but no intrinsic activity
c. Affinity with sub maximal intrinsic activity
d. Affinity but intrinsic activity with minus sign

24. Which branch of pharmacology is related to the detection, assessment understanding and prevention of adverse effect or any drug-related problem? *(MH 2011)*
a. Pharmacogenetics
b. Pharmacogenomics
c. Pharmacovigilance
d. Pharmacokinetics

SYSTEMIC PHARMACOLOGY

25. The adverse effect of valproic acid derivatives include the following, *except*: *(AIIMS May 2011)*
a. Alopecia b. Liver failure
c. Weight gain d. Osteomalacia

26. Which of the following drugs is both antiresorptive and bone formative? *(AIIMS May 2011)*
a. Strontium ranelate
b. Calcitonin
c. Ibandronate
d. Teriparatide

27. All of the following causes hypoglycemia, *except*: (AIIMS May 2011)
a. Nateglinide
b. Glimepiride
c. Insulin
d. Acarbose

28. Which of the following is not true about pioglitazone? (AIIMS May 2011)
a. It acts on nuclear peroxisome proliferator-activated receptor (PPAR-r)
b. Acts by inducing transcription of gene responsible for carbohydrate and lipid catabolism in the absence of insulin
c. It is metabolized in the liver
d. It is not to be used in patient with cardiac diastolic dysfunction

29. Which of the following is not true about exenatide? (AIIMS May 2011)
a. Glucoregulatory actions similar to GLP-1
b. Suppressed inappropriate glucagon secretion
c. Helps slow down gastric emptying
d. Used in type 2 diabetes mellitus subcutaneously

30. All of the following are true about ifosfamide alkylating agent, *except*: (AIIMS May 2011)
a. Acetaldehyde conversion to chloroacetaldehyde
b. It is a nitrogen mustard
c. It is metabolized by CPY
d. It causes less neurotoxicity than cyclophosphamide

31. Which of the following is associated with thiazide diuretics? (AIIMS Nov 2010)
a. Hyperkalemic paralysis
b. Hypouricemia
c. Hypolipidemia
d. Impotence

32. Drug used for heparin overdose is: (AIIMS Nov 2010)
a. Protamine sulphate
b. Phylloquinone
c. Ticlopidine
d. Clopidogrel

33. Reverse steal phenomenon causing cerebral ischemia is shown by which anesthetic agent? (AIIMS Nov 2010)
a. Isoflurane b. Opioid
c. Benzodiazepine d. Barbiturate

34. All of the following are atypical antipsychotic drugs, *except*: (AIIMS May 2010)
a. Olanzapine
b. Clozapine
c. Risperidone
d. Thioridazine

35. The drug that is used for long-term maintenance in opioid addiction is: (AIIMS May 2010, AIPG 2010)
a. Naloxone
b. Nalorphine
c. Butorphanol
d. Methadone

36. Antiepileptic that is not associated with congenital malformation when used in pregnant women is: (AIIMS May 2010)
a. Phenytoin
b. Phenobarbitone
c. Carbamazepine
d. Valproate
e. None of the above

37. Drug of choice in absence seizures is: (AIIMS May 2010, AIPG 2010)
a. Phenytoin b. BZD
c. Valproate d. Carbamazepine

38. Sildenafil is a selective inhibitor of: (AIIMS Nov 2009)
a. Phosphodiesterase (PDE-5)
b. PGI2
c. cGMP
d. cAMP

39. Which drug is not acetylated? (AIIMS May 2009, AIPG 2010)
a. INH
b. Dapsone
c. Hydralazine
d. Metoclopramide

40. Which is not a second-generation antihistaminic? (AIIMS May 2009, AIPG 2010)
a. Loratadine b. Acrivastine
c. Cyclizine d. Terfenadine

41. Which of the following is a benzodiazepine (BZP) antagonist? (AIIMS May 2009, Nov 2008, AIPG 2010)
a. Flumazenil b. Naloxone
c. Furazolidone d. Naltrexone

42. In case of renal failure, the clearance of which of the following drugs is not affected by hemodialysis? *(AIIMS May 2009)*
a. Calcium channel blockers (CCBs)
b. Vancomycin
c. Aminoglycosides
d. Pancuronium

43. Which of the following four anesthetic agents is characterized by rapid recovery from sedation and excellent postoperative clear headedness after anesthesia? *(AIIMS Nov 2008)*
a. Propofol b. Ketamine
c. Sevoflurane d. Halothane

44. Which of the following is used in long-term treatment for opioid withdrawal? *(AIIMS Nov 2008)*
a. Pethidine b. Nalorphine
c. Methadone d. Fentanyl

45. Nitrous oxide alone is not used as a general anesthetic agent because of the: *(AIIMS Nov 2008)*
a. Difficulty in maintaining an adequate oxygen concentration
b. Expense of the agent
c. Poor analgesic properties
d. Explosive hazard of the agent

46. Which of the following is an antifibrinolytic? *(AIIMS May 2008)*
a. Aspirin
b. Tranexamic acid
c. Abciximab
d. Danaparoid sodium

47. Which of the following NSAIDs undergoes enterohepatic cycling? *(AIIMS May 2008, AIPG 2010)*
a. Phenylbutazone
b. Piroxicam
c. Aspirin
d. Ibuprofen

48. All are true about heparin, *except*: *(AIIMS May 2008, AIPG 2013)*
a. It is a heterogeneous mixture of sulphates and polypeptides
b. It potentiates the action of antithrombin-3
c. Its action can be stopped by protamine sulphate
d. It can cause idiopathic thrombocytopenia

49. All of the following drugs are used as antiemetics, *except*: *(AIIMS May 2008)*
a. Cyclizine
b. Phenazocine
c. Ondansetron
d. Domperidone

50. The action of epinephrine is potentiated by: *(AIIMS May 2008)*
a. MAO inhibitors
b. Isoprenaline
c. Dopamine
d. Beta-blockers

51. Long-term use of aspirin causes: *(AIIMS Nov 2007)*
a. Decreased platelet adhesion
b. A decrease in fibrinogen formation
c. Hypoprothrombinemia
d. None of the above

52. Which of the following is true about BZPs? *(AIIMS Nov 2007)*
a. In higher quantities, it is relatively safer than other hypnotics
b. Alters the sleep pattern to a great extent
c. Stimulates hepatic metabolic enzymes
d. All have metabolically active substrates

53. IV diazepam in a patient on the dental chair can cause: *(AIIMS Nov 2007, 2006)*
a. Tinel's sign
b. Verrill's sign
c. Bell's sign
d. Corman's sign

54. Drug that can result in hyperglycemia is: *(AIIMS Nov 2007)*
a. Beta-blockers
b. ACE inhibitors
c. Glucocorticoids
d. NSAIDs

55. Folic acid deficiency occurs in: *(AIIMS Nov 2006)*
a. Aspirin
b. Phenytoin
c. Chloramphenicol
d. Cyclosporine

56. Which of the following general anesthetics is given by the IV route? *(AIIMS Nov 2006)*
a. Propofol b. Sevoflurane
c. Naloxone d. Isoflurane

57. An anesthetist orders a new attendant to bring the oxygen cylinder. He will ask the attendant to identify the correct cylinder by the following color code: *(AIIMS Nov 2006)*

a. Black cylinder with white shoulder
b. Black cylinder with grey shoulders
c. White cylinders with black shoulders
d. Grey cylinder with white shoulders

58. In treatment of papillary carcinoma thyroid, radio-iodine destroys the neoplastic cells predominantly by: *(AIIMS Nov 2005)*

a. X-rays b. β-rays
c. W-rays d. α-particles

59. Which one of the following statements is not true about NSAIDs? *(AIIMS Nov 2005)*

a. Acetyl salicylic acid is an irreversible inhibitor of COX enzyme
b. Salicylic acid reduces in vivo synthesis of prostaglandins
c. Duration of action of aspirin is primarily related to the pharmacokinetic clearance of the drug from the body
d. Antiplatelet effect of low-dose aspirin is related to presystemic COX inhibition

60. Drug of choice in trigeminal neuralgia: *(AIPG 2011)*

a. Carbamazepine b. Phenytoin
c. Verapamil d. Ethosuximide

61. Postural hypotension as first dose effect is seen in: *(AIPG 2011)*

a. Prazosin b. Captopril
c. Clonidine d. Nitroglycerine

62. Which of the following does not cause postural hypotension? *(AIPG 2011)*

a. Prazosin b. Phentolamine
c. Tamsulosin d. Ergotamine

63. Which of the following is not an Alpha 2 blocker? *(AIPG 2011)*

a. Yohimbine b. Phenoxybenzamine
c. Phentolamine d. Prazosin

64. Which of these drugs interacts with warfarin but doesn't increase INR? *(AIPG 2011)*

a. OCP b. Metoclopramide
c. Erythromycin d. Phenytoin

65. True about ACE inhibitors: *(AIPG 2011)*

a. Adverse effect is hypokalemia
b. Secondary hyperaldosteronism and K^+ loss due to diuretics
c. Rebound hypertension on withdrawal
d. Used safely in asthmatics

66. Which of the following is not a prodrug? *(AIPG 2011)*

a. Quinapril
b. Fosinopril
c. Benazepril
d. Lisinopril

67. Regarding Propofol all are true *except*: *(AIPG 2011)*

a. Has a rapid recovery rate
b. Used for induction of anesthesia
c. Causes vomiting after use
d. none of the above

68. Less light headedness and early recovery and ambulation is due to: *(AIPG 2011)*

a. Propofol
b. Thiopentone
c. N20
d. Halothane

69. Intravenous Anesthetic agent with bronchodilator activity: *(AIPG 2011)*

a. Propofol b. Halothane
c. Ketamine d. Thiopentone Na

70. Which does not cause sedation? *(AIPG 2011)*

a. Buspirone b. Diazepam
c. Lorazepam d. Alprazolam

71. Oral Contraceptive failure occurs in a patient on Rifampicin because of: *(AIPG 2011)*

a. Rifampicin induce the metabolism of contraceptive
b. Rifampicin simulates gonadotropin release from pituitary
c. Rifampicin decrease the secretion of progestin
d. Rifampicin antagonize the action of oral contraceptive

72. Least efficient antiemetic drug: *(AIPG 2011)*

a. Domperidone
b. Cisapride
c. Chlorpromazine
d. Metoclopramide

73. General anesthetic agent intrathecal application is contraindicated: *(AIPG 2011)*
a. Fentanyl
b. Remifentanil
c. Sufentanil
d. Alfentanil

74. The antiviral mechanism of interferon therapy can be best described as: *(AIPG 2011)*
a. Phagocytosis of virus when it enters the cell
b. Prevention of viral DNA/RNA replication
c. Inhibited protein synthesis of virus
d. Prevents uncoating of virus in the host cell

75. Nitrates are not used in the management of: *(AIPG 2011)*
a. CCF
b. Esophageal spasm
c. Renal colic
d. Cyanide poisoning

76. All are true about sitagliptin, *except*: *(AIPG 2011)*
a. It is not given alone. It is given always with sulphonylureas
b. It is given in Class II diabetics only and not in Type I
c. It can be taken with or without food
d. It causes some adverse effects

77. Cross resistance of isoniazid is seen with: *(AIPG 2011)*
a. Rifampicin
b. Ethionamide
c. Cycloserine
d. Ethambutol

78. True about aminoglycosides are all, *except*: *(AIPG 2010)*
a. Are bacteriostatic
b. Distributed only extracellularly
c. Excreted unchanged in urine
d. Teratogenic

79. Dopa and 5-hydroxy tryptophan have which of the following characteristic? *(AIPG 2010)*
a. They are acid precursor of brain amine
b. They can cross blood brain barrier
c. They control neuromodulator
d. They are metabolites of brain amine

80. Which of the following is a leukotriene antagonist? *(AIPG 2010)*
a. Montelukast b. Zileuton
c. Omalizumab d. Nedocromil

81. Filgrastim is used in treatment of: *(AIPG 2010)*
a. Anemia
b. Neutropenia
c. Malaria
d. Filarial

82. Which of the following is a long-acting beta-2 agonist? *(AIPG 2010)*
a. Albuterol
b. Salmeterol
c. Pirbuterol
d. Orciprenaline

83. All are true about glutathione, *except*: *(AIPG 2010)*
a. It is a tripeptide
b. It converts hemoglobin to methemoglobin
c. It conjugates xenobiotics
d. It scavenges free radicals and superoxide ions

84. Finasteride 5-alpha hydroxylase inhibition: *(AIPG 2010)*
a. Inhibits steroidogenic SYP-450 enzymes
b. Phosphodiesterase-5 (PDE-5) inhibitors
c. Competitive inhibitor of the enzyme 5-alpha reductase
d. All of the above

85. In hemophilia, the drug administered before a surgical procedure is: *(AIPG 2010)*
a. Vitamin K
b. Aspirin
c. Epsilon caproic acid
d. Chloral hydrate

86. The most common cause of xerostomia in adults is: *(AIPG 2010)*
a. Tranquilizers b. Antihistamines
c. Insulin d. OCP

87. One-year-old child is suffering from asthma. Treatment is: *(AIPG 2009)*
a. Short-acting beta-2 agonist
b. Inhalational steroid
c. Sustained slow-release theophylline
d. Long-acting beta-2 agonist

88. Clonidine is a: *(AIPG 2009)*
a. α-receptor agonist
b. α2-receptor agonist
c. aα2-receptor antagonist
d. bα-receptor antagonist

89. Which one of the following is not an analgesic? *(AIPG 2008)*

a. Flumazenil b. Midazolam
c. Thiopentone d. Propofol

90. Which one of the following drugs does not cause pulmonary fibrosis? *(AIPG 2008)*

a. Busulfan
b. Bleomycin
c. Methotrexate
d. Methysergide
e. None of the above

91. Aminoglycosides cause all of the following, *except*: *(AIPG 2008)*

a. Ototoxicity
b. Cardiotoxicity
c. Nephrotoxicity
d. Neuromuscular blockade

92. Which one of the following antimalarial agents is not used in prophylaxis against P. falciparum? *(AIPG 2008)*

a. Doxycycline b. Mefloquine
c. Chloroquine d. Atabrine

93. Antibiotic prophylaxis is indicated in which one of the following conditions? *(AIPG 2008)*

a. Congestive cardiac failure
b. Congenital heart diseases
c. Prosthetic valve in the heart
d. Atherosclerosis

94. Which of the following agents causes interstitial nephritis? *(AIPG 2008)*

a. Ampicillin b. Amoxicillin
c. Methicillin d. Cloxacillin

95. Melphalan is used in the treatment of: *(AIPG 2008)*

a. Multiple myeloma
b. CML
c. Renal cell carcinoma
d. Hepatic cell carcinoma

96. Which of the following is responsible for causing myocardial depression? *(AIPG 2008)*

a. Isoflurane b. Halothane
c. Desflurane d. Sevoflurane

97. All are symptoms of opiate withdrawals, *except*: *(AIPG 2006)*

a. Diarrhea b. Lacrimation
c. Mydriasis d. Excessive speech

98. Nevirapine is a: *(AIPG 2006)*

a. Protease inhibitor
b. Nucleoside reverse transcriptase inhibitor
c. Non-nucleoside reverse transcriptase inhibitor
d. Fusion inhibitor

99. Bisphosphonates act by: *(AIPG 2006)*

a. Increasing the osteoid formation
b. Increasing the mineralization of osteoid
c. Decreasing the osteoclast-mediated resorption of bone
d. Decreasing the parathyroid hormone secretion

100. A person with glaucoma should not receive: *(AIPG 2005)*

a. Sedatives
b. Vasoconstrictors
c. Antisialagogues
d. Local anesthetics

101. All of the following causes seizures, *except*: *(AIPG 2013)*

a. Tramadol b. Lamotrigine
c. Morphine d. Aspirin

102. Aspirin will cause: *(AIPG 2013)*

a. Increase in BT b. Increase in CT
c. Increase in PT d. Increase in PTT

103. True about use of midazolam over diazepam in sedation is all, *except*: *(AIPG 2012)*

a. Less thrombophlebitis due to low solubility in blood
b. More plasma binding and less toxicity
c. More potent than diazepam
d. Binds to benzodiazepine receptors with 3 to 4 times more avidity

104. A patient with bronchodilation, increased temperature, tachycardia, and constipation is seen. The diagnosis is which poisoning? *(AIPG 2012)*

a. Opiate poisoning
b. Atropine poisoning
c. Mushroom poisoning
d. Paracetamol poisoning

105. A patient developed hemolytic reaction after a dose of primaquine. Which enzyme can be deficient in the patient? *(AIPG 2012)*

a. Glucose-6-phosphatase
b. Glucose-6-phosphate dehydrogenase
c. Galactose -6-phosphate dehydrogenase
d. Galactose-6-phosphatase

106. All can cause SLE like reaction *except*: *(AIPG 2012)*
a. Hydralazine b. Penicillin
c. INH d. Sulfonamide

107. All of the following drugs are the components of the MOPP cancer chemotherapy regimen, *except*: *(COMED 2005)*
a. Procarbazine b. Vincristine
c. Mechlorethamine d. Methotrexate

108. Granulocytopenia, GI tract irritation, gingival hyperplasia, and facial hirsutism are all possible side effects of which one of the following anticonvulsant drugs? *(COMED 2005)*
a. Phenobarbital
c. Acetazolamide
b. Carbamazepine
d. Phenytoin sodium

109. Heparin acts by: *(COMED 2006)*
a. Blocking thrombin formation
b. A fibrinolytic action
c. Preventing thrombin synthesis
d. Potentiating antithrombin III activity

110. Which of the following drugs will not produce allergic reaction? *(COMED 2006)*
a. Penicillins b. Sulfonamides
c. Cetirizine d. Cephalosporins

111. Which one of the following drugs is not a reversible anticholinesterase drug? *(COMED 2006)*
a. Edrophonium b. Demecarium
c. Carbaryl d. Tacrine

112. Which one of the following drugs is not a non depolarizing competitive neuromuscular blockers? *(COMED 2006)*
a. Doxacurium b. Decamethonium
c. Rocuronium d. Mivacurium

113. D-tubocurarine blocks neuromuscular transmission by: *(COMED 2007)*
a. Blocking acetylcholine receptors
b. Preventing release of acetylcholine
c. Destroying acetylcholine
d. Inactivating acetylcholine esterase

114. Digitalis induced automaticity is enhanced by: *(COMED 2007)*
a. High K^+ levels b. High Ca^+ levels
c. High Na^+ levels d. Low K^+ levels

115. The most common cause of antibiotic related diarrhea is: *(COMED 2007)*
a. H. pylori
b. C. difficile
c. P. pneumonia
d. Shigella

116. Intramuscular route is precluded during the medication of: *(COMED 2007)*
a. Antihypertensives
b. Antidiabetics
c. Anticoagulants
d. Antifibrinolytics

117. Therapeutic uses of alpha-adrenoreceptors blockers include all of the following, *except*: *(COMED 2007)*
a. Hypertension
b. Anxiety
c. Peripheral vascular disease
d. Benign prostatic hypertrophy

118. Activation of which of the following receptors would be expected to decrease anxiety? *(COMED 2007)*
a. Nicotinic cholinergic receptors
b. Glutamate receptors
c. GABA receptors
d. Glucocorticoid receptors

119. Which one of the following does not act by increasing insulin secretion? *(COMED 2008)*
a. Glyburide
b. Repaglinide
c. Tolbutamide
d. Biguanide

120. Which of the following can be given as a single dose antimalarial for P. vivax malaria? *(COMED 2008)*
a. Atovaquone + Proguanil
b. Artemisinin
c. Quinine + Tetracycline
d. Pyrimethamine + Sulfadoxin

121. Which among the following may be used as a sedative hypnotic? *(COMED 2008)*
a. Zolmitriptan
b. Zileuton
c. Zolpidem
d. Zalcitabine

122. Which one of the following is NOT an ergot alkaloid? *(COMED 2008)*

a. Bromocriptine
b. Lysergic acid diethylamide (LSD)
c. Ketanserin
d. Methysergide

123. Which among the following is a pure antagonist of opioid receptors? *(COMED 2008)*

a. Naltrexone
b. Nalbuphine
c. Butorphanol
d. Pentazocine

124. Which among the following anti-histamines is LEAST likely to cause sedation? *(COMED 2009)*

a. Promethazine
b. Diphenhydramine
c. Hydroxyzine
d. Loratadine

125. Which among the following is NOT a pharmacological action of opioids? *(COMED 2009)*

a. Cough suppression
b. Antiemesis
c. Miosis
d. Truncal rigidity

126. Which among the following would be most effective in absence seizures? *(COMED 2009)*

a. Phenytoin
b. Carbamazepine
c. Valproic acid
d. Phenobarbitone

127. All of the given drugs may be useful in acute exacerbation of bronchial asthma, *except*: *(COMED 2010)*

a. Cromolyn sodium
b. Hydrocortisone
c. Salbutamol
d. Ipratropium

128. Inhaled GA with low blood gas partial coefficient are characterized by: *(COMED 2010)*

a. Rapid induction and quick recovery from anesthesia
b. Rapid induction and slow recovery from anesthesia
c. Slow induction and slow recovery from anesthesia
d. Slow induction and quick recovery from anesthesia

129. Which among the following is also called "peakless" insulin analog? *(COMED 2010)*

a. Insulin lispro
b. Insulin glargine
c. Insulin aspart
d. Lente insulin

130. Which among the following is not used for surface anesthesia? *(COMED 2010)*

a. Lignocaine
b. Procaine
c. Tetracaine
d. Benzocaine

131. Hyperthyroidism can be caused by: *(COMED 2010)*

a. Clonidine
b. Amiodarone
c. Hydralazine
d. Penicillamine

132. Which among the following is a cell-cycle specific anti-neoplastic drug? *(COMED 2010)*

a. Cyclophosphamide
b. Doxorubicin
c. Methotrexate
d. Cisplatin

133. The following chemical mediator is a product of arachidonic acid metabolite by cyclooxygenase pathway: *(COMED 2010)*

a. LXA4 b. LxB4
c. 5HETE d. PGH2

134. During the cell cycle, Colchicine is known to act in: *(COMED 2011)*

a. G1 phase b. S phase
c. G2 phase d. M phase

135. Which among the following is used as an Immunosuppressant? *(COMED 2011)*

a. Cyclosporine
b. Cycloserine
c. Cyclopentolate
d. Cyclizine

136. All of the given drugs are positive inotropes, *except*: *(COMED 2011)*

a. Dopamine
b. Dobutamine
c. Digoxin
d. Doxepin

137. Thyroid storm can be treated by all the following drugs, *except*: *(COMED 2012)*
a. Propylthiouracil
b. Dexamethasone
c. Propranolol
d. Aspirin

138. Ligand for peroxisome proliferation activating receptor (PPAR) receptors, a group of nuclear hormone receptors that are involved in the regulation of genes related to glucose and lipid metabolism is: *(COMED 2013)*
a. Repaglinide
b. Voglibose
c. Exenatide
d. Rosiglitazone

139. Infection with Helicobacter pylori is associated with: *(COMED 2014)*
a. Acute gastritis
b. Chronic gastritis
c. Eosinophilic gastritis
d. Recurrent esophagitis

140. Which of the following statements regarding nitroglycerin is true? *(KCET 2014)*
a. The effect is more pronounced in venous
b. High membrane penetrability
c. Poorly suited for oral administration
d. All of the above

141. Which of the following is the drug of choice for treating anaphylactic reaction? *(KCET 2014)*
a. Epinephrine 2.5 ml of 1:10,000(IV)
b. Diphenhydramine 50 to 100 mg (IM or IV)
c. Aminophylline 0.25 to 0.5 g (IV)
d. Medrol 0.5 to 1.0 mg/kg (IV)

142. Indirect sympathomimetics can: *(KCET 2013)*
a. Penetrate the blood brain barrier
b. Cause euphoria
c. Both of the above
d. None of the above

143. Progestin compound that does not alter lipid profile is: *(KCET 2012)*
a. Medroxyprogesterone
b. Norethindrone
c. G estodene
d. Levonorgestrel

144. Drug of choice for anaphylactic shock is: *(KCET 2012)*
a. Atropine
b. Dopamine
c. Adrenaline
d. Dobutamine

145. Which of these drugs can be given safely to a patient with renal disease? *(KCET 2012)*
a. Phenacetin
b. Tetracycline
c. Aminoglycoside
d. Diazepam

146. A patient presents with congestive cardiac failure with depressed ejection fraction. Which drug may be effective in reducing mortality? *(KCET 2011)*
a. Digoxin
b. Furosemide
c. Lidocaine
d. Enalapril

147. Most common adverse effect associated with phenytoin is: *(KCET 2011)*
a. Megaloblastic anemia
b. Gum hypertrophy
c. Hirsutism
d. Drowsiness

148. Morphine withdrawal is characterized by all, *except*: *(KCET 2011)*
a. Miosis
b. Yawning
c. Lacrimation
d. Diarrhea

149. Ethambutol causes: *(KCET 2011)*
a. Red discoloration of urine
b. Psychosis
c. Optic neuritis
d. Flu like s`yndrome

150. Ipratropium bromide is used for: *(KCET 2011)*
a. Renal colic
b. Organophosphorus poisoning
c. Bronchial asthma
d. Miosis

151. Drug used in treatment of malignant hyperthermia is: *(KCET 2011)*
a. Baclofen
b. Diazepam
c. Dantrolene
d. Halothane

152. Which of these drugs can be given safely to patient with renal disease? *(KCET 2011)*
a. Phenacetin
b. Tetracycline
c. Aminoglycoside
d. Diazepam

153. A 70-year-old male is admitted to the hospital with a left hemiparesis and altered consciousness. He is on aspirin 75 mg OD and glibenclamide 15 mg daily. His wife says he has been unwell for a couple of days and he has been off food. He has however, still been giving him all his medications. Which of the following tests is going to be most useful in finding an immediately reversible cause for his symptoms? *(KCET 2011)*
a. Blood glucose levels
b. CT brain
c. ECG
d. Troponin levels

154. A 50-year-old female with end stage renal disease (ESRD), develops pulmonary tuberculosis. Which one of the following drugs should be used in a reduced dose? *(KCET 2011)*
a. Rifampicin
b. Isoniazidina
c. Pyrazinamide
d. Ethambutol

155. The beneficial effect of drug neostigmine in the treatment of myasthenia gravis is due to the following action: *(KCET 2010)*
a. It produces more acetylcholine
b. It inhibits the action of cholinesterase
c. It produces more acetylcholine
d. It increases the action of cholinesterase

156. All the following drugs reduced the gastric acid secretion, *except*: *(KCET 2010)*
a. Ranitidine
b. Sucralfate
c. Misoprostol
d. Pantoprazole

157. Which of the following will cause post-operative hemorrhage? *(KCET 2010)*
a. Salicylates
b. Liver cirrhosis
c. Prolonged antibiotic administration
d. All of the above

158. Beta-blocker with additional blocking property is: *(KCET 2009)*
a. Propranolol b. Timolol
c. Metoprolol d. Labetalol

159. The most preferred acute emetic for emesis induced by anticancer drugs is: *(KCET 2009)*
a. Ondansetron
b. Metoclopramide
c. Chlorpromazine
d. Dicyclomine

160. All of the following glucocorticoids can be given by inhalation, *except*: *(KCET 2009)*
a. Dexamethasone
b. Beclomethasone
c. Budesonide
d. Fluticasone

161. Drugs exhibit first-pass metabolism are all, except one: *(KCET 2009)*
a. Morphine b. Nitroglycerine
c. Propranolol d. Salicylates

162. Which one of the following is not true of angiotensin enzyme inhibitor (ACE inhibitor)? *(KCET 2009)*
a. May cause hyperkalemia in diabetic patient
b. Contraindicated in pregnancy
c. Contraindicated in diabetic nephropathy
d. NSAID may impair its hypotensive effect

163. Most important drug used in the treatment of coronary artery disease is: *(KCET 2009)*
a. Aspirin
b. Digoxin
c. Streptokinase
d. Nifedipine

164. Which calcium channel blocker can cause excessive growth of gingival tissue? *(KCET 2009)*
a. Cyclosporine
b. Nifedipine
c. Phenytoin
d. Corticosteroid

165. Which of the following statement about azoles is false? *(KCET 2009)*
a. They are fungistatic
b. They are hepatotoxic
c. Resistance to the drug is common
d. They affect the metabolism of drugs such as cyclosporine necessitating an increase in the dosage

166. Which of the following synthetic steroids shows predominantly mineralocorticoid action? *(KCET 2008)*
a. Hydrocortisone
b. Spironolactone
c. Dexamethasone
d. Fludrocortisone

167. An anxiolytic, not interacting with GABAergic system and used in generalized anxiety is: *(KCET 2008)*
a. Alprazolam
b. Buspirone
c. Diazepam
d. Phenobarbital

168. The toxic effect of beta-receptor antagonist includes all the following, *except*: *(KCET 2008)*
a. Hypoglycemic episodes in diabetes
b. Worsening of preexisting asthma
c. Ischemic cardiac episode on abrupt discontinuation
d. Precipitate migrainic effect

169. Clopidogrel is an: *(KCET 2008)*
a. Antihypertensive
b. Antidiabetic
c. Antiplatelet
d. Anticoagulant

170. Following administration, nitrous oxide will become saturated in blood and dissolved in serum fraction of blood within: *(KCET 2008)*
a. 3–5 mins
b. 10 mins
c. 10–15 mins
d. 6–8 mins

171. Which of these is not a Glycoside? *(KCET 2008)*
a. Digoxin
b. Digitoxin
c. Ergotoxine
d. Gitoxin

172. The statement, NOT true of selective COX2 inhibitor is: *(KCET 2007)*
a. The analgesic and anti-inflammatory effects identical to that of Non-selective NSAID
b. They do not offer the cardio-protective effect
c. Safe in patients with renal insufficiency
d. Fewer incidence of gastrointestinal side effect

173. Following are the prodrugs except one:
a. Levodopa *(KCET 2006)*
b. Enalapril
c. Epinephrine
d. Proguanil

174. Which one of the following drugs is not a cardio-selective (al) beta blocker? *(KCET 2006)*
a. Metoprolol
b. Alprenolol
c. Atenolol
d. Esmolol

175. Antispastic drug used in treating trigeminal neuralgia is: *(KCET 2006)*
a. Gabapentin
b. Nortriptyline
c. Clonazepam
d. Baclofen

176. Among the following drugs which is not an immunosuppressive agent? *(KCET 2006)*
a. Levamisole
b. Azathioprine
c. Cyclosporin
d. Corticosteroid

177. Contraindications for the use of corticosteroids are the following, *except*: *(KCET 2005)*
a. Peptic ulcer
b. Herpes simplex Infection
c. Diabetes mellitus
d. Severe acute bronchial asthma

178. Malignant hyperthermia is caused by: *(KCET 2005)*
a. Atropine b. Aspirin
c. Succinylcholine d. None of the above

OTHERS

179. Drug that is used for both diabetes mellitus and diabetes insipidus is: *(MH 2009)*
a. Chlorpropamide
b. Tolbutamide
c. Acetazolamide
d. Glipizide

180. Ondansetron is: *(MH 2009)*
a. 5-HT1 antagonist
b. 5-HT2 antagonist
c. 5-HT3 antagonist
d. 5-HT 2B antagonist

181. Steroid that can be used topically for bronchial asthma is: *(MH 2009)*
a. Beclomethasone
b. Triamcinolone
c. Budesonide
d. Betamethasone

182. Antidote for overdose of heparin is: *(MH 2009)*
a. Protamine sulphate
b. Vitamin K
c. Hemodialysis
d. Activated charcoal

183. Which of the following drug inhibits cytochrome P-450? *(MH 2010)*
a. Omeprazole
b. Sucralfate
c. Pantoprazole
d. Cimetidine

184. Out of the following which is proton pump inhibitor? *(MH 2010)*
a. Cimetidine
b. Omeprazole
c. Pirenzepine
d. Doxepin

185. Drug used both in diabetes mellitus and diabetes insipidus: *(MH 2010)*
a. Insulin
b. Glyburide
c. Tolbutamide
d. Chlorpropamide

186. Drug of choice for malignant hyperthermia treatment: *(MH 2010)*
a. Succinylcholine
b. Dantrolene sodium
c. D-tubocurarine
d. Diazepam

187. Which of the following is an alpha 1 selective blocker? *(MH 2011)*
a. Phentolamine
b. Prazosin
c. Clonidine
d. Yohimbine

188. Which of the following is a Cardioselective beta blocker? *(MH 2011)*
a. Atenolol b. Pindolol
c. Timolol d. Carvedilol

189. An anti-spasmodic anti-secretory used for the treatment of peptic ulcer patient: *(MH 2011)*
a. Dicyclomine
b. Sucralfate
c. Ondansetron
d. Pirenzepine

190. Therapeutic agent that causes lysis of clot is: *(MH 2012)*
a. Urokinase
b. Hyaluronidase
c. Aspirin
d. Warfarin

191. Halothane is: *(MH 2012)*
a. 2-bromo 2-chloro 1, 1, 1 trifluoroethane
b. 2-bromo 2-iodo 1, 1, 1 trifluoroethane
c. 2- bromo 2-fluoro 1, 1, 1 trifluoroethane
d. 2-iodo 2-chloro 1, 1, 1 trifluoroethane

192. Aspirin is teratogenic and can cause: *(MH 2012)*
a. Premature closure of ductus arteriosus
b. Cleft lip and palate
c. Both of the above
d. None of the above

193. Drug of choice for moderate-to-severe Alzheimer's disease: *(MH 2012)*
a. Memantine
b. Selegiline
c. Vitamin E
d. All of the above

194. Which of the following decreases the rate of recovery from hypoglycemia if insulin is given with oral anti diabetics? *(MH 2012)*
a. Propofol
b. Atenolol
c. Propranolol
d. Acebutolol

195. All of the following drugs are unsafe in pregnancy, *except*: *(MH 2012)*
a. Hydralazine
b. Hydrochlorothiazide
c. Propranolol
d. Enalapril

196. Which of the following drug is contraindicated in patient with liver disease? *(MH 2012)*
a. Pyrazinamide b. Rifampicin
c. Streptomycin d. Ethambutol

DRUGS IMPORTANT IN DENTAL THERAPEUTICS

197. Which of the following cephalosporins do not need dose modifications even in the presence of raised levels of GFR? *(AIIMS May 2011)*
a. Cefepime
b. Cefoperazone
c. Cefotaxime
d. Cefuroxime

198. The ideal analgesic for Patient-Controlled Analgesia (PCA) should have: *(AIIMS May 2011)*
a. Early onset, average efficacy, short duration
b. Late onset, high efficacy, long duration
c. Delayed onset, intermediate efficacy, short duration
d. Early onset, high efficacy, intermediate duration

199. If bacteria were susceptible to both penicillin and erythromycin, then it would not be appropriate to treat the patient with both the antibiotics at the same time, because: *(AIIMS Nov 2010)*
a. Penicillin is inactivated by erythromycin
b. Erythromycin exerts its effects extracellularly
c. Penicillin acts only on growing bacterial population
d. Erythromycin increases beta-lactamase activity

200. Antipseudomonal cephalosporin is: *(AIIMS Nov 2010, 2009, AIPG 2011)*
a. Cefoperazone
b. Cefuroxime
c. Cefadroxil
d. Cefoxitin

201. True about penicillin G is: *(AIIMS Nov 2010, 2009)*
a. Acid resistant
b. Broad-spectrum antibiotic
c. Mainly excreted by kidney
d. Resistance to penicillinase

202. First local anesthesia to be used clinically was: *(AIIMS Nov 2010, 2009)*
a. Cocaine b. Bupivacaine
c. Procaine d. Lignocaine

203. Antanalgesia is seen with: *(AIIMS Nov 2010)*
a. Nitrous oxide b. Thiopentone
c. Etomidate d. Propofol

204. All structures are pierced in epidural anesthesia, *except*: *(AIIMS Nov 2010)*
a. Ligamentum flavum
b. Interspinous ligament
c. Supraspinous ligament
d. Posterior longitudinal ligament

205. Which of the following drug is not useful for MRSA? *(AIIMS May 2010)*
a. Cefaclor
b. Cotrimoxazole
c. Ciprofloxacin
d. Vancomycin

206. The most commonly employed route for preoperative sedation in children younger than 6 years is: *(AIIMS May 2010)*
a. Oral
b. Nasal
c. Submucosal
d. Intravenous

207. The first local anesthetic agent to be used clinically is: *(AIIMS Nov 2009)*
a. Lignocaine
b. Bupivacaine
c. Cocaine
d. Procaine

208. For propofol, all are true, *except*: *(AIIMS Nov 2009)*
a. It has a rapid recovery rate
b. It is used for induction and maintenance of anesthesia
c. It causes vomiting after use
d. It causes sedation

209. Which of the following inducing agents has analgesic property? *(AIIMS May 2009)*
a. Nitrous oxide
b. Halothane
c. Enflurane
d. Sevoflurane

210. Which drug is not used in H. pylori? *(AIIMS May 2009, AIPG 2010)*
a. Metronidazole
b. Omeprazole
c. Mosapride
d. Amoxicillin

211. Antiemetic is: *(AIIMS May 2009)*
a. Propofol
b. Thiopentone
c. Ketamine
d. Midazolam

212. Penicillin and erythromycin cannot be administrated simultaneously because: *(AIIMS Nov 2008)*
a. Penicillin is inhibited by erythromycin
b. Erythromycin acts extracellularly
c. Penicillin acts only on growing bacterial population
d. Erythromycin increases β-lactamase activity

213. False about penicillin G is that: *(AIIMS Nov 2008, AIPG 2010)*
a. It is active against gram-positive organisms
b. Gastric acid destroys it
c. It is found in intraocular and prostatic secretions
d. It is given in meningococcal meningitis

214. Which of the following is a first-generation cephalosporin? *(AIIMS May 2008, AIPG 2010)*
a. Cefotaxime
b. Cefaclor
c. Cefadroxil
d. Cefuroxime

215. Which of the following antibiotics is useful against Pseudomonas aeruginosa? *(AIIMS May 2008, AIPG 2010)*
a. Cefeperazone
b. Oxytetracycline
c. Doxycycline
d. Penicillin

216. Which of the following is a third-generation cephalosporin? *(AIIMS Nov 2006)*
a. Cefeperazone
b. Cefuroxime
c. Cefoxitin
d. Cefadroxil

217. Tetracycline inhibits protein synthesis by: *(AIIMS Nov 2006)*
a. Inhibiting initiation and causing misreading of m-RNA
b. Binding to 30S subunit and inhibits binding of aminoacyl tRNA
c. Inhibiting peptidyl transferase activity
d. Inhibiting translocation

218. Which of the following is true about Penicillin? *(AIPG 2011)*
a. Acid resistant
b. Excreted mainly through kidney
c. Anaphylaxis never occurs
d. more concentrated in prostatic secretions and intraocular fluid

219. When patient has vancomycin resistant infection, tablet to be given is: *(AIPG 2011)*
a. Ofloxacin
b. Clarithromycin
c. Cefatrime
d. Linezolid

220. Which ATT cause transient memory loss? *(AIPG 2010)*
a. Ethionamide
b. INH
c. Ethambutol
d. Pyrazinamide

221. Which of the following antibiotic acts by inhibiting cell wall synthesis? *(AIPG 2010)*
a. Cefepime
b. Aminoglycosides
c. Erythromycin
d. Doxycycline

222. Which one of the following is not an antifungal agent? *(AIPG 2009)*
a. Ketoconazole
b. Ciclopirox
c. Clofazimine
d. Undecylenic acid

223. Prolonged administration of streptomycin may result in damage to the: *(AIPG 2005)*
a. Optic nerve
b. Facial nerve
c. Auditory nerve
d. Trigeminal nerve

224. LA with adrenaline is injected in artery then it causes: *(AIPG 2013)*
a. Hypertension with tachycardia
b. Hypertension with bradycardia
c. Hypotension and tachycardia
d. Hypotension and bradycardia

225. Least transplacental transfer LA is: *(AIPG 2013)*
a. Chloroprocaine
b. Mepivacaine
c. Lidocaine
d. Bupivacaine

226. All are beta lactams, *except*: *(H.P. 2010, AIPG 2013)*
a. Carbapenem
b. Imipenem
c. Cephalosporin
d. Sulfonamides

227. General anesthetic unsafe for children in dentistry is: *(AIPG 2013)*
a. Halothane b. Sevoflurane
c. Isoflurane d. Desflurane

228. Over usage of isoniazid leads to deficiency of: *(AIPG 2012)*
a. Pyridoxine b. Thiamine
c. Pantothenic acid d. Niacin

229. Clavulanic acid is given in combination with amoxicillin in order to: *(COMED 2005)*
a. Reduce the risk of allergic reactions
b. Prolong half life of amoxicillin
c. Reduces the severity of diarrhea
d. Extend amoxicillin's antibacterial spectrum

230. Which of the following drugs is not a long acting local anesthetic? *(COMED 2006)*
a. Tetracaine
b. Procaine
c. Bupivacaine
d. Dibucaine

231. Which among the following class of antibiotics are relatively safer to use in patients on warfarin therapy? *(COMED 2007)*
a. Cephalosporins b. Imidazoles
c. Penicillins d. Macrolides

232. Which drug can be safely used in lactating mothers? *(COMED 2007)*
a. Ampicillin
b. Chloramphenicol
c. Ciprofloxacin
d. Erythromycin

233. Which of the following commonly used topical antiseptic has antifungal activity? *(COMED 2008)*
a. Povidone iodine b. Cetrimide
c. Chlorhexidine d. Alcohol

234. Combination of ampicillin and gentamicin is an example of: *(COMED 2009)*
a. Indifference b. Synergism
c. Antagonism d. Bacterial symbiosis

235. All of the following are adverse effects of long term corticosteroids, *except*: *(COMED 2009)*
a. Hypoglycemia b. Psychosis
c. Peptic ulcers d. Osteoporosis

236. Which among the following antibiotics should be avoided in pregnancy? *(COMED 2009)*
a. Erythromycin b. Tetracycline
c. Cephalexin d. Amoxicillin

237. Pseudomembranous colitis is an adverse effect following the long term use of: *(COMED 2010)*
a. Tetracycline
b. Clindamycin
c. Metronidazole
d. Erythromycin

238. The drug which has an abusive effect when alcohol is ingested is? *(COMED 2010)*
a. Penicillin-G
b. Clindamycin
c. Metronidazole
d. Doxycycline

239. Among the drugs given below, which is LEAST likely to be implicated in drug induced hepatitis? *(COMED 2011)*
a. Isoniazid
b. Streptomycin
c. Rifampicin
d. Pyrazinamide

240. Which of the following drugs given below does not act by protease inhibition? *(COMED 2011)*
a. Ritonavir
b. Saquinavir
c. Nelfinavir
d. Zanamivir

241. Which among the following is the drug of choice for Clostridium Difficile-induced colitis? *(COMED 2011)*
a. Gentamicin
b. Ciprofloxacin
c. Metronidazole
d. Linezolid

242. Which of the following anti-tubercular drug is bacteriostatic? *(COMED 2011)*
a. INH
b. Ethambutol
c. Pyrazinamide
d. Streptomycin

243. Which among the following drugs is NOT used orally? *(COMED 2011)*
a. Quinidine
b. Verapamil
c. Lignocaine
d. Phenytoin

244. Which among the following anti HIV drugs is also used to treat viral hepatitis B? *(COMED 2012)*
a. Enfuvirtide
b. Lamivudine
c. Efavirenz
d. Ritonavir

245. Which among the following antibiotics should be avoided in pregnancy? *(COMED 2012)*
a. Erythromycin
b. Tetracycline
c. Cephalexin
d. Amoxicillin

246. All of the following drugs may be effective against methicillin resistant staphylococcus aureus (MRSA), *except*: *(COMED 2012)*
a. Vancomycin
b. Streptogramins
c. Imipenem
d. Linezolid

247. Epinephrine should not be combined with one of the following local anesthetic: *(COMED 2014)*
a. Cocaine
b. Lignocaine
c. Procaine
d. Mepivacaine

248. To minimize the effects of diffusion hypoxia during N_2O- O_2 analgesia, the patient should be oxygenated for: *(COMED 2014)*
a. 30 seconds to 1 minute
b. 3 to 5 minutes
c. 10 to 30 minutes
d. 30 to 45 minutes

249. DOTS is a community based treatment and care strategy for: *(COMED 2014)*
a. Filaria
b. Leprosy
c. Tuberculosis
d. Malaria

250. Long acting local anesthetic agent: *(COMED 2014)*
a. Lidocaine
b. Prilocaine
c. Bupivacaine
d. Procaine

251. Mechanism of action of beta lactam antibiotics would be: *(KCET 2013)*
a. Inhibition of bacterial protein synthesis by binding to subunits of bacterial ribosomes
b. Inhibition of cell wall peptidoglycan synthesis by competitive inhibition of transpeptidases
c. Reduced drug causes breaks n DNA strands
d. Inhibition of DNA synthesis by inhibiting DNA dependent RNA polymerase

252. Which of the following anesthetic agent is frequently used for conscious sedation? *(KCET 2013)*
a. Nitrous oxide and oxygen
b. Chloral hydrate
c. Diazepam
d. Ether

253. Which of the following is false about conscious sedation? *(KCET 2013)*
a. Patients retains ability maintain a patent airway
b. Responds appropriately to physical stimulation
c. Responds appropriately to verbal commands
d. None of the above

254. All of the following are inhalational anesthetic agents *except*: *(KCET 2013)*
a. Halothane
b. Ketamine
c. Enflurane
d. Isoflurane

255. The incidence of allergy to penicillin among various population ranges from: *(KCET 2012)*
a. 1–10%
b. 10–20%
c. 20–30%
d. 30–40%

256. Redman syndrome is side effect of: *(KCET 2012)*
a. Rifampicin
b. Vancomycin
c. Chloramphenicol
d. Tetracycline

257. Tetracyclines act by: *(KCET 2012)*
a. Inhibiting the binding of aminoacyl tRNA to the ribosomal complex
b. Inhibiting peptidyl transferase
c. Inactivating elongation factors
d. Causing misreading of mRNA

258. An antibiotic that achieves high concentration in hard tissue, because of its molecular size is? *(KCET 2011)*
a. Ceftum b. Ciprotloxacin
c. Clindamycin d. Erythromycin

259. Each of the following statement is correct about Metronidazole except that it: *(KCET 2011)*
a. Is a broad spectrum antiprotozoal drug
b. Is active against bacteroides and clostridium
c. Is an effective alternative for infection caused by aerobic gram positive cocci
d. May cause peripheral neuropathy on prolonged use

260. All of the following statements about ketorolac are incorrect, *except*: *(KCET 2011)*
a. An effective analgesic for mild to moderate post operative dental pain
b. Like morphine it interacts with opioid receptors
c. Administered only be intravenous route
d. Safe even in chronic use

261. Penicillin exerts its effect on bacteria by interfering with: *(KCET 2011)*
a. Cellular respiration
b. Cellular oxidation
c. Cell wall synthesis
d. Cellular division

262. Optic neuritis is the side effect of: *(KCET 2006)*
a. Rifampicin b. Isoniazid
c. Ethambutol d. Pyrazinamide

263. Which one of the following drugs is not an amino-glycoside? *(KCET 2006)*
a. Kanamycin
b. Tobramycin
c. Erythromycin
d. Streptomycin

264. 'Second gas effect' is exerted by the following gas when co-administered with halothane: *(KCET 2006)*
a. Nitrogen b. Cyclopropane
c. Nitrous oxide d. Helium

265. Amphotericin B is not effective in the following fungal disease: *(KCET 2006)*
a. Cryptococcosis
b. Histoplasmosis
c. Blastomycosis
d. Dermatophytosis

266. Dissociative anesthesia is produced by: *(KCET 2005, AIPG 2010)*
a. Lignocaine
b. Nitrous Oxide
c. Diazepam
d. Ketamine

267. Drug with poor peripheral anti-inflammatory activity is: *(MH 2009)*
a. Indomethacin b. Paracetamol
c. Aspirin d. Piroxicam

268. Clavulanic acid is known for: *(MH 2010)*
a. Sucide bag
b. Antibacterial activity
c. Progressive sucide inhibitor
d. DNA gyrase inhibitor

269. Ototoxicity is seen with: *(MH 2010)*
a. Chloramphenicol
b. Streptomycin
c. Clindamycin
d. Cefixime

270. Mechanism of action of Tetracycline's: *(MH 2011)*
a. Binds to 30s ribosome
b. Binds to 50s ribosome
c. Freeze initiation
d. Prevents transfer of the peptide chain

271. Mechanism of action of sulfonamides is by: *(MH 2011)*
a. Allosteric inhibition
b. Competitive inhibition
c. Non competitive inhibition
d. None of the above

272. Anti-hypertensive of choice during pregnancy is: *(MH 2011)*
a. Propoanolol b. Pindolol
c. Carvedilol d. Methyldopa

Answers with Explanations

GENERAL PHARMACOLOGICAL PRINCIPLES

1. Ans. (c) Salmeterol *Ref: KDT, 6th ed. p 23, 24*

Prodrug	*Active form*
• Levodopa	Dopamine
• Enalapril	Enalaprilat
• Alpha methyldopa	Alpha-methylnorepinephrine
• Dipivefrine	Epinephrine
• Sulindac	Sulphide metabolites
• Hydrazide, MAO inhibitors	Hydrazine derivatives
• Proguanil	Proguanil triazine
• Prednisone	Prednisolone
• Bacampicillin	Ampicillin
• Sulfasalazine	5-aminosalicylate
• Cyclophosphamide	Aldophosphamide, phosphoramide mustard, acrolein
• Fluorouracil	Fluorouridine monophosphate
• Acyclovir	Acyclovir triphosphate
• Mercaptopurine	Methylmercaptopurine ribonucleotide

- Enalapril maleate is a prodrug that is hydrolyzed by esterases in the liver to produce the active dicarboxylic acid, enalaprilat.
- Enalaprilat is a highly potent inhibitor of ACE.

2. Ans. (a) The volume of distribution *Ref: KDT, 6th ed. p 18, 19*

- A loading dose is an initial higher dose of a drug that may be given at the beginning of a course of treatment before dropping down to a lower maintenance dose.
- A loading dose is most useful for drugs that are eliminated from the body relatively slowly, i.e. have a long systemic half-life. Such drugs need only a low maintenance dose in order to keep the amount of the drug in the body at the appropriate therapeutic level, but this also means that, without an initial higher dose, it would take a long time for the amount of the drug in the body to reach that level.
- The volume of distribution (V_D) It is defined as the distribution of a medication between plasma and the rest of the body after oral or parenteral dosing. It is defined as the theoretical volume in which the total amount of drug would need to be uniformly distributed to produce the desired blood concentration of a drug.
- The volume of distribution is given by the following equation:

$$V_D = \frac{\text{Total amount of drug in the body}}{\text{Drug blood plasma concentration}}$$

Also remember

- The volume of distribution (V_D) is the proportionality factor that relates the total amount of drug in the body to the concentration in the plasma (Cp); if a loading dose is to achieve the target concentration, Tc
- Loading dose = $V_D \times Tc$
- Maintenance dose = $Cl \times Cp$

  Where Cp = target plasma concentration and Cl = clearance. In patients with impaired renal or hepatic function, the loading dose remains the same, although the maintenance dose is decreased.

Factors governing the volume of drug distribution:

- Lipid: water partition coefficient of the drug
- pKa value of the drug
- Degree of plasma protein binding
- Affinity for different tissues
- Fat: lean body mass ratio, which can vary with age, sex, obesity, etc.
- Diseases like CHF, uremia and cirrhosis.

3. Ans. (c) Low oral bioavailability always and necessarily means poor absorption *Ref: KDT, 6th ed. p 18*

- Bioavailability refers to the extent and rate at which the active moiety (drug or metabolite) enters systemic circulation, thereby accessing the site of action.
- Bioavailability of a drug is largely determined by the properties of the dosage form, which depend partly on its design and manufacture.
- Differences in bioavailability among formulations of a given drug can have clinical significance; thus, knowing whether drug formulations are equivalent is essential.

Causes of low bioavailability:

Orally administered drugs must pass through the intestinal wall and then the portal circulation to the liver; both are common sites of first-pass metabolism (metabolism that occurs before a drug reaches systemic circulation). Thus, many drugs may be metabolized before adequate plasma concentrations are reached. Low bioavailability is most common with oral dosage forms of poorly water-soluble, slowly absorbed drugs.

- The area under the blood concentration time curve (AUC) is a common measure of the extent of bioavailability for a drug given by a particular route.

Also remember

Luminal effect: Absorption of drug affected by other concurrently ingested drug by the formation of insoluble complexes, e.g. tetracycline with iron preparation.

Gut wall effect: Drug can alter absorption by either altering motility (anticholinergics, TCA, opioids and metoclopramide) or causing mucosal damage (neomycin, methotrexate and vinblastine).

4. Ans. (a) High affinity *Ref: KDT, 6th ed. p 42*

- Affinity is defined as the ability of the drug to bind with the receptor and it is determined by the interaction of the drug with the molecular structure of the receptor.
- Affinity relates the drug concentration to the functional receptor occupancy.
- Affinity will enable drug to be used in low concentration process.
- The drug with more affinity will occupy more receptor at given concentration and same for the reverse (vice versa).

5. Ans. (a) Context half life *Ref: Essential Equations for Anesthesia by Edward T Gilbert Kawai, 1st ed. p 68*

The context-sensitive half-time is the time required for blood or plasma concentrations of a drug to decrease by 50% after discontinuation of drug administration. The context-sensitive half-time often cannot be predicted by the elimination half-life (a measure of the time needed for actual drug metabolism or elimination) because it also depends on drug distribution. It is a useful concept because it helps explain the duration of action of a drug given by infusion after stopping the infusion. It reflects several pharmacokinetic principles:

- First, as any drug is infused into the body more of the drug will deposit in the body's tissues (i.e., accumulate) the longer the duration of infusion (or 'context' as it is known) until the body's tissues are completely saturated. Once the drug infusion is stopped this stored drug will then redistribute back into the blood and maintain its effects.
- Second, every drug accumulates to differing extents, which is largely influenced by the physicochemical properties of the drug.

- Third, drugs are removed from the blood through two major mechanisms:
  - **Distribution**: Where the drug moves from the blood into the tissues, e.g. fat.
  - **Excretion**: Where the drug is either metabolized (e.g. by the liver) or excreted from the body unchanged (e.g. in urine). Whether or not the metabolites are active is also important.

6. Ans. (b) Body weight of child *Ref: KDT, 6th ed. p 42*

- Most drugs approved for use in children have recommended pediatric doses, generally stated as milligrams per kilogram or per pound.
- Doses based on surface area are also more likely to be adequate.
- The pediatric dose should never exceed the adult dose.
- Calculations of dosage based on age or weight are conservative and tend to underestimate the required dose.

7. Ans. (d) 1 gm of drug A produces more effect that can't be produced by 1 gm drug B so drug A is more efficacious than drug B *Ref: http://aimmds.org/forum/viewtopic.php?f=12 and t = 944*

Potency and Efficacy

Potency is the amount of a drug needed for it to have the maximum effect. So, when one drug produce more effect with less dose its potency is better. So option (A) is true.

Efficacy is the maximum effect that a drug can produce. It does not depend on dosage.
If both drugs do bring about same effect with different dosages, their efficacy is same, e.g: 1 gm drug A and 4 gm of drug B bring about same effect.

However if one drug does not bring about same effect with its maximum tolerated dose, then its less efficacious, e.g. 1 gm of drug A brings about more effect than 3 gm of drug B (max tolerated dose) then A is more efficacious than drug B. So option (B) and (C) are also true.

Option D says 1 gm of both drugs do not bring same effect. 1 gm of drug A brings more effect than 1 gm of drug B. This does not decide whether one is less efficacious or not. So this is false.

8. Ans. (a) Synergism *Ref: KDT, 6th ed. p 702, 703*

Several naturally occurring and semisynthetic compounds can inhibit many of the β-lactamase enzymes produced by penicillin-resistant bacteria. When used in combination with broad-spectrum penicillins, there is a notable synergistic effect because the active penicillin is protected from enzymatic hydrolysis and thus is fully active against a wide variety of previously resistant bacteria. Examples of this chemotherapeutic approach include clavulanate-potentiated amoxicillin and ticarcillin as well as sulbactam-potentiated ampicillin and tazobactam-potentiated piperacillin.

Clavulanate-potentiated amoxicillin is an excellent example of such a synergistic association.

9. Ans. (a) Thalidomide *Ref: KDT, 6th ed. p 85*

Human teratogenic drugs

Drug	*Abnormality*
Thalidomide	Phocomelia, multiple defects
Carbamazepine	Neural tube defects
Androgens	Virilization; limb oesophageal, cardiac defect
Progestins	Virilization of female fetus
Stilboestrol	Vaginal carcinoma in teenage female offspring
Phenytoin	Hypoplastic phalanges, cleft lip and palate, microcephaly
Valproate sod.	Spina bifida
ACE inhibitor	Hypoplasia of organs, foetal loss

10. Ans. (a) At bed time *Ref: Medical Terminology - By Marjorie Canfield Willis - 1st ed. p 76*

Most common abbreviations used in prescription:

- Rx: Take
- Tab: tablet
- Cap: capsule
- Top: topically
- po: by mouth
- prn: as method
- hs: at bedtime
- pc: after meal
- ac: before meal
- q4h: every four hour
- qd: every day
- bid: twice a day
- tid: thrice in a day
- qid: four times in a day
- disp#60: dispense 60 pills

11. Ans. (b) Maximal intensity of response that can be reduced by the drug *Ref: Essentials of Pharmacology for Dentistry, KD Tripathi, 2nd ed. p 44*

- Drug efficacy refers to the maximal response that can be produced by the drug.
- Efficacy is the more decisive factor in the choice of drug.
- Drug potency refers to the amount of drug requires to produce a certain response.

12. Ans. (b) Acute alcohol ingestion *Ref: Introduction to Drug Metabolism by G. Gordon Gibson p 236.*

- Drug metabolism can be induced by cigarette smoking or by consuming charcoal boiled meat as they have been shown to be potent inducess of drug metabolism polycyclic hydrocarbons [e.g. benzo (a) pyrene)
- At time of exposure to insecticides, our enzyme system respond by increasing in amount and in activity, i.e. they become induced
- Acute alcohol ingestion can inhibits drug metabolism, thus increasing serum drug concentration.

13. Ans. (d) Ed50 *Ref: Lange, 11th ed. p 32*

- Median effective dose (ED50)—dose at which 50% of individuals exhibit quantal effect.
- Median toxic dose (TD50)—dose required to produce a particular toxic effect in 50% of animals.
- Median lethal dose (LD50)—If toxic effect is death of animal.

14. Ans. (c) Ioliosyneratic effect *Ref: KDT, 6th ed. p 81*

- A drug create an unpredictable effect and shows unique feature of the individuals termed as Idiosyncratic effect.
- Their effects are not found in majority of subjects.
- Barbiturates cause excitement and mental confusion in some individuals.
- Quinine/quinidine cause cramps, diarrhea, purpura, asthma and vascular collapse in some patients.
- Chloramphenicol produces nondose related serious aplastic anemia in rare individuals.

15. Ans. (c) Bioassay *Ref: Bronwen Bryant- 3rd ed. p 97*

- The design of bioassays usually involves comparison of two preparations, a standard and an unknown, by testing many concentrations of each on the same model and constructing log dose response curves.
- If the substances act by similar mechanisms, the curves will be roughly parallel in the mid sections and so the potency ratio can be determined, allowing the strength of the unknown compared to the known standard.

16. Ans. (b) Sequential blockade in folate metabolism *Ref: Essentials of Pharmacology for Dentistry, KD Tripathi, 2nd ed. p 46*

Synergism

When two drugs used together result in a response that is greater than their individual responses (1 + 1 > 2), it is called drug synergism.

Examples

1. Sulfamethoxazole + trimethoprim: It is the synergistic drug due to sequential blockade in folate metabolism as their t ½ is similar. There is the inhibition of two different enzyme in the same metabolic pathway.
2. Levodopa + Carbidopa—Here the carbidopa prevents peripheral conversion of LD.
3. Addition of adrenaline to lignocaine increases duration of action of lignocaine. This is known as 'time synergism'.

17. Ans. (d) Suspensions can be administered *Ref: KDT, 6th ed. p 10*

Intravenous (iv)

- The drugs are injected into the superficial vein and reaches to the blood stream.
- If extravasation occurs, It may cause thrombophlebitis of the injected vein and necrosis of adjoining tissue.
- Only aqueous solution (not suspension) can be injected i.v. and are no depot preparation for this route.
- Bioavailability is 100%.

18. Ans. (a) Weight *Ref: Tripathi's, 1st ed. p 49*

- The safer way of calculating drug dosage in children is based on weight.

19. Ans. (d) Bypasses first-pass metabolism *Ref: K.D. Tripathi, 6th ed. p 7*

The chief advantage of sublingual route is that liver is bypassed and drugs with high first pass metabolism can be absorbed directly into systemic circulation. Drugs given sublingually are GTN, buprenorphine, desaminooxytocin.

20. Ans. (c) Hyper sensitivity *Ref: KDT, 6th ed. p 81*

- Super sensitivity—increased response of a drug.
- Hyper-sensitivity—immune mediated qualitative drug intolerance.
- Idiosyncrasy—it defined as the genetically determined abnormal reaction of a chemical.

21. Ans. (a) Safety of a drug *Ref: KD Tripathi, 6th ed. p 55*

Therapeutic index

The therapeutic index (TI) of a drug is the ratio of the dose that produces toxicity to the dose that produces a clinically desired or effective response in a population of individuals.

Therapeutic index = TD50/ED50

Where,

TD50 = the drug dose that produces a toxic effect in half the population, and

ED50 = the drug dose that produces a therapeutic or desired response in half the population.

The therapeutic index is a measure of a drug's safety because a larger value indicates a wide margin between doses that are effective and doses that are toxic.

22. Ans. (d) Dentine desensitizers *Ref: Short Textbook of Pharmacology for Dental and Allied Health Sciences by Padmaja Udaykumar p 390*

Obtundents are the dentin desensitizing agents.

It acts by three process:

- Paralyzing the sensory nerve
- Precipitating agents
- Destruction of nervous tissue.

23. Ans. (a) Affinity with intrinsic activity *Ref: K.D. Tripathi, 5th ed. p 37*

Agonist—has both affinity and maximal intrinsic activity
- Adrenaline, histamine, morphine

Competitive antagonist has affinity but no intrinsic activity
- Propranolol, atropine, naloxone

Partial agonist has affinity and submaximal intrinsic activity.
- Nalorphine, dichloroisoproterenol

Inverse agonist has affinity but intrinsic activity with minus sign
- DMDC

24. Ans. (c) Pharmacovigilance *Ref: KDT, 6th ed. p 79*

- Pharmacovigilance has been defined by the WHO as the 'science and activities relating in the detection, assessment, understanding and prevention of adverse effect or any other drug related problems.'
- It has an important role in rational use of medicines, as it provides the basis for assessing safety of medicines.

SYSTEMIC PHARMACOLOGY

25. Ans. (d) Osteomalacia *Ref: Essentials of Medical Pharmacology, KD Tripathi, 6th ed. p 407*

Valproic acid (VPA, Valproate)
- It is an acidic chemical compound, has found clinical use as an anticonvulsant and mood-stabilizing drug, primarily in the treatment of epilepsy, bipolar disorder and prevention of migraine headaches.
- It has also been successfully given intravenously to treat status epilepticus.
- The most common adverse effects of valproic acid are digestive complaints like diarrhea, nausea, vomiting and indigestion; vision problems like seeing double or lazy eye; hormonal disturbances (increased testosterone production in females and menstrual irregularities), hair loss, memory problems, weight gain, infections, low platelet count (which can make one bleed more easily), infection, dizziness, drowsiness, tremor and headache.
- Less common, yet serious side effects include liver damage, brittle bones (becomes far more common with long-term use), polycystic ovaries, movement disorders (which may be irreversible like tardive dyskinesia), psychiatric/neurologic disturbances like hallucinations, anxiety and confusion; swollen pancreas, low body temperature and potentially life-threatening blood abnormalities.

26. Ans. (a) Strontium ranelate *Ref: Osteoporosis - Diagnosis, Prevention, Therapy by Reiner Barti, 1st ed. p 152*

- Strontium ranelate, a new orally active drug which is soon to be released in this country, has been shown in animal and in-vitro studies to have a dual action it decreases bone resorption and stimulates bone formation.
- Strontium ranelate also stimulates the proliferation of pre-osteoblasts and its differentiation into mature osteoblasts. The net result is an increase in bone volume, mass, diameter and strength.
- Strontium ranelate appears to be safe and well tolerated.

27. Ans. (d) Acarbose *Ref: Essentials of Medical Pharmacology, KD Tripathi, 6th ed. p 270*

Acarbose:
- Acarbose must be taken at the beginning of a meal to be fully effective.
- Acarbose works only when taken at the beginning of a meal. If it is not taken at that time, it should not be taken until the next meal.
- Acarbose does not cause hypoglycemia when given alone. However, low blood sugar can occur if you take acarbose with another type of diabetes medicine, delay or miss a meal, drunk alcohol etc.
- Acarbose tablets are an oral alpha-glucosidase inhibitor for use in the management of type 2 diabetes mellitus.
- Acarbose is an oligosaccharide which is obtained from fermentation processes of a microorganism.

28. Ans. (b) Acts by inducing transcription of gene responsible for carbohydrate and lipid catabolism in the absence of insulin *Ref: Essentials of Medical Pharmacology, KD Tripathi, 6th ed. p 269*

- Peroxisomes proliferator- activated receptor (PPAR)-γ is a member of the nuclear receptor superfamily that appears to have an important role in insulin sensitivity.
- The thiaszolidinediones such as troglitazone and pioglitazone, are high affinity ligands for PPAR-γ that can be used clinically as insulin sensitizing agents.
- It modulates the transcription of the insulin-sensitive genes concerned with the control of glucose and lipid metabolism in the muscle, adipose tissue and the liver.
- It means that at least some insulin produced by the pancreas must be present for pioglitazone to work upon the cell receptors. Hence it can be used only in type II diabetes. Hence option (b) is not true.

29. Ans. (a) Glucoregulatory actions similar to GLP-1 *Ref: Essentials of Medical Pharmacology, KD Tripathi, 6th ed. p 273*

Exenatide:

- Exenatide is the first member of a new class of agents.
- Exenatide exhibits many of the same glucoregulatory properties of GLP-1
- Exenatide may also preserve β-cell function.
- Exenatide enhanced glucose dependent insulin secretion, suppressed the inappropriate glucagon secretion seen in T2 DM in a glucose dependent manner and slowed gastric emptying.

30. Ans. (d) It causes less neurotoxicity than cyclophosphamide *Ref: Essentials of Medical Pharmacology, KD Tripathi, 6th ed. p 273*

- The most frequently used alkylating agents are the nitrogen mustards such as mechlorethamine (the original 'nitrogen mustard'), cyclophosphamide, ifosfamide, melphalan, and chlorambucil.
- Ifosfamide is a structural isomer of cyclophosphamide that is used particularly in the treatment of testicular tumors and sarcomas.
- The increased production of chloroacetaldehyde has been implicated in the neurotoxicity of ifosfamide, and may also contribute to the greater renal and bladder toxicity of ifosfamide.
- Metabolism of ifosfamide by CPY.
- Renal damage following chemotherapy with ifosfamide is attributed to the metabolic activation of the drug and the generation of chloroacetaldehyde (CAA).

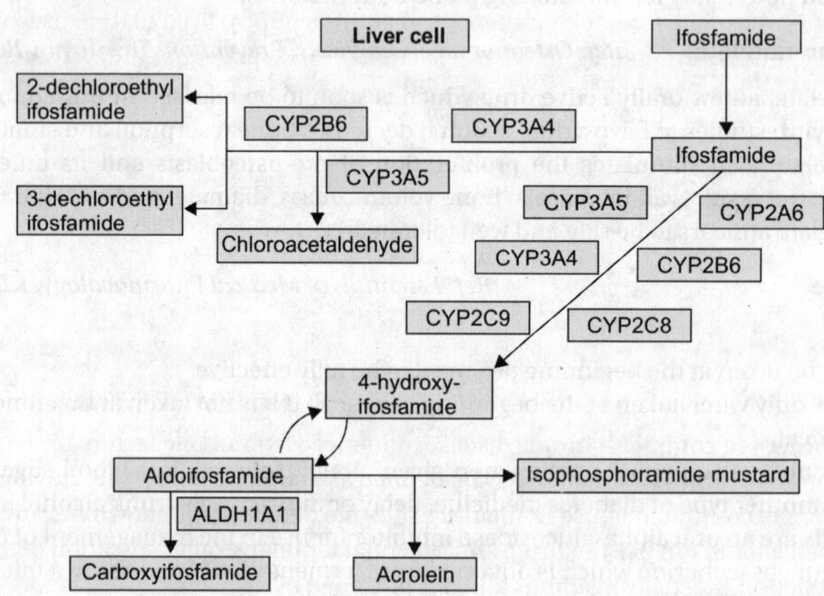

31. Ans. (d) Impotence *Ref: Essentials of Medical Pharmacology, KD Tripathi, 6th ed. p 566, 567*

- The most commonly cited diuretics associated with sexual difficulties include thiazide diuretics, chlorthalidone, acetazolamide, indapamide and spironolactone.
- Side effects of thiazide diuretics includes stomach upset, dizziness on standing (due to low blood pressure), impotence (often reversible on stopping treatment) and skin sensitivity to sunlight.

32. Ans. (a) Protamine sulphate *Ref: Essentials of Medical Pharmacology, KD Tripathi, 6th ed. p 564*

- Protamine sulphate is used to stop the effects of a medicine called heparin.
- Heparin is used to prevent blood from clotting but too much heparin can increase the risks of serious bleeding.
- Protamine sulphate reduces the risk of serious bleeding by stopping the effect of heparin on the blood.
- Bleeding is the chief sign of heparin overdosage.
- Each mg of protamine sulfate neutralizes approximately 100 USP heparin units.

33. Ans. (d) Barbiturate *Ref: A Practical Approach to Anesthesia for Emergency Surgery, 1st ed. p 416*

Barbiturates

Barbiturates have four major actions on the CNS: (1) hypnosis, (2) depression of cerebral metabolic rate (CMR), (3) reduction of cerebral blood flow (CBF) due to increased cerebral vascular resistance, and (4) anticonvulsant activity. These properties make barbiturates, particularly thiopental, the most commonly used induction agents in neuroanesthesia. Barbiturates produce dose-dependent decreases in CMR and CBF until the EEG becomes isoelectric. At that point, maximum reductions of nearly 50% are observed; additional barbiturate does not further reduce metabolic rate. Unlike isoflurane, however, barbiturates reduce metabolic rate uniformly throughout the brain. CMR is depressed slightly more than CBF, such that metabolic supply exceeds metabolic demand (as long as CPP is maintained). Because barbiturate- induced cerebral vasoconstriction occurs only in normal areas, these agents tend to redistribute blood flow from normal to ischemic areas in the brain (Robin Hood, or reverse steal phenomenon). The cerebral vasculature in ischemic areas remains maximally dilated and is unaffected by the barbiturate because of ischemic vasomotor paralysis.

34. Ans. (d) Thioridazine *Ref: Essentials of Medical Pharmacology, KD Tripathi, 6th ed. p 425*

- The atypical antipsychotics (AAP) [also known as second generation antipsychotics (SGAs)] are a group of antipsychotic drugs (antipsychotic drugs in general are also known as major tranquilizers and neuroleptics although the latter is usually reserved for the typical antipsychotics) used to treat psychiatric conditions.
- Atypical antipsychotics exert their main effect by acting on 5H2 receptors. They have weak D2 blocking activity.
- They have no extra pyramidal effects.
- It includes:
  - Clozapine
  - Olanzapine
  - Quetiapine
  - Aripiprazole
  - Ziprasidone
  - Risperidone.

35. Ans. (d) Methadone *Ref: Essentials of Medical Pharmacology, KD Tripathi, 6th ed. p 460*

- Opioid use disorder is a complex, chronic disease influenced by multiple factors.
- Common symptoms of opioid addiction may be defined as a compulsion to 'use', craving of the individual's drug (or drugs) of choice, continued abuse of the drugs despite perceived or known negative consequences, loss of control of the behavior to not use the drug, and potential for relapse after cessation of the drugs of choice.
- The onset of addiction is usually insidious and not preceded by any single event before diagnosis or treatment.

- Common risks for addiction may include self-medication to treat health-related disorders, such as somatic or neuropathic pain, anxiety, or depression.
- Both methadone and buprenorphine have US Food and Drug Administration approval for the treatment of opioid addiction.
- Opioid withdrawal reactions are very uncomfortable but are not life threatening. Symptoms usually start within 12 hours of last heroin usage and within 30 hours of last methadone exposure.

36. Ans. (e) None of the above *Ref: Essentials of Medical Pharmacology, KD Tripathi, 6th ed. p 85*

Here, all of the given drugs can cause the congenital malformation when used in a pregnant women so the answer is none of the above:
- Phenytoin—Hypoplastic phalanges, cleft lip/cleft palate, Microcephaly.
- Phenobarbitone—Various malformation.
- Carbamazepine—Neural tube defects.
- Valproate—Spina bifida and neural tube defects.

37. Ans. (c) Valproate *Ref: Essentials of Medical Pharmacology, KD Tripathi, 6th ed. p 408*

	1st line drug	*2nd line drug*	*3rd line drug*
Absence seizure (Petit Mal)	Ethosuximide • Zarontin • Emeside Valporic acid	Lamotrigine Clonazepam	Phenobarbital Primidone Tiagabine Topiramate Felbamate

38. Ans. (a) Phosphodiesterase (PDE-5) *Ref: Molecules and Medicine by E.J. Corey*

Sildenafil
- It is the first selective type 5 phosphodiester inhibitor (PDE-5).
- It is used as a potent therapy for erectile dysfunction.
- It increases cGMP levels and improves erectile function.

Remember
- Phosphodiester inhibitor 5 are—Sildenafil, tadalafil, Vardenafil.
- Phosphodiester inhibitor 4 are—Cilomilast, Roflumilast.

39. Ans. (d) Metoclopramide *Ref: Essentials of Medical Pharmacology, KD Tripathi, 6th ed. p 25*

Drugs metabolized by acetylation: N-acetyl conjugation:
- All the drugs having amino or hydrazine residues, e.g. sulfonamide, isoniazid (INH), hydralazine, PAS, clonazepam, procainamide, histamine.
- Metoclopramide does not undergo acetylation.

40. Ans. (c) Cyclizine *Ref: Essentials of Medical Pharmacology, KD Tripathi, 6th ed. p 156*

- Second-generation histamine H1 receptor antagonists (antihistamines) have been developed to reduce or eliminate the sedation and anticholinergic adverse effects that occur with older H1 receptor antagonists.
- Second-generation antihistamines are 'Red FLAME':
  - Rupatadine
  - Fexofenadine
  - Loratadine/levocetirizine/levocabastine
  - Acrivastine/azelastine

- Mizolastine
- Ebastine

Cyclizine is a mild sedative antihistamine drug used to treat nausea, vomiting and dizziness associated with motion sickness, vertigo and post-operatively following administration of general anesthesia and opioids.

41. Ans. (a) Flumazenil *Ref: Essentials of Medical Pharmacology, KD Tripathi, 6th ed. p 399*

- Flumazenil is a recently discovered pharmacologic antagonist of the CNS effects of benzodiazepines.
- It acts by binding CNS benzodiazepine receptors and competitively blocking benzodiazepine activation of inhibitory GABAergic synapses.
- Flumazenil is of benefit in patients who become excessively drowsy after benzodiazepines are used for either diagnostic or therapeutic procedures.
- It has been used as an antidote in the treatment of benzodiazepine overdoses. GAB_A It reverses the effects of benzodiazepines by competitive inhibition at the benzodiazepine binding site on the $GABA_A$ receptor. There are many complications that must be taken into consideration when used in the acute care setting.

42. Ans. (a) Calcium channel blockers (CCBs) *Ref: Essentials of Medical Pharmacology, KD Tripathi, 6th ed. p 528, 543*

- In dialysis patients, renal clearance is largely replaced by dialysate clearance.
- If, for a particular drug, nonrenal clearance is large compared to renal clearance, the total clearance of that drug is not affected by hemodialysis.
- In this case, the clearance of all except CCBs is dependent mainly on renal.

43. Ans. (c) Sevoflurane *Ref: KDT, 6th ed. p 373, 374*

Sevoflurane:

- It is a polyfluoridated anesthetic drug.
- Solubility of this drug in blood as well as tissue and potency are more than desflurane but less than isoflurane.
- Recovery is rapid, smooth and clear headed.
- Orientation, cognitive and motor function are regained quickly.
- It does not cause sympathetic stimulation and airway irritation.
- As it is degraded by sodalime, it is not used in closed circuit.

44. Ans. (c) Methadone *Ref: Essentials of Medical Pharmacology, KD Tripathi, 6th ed. p 460*

Refer Ans no. 35

45. Ans. (a) Difficulty in maintaining an adequate oxygen concentration *Ref: Essentials of Medical Pharmacology, KD Tripathi, 6th ed. p 371*

Nitrous oxide

- Insoluble in blood as well as other tissues.
- Second gas effect: The rapid uptake of N_2O from alveolar gas serves to concentrate coadministered halogenated anesthetics. It speeds the induction of anesthesia.
- The N_2O gas can diffuse from the blood to the alveoli, and hence diluting O_2 in the lungs during discontinuation of N_2O administration. In order to avoid hypoxia 100% O_2 should be administered when N_2O is discontinued.
- Nitrous oxide is not a flammable or explosive gas.
- So, nitrous oxide is always used as a mixture of 70% N_2O and 25 to 30% O_2 and 0.2 + 2% of another potent anesthetic.

46. Ans. (b) Tranexamic acid *Ref: Essentials of Medical Pharmacology, KD Tripathi, 6th ed. p 608*

- Antifibrinolytics, such as aminocaproic acid (ε-aminocaproic acid) and tranexamic acid are used as inhibitors of fibrinolysis.

- These lysine-like drugs interfere with the formation of the fibrinolytic enzyme plasmin from its precursor plasminogen by plasminogen activators which takes place mainly in lysine rich areas on the surface of fibrin.
- These drugs block the binding sites of the enzymes or plasminogen respectively and thus stop plasmin formation.
- They are used in menorrhagia and bleeding tendency due to various causes. Their application may be beneficial in patients with hyperfibrinolysis because they arrest bleeding rapidly if the other components of the hemostatic system are not severely affected. This may help to avoid the use of blood products such as fresh frozen plasma (FFP) with its associated risks of infections or anaphylactic reactions.

47. Ans. (b) Piroxicam *Ref: Essentials of Medical Pharmacology, KD Tripathi, 6th ed. p 194*

- Piroxicam is a non-steroidal anti-inflammatory drug (NSAID) of the oxicam class used to relieve the symptoms of rheumatoid and osteoarthritis, primary dysmenorrhea, postoperative pain; and act as an analgesic, especially where there is an inflammatory component.
- Piroxicam works by preventing the establishment of a certain type of body chemicals which contributes to inflammation, pain, stiffness, tenderness and swelling.
- Piroxicam is an NSAID and, as such, is a non-selective COX inhibitor possessing both analgesic and antipyretic properties. It undergoes enterohepatic circulation.
- Piroxicam use can result in gastrointestinal toxicity, tinnitus, dizziness, headache, rash, and pruritus. The most severe adverse reactions are peptic ulceration, gastrointestinal bleeding, and severe skin reactions including Stevens-Johnson syndrome and toxic epidermal necrolysis. Approximately 30% of all patients receiving daily doses of 20 mg of piroxicam experience side effects.

48. Ans. (a) It is a heterogeneous mixture of sulphates and polypeptides *Ref: Essentials of Medical Pharmacology, KD Tripathi, 6th ed. p 597*

Heparin

- The anticoagulant effect of heparin is directly related to its activation of antithrombin III, which rapidly inactivates the thrombin and Factor Xa in the coagulation process.
- Unfractionate heparin (UFH) or IV heparin potentiates the action of antithrombin III and this rapidly inactivates thrombin and Factor Xa in the coagulation process.
- IV heparin also inactivates factor IX, X, XI, XII and plasmin. It also inhibit the conversion of fibrinogen to fibrin.
- Excessive bleeding associated with heparin can be reversed by protamine sulphate; 1 mg protamine sulphate neutralizes 100 units of heparin.
- Heparin-induced thrombocytopenia (HIT) is an important and life-threatening complication of heparin therapy. Heparin-induced thrombocytopenia (HIT) must be suspected when a patient has a fall in thrombocyte count while receiving heparin.

49. Ans. (b) Phenazocine *Ref: Essentials of Medical Pharmacology, KD Tripathi, 6th ed. p 641*

- Phenazocine is an opioid analgesic drug, which is related to pentazocine and has a similar profile of effects.
- Effects of phenazocine include analgesia and euphoria, also may include dysphoria and hallucinations at high doses, most likely due to action at κ-opioid and σ receptors.
- Phenazocine appears to be a much stronger analgesic with fewer side effects than pentazocine.
- It causes emesis and is not used as an antiemetic.

50. Ans. (a) MAO inhibitors *Ref: Essentials of Medical Pharmacology, KD Tripathi, 6th ed. p 121*

- Epinephrine is ultimately metabolized by COMT and MAO and 3-methoxy-4-hydroxy-mandelic acid.
- Tricyclic antidepressants and MAO inhibitors will potentiate the effects of epinephrine.
- Some of MAO (Monoamine oxidase) inhibitors are:
  - Isocarboxazid.
  - Phenezine.
  - Nialamide.
  - Tranylcypromine.

51. Ans. (c) Hypoprothrombinemia *Ref: Essentials of Medical Pharmacology, KD Tripathi, 6th ed. p 189*

- Aspirin also known as acetylsalicylic acid (ASA), is a salicylate drug, often used as an analgesic to relieve minor aches and pains, as an antipyretic to reduce fever, and as an anti-inflammatory medication.
- Aspirin also has an antiplatelet effect by inhibiting the production of thromboxane, which under normal circumstances binds platelet molecules together to create a patch over damaged walls of blood vessels.
- Blood and lymphatic system disorders: Aspirin increases bleeding time, decreases platelet adhesiveness and, in large doses, may cause hypoprothrombinemia. It may also cause other blood disorders including anemia, thrombocytopenia, aplastic anemia, pancytopenia. Hemolytic anemia can occur in patients with glucose 6-phosphate dehydrogenase deficiency (G6PD).

52. Ans. (a) In higher quantities, it is relatively safer than other hypnotics *Ref: KDT, 6th ed. p 393*

Benzodiazepines

- Possess high therapeutic index. Even 20 hypnotic doses of BZD will not endanger life.
- Even respiration and cardiovascular functions are not affected by the hypnotic dose of BZD.
- It does not alter disposition of other drugs by microsomal enzyme induction.

53. Ans. (b) Verrill's sign *Ref: Principles of Oral Surgery by GV Gillbe p 44*

- When the patient lying in supine position, slow IV dose of diazepam is injected at a rate of 2 mg/30 secs. This correct dose will cause the drooping of the upper lid (ptosis) occurs and this half covers the pupil. This is known as Verrill's sign.
- 20 ml is the maximum dose for adult.

54. Ans. (c) Glucocorticoids *Ref: Essentials of Medical Pharmacology KD Tripathi, 6th ed. p 286*

Drugs causing hyperglycemia are:

- Asparaginase
- Niacin
- Oral contraceptives
- Phenytoin
- Thiazides
- Pentamidine
- Chlorthalidone
- Diazoxide
- Encainide
- Ethacrynic acid
- Furosemide
- Glucocorticoids
- HIV protease inhibitors.

55. Ans. (b) Phenytoin *Ref: Essentials of Medical Pharmacology, KD Tripathi, 6th ed. p 405*

Drug interaction with folic acid:

- Aminosalicylic acid—Decreased serum folate levels.
- Corticosteroid—Increased folic acid requirement.
- Oral contraceptive—Increased risk of folate deficiency.
- Phenytoin—Decreased folic acid level, thus leading to folic acid deficiency.
- Pyrimethamine—A folic acid antagonist.
- Sulfonamide—Decreased absorption of folic acid.
- Triamterene—Decreased utilization of folic acid.
- Trimethoprim—Decreased utilization of folic acid.

56. Ans. (a) Propofol *Ref: Essentials of Medical Pharmacology, KD Tripathi, 6th ed. p 370*

General anesthetics that can be given intravenously are divided into:

- Fast-acting agents: thiopentone, methohexitone, propofol and etomidate.
- Slow-acting agents: benzodiazepines, ketamine and fentanyl.

Propofol

- Propofol is a short-acting, intravenously administered hypnotic/amnestic agent.
- Its uses include the induction and maintenance of general anesthesia, sedation for mechanically ventilated adults, and procedural sedation.
- Propofol is also commonly used in veterinary medicine.

57. Ans. (a) Black cylinder with white shoulder *Ref: Modern Trends in Planning and Designing of Hospitals: Principles and Practice by Kant Gupta, p 187*

- Oxygen (O_2): Black body with white shoulder
- Nitrous oxide (N_2O): French blue
- Cyclopropane: Orange
- Carbon dioxide (CO_2): Grey
- Halothane bottle: Amber (purple red)
- Ethylene bottle: Red
- Helium (He): Brown
- Air: Grey body with black-and-white shoulder.

58. Ans. (b) β-rays *Ref: Essentials of Medical Pharmacology, KD Tripathi, 6th ed. p 252*

- I_{131} emits X rays as well as β-rays.
- X rays used in traces while beta particle for destructive action on thyroid cells.
- I_{131} has a half-life of 8 days.
- The most common indication of I_{131} is hyperthyroidism due to Graves' disease or toxic nodular goiter.
- Radioactive iodine (I_{131}) treatment of choice after 25 years of age and if congestive heart failure, angina or any other contraindication to surgery is present.

59. Ans. (c) Duration of action of aspirin is primarily related to the pharmacokinetic clearance of the drug from the body *Ref: Essentials of Medical Pharmacology, KD Tripathi, 6th ed. p 185*

Aspirin is part of a group of medications called nonsteroidal anti-inflammatory drugs (NSAIDs), but differs from most other NSAIDs in the mechanism of action. Though it, and others with similar structure called the salicylates, have similar effects (antipyretic, anti-inflammatory, analgesic) to the other NSAIDs and inhibit the same enzyme cyclooxygenase (COX). Aspirin does so in an irreversible manner and, unlike others, affects more the COX-1 variant than the COX-2 variant of the enzyme.

- Due to inhibition of cyclo-oxygenase, prostaglandin synthesis is reduced.
- The ability of platelets to be inhibited by low doses of aspirin is related to the presystemic inhibition of the cyclooxygenase in the portal circulation before the aspirin is deacetylated to salicylate in the liver.
- Other NSAIDs are competitive and reversible inhibitor of COX, the return of activity depends on their dissociation.

60. Ans. (a) Carbamazepine *Ref: Essentials of Medical Pharmacology, KD Tripathi, 6th ed. p 406, 407*

Trigeminal neuralgia is among the most common facial pain syndromes and has also been called tic douloureux. While it may be caused by compressive blood vessels, tumors and vascular malformations, its basic pathophysiology (or pain mechanism) remains unknown. What is known is the sudden, stabbing, excruciating pain that it produces, which lasts only a few seconds and affects the face. In most cases, treatment for trigeminal neuralgia begins with anticonvulsant drug therapy that seeks to suppress the transmission of impulses by the trigeminal nerve. Carbamazepine is the first drug of choice. It should be started at low doses. A small number of patients do not respond well or at all to anticonvulsants and should be put on a drug called baclofen. Although baclofen has fewer and less serious side effects than carbamazepine, it too can lose its effectiveness over time. Additionally, it can cause drowsiness, dizziness and fatigue. Baclofen may provide enhanced relief when used in combination with an anticonvulsant.

61. Ans. (a) Prazosin *Ref: Essentials of Medical Pharmacology, KD Tripathi, 6th ed. p 132*

- The first-dose phenomenon is a sudden and severe fall in blood pressure that can occur when changing from a lying to a standing position the first time that an alpha blocker drug is used or when resuming the drug after many months off.
- This postural hypotension usually happens shortly after the first dose is absorbed into the blood and can result in syncope (fainting).
- Syncope occurs in approximately 1% of patients given an initial dose of 2 mg prazosin or greater. This adverse effect is self-limiting and in most cases does not recur after the initial period of therapy or during subsequent dose titration.
- The alpha blocker prazosin (Minipress) is most notorious for producing a first dose phenomenon. Other drugs of the same family, doxazosin (Cardura) and terazosin (Hytrin), can also cause this phenomenon, though less frequently.
- The cause is not clear. It occurs more commonly in patients who are salt and fluid volume depleted (as happens due to the use of diuretics), or were using beta blockers. Diuretics and beta blockers are frequently used to control hypertension. For this reason, treatment with prazosin (Minipress) should always be initiated with a low dose and should be taken at bedtime to avoid standing position.

62. Ans. (c) Tamsulosin *Ref: KDT 6th ed. p 135*

Tamsulosin

- A uroselective α 1A/ 1D blocker.
- Doesn't have any significant action on BP and HR. So, it does not cause postural hypotension.
- Dizziness, retrograde ejaculation are the only ADR.
- Dosage is 0.2 to 2 mg.
- Tamsulosin have fewer vascular side effects because of relative α 1A/1D sensitivity.

63. Ans. (d) Prazosin *Ref: Essentials of Medical Pharmacology, KD Tripathi, 6th ed. p 132*

Classification of Alpha Adrenergic Blocking agents:

- Nonequilibrium Type
  Beta-Haloalkylamines Phenoxybenzamine
- Equilibrium type (Competitive)
- Nonselective

Ergot Alkaloids Ergotamine, Ergotoxine

Hydrogenerated ergot alkaloid Dihydroergotamine, Dihydroergotoxine Imidazolines- Tolazoline, Phentolamine

Miscellaneous-Chloropromazine Ketanserin

- Alpha-1 selective Prazosin, Terazosin, Doxazosin
- Alpha-2 selective Yohimbine

64. Ans. (a) OCP *Ref: KDT, 6th ed. p 603*

- Oral contraceptive pills decrease the efficiency of Warfarin and INR as well.
- Oral contraceptive also increases the level of clotting factor in blood.

65. Ans. (d) Used safely in asthmatics *Ref: Pharmacology for Nursing Care by Richard A. Lehne, 8th ed. p 504*

ACE inhibitor

- Almost all administered orally except enalapril.
- All have prolonged half lives so they administered as once or twice in a day except captopril which is given 2 to 3 times in a day.
- All ACE inhibitors are prodrugs except lisinopril.
- All ACE inhibitors are excreted by the kidneys.
- They do not interfere with the cardiovascular reflex.
- ACE inhibitors used safely in asthmatics.

66. Ans. (d) Lisinopril *Ref: Essentials of Medical Pharmacology, KD Tripathi, 6th ed. p 485*

Refer Ans 65 from the same section and Ans No. 1 from general pharmacy also.

67. Ans. (c) Causes vomiting after use *Ref: Essentials of Medical Pharmacology, KD Tripathi, 6th ed. p 375*

- Commonly used as a parenteral anesthetic agent.
- It possess rapid post anesthetic recovery with clear-headedness.
- It does not cause nausea and vomiting.
- Propofol can cause respiratory depression and results apnea.

68. Ans. (a) Propofol *Ref: Essentials of Medical Pharmacology, KD Tripathi, 6th ed. p 375*

Refer Ans No. 67

69. Ans. (c) Ketamine *Ref: Essentials of Medical Pharmacology, KD Tripathi, 6th ed. p 376*

Ketamine

- It is an intravenous anesthetic agent.
- It is a dissociative anesthesia, i.e. it produce profound analgesia, immobility, amnesia with light sleep and feeling of dissociation from ones own body and the surroundings.
- It is the only intravenous agent with bronchodilator activity.
- Ketamine has a bronchodilator action that may be mediated either via an increase in blood catecholamines or by its direct smooth muscle relaxant effect.

70. Ans. (a) Buspirone *Ref: Essentials of Medical Pharmacology, KD Tripathi, 6th ed. p 451*

- Buspirone is a medication that is used for the treatment of anxiety.
- Its mechanism of action is not clearly understood but may involve effects on neurotransmitters, chemicals that nerves use to communicate with one another.
- Serotonin and dopamine are two of these neurotransmitters.
- Buspirone may work by stimulating serotonin type 1A receptors on nerves, thereby altering the chemical messages that nerves receive.
- It also has minor effects on dopamine receptors, but this does not contribute much to its action. Unlike medications for anxiety of the benzodiazepine class, for example, diazepam (Valium), lorazepam (Ativan), alprazolam (Xanax), and clonazepam (Klonopin).
- Buspirone does not cause sedation.

71. Ans. (a) Rifampicin induce the metabolism of contraceptive *Ref: Essentials of Medical Pharmacology, KD Tripathi, 6th ed. p 741*

Cytochrome P-450 enzyme induction by rifampicin (and phenytoin) also increases the metabolism of oestrogens so that the efficacy of the combined oral contraceptive pill is reduced. Break through bleeding or contraceptive failure may occur.

72. Ans. (b) Cisapride *Ref: KDT, 6th ed. p 645*

Cisapride

- It is least efficient antiemetic property.
- It lacks D2 receptor antagonism.
- It is a prokinetic drug.
- It does not possess anti-dopaminergic side effect, but abdominal cramps and diarrhea can occur.

73. Ans. (b) Remifentanil *Ref: Handbook of Anesthesia by John 5th ed. p 692*

- Remifentanil is a unique μ opioid agonist that has a rapid blood brain equilibration.
- Remifentanil crosses the placenta.
- Neonates can metabolizes remifentanil.
- It is a contraindicated for epidural and intrathecal use, due to glycine in the formulation.
- Remifentanil is only available for parenteral administration either as a bolus or infusion.
- Remifentanil is synergistic with thiopental and propofol.

74. Ans. (c) Inhibited protein synthesis of virus *Ref: Fundamentals of Human Physiology by Lauralee Sherwood 4th ed. p 317*

Interferons (IFNs) are proteins made and released by host cells in response to the presence of pathogens such as viruses, bacteria, parasites or tumor cells. They allow for communication between cells to trigger the protective defenses of the immune system that eradicate pathogens or tumors. Interferon inhibited protein synthesis destroys both the virus and infected host cells. In addition, interferons induce production of hundreds of other proteins collectively known as interferon-stimulated genes (ISGs) that have roles in combating viruses.

75. Ans. (c) Renal colic *Ref: Essentials of Medical Pharmacology, KD Tripathi, 6th ed. p 527*

Uses of Nitrates are:

- Angina pectoris
- Acute coronary syndromes
- Myocardial infarction
- Chronic heart failure and acute LVF
- Biliary colic
- Esophageal spasm
- Cyanide poisoning.

76. Ans. (a) It is not given alone. It is given always with sulphonylureas *Ref: KDT, 6th ed. p 273*

- Sitagliptin can be used as triple therapy with metformin and a sulphonylurea.
- Only sitagliptin is licenced for triple therapy.
- It can be given in initial therapy as an adjunct to exercise and diet or it can be given monotherapy or combination therapy with oral antidiabetics or insulin.
- It is given in Type II diabetes only. It is not used in Type I doses.
- It can be given with or without food.

77. Ans. (b) Ethionamide *Ref:Tuberculosis: Diagnosis and Treatment by Timothy DMcHugh p 117*

InhA have cross resistance with isoniazid and ethionamide.

78. Ans. (a) Are bacteriostatic *Ref: Essentials of Medical Pharmacology, KD Tripathi, 6th ed. p 718*

Aminoglycosides are potent bactericidal antibiotics that act by creating fissures in the outer membrane of the bacterial cell. They are particularly active against aerobic, gram-negative bacteria and act synergistically against certain gram-positive organisms. Gentamicin is the most commonly used aminoglycoside, but amikacin may be particularly effective against resistant organisms. Aminoglycosides are used in the treatment of severe infections of the abdomen and urinary tract, as well as bacteremia and endocarditis. They are also used for prophylaxis, especially against endocarditis. Resistance is rare but increasing in frequency. Avoiding prolonged use, volume depletion and concomitant administration of other potentially nephrotoxic agents decreases the risk of toxicity.

79. Ans. (a) They are acid precursor of brain amine *Ref: Essentials of Medical Pharmacology, KD Tripathi, 6th ed. p 165*

In all probability the amines occur in the brain as the result of local formation by decarboxylation of their amino acid precursor, 3-4 dihydroxyphenylalanine (DOPA) and 5-hydroxytryptophan (HTP). Enzyme performing this decarboxylating reaction are present in the brain and in the case of HTP, the distribution of the decarboxylase parallels of serotonin. DOPA is the acid precursor of dopamine and 5-HTP is the acid precursor of 5-hydroxyl tryptamine.

80. Ans. (a) Montelukast *Ref: Essentials of Medical Pharmacology, KD Tripathi, 6th ed. p 217*

Montelukast is a leukotriene receptor antagonist (LTRA) used for the maintenance treatment of asthma and to relieve symptoms of seasonal allergies. It is usually administered orally once a day. Montelukast is a CysLT1 antagonist; it blocks the action of leukotriene D4 and secondary ligands LTC4 and LTE4 on the cysteinyl leukotriene receptor, CysLT1 in the lungs and bronchial tubes by binding to it. This reduces the bronchoconstriction otherwise caused by the leukotriene and results in less inflammation. Because of its method of operation, it is not useful for the treatment of acute asthma attacks. Again because of its very specific mechanism of action, it does not interact with other asthma medications such as theophylline. Another leukotriene receptor antagonist is zafirlukast (Accolate), taken twice daily. Zileuton (Zyflo), an asthma drug taken four times per day, blocks leukotriene synthesis by inhibiting 5-lipoxygenase, an enzyme of the eicosanoid synthesis pathway.

81. Ans. (b) Neutropenia *Ref: Pharmacology by George 4th ed. p 172*

Filgrastim is used to prevent or treat neutropenia, a condition in which the number of white blood cells is very low. Neutropenia can result from cancer chemotherapy or other conditions. Patients with neutropenia are more prone to serious infections. Filgrastim promotes white blood cell growth, which helps the immune system fight infections. Filgrastim is also sometimes used to stimulate the bone marrow to make more young white blood cells (stem cells) and release them into the bloodstream, where they can be collected for a peripheral blood stem cell transplant (PBSCT).

82. Ans. (b) Salmeterol *Ref: Essentials of Medical Pharmacology, KD Tripathi, 6th ed. p 216, 217*

- Salmeterol is a long-acting beta2-adrenergic receptor agonist drug that is prescribed for the treatment of asthma and chronic obstructive pulmonary disease (COPD).
- It is available as a dry powder inhaler that releases a powdered form of the drug. Before 2008, it was also available as a metered-dose inhaler (MDI). It is still available as a MDI in the UK as of 2013.
- It is a long-acting beta-adrenoceptor agonist (LABA), usually prescribed only for severe persistent asthma following previous treatment with a short-acting beta agonist such as salbutamol and is prescribed concurrently with a corticosteroid, such as beclometasone.
- The primary noticeable difference of salmeterol to salbutamol is that the duration of action lasts approximately 12 hours in comparison with 46 hours of salbutamol.

83. Ans. (b) It converts hemoglobin to methemoglobin *Ref: Internet*

- Glutathione (GSH) is an important antioxidant in plants, animals, fungi and some bacteria and archaea, preventing damage to important cellular components caused by reactive oxygen species such as free radicals and peroxides. It is a tripeptide with a gamma peptide linkage between the carboxyl group of the glutamate side-chain and the amine group of cysteine (which is attached by normal peptide linkage to a glycine).

- The enzymes of xenobiotic metabolism, particularly the glutathione S-transferases are important in agriculture, since they may produce resistance to pesticides and herbicides.
- Antioxidants (e.g. glutathione, arginine, citrulline, taurine, creatine, selenium, zinc, vitamin E, vitamin C, vitamin A, and tea polyphenols) and antioxidant enzymes (e.g. superoxide dismutase, catalase, glutathione reductase, and glutathione peroxidases) exert synergistic actions in scavenging free radicals.

84. Ans. (c) Competitive inhibitor of the enzyme 5-alpha reductase *Ref: Essentials of Medical Pharmacology, KD Tripathi, 6th ed. p 294*

Finasteride is a competitive and specific inhibitor of Type II 5 alpha-reductase, an intracellular enzyme that converts the androgen testosterone into dihydrotestosterone (DHT). Two distinct isozymes of 5 alpha-reductase are found in mice, rats, monkeys, and humans: Type I and II. Each of these isozymes is differentially expressed in tissues and developmental stages. In humans, Type I 5 alpha-reductase is predominant in the sebaceous glands of most regions of skin, including scalp and liver. Type I 5 alpha- reductase is responsible for approximately one-third of circulating DHT. The Type II 5 alpha-reductase isozyme is primarily found in prostate, seminal vesicles, epididymides and hair follicles as well as liver, and is responsible for two-thirds of circulating DHT Finasteride has been used successfully in the treatment of hirsutism in women and early male pattern baldness in men (1 mg/day).

85. Ans (c) Epsilon caproic acid *Ref: Essentials of Medical Pharmacology, KD Tripathi, 6th ed. p 608*

Aminocaproic acid is used to treat excessive postoperative bleeding, especially after procedures in which a great amount of bleeding is expected, such as cardiac surgery. It can be given orally or intravenously. A meta-analysis found that lysine analogs like aminocaproic acid significantly reduced blood loss in patients undergoing coronary artery bypass grafting. Aminocaproic acid can also be used to treat the overdose and/or toxic effects of the thrombolytic pharmacologic agents tissue plasminogen activator (commonly known as tPA) and streptokinase.

86. Ans. (b) Antihistames *Ref: Essentials of Medical Pharmacology, KD Tripathi, 6th ed. p 157*

Xerostomia is defined as dry mouth resulting from reduced or absent saliva flow. Xerostomia is not a disease, but it may be a symptom of various medical conditions, a side effect of a radiation to the head and neck, or a side effect of a wide variety of medications. It may or may not be associated with decreased salivary gland function. Xerostomia is often a contributing factor for both minor and serious health problems. It can affect nutrition and dental, as well as psychological health. Some common problems associated with xerostomia include a constant sore throat, burning sensation, difficulty in speaking and swallowing, hoarseness and/or dry nasal passages. More than 400 commonly used drugs can cause xerostomia. The main culprits are antihistamines, antidepressants, anticholinergics, anorexiants, antihypertensives, antipsychotics, anti-Parkinson agents, diuretics and sedatives.

87. Ans. (a) Short-acting beta-2 agonist *Ref: Asthma in Children by Dr. O.P. Jaggi, 2nd ed. p 124*

Short-acting beta2-agonists are bronchodilators. They relax the muscles lining the airways that carry air to the lungs (bronchial tubes) within 5 minutes. This increases airflow and makes it easier to breathe. They relieve asthma symptoms for 3 to 6 hours. They do not control inflammation.

Short-acting beta-2-agonists are used to:

- Provide quick relief of symptoms during asthma attacks.
- Prevent asthma symptoms before exercise.
- Treat symptoms in intermittent asthma.

One-year-old child suffering from asthma should be treated with inhaled Short-acting beta2-agonists.

88. Ans. (b) α2-receptor agonist *Ref: Essentials of Medical Pharmacology, KD Tripathi, 6th ed. p 546*

- Clonidine is an α2-adrenergic receptor agonist prescribed historically as a centrally acting antihypertensive agent.
- Several clinical studies demonstrated the efficacy of intrathecal clonidine for the treatment of postoperative, neuropathic or cancer-associated pain.

89. Ans. (d) Propofol *Ref: Essentials of Medical Pharmacology, KD Tripathi, 6th ed. p 375*

- Propofol is a short-acting, intravenously administered hypnotic/amnestic agent.
- Its uses include the induction and maintenance of general anesthesia, sedation for mechanically ventilated adults, and procedural sedation.
- Propofol is not considered an analgesic, so opioids such as fentanyl may be combined with propofol to alleviate pain.
- Propofol has been referred to as milk of amnesia (a play on words of milk of magnesia), because of the milk-like appearance of its intravenous preparation.

90. Ans. (e) None of the above *Ref: Drug induced diseases fibrosis by James E. Tisdale, 2nd ed. p 360*

Drugs causing pulmonary fibrosis:

- Bleomycin
- Apomorphine
- Mitomycin
- Amiodarone
- Busulfan
- Chlorambucil
- Cyclophosphamide
- Methysergide vinblastine
- Methotrexate

91. Ans. (b) Cardiotoxicity *Ref: Essentials of Medical Pharmacology, KD Tripathi, 6th ed. p 721*

- Ototoxicity, neuromuscular blockade, and nephrotoxicity are reported most frequently due to the use of aminoglycosides.
- These effects may vary with the aminoglycoside and dose or interval used, but all members of the group are potentially toxic.
- Nephrotoxicity is of major concern and may result in renal failure due to acute tubular necrosis with secondary interstitial damage.

92. Ans. (d) Atabrine *Ref: Essentials of Medical Pharmacology, KD Tripathi, 6th ed. p 784*

Drugs currently used for prophylaxis:

- Mefloquine
- Chloroquine
- Proguanil
- Pyrimethamine
- Doxycycline
- Hydroxychloroquine

93. Ans. (c) Prosthetic valve in the heart *Ref: Heart Disease in Pregnancy by Celia Oakley, 2nd ed. p 117*

The current recommendations cite that use of preventive antibiotics before certain dental procedures might be useful for patients with:

- Artificial heart valves
- A history of infective endocarditis
- A cardiac transplant that develops a heart valve problem
- The following congenital (present from birth) heart conditions:
  - Unrepaired or incompletely repaired cyanotic congenital heart disease, including those with palliative shunts and conduits

- A completely repaired congenital heart defect with prosthetic material or device, whether placed by surgery or by catheter intervention, during the first six months after the procedure
- Any repaired congenital heart defect with residual defect at the site or adjacent to the site of a prosthetic patch or a prosthetic device.

94. Ans. (c) Methicillin *Ref: Essentials of Medical Pharmacology, KD Tripathi, 6th ed. p 700*

- Methicillin can cause interstitial nephritis.
- Oxacillin and nafcillin can cause hepatitis.
- Nafcillin can cause neutropenia.

95. Ans. (a) Multiple myeloma *Ref: Essentials of Medical Pharmacology, KD Tripathi, 6th ed. p 832*

The treatment of multiple myeloma (MM) is complex because of rapid advances in stem cell transplantation, medications, and better supportive care, which have led to improved survival for patients with multiple myeloma over the past thirty years.

The main options for therapy include:

- Standard chemotherapy drugs such as melphalan (Alkeran), cyclophosphamide (Cytoxan), Doxorubicin (Adriamycin) and liposomal doxorubicin (Doxil)
- Newer drugs such as thalidomide (Thalomid), lenalidomide (Revlimid), bortezomib (Velcade), carfilzomib (Kyprolis), and pomalidomide (Pomalyst)
- Corticosteroids such as prednisone or dexamethasone (Decadron)
- Stem cell (bone marrow) transplantation.

96. Ans. (b) Halothane *Ref: Essentials of Medical Pharmacology, KD Tripathi, 6th ed. p 372*

- Halothane cause direct depression of myocardial muscle by reducing intracellular Ca^+ concentration.
- Heart rate is reduced by vagal stimulation and direct depression of SA nodal automacity.
- It tends to sensitize heart to arrhythmogenic action of adrenaline.

97. Ans. (d) Excessive speech *Ref: Essentials of Medical Pharmacology, KD Tripathi, 6th ed. p 457*

Symptoms of opiate withdrawals are:

- Lacrimation
- Sweating
- Yawning
- Anxiety
- Fear
- Goose flesh
- Mydriasis
- Tremors
- Insomnia
- Abdominal colic
- Diarrhea
- Dehydration
- Rise in BP
- Palpitation and rapid weight loss.

98. Ans. (c) Non-nucleoside reverse transcriptase inhibitor *Ref: Essentials of Medical Pharmacology, KD Tripathi, 6th ed. p 767*

- Nevirapine (NVP) is a non-nucleoside reverse transcriptase inhibitor widely used in combination with other antiretroviral agents for the treatment of human immunodeficiency virus disease.
- NVP has been shown to be well tolerated in both adult and pediatric patients.

99. Ans. (c) Decreasing the osteoclast-mediated resorption of bone *Ref: Essentials of Medical Pharmacology, KD Tripathi, 6th ed. p 334*

Bisphosphonates are potent inhibitors of osteoclast-mediated bone resorption. They are widely used in the management of osteoporosis and other diseases of high bone turnover. Bisphosphonates' pronounced affinity for bone, but not other tissues, makes them the ideal candidates for treatment of bone diseases. Bisphosphonates have been shown to increase bone mineral density (BMD), reduce bone turnover markers, and reduce the risk of osteoporotic fractures. They are currently the most important and effective class of drugs for metabolic bone disorders such as osteoporosis, Paget's disease, and osteogenesis imperfect.

100. Ans. (c) Antisialagogues *Ref: Essentials of Medical Pharmacology, KD Tripathi, 6th ed. p 114*

Person with glaucoma especially angle-closure glaucoma should not receive antisialagogues because it have antimuscarinic properties.

101. Ans. (b) Lamotrigine *Ref: Essentials of Medical Pharmacology, KD Tripathi, 6th ed. p 409*

- Lamotrigine is an anticonvulsant drug used in the treatment of epilepsy and bipolar disorder.
- It is a drug used to treat the seizure. It is used to treat focal seizures, primary and secondary tonic-clonic seizures, and seizures associated with Lennox-Gastaut syndrome.
- Lamotrigine prescribing information has a black box warning about life-threatening skin reactions, including Stevens-Johnson syndrome, DRESS syndrome and toxic epidermal necrolysis.
- Other side-effects include loss of balance or coordination, double vision, crossed eyes, pupil constriction, blurred vision, dizziness and lack of coordination, drowsiness, insomnia, anxiety, vivid dreams or nightmares, dry mouth.

102. Ans. (a) Increase in BT *Ref: Essentials of Medical Pharmacology, KD Tripathi, 6th ed. p 609*

Conditions in which Bleeding time is prolonged.

- Disseminated intravascular coagulation
- Von willebrand disease
- Aspirin therapy
- Thrombocytopenia
- Uremia
- Liver failure (end stage)
- Congenital fibrinogenemia
- Bernard-Soulier syndrome
- Glanzmann's thrombasthenia

103. Ans. (b) More plasma binding and less toxicity *Ref: Essentials of Medical Pharmacology, KD Tripathi, 6th ed. p 376*

- It is 3-4 times more potent than diazepam.
- It is water soluble in nature and non irritating to vein.
- It has twice the affinity for the benzodiazepine receptors.
- It is less plasma protein bound in compare to diazepam.
- The incidence of injection pain and thrombophlebitis is low.

104. Ans. (b) Atropine poisoning *Ref: Essentials of Medical Pharmacology, KD Tripathi, 6th ed. p 107-110*

Atropine can cause:

- Bronchodilation
- Rise in body temperature

- Tachycardia
- Constipation
- Lower BP
- Relaxation of smooth muscle.

105. Ans. (b) Glucose-6-phosphate dehydrogenase *Ref: Professional Guide to Disease by Lippincott, 10th ed., p 908*

- Primaquine (or primaquine phosphate) is a medication used in the treatment of malaria and Pneumocystis pneumonia.
- Common side effects of primaquine administration include nausea, vomiting and stomach cramps. Other known adverse effects that occasionally occur are headache, visual disturbances and intense itching.
- The most dangerous adverse effect of primaquine is hemolysis in patients with G6PD deficiency (Africans or Caucasians of Mediterranean descent). This is associated with the administration of large doses over several days and can be fatal, although the number of reports remains small.
- Primaquine causes methemoglobinemia in all patients who take it (levels of up to 18% are reported, normal level is <1%), but this seldom causes symptoms and is always self-limiting.There may be an association with NADH methemoglobin reductase deficiency.

106. Ans. (b) Penicillin *Ref: Harrison's, 17th ed. p 2077*

SLE is associated with the following drugs:

- Antibiotics - INH, minocycline, and macrodantin
- Diuretics Hydrochlorothiazide
- Antirheumatic sulfasalizine
- Antihypertensives Hydralazine, ACE inhibitors, and beta-blockers
- Antipsychotic Chlorpromazine, lithium
- Anti-thyroid Propylthiouracil
- Anti-convulsants Carbamazepine and phenytoin
- Anti-Hyperlipidemic Lovastatin, simvastatin.

107. Ans. (d) Methotrexate *Ref: Essentials of Medical Pharmacology, KD Tripathi, 6th ed. p 831*

MOPP is a combination chemotherapy regimen used to treat Hodgkin's disease.

The acronym is derived from the component drugs of the regimen:

- Mustargen (also known as mechlorethamine, mustine, nitrogen mustard, or MSD)
- Oncovin (also known as Vincristine or VCR)
- Procarbazine (also known as Matulane or Natulan)
- Prednisone (also known as Deltasone or Orasone)

The treatment is usually administered in four week cycles, often for six cycles. MSD and VCR are administered intravenously, while procarbazine and prednisone are pills taken orally.

108. Ans. (d) Phenytoin sodium *Ref: Essentials of Pharmacology for Dentistry, KD Tripathi, 2nd ed. p 142*

- Phenytoin is a hydantoin-derivative anticonvulsant drug used primarily in the management of complex partial seizures and generalized tonic-clonic seizures.
- Phenytoin is also used to prevent seizures following neurosurgery.
- Phenytoin is believed to protect against seizures by causing voltage-dependent block of voltage-gated sodium channels.
- Additionally, phenytoin is a class 1b antiarrhythmic that can be used to treat cardiac arrhythmias when conventional options have failed or after cardiac glycoside intoxication.

Adverse effects of phenytoin sodium are:

- Cardiovascular: Severe hypotension and cardiac arrhythmias seen with rapid infusion of IV phenytoin. IV infusion should not exceed 50 mg/min in adults.
- Neurologic: At therapeutic doses, phenytoin may produce nystagmus on lateral gaze. At toxic doses, patients experience vertical nystagmus, diplopia, sedation, slurred speech, cerebellar ataxia, and tremor. Abrupt discontinuation of phenytoin may result in increased seizure frequency, including status epilepticus.
- Hematologic: It has been suggested that phenytoin causes a reduction in folic acid levels, predisposing patients to megaloblastic anemia. Folic acid is presented in foods as polyglutamate, which is then converted into monoglutamates by intestinal conjugase. Phenytoin acts by inhibiting this enzyme, thereby causing folate deficiency. Other side effects may include: agranulocytosis, aplastic anemia, leucopenia, thrombocytopenia.
- Teratogenicity: Phenytoin is a known teratogen. The syndrome consists of craniofacial anomalies (broad nasal bridge, cleft lip and palate, microcephaly) and a mild form of mental retardation.
- Gingival: Phenytoin has been associated with drug-induced gingival enlargement (overgrowth of the gums).
- Dermatologic: Hypertrichosis, purple glove syndrome, rash, exfoliative dermatitis, pruritus, hirsutism, and coarsening of facial features.
- Immunodeficiency disease: Phenytoin is also associated with induction of reversible IgA deficiency.

109. Ans. (d) Potentiating antithrombin III activity *Ref: Essentials of Pharmacology for Dentistry, KD Tripathi, 2nd ed. p 256*

Heparin:

- Heparin is a polymer of acidic sulfated disaccharide, derived from porcine or bovine mucosa.
- Heparin acts to potentiate antithrombin III, an endogenous substance that inhibits the conversion of fibrinogen to fibrin.
- The drug induces a conformational change in antithrombin III and binds simultaneously to thrombin and antithrombin III, facilitating the inactivation of thrombin.
- Heparin should be given by parenteral route as it is destroyed by digestive enzyme.
- Heparin inhibits the carboxylation of bone proteins, and decreases the activity of vitamin K in osteoblast.
- In high dose of heparin, platelet aggregation is affected and bleeding time is prolonged.
- The elimination rate of higher molecular weight forms of heparin is faster than that of lower molecular weight forms.
- Heparin eliminates in the form of urine.

110. Ans. (c) Cetirizine *Ref: Essentials of Pharmacology for Dentistry, KD Tripathi, 2nd ed. p 102*

- Cetirizine is an antihistamine that reduces the effects of natural chemical histamine in the body. Histamine can produce symptoms of sneezing, itching, watery eyes, and runny nose.
- Cetirizine is used to treat cold or allergy symptoms such as sneezing, itching, watery eyes, or runny nose.
- Cetirizine is also used to treat itching and swelling caused by chronic urticaria (hives).
- Drinking alcohol can increase certain side effects of cetirizine.

111. Ans. (c) Carbaryl *Ref: Essentials of Medical Pharmacology, KD Tripathi, 6th ed. p 99*

Classification of anticholinesterases:

- **Reversible:**
  - **Carbonates:**
    - Physostigmine
    - Neostigmine
    - Pyridostigmine
    - Edrophonium
    - Rivastigmine

- Donepezil
- Galantamine
- **Acridine:**
  - Tacrine
- **Irreversible:**
  - **Organophosphates:**
    - Dyflos
    - Echothiophate
    - Parathion
    - Diazinon
    - Tabun
  - **Carbamates**
    - Carbaryl
    - Propoxur

112. Ans. (b) Decamethonium *Ref: Essentials of Pharmacology for Dentistry, KD Tripathi, 2nd ed. p 124-125*

Neuromuscular blocking agents fall into two groups:

- Non-depolarizing blocking agents: These agents constitute the majority of the clinically relevant neuromuscular blockers. They act by competitively blocking the binding of ACh to its receptors, and in some cases, they also directly block the ionotropic activity of the ACh receptors.
  Long acting: d-Tubocurarine, Pancuronium, Doxacurium, Pipecuronium
  Intermediate acting: Vecuronium, Atracurium, Rocuronium, Rapacuronium
  Short acting: Mivacurium
- Depolarizing blocking agents: These agents act by depolarizing the plasma membrane of the skeletal muscle fiber. This persistent depolarization makes the muscle fiber resistant to further stimulation by Ach.
  Succinylcholine (SCh., Suxamethonium),
  Decamethonium (C-10)

113. Ans. (a) Blocking acetylcholine receptors *Ref: Essentials of Pharmacology for Dentistry, KD Tripathi, 2nd ed. p 125*

- Neuromuscular-blocking drugs block neuromuscular transmission at the neuromuscular junction, causing paralysis of the affected skeletal muscles.
- This is accomplished either by acting presynaptically via the inhibition of acetylcholine (ACh) synthesis or release or by acting postsynaptically at the acetylcholine receptors of the motor nerve end-plate.
- While some drugs act presynaptically (such as botulinum toxin and tetanus toxin), those of current clinical importance work postsynaptically.
- D-Tubocurarine is a non-depolarizing blocker, it acts by blocking acetylcholine receptors.

114. Ans. (d) Low K^+ levels

115. Ans. (b) C. difficile *Ref: Essentials of Pharmacology for Dentistry, KD Tripathi, 2nd ed. p 280*

- Antibiotic-associated diarrhea refers to diarrhea that develops in a person who is taking or recently took antibiotics.
- One of the most serious causes of antibiotic-associated diarrhea is infection with a bacterium, Clostridium difficile.
- C. difficile infections are most common in people who are hospitalized.
- C. difficile is a disease-causing bacterium that can infect the large bowel and cause colitis.

- C. difficile infections have become more frequent, more severe, more difficult to treat, and more likely to recur after initial treatment. Although most people become infected with C. difficile in the hospital, the infection has also become more common in patients who have not been hospitalized or through community-acquired infection.

116. Ans. (c) Anticoagulants *Ref: Essentials of Medical Pharmacology by, KD Tripathi, 6th ed. p 9*

Intramuscular injection should be avoided in anticoagulant treated patients, because it can produce local haematoma

117. Ans. (b) Anxiety *Ref: Essentials of Medical Pharmacology by KD Tripathi, 6th ed. p 135*

Enteral	*Special utility*	*Limitations/risks*
Oral (p.o.)	• Easy • Usually safe • Economical	• Relatively slow • Less predictable • First pass effect • Patient compliance
Sublingual	• Rapid response • No first pass effect • Bypasses gi acids and enzymes	• Many molecules do not penetrate oral mucosa • Not used for irritating substances
Rectal	• Unconscious patients • Vomiting patients • Small children • Minimal first pass effect • Bypasses gi acids and enzymes	• Irregular and incomplete absorption • Not used for irritating substances • Solutions must be isotonic
Parenteral		
Intravenous (i.v.)	• Most rapid response (emergencies) • Permits titration of dosage • Most suitable for irritating substances and large volumes • Lowest intra-individual variability	• Greatest risks: overdose, anaphylaxis, infection, embolism, vascular injury, extravasion
Intramuscular (i.m.)	• Moderate volumes • Faster absorption than s.c.	• Not used for irritating substances • Sterile abscesses • May interfere with diagnostic tests • **Precluded during anticoagulant therapy**
Subcutaneous (s.c.)	• Slower absorption than i.m. • Absorption slowed by vasoconstriction	• Not used for irritating substances • Large volumes are painful
Intraperitoneal (i.p.)	• Provides large absorbing surface • Primarily used on lab animals	• First pass effect • Risks: adhesions, infection, injury
Topical	• Useful for local effects • Poisons and toxins	• Least effective for systemic absorption
Intrathecal	• Local anesthetics/antibiotics	• Risks: infection, headaches

Uses of α-adrenoceptors blockers are:

Pheochromocytoma

- Hypertension
- Benign hypertrophy of prostate (BHP)

- Secondary shock
- Peripheral vascular disease
- Congestive heart failure
- Papaverine induced penile erection (PIPE) therapy for impotence.

Uses of β-adrenoceptors blockers are:

- Hypertension
- Angina pectoris
- Cardiac arrhythmias
- Myocardial infarction (MI)
- Congestive heart failure
- Dissecting aortic aneurysm
- Pheochromocytoma
- Thyrotoxicosis
- Migraine
- Anxiety
- Essential tremors
- Glaucoma
- Hypertrophic obstructive cardiomyopathy.

118. Ans. (c) GABA receptors *Ref: Essentials of Pharmacology for Dentistry, KD Tripathi, 2nd ed. p 449*

- Anxiolytic medications have been used for the treatment of anxiety and its related psychological and physical symptoms. Anxiolytics have been shown to be useful in the treatment of anxiety disorders.
- Anxiolytics are also known as minor tranquilizers.
- Activation of GABA receptors would be expected to decrease anxiety.

119. Ans. (d) Biguanide *Ref: K.D. Tripathi—Essentials of Pharmacology for Dentistry, p 219,220,22*

- Sulfonylureas provoke a brisk release of insulin from pancreas.
- Mechanism of action of biguanides is not clearly understood. They do not cause insulin release but presence of some insulin is essential for their action.
- Repaglinide induces rapid onset short-lasting insulin release.

120. Ans. (d) Pyrimethamine + Sulfadoxine *Ref: K.D. Tripathi, 6th ed. p 790-791*

- Sulfonamides/dapsone are not particularly effective antimalarial drugs in their own right; have some inhibitory influence on the erythrocytic phase, especially of P. falciparum. However, they form supra-additive synergistic combination with pyrimethamine due to sequential block (as in case of cotrimoxazole). Though, both components are slow acting, the combination acts faster, so that it can be employed as a clinical curative, particularly for P. falciparum. Efficacy against P. vivax is rather low. By the addition of sulfonamide, development of resistance to pyrimethamine is retarded. There is no cross-resistance with other groups of antimalarial drugs.
- As clinical curative: Sulfadoxine 1500 mg + pyrimethamine 75 mg (3 tab) single dose (children 9–14 year 2 tab, 4–8 year 1 tab, 1–4 year ½ tab).

121. Ans. (c) Zolpidem *Ref: K.D. Tripathi, 6th ed. p 398*

- Zolpidem—An imidazopyridine which preferentially acts on the α1 subunit containing subtype of BZD receptors those are important in mediating the hypnotic effect. Hypnotic effect is pronounced: sleep latency is shortened, sleep duration is prolonged in insomniacs but anticonvulsant, muscle relaxant and antianxiety effects are not evident. Its advantages are: relative lack of effect on sleep stages (REM suppression is slight); minimal residual day time sedation or fading of hypnotic action on repeated nightly use; no/little rebound insomnia on discontinuation; near absence of tolerance or physical dependence and low abuse potential combined with safety in overdose like BZDs.

122. Ans. (c) Ketanserin *Ref: K.D. Tripathi, 4th ed. p 190*

- Ketanserin is a selective 5HT2 receptor blocker; it is an effective antihypertensive.
- Bromocriptine:
  - It is a synthetic ergot derivative and a potent dopamine agonist.
  - It has greater action on D2 receptors.
  - It is used in Hyperprolactinemia, Suppression of Lactation and Breast Engorgement, Acromegaly, Parkinsonism and hepatic coma.
- Lysergic Acid Diethylamide (LSD) is an ergot derivative; found to be an extremely potent hallucinogen.
- Methysergide:
  - Chemically related to ergot alkaloids, it antagonizes the action of 5HT on smooth muscles.
  - It has been used for Migraine prophylaxis, Carcinoid and Post-gastrectomy dumping syndrome.

123. Ans. (a) Naltrexone *Ref: K.D. Tripathi, 4th ed. p 445*

- Complex action opioids and opioid antagonists are as follows:
  - Agonist Antagonist-
    - Not used as analgesic—Nalorphine, Levallorphan
    - Used as analgesic—Pentazocine, Nalbuphine
  - Partial/Weak Agonists—Buprenorphine, Butorphanol
  - Pure Antagonists—Naloxone, Naltrexone

124. Ans. (d) Loratadine *Ref: K.D. Tripathi, 6th ed. p 156*

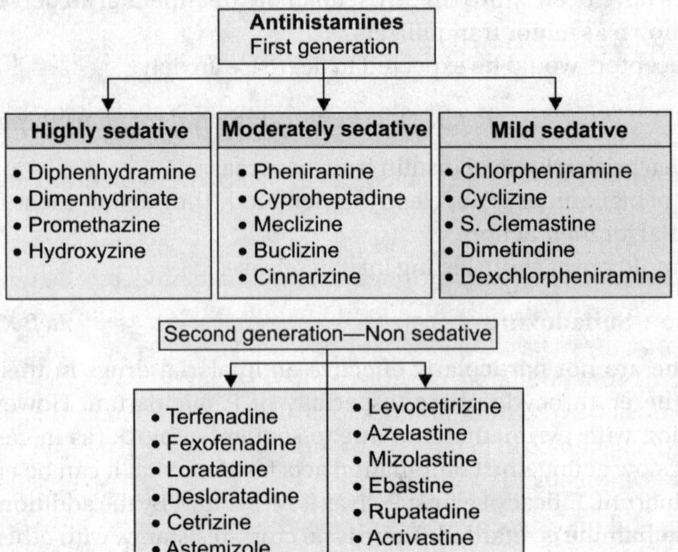

125. Ans. (b) Antiemesis *Ref: K.D. Tripathi, 6th ed. p 454-456*

'Opioids induce nausea and vomiting by stimulating CTZ.'

Pharmacological action of morphine

- **CNS**
  - **Stimulation action**
    - CTZ nausea and vomiting
    - Edinger-westphal nucleus Miosis
    - Vagal center Bradycardia
    - Muscular rigidity and convulsions

- **Depressant action**
  - Analgesia, sedation, respiratory depression
  - Antitussive, hypothermia, fall in BP
- **CVS causes vasodilation**
- **GIT causes constipation**
- **Smooth muscle cause bronchoconstriction due to histamine release**
  - Spasm of sphincter of oddi-biliary colic
- **ANS causes mild hyperglycemia**
  Weak anti-cholinesterase action
- **Morphine causes antidiuresis by releasing ADH**

126. Ans. (c) Valproic acid *Ref: Harrison, 17th ed. p 2507-2508*

Conditions	*Drug of choice*
• Partial seizure	Carbamazepine, phenytoin
• Generalized tonic clonic seizure	Valproate, lamotrigine, Phenytoin
• Absence seizure	Valproate, ethosuximide
• Myoclonic	Valproate, lamotrigine, topiramate
• Atonic	Valproate, lamotrigine, topiramate
• Febrile	Diazepam (rectal)
• Status epilepticus	IV lorazepam, IV Diazepam

127. Ans. (d) Ipratropium *Ref: K.D. Tripathi, 6th ed. p 222-223*

- Atropinic drugs cause bronchodilation by blocking cholinergic constrictor tone; act primarily in the large airways.
- Inhaled ipratropium bromide is less efficacious than sympathomimetics. Patients of asthmatic bronchitis, COPD and psychogenic asthma respond better to anticholinergics. Inhaled ipratropium/tiotropium is the bronchodilators of choice in COPD.
- Sod. cromoglycate is used as a long term prophylactic in mild to moderate asthma.
- Anticholinergic bronchodilation inhibit only the cholinergic reflex component of bronchoconstriction while β2 agonists prevent all bronchoconstriction mechanisms.
- Inhaled ipratropium are bronchodilators of choice in COPD.
- They are less efficacious than sympathomimetics for asthma.
- They are bronchodilators of choice in patients of bronchial asthma of β blocker or β2 agonists will be ineffective due to blockage of β2 receptors.

128. Ans. (a) Rapid induction and quick recovery from anesthesia *Ref: K.D. Tripathi, 6th ed. p 365*

Blood-gas partition coefficient: Given by the ratio of the concentration of the anesthetic in blood in that in the gas phase at equilibrium is the index of solubility of the GA in blood.

- It is the measure of solubility of agent in blood.
- It determines the speed of onset and recovery.
- Higher the blood-gas partition coefficient, lesser the speed of induction and recovery. More blood soluble agents have slower induction and recovery.

Remember

- Max MAC → N_2O.
- Min MAC → Halothane.
- Max blood gas coefficient → Ether.
- Min blood gas coefficient → Desflurane.

129. Ans. (b) Insulin glargine *Ref: Lawrence, 9th ed. p 682*

There are four type of insulin preparation:

- Conventional.
- Insulin analogues.
- Human insulin.
- Highly purified—monocomponent insulins.

Insulin analogues produced by recombinant DNA technology

- Preparations are—Insulin lispro, insulin aspart, insulin glulisine, insulin glargine.
  Insulin glargine is longer acting and has lower incidence of night time hypoglycemic episodes (all other insulin analogues are repaid and short acting).
- However insulin glargine has delayed onset of action. It does not control meal time glycemia, for which a rapid acting insulin or an oral hypoglycemia is used concurrently, i.e. it is also referred as 'peakless' insulin analogue.

130. Ans. (b) Procaine *Ref: K.D Tripathi, 6th ed. p 356, 359 and K.D. Tripathi, 5th ed. p 325*

Surface anesthetics are:

- Dibucaine
- Lignocaine
- Tetracaine
- Benzocaine
- Cocaine.
- Benoxinate.
- Oxethazaine.
- Prilocaine.
- Butamben.
- Procaine has very less potent surface anesthetic action, hence not used as surface anesthetic.

131. Ans. (b) Amiodarone *Ref: K.D. Tripathi, 6th ed. p 511, 515 and K.D. Tripathi, 5th ed. p 475*

Amiodarone - Class III antiarrhythmic drug

- It is most powerful antiarrhythmic drug available for the treatment and prevention of both atrial and ventricular arrhythmias.
- It posses all classes antiarrhythmic action.

i.e., Class I → Na^+ channel blockade
Class II → β-blockade
Class III → K^+ channel blockade
Class IV → Ca^{2+} channel blockade

Adverse effects

→ Hypothyroidism and Hyperthyroidism
→ Peripheral neuropathy, pulmonary fibrosis, hepatitis
→ Myocardial depression, corneal deposits
→ Photosensitivity, bluish discoloration of exposed skin
→ Amiodarone can be used for all arrhythmia except for torsades de pointes and digitalis induced arrhythmia.

132. Ans. (c) Methotrexate *Ref: K.D. Tripathi, 6th ed. p 823 and K.D. Tripathi, 5th ed. p 772*

- Methotrexate is folate antagonist—inhibits dihydrofolate reductase by blocking the conversion of dihydrofolic acid to tetrahydrofolic acid.
- The toxicity of methotrexate is antagonized by folinic acid.
- Methotrexate has cell cycle specific action-kills cells in 'S' phase primarily inhibits DNA synthesize but also affects RNA and protein synthesis.
- It exerts major toxicity on bone marrow. Low dose cause megaloblastic anemia, but high dose produce pancytopenia.
- Methotrexate is used in choriocarcinoma, leukemia, IBD, RA, Psoriasis and is immunosuppressant.

133. Ans. (d) PGH2 *Ref: K.D. Tripathi, 6th ed. p 174*

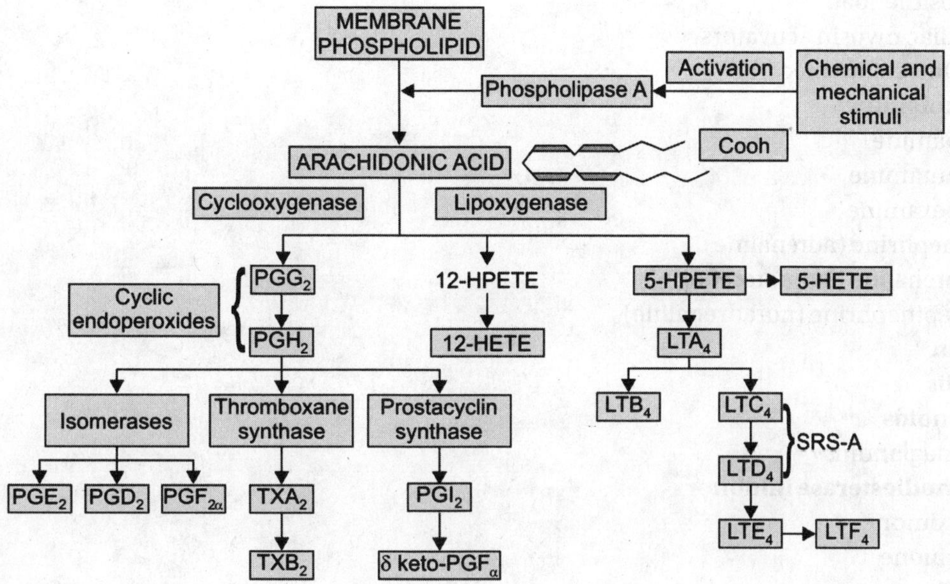

Biosynthesis of prostaglandins (PG) and leukotrienes (LT). Less active metabolites are shown in italics TX-Thromboxane, PGI-Prostacyclin; HPETE-Hydroperoxyeicosatetraenoic acid (Hydroperoxy arachidonic acid); HETE-Hydroxyeicosatetraenoic acid (Hydroxy arachidonic acid); SRS—a slow reacting substance of anaphylaxis.

134. Ans. (d) M phase *Ref: Goodman and Glickmans, 10th ed. p 718, Robbins, 8th ed. p 45*

- Colchicine is an effective anti-inflammatory agent mainly used to treat acute attacks of Gout.
- Colchicine prevents the cycle of inflammatory response.
- It can arrest mitosis in metaphase (M phase) in which it prevents spindle formation.

135. Ans. (a) Cyclosporine *Ref: K.D. Tripathi, 5th ed. p 787*

Cyclosporine
- Specific T cell (or calcineurin) inhibitor.
- Selectively inhibits T lymphocyte proliferation IL 2 and other cytokines production and response of inducer T cells to IL 2 without any effect on suppressor T cells.
- Lymphocytes get arrested in G0 or G1 phase.
- Most effective drug for treatment and as a preventive measure for graft rejection reaction.
- Used in renal cardiac bone marrow and other transplantation cases.
- Induction time is 12 hours before any process and continued till it is needed.
- Concentrated in RBCs and WBCs.
- Metabolized in liver and excreted via bile.
- Biphasic plasma half life i.e. 4-6 hr and 12-18 hr.

136. Ans. (d) Doxepin *Ref: K.D. Tripathi, 5th ed. p 112, 405, 458*

- An inotrope is an agent that alters the force or energy of muscular contractions. Negatively inotropic agents weaken the force of muscular contractions. Positively inotropic agents increase the strength of muscular contraction.
- **Examples of positive inotropic agents include:**
  - Berberine
  - Calcium

- Calcium sensitizers
- Levosimendan
- Cardiac myosin activators
  - Omecamtivmecarbil
- **Catecholamines**
  - Dopamine
  - Dobutamine
  - Dopexamine
  - Epinephrine (adrenaline)
  - Isoprenaline (isoproterenol)
  - Norepinephrine (noradrenaline)
- **Digoxin**
- **Digitalis**
- **Eicosanoids**
  - Prostaglandins
- **Phosphodiesterase inhibitors**
  - Enoximone
  - Milrinone
  - Amrinone
  - Theophylline
- **Glucagon**
- **Insulin**
- Doxepin is tricyclic antidepressant which causes postural hypotension.
- All other drugs have positive inotropic action.

137. Ans. (d) Aspirin *Ref: KDT, 6th ed. p 249*

- Thyroid storm is also known as thyrotoxicosis.
- Thyroid storm is due to increase in secretion of thyroid hormone so drugs used to lower the secreation is:

The following drugs are used in thyroid storm:

- Inhibits thyroid hormone synthesis:
  - Propylthiouracil
  - Methimazole
  - Carbimazole
- Inhibit hormone release
  - Iodine
  - Iodides
- Destroy thyroid tissue
  - Radioactive iodine (131I, 125I, 123I)
- In counteract adrenal insufficiency (if there is)
  - Corticosteroids
- To control sympathetic symptoms
  - Propranolol

138. Ans. (d) Rosiglitazone *Ref: K.D. Tripathi Medical, p 269*

- Two thiazolidinediones rosiglitazone and pioglitazone are available. These oral antidiabetic drugs are selective agonists for the nuclear peroxisome proliferator activated receptor γ (PPAR γ) which enhances the transcription of several insulin responsive genes. Hepatic gluconeogenesis is suppressed. Activated genes regulate fatty acid metabolism and lipogenesis in adipose tissue.
- The risk of fractures especially in elderly women may increase.

139. Ans. (b) Chronic gastritis *Ref: KDT, 6th ed. p 637*

- Helicobacter pylori, previously named Campylobacter pylori, is a Gram-negative, microaerophilic bacterium found in the stomach.
- It was identified in 1982 by Australian scientists Barry Marshall and Robin Warren, who found that it was present in patients with chronic gastritis and gastric ulcers, conditions that were not previously believed to have a microbial cause.
- It is also linked to the development of duodenal ulcers and stomach cancer.
- More than 50% of the world's population harbor H. pylori in their upper gastrointestinal tract.
- Colonization of the stomach by H. pylori can result in chronic gastritis, an inflammation of the stomach lining at the site of infection. Helicobacter cysteine-rich proteins (Hcp), particularly HcpA (hp0211) are known to trigger an immune response causing inflammation. Chronic gastritis is likely to underlie H. pylori-related diseases.
- The most reliable method for detecting H. pylori infection is a biopsy check during endoscopy with a rapid urease test, histological examination, and microbial culture.
- Once H. pylori is detected in a person with a peptic ulcer, the normal procedure is to eradicate it and allow the ulcer to heal. The standard first-line therapy is a one week 'triple therapy' consisting of proton pump inhibitors such as omeprazole and the antibiotics clarithromycin and amoxicillin.
- Variations of the triple therapy have been developed over the years, such as using a different proton pump inhibitor, as with pantoprazole or rabeprazole, or replacing amoxicillin with metronidazole for people who are allergic to penicillin.

140. Ans. (d) All of the above *Ref: KDT, 6th ed. p 523, 524, 525*

Nitroglycerin:

- The effect is more pronounced in venous. The sublingual route is used when terminating an attack or aborting an imminent one is the aim. IV infusion provides rapid, steady, titratable plasma concentration for as long as desired. High membrane permeability. Nitroglycerin is readily absorbed from skin.

141. Ans. (a) Epinephrine 2.5 ml of 1:10,000(IV) *Ref: KDT, 6th ed. p 82*

Inject epinephrine 0.5 mg (0.5 ml of 1 in 1000 solution) i.m; repeat every 5-10 min in case patient does not improve or improvement is transient. This is the only life saving measure.

142. Ans. (c) Both of the above *Ref: Color Atlas of Pharmacology, p 92*

Sympathomimetics are drugs with action similar to adrenaline or of sympathetic stimulation.

- **Direct:** Act directly on alpha and beta adrenoceptors, e.g. Adrenaline, Noradrenaline, Isoprenaline
- **Indirect:** Action adrenergic neuron to release noradrenaline, which then acts on the adrenoceptors, e.g. Tyramine, Amphetamine
- **Mixed action:** Act directly as well as Indirectly, e.g. Ephedrine, Dopamine.

143. Ans. (c) Gestodene *Ref: Harrison's, 16th ed. p 282*

- Gestodene is a progestogen hormonal contraceptive.
- Gestodene is androgenically neutral, meaning that contraceptive pills containing gestodene do not exhibit the androgenic side effects, e.g. acne, hirsutism, weight gain.
- The synthetic estrogen dosage in third-generation contraceptive pills (including those containing gestodene) is lower than that in second-generation oral contraceptives.
- Third-generation oral contraceptives are also suitable for use in patients with diabetes or lipid disorders because they have minimal impact on blood glucose levels and the lipid profile.

144. Ans. (c) Adrenaline *Ref: Balaji, 1st ed. p 660*

- Adrenaline is the drug of choice for the emergency treatment of severe allergic reactions to food, insect stings, medication, latex, exercise, and other allergens. It should be administered as soon as anaphylaxis is suspected, as there is clear evidence that failure to do so has contributed to fatal outcomes.

- Adrenaline rapidly treats all of the most dangerous symptoms of anaphylaxis including throat swelling, difficulty in breathing, and low blood pressure. It also helps alleviate itching, rash, swelling, gastrointestinal and genitourinary symptoms.

145. Ans. (d) Diazepam *Ref: Tripathi's, 5th ed. p 365*

- Diazepam drug can be given safely to the patient suffering from renal disease.
- Diazepam is often used clinically to treat anxiety and insomnia in patients with renal insufficiency or thyroid disease.

146. Ans. (d) Enalapril *Ref: KDT, 6th ed. p 484,486*

Enalapril is an angiotensin converting enzyme (ACE) inhibitor used in the treatment of hypertension diabetic nephropathy, and some types of chronic heart failure. ACE converts the peptide hormone angiotensin I to angiotensin II. One of the actions of angiotensin II is the vasoconstriction of blood vessels resulting in an increase in blood pressure. ACE inhibitors such as enalapril prevent this effect. Enalapril has been shown to lower the death rate in systolic heart failure. Enalapril is an ACE inhibitor used for long term CHF cases. They have been found to be effective in reducing mortality in these patients.

147. Ans. (b) Gum hypertrophy *Ref: KDT, 6th ed. p 404*

Phenytoin has been associated with drug-induced gingival enlargement (overgrowth of the gums), probably due to above-mentioned folate deficiency; indeed, evidence from a randomized controlled trial suggests that folic acid supplementation can prevent gingival enlargement in children who take phenytoin. Plasma concentrations needed to induce gingival lesions have not been clearly defined. Effects consist of the following: bleeding upon probing, increased gingival exudate, pronounced gingival inflammatory response to plaque levels, associated in some instances with bone loss but without tooth detachment.

Also note other side effects of phenytoin:

Gum hypertrophy commonest (20%)	Megaloblastic anemia
Hirsutism	Osteomalacia
Acne	Fetal hydantoin syndrome
Hypersensitivity reaction	

148. Ans. (a) Miosis *Ref: KDT, 6th ed. p 457*

Cessation of dosing with morphine creates the prototypical opioid withdrawal syndrome, which, unlike that of barbiturates, benzodiazepines, alcohol, or sedative-hypnotics, is not fatal by itself in neurologically healthy patients without heart or lung problems. Acute morphine along with and other opioid withdrawal proceeds through a number of stages. Other opioids differ in the intensity and length of each, and weak opioids and mixed agonist-antagonists may have acute withdrawal syndromes that do not reach the highest level. As commonly cited, they are:

- **Stage I:** Six to fourteen hours after last dose: Drug craving, anxiety, irritability, perspiration, and mild to moderate dysphoria.
- **Stage II:** Fourteen to eighteen hours after last dose: Yawning, heavy perspiration, mild depression, lacrimation, crying, running nose, dysphoria, also intensification of the above symptoms. 'Yen sleep' (a waking trance-like state).
- **Stage III:** Sixteen to twenty-four hours after last dose: Rhinorrhea (runny nose) and increase in other of the above, dilated pupils, piloerection (goosebumps giving the name 'cold turkey'), muscle twitches, hot flashes, cold flashes, aching bones and muscles, loss of appetite and the beginning of intestinal cramping.
- **Stage IV:** Twenty-four to thirty-six hours after last dose: Increase in all of the above including severe cramping and involuntary leg movements ('kicking the habit' also called restless leg syndrome), loose stool, insomnia, elevation of blood pressure, moderate elevation in body temperature, increase in frequency of breathing and tidal volume, tachycardia (elevated pulse), restlessness, nausea.

- **Stage V:** Thirty-six to seventy-two hours after last dose: Increase in the above, fetal position, vomiting, free and frequent liquid diarrhea, which sometimes can accelerate the time of passage of food from mouth to out of system to an hour or less, weight loss of two to five kilos per 24 hours, increased white cell count and other blood changes.
- **Stage VI:** After completion of above: Recovery of appetite and normal bowel function, beginning of transition to post-acute and chronic symptoms that are mainly psychological but that may also include increased sensitivity to pain, hypertension, colitis or other gastrointestinal afflictions related to motility, and problems with weight control in either direction.

Withdrawal symptoms of morphine:

Lacrimation	Dehydration
Sweating	Rise in B.P.
Yawning	Palpitation
Anxiety	Rapid weight loss
Gooseflesh	Absence of delirium
Mydriasis	and convulsion

Also note contraindications for morphine:

- The following conditions are relative contraindications for morphine:
  - Acute respiratory depression
  - Renal failure (due to accumulation of the metabolites morphine-3-glucuronide and morphine-6 glucuronide)
  - Chemical toxicity (potentially lethal in low tolerance subjects)
  - Raised intracranial pressure including head injury (risk of worsening respiratory depression)
- Biliary colic

149. Ans. (c) Optic neuritis *Ref: KDT, 6th ed. p 421*

Side effects of Ethambutol

- Optic neuritis (hence contraindicated in children below six years of age)
- Red-green color blindness
- Peripheral neuropathy
- Arthralgia
- Hyperuricemia
- Vertical nystagmus
- Milk skin reaction

150. Ans. (c) Bronchial asthma *Ref: KDT, 6th ed. p 108*

- Ipratropium bromide is an anti-cholinergic drug used for the treatment of chronic obstructive pulmonary disease and acute asthma. It blocks the muscarinic acetylcholine receptors in the smooth muscles of the bronchi in the lungs, opening the bronchi
- In contrast to sympathomimetic which acts on peripheral bronchioles, ipratropium bromide mainly acts on larger central airways but does not affect respiratory secretion
- Although it is used for treatment of bronchial asthma but is more effective in COPD.
- Ipratropium is administered by inhalation for the treatment of chronic obstructive pulmonary disease (COPD). For that purpose it is supplied in a canister for use in an inhaler or in single dose vials for use in a nebulizer.
- There are no contraindications for inhaled ipratropium, apart from hypersensitivity to atropine and related substances. For oral administration, contraindications are similar to other anticholinergics; they include narrow angle glaucoma and obstructions in the gastrointestinal tract and urinary system.

- Combination with beta-adrenergic agonists, as well as theophylline and other xanthine derivatives, increases the dilating effect on the bronchi. Interactions with other anticholinergics like tricyclic antidepressants, anti-parkinson drugs and quinidine, which theoretically increase side effects, are clinically irrelevant when ipratropium is administered as an inhalant.
- If ipratropium is inhaled, side effects resembling those of other anticholinergics are minimal. However, dry mouth and sedation have been reported. Also, effects such as skin flushing, tachycardia, acute angle-closure glaucoma, nausea, palpitations and headache have been observed. Inhaled ipratropium does not decrease mucociliary clearance. The inhalation itself can cause headache and irritation of the throat in a few percent of patients.

151. Ans. (c) Dantrolene *Ref: KDT, 6th ed. p 347*

- Malignant hyperthermia (MH) or malignant hyperpyrexia is a rare life-threatening condition that is usually triggered by exposure to certain drugs used for general anesthesia, specifically the volatile anesthetic agents and the neuromuscular blocking agent, succinylcholine. In susceptible individuals, these drugs can induce a drastic and uncontrolled increase in skeletal muscle oxidative metabolism, which overwhelms the body's capacity to supply oxygen, remove carbon dioxide, and regulate body temperature, eventually leading to circulatory collapse and death if not treated quickly.
- The current treatment of choice is the intravenous administration of dantrolene, the only known antidote, discontinuation of triggering agents, and supportive therapy directed at correcting hyperthermia, acidosis, and organ dysfunction. Treatment must be instituted rapidly on clinical suspicion of the onset of malignant hyperthermia.
- Dantrolene is a muscle relaxant that appears to work directly on the ryanodine receptor to prevent the release of calcium. After the widespread introduction of treatment with dantrolene, the mortality of malignant hyperthermia fell from 80% in the 1960s to less than 10%. Dantrolene remains the only drug known to be effective in the treatment of MH.

152. Ans. (d) Diazepam *Ref: KDT, 5th ed. p 365*

- Phenacetin causes analgesic nephropathy.
- Tetracycline causes kidney damage except doxycycline which is named as Fanconi's syndrome.
- Aminoglycosides results in nephrotoxicity due to tubular damage.
- Diazepam is a BZD which is relatively a safe drug.

Also know about diazepam

- It possesses anxiolytic, anticonvulsant, hypnotic, sedative, skeletal muscle relaxant, and amnestic properties. The pharmacological action of diazepam enhances the effect of the neurotransmitter GABA by binding to the benzodiazepine site on the GABA receptor (via the constituent chlorine atom) leading to central nervous system depression.
- It is commonly used to treat anxiety, panic attacks, insomnia, seizures (including status epilepticus), muscle spasms (such as in tetanus cases), restless legs syndrome, alcohol withdrawal, benzodiazepine withdrawal, opiate withdrawal syndrome and Ménière's disease. It may also be used before certain medical procedures (such as endoscopies) to reduce tension and anxiety, and in some surgical procedures to induce amnesia.
- Adverse effects of diazepam include anterograde amnesia (especially at higher doses) and sedation, as well as paradoxical effects such as excitement, rage or worsening of seizures in epileptics. Benzodiazepines also can cause or worsen depression. Long-term effects of benzodiazepines such as diazepam include tolerance, benzodiazepine dependence and benzodiazepine withdrawal syndrome upon dose reduction. After cessation of benzodiazepines, cognitive deficits may persist for at least six months and it was suggested that longer than six months may be needed for recovery from some deficits.

153. Ans. (a) Blood glucose levels *Ref: K.D. Tripathi, 5th ed. p 248*

- In the given case the patient is on Glibenclamide which is a second generation sulfonylureas—an oral anti-diabetic drug.

- The most common adverse effect with these drugs is said to be hypoglycemia which leads to altered consciousness and in the above case the patient has been taking aspirin which is contraindicated in both diabetic patients and those taking sulfonylureas as it increases the toxicity of these drugs by its displacement from plasma proteins.
- Also he has been off from food for few days which may lead to hypoglycemia easily but it surely can be reversed. Hence the blood glucose level should be estimated first.
- Normal value ranges may vary slightly among different laboratories. Many factors affect a person's blood sugar level. A body's homeostatic mechanism, when operating normally, restores the blood sugar level to a narrow range of about 4.4 to 6.1 mmol/L (79.2 to 110 mg/dL) (as measured by a fasting blood glucose test).
- Despite widely variable intervals between meals or the occasional consumption of meals with a substantial carbohydrate load, human blood glucose levels tend to remain within the normal range. However, shortly after eating, the blood glucose level may rise, in non-diabetics, temporarily up to 7.8 mmol/L (140 mg/dL) or slightly more.
- The American Diabetes Association recommends a post-meal glucose level of less than 10 mmol/L (180 mg/dL) and fasting plasma glucose of 5 to 7.2 mmol/L (90 to 130 mg/dL).
- The actual amount of glucose in the blood and body fluids is very small. In a healthy adult male of 75 kg with a blood volume of 5 liters, a blood glucose level of 5.5 mmol/L (100 mg/dL) amounts to 5 grams, slightly less than two typical American restaurant sugar packets for coffee or tea. Part of the reason why this amount is so small is that, to maintain an influx of glucose into cells, enzymes modify glucose by adding phosphate or other groups to it.

154. Ans. (d) Ethambutol *Ref: K.D. Tripathi, 5th ed. p 699-701*

- A side effect of ethambutol is hyperuricemia due to its interference with rate excretion. Hence it should be used in reduced doses in end stage renal diseases as its excretion is mainly dependent on glomerular filtration.
- In case of reduced renal function, the main side effect optic neuritis will occur rapidly as this adverse effect is dose dependent

155. Ans. (b) It inhibits the action of cholinesterase *Ref: K.D. Tripathi, Essentials of Pharmacology for Dentistry, p 73, 75*

Anticholinesterases: (Anti-ChEs) are agents which inhibit ChE, protect ACh from hydrolysis produce cholinergic effecting vivo and potentiate ACh both in vivo and in vitro. Some anti- ChE has additional direct action on cholinergic receptors.

Reversible	
Carbamates Physostigmine (Eserine) Neostigmine Pyridostigmine Edrophonium Rivastigmine, Donepezil	Acridine Tacrine
Irreversible	
Organophosphates Dyflos (DFP) Echothiophate Parathion*, Malathion* Diazinon* (TIK-20) —	Carbamates Carbaryl* (SEVIN) Propoxur* (BAYGON) *Insecticides £Nerve gases for chemical warfare

Myasthenia gravis is an autoimmune disorder due to development of antibodies to the muscle endplate nicotinic receptors (NR) resulting in weakness and easy fatigability. Neostigmine and its congeners improve muscle contraction by preserving ACh as well as by directly depolarizing the endplate.

156. Ans. (b) Sucralfate *Ref: K.D. Tripathi, Essentials of Pharmacology for Dentistry, p 265*

Approaches for the treatment of peptic ulcer are:

- Reduction of gastric acid secretion
  - H2 antihistamines: Cimetidine, Ranitidine, Famotidine, Roxatidine, Loxatidine
  - Proton pump inhibitors: Omeprazole, Lansoprazole, Pantoprazole, Rabeprazole, Esomeprazole
  - Anticholinergics: Pirenzepine, Propantheline, Oxyphenonium
  - Prostaglandin analogues: Misoprostol
- Neutralization of gastric acid (Antacids)
  - Systemic: Sodium bicarbonate, Sodium citrate
  - Nonsystemic: Magnesium hydroxide, Magnesium trisilicate, Aluminium hydroxide gel, Magaldrate, Calcium carbonate.
- Ulcer protectives: Sucralfate, Colloidal bismuth subcitrate (CBS)
- Anti-H. pylori drugs: Amoxicillin, Clarithromycin, Metronidazole, Tinidazole, Tetracycline

157. Ans. (d) All of the above *Ref: Davidson, 20th ed. p 1056 and Harsh Mohan, 3rd ed. p 511*

Drugs inhibiting platelet function	
NSAIDs	
• Aspirin	• Phenylbutazone
• Indomethacin	• Sulfinpyrazone
Antibiotics	
• Penicillins	• Cephalosporins
Dextran	
Heparin	
B-blockers	

Coagulation Disorders in Liver Disease

Since liver is the major site for synthesis and metabolism of coagulation factors, liver disease often leads to multiple hemostatic abnormalities. The liver also produces inhibitors of coagulation such as antithrombin III and protein C and S and plays a role in the clearance of activated factors and fibrinolytic enzymes. Thus, patients with liver disease may develop hypercoagulability and are predisposed to develop DIC and systemic fibrinolysis.

The major causes of bleeding in liver diseases are as under:

- Anatomic lesions. These include:
  - Portal hypertension, e.g. varices, splenomegaly with secondary thrombocytopenia.
  - Peptic ulceration.
  - Gastritis.
- Hepatic dysfunctions, e.g.
  - Impaired hepatic synthesis of coagulation factors.
  - Impaired hepatic synthesis of coagulation inhibitors: protein C, protein S and antithrombin III.
  - Impaired absorption and metabolism of vitamin K.
  - Failure to clear activated coagulation factors causing DIC and systemic fibrinolysis.
- Complications of therapy. These causes are:
  - Following massive transfusion leading to dilution of platelets and coagulation factors.
  - Infusion of activated coagulation proteins.
  - Following heparin therapy.

Many a times, the hemostatic abnormality in liver disease is complex but most patients have prolonged PT and PTTK, mild thrombocytopenia, normal fibrinogen level and decreased hepatic stores of vitamin K.

158. Ans. (d) Labetalol *Ref: Essentials of Pharmacology for Dentistry, KD Tripathi p 92*

Classification of β blockers: Nonselective (β1 and β2)

- Without intrinsic sympathomimetic activity → propranolol, Sotalol, Timolol.
- With intrinsic sympathomimetic activity → Pindolol, Oxprenolol.
- With additional α blocking property → Labetalol, Carvedilol.

Cardioselective (β1)

Metoprolol, Atenolol, Acebutolol, Bisoprolol, Esmolol, Betaxolol, Celiprolol, Nebivolol.

159. Ans. (a) Ondansetron *Ref: Essentials of Pharmacology for Dentistry, KD Tripathi p 276*

5-HT3 Antagonists

- Ondansetron is the prototype of a new class of antiemetic drugs developed to control cancer chemotherapy/ radiotherapy induced vomiting and later found to be highly effective in postoperative nausea and vomiting as well. It blocks the depolarizing action of 5-HT through 5-HT3 receptors on vagal afferents in the G.I.T. as well as in NTS and CTZ.
- Cytotoxic drugs/ radiation produce nausea and vomiting by causing cellular damage → release of mediators including 5-HT from intestinal mucosa → activation of vagal afferents in the gut → emetogenic impulses to the NTS and CTZ.
- Ondansetron blocks emetogenic impulses both at their peripheral origin and their central relay.

160. Ans. (a) Dexamethasone *Ref: Essentials of Pharmacology for Dentistry/KD Tripathi p 289-290*

Inhaled steroids: These have high topical and low systemic activity (due to poor absorption and/or marked first pass metabolism).

Beclomethasone dipropionate, budesonide and fluticasone have similar properties.

161. Ans. (d) Salicylates *Ref: Essentials of Pharmacology for Dentistry, KD Tripathi p 23, 333, 182, 93, 320*

Extent of first pass metabolism of some important drugs

		High	
Low	*Intermediate*	*Not given orally*	*High oral dose*
Phenobarbitone	Aspirin	Isoprenaline	Propranolol
Tolbutamide	Quinidine	Lignocaine	Alprenolol
Theophylline	Desipramine	Hydrocortisone	Verapamil
Pindolol	Northriptyline	Testosterone	Salbutamol
Isosorbide mononitrate	Chlorpromazine		Glyceryl trinitrate
	Pentazocine		Morphine
	Metoprolol		Pethidine

- **Morphine:** The oral absorption of morphine is unreliable because of high and variable first pass metabolism: oral bioavailability is 1/6 to 1/4th of parenterally administered drug. About 30% is bound to plasma proteins. Only a small fraction enters brain rather slowly. Morphine freely crosses placenta and can affect the fetus more than the mother. It is primarily metabolized in liver by glucuronide is an active metabolite (inherently more potent than morphine) which accumulates during chronic dosing and contributes to analgesia, despite its restricted passage across blood-brain barrier.

- **Nitrates:** Organic nitrates are lipid soluble; well absorbed from buccal mucosa, intestines and skin. All except isosorbide mononitrate undergo extensive but variable first pass metabolism in liver. They are rapidly denitrated by a glutathione reductase.
- **Propranolol** is well absorbed after oral administration, but has low bioavailability due to high first pass metabolism in liver. Oral parenteral dose ratio of up to 40:1 has been found.
- **Aspirin** is absorbed from stomach and small intestines. Its poor water solubility is the limiting factor in absorption: microfining the drug-particles and inclusion of an alkali (solubility is more at higher pH) enhances absorption. However, higher pH also favors ionization, thus decreasing the diffusible form.
- **Among the given option, Aspirin/Salicylates has intermediated first pass metabolism. Hence the correct option is 4.**

162. Ans. (c) Contraindicated in diabetic nephropathy *Ref: Essentials of Pharmacology for Dentistry, K.D Tripathi p 169,170*

- ACE inhibitors are contraindicated in bilateral renal artery stenosis and pregnancy.
- In patients with type 1 diabetes mellitus and diabetic nephropathy, captopril prevents or delays the progression of renal disease. Several mechanism participate in the renal protection afforded by ACE inhibitors. Increased glomerular capillary pressure induces glomerular injury and ACE inhibitors reduce this parameter both by decreasing arterial blood pressure and by dilating renal efferent arterioles. ACE inhibitors increase the permeability selectivity of the filtering membrane, thereby diminishing exposure of the mesangium to proteinaceous factors that may stimulate mesangial cell proliferation and matrix production, two processes that contribute to expansion of the mesangium in diabetic nephropathy. Since angiotensin II is a growth factor, reductions in the intrarenal levels of angiotensin II may further attenuate mesangial cell growth and matrix production.
- NSAIDs, including aspirin, may reduce the antihypertensive response to ACE inhibitors.

163. Ans. (d) Nifedipine *Ref: Essentials of Pharmacology for Dentistry, K.D. Tripathi, p 173, 319, 322, 188*

As per the key correct answer is given to be (1) i.e. Aspirin. However according to reference nifedipine should be the most correct option.

- CVS: Aspirin has no direct effect in therapeutic doses. Larger doses increase cardiac output to meet increased peripheral O_2 demand and cause direct vasodilatation. Toxic doses depress vasomotor center: BP may fall. Because of increased cardiac work as well as Na^+ and water retention, CHF may be precipitated in patients with low cardiac reserve.
- Aspirin is absorbed from stomach and small intestines. Its poor water solubility is the limiting factor in absorption: microfining the drug-particles and inclusion of an alkali (solubility is more at higher pH) enhances absorption. However, higher pH also favors ionization, thus decreasing the diffusible form.
- Blood vessels: Digitalis has mild direct vasoconstrictor action peripheral resistance is increased in normal individuals. However, in CHF patients this is more than compensated by the indirect effect of improvement in circulation.
- Digitalis has no prominent effect on BP. Hypertension is no contraindication to the use of digitalis. Therapeutic doses of digitalis have no significant effect on coronary circulation. Coronary insufficiency is no contraindication to its use.
- Angina pectoris: All CCBs are effective in reducing frequency and severity of classical as well as variant angina. Benefit in classical angina appears to be primarily due to reduction in cardiac work: mainly as a result of reduced afterload. Though they can increase coronary flow in normal individuals, this is unlikely to be significant in patients with fixed arterial obstruction. Exercise tolerance is increased.
- The capacity of CCBs to prevent arterial spasm is undoubtedly responsible for the beneficial effect in variant angina.

164. Ans. (b) Nifedipine *Ref: Carranza's, 10th ed. p 377-379*

Drug causing gum hypertrophy:

- Calcium antagonist nifedipine
- Cyclosporine
- Phenytoin

1. **Anticonvulsants:** The first drug induced gingival enlargements reported were those produced by phenytoin (dilantin). Dilantin is a hydantoin, introduced by Merritt and Putnam in 1938 for the treatment of all forms of epilepsy, except petit mal. Shortly thereafter, its relationship with gingival enlargement was reported.
2. **Immunosuppressants:** Cyclosporine is a potent immunosuppressive agent used to prevent organ transplant rejection and to treat several diseases of autoimmune origin. Its exact mechanism of action is not well known, but it appears to selectively and reversibly inhibit helper T cells, which play a role in cellular and humoral immune responses. Cyclosporine A (Sandimmune, Neoral) is administered intravenously or by mouth and dosages greater than 500 mg/day have been reported to induce gingival overgrowth.
3. **Cyclosporine** induced gingival enlargement is more vascularized than phenytoin enlargement.
4. **Calcium channel blockers:** These drugs are the dihydropyridine derivatives (amlodipine, felodipine, nicardipine, nifedipine, the benzothiazine derivatives (diltiazem) and the phenylalkylamine derivatives (verapamil calan, isoptin, verelan, covera-HS)].
5. Some of these drugs can induce gingival enlargement. Nifedipine, one of the most often used, induces gingival enlargement in 20% of patients. Diltiazem, felodipine, nitrendipine, and verapamil also induce gingival enlargement. The dihydropyridine derivative isradipine can replace nifedipine in some cases and doses not induce gingival overgrowth.

165. Ans. (d) They affect the metabolism of drugs such as cyclosporine necessitating an increase in the dosage

Ref: Davidson's, 20th ed. pg 155 and Essentials of Pharmacology for Dentistry KD Tripathi p 428, 431

- Azoles are fungostatic.
- Azoles are enzyme inhibitors; they inhibit the metabolism of many drugs. Dose of the concomitant drug needs to be reduced with the azoles.
- Azole resistance has emerged gradually during prolonged azole therapy.
- Serious hepatotoxicity has rarely led to hepatic failure and death. If symptoms of hepatotoxicity occur, the drug should be discontinued and liver function assessed.

166. Ans. (d) Fludrocortisone *Ref: K.D. Tripathi, 6th ed. p 282*

Fludrocortisone is a potent mineralocorticoid having some glucocorticoid activity as well, orally active, used for:

- Replacement therapy in Addison's disease 50-200 μg daily. Congenital adrenal hyperplasia in patients with salt wasting 50-200 μg/day.
- Idiopathic postural hypotension 100-200 μg/day.

167. Ans. (b) Buspirone *Ref: K.D. Tripathi, 6th ed. p 451*

- Buspirone is the first azapirone, a new class of antianxiety drugs distinctly different from BZDs.
- Does not interact with BZD receptor or modify GABAergic transmission.
- Buspirone relieves mild-to-moderate generalized anxiety.

168. Ans. (d) Precipitate migrainic effect *Ref: K.D Tripathi, 6th ed. p 138,139*

- Beta-blockers are used in prophylaxis of migraine.
- Abrupt discontinuation of beta-receptor antagonists after long-term treatment can exacerbate angina and may increase the risk of sudden death.

- Beta-blockade may blunt recognition of hypoglycemia by patients; it also may delay recovery from insulin-induced hypoglycemia.
- A major adverse effect of beta-receptor antagonists is caused by blockade of β2 receptors in bronchial smooth muscle. These receptors are particularly important for promoting bronchodilation in patients with bronchospastic disease, and beta-clockers may cause a life-threatening increase in airway resistance in such patients.

169. Ans. (c) Antiplatelet *Ref: K.D. Tripathi, 6th ed. p 610*

- Clopidogrel: This newer congener of ticlopidine has similar mechanism of action, ability to inhibit platelet function and therapeutic efficacy, but appears to be safer and better tolerated (CLASSICS study).

170. Ans. (a) 3-5 mins *Ref: K.D. Tripathi, 6th ed. p 371*

Following administration, nitrous oxide will become saturated in blood and dissolved in serum fraction of blood within 3-5 mins.

171. Ans. (c) Ergotoxine *Ref: KDT, 6th ed. p493, 132*

- Cardiac glycoside are digitoxin, gitoxin, gitalin, digoxin, strophanthin-G (Ouabain), procillaridin-A, thevetin, convallotoxin, bufotoxin.
- Ergotoxine is a nonselective ergot alkaloid alpha adrenergic blocking agent.

172. Ans. (c) Safe in patients with renal insufficiency *Ref: KDT, 6th ed. p 197*

Selective COX-2 inhibitors:

- It is generally used in a patient who are at risk of peptic ulcer, perforation or bleeds.
- It should be avoided in a patient having heart diseases such as hypertension, cardiac failure, ischaemic heart disease, cerebrovascular disease.
- It does not depress thromboxane A2 production and reduces PGI2 production by vascular endothelium.
- It is not safe in cardiac as well as renal insufficiency.

173. Ans. (c) Epinephrine *Ref: KDT, 6th ed. p 24*

Prodrug	*Active form*
Levodopa	Dopamine
Enalapril	Enalaprilat
Proguanil	Cycloguanil
A-methyldopa	A-methyl norepinephrine
Prednisone	Prednisolone
Bacampicillin	Ampicillin

174. Ans. (b) Alprenolol *Ref: KDT, 6th ed. p 136*

Classification of β-adrenergic blocking drugs-

Non selective (β1 and β2)			*Cardioselective* β_1
Without intrinsic sympathomimetic activity	**With intrinsic sympathomimetic activity**	**With additional α-blocking property**	• Metoprolol • Atenolol • Acebutolol • Bisoprolol • Esmolol • Betaxolol • Celiprolol • Nebivolol
• Propranolol • Sotalol • Timolol	• Pindolol	• Labetalol • Carvedilol	

175. Ans. (d) Baclofen *Ref: KDT, 6th ed. p 349*

Baclofen:

- It depresses both polysynaptic and monosynaptic reflexes of spinal cord.
- It is used as an antispasmatic drug in many neurological disorders like multiple sclerosis, spinal injury, and trigeminal neuralgia.

176. Ans. (a) Levamizole *Ref: KDT, 6th ed. p 837*

Classification of immunosuppressant drugs:

Calcineurin inhibitors	*Anti proliferative drugs*	*Glucocorticoids*	*Antibodies*
Cyclosporine Tacrolimus	Azathioprine Cyclophosphamide Methotrexate Chlorambucil Mycophenolate mofetil (MMF)	Prednisolone	Muromonals Rho (D) Immunoglobulin ATG

177. Ans. (d) Severe acute Bronchial asthma *Ref: K.D. Tripathi, 6th ed. p 287*

Contraindications of corticosteroids:

- Peptic ulcer
- Hypertension
- Osteoporosis
- Psychosis
- Epilepsy
- CHF
- Diabetes mellitus
- Renal failure
- Herpes simplex keratitis
- Viral and fungal infection
- Tuberculosis and other infection

178. Ans. (c) Succinylcholine *Ref: K.D. Tripathi, 6th ed. p 372*

Malignant hyperthermia (MH)

- It is a life-threatening clinical syndrome of hypermetabolism involving the skeletal muscle.
- It is triggered in susceptible individuals primarily by the volatile inhalational anesthetic agents and the muscle relaxant succinylcholine, though other drugs have also been implicated as potential triggers.
- MH is not an allergy but an inherited disorder that is found both in humans and in swine.
- In persons susceptible to MH, the ryanodine receptor in skeletal muscle is abnormal, and this abnormality interferes with regulation of calcium in the muscle. An abnormal ryanodine receptor that controls calcium release causes a buildup of calcium in skeletal muscle, resulting in a massive metabolic reaction.

OTHERS

179. Ans. (a) Chlorpropamide *Ref: KDT, 5th ed. p 246-542*

Chlorpropamide:

- It is first generation sulfonylurea's Sole significant action being lowering of blood glucose level in normal subjects and in type 2 diabetics, but not in type 1 diabetics.
- It is a long acting oral hypoglycemic, found to reduce urine volume in diabetes insipidus of pituitary origin, but not in diabetes insipidus.
- It sensitizes kidney to ADH actions, thus its efficacy depends on small amounts of the circulating hormone.

180. Ans. (c) 5HT3 antagonist *Ref: KDT, 5th ed. p 150*

Odansetron:

- It is the proto type of the new class of selective 5HT3 antagonist that have shown remarkable efficacy in controlling nausea and vomiting following administration of highly emetic anti-cancer drug and Radiotherapy.
- Granisetron and Tropisetron are the other selective 5HT3 antagonist.

181. Ans. (a) Beclomethasone and (c) Budesonide *Ref: KDT, 5th ed. p 207*

- Inhaled Steroids: These are steroids with high topical and low systemic activity (due to poor absorption and/or marked first pass metabolism)
- Beclomethasone dipropionate, Budesonide, and fluticasone are available in India.
- Inhaled steroids suppress bronchial inflammation, increase peak expiratory flow rate, reduce need for rescue β_2- agonist inhalations and prevent episodes of acute asthma.

182. Ans. (a) Protamine sulphate *Ref: KDT, 5th ed. p 564*

Protamine sulphate

- It is a strongly basic, low molecular weight protein obtained from the sperm of certain fish
- Given i.v. it neutralizes heparin weight for weight, i.e. 1mg is needed for every 100u of heparin

183. Ans. (d) Cimetidine *Ref: KDT, 3rd ed. p 580*

- Cimetidine inhibits cytochrome P-450 and reduces hepatic blood flow
- It inhibits the metabolism of many drugs so that they can accumulate to toxic levels, e.g. Warfarin, Lignocaine, Nifedipine etc.

184. Ans. (b) Omeprazole *Ref: KDT, 3rd ed. p 583*

- It is inactive at neutral pH, but pH <5.0 rearranges to two charged cationic forms (a sulfenic acid and a sulfenamide configurations) that react covalently with the SH groups of the H^+K^+ ATPase enzyme and inactivate irreversibly
- It gets concentrated in the acidic pH of parietal cell canaliculi because the charged forms generated there at the acidic pH are unable to diffuse back and get tightly bound to the enzyme
- HCl secretion resumes only when new H^+K^+ ATPase molecules are synthesized

185. Ans. (d) Chlorpropramide *Ref: KDT, 3rd ed. p 249, 527*

- Introduced in the pre-diabetic 'impaired glucose tolerance phase', sulfonylurea + dietary regulation has been shown to postpone manifest NIDDM
- This may be due to the fact that hyperglycemia is a self perpetuating condition
- Also, it is found to reduce urine volume in DI of pituitary origin but not renal DI
- It sensitizes kidney to ADH action, thus its efficacy depends on small amount of circulating hormone
- It directly promotes salt re-absorption in the ascending limb which may contribute to its anti-diuretic action

186. Ans. (b) Dantrolene sodium *Ref: KDT, 3rd ed. p 249, 527*

- It is used i.v. (1 mg/kg repeated as required) is DOC for malignant hyperthermia
- Malignant hyperthermia is due to persistent release of Ca^{2+} from sarcoplasmic reticulum (induced by fluorinated anesthetics in genetically susceptible individuals
- Also used in Neuroleptic malignant syndrome

187. Ans. (b) Prazosin *Ref: K.D. Tripathi, 5th ed. p 119*

Classification of alpha adrenergic blocking agents

- **Nonequilibrium type**
  - Beta haloalkylamines phenoxybenzamine

- **Equilibrium type (competitive)**
  - **Nonselective**
    - Ergot alkaloids—ergotamine, ergotoxine
    - Hydrogenated ergot alkaloid dihydroergotamine, dihydroergotoxine
    - Imidazolines, tolazoline, phentolamine
    - Miscellaneous—chloropromazine, ketanserin
  - **Alpha 1 selective**—prazosin terazosin, doxazosin
  - **Alpha 2 selective**—yohimbine

188. Ans. (a) Atenolol *Ref: K.D. Tripathi, 5th ed. p 125*

Non selective Beta Blockers (Beta 1 and Beta 2)

- Without intrinsic sympathomimetic activity—Propranalol, Sotalol, Timolol
- With intrinsic sympathomimetic activity—pindolol.
- With additional alpha blocking labelolol—carvedilol.

Cardioselective (beta 1)

Atenolol, metoprolol, acebutolol, bisoprolol, betaxolol, celiprolol, esmolol.

Selective (beta 2)

Butoamine

189. Ans. (d) Pirenzepine *Ref: K.D. Tripathi, 5th ed. p 94, 97-98*

- Pirenzepine (Gastrozepin), an M1 selective antagonist, is used in the treatment of peptic ulcers, as it reduces gastric acid secretion and reduces muscle spasm.
- It is in a class of drugs known as muscarinic receptor antagonists - acetylcholine being the neurotransmitter of the parasympathetic nervous system which initiates the rest-and-digest state (as opposed to fight-or-flight), the result being an increase in gastric motility and digestion.
- It has no effects on the brain and spinal cord as it cannot diffuse through the blood-brain barrier. Pirenzepine has been investigated for use in myopia control.

190. Ans. (a) Urokinase *Ref: KDT, 6th ed. p 605-606*

- Fibrinolytics are drugs used to lyse thrombi/clot to recanalize occluded blood vessels (mainly coronary artery). They are curative rather than prophylactic, work by activating the natural fibrinolytic system.
- Venous thrombi are lysed more easily than arterial and recent thrombi respond better.
- The clinically important fibrinolytics are:

Streptokinase	Alteplase (rt PA)
Urokinase	Reteplase
	Tenecteplase

191. Ans. (a) 2-bromo 2-chloro 1, 1, 1 trifluroethane *Ref: KDT, 6th ed. p 372*

Halothane

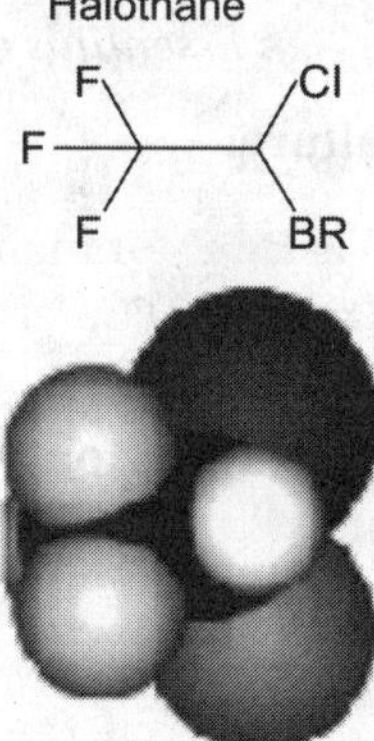

Systematic (IUPAC) name 2-bromo-2-chloro-1,1,1-trifluoroethane

It is an inhalational general anesthetic. Its IUPAC name is 2-bromo-2-chloro-1,1,1- trifluoroethane. It is the only inhalational anesthetic agent containing a bromine atom.

- Its use in developed countries, however, has been almost entirely superseded by newer inhalational anesthetic agents.
- It is a volatile liquid with sweet odor, non-irritant and non-inflammable. Solubility in blood is intermediate induction is reasonably quick and pleasant.

192. Ans. (c) Both of the above *Ref: Internet*

- During pregnancy it may cause premature closure of ductus arteriosus
- Aspirin birth defects include such as amniotic band syndrome, cleft lip, cleft palate, spina bifida, anophthalmia, microphthalmia, and clubfoot.

Saxen noted an association between aspirin ingestion in the first trimester and cleft palate/lip in a retrospective, controlled study involving 599 children. The incidence of combined cleft lip and palate was 19.8%, nearly 4 times the rate in the control group.

193. Ans. (c) Vitamin E *Ref: Davidson's, 20th ed. p 1217*

- Memantine in DOC of moderate to severe Alzheimer's Disease (AD)
- But its use in milder case are unclear
- It blocks excitotoxicity of the transmitter glutamate in a non-competitive and use depended manner.

194. Ans. (c) Propranolol *Ref: KDT, 5th ed. p 127*

- Propranolol delays recovery from hypoglycemia due to insulin and oral antidiabetics.
- Warning signs of hypoglycemia mediated through sympathetic stimulation (tachycardia, tremor) are suppressed.
- In some cases BP raised due to unopposed β action of released adrenaline.

195. Ans. (a) Hydralazine *Ref: KDT, 6th ed. p 910*

Antihypertensives during pregnancy

Drug not safe: ACE inhibitors (X), angiotensin antagonists (X)< Thiazide diuretics, Furosemide, propranolol, Nitroprusside.

Safe: Methyldopa, hydralazine, atenolol, metoprolol, pindolol, nifedipine, prazosin, clonidine.

196. Ans. (a) Pyrezenamide *Ref: KDT, 6th ed. p 742*

- Pyrazinamide is the most hepatotoxic drug hence it is contraindicated in patients with liver disease.
- Hyperuricemia is common and is due to inhibition of uric acid secretion in kidney gout can occur.
- Other adverse effects are arthralgia, flushing, rashes, fever and loss of diabetes control.

DRUGS IMPORTANT IN DENTAL THERAPEUTICS

197. Ans. (b) Cefoperazone *Ref: Essentials of Medical Pharmacology, KD Tripathi, 6th ed. p 706*

Cephalosporins that can be given in renal failure:

- Cefoperazone
- Ceftriaxone
- Cefpiramide

198. Ans. (d) Early onset, high efficacy, intermediate duration *Ref: Fundamentals of Perioperative Management by David Green p 141*

Patient controlled by analgesia:

- Introduced in 1970
- PCA rationale to improve the efficiency of analgesics by allowing the patient to manage the requirement of analgesics.

- It possess early onset, high efficacy, intermediate duration.
- Most commonly used opioid analgesics are morphine and meperidine.

199. Ans. (c) Penicillin acts only on growing bacterial population *Ref: Essentials of Medical Pharmacology, KD Tripathi, 6th ed. p 677*

- Two bacteriostatic agents are rarely synergistic, often additive in nature.
- Two bactericidal agents sometimes synergistic and frequently additive in nature.
- Combination of cidal and static anti-microbial agents either be synergistic or antagonistic.
- In the given condition penicillin is a bactericidal drug which act primarily on growing bacteria and erythromycin is a bacteriostatic drug which acts by retarding the growth of bacteria.
- So, together (Penicillin + Erythromycin) they act as apparent antagonism.

200. Ans. (a) Cefoperazone *Ref: Essentials of Medical Pharmacology, KD Tripathi, 6th ed. p 706*

Antibiotics showing antipseudomonal activity
- Penicillin: Piperacillin, mezlocillin and ticarcillin
- Cephalosporin: Ceftazidime, cefoperazone, cefepime, cefpirome, monobactam and aztreonam
- Carbapenem: Imipenem/cilastatin and meropenem
- Aminoglycosides: TAG (tobramycin, amikacin, gentamycin)
- Fluoroquinolones: Ciprofloxacin and levofloxacin
- Others: Polymyxin and colistin

201. Ans. (c) Mainly excreted by kidney *Ref: Essentials of Medical Pharmacology, KD Tripathi, 6th ed. p 696-699*

- Penicillin G exerts a bactericidal action against penicillin-susceptible microorganisms during the stage of active multiplication. It acts through the inhibition of biosynthesis of cell wall mucopeptide rendering the cell wall osmotically unstable.
- It is not active against the penicillinase-producing bacteria, which include many strains of staphylococci.
- Penicillin acts synergistically with gentamicin or tobramycin against many strains of enterococci.
- Aqueous penicillin G is rapidly absorbed following both intramuscular and subcutaneous Injection.
- Penicillins are rapidly excreted in the urine by glomerular filtration and active tubular secretion, primarily as unchanged drug.

202. Ans. (a) Cocaine *Ref: Principles and Practice of Pharmacology, 5th ed. p 149*

- Cocaine was the first local anesthetic used in clinical practice. It is a natural alkaloid obtained from erythroxylum coca. Cocaine introduced by Neimann 1860.
- Karl Koller initially used cocaine to produce corneal anesthesia in animals.
- Procaine is the first synthetic local anesthetic, introduced by Einhorn in 1905.
- Articaine and mepivacaine are only used in dental practice.
- Lidocaine was developed by Lofgren in 1943.

203. Ans. (b) Thiopentone *Ref: Drugs and Equipment in Anesthetic Practice by Arun Kumar, 6th ed.*

- Thiopentone does not possess analgesic property, so pain perception and its reaction are relatively unimpaired, until the final and very deep stage of anesthesia is reached.
- Contrary in small doses the barbiturate increases the reaction to painful stimuli.
- So, thiopentone has the hyperalgesic affect by subanesthetic dose. This hyperalgesic effect by subanesthetic dose. This hyperalgesia or antanalgesia effect of sub-anesthetic dose of thiopentone may result only from the depression effect of barbiturate on some inhibitory system of brain.

204. Ans. (d) Posterior longitudinal ligament *Ref: Neural Blockade by Michael J Cousins, 4th ed. p 496*

Structure encountered during epidural block with correct procedure:
- Skin
- Supraspinous ligament

- Interspinous ligament
- Ligament flavum
- Epidural space.

205. Ans. (a) Cefaclor *Ref: Harrison, 16th ed. p 821, 822*

MRSAs (methicillin-resistant Staphylococcus aureus) are resistant to all cephalosporins.

206. Ans. (a) Oral *Ref: Anesthesiology by Raj K. Modak, 2nd ed. p 474*

- Oral is the most acceptable route for preoperative sedative of choice for children in 90%.
- Midazolam is generally used with a wide margin of safety.
- A dose of 0.5 mg/kg to a maximum of 15 to 20 mg produce consistent preoperative anxiolysis with a wide margin of safety.

207. Ans. (c) Cocaine *Ref: Nursing Care by Laura, 3rd ed. p 72*

- In long term pain management patients, the most preferred route of drug administration is subdermal.
- The subcutaneous route is often used for long term opioid therapy who lacks intravenous access.
- Continuous subcutaneous infusion is preferred in cancer patient who requires long term drug administration.
- Subcutaneous infusion is also a preferred route in the patient who requires continuous parenteral morphine.

208. Ans. (c) It causes vomiting after use *Ref: Textbook of Oral and Maxillofacial Surgery by Malik p 173*

Propofol

- It is IV anesthetic agent
- It is used for induction and maintenance of anesthesia
- It has a rapid recovery rate.
- It is used for sedation in dental procedures which is done under local anesthetics.

209. Ans. (a) Nitrous oxide *Ref: Pharmacology by Bhattacharya, 2nd ed. p 228*

Introduction of general anesthesia

- Induction of general anesthetic is induced by intravenous anesthetic, it will produces the unconsciousness smoothly within 15 to 20 seconds.
- Drug used for induction of anesthesia are:
- Thiopentone sodium
  - Ketamine.
  - Methohexitone
  - Etomidate
  - Propofol.
  - Midazolam.
  - Nitrous oxide
  - Nitrous oxide is an inhalational anesthetic which is often used as inducing agent.

210. Ans. (c) Mosapride *Ref: Essentials of Medical Pharmacology, KD Tripathi, 6th ed. p 637*

- Helicobacter pylori, also known as H. pylori, is a bacterium that is commonly found in the stomach. It is present in approximately one-half of the world's population.
- H. pylori is probably spread by consuming food or water contaminated with fecal matter. H. pylori causes changes to the stomach and duodenum (the first part of the small intestine). The bacteria infect the protective tissue that lines the stomach. This leads to the release of certain enzymes and toxins and activation of the immune system. Together, these factors may directly or indirectly injure the cells of the stomach or duodenum.

This causes chronic inflammation in the walls of the stomach (gastritis) or duodenum (duodenitis).
- People with a history of peptic ulcer disease, active gastric ulcer, or active duodenal ulcer associated with H. pylori infection should be treated. Successful treatment of H. pylori can help the ulcer to heal, prevent ulcers from coming back, and reduce the risk of ulcer complications (like bleeding).

Drugs used in H. pylori are
- Amoxicillin
- Bismuth
- Clarithromycin
- Proton-pump inhibitors
- Metronidazole
- Tetracycline

211. Ans. (a) Propofol *Ref: Pharmacology for Nurse Anesthesiology by Richard, 1st ed. p 224*

- Propofol is known to possess direct antiemetic effects. Propofol antiemetic use for induction and maintenance of anesthesia has been shown to be associated with a lower incidence of postoperative nausea and vomiting (PONV) when compared to any other anesthetic drug or technique.
- Subhypnotic doses of propofol (10 to 15 mg IV) may be used in the postanesthesia care unit to treat nausea and vomiting, particularly if it is not of vagal origin.
- In the postoperative period, the advantage of propofol antiemetic is its rapid onset of action and the absence of serious side effects.
- When used as an adjuvant propofol in subhypnotic doses is effective against chemotherapy-induced nausea and vomiting.

212. Ans. (c) Penicillin acts only on growing bacterial population *Ref: Essentials of Medical Pharmacology, KD Tripathi, 6th ed. p 694, 695*

- Penicillin inhibits the cross linking of peptidoglycan strands, an important component in the cell wall of bacteria. This cross linking (linking strands to adjacent strands) gives the cell wall mechanical strength.
- When susceptible bacteria divide in the presence of β-lactam antibiotic—cell wall deficient (CWD) forms are produced.
- CWD bacteria swell and burst in hyperosmotic environment and in this way penicillin acts on growing bacteria.

213. Ans. (c) It is found in intraocular and prostatic secretions *Ref: Essentials of Medical Pharmacology KD Tripathi, 6th ed. p 697*

Penicillin G
- Narrow spectrum antibiotic.
- It is active against gram positive bacteria.
- Therapeutic concentration of penicillin is in tissues and in secretion, e.g. joint fluid, pleural fluid, pericardial fluid, and bile.
- Penicillin is destroyed by gastric acid due to its highly acidic nature that is pH-2.
- IV of high doses is recommended for meningococcal meningitis.

214. Ans. (c) Cefadroxil *Ref: Essentials of Medical Pharmacology, KD Tripathi, 6th ed. p 704*

First Generation
- Are moderate spectrum agents.
- Effective for treating staphylococcal and streptococcal infections and for skin and soft-tissue infections, as well as for streptococcal pharyngitis.
- Have activity against some Escherichia coli, Klebsiella pneumoniae and Proteus mirabilis

Medscape®	www.medscape.com		
First generation	*Second generation*	*Third generation*	*Fourth generation*
Cefadroxil	Cefactor	Cefdinir	Cefepime
Cefatrizine	Cefamandole	Cefetamet	Cefpirome
Cefazolin	Cefmetazole	Cefixime	
Cephalexin	Cefonicid	Cefoperazone	
Cephaloridine	Cefotetan	Cefotaxime	
Cephalothin	Cefoxitin	Cefotiam	
Cephapirin	Cefprozil	Cefpodoxime	
Cephradine	Cefuroxime	Cefsulodin	
	Loracarbef	Ceftazidime	
		Ceftibuten	
		Ceftizoxime	
		Ceftriaxone	
		Moxalactam	
Source: J Am Pham Assocc 2008 American Pharmacists Association			

Second Generation

- Have a greater gram-negative spectrum.
- More resistant to beta-lactamase.
- Useful agents for treating upper and lower respiratory tract infections, sinusitis and otitis media.
- Cefoxitin is a second generation cephalosporin with anaerobic activity.

Third Generation

- Have a broad spectrum of activity and increased activity against gram-negative organisms.
- Have excellent activity against most strains of Streptococcus pneumoniae.
- Have activity against Neisseria gonorrhoeae.

Fourth Generation

- Have a greater resistance to beta-lactamases than the third generation cephalosporins.
- Can cross blood brain barrier and are effective in meningitis.
- Cefpirome is more active against pneumococci.
- Activity against nosocomial pathogens such as Enterobacter and Acinetobacte

Other Cephalosporins Carbapenems

- Bactericidal antibiotic
- Active against gram-positive and gram-negative aerobic and anaerobic pathogenic bacteria.
- Resist the hydrolysis by most beta-lactamases

Imipenem

- Used to treat septicemia

215. Ans. (a) Cefaperazone *Ref: Essentials of Medical Pharmacology, KD Tripathi, 6th ed. p 706*

- Pseudomonas aeruginosa is termed as an opportunistic pathogen belonging to the family pseudomonacae which have a large number of species and are able to cause oportunistic infections in humans.
- Several resistance mechanism may be developed by pseudomonas aeruginosa against different antibiotic, beta lactamase production is the major mechanisms of resistance to beta lactam antibiotic.
- Mostly 3rd generation cephalosporin are hydrolyzed by ESBL enzymes.

- Cefoperazone and ceftazidime are most effective against pseudomonas aeruginosa and, they are also stable to breakdown effect of most beta lactamases.
- Cefperazone is the DOC for Pseudomonas aeruginosa.

216. Ans. (a) Cefoperazone *Ref: Essentials of Medical Pharmacology, KD Tripathi, 6th ed. p 704*

Refer Ans No. 214

217. Ans. (b) Binding to 30S subunit and inhibits binding of aminoacyl tRNA *Ref: Essentials of Medical Pharmacology, KD Tripathi, 6th ed. p 710*

Protein synthesis inhibition is a simple concept. There are a few key points:

- Chloramphenicol: Inhibits peptide bond formation.
- Erythromycin, clindamycin: Inhibition of translocation
- ATT: Aminoglycoside tetracyclines bind to 30S subunit; rest all bind to 50S subunit of ribosome.
- Puromycin: tRNA analogue.
- Aminoglycosides: Misreading of mRNA, initiation freezing, no polysome formation.
- Tetracycline: Prevents tRNA attachment to a site.

218. Ans. (b) Excreted mainly through kidney *Ref: KDT, 6th ed. p 697*

Penicillin

- 1st antibiotic to be used clinically in 1941.
- PnGs is thermo and acid labile in nature.
- Interferes in the synthesis of cell wall.
- Plasma t ½ of PnG is 30 min.
- Penetration capacity of PnG in CSF and serous cavity is poor.
- Plasma protein bound is about 60%.
- Excreted mainly through kidney.

219. Ans. (d) Linezolid *Ref: Essentials of Medical Pharmacology, KD Tripathi, 6th ed. p 733*

- It is a synthetic AMA's
- Linezolid active against methicillin resistant and some vancomycin resistant Staph aureus (VRSA), VRE, penicillin resistant etc.
- Vancomycin is the drug of choice in MRSA and MRSE
- Newer drugs are developed to treat vancomycin resistant infections like Linezolid, dalfopristin/quinupristin, daptomycin.

220. Ans. (b) INH *Ref: KDT-6th ed. p 741*

Adverse reaction of INH:

On peripheral nervous system:

- Peripheral neuritis.
- Deficiency of Vitamin B6.

On central nervous system:

- Convulsion
- Psychotic behavior.
- Euphoria.
- Transient loss of memory.
- Loss of self control.

Hepatitis is a major adverse effect of INH

221. Ans. (a) Cefepime *Ref: Essentials of Medical Pharmacology, KD Tripathi, 6th ed. p 669*

Antimicrobial agents are classified based on the mechanism of action, as follows:

- Agents that inhibit the synthesis of bacterial cell walls, including the beta-lactam class (e.g. penicillins, cephalosporins and carbapenems), and dissimilar agents such as cycloserine, vancomycin and bacitracin.
- Agents that act directly on the cell membrane of the microorganism, increasing permeability and leading to leakage of intracellular compounds, including detergents, such as polymyxin, polyene antifungal agents (e.g. nystatin and amphotericin B) and the lipopeptide daptomycin.
- Agents that reversibly inhibit protein synthesis (for example, chloramphenicol, tetracyclines, erythromycin, clindamycin, streptogramins, linezolid and aminoglycosides).
- Agents that affect bacterial nucleic acid metabolism, such as the rifamycins (for example, rifampin and rifabutin), which inhibit RNA polymerase, and the quinolones, which inhibit topoisomerases.
- Antimetabolites, including trimethoprim and the sulfonamides, which block essential enzymes of folate metabolism.

222. Ans. (c) Clofazimine *Ref: Essentials of Medical Pharmacology, KD Tripathi, 6th ed. p 757*

- Clofazimine is a fat-soluble riminophenazine dye used in combination with rifampicin and dapsone as multi-drug therapy (MDT) for the treatment of leprosy.
- It has been used investigationally in combination with other antimycobacterial drugs to treat Mycobacterium avium infections in AIDS patients and Mycobacterium avium paratuberculosis infection in Crohn's disease patients.
- Clofazimine also has a marked anti-inflammatory effect and is given to control the leprosy reaction, erythema nodosum leprosum (ENL).

223. Ans. (c) Auditory nerve *Ref: Essentials of Medical Pharmacology, KD Tripathi, 6th ed. p 722*

Streptomycin is not absorbed from the gastrointestinal tract but, after intramuscular administration, it diffuses readily into the extracellular component of most body tissues and it attains bactericidal concentrations, particularly in tuberculous cavities. Little normally enters the cerebrospinal fluid, although penetration increases when the meninges are inflamed. The plasma half-life, which is normally 2-3 hours, is considerably extended in the newborn, in the elderly and in patients with severe renal impairment. It is excreted unchanged in the urine. Streptomycin should be avoided, when possible, in children because the injections are painful and irreversible auditory nerve damage may occur. Both the elderly and patients with renal impairment are also vulnerable to dose-related toxic effects resulting from accumulation. Streptomycin should not be used in pregnancy. It crosses the placenta and can cause auditory nerve impairment and nephrotoxicity in the fetus.

224. Ans. (a) Hypertension with tachycardia *Ref: Essentials of Medical Pharmacology, KD Tripathi, 6th ed. p 122*

Lidocaine with epinephrine is the most common local anesthetic drug used in Dentistry. Epinephrine is added to lidocaine to:

- Minimize the hemorrhage,
- Minimize systemic absorption of lidocaine, and
- Increase duration of anesthesia

Systemic absorption of epinephrine causes cardiovascular effects such as hypertension, chest pain, tachycardia, and other cardiac arrhythmia. Maximum dose of epinephrine in healthy dental patients is 200 micrograms of 1/250000 solution.

225. Ans. (a) Chloroprocaine *Ref: Anesthesia for Obstetrics and Gynecology by Robin Russell, 1st ed. p. 49*

- In maternal blood, chloroprocaine is rapidly hydrolyzed.
- It possess minimum transfer to fetus.
- Virtually it is non-existence in fetus.

226. Ans. (d) Sulfonamides *Ref: Essentials of Medical Pharmacology, KD Tripathi, 6th ed. p 682*

Sulfonamide is the basis of several groups of drugs. The original antibacterial sulfonamides (sometimes called sulfa drugs or sulpha drugs) are synthetic antimicrobial agents that contain the sulfonamide group. Many sulphonamides are rapidly excreted and very soluble in urine so they are used to treat infections of the urinary tract. β-Lactam antibiotics (beta-lactam antibiotics) are a broad class of antibiotics, consisting of all antibiotic agents that contains a β-lactam ring in their molecular structures. This includes penicillin derivatives (penams), cephalosporins (cephems), monobactams, and carbapenems. Most β-lactam antibiotics work by inhibiting cell wall biosynthesis in the bacterial organism and are the most widely used group of antibiotics.

227. Ans. (d) Desflurane *Ref:Fundamentals of Anesthesia edited by Tim Smith p 113*

- Desflurane is unsafe for children in dentistry because it can cause airway irritation in children

228. Ans. (a) Pyridoxine *Ref: Essentials of Medical Pharmacology, KD Tripathi, 6th ed. p 740*

The main cause of pyridoxine deficiency is a lack of pyridoxine in the diet. Another cause of vitamin B6 deficiency is the use of the tuberculostatic medication isoniazid.

229. Ans. (d) Extend amoxicillin's antibacterial spectrum *Ref: Essentials of Medical Pharmacology, KD Tripathi, 6th ed. p 702*

Amoxicillin:
- It has a similar spectrum of activity to ampicillin and also inactivated by penicillinase.
- Amoxicillin is preferred to ampicillin.
- Amoxicillin can be used in a patient with both kidney and liver disease with dose adjustment.
- Clavulanic acid is the beta lactamase inhibitor. It has no significant antibacterial activity but in combination with amoxicillin widens amoxicillin's spectrum of activity and also allows its use against amoxicillin resistant strains of bacteria.

230. Ans. (b) Procaine *Ref: Essentials of Medical Pharmacology, KD Tripathi, 6th ed. p 344*

I. Classification of local anesthetics based on chemistry:

Esters	*Amides*	*Quinoline*	*Para-amino benzoic acid*
Butacaine Cocaine Benzocaine Tetracaine Piperocaine	Prilocaine Bupivacaine Etidocaine Articaine Lidocaine Mepivacaine	Centbucridine	Procaine Chloroprocaine Propoxycaine

II. Classification based on duration of action:

Duration on pulpal (mins)	*Duration on soft tissue (mins)*	*LA*
Ultrashort (10 to 15)	30 to 45 min	Lignocaine 2% (plain) Mepivacaine 3% (plain) Prilocaine 4% (infilteration)
Short (45 to 60)	120 to 180 min	Procaine Chloroprocaine
Intermediate (60 to 90)	180 to 270 min	Lignocaine Prilocaine (block) Mepivacaine
Long (>90)	>270 min	Tetracaine Bupivacaine Ropivacaine Dibucaine

III. Classification based on mode of administration:

Mode of administration	*LA*
1. Injectable	
• Low potency	Procaine, Chloroprocaine
• Intermediate potency	Lidocaine, Prilocaine
• High potency	Tetracaine, bupivacaine, ropivacaine, dibuvacaine
2. Surface	
• Soluble	Cocaine, lidocaine, tetracaine
• Insoluble	Benzocaine, butylaminobenzoate, oxythazaine

231. Ans. (c) Penicillins *Ref: Scully's Medical Problem in Dentistry by C. Scully*

The usage of penicillin is justified in patients taking warfarin.

232. Ans. (d) Erythromycin *Ref: Essentials of Medical Pharmacology, KD Tripathi, 6th ed. p 911*

- Erythromycin can be safely used in lactating mothers

233. Ans. (a) Povidone iodine *Ref: K.D. Tripathi, 4th ed. p 865*

- Povidone (Polyvinylpyrrolidone) Iodine-
  - They are soluble complexes of iodine with large molecular organic compounds that serve as carriers and release free iodine slowly
  - It is used on foils, furunculosis, burns, otitis externa, ulcers, tinea, monilial/trichomonal/non-specific vaginitis, and for surgical scrubbing, disinfection of endoscopes and instruments.
- Cetrimide
  - It is a quaternary ammonium (cationic) antiseptic
  - It has good cleansing action, efficiently removes dirt, grease, tar and congealed blood from roadside accident wounds.
  - Alone or in combination with chlorhexidine, it is a popular hospital antiseptic and disinfectant for surgical instruments, utensils, baths etc.
- Chlorhexidine
  - It is biguanide, non-irritating antiseptic that disrupts bacterial cell membrane.
  - It is relatively more active against gram positive bacteria.
  - Persists on skin
  - It is present in SAVLON
  - Extensively used for surgical scrubs, neonatal baths, in mouthwashes, in obstetrics and as a general skin antiseptic.
- Alcohol
  - Ethanol is an effective antiseptic and cleansing agent at 40–90% concentration.
  - The rapidity of action increases with concentration upto 70% and decreases above 90%.
  - Acts by precipitating bacterial proteins.
  - It is an irritant and should not be applied to mucus membranes or to delicate skin.
  - On open wounds it produces a burning sensation, injures the surface and forms a coagulum under which bacteria could grow.

234. Ans. (b) Synergism *Ref: K.D. Tripathi, 6th ed. p 677*

Two bactericidal drugs are frequently additive and sometimes synergistic if the organism is sensitive to both, e.g.:

- Penicillin/ampicillin + streptomycin/gentamicin or vancomycin + gentamicin for enterococcal SABE. Penicillins by acting on the cell wall may enhance the penetration of the aminoglycoside into the bacterium.

- Carbenicillin/ticarcillin + gentamicin for Pseudomonas infection, especially in neutropenic patients.
- Ceftazidime + ciprofloxacin for Pseudomonas infected orthopedic prosthesis.
- Rifampin + isoniazid in tuberculosis.

235. Ans. (a) Hypoglycemia *Ref: K.D. Tripathi, 6th ed. p 285-286*

Adverse effects of Glucocorticoids:

1. Cushing's habitus
2. Delayed wound healing
3. Glaucoma
4. Fragile skin, purple striae
5. Muscular weakness
6. Hyperglycemia
7. Peptic ulceration
8. Osteoporosis
9. Growth retardation
10. Fetal abnormalities
11. Psychiatric disturbance
12. AVN of femoral head
13. Post subcapsular cataract

236. Ans. (b) Tetracycline *Ref: K.D. Tripathi, 6th ed. p 85*

- Tetracycline is teratogenic causes discoloration and defects of teeth and altered bone growth of the fetus
- Tetracycline can cause super infection (including pseudomembranous colitis)
- Erythromycin, ampicillin, chloroquine, cephalexin do not have teratogenic effect.

Human teratogenic drugs

Drug	*Abnormality*
Thalidomide	Phocomelia, multiple defects
Anticancer drugs (methotrexate)	Cleft palate, hydrocephalus, multiple defects, foetal death
Androgens	Virilization; limb, esophageal, cardiac defects
Progestins	Virilization of female foetus
Stilboestrol	Vaginal carcinoma in teenage female offspring
Tetracyclines	Discolored and deformed teeth, retarded bone growth
Warfarin	Depressed nose; eye and hand defects, growth retardation
Phenytoin	Hypoplastic phalanges, cleft lip/palate, microcephaly
Phenobarbitone	Various malformations
Carbamazepine	Neural tube defects, other abnormalities
Valproate sod.	Spina bifida and other neural tube defects
Alcohol	Low IQ baby, growth retardation, foetal alcohol syndrome
ACE inhibitors	Hypoplasia of organs, growth retardation, foetal loss
Lithium	Foetal goiter, cardiac and other abnormalities
Antithyroid drugs causes	Foetal goiter and hypothyroidism
Indomethacin/aspirin	Premature closure of ductus arteriosus
Isotretinoin	Craniofacial, heart and CNS defects

237. Ans. (b) Clindamycin *Ref: K.D. Tripathi, 6th ed. p 731*

Side effects are rashes, urticaria, abdominal pain, but the major problem is diarrhea and pseudomembranous enterocolitis due to Clostridium difficile superinfection which is potentially fatal. The drug should be promptly stopped and metronidazole (alternatively vancomycin) given to treat it.

238. Ans. (c) Metronidazole *Ref: K.D. Tripathi, 6th ed. p 351*

Chlorpropamide, Metronidazole, griseofulvin, tolbutamide, cephalosporins (cefoperazone, moxalactam, cefamandole) and phenylbutazone can cause a mild disulfiram like reaction when administered with ethylalcohol.

239. Ans. (b) Streptomycin *Ref: K.D. Tripathi, 6th ed. p 741-743*

Hepatotoxicity of antitubercular drugs is most common with

- Isoniazid
- Rifampicin
- Pyrazinamide

Least hepatotoxic

- Streptomycin
- Ethambutol

240. Ans. (d) Zanamivir *Ref: K.D. Tripathi, 5th ed. p 725*

Classification of antiviral drugs:

Anti-herpes virus	**Anti-influenza virus**	**Nonselective Antiviral drugs**
• Acyclovir • Valacicovir • Famciclovir • Idoxuridine • Ganciclovir • Foscarnet	• Amantadine • Rimantadine • Zanamivir	• Ribavirin • Lamivudine • Interferon alfa
Anti-retroviral drugs		
Nucleoside reverse transcriptase inhibitors (NRTIs) • Zidovudine (AZT) • Didanozine • Stavudine • Lamivudine • Zalcitabine • Abacavir	**Nonnucleoside reverse transcriptase inhibitors (NNRTIs)** • Nevirapine • Efaverenze • Delaviridine	**Protease inhibitors** • Saquinavir • Indinavir • Amprenavir • Ritonavir • Nelfinavir • Lopinavir

241. Ans. (c) Metronidazole *Ref: K.D. Tripathi, 6th ed. p 799*

- Antibiotic-associated (C. difficile) colitis is an infection of the colon caused by C. difficile that occurs primarily among individuals who have been using antibiotics. It is the most common infection acquired by patients while they are in the hospital. More than three million C. difficile infections occur in hospitals in the US each year. After a stay of only two days in a hospital, 10% of patients will develop infection with C. difficile. C. difficile also may be acquired outside of hospitals in the community.
- Oral metronidazole 800 mg TDC is preferred over Vancomycin for treatment of Clostridium difficile induced colitis because it is more effective, more convenient and less toxic.

242. Ans. (b) Ethambutol *Ref: K.D. Tripathi, 5th ed. p 701*

Ethambutol
- Selectively bacteriostatic
- Inhibits arabinogalactan synthesis and interferes with mycolic acid incorporation into bacterial cell wall.
- Plasma half life is 4 hours and is excreted in urine via glomerular filtration and tubular secretion.
- Dose and duration of therapy dependent toxicity includes loss of visual acuity and color vision due to optic neuritis.
- Not to be used below 6 years of age
- Causes hyperuricemia.

243. Ans. (c) Lignocaine *Ref: K.D. Tripathi, 5th ed. p 476*

- Lignocaine is absorbed orally but has very high first pass metabolism in liver therefore it will not attain a proper and consistent blood level and hence it is ineffective by this route.
- Channels in the neuronal cell membrane that are responsible for signal propagation. With sufficient blockage the membrane of the postsynaptic neuron will not depolarize and will thus fail to transmit an action potential. This creates the anesthetic effect by not merely preventing pain signals from propagating to the brain but by stopping them before they begin. Careful titration allows for a high degree of selectivity in the blockage of sensory neurons, whereas higher concentrations will also affect other modalities of neuron signaling.

244. Ans. (b) Lamivudine *Ref: KDT, 6th ed. p 771*

- Lamivudine (3TC) inhibits HIV reverse transcriptase as well as hepatitis B virus DNA polymerase.
- Its uncorporation into DNA results chain termination.
- It is frequently used for HBV.

245. Ans. (b) Tetracycline *Ref: KDT, 6th ed. p 85*

- There are some drugs which are known to cause fatal abnormalities when administered to the pregnant women, these are termed as teratogenic drugs.
- Drugs can affect the foetus at 3 stage:
  - During fertilization and implantation
  - During organogenesis
  - During growth and development
- Tetracycline is the antibiotic which should not be given during pregnancy as it cause discolored and deformed tooth and retarded bone growth in fetus.

246. Ans. (c) Imipenem *Ref: KDT, 6th ed. p 700-708*

The drug choice of MRSA is
- First line of drug—Vancomycin/rifampicin
- Alternatives—Streptogramins
  - Linezolid
  - Ciprofloxacin can also be used.
- Imipenem inhibits penicillinase producing staphylococci and some MRSA.

247. Ans. (d) Mepivacaine *Ref: Endodontics by Richard E Walton, 1st ed. p 137*

Mepivacaine:
- Mepivacaine is widely used as an emergency wound anesthetic.
- Mepivacaine has a less vasodilatory effect than lidocaine and usually does not require the use of epinephrine.
- Mepivacaine stabilizes the neuronal membrane and prevents the initiation and transmission of nerve impulses.

- Mepivacaine with epinephrine or other vasopressors should not be used concomitantly with ergot type oxytocic drugs because a severe persistent hypertension may occur.

248. Ans. (b) 3 to 5 minutes *Ref: Principles and Practice of Pedodontics by Arathi Rao, 3rd ed. p 123*

- Nitrous oxide (N_2O) has long been a valuable analgesic in both adult and pediatric dental practice.
- In pediatric practice, N_2O/O_2 is especially effective when caring for mildly to moderately anxious children.
- The adverse side effects of N_2O/O_2 analgesia, which appear to be minor, include intra-administration dreams and postadministration headache, nausea, vomiting, and possibly diffusion hypoxia.
- Once the nitrous oxide flow is terminated, 100% oxygen should be delivered for 3 to 5 minutes. The patient must return to pre-treatment responsiveness before discharge.

249. Ans. (c) Tuberculosis *Ref: Essentials of Pharmacology for Dentistry, KD Tripathi, 2nd ed. p 423*

DOTS (Direct Observe Treatment Short course)

- It is the recommended strategy for global tuberculosis control.
- All the drugs are administered under direct supervision during the intensive phase of chemotherapy.
- It is a community based tuberculosis treatment and care strategy which provide combine benefits of supervised treatment as well as community base care and support.

250. Ans. (c) Bupivacaine *Ref: Essentials of Medical Pharmacology, KD Tripathi, 6th ed. p 344*

Refer Ans no. 198

251. Ans. (b) Inhibition of cell wall peptidoglycan synthesis by competitive inhibition of transpeptidases
Ref: Essentials of Pharmacology for Dentistry, KD Tripathi, 2nd ed. p 380-382

- All β-lactam antibiotics interfere with the synthesis of bacterial cell wall
- The β-lactam antibiotics inhibit the transpeptidases so that cross linking (which maintains the close knit structure of the cell wall) does not take place
- When bacteria divide in the presence of a β-lactam antibiotic, cell wall deficient (CWD) forms are produced. Because the interior of the bacterium is hyperosmotic the CWD forms swell and burst → bacterial lysis. This is how β-lactam antibiotics exert bactericidal action.

252. Ans. (a) Nitrous oxide and oxygen *Ref: Essentials of Medical Pharmacology, KD Tripathi, 6th ed. p 371*

- Nitrous oxide is generally used as a carrier and adjuvant to other anaesthetics.
- A mixture of 70% N_2O + 25–30% O_2 + 0.2–2% another potent anesthetic is employed for most surgical procedures.
- In this way concentration of the other anesthetic can be reduced to 1/3 for the same level of anesthesia. Because N_2O has little effect on respiration, heart and BP: breathing and circulation are better maintained with the mixer than with the potent anesthetic given alone in full doses.
- As the sole agent, N_2O (50%) has been used with O_2 for dental and obstetric analgesia.
- It is nontoxic to liver, kidney and brain.

253. Ans. (a) Patients retains ability maintain a patent airway *Ref: Shobha Tondon, 2nd ed. p 160*

Conscious sedation:

1. At several visits the procedure may be performed.
2. Patient is cooperative, but anxious and fearful.
3. Airway is maintained
4. Responds appropriately to verbal commands
5. No mortality
6. Recuperation period is 1–2 minutes
7. Patient feels he is in control of the situation

8. NPO is required.
9. Patient is conscious and contact is maintained.

254. Ans. (b) Ketamine *Ref: KDT, 6th ed. p 370*

Ketamine is intravenous slow acting anesthetic.

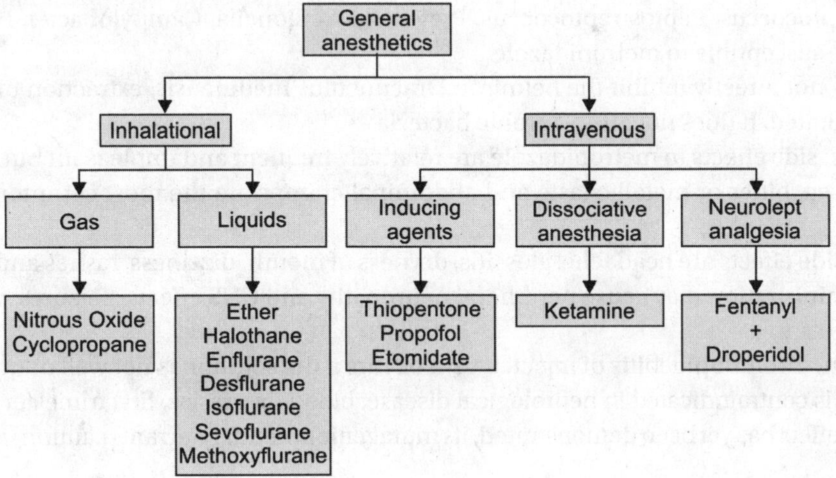

255. Ans. (a) 1–10% *Ref: Tripathi's, 1st ed. p 383*

- Allergies to penicillin are common, with about 10 percent of people reporting an allergy
- Anyone who is allergic to one of the penicillins should be presumed to be allergic to all penicillins and should avoid the entire group, unless they have been specifically evaluated for this problem
- An allergic reaction occurs when the immune system begins to recognize a drug as something 'foreign'. Several different symptoms can indicate that a person is allergic to penicillin. These include hives (raised, intensely itchy spots that come and go over hours), angioedema (swelling of the tissue under the skin, commonly around the face), throat tightness, wheezing, coughing, and trouble breathing from asthma-like reactions (narrowing of the airways into the lungs).

256. Ans. (b) Vancomycin *Ref: Tripathi's, 1st ed. p 415*

- Vancomycin can cause two types of hypersensitivity reactions, the red man syndrome and anaphylaxis. Red man syndrome has often been associated with rapid infusion of the drug.
- Vancomycin is recommended to be administered in a dilute solution slowly, over at least 60 minutes (maximum rate of 10 mg/minute for doses >500 mg). This is due to the high incidence of pain and thrombophlebitis and to avoid an infusion reaction known as the red man syndrome or red neck syndrome. This syndrome, usually appearing within 4–10 minutes after the commencement or soon after the completion of an infusion
- Symptoms may be treated or prevented with antihistamines, including diphenhydramine, and are less likely to occur with slow infusion.

257. Ans. (a) Inhibiting the binding of aminoacyl tRNA to the ribosomal complex *Ref: KDT, 6th ed. p 710*

- Tetracyclines are primary bacteriostatic, inhibit protein synthesis by binding to 30S ribosome in susceptible organisms.
- Tetracycline acts by inhibiting the binding of aminoacyl tRNA to the mRNA ribosomal complex.
- Finally, the peptide chain fails to grow.

258. Ans. (c) Clindamycin *Ref: KDT, 6th ed. p 731*

- Clindamycin is known to achieve high concentration in hard tissue because of its molecular size.

259. Ans. (c) Is an effective alternative for infection caused by aerobic gram positive cocci

Ref: KD Tripathi, Essentials of Pharmacology for Dentistry, p 377-378

- Metronidazole, the prototype member of this class was introduced in 1959 for trichomonas vaginalis and later found to be a broad spectrum antiprotozoal drug against Entamoeba histolytica and Giardia lamblia.
- Many anaerobic bacteria such as Bact. fragilis, Bact. melaninogenicus, fusobacterium, Clostridium perfringens, Cl. difficile, Peptococcus, Peptostreptococcus, Prevotella, Veillonella, Campylobacter, Helicobacter Pylori and spirochetes are susceptible to metronidazole.
- Though it does not directly inhibit the helminth Dracunculus medinensis, extraction of the worm from under the skin is facilitated. It does not affect aerobic bacteria.
- Adverse effects: side effects to metronidazole are relatively frequent and unpleasant but mostly non serious.
- Anorexia, nausea, bitter or metallic taste and abdominal cramps are the most common. Looseness of stool is occasional.
- Less frequent side effects are headache, glossitis, dryness of mouth, dizziness, rashes and transient neutropenia
- Prolonged administration may cause peripheral neuropathy and CNS effects. Seizures have followed very high doses.
- On i.v. injection, thrombophlebitis of injected vein occurs if the solution is not well diluted.
- Metronidazole is contraindicated in neurological disease, blood dyscrasias, first trimester of pregnancy (theough no teratogenic effect has yet been demonstrated, its mutagenic potential warrants caution) and chronic alcoholism.

260. Ans. (a) An effective analgesic for mild to moderate post operative dental pain *Ref: K.D. Tripathi, Essentials of Pharmacology for Dentistry, p 324-325*

Pyrrolo-Pyrrole Derivative

Ketorolac:

- A novel NSAID with potent analgesic and modest anti-inflammatory activity. In postoperative pain it has equaled the efficacy of morphine, but does not interact with opioid receptors and is free of opioid side effects. Like other NSAIDs, it inhibits PG synthesis and relieves pain by a peripheral mechanism. In short-lasting pain, it has compared favorably with aspirin.
- Ketorolac is rapidly absorbed after oral and i.m. administration. It is highly plasma protein bound and 60% excreted unchanged in urine. Major metabolic pathway is glucuronidation plasma t½ is 5–7 hours.

Adverse effects:

- Nausea, abdominal pain, dyspepsia, ulceration, loose stools, drowsiness, headache, dizziness, nervousness, pruritus, pain at injection site, rise in serum transaminase and fluid retention have been noted.
- Use Ketorolac is frequently used in postoperative, dental and acute musculoskeletal pain: 1530 mg i.m or i.v. is comparable to 10–12 mg morphine, and can be repeated every 4–6 hours (max 90 mg/day). It can also be used for renal colic, migraine and pain due to bony metastasis.
- Orally it is used in a dose of 10–20 mg 6 hourly for short-term management of moderate pain. In postoperative dental pain ketorolac has been rated superior to aspirin 650 mg, paracetamol 600 mg and equivalent to ibuprofen 400 mg. Continuous use for more than 5 days is not recommended.

261. Ans. (c) Cell wall synthesis *Ref: K.D. Tripathi, 6th ed. p 694*

Penicillins interfere with the synthesis of bacterial cell wall.

262. Ans. (c) Ethambutol *Ref: KDT, 6th ed. p 742*

Ethambutol:

- It is first line anti-tubercular drug.
- It inhibits arabinosyltransferases in arabinogalactan synthesis and interferes with mycolic acid incorporation.
- It is excreted through urine.

- Side effect of ethambutol is optic neuritis.
- It should not be prescribed below 6 years of age.

263. Ans. (c) Erythromycin *Ref: KDT, 6th ed. p 719*

Systemic aminoglycosides	*Topical aminoglycosides*
Streptomycin	Neomycin
Amikacin	Framycetin
Gentamycin	
Sisomicin	
Kanamycin	
Tobramycin	
Netilmicin	

264. Ans. (c) Nitrous oxide *Ref: KDT, 6th ed. p 369*

Second gas effect

During induction of general anesthesia when a large volume of nitrous oxide is taken up from alveoli into pulmonary capillary blood, the concentration of gases remaining in the alveoli is increased. This results in effects known as the 'concentration effect' and the 'second gas effect.' These effects occur because of the contraction in volume associated with the uptake of the nitrous oxide.

265. Ans. (d) Dermatophytosis *Ref: KDT, 6th ed. p 758*

- Amphotericin B is an antifungal drug
- It is widely used for many fungal diseases such as cryptococcosis, histoplasmosis, blastomycosis, torulopsis, candidiasis, aspergillosis etc.
- It is not used for dermatophytosis because in infected skin it is used in low concentration.
- New amphotericin B formulation:
  - Amphotericin B lipid complex.
  - Amphotericin B colloidal dispersion.
  - Liposomal amphotericin B.

266. Ans. (d) Ketamine *Ref: K.D. Tripathi, 6th ed. p 376*

Ketamine

- It is a drug used in human and veterinary medicine, mainly for starting and maintaining general anesthesia.
- Other uses include sedation in intensive care, as a pain killer (particularly in emergency medicine and patients with potentially compromised respiration and/or allergies to opiate and barbiturate analgesics), and treatment of bronchospasm.
- Ketamine is classified as a dissociative agent.
- The dissociative anesthetic effects of ketamine have also been applied for postoperative pain management. Low doses of ketamine have been found to significantly reduce morphine consumption, as well as reports of nausea following abdominal surgery.

267. Ans. (b) Paracetamol *Ref: KDT, 5th ed. p 181*

- The central analgesic action of paracetamol is like aspirin, i.e. it raises pain threshold, but has weak peripheral anti-inflammatory component.
- Paracetamol has negligible anti-inflammatory action. It is poor inhibitor of PG synthesis in peripheral tissue, but more active on Cyclooxygenase in brain.

268. Ans. (c) Progressive succide inhibitor *Ref: KDT, 3rd ed. p 648*

- Clavulanic acid has β-Lactam ring but no antibacterial activity of its own
- It inhibits wide variety of β-Lactamases (except class I cephalosporinase) produced by both gram +ve and –ve bacteria
- It is a 'progressive' inhibitor: binding with β-Lactamase is reversible initially but becomes covalent later
- It is called 'Suicide' inhibitor because it gets inactivated after binding to the enzyme.

269. Ans. (b) Streptomycin *Ref: KDT, 3rd ed. p 668*

- It is the most important, dose and duration of treatment related adverse effect of streptomycin
- The vestibular or cochlear part may be primarily affected by it
- Drug is concentrated in the labyrinthine fluid and are slowly removed from it when the plasma concentration falls.

270. Ans. (a) Binds to 30s ribosome *Ref: K.D. Tripathi, 5th ed. p 669*

- Tetracycline binds to the 30s subunit of microbial ribosomes. It inhibits protein synthesis by blocking the attachment of charged aminoacyl-tRNA to the A site on the ribosome. Thus, it prevents introduction of new amino acids to the nascent peptide chain.
- The action is usually inhibitory and reversible upon withdrawal of the drug. Mammalian cells are less vulnerable to the effect of tetracyclines, despite the fact that tetracycline binds to the small ribosomal subunit of both prokaryotes and eukaryotes (30s and 40s respectively). This is because bacteria actively pump tetracycline into their cytoplasm, even against a concentration gradient, whereas mammalian cells do not. This accounts for the relatively small off-site effect of tetracycline on human cells.
- Tetracyclines have a broad spectrum of antibiotic action. Originally, they possessed some level of bacteriostatic activity against almost all medically relevant aerobic and anaerobic bacterial genera, both Gram-positive and Gram-negative, with a few exceptions, such as Pseudomonas aeruginosa and Proteus spp., which display intrinsic resistance. However, acquired (as opposed to inherent) resistance has proliferated in many pathogenic organisms and greatly eroded the formerly vast versatility of this group of antibiotics. Resistance amongst Staphylococcus spp., Streptococcus spp., Neisseria gonorrhoeae, anaerobes, members of the Enterobacteriaceae and several other previously sensitive organisms is now quite common. Tetracyclines remain especially useful in the management of infections by certain obligately intracellular bacterial pathogens such as Chlamydia, Mycoplasma and Rickettsia. They are also of value in spirochetal infections, such as syphilis, leptospirosis and Lyme disease. Certain rare or exotic infections, including anthrax, plague and brucellosis, are also susceptible to tetracyclines. These agents also have activity against certain eukaryotic parasites, including those responsible for diseases such as malaria and balantidiasis.
- It is first-line therapy for Rocky Mountain spotted fever (Rickettsia), Lyme disease (Borellia burgdorferi), Q fever (Coxiella), psittacosis and lymphogranuloma venereum (Chlamydia), and to eradicate nasal carriage of meningococci. Tetracycline tablets were used in the plague outbreak in India in 1992
- Side-effects and contra-indications:
  - Stain developing teeth (even when taken by the mother during pregnancy)
  - Discolor permanent teeth (yellow-gray-brown), from infancy and childhood to eight years old
  - Be inactivated by Ca^{2+} ion, so are not to be taken with milk, yogurt, and other dairy products
  - Be inactivated by aluminium, iron and zinc, not to be taken at the same time as indigestion remedies (common antacids and over-the-counter heartburn medicines)
  - Cause skin photosensitivity, sso exposure to the sun or intense light is not recommended
  - Cause drug-induced lupus, and hepatitis
  - Cause microvesicular fatty liver
  - Cause tinnitus
  - Suppress sperm production

- Interfere with methotrexate by displacing it from the various protein binding sites
- Cause breathing complications, as well as anaphylactic shock, in some individuals
- Affect bone growth of the fetus, so should be avoided during pregnancy
- Caution should be exercised in long-term use with breastfeeding. Short-term use is safe; bioavailability in milk is low to nil.
- In 2010, the FDA added tetracycline to its Adverse Event Reporting System (AERS).
- The AERS contains a list of medications under investigation by the FDA for potential safety issues. The list is published quarterly and available online. The AERS cites a potential link between the use of tetracycline products and Stevens-Johnson syndrome, toxic epidermal necrolysis and erythema multiforme.

271. Ans. (b) Competitive inhibition *Ref: K.D. Tripathi, 5th ed. p 34*

Inhibition of enzymes by drugs takes place in two types:

- Nonspecific inhibition
  - After tertiary structure of any enzyme formaldehyde phenol alkalies.
- Specific inhibition - affect a particular enzyme in two ways:
- **Competitive**
  - (Equilibrium type)
  - Drug competes with normal substrate or the co enzyme.
  - K_m increased but V_{max} not changed. (K_m = Michaclis constant and V_{max} = Maximal Velocity)
  - Physostigmine and neostigmine on acetylecholine.
  - Sulfonamides with PABA for bacterial folate synthesis.
  - Aflopunnot with hypoxantine for xanthine oxidase.
  - Carbidopa and methyldopa with Levodopa for dopa decarboxylase
  - Nonequilibrium type
  - Drugs acts on same catalytic site of enzyme
  - Organophosphates with esteric site of cholinesterase
- **Noncompetitive**
  - Inhibitors acts on adjacent site
  - K_m unchanged, V_{max} reduced
  - Aspirin Cyclooxygenase

272. Ans. (d) Methyldopa *Ref: K.D. Tripathi, 5th ed. p 511*

- Methyldopa is an alpha-adrenergic agonist (selective for α2-adrenergic receptors) psychoactive drug used as a sympatholytic or antihypertensive.
- Its use is now mostly deprecated following the introduction of alternative safer classes of agents. However, it continues to have a role in otherwise difficult to treat hypertension and gestational hypertension [also known as pregnancy-induced hypertension (PIH)]
- Methyldopa is used in the clinical treatment of the following disorders:
  - Hypertension (or high blood pressure)
  - Gestational hypertension (or pregnancy-induced hypertension) and pre-eclampsia.